Birkner · Normal Radiologic Patterns and Variances of the Human Skeleton

Rudolf Birkner M.D.

Normal Radiologic Patterns and Variances of the Human Skeleton

An X-Ray Atlas of Adults and Children

With 1227 Illustrations,
including 803 full-size Radiographs

Urban & Schwarzenberg · Baltimore-Munich 1978

Urban & Schwarzenberg, Inc.
7 East Redwood Street
Baltimore, Maryland 21202
U.S.A.

Urban & Schwarzenberg
Pettenkoferstrasse 18
D-8000 München 2
Germany

A translation of Birkner, Das typische Röntgenbild des Skeletts
Urban & Schwarzenberg, München–Wien–Baltimore 1977

Translated by Magal, Translation Agency

Library of Congress Cataloging in Publication Data

Birkner, Rudolf, 1911–
Normal radiologic patterns and variances of the human skeleton.

Translation of Das typische Röntgenbild des Skeletts.
Bibliography: p.
Includes index.
1. Radiography, Medical--Atlases. I. Title.
[DNLM: 1. Radiography--Atlases. WN17 B619n]
RC78.2.B5713 611'.71'0222 78-692
ISBN 0-8067-0211-7

ISBN 0-8067-0211-7 Urban & Schwarzenberg Baltimore
ISBN 3-541-70211-7 Urban & Schwarzenberg München

Printed in Germany by Kastner & Callwey, München

Introduction

This new material is based on the pioneering work of my honored teacher, Rudolf Grashey.

I wish to thank the eminent surgeon, Rudolf Zenker, for his suggestion that the material of the "Atlas typischer Röntgenbilder vom normalen Menschen" (Grashey–Birkner) be arranged in such a form that not only roentgenologists but also medical students and X-ray technicians will benefit from its comprehensive information on the roentgenology of the skeleton.

In this era of short handbooks, the author has set himself the task of presenting the subject in 1,000 pages in such manner that an increase in information can be obtained from the newly added radiographs and, in particular, from the clinically oriented analysis, without losing existing material. This is important as the roentgenology of the skeleton is a crucial link between anatomy and the mechanics of the joints and muscles, anthropology and clinical medicine.

Because of the broad range of roentgenologic procedures, from X-rays following accidents to criminology, the medical expert in court, for example, now has an important tool at his disposal. The development of the child's skeleton also has an important place in this book.

It should be taken into consideration that in our fast-paced era the knowledge of anthropologists and anatomists has already been partly forgotten. Therefore, roentgenologic anatomy offers virtually the only opportunity to carry out comparative anthropological and phylogenetic research on a large scale *(Neiss)*. Moreover, through analyses of radiographs the research on variants in man can be further developed. Therefore, an extended representation of variants is one of the main subjects of this work.

For the English publication, the publisher and author have agreed to reproduce positives of the radiographs. Although in Anglo-American literature radiographs are also reproduced as negatives, the reproduction of positives was chosen because details, subtleties and variations can be better recognized.

I would particularly like to thank Dr. Kathrin Consentius. Through her knowledge of radiology, general medicine and anatomy, she has made valuable contributions by her analyses.

My former collaborator, Dr. F. Kossel, agreed to the reproduction in Part A of his excellent physical article in "Atlas typischer Röntgenbilder von normalen Menschen" in an abbreviated and modified form. I therefore owe him particularly warm thanks.

I thank Lucie Vlachy, my close collaborator and consultant on scientific questions for over 25 years, for her work with regard to the arrangement of this book.

I should also like to thank my former first assistant, Gertrude Kothe, who until September 1974 took care of the technical arrangements.

And, finally, my thanks to Urban & Schwarzenberg, and in particular Mr. Michael Urban and the chief editor, Dr. H. J. Clemens, and the production manager, Mr. G. Herwig, for their understanding and care in the production of this book.

Berlin, Summer 1978 *Rudolf Birkner*

Contents

A. Fundamentals of Radiation Physics, Picture Formation and Radiation Protection

B. Radiographic View of the Normal Adult Skeleton

This book uses Parisian nomenclature (PNA) exclusively. However, it has not been possible to be altogether consistent, since there are still differences in the various editions of the PNA. In addition, anatomic and roentgenologic handbooks, atlases and encyclopedias have until recently also been using Jenaer and Basel nomenclature and this tradition has been carried on by showing these terms in brackets wherever the author thought necessary.

A. Fundamentals of Radiation Physics, Picture Formation and Radiation Protection

General Principles

Radiographs and Photographs

Any interpretation of X-ray pictures which is intended to be of assistance to persons interested or active in radiology, be they physicians, students or radiology assistants, would be incomplete without mention of the physico-technical potentialities and limits of the radiographic method. However, fulfillment of this important precondition for the analysis of radiographs is often thwarted by tedious, long-winded explanations, which make it difficult for the reader to gain an overall understanding of the field.

For this reason, in the following sections we will focus on general principles. Moreover, and again to facilitate a better understanding, we will consciously simplify the problems.

To begin, let us explain some essential physical differences between radiographs and photographs.

The photographic image is, as a rule, formed by illuminating the object and producing, with the object-reflected light, a picture on a screen or film by means of an optical system, e.g., photographic object lenses (Fig. 1).

On the other hand, the X-ray picture or radiograph is always a ray-penetration image, regardless of whether it is presented on a fluorescent screen or on film. The object is placed between the radiation source and the film (Fig. 2).

This difference is due to the fact that most objects are impenetrable to light rays, meaning that their image must be formed by reflected light, unless only the object's contours are to be recognized. The light is not reflected as it is by a mirror-like source (e.g., a mirror, a water surface or a pane of glass) in narrow beams in a certain direction, but rather by the comparatively rough surface in a diffuse manner. Light is scattered over all sides. This scattered light is used for forming the image and provides an impression of the shape of the object. The scattered reflection by the generally turbid and inhomogeneous media prevents the penetration of visible light. X-rays, on the other hand, are not subjected to scattered reflection in turbid, inhomogeneous substances, as are body tissues, bones or wood. They are not affected by the many, irregularly distributed interfaces. For this reason, most substances are permeable by X-rays.

An example of the impermeability of a substance with many interfaces, causing scattered reflection of light, is illustrated in Figures 3 to 5. Figure 3 shows the photographic image of a glass of light beer in incident and then in reflected light. This image corresponds to what is seen. The path of the ray, starting from Q_1, is shown in Figure 4. In transmitted light, the foam crown is completely impermeable. The arrangement of the light source (Q_1) for this photograph is shown by dotted lines. Scattered reflection takes place on the countless irregular interfaces of the foam. If an X-ray source is substituted for the light source, and the picture is taken according to the arrangement in Figure 2, Figure 5 results. The foam is completely penetrable by X-rays. The numerous interfaces show no effect. Yet, the same substance in the homogeneous state is more penetrable to light than to X-rays.

A substance which is penetrable both to light and X-rays was intentionally selected. However, most substances are turbid and light-penetrable only when in thin sections. This fact is known to all those involved in microscopy. Thus, for observation in transmitted light, thin sections must be prepared.

In order to demonstrate the effect of turbidity on penetrability, water was mixed with milk (Fig. 6). In the top photograph (a), there are four plexiglass beakers photographed in incident and reflected light. The far-left beaker contains only milk and the far-right one only water. In between are two beakers with water, which in one case is made strongly and in the other weakly turbid with milk.

The middle photograph (b) shows the same arrangement photographed with transmitted light. Water is very light-penetrable. With turbidity, penetrability decreases.

In the picture taken with X-rays (c), no increase in turbidity is observed. The X-rays are not affected by the

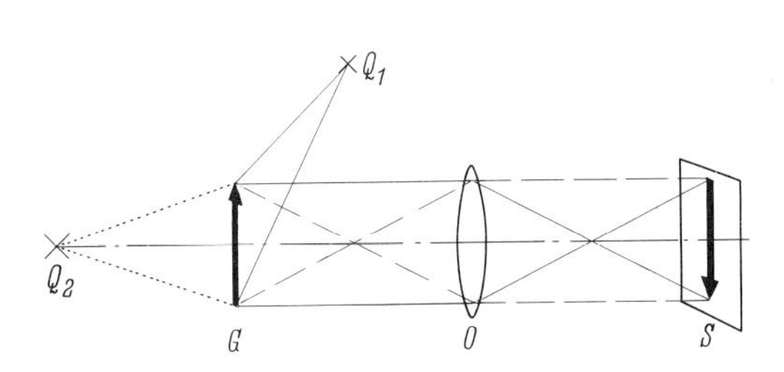

Fig. 1. With visible light, the image of the object (G) is projected onto a screen (S) in the plane of projection, with the light reflected from G via an optical system (O). The light is emitted from the light source. Transparent objects are illuminated by Q_2.

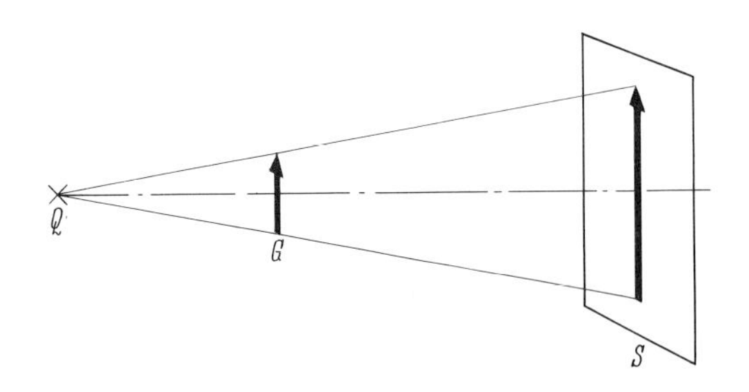

Fig. 2. X-rays emitted from the radiation source (Q) penetrate the object (G), and the image is projected onto a screen (S). There is no image-forming optical system.

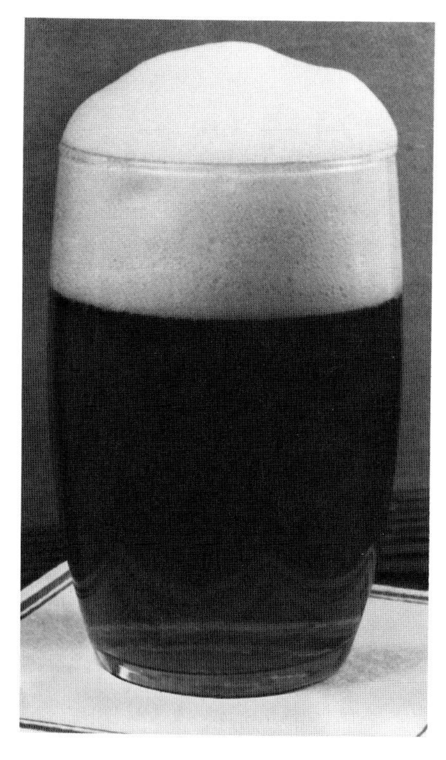

Fig. 3. A glass of light beer photographed first in incident and then in reflected light. The foam crown reflects the light, giving it a whitish appearance.

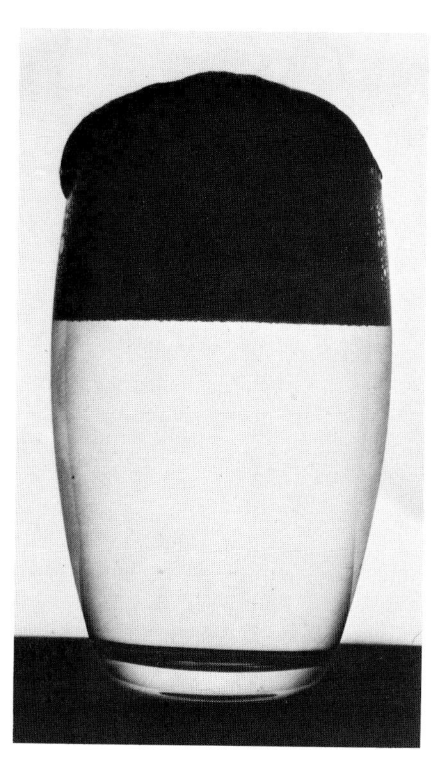

Fig. 4. The same glass of beer photographed in transmitted light. The foam crown is light-inpenetrable because of scattered reflection of the light on the countless foam bubbles, while the beer itself is light-penetrable.

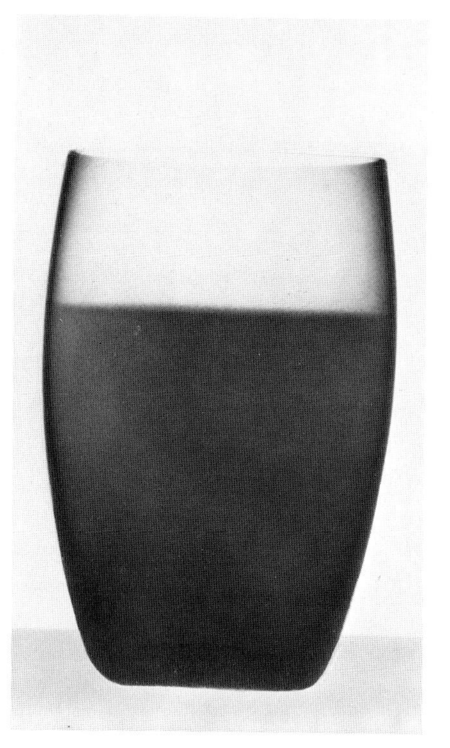

Fig. 5. The same glass of beer taken with X-rays. The foam crown is not perceptible because it does not appreciably attenuate the X-rays. Foam substances, e. g., those made from plastics, are therefore very suitable for mobilizing the patient when taking radiographs.

Figs. 3–5. Comparisons between photographic and X-ray pictures (suggested by *Pohl*).

milk particles; particles the size of a molecule or larger, having about the same density as the water molecules, do not produce turbidity. Turbidity occurs only with considerable differences in density.

The attenuation of X-rays is even stronger when atoms of a higher atomic number are present. Figure 7, showing barium bromide solutions in water, provides an example of turbidity produced by atoms having a higher atomic number.

The solutions having different concentrations of barium bromide show no difference, whether photographed in incident light (a) or transmitted light (b). With X-radiation (c), the penetrability increases with decreasing concentration of barium bromide. Barium has a high atomic number (56) in comparison with water (whose effective total atomic number is 7.4). Chambers with aqueous barium bromide solutions are also used as radiation protection windows because of the strong attenuation of X-rays and the high penetrability for light rays.

The individual differences between the substances, due to their structures, are not decisive for scattering or absorptional attenuation of X-rays. Chemical bonds and states of aggregation also have no effect. Only thickness, density and atomic number are decisive.

X-ray diagnostics are based on the fact that body tissues are more or less transparent for X-rays, while the scattered reflection on the interfaces of the inhomogeneous media of the body and the turbidity are insignificant if compared with visible light.

There is no image-forming system for X-rays comparable to the object lenses for light. For this reason, only the shadow of an object can be projected upon a screen. Radiographs are thus silhouettes, projected one over the other, of the spatially distributed, more or less transparent details of the object.

The geometric configuration of the rays makes possible the production of such silhouettes. The object should transmit radiation. Sharp shadows are possible only when the rays either fall parallelly upon the object (parallel projection, Fig. 8a) or are emitted from a point-like radiation source (central projection, Fig. 8b).

Parallel projection has the advantage that the image and object always have the same size, independently of their spatial position, as is shown in Figure 8a. The source supplies parallel rays only when infinitely distant from the object. The sun is an example of such a light source. Shadows in sunlight are sharp because they are produced by parallel rays. Since the intensity of rays strongly decreases with distance, the radiation intensity from a very remote source, e.g., the sun, must be extremely strong. Both for spatial reasons and the limited intensity, parallel projection cannot be used for X-ray sources. Thus, only central projection can be used.

In this case, the shadow is increased by the ray di-

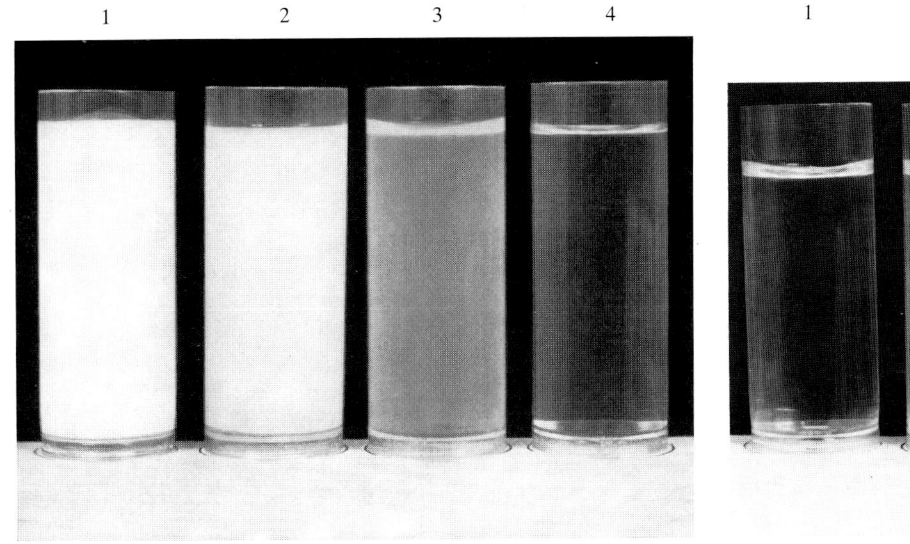

a) Obtained with reflected light

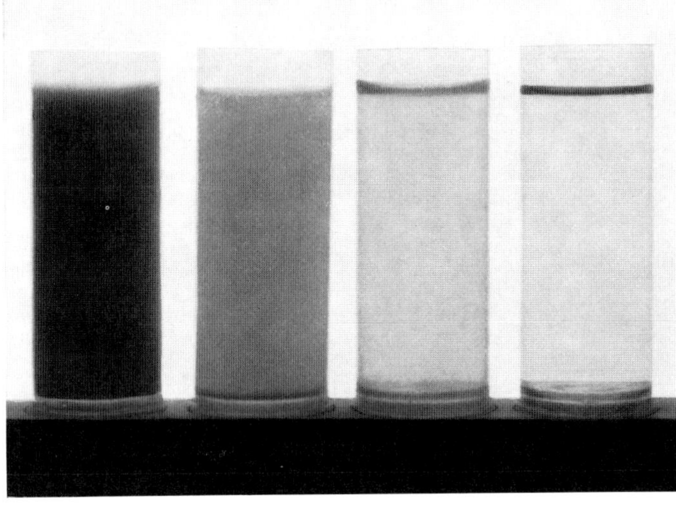

b) Obtained with transmitted light

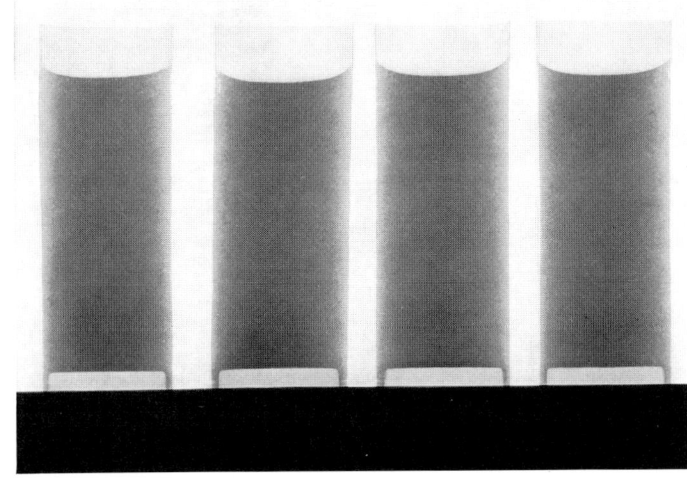

c) Obtained with soft X-radiation

Fig. 6. Milk-water mixtures. The milk concentration decreases from 1 to 4.

1 2 3 4

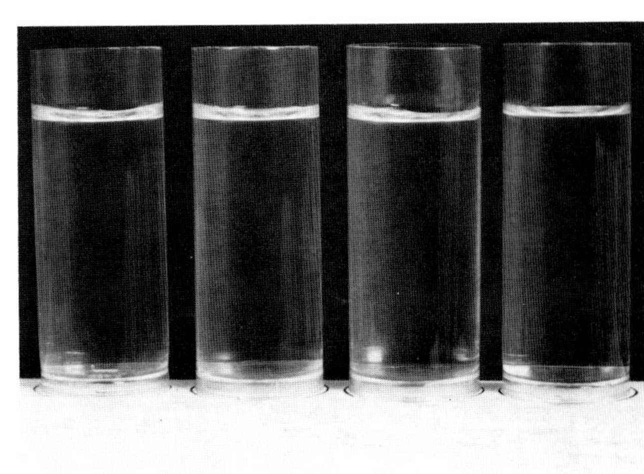

a) Obtained in reflected light

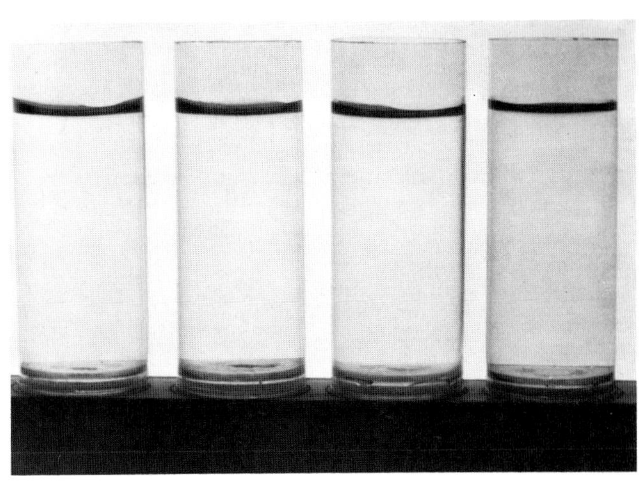

b) Obtained in transmitted light

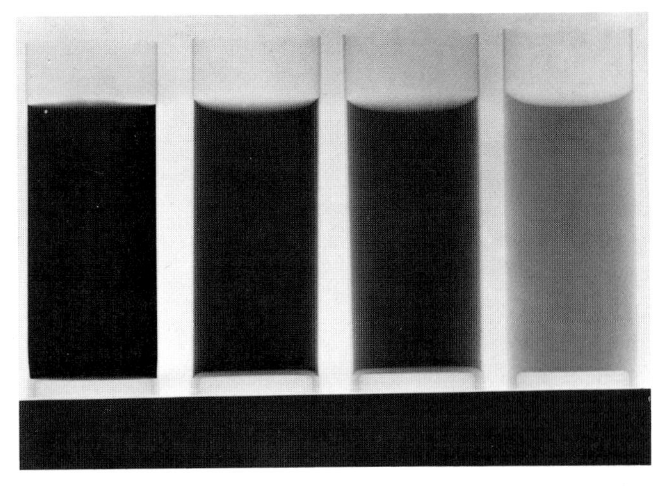

c) Obtained with soft X-radiation

Fig. 7. Solutions of barium bromide in water. The $BaBr_2$ concentration decreases from 1 to 4.

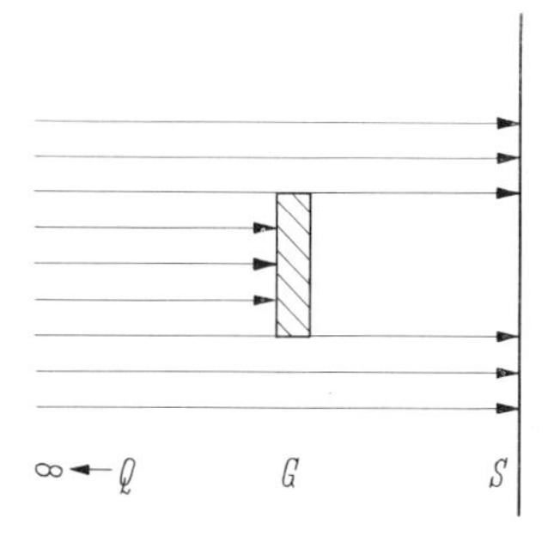

Fig. 8a. Parallel projection. The rays are strictly parallel. The radiation source is infinitely remote. The shadow is the size of the object, regardless of the object's distance. Q = source, G = object, S = screen.

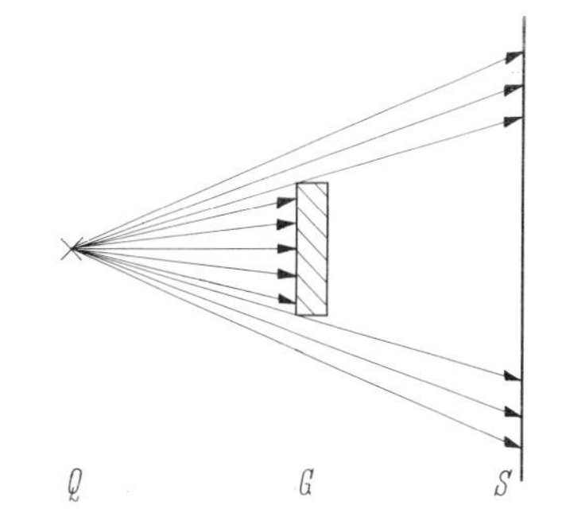

Fig. 8b. Central projection. The beam is divergent. The size of the shadow increases with decreasing distance between G and Q and increasing distance between G and S. The contours of the shadow are sharper the less extended the light source.

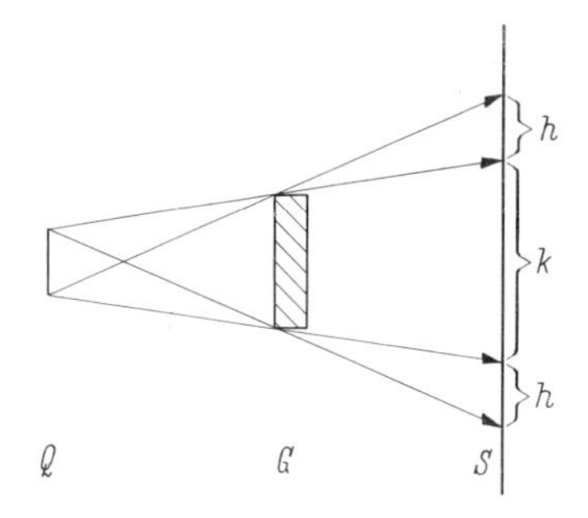

Fig. 8c. Extended radiation source. (Only the rays on the edge are shown.) There are two shadow regions: the umbra (k), into which no radiation enters, and the penumbra (h), into which only the rays from a part of the source arrive. The contours of the shadow are blurred.

vergence. This increment is larger with reduced distance between object and radiation source and increased distance between object and screen. A non-optical, point-like radiation source leads to a blurred shadow. Figure 8c shows the edge rays from the point source (Q). A region (umbra) can be observed behind the object where no radiation enters. This is followed by another region (penumbra) which is only partially illuminated by the radiation source. Thus, there is no sharp division between complete brightness and the darkness of the shadow, but rather a continuous transition. In other words, the shade contour is blurred.

As has been explained, there is no image-forming system for X-rays comparable to the optical system for light rays. Depending on the penetrability of the individual parts of the object, more or less dense silhouettes can be projected. For this purpose, a radiation source, which must be as point-like as possible, is required. In central projection (Fig. 8b), the image is most favorable, i.e., equal to or larger than the size of the object, when the object is placed directly in front of the screen. All objects lying in horizontal sequence are projected in vertical sequence.

With visible light and an image-forming lens system,

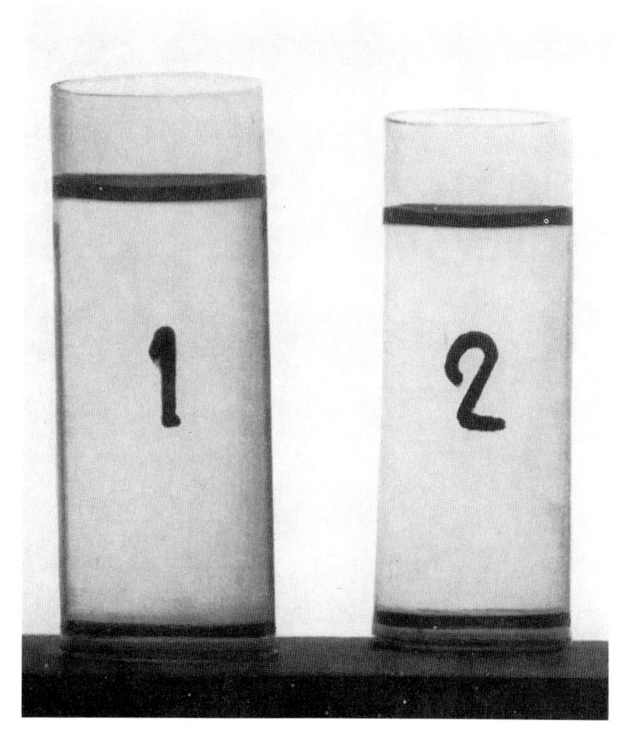

Fig. 9. Two water-filled plexiglass beakers photographed in transmitted light. The beaker nearer to the screen is designated with metal number 1, and the rear beaker with 2. The beaker farther from the screen (2) is smaller in the picture than the beaker nearer to the screen (1).

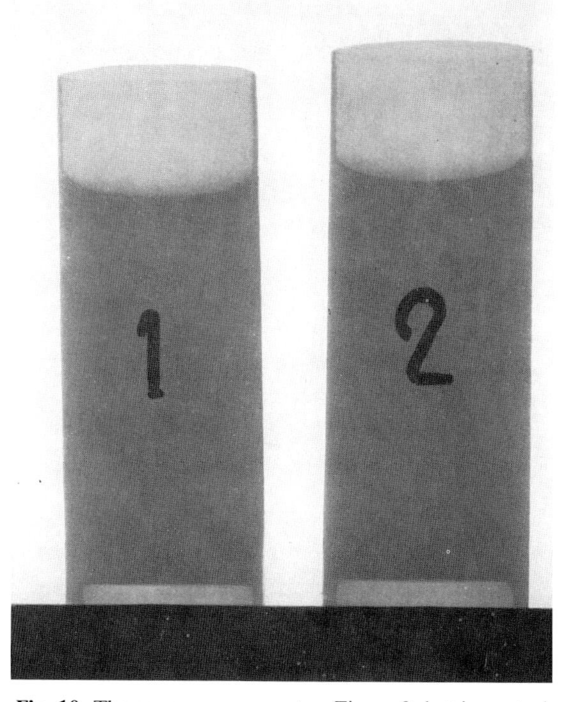

Fig. 10. The same arrangement as Figure 9, but in central projection with X-rays. Beaker farther from the screen is now larger than beaker 1, nearer to the screen.

uniform illumination of the object is sufficient. By manipulating the image-forming conditions and the optical system, pictures can be made either smaller or larger than the object. Moreover, appropriate selection of the image-forming system can ensure that close objects do not interfere with the image production of remote objects. They must not cover the whole field of view, and must be, to the extent possible, within the focal distance of the object lens. This phenomenon is easily grasped by holding spread fingers in front of a telescope objective. The fingers are not perceived at all; they only reduce the light intensity. It is known from microscopy that superimposed parts of a preparation can be observed without mutual interference by successively adjusting the resolving power. If, on the other hand, no image is produced and the object is projected without an optical system, any object which stands between the radiation source and screen will appear on the latter as a silhouette.

Because of this type of projection, in the radiograph all dimensional relations and light and shadow distributions, which are used in a photographic image for orientation and to which we are accustomed through vision, are lost. In the photograph of two equal-sized objects, the closer images are larger than the more distant ones.

Figure 9 shows photographs of two water-filled plexiglass beakers taken with transmitted light. The front beaker is designated as beaker 1; the rear one as beaker 2. In the photographs, the beaker farther from the screen (2) is smaller than the beaker nearer to the screen (1). Using X-rays in central projection, however, the object farther from the screen (2) is larger than the object nearer to the screen (1) (Figs. 10 and 11). Thus, in radiographs an entirely different spatial impression is produced. But here also, observer reorientation is necessary. For complicated shapes of the object, this perspective reversal is so potentially confusing that it is impossible to interpret the radiograph without stipulating which part of the object is closer to the screen and which is farther from it.

As we have mentioned above, the radiograph as a silhouette in central projection is entirely different from a picture obtained by visible light with the aid of an optical system. Thus, the ordinary visual experience, which is also produced by a light optical system, may easily lead to an erroneous interpretation. The "roentgenologic vision" is acquired only through long-term experience in the comparison of numerous radiographs.

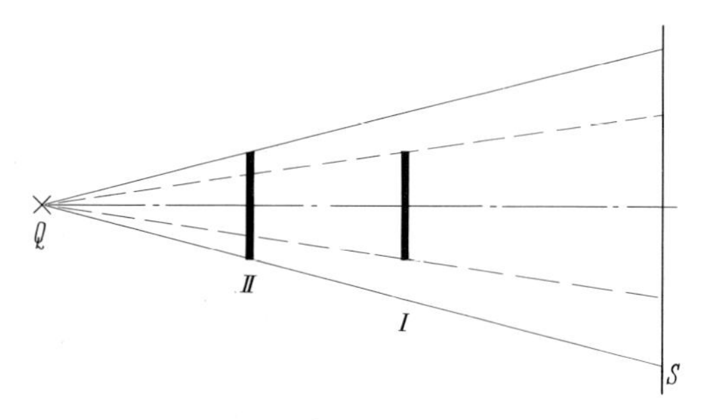

Fig. 11. Given two equal-sized objects, the image of the object farther from the screen (II) is larger in central projection than the image of the object nearer to the screen (I).

The reasons radiographs must be produced by procedures other than photographic images will be explained in detail in the following sections, as will the laws governing central projection. The rules which must be observed in this case are far simpler and clearer than the laws of geometric optics.

The Physical Nature of X-Rays

The following is a short and necessarily simplified presentation of the physical nature of X-rays from the vantage point of atomic physics. The discussion does not contain any physical refinements; these were consciously dispensed with for the sake of clarity and to avoid confusion.

To begin, we must challenge the impression that matter is dense because it consists predominantly of wide, mass-free spaces.

Dispersed, but with uniform distances, the mass is concentrated, in almost unimaginable density, in the atomic nuclei. The latter have an average density of 2×10^{14} g/cm^3. Thus, a small cube of 1 cm edge, if it had the density of the nucleus, would have a mass of 200 million tons. The spaces between the nuclei are occupied by electrical and magnetic fields, which are very strong in the close vicinity of the nucleus and drive the electrons around the nucleus on fixed orbitals. The electrons far from the nucleus on the outermost orbital are no longer as strongly bound, and therefore, very readily interact with neighboring atoms. They are responsible for the cohesion of the atom groups, both in the individual molecule and the solid body. Electromagnetic waves enter this matter.

Electromagnetic waves consist of electrical and magnetic rotational fields. When an electrical field is rapidly built up, a magnetic field is formed. This magnetic field in turn produces another electrical field. Such rapidly forming fields can be detached from their site of origin. Because of the continuous and repetitive building up of both fields, whereby any change of one field leads to the building up of the other, waves propagate through space. These interlinked, rapidly propagating fields are the electromagnetic waves. When entering matter, they produce a disturbance of the fields present between the individual atomic nuclei, corresponding to the rhythm of a wave. In this way, the molecular bonds of the individual atoms and the electron orbitals in the atoms are also disturbed. The molecules and atoms are excited to forced vibration by the electromagnetic waves. These forced vibrations of the molecular and atomic components, all of which are carriers of an electrical charge, in turn produce electromagnetic waves. These waves repenetrate the matter and again excite molecules and atoms, which are in turn points of origin for new elementary waves. (This principle of wave propagation was stated as early as 1678 by *Huygens,* although without knowledge of the atomic

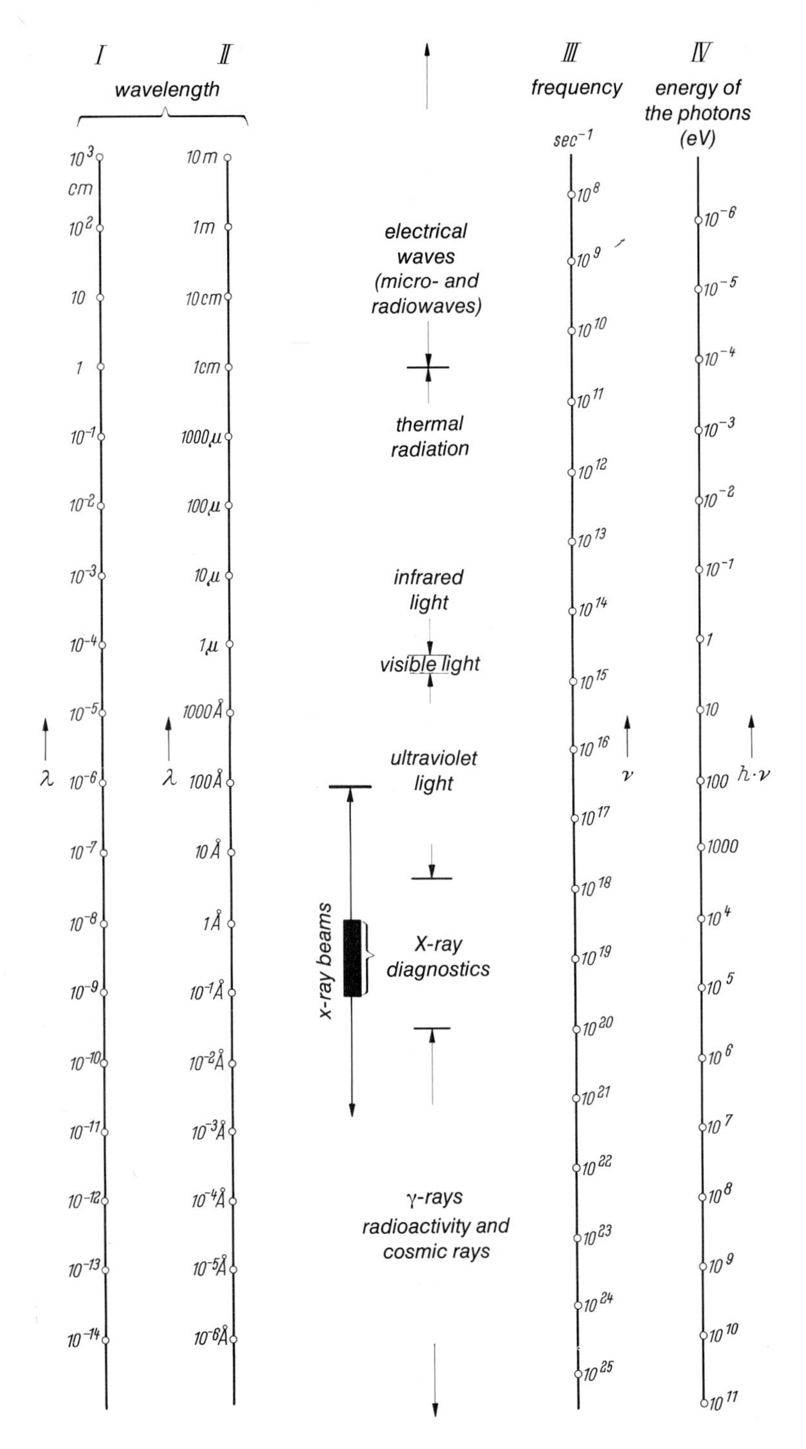

Fig. 12. Chart of the total electromagnetic spectrum (based on *Finkelnburg).* Wavelength scales (scale I in cm, scale II in conventional subunits), frequency (III) and energy scales (IV).

structure of matter.) Thus, every site excited by a wave is the starting point of new waves.

As can be seen from scale IV on Figure 12, the energy of visible light is a few electronvolts. Thus, when penetrating matter, light excites the outer valence electrons or ejects them from the atom. Such a separation is termed ionization of the atoms. However, this energy is insufficient for affecting the electrons of the atom shell, which are 1000 times more strongly bound. The energy of the X-rays, on the other hand, is of the order of 10^4 eV. An X-ray photon loses an appreciable part of its energy only when an electron near the nucleus is ejected. The ionizing action here is much stronger and, as a rule, takes place in several stages. Such high-energy electromagnetic waves and high-energy corpuscular radiation (fast electrons and β-rays) are called ionizing rays in medicine. Physically, however, this term is not accurate because the energy of light is also sufficient to ionize atoms.

Whether the electromagnetic waves readily penetrate the matter, or are more or less scattered and absorbed depends on the structure of the matter. The atomic representation of matter shows quite clearly that an appreciable interaction can occur only between the high-energy X-rays and the fields surrounding the atom's nucleus.

The interaction will increase with the number of atoms, i.e., with the density of matter, and the strength of the nuclear fields. In other words, the effect of X-rays on matter increases with the atomic number, which is equal to the number of positive charges. For light, whose energy is of the same order of magnitude as the molecular bond energy, there are more possibilities to influence matter because far more molecular species than atomic species exist. The molecular structure and the arrangement of the atoms in larger regions of uniform solid bodies create excitation and propagation conditions for light, which vary strongly from substance to substance.

The difference between radiographs and photographs is caused by the differing interaction between radiation and matter. The energy of X-rays is so much larger than the energy of light radiation that only processes in the atomic region show a considerable effect upon the mode of propagation of the X-rays. On the other hand, the energy of light is insufficient to affect the atom more profoundly.

Formation of the Radiograph

The Path of the Rays

The radiograph is a picture produced by penetration of radiation. The rays come from the radiation source, penetrate the object, and fall either upon the fluorescent screen or upon a film, which is thus exposed (Fig. 13). In order to obtain sharp silhouettes, the radiation source (Q) must be as point-like as possible. The rays emitted by the source propagate linearly. The intensity of the beam is uniform throughout. Only the object, e.g., the irradiated body organ, changes this distribution. Depending on the structure of the irradiated parts of the body, larger or smaller amounts of radiation are transmitted. Bones absorb more radiation than do soft tissues such as fat, muscles, etc.

Thus, every part of the screen (S) is more or less illuminated. In other words, the structure of the beam behind the object, the radiation relief, corresponds to the structure of the irradiated region of the body. The conversion of the radiation relief into values visible to us either by fluorescence, i.e., light excitation of the fluorescent screen, or by blackening of the photographic layer, yields the radiograph.

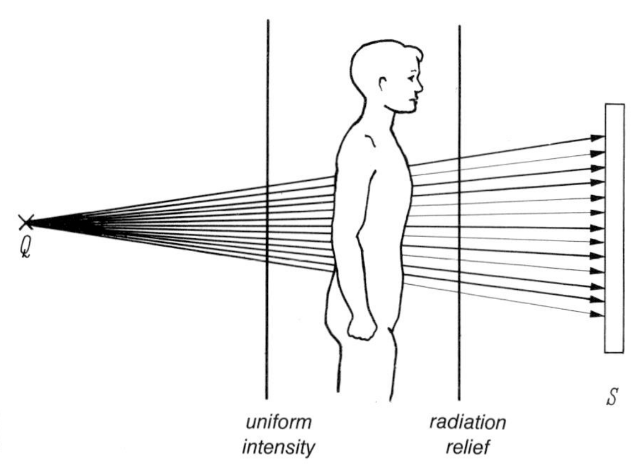

Fig. 13. The path of the rays in the radiograph. Before penetrating the object, the intensity of the beam is uniform; after penetration, the intensity varies depending upon the irradiated part of the body and absorption by the body.

The Production of X-rays

Put most simply, the electrons emitted from the cathode of the X-ray tube are accelerated on their way to the anode and then braked in the material of the anode (anticathode), producing X-rays.

The electrons, minute, negatively charged particles which are considerably smaller than the individual atomic nuclei, penetrate the wide spaces, free of mass but full of fields, between the lattice atoms of the solid anode substance. Electrons which, for example, are accelerated by a voltage of 50,000 V (50 kV), a voltage widely used in X-ray diagnostics, are already very fast. They reach a velocity of 133,000 km/sec (one-third the velocity of light) prior to their entrance into matter. Though the electrons penetrate only fractions of a millimeter, they travel through 10,000 to 100,000 layers of the atom lattice.

During their travel, these small electric particles are ejected from their linear trajectory by the effect of the fields and decelerated, i.e., they lose kinetic energy. A few electrons fly through the space between the electrons of the atom shell and perturb the strong fields near the atomic nuclei. This perturbation can, as was mentioned before, be shed from the site of its origin and propagate to the outside. The majority of the electrons, however, transfer their energy in many small portions onto the matter and excite the lattice atoms to vibration.

Less than 1% of the energy of the electron flux is converted into X-rays, while more than 99% is converted into heat. Because this type of X-ray is produced by the braking of the electrons, it is called "Bremsstrahlung".

Braking of a single electron is stronger the closer its trajectory is to the nucleus. Occasionally, the electron loses all its kinetic energy at once in this way. Such electrons produce very high-energy X-rays. From the "atomic point of view," the genesis of the Bremsstrahlung is easy to understand. It is clear that because of the relatively large internuclear distance, not many electrons reach the vicinity of the nucleus and therefore the X-ray yield is low. Because the electrons, depending on their trajectory through the material, are braked to dif-

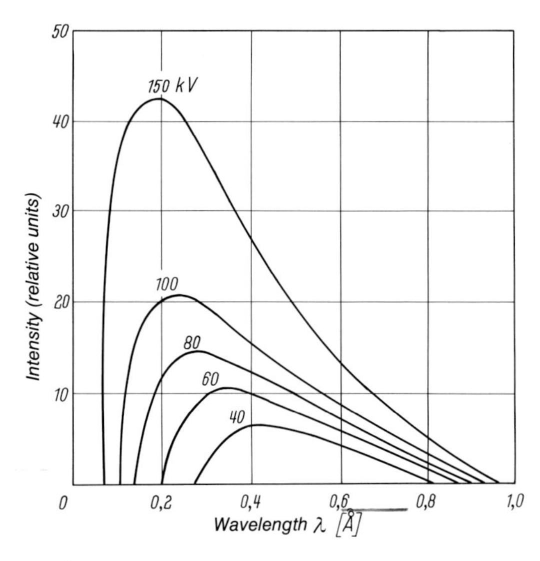

Fig. 14. Spectral intensity distribution of the Bremsstrahlung for different generating voltages in kilovolts (kV). Intensity is plotted as a function of wavelength.

ferent extents, the composition of the Bremsstrahlung is heterogeneous. A typical picture of the wavelength distribution is shown in Figure 14.

The higher the voltage, the greater the frequency of electron-strong field interaction and the farther the spectrum reaches into the shorter wavelength region. As Figure 12 shows, a shorter wavelength also implies a higher energy of the photons. The sharp short-wave boundary is produced by electrons which, as has been described above, lose all their kinetic energy in a single braking process.

When penetrating matter, the electrons may also collide with the electrons of the atom cloud. The electrons arrive close to the atomic nucleus or even penetrate into it only when they possess a very high energy. Such fast electrons cannot be produced in the X-ray tube. If an atom loses an electron by collision, i.e., it is ionized, the missing electron is replaced by another electron from the surroundings in a period as short as 10^{-6} sec. During this process, the binding energy is released in the form of electromagnetic radiation. Since the electrons move over certain orbitals around the atoms, the binding energy has a certain value for each orbital, which is characteristic for the atoms of the material in question. In this case, in addition to the Bremsstrahlung, a so-called characteristic X-radiation is generated. This, however, is not continuously distributed over all wavelengths. It consists of some typical wavelength values which can be assigned uniquely to the different electron orbitals of the atom species in question.

Thus, the whole X-ray spectrum consists of a continuous Bremsstrahlung spectrum with voltage-dependent wavelength distribution (Fig. 14). Onto these curves, the individual peaks of the characteristic X-radiation are superimposed. These are typical for the used material in their distribution and size (Fig. 15). Each wavelength is represented by an intensity, determined by the spectral distribution curve. Integration of the individual intensity values for each wavelength gives the total intensity of the X-ray source. Thus, the total intensity is given by the area under the curve. It immediately becomes clear that the contribution of the individual peaks to the total radiation is small when compared to the large area under the curve of the Bremsstrahlung spectrum. This fact is very important.

In summary, the X-rays are generated by the braking of fast electrons in matter. The energy and wavelength of the radiation are not homogeneous, just as the white light in the visual region is composed of waves of different lengths (color). For every voltage, there is a minimum wavelength. To this wavelength, the radiant energy produced by the fastest electron must be assigned. The Bremsstrahlung supplies the main contribution to the intensity of the X-ray source. Only a minute fraction of the total energy of the electrons is converted into X-rays, while the larger part is converted into heat, and this leads to a very strong heating up of the material. An increase in the accelerating voltage increases both the intensity and the energy (penetrating power) of the X-rays. The structure of an X-ray tube is shown in Figure 16.

The thoroughly evacuated glass vessel contains a cathode (K) and an anode (A). The voltage (U) between anode and cathode is of the order of several 10,000 volts. The cathode consists of a wire, which is heated by an electric current and thus excited to emit electrons. The filament current required for this purpose is produced by the filament voltage (U_H). The electrons are accelerated during their travel from the cathode to the anode by high voltage. Since electrons carry a negative charge, they are attracted by the positive anode. In the anode material, the electrons are braked and produce X-rays (R). To ensure unimpeded travel, i.e., without collision with air molecules, from the cathode to the anode, the glass vessel must be evacuated. To ensure sharp pictures, the radiation source must be as point-like as possible (Fig. 8b).

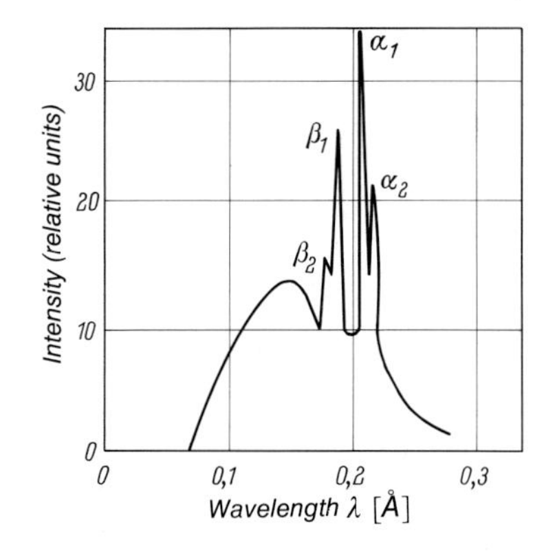

Fig. 15. Intensity distribution of the X-ray spectrum of an X-ray tube with tungsten anode (generating voltage: 168 kV). The spectrum of the continuous Bremsstrahlung is shown with some sharp peaks ($\alpha_1, \alpha_2, \beta_1, \beta_2$) of the characteristic tungsten radiation *(Pohl)*.

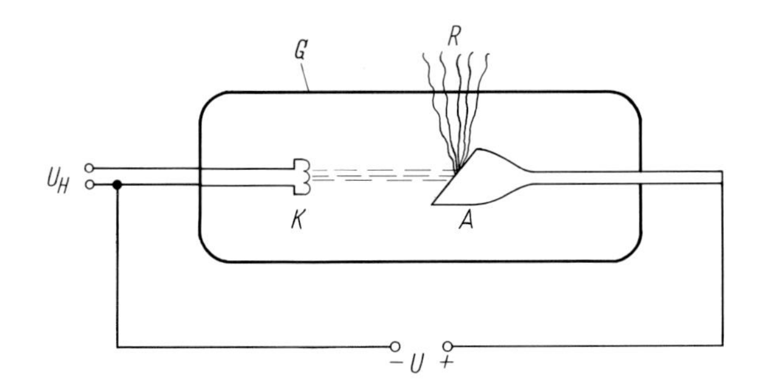

Fig. 16. Schematic diagram of an X-ray tube. G = Evacuated glass vessel, K = Cathode, A = Anode, U_H = Filament voltage, U = High voltage, R = X-Rays.

That is, the place where the rays are produced, the focus, must be kept very small. On the other hand, certain minimum dimensions of the focus are necessary, mainly because the X-ray yield is low and the evolved heat must be removed to prevent destruction of the anode.

Thus, it is apparent that a compromise is necessary in order to obtain the minimum possible focus. With very small foci, the intensity of the X-rays becomes very low. If moving objects, e.g., the lungs or the heart, are to be examined, very short exposure times are necessary, and these are possible under certain circumstances only by using a larger focus. Thus, the resulting picture is not very clear. On the other hand, if it is possible for the patient to keep his body organ, e.g., his hand, at rest for a sufficiently long period, a smaller focus and longer exposure time can be used. The foci of the X-ray tubes used in diagnostics range in size from 0.09 mm^2 in the direction of the emitted X-rays up to 4 mm^2. (At a later point in our discussion, when the possibility exists for comparison with other sources of error, the effect of the size of the focus will be quantitatively estimated.)

The Radiation Relief (or Picture) as a Preliminary Stage of the X-Ray Picture[1])

After leaving the anode (anticathode), the X-rays penetrate the glass wall of the tube, the oil with which the protective hood of the X-ray tube is filled (to insulate the high voltage and remove the radiant heat of the anode), and the radiation outlet window of the protective hood. Here, the long-wave and low-energy portions of the X-radiation are absorbed. That is, the radiation is "filtered" on the first part of its path through the materials of the tube and hood. Thus, a portion of the heterogeneous radiation is not very penetrating, leading us to refer to "soft" rays. The so-called "hard" rays are the high-energy, short-wave portions of the X-ray spectrum (see Fig. 14). These conventional terms, taken from colloquial speech, should be clear without the necessity of analyzing the physical process of the absorption in any more detail.

The filtering of the radiation through the X-ray tube and the protective hood is advantageous since the absorbed radiation would not contribute to the formation of the X-ray picture in any way. Rather, it would be totally absorbed as immediately as in the skin or in the first few centimeters of body tissue, and cause a potential radiation load to the patient. For this reason, a certain supplementary prefiltering of the diagnostic X-ray radiation is prescribed.

On its path through the air to the skin of the patient, the composition of the radiation no longer changes. This is because the attenuation of the prefiltered and soft-ray free radiation is very small, owing to the very low density of the air. Only in the body do processes occur which are decisive for the formation of the radiation relief.

The importance of the ray-matter interaction for the formation of the radiograph from the vantage point of atomic physics has already been emphasized. The same interaction modulates the intensity, which before penetration of the object is homogeneously distributed over the cross section of the beam. The structure of the object changes the intensity distribution in a typical manner, depending on whether bones, soft tissues, cavities, etc. are irradiated. By making the intensity distribution, i.e., the radiation relief, produced in this way visible on a fluorescent screen or film, the structure of the object can be determined. The structure of the object is transformed into a structure of the radiation, and thus made visible to the eye. If we want to evaluate the structure of the object from the visualized radiation relief, we must be aware of the exact transformation process, i.e., the production of the radiation relief.

Again as has been mentioned, the intensity distribution over the cross section of the beam is homogeneous (Fig. 17). The degree of intensity is indicated by the length of the arrows. The object should have some structure. In this case, the intensity distribution is no longer homogeneous; we speak about a radiation relief. An object which is structureless, and thus homogeneous for X-rays, does not change the intensity distribution. The rays are only uniformly attenuated and no radiation relief is formed (Fig. 18).

A layer of homogeneous material can easily be inserted somewhere in the path of the rays, without thereby changing the form of the radiation relief, which gives us information about conditions in the body. Such layers include, for example, the plate of the table on which the patient is placed or the X-ray film holder. For practical reasons, substances are selected for this material which do not excessively attenuate the X-rays; otherwise, unnecessary intensity losses occur. Materials with low molecular or atomic number, such as wood, aluminum,

[1]) Since a relief denotes a spatial formation, while here the two-dimensional distribution of the X-ray quanta behind an object is meant, we speak, with *Angerstein,* of a ray picture.

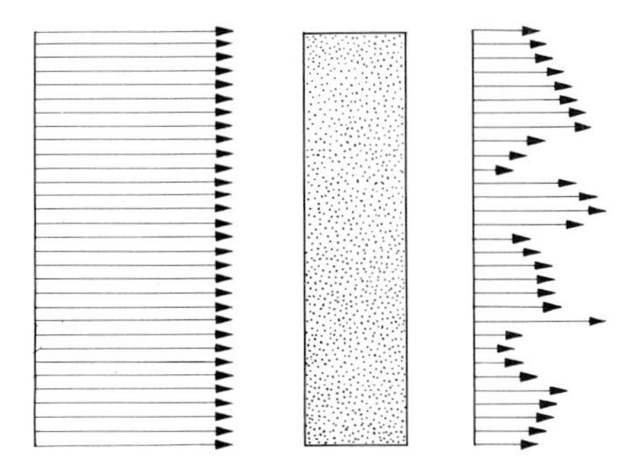

Fig. 17. The homogeneous intensity distribution is altered by an inhomogeneous object. The length of the arrows indicates the intensity.

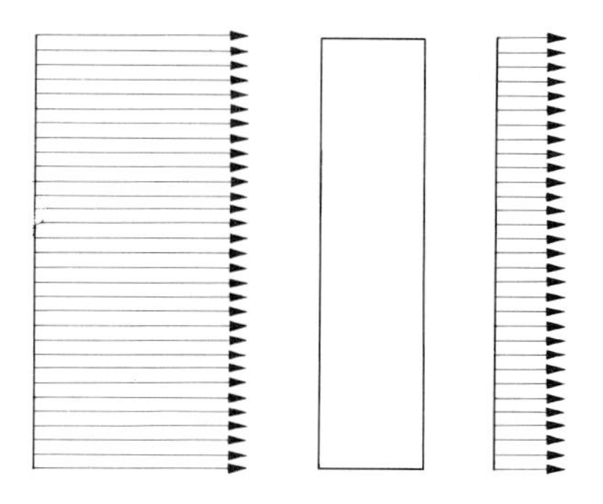

Fig. 18. The homogeneous intensity distribution is only attenuated by a homogeneous object.

many plastics (plexiglass), etc., are therefore suitable. The extent of the attenuation also depends on the thickness of the homogeneous layer of the material.

Attenuation of the Primary Ray Beam

Matter attenuates the primary beam by absorption and scattering. Radiant energy is absorbed because of the fact that atoms and molecules are excited or ionized by radiation. Through ionization, the electrons are ejected from the atom cluster. These electrons can, in turn, excite or ionize atoms, which are not directly impacted by the primary X-rays. These newly released electrons again affect other atoms, until all the energy has been used up in stages.

Because the atoms and molecules are excited to vibration, molecular conversions may occur, in turn producing chemical changes. These processes may harm cells in the living tissue. This property of ionizing radiation is used to destroy malignant cells. In X-ray diagnostics, however, this leads to a radiation load of the patient, which is always undesirable. By suitable steps, this load can and must be reduced to a minimum. Generally, the extent of this "lesion" is unimportant in X-ray diagnostics, and must be endured given the necessity of X-ray examination.

The absorption differences lead to the formation of the radiation relief. Without absorption, no radiograph is possible.

In the second process, also leading to an attenuation of the incident radiation, a part of the primary beam is scattered to all sides by the matter. This scattered radiation is problematic in X-ray diagnostics. It is superimposed over the radiation relief, thereby, reducing the intensity differences which give us information about the structure of the object. Its final effect is the veiling of the X-ray picture. Therefore, special measures must be used to prevent this undesirable effect.

Since the beam is scattered over all directions, the scattered radiation also penetrates into those body regions of the patient which were not struck by the primary beam, and, through its ionizing and excitational effects, increases the radiation load of the patient. Moreover, the scattered radiation, reflected from the patient or from parts of the X-ray instrument, also leads to a radiation load in the investigator. The protection of the physician against such scattered radiation is technically far more difficult than protection against primary radiation.

Origin and Elimination of Scattered Radiation

Scattered radiation always occurs when electromagnetic waves penetrate matter. The amount and distribution of the direction of the scattered radiation depend on the size of the scattering particle of matter in comparison with the wavelength of the primary radiation. The scattered radiation emerges from all particles of matter which were hit by the primary radiation and were excited to vibration and emission of secondary waves. Since the scattering particles (the electrons of the atom group) are of constant size, the distribution of the direction and the extent of scattering depend only on the wavelength, i.e., on the energy of the primary radiation.

A representation of this process is given in Figure 19. An X-ray (R) passes the plane of the drawing from the left-hand to the right-hand side. A piece of matter, in which scattered radiation is produced, is present at point A. The distribution of the scattered radiation in accordance with size and direction around point A is clearly represented for different generating voltages. The distance between point A and the circumference of the curve enclosing point A is a measure for the size of the scattered radiation in a certain direction. Thus, the scattered radiation for 10 kV, for example, is not very large. Moreover, it is in the direction of the primary beam and in opposite direction almost as large and stronger as it is perpendicularly to the direction of the primary beam. With increasing voltage, the scattered radiation becomes much more intensive, attaining a peak at 100 kV. The rays are increasingly scattered in the direction of the primary ray. For very high voltages, the scattered radiation is again reduced, as shown by the 500 kV curve. Also, back scattering is reduced.

The proportion of scattering is small for relatively

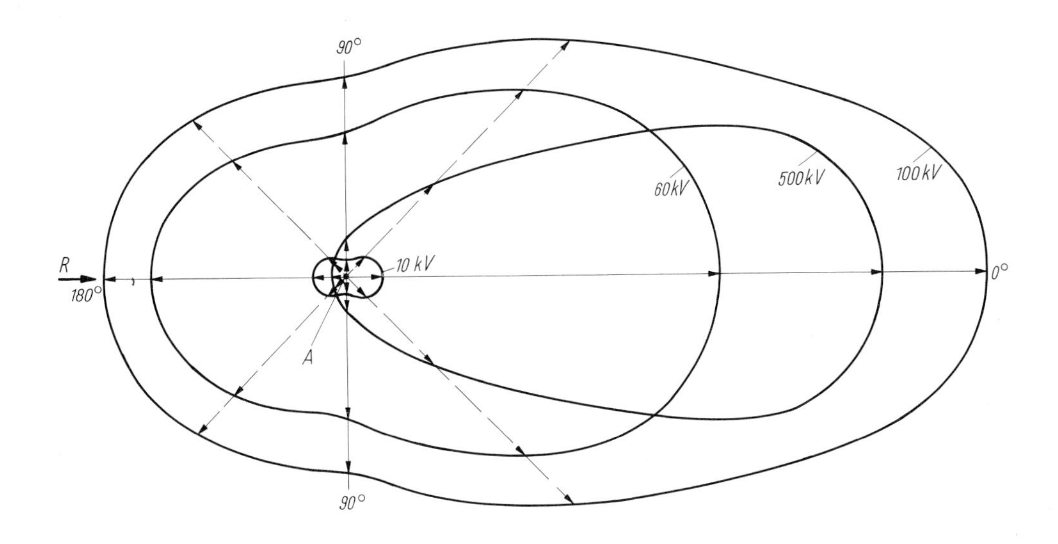

Fig. 19. Schematic diagram (after *Rump*) of the distribution of the scattered radiation, in accordance with direction and size for different generating voltages of the primary X-rays (very narrow beam). R=Direction of the primary X-ray, A=Piece of matter.

long-wave soft X-rays when compared with the proportion of absorption. The long-wave X-radiation produces a scattered radiation (the so-called coherent radiation, also termed classical or photoradiation), whose wavelength and energy are unchanged relative to the primary beam. With higher energy, another process becomes increasingly important – the so-called Compton scattering. Here, the primary X-ray quantum transfers a part of its energy onto an electron. The latter leaves the atom formation with a relatively low energy. The residual energy remains at the X-ray quantum, travelling in another direction, with a lower energy, i.e., longer wavelength. The scattered radiation produced by the Compton process is softer than the primary radiation, and the scattering is said to be incoherent. The shift of the wavelength is independent of the energy of the primary radiation, dependent only on the direction of scattering. At 10 kV, the Compton process is negligibly small. For 40 and 200 kV, the process makes up 25 and 99% of the interaction, respectively. Coherent scattering very rapidly decreases at voltages above 100 kV. At the same time, the number of interactions between matter and radiation becomes smaller because the radiation becomes increasingly penetrating. For this reason, there is actually less scattered radiation at 50 kV than at 100 kV.

The contributions of absorption and scattering to the total attenuation of the radiation depend, not only on the wavelength of the radiation, but also on the irradiated material. With energy, i.e., shorter wavelengths, the contribution of scattering strongly increases, while for lower energy and longer waves, absorption predominates. Figure 20 shows both contributions in percentages of the total attentuation for substances with a smaller atomic number, e.g., water (total effective atomic number 7.4) and for substances with a medium atomic number, e.g., copper (atomic number 29).

In summary, when X-rays penetrate matter, the radiation is attenuated by absorption and scattering. This scattering is noxious because, as is seen from Figure 19, it can assume considerable values in the direction of the primary radiation. Thus, ways must be found to keep scattered radiation away. Both scattered radiation and the absorption by tissues lead to a certain radiation hazard; it must be taken into account in all X-ray investigations. The formation of a radiation relief is a very involved process, since several physical factors are simultaneously effective.

The X-rays have a heterogeneous composition prior to their entrance into matter. The primary radiation beam is the Bremsstrahlung with a certain distribution according to quality and quantity (see Fig. 14).

The beam has, after penetrating matter, a new distribution in quality and quantity. The primary beam becomes significantly weaker. The soft, long-wave portions of the primary beam are much more strongly absorbed than are the short-wave, high-energy portions (Fig. 20).

To this reduced amount of primary radiation, the secondary scattered radiation is added (Fig. 19). The scattered rays of the soft primary radiation now have the same energy as the primary radiation itself. For harder primary radiation, the generated scattered radiation has longer waves and less energy. This is another reason, for the fact, that the composition of the beam is entirely different after it has passed through matter.

The conditions become even more complicated by the fact that, in practice, homogeneous matter is never investigated, meaning that the composition of the outlet radiation depends on whether bones or air-containing lung tissues, for instance, or a series of various materials have been irradiated one after the other. The composition of the outlet radiation is affected by the thickness, density and total atomic number of the irradiated layers. Under

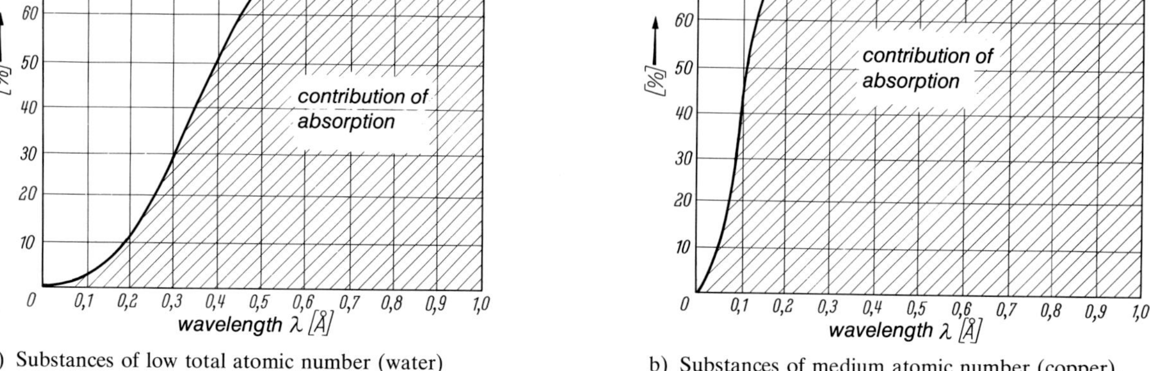
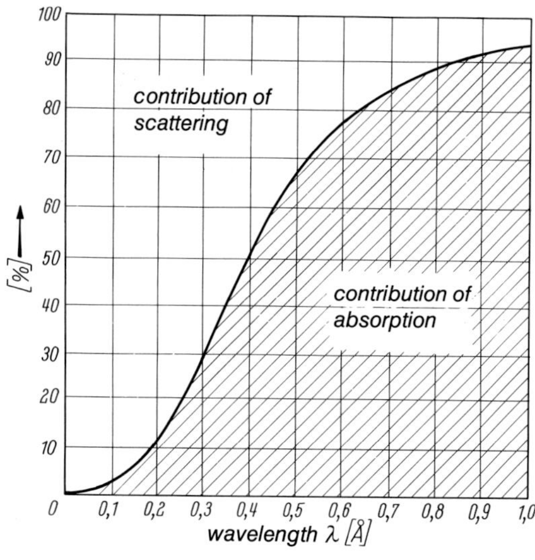

a) Substances of low total atomic number (water)

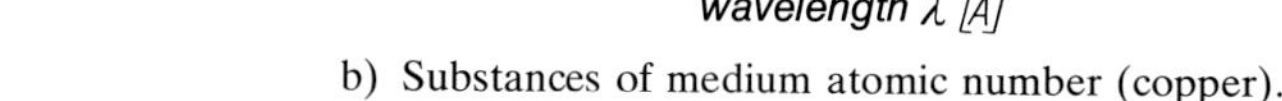

b) Substances of medium atomic number (copper).

Fig. 20. Contributions of absorption and scattering to the attenuation of X-rays (100%) in various substances (after *Holthusen*).

certain circumstances, a thick layer of material with a low total atomic number or thickness may produce the same attenuation as a thin layer with a high total atomic number or high density. In this case, we cannot distinguish both these layers by their silhouettes in the radiograph.

The physical reasons which lead to this complicated result have already been discussed. It is our task to show how the individual factors can be influenced in such a way as to permit us to obtain the clearest possible radiation relief and thereby the optimal radiograph.

Let us first investigate an object (O) which consists of homogeneous material but is of different thicknesses (Fig. 21). The upper part is very thick and the lower part comparatively thin. In front of the object, the intensity of the radiation is uniform. In the thick material, the primary beam is more attenuated by scattering and absorption than it is in the thin part with the lower attenuating power. The intensity (in the first instance, without taking into account the scattering) is smaller behind the thick part of the object than behind the thin part, as is indicated in Figure 21 by the length of the arrows. Outside the object, the intensity remains unchanged. The dotted line (K) is the radiation relief. On the basis of the intensity difference, it can be concluded which part of the object is thicker and where the boundary between both of the parts lies.

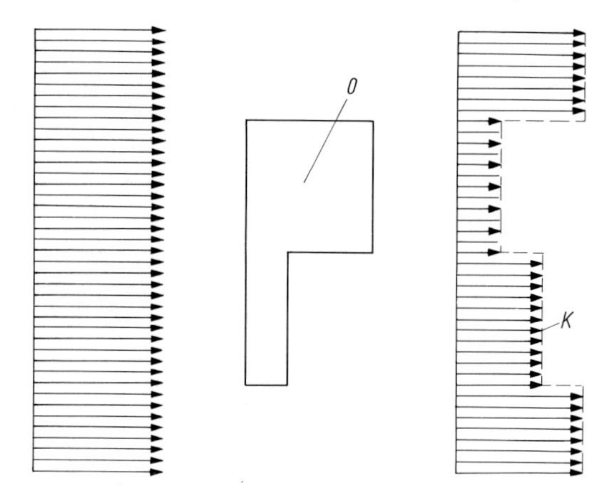

Fig. 21. Formation of the radiation relief.

The object (O) is homogeneous for X-rays, but it is of different thicknesses. In front of the object, the intensity (length of the arrows) is uniform. Behind the object, the intensity above and below the object remains unchanged. Behind the thick part of the object, the attenuation is stronger than behind the thin part. The dotted line (K) is the contour of the radiation relief.

The effect of the scattered radiation upon the form of the radiation relief must also be taken into account. The scattering takes place to all sides and, because of the greater thickness, is stronger in the upper than in the lower part. Thus, the radiation relief is changed. The proportion of the scattered radiation which passes in the direction of the direct beam strengthens the intensity in the upper section more than in the lower section because less radiation is produced at the bottom. Thus, the difference in intensity between the top and bottom becomes smaller (Fig. 22b).

The scattered radiation obliquely leaving the thick piece of material arrives in the lower section and also reaches the edge regions outside the object. The same applies to the oblique scattered radiation which emerges from the lower, thinner part of the object. Thus, the radiation relief is distorted. The oblique, scattered radiation blurs the sharp boundaries on the edge of the object and between both parts. The unattenuated intensity above the object is increased by the relatively stronger scattered radiation of the thicker part of the object to a larger extent than on the lower boundary (Fig. 22c).

Thus, under certain circumstances, it is difficult to draw conclusions on the form of an object from the form of the radiation relief.

The extent of the distortion of the contour depends on the type of material and the composition of the primary radiation. The scattered radiation, especially the Compton process, will be stronger for hard than for soft radiation. The scattering is also greater when the object consists of atomic materials with a low atomic number. Under certain circumstances, small absorption differences in large objects, where much scattered radiation is generated, are not recognizable in the radiation relief. For these reasons, the effect of scattered radiation on the radiation relief must be reduced to a minimum. Absorption must predominate.

In the following section, the practical possibilities for limiting the effect of scattered radiation on radiation relief will be discussed. Theoretically, a reduction of the scattered radiation would be possible if the elements of the irradiated body region could be converted to elements with higher atomic numbers, for which, according to Figure 20b, the scattering is weaker. However, the composition of the human body cannot be changed. Most of the body substances and lung tissues, excepting the bones, behave like water (see Table 1), and thus their distribution of absorption and scattering is governed by the pattern shown in Figure 20a.

Also, the production of scattered radiation cannot be prevented by using maximum wavelength X-rays (about 1 Å). The absorption-scattering ratio uniquely shifts in favor of absorption (Fig. 20); this means, however, that the radiation has a very low penetrating power because of the strong absorption. Such a strong absorption causes an impermissibly high radiation load to the patient. Only for thin parts of the body, e.g., the fingers, can the effect of scattered radiation be reduced by taking the picture with long-wave X-rays produced with low generating voltage.

For thicker objects, the reduction of scattered radiation is possible only by sharply "diaphragming out" the body part which has to be investigated with short-wave

Table 1. Density and effective total atomic numbers of selected body substances (calculated according to the weight fractions of their component parts).

Substances	*Density g/cm³*	*Effective total atomic number*
Blood, muscles	1	7.5
Fat	0.92	6.0
Air-containing lung tissues	0.2	7.7
Bones	1.9	15.0
Water	1	7.4
Air	0.0013	7.7

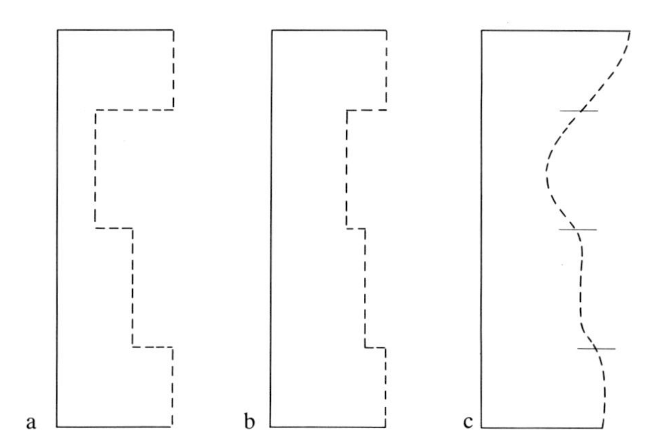

Fig. 22. Radiation relief of the object (O) in Figure 21.
a) Without scattered radiation.
b) Under the influence of scattering in the direction of the direct beam. The total contrast and the contrast between both parts is smaller.
c) Under the influence of lateral scattering; the contours are blurred, and the whole radiation relief, especially on the edges, is distorted.

radiation. A narrow primary beam produces few scattered rays. Moreover, by narrowing the beam, the radiation load is also reduced.

Since the formation of scattered radiation cannot be prevented, its effect on the radiation relief must be minimized through technical means. The simplest way is to increase the distance between object and screen (distance techniques). With distance, the fraction of the oblique scattered rays which are superimposed over the primary beam decreases.

Figure 23 illustrates this process. The segment of the scattered ray beam emitted to all sites, which is superimposed over the picture (B_1) for a short distance between object (O) and screen (S_1), is spread with increasing object (O) – screen (S_2) distance over a much larger area, so that picture B_2 is hit by lesser amounts of scattered radiation than is picture B_1. In this way, the intensity of scattered radiation referred to the same area becomes smaller. This technique has the disadvantage that the magnification of the picture rapidly increases with distance.

Another relatively simple, though not very popular, procedure for eliminating scattered radiation is the filtering of the rays behind the object by, for example, a thin lead foil. The scattered radiation is mainly caused by Compton processes, especially when the generating voltage of the primary X-radiation is high. Compton radiation is softer than primary radiation. The softer Compton radiation is more strongly absorbed by thin lead foils (which themselves, because of their high atomic number and small thickness, produce few scattered rays) than is direct radiation. Another decrease in the amount of scattered radiation is achieved by the fact that the oblique scattered rays travel longer paths through the filter material than does direct radiation.

Scattering is most efficiently eliminated by arranging scanning diaphragms, e.g., Bucky diaphragms, behind the object. Such diaphragms consist of thin lead bars, arranged as closely as possible to one another, which are

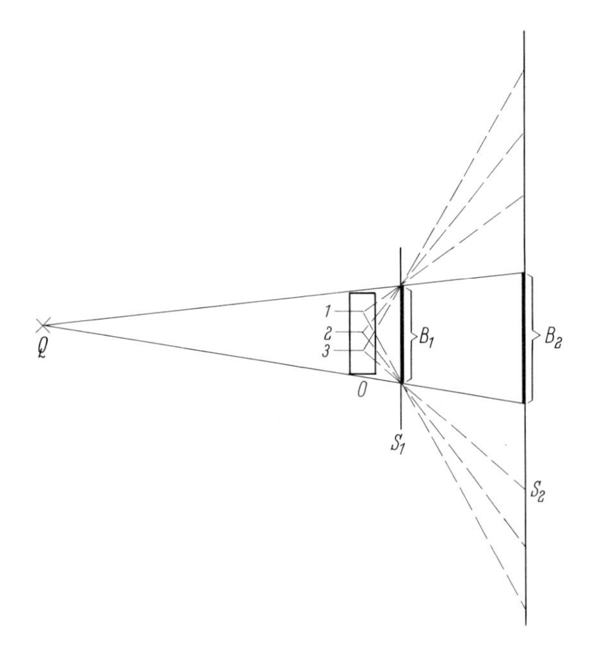

Fig. 23. The distance technique. By increasing the distance between object (O) and screen (A), the scattered ray cone superimposed on picture B_1 is spread over a much larger area, so picture B_2 is hit by far less radiation than B_1.
O = radiation source. (Only three of the scattering centers are shown in the figure.)

aligned mostly in the direction of the primary beam (focused diaphragm). The direct radiation can pass through the diaphragm cells without obstacles, while the oblique scattered rays are absorbed by the lead bars. Figure 24 schematically shows the effect of the diaphragm. The scattered radiation of only one scattering center is drawn.

The diaphragm is more effective the higher the individual cell in comparison with the distance between two lead bars. The so-called leaf ratio is characteristic for the quality of the aperture. If large amounts of scattered radiation are to be expected, the requirements set forth for the diaphragms are higher. The diaphragm contour is represented on the radiograph as any other object. Therefore, the diaphragm must be very fine in order not to interfere with the recognizability of the picture. In many instruments, the diaphragm is moved transversely during the exposure to the direction of the rays, and thus the image of the diaphragm is obliterated. As a matter of fact, the diaphragm should have a grid-like structure. But because the diaphragm is moved crosswise in the direction of the bar, the cross-like arrangement of the bars can be dispensed with. Naturally, a diaphragm attenuates the total intensity since the portions which strike upon the bars are lost. This disadvantage is small, however, if one takes into account the fact that, because of the elimination of scattered radiation, the original form of the radiation relief, predominantly caused by absorption (as in Fig. 22a), is reconstituted.

Especially when exposing larger body parts, by which a large amount of scattered radiation is produced, this radiation complicating and distorting the radiation relief must be eliminated as much as possible. This is best achieved, as has been shown, by arranging a scanning diaphragm behind the object.

Influencing the Radiation Relief through Absorption Differences

When irradiating the human body, we do not deal with homogeneous media; rather, several tissue layers which differ in thickness, density and total atomic number from place to place are irradiated one after the other.

The natural difference in the thicknesses of the individual body sections of man have an interfering effect in some X-ray investigations. This is especially seen by total exposures of the vertebral column. In lateral exposures, the irradiated body layer varies from 10 cm in the region

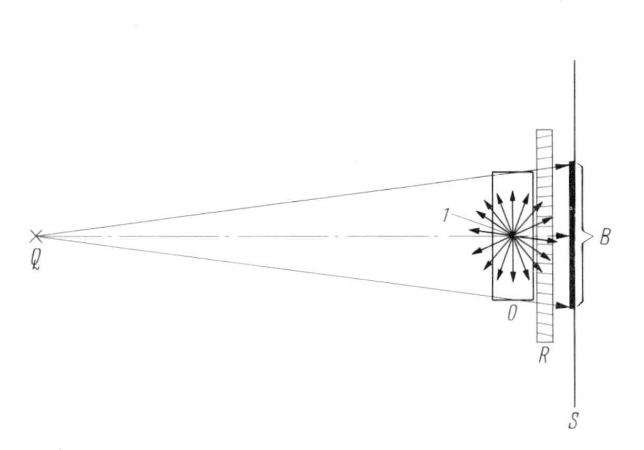

Fig. 24. Elimination of scattered radiation by a scanning diaphragm. Q=Radiation source, O=Object, R=Diaphragm focused onto Q, S=Screen, B=Picture, l=Scattering center.

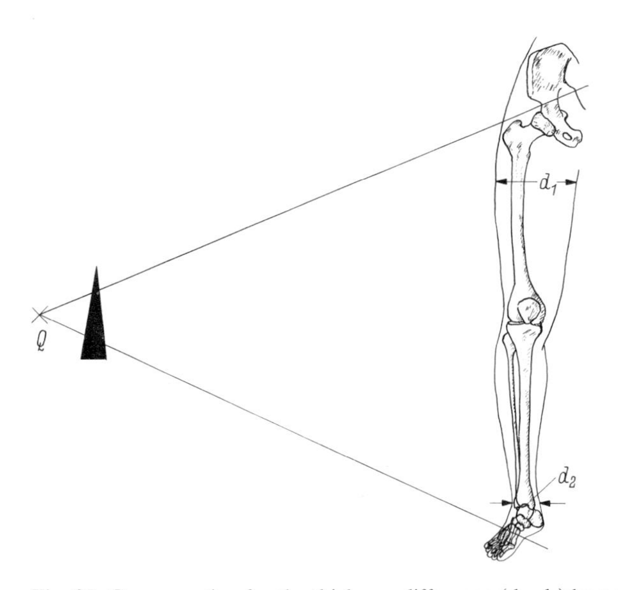

Fig. 25. Compensation for the thickness difference (d_1, d_2) by a small wedge filter in the vicinity of the radiation source (Q).

of the neck to 35–45 cm in the pelvic region. This large difference in the attenuation is superimposed over the contrast differences, determined by the structure of the vertebral column, and complicates the interpretation of the radiograph. In such cases, equalizing filters may be inserted into the path of the rays. These filters consist of homogeneous material of different thicknesses. Such a filter should be, in exposures of the vertebral column, especially thick in the region of the neck. In total exposures of the leg, wedge-shaped filters are used. These filters are arranged near the focus, because here the divergent radiation beam is still narrow and a correspondingly small filter can be used (Fig. 25).

The human body considerably attenuates the radiation. From the whole intensity, at 60 kV only 1% remains. Thus, the question arises as to whether this undesirable state can be corrected by using X-radiation (more penetrating than the radiation produced at 60 kV, which was the basis of our calculations). With increasing voltage, absorption decreases. Unfortunately, however, the absorption differences between the individual tissue types also become smaller. This decrement of the absorption in different tissues, related to the absorption in water, is shown as a function of the X-ray tube voltage in Figure 26.

At lower voltages (40 kV), there are still differences between the absorption of fat and muscular tissues, which disappear at voltages exceeding 126 kV. Also, absorption by bones amounts to only one-third of the absorption at 40 kV.

Practically, the curves of Figure 26 determine the voltage range useful for X-ray diagnostics. It ranges from 40–125 kV. In exceptional cases, using soft radiation (when the difference between muscular and fat tissues, for example, can be recognized), voltages as low as 30 kV (Fig. 27) can be used. Voltages between 125 and 200 kV are used for special hard radiation exposures. Such exposures, however, are used when the radiation is more strongly prefiltered, so that only the hard rays determine the form of the radiation relief. In high-voltage exposures of the thorax, for instance, the ribs are relatively transparent because of the low absorption by bones. Thus, under certain circumstances, details of the lungs, which are otherwise superposed by the ribs, can be recognized.

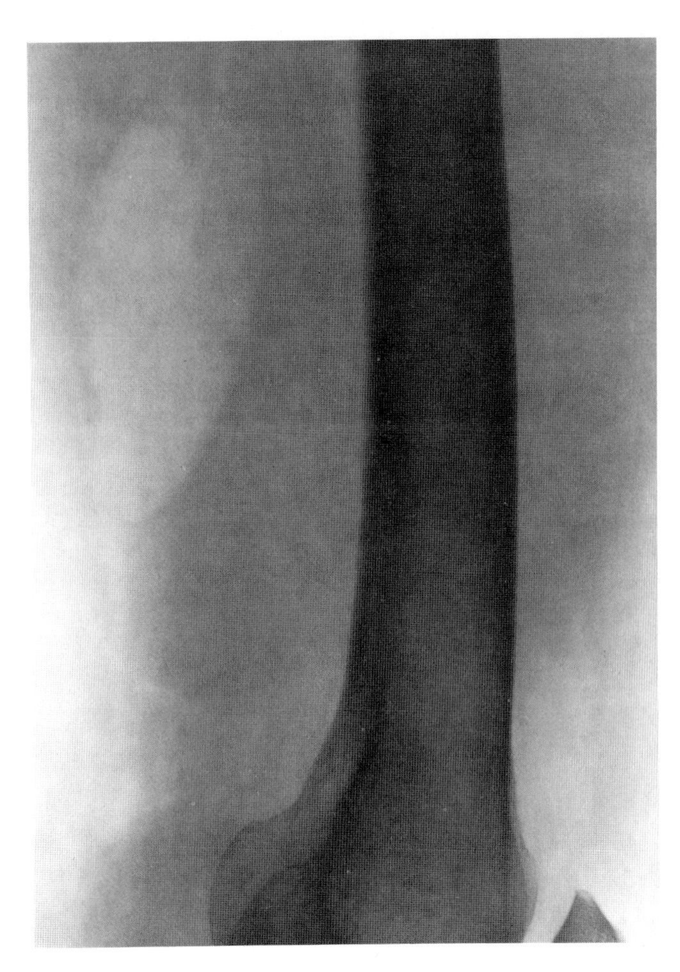

Fig. 27. Soft-ray exposure of a lipoma in the muscles of the thigh.

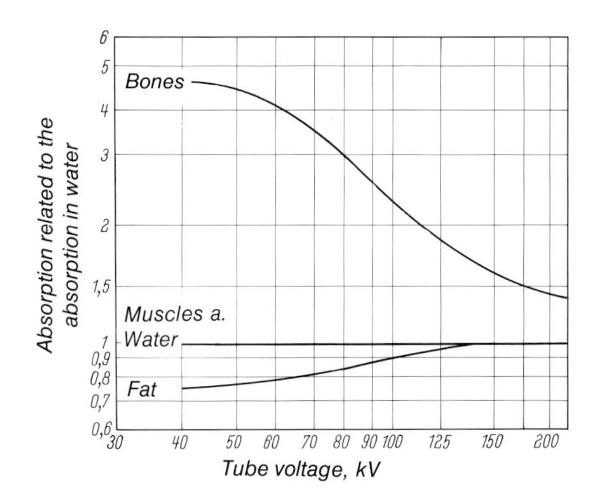

Fig. 26. Relative absorption of different tissues (related to the absorption of water = 1) versus voltage *(Balz, Birkner* and *Wachsmann).*

Heterogeneous Radiation and the Radiation Relief

In the preceding discussion of influencing the radiation relief by differences in absorption, we dealt only with the significance of the absorption properties of different body tissues during homogeneous irradiation and neglected the heterogeneous composition of the X-rays.

Moreover, we have discussed only the attenuation of uniform-energy radiation, and thus the attenuation of just a certain part of the total spectrum, e.g., of part I (Fig. 28). Now, however, the Bremsstrahlung is a mixture of rays possessing various energies. The highest-energy, short-wave portion of this mixture (short-wave boundary) is determined by the value of the generating voltage. Then follows a continuum, the intensity distribution of which is shown in Figure 14.

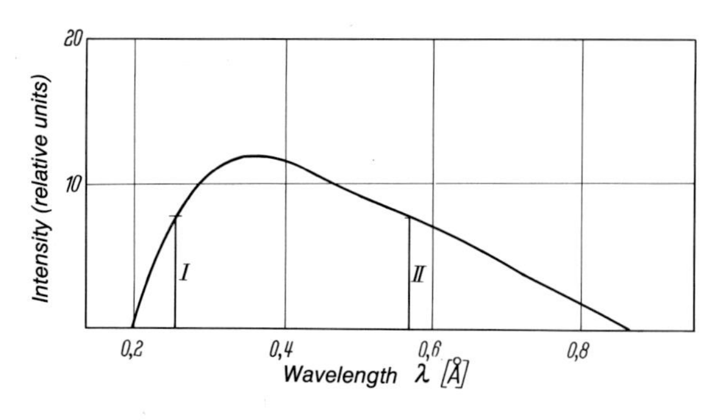

Fig. 28. Spectral intensity distribution of the Bremsstrahlung of 60 kV. Intensity, relative units. Wavelength λ (Å).

One of these curves, applying to 60 kV, is shown again in Figure 29.

Every substance has a certain layer thickness, which reduces the intensity to half of its value, the so-called half-value layer (HVL). For another part of the total spectrum, for instance part II (Fig. 28), which is lower in energy and thus less penetrating, there is a smaller HVL. A body, in accordance with its thickness, attenuates all the intensities occurring in the spectrum. The curve (Fig. 28) becomes flatter. Moreover, the long-wave part of the spectrum is attenuated to a larger degree than is the high-energy, short-wave part. The peak of the distribution curve is shifted towards shorter wavelengths. In Figure 29, this process is schematically shown in a sequence of material layers of equal thickness. With increasing thickness of the material, the soft portions of the radiation are increasingly diminished. In this case, the radiation is said to be filtered or hardened by the material.

It should be emphasized that the radiation is indeed hardened. However, the scattered radiation again increases the proportion of soft radiation, especially when Compton processes have an appreciable influence. Thus, the way in which the quantitative changes of the spectrum will proceed cannot readily be predicted. This is not essential, however, because, to the extent possible, scattered radiation is eliminated in X-ray examinations. Therefore, only the alteration in the radiation due to absorption is predicted.

The absorption depends on the thickness, density and total atomic number of the object. The density differences of the individual body tissues and their effect on absorption are relatively small. On the other hand, the total atomic number considerably affects absorption. This is favorable for the representation of the skeleton, because the bone tissues have a relatively high total atomic number. In order to differentiate the other tissues, contrast agents with a high total atomic number are used under certain circumstances.

With penetrating power of the radiation, the contrasts decrease. It is therefore recommended that the lowest possible voltage be selected. However, the fact that the considerable total absorption by the human body attenuates the radiation to 1% of its initial value poses a lower limit to the selection of the voltage. Thick parts of the body which are irradiated with higher voltages cannot be represented as richly in terms of contrasts and details as can thin parts.

For equal generating voltages, the quality of the radiation relief also depends on the heterogeneity of the X-radiation. When examining thick objects, high-output instruments should be used so that the spectrum of the Bremsstrahlung contains sufficient amounts of hard rays.

The Conversion of the Radiation Relief into a Visible Picture

X-rays are invisible. The visible range of the electromagnetic spectrum (Fig. 12) is in the region of the longer waves. Therefore, the properties of the X-rays are used and, by converting the radiation relief, produce a visible image. Any procedure is suitable in which X-radiation produces a visible effect, either by direct or indirect means. Following the conversion process, the form and size of the radiation relief must be retained. The procedures most widely used today, i.e., scanning with fluorescent screen and fixation with photographic emulsion, were used by Röntgen. The techniques of both methods have since been improved, however. X-ray scanning makes it possible to observe the phenomenon of motion within the body. Since the intensity of the radiation following penetration through the body is low, the pictures on the fluorescent screen are weak and can only be recognized in total darkness and with good adaptation of the eye.

In modern picture-intensifier-television irradiation, the picture on the fluorescent screen is so intense and bright that viewing with the cone apparatus is again possible and adaptation is no longer necessary.

X-ray photography makes the fixation of the radiograph possible. In this way, information of documentary value is obtained. Changes in the tissues and course of disease can be observed over long periods at arbitrary intervals. The possibility of comparing a present state with previous investigation is especially valuable.

X-ray Photographs with Intensifying Screens

The X-ray film makes it possible to compare exposures which were prepared at various periods. Also, reproductions of the same body section from various directions (e.g., anteroposteriorly or laterally) can be compared.

The constant film properties are important for this practice. The only serviceable film material is that which can over the years be correctly exposed with the same light exposure data. Differences in the quality from lot to lot, from film packing to film packing, or among various sizes complicate work and increase the number of incorrect exposures, and thus the number of repeat examinations (radiation load). The consumer must be careful not to use old film which has been stored for an excessively long time. For storage, adherence to the instructions of the manufacturer is recommended.

Good X-ray film has a slight veil, with a small veil being, of course, preferable. Inexpert or excessively long storage prior to exposure can strengthen the veil and affect the quality of the film. The suitability of an X-ray film can be determined by whether unexposed or only slightly exposed places (e.g., behind marks such as lead letters) appear greyish or not.

The X-ray film must be very sensitive and provide as much contrast as possible. Film sensitivity depends on the grain size of the silver salts uniformly distributed in the emulsion (mainly silver bromide). With increases in the size of the radiation-sensitive centers, the sensitivity of the film also increases. The grain size must not be so large, however, that recognizability of details is jeopardized. A higher sensitivity can be achieved only with an increase in the grain size and with little contrast. A serviceable film, however, must have the properties of both contrast and sensitivity. Since X-radiation is only slightly absorbed by the thin emulsion, the film is provided with emulsion on both sides (double-coated film). The blackening is then twice as large in each place.

In many cases, it is useful to intensify the effect of the X-rays by fluorescent intensifying screens. These screens are fixed on the inside of the front and rear walls of the X-ray film holder. The film is placed between the two screens and both sides are exposed by the X-rays. Additionally, each side is subject to exposure by the fluorescent light of the screens placed on the corresponding side. The film is more sensitive to the light of the screen than to the X-rays. Only 5% of the blackening is produced by direct X-rays, with the remaining 95% produced by screens containing calcium tungstate as phosphor. Screens which contain the so-called rare earths as phosphors have recently been developed. At the same resolving power, these screens are able to provide less lack of definition due to motion, excellent contrast, and thus an enormous improvement in the exposure technique. Their most important achievement, however, is their excellent radiation protection, due to the fact that only one-fourth to one-sixth of the previously used radiation dose is necessary. Thus, phosphor-containing screens are very useful and could be used as standard equipment. The extraordinary reduction of the radiation load alone would seem to justify their exclusive use in the future.

For examination of the skeleton, however, fluorescent intensifying screens are frequently useless. When evaluating changes in bones, for example, the most minute details are important. In order to recognize inflammations, fine infractions or structural changes of the bones, the highest order of recognizability of details is required.

Therefore, where possible, films without screens are used for radiographs of the bones and their lower sensitivity is tolerated. If intensification is necessary, only finely representing screens can be used. These intensify less than other screens, but lead to good recognizability of details. The production of X-ray pictures in light-impermeable packing (e.g., X-ray film holder) is comparatively simple. Since the photographic layer is light sensitive, the X-ray film is placed in the path of the rays behind the scattered radiation diaphragm and exposed. The film is further processed to the finished picture in conventional ways, using the standard dark room procedures.

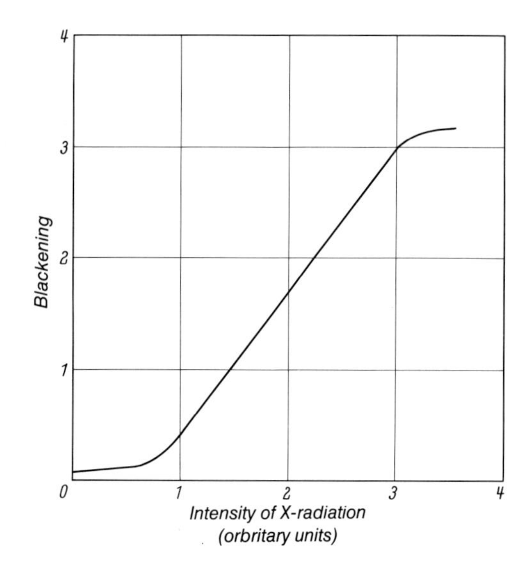

Fig. 29. Blackening curve (schematic representation).

The utilization of the development machine is becoming increasingly popular, even in smaller X-ray clinics and practices. The X-ray film reproduces for each intensity occurring in the radiation relief a corresponding intensity. It is unimportant whether the blackening is produced by the fluorescent light of the screens or by direct absorption of X-rays. The blackening of a given area is the visible reference value for the X-ray intensity on that place, invisible to our eye. If the X-ray exposure is to be a useful procedure, the blackening-intensity curve must have a shape, satisfying the requirement for proportionality between intensity and visible reference value. Indeed, a blackening curve can be plotted, the shape of which is shown in Figure 29.

The correct exposure times for every adjustment and every working place cannot be obtained by theoretical considerations alone; a certain amount of experience is also necessary. Thus, many factors must be taken into account, including the film or screen sensitivity, the exposed object, etc. Using an automatic illuminating device (which, after reaching a medium intensity, automatically interrupts the exposure), we can use the same adjustment to compensate for differences, e.g., different body thicknesses, from patient to patient.

The path of the X-ray has now been followed from the source to the finished radiograph. Though attempts are made to absorb the major part of the radiation in the film and screens in order to attain the maximum possible intensity, a part of the rays penetrates through the X-ray film holder and strikes parts of the X-ray equipment, e.g., the mounting of the holder, etc. The scattered radiation from the rear wall of the holder and from parts of the instrument can also expose the film directly behind the holder. Since the scattering is entirely diffuse, this additional exposure is seen as a grey veil. In order to prevent exposure by scattered radiation from behind, the rear wall of the holder is protected with lead.

Fluorescent Screen and Picture-Intensifier Television Chain

The fluorescent screen is the simplest and most inexpensive means to observe motion processes such as the movement of the diaphragm during respiration or the stomach-intestine peristalsis. It consists of a homogeneous cardboard support, onto which the fluorescent layer is applied. In order to protect the examiner against rays, a lead glass plate is mounted behind this layer. The composition of a phosphor fluorescent screen is chosen so that the spectral composition of the fluorescent light lies in a region (yellow-green) in which the eye is very sensitive.

The coarser the grain of the fluorescent layer, the brighter the picture and the less recognizable the details. The dimensions of the radiation-sensitive grains of the phosphor in the layer are termed grain size. In the X-ray film, the diameter of the AgBr grains is 1–2 μ. Fluorescent screens have a grain size between 5 and 50 μ diameter. Thus, it is clear that details can be recognized to a lesser degree on screens than on film. Moreover, in the picture-intensifier television chain, the X-rays are first absorbed by a fluorescent screen (inlet luminescent screen) and then converted into light quanta (photons). These photons eject the electrons of a photocathode, which are released and accelerated in a magnetic field, before they strike a second fluorescent screen (outlet screen). The fluorescence which is thus produced is about 1000 times larger than that of the inlet screen. The picture is then taken with a television camera and transferred onto a television monitoring device.

This method, however, does not enable the essential reduction of the radiation dose that conventional radiographs do. Its advantages are due to the fact that the examiner needs not be adapted and the picture can simultaneously be observed by more than one examiner.

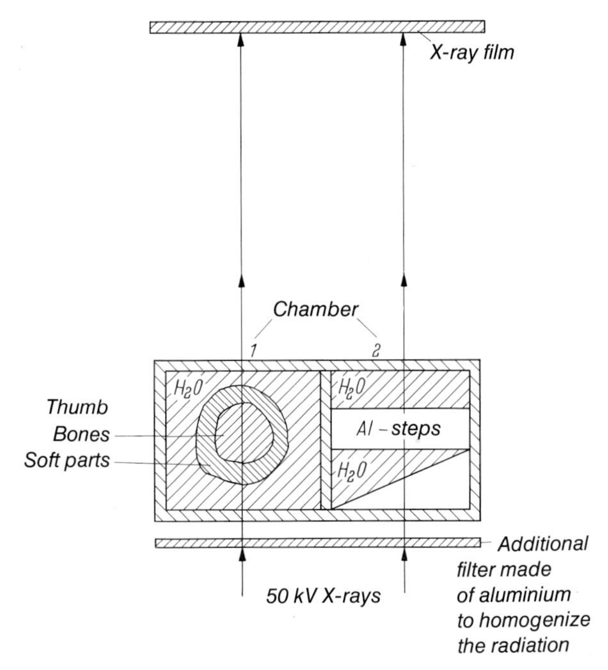

a) Schematic diagram (top view).

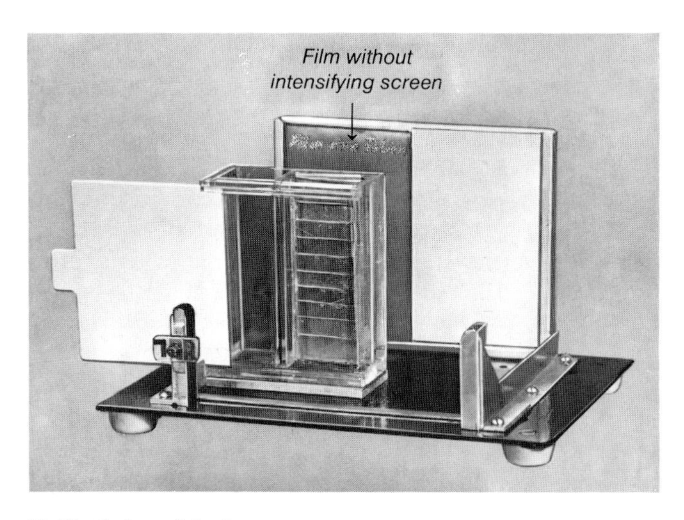

b) Total view of the instrument.

Fig. 30. Setup for the quantitative evaluation of changes in the bone substance (after *Balz* and *Birkner).*

Example of a Quantitative X-Ray Procedure

Most radiographs are only qualitatively evaluated. The picture is interpreted by subjective means, e.g., with the eye, in order to detect deviations from the norm. Several attempts have been made, however, to quantitatively determine the extent of this deviation *(Heuck* and *Schmidt; Krokowski* and *Haasner).* In this book, the typical radiograph of a skeleton is shown in order to determine the limits of the norm. The practical purpose of such comparison is to detect deviations in form and structure. It is possible, however, that deviations in the chemical composition of the bone substance occur whose extent cannot be determined by the eye.

Balz and *Birkner* reported a comparatively simple procedure, which one can judge the mineral level in the bones by a quantitative evaluation of the radiation absorption. The procedure was found to be valuable because any defects which may occur through conversion of the radiation relief into blackenings are eliminated by simultaneous X-ray exposure of aluminum stairs. Let us now briefly describe this procedure in order to provide guidelines for the quantitative evaluation of the radiograph.

This small instrument is suitable for measurements on thumbs and finger joints. Figure 30a is a schematic representation in top view, while Figure 30b shows the total view. The X-rays pass through two plexiglass chambers of equal size and strike an X-ray film behind them. The distance between chamber and film reduces the effect of

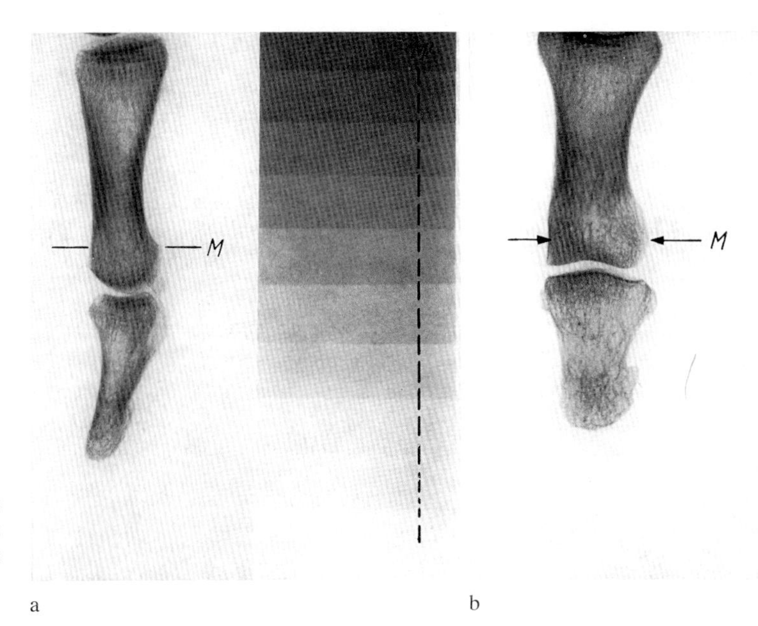

Fig. 31. a) Radiograph for photometric comparison of the blackening by the thumb and by the aluminum stairs. b) Radiograph of a thumb for the determination of the bone thickness.

scattered radiation. The finger or thumb is immersed from the top into the water-filled, left-hand chamber (1) so that a lateral picture is formed. In the center of the right-hand chamber, there are 10-step aluminum stairs, which are simultaneously photographed with the thumb on the same film. In front of the aluminum stairs, there is a wedge-shaped water layer, and behind it a uniform water layer. The water in chamber 1 has to compensate for differences in the thickness of the enveloping muscle layer. The absorbing muscle layer plus the water are equal to the thickness of the chamber minus the thickness of the bone. The additional bone-independent absorption by the muscular tissue and water is simulated in chamber 2 by a water layer consisting of uniform and wedge-shaped water sublayers. The blackening produced by the absorption in the bones can be directly and photometrically compared with the blackening produced by absorption in the aluminum stairs. However, the measuring point on the radiograph of the aluminum stairs must be chosen so that the uniform and wedge-shaped water sublayers together have exactly the same thickness as have the muscles surrounding the bone and the water layer in chamber 1.

Figure 31a shows a radiograph obtained with this setup. The measured value is marked on the lateral permanent radiograph and on the aluminum stairs. The thickness of the bones is determined with the aid of an anteroposterior exposure of the thumb (Fig. 31b).

Thus, the bone absorption is in direct proportion to the absorption of a step of the aluminum stairs. In order to achieve relatively large differences in blackening, low voltage (50 kV) is used. The radiation is homogenized by an additional aluminum filter.

The simultaneous photographing of the thumb and the aluminum stairs on the same X-ray film has the advantage that both pictures are prepared and processed in the dark chamber under the same conditions. Thus, any defects which may be produced by conversion of the radiation relief into visible values are eliminated.

Using the results of the examination of a large number of healthy individuals of all ages, a curve (Fig. 888, p. 368) can be plotted, from which one can determine which of the so-called aluminum attenuation values can be considered normal. On the basis of deviations from this curve, conclusions can be drawn as to pathological states of bones, e.g., generalized osteopathy, which involve disturbances in their mineral content (see *Balz, Birkner* and *Schmitt-Rhode).*

Central Projection in X-Ray Technique

The radiograph is formed by projection of the object, more or less transparent for X-rays, onto a film or fluorescent screen. Radiographs are silhouettes. They are also produced as silhouettes by placing the object between the source, which must be as point-like as possible, and the plane of the projection (see Fig. 2). The projection of a divergent beam emerging from a point is termed central projection. The projection conditions can be described by relatively simple geometric laws.

The Law of Distances

The intensity of radiation which strikes a certain area at distance a = 1 from the focus (F) is distributed at a = 2 over the fourfold area because of divergence of the beam. Related to equal-size areas, the intensity at a double distance from F decreases to $^1/_4$.

The decrease in intensity is the result of the geometry

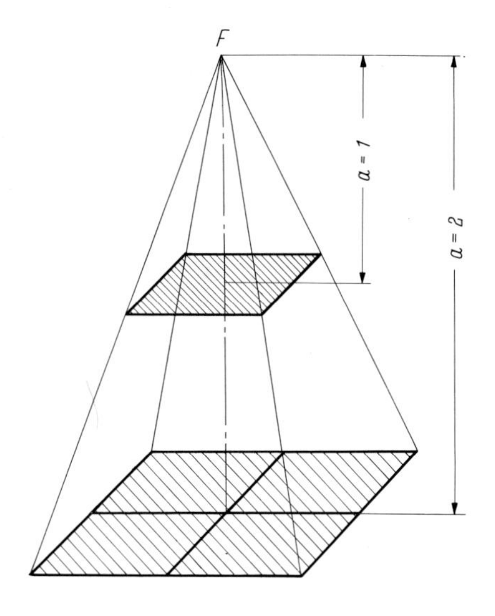

Fig. 32. Distribution of the intensity over the fourfold area due to doubling of the distance. The intensity per unit area decreases to $^1/_4$.

Table 2.

Distance	*Intensity*
a_1 = 1	I_1 = 1
a_2 = 2	I_2 = $^1/_4$
a_3 = 3	I_3 = $^1/_9$
a_4 = 4	I_4 = $^1/_{16}$
a_{10} = 10	I_{10} = $^1/_{100}$

of the path of the rays (Fig. 32). With distance from the point source, the intensity very rapidly decreases (Table 2).

The law of distances can be formulated as follows:

1. The intensity (I) per unit area is inversely proportionate to the square of the distance (a) or, mathematically, $1 \sim 1 a^2$.
2. The ratio of the intensity per unit area at different distances is equal to the ratio reciprocal squares of the distances, or $I_1/II_2 = a_2{}^2/a_1{}^2$.

In practice, the milliampere second product (intensity) for the correctly exposed radiograph at a certain distance is known. For a radiograph taken at double distance, the milliampere second product must be multiplied by a factor of four.

This strong decrease in intensity shows that photographs can be made over large distances only when the output of the X-ray equipment is adequate.

Magnification

All objects are projected following the laws of central projection (see Fig. 2). The extent of magnification depends on the divergence of the beam, i.e., on the size of the selected focus-object and object-picture distances. The geometry of picture magnification is shown in Figures 33 and 34. In Figure 33, the distance between object and plane of projection remains the same. With decreasing focus-object distance, the picture becomes larger.

The agreement between the size of the object and the size of the picture improves with increasing focus-object distance. Thus, when it is important to obtain a reproduction of the object in the natural scale, photographs should be made from large distances. The distance cannot be ar-

Fig. 33. Increase in the size of the picture when the focus is brought closer to the object. The object-plane of projection distance remains the same.

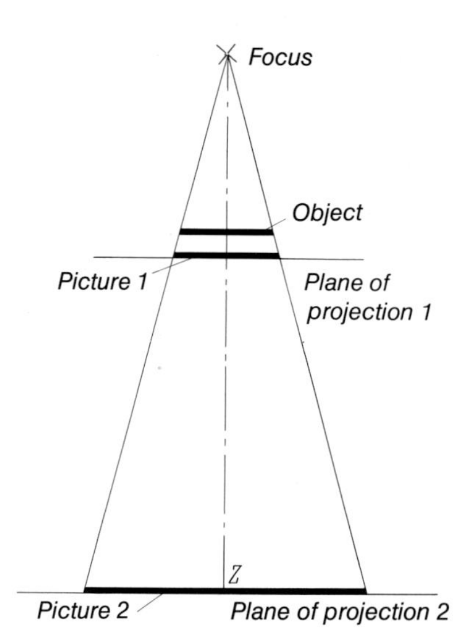

Fig. 34. Increase in the size of the picture with increase in the object-plane of projection distance. The focus-object distance remains the same.

bitrarily increased, however, because otherwise the intensity very strongly decreases.

The magnification of the picture is small when the distance between object and plane of projection is reduced to a minimum. Figure 34 shows the size of the picture in two different planes of projection for the same focus-object distances.

When the plane of projection is right behind the object, the sizes of the object and the picture nearly coincide. The size of the projected picture is larger, the larger the object-picture distance (plane of projection 2). In some cases, this is desirable. Such magnified photographs are made with the minimum possible focus (finest focus exposures) in order to obtain good resolution. In other cases, however, the magnification due to an additional object-plane of projection distance is an undesirable side effect, as, for example, when this distance is increased in order to reduce the effect of scattered radiation (distance techniques, Fig. 23).

It can be concluded from the geometry of the path of the rays that the size of an organ can be evaluated only when the X-ray film is exposed from the maximum possible distance and the distance between patient and film is kept at a minimum. In special cases, a scale can be placed in the plane of the object on lead marks. With this scale, which is also represented on the X-ray picture, the size of the organ can be determined.

The objects from which radiographs are to be obtained are spatially extended, in contrast to the schematic representation in Figures 33 and 34. The object parts near to the focus and far from the picture are represented in much larger size than are the parts far from the focus, which are very close to the plane of projection. This is also a consequence of the beam divergence and must be taken into account when interpreting radiographs (see Fig. 11). In fact, a spatial impression is formed in which the perspective is the reverse of our ordinary visual perception. Moreover, the parts of the object which are remote from the plane of projection are projected in a blurred fashion. It is thus recommended, that patients be positioned in such a way that the organs to be examined are as close to the plane of projection as possible. If this is not feasible because, for instance, the organs are in the middle of the body, a large distance should be placed between focus and object in order to reduce the magnification of the picture as much as possible. In certain cases, because of the spatial structure of the object, a superposition of the radiograph takes place, so-called contact exposure can be used to produce a radiograph of the part of the body which is close to the plane of projection (Fig. 35). In this case, the part far from this plane appears very large and blurred.

As Figure 35 shows, in a remote exposure, two regions of equal size on the upper and lower sides of the object are reproduced one over the other in virtually natural dimensions. In contact exposures, the hood of the tube contacts the upper side of the object. Thus, the upper part of the object yields a strongly magnified reproduction. Within the region of this extended projection, the lower part of the object is reproduced in natural size. In the contact exposure, the intensity per unit area is very high at the side where the radiation enters, owing to the low focal distance (the square law of distances). The part of the body on this side is subjected to a considerable radiation load. It must be carefully considered whether such exposure is justified. Especially to be avoided are repeated exposures over short time intervals.

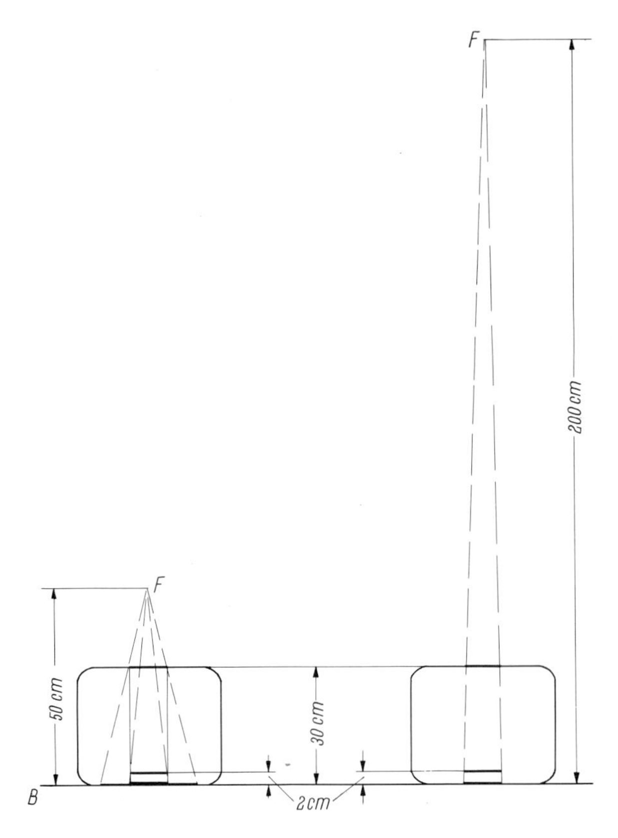

Fig. 35. Comparison between contact and remote exposure (after *Schoen*).

It is a general rule, that the focus-film distance should be five times as large as the thickness of the object in the direction of the rays. In these cases, the magnification remains within tolerable limits (10–20%). When a reproduction in natural size is important (e.g., radiographs of the heart), the focus-film distance must be at least 2 m (the magnification is no more than 5% in this case).

Distortion

In all our prior representations of the path of the rays, the object was drawn parallelly to the plane of projection and vertically to the central ray of the beam. Moreover, care was taken that the central ray pass through the center of the object. In practice, it is not so simple to align the object. Most objects are uneven and cannot be arranged parallel to the plane of projection.

Figure 36 sets forth the effects of centering and the slope of the plane of projection on the form of the picture.

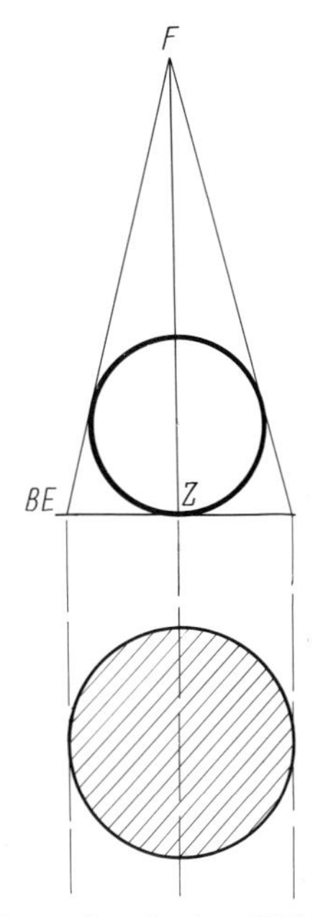

a) Plane of projection (BE) vertical to the central ray (Z). A somewhat magnified, undistorted reproduction of the sphere as circle is obtained.

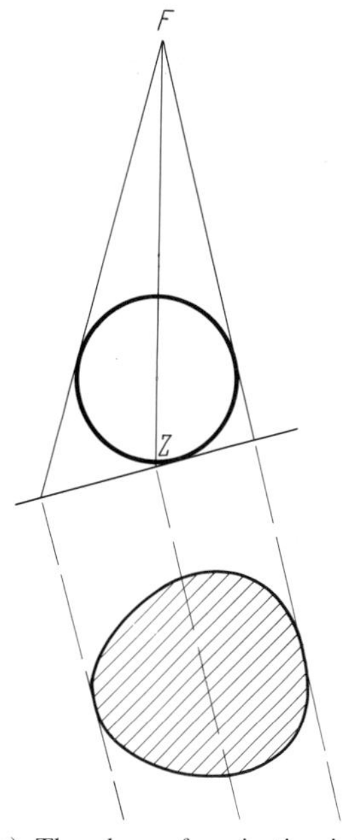

b) The plane of projection is inclined. The circle is distorted to an ellipse.

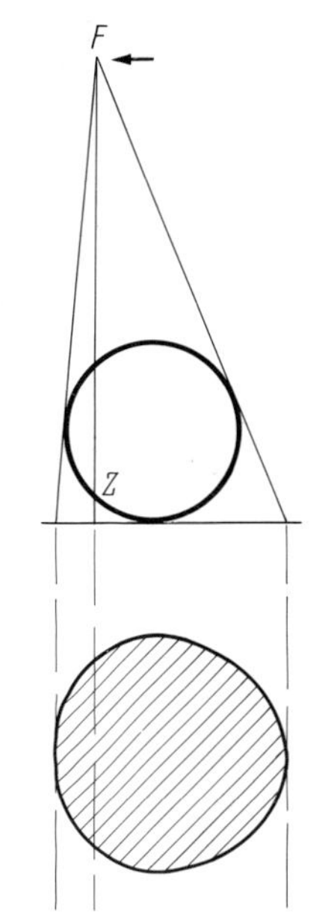

c) The focus is displaced in the direction of the arrow. The central beam does not pass through the center of the sphere; an ellipse-like distortion results.

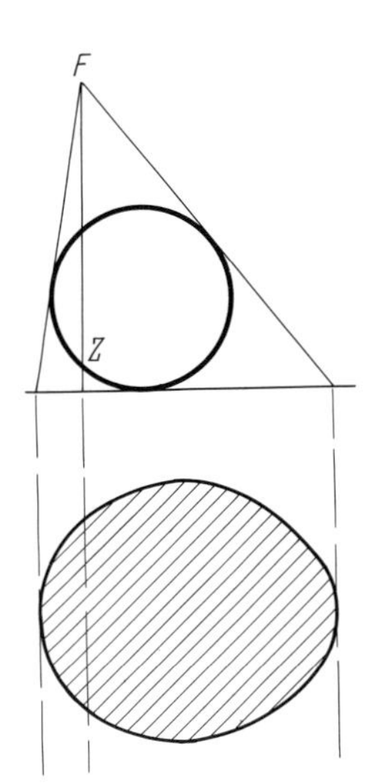

d) With additional approach of the focus to the object, the picture and the distortion increase.

Fig. 36. Representation of a compact sphere in central projection.

The position of the object in the path of the rays and below a top view of the central projection is shown just as the object is reproduced on the radiograph. The object is a compact sphere.

In Figure 36a, the central ray passes right through the center of the sphere. The plane of projection is vertical to the central ray (Z). The sphere is projected as a circle. If, however, an angle is formed between the plane of projection and the central ray, the result is an ellipse-like distortion (Fig. 36b). Such a distortion can also be expected when the ray does not pass through the center of the sphere (Fig. 36c). If the focus is placed nearer to the object, both the picture and the distortion become larger (Fig. 36d).

A sphere was selected as the object (Fig. 36) because it has no defined axis of the body. That is, when adjusting a sphere, there is no preferable position relative to the plane of projection is vertical to the central ray, and the optimum position of the plane of projection and the central ray can be fixed without taking into account the object's shape.

It should now be clear that an object-similar reproduction of the radiograph can be achieved only when the plane of projection is vertical to the central ray and the central ray is directed to the center of the irradiated region of the body. There are several adjustment aids, e.g., telescopic adjustment rods or optical systems, which, with a light beam, reproduce the X-ray beam and are mounted on the field diaphragms (light sights). Through their use, the center of the field and the lateral boundaries of the ray beam can be fixed. As a rule, the X-ray equipment is so constructed that the plane of projection is vertical to the direction of the central ray. Deviations can be read from the scales on the X-ray tube hood and then corrected. Good X-ray equipment has adequate adjustment devices making it possible to carefully align the tube and film holder.

The correct arrangement of the object in the path of the rays is far more complicated because, here, human anatomy must be taken into account. The prerequisite for a distortion-free reproduction is that the plane of the body, in which the object preferably lies, is arranged vertically to the central ray and parallelly to the plane of projection. It is frequently necessary to represent the object in several (at least two) planes in order to prevent incorrect interpretations. The correct adjustments for this purpose are reported here. In difficult cases, it may be necessary to dispense with vertical centering in order to obtain any reproduction at all, and therefore distortion must be tolerated.

Free Projection through Parallax

With vertical centering, the shadow of the sternum is masked by the stronger shadow of the vertebral column (Fig. 37). The pictures of objects which lie spatially one before the other are shifted in the plane of projection relative to each other when the direction of the beam is changed. This shift is termed parallactic deviation or, in short, parallax.

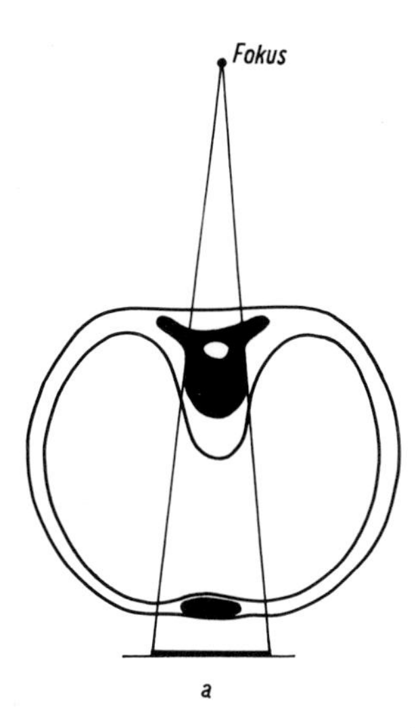

Fig. 37. In vertical projection, the shadow of the vertebral column overlaps with the shadow of the sternum.

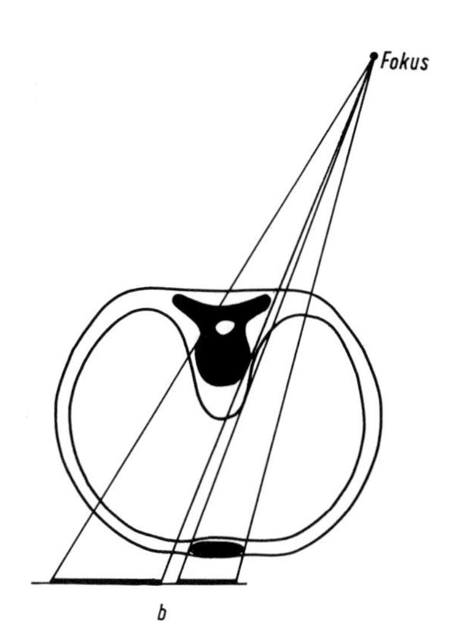

Fig. 38. In steep projection, the shadows of the object lie near each other.

The picture of a part of the object which is close to the plane of projection is shifted to a lesser extent than is the picture of a more remote part of the object. Thus, by lateral shifting of the focus, the free projection of the sternum can be obtained. Although both objects are distorted, the distortion of the sternum placed near the film is not critical. The strong distortion of the vertebral column is without significance, since only the reproduction of the sternum is important. And, because of the lateral tube displacement, the sternum is thus freely projected (Fig. 38).

Parallax is also used in irradiation in order to obtain spatial orientation by rotating the patient in front of the luminescent screen.

Summary

The representation of objects in central projection, as used in X-ray exposures, requires, for a realistic reproduction, the centering of the object and the plane of projection vertically to the central ray. With strongly divergent beams, the picture is greatly magnified and distorted. In order to obtain a reproduction true in size and form, large distances between focus and plane of projection and small distances between object and plane of projection are recommended. Since intensity strongly decreases with distance, one cannot work with arbitrarily large distances between focus and picture, especially because the output of the X-ray equipment is limited.

Lack of Resolution and Recognizability of Detail

The physician who has to analyze a radiograph wants, of course, a picture on which every detail can be distinctly recognized. In the preceding description of the processes taking place when the radiograph is formed, several physical and technical factors which limit the recognizability of details were discussed.

It may happen that the parts of the object are, by nature, not sharply bounded from one another, or the transitions between the different chemical components of the material (for instance, because of small differences in their density) may not be recognizable in the radiograph. Also, when irradiating parts of the skeleton, which tend to show good contrast against soft part tissues, such diffuse transitions may occur within larger skull regions, for example. In this case, the requirement for good detail recognizability is not fulfilled. Nonetheless, under certain circumstances, such a hazy, blurred reproduction of detail may provide an important diagnostic indication.

In addition to the blurred reproduction of detail inherent in the irradiated object, there are other factors which lead to lack of resolution in the X-ray picture. The most important is geometric lack of resolution caused by film, screen or movement.

In our discussion of the geometric conditions for projection, it was assumed that the radiation source is pointlike. Relative to the large distances between focus and plane of projection, the dimensions of the focus are small. However, as was pointed out in the discussion of the spatial origin of X-rays, certain spatial extensions of the focal spot cannot be avoided. The minimum size of the focus is determined by the strong heating which occurs in the place where the electrons, after striking the material of the anode, are braked and X-rays are produced. An extended radiation source does not yield sharp silhouettes in central projection (see Fig. 8c).

The lack of resolution depends on the extension of the

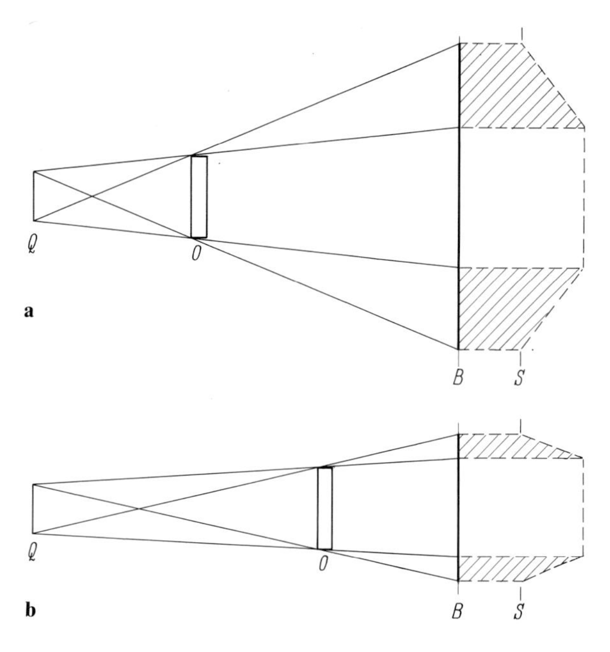

Fig. 39. The extension of the penumbra. Behind the plane of projection the course of the radiation relief is indicated. The zone of the penumbra is dotted.
Q = Radiation source, O = Object, S = Radiation relief.

radiation source and the geometry of the path of the rays (Fig. 39). The shadow of the picture is no longer sharply bounded when the radiation source is spatially extended. The edge zone, which is only partially hit by the radiation, is termed penumbra. The size of the penumbra mainly depends on the extension of the source, and the zone of the penumbra increases with focal size. The lack of resolution caused by the zone of the penumbra also depends on the distance between object and plane of projection. If the object is close to the plane of projection (Fig. 39b), a small zone of penumbra is formed, and thus a less blurred boundary is produced in the radiation relief than is the case for objects far from the plane of projection (Fig. 39a). Therefore, the lack of resolution produced by the penumbra is called geometric lack of resolution.

Figure 40 shows a nomogram on which both the geometric lack of resolution (U) and the picture magnification (V) can be determined. For example, a focus-film distance of 75 cm and an object-film distance of 15 cm give a lack of resolution of 0.25 mm, when the focal diameter is 1 mm. For other focal sizes, U must be multiplied by the focal diameter.

As Figure 40 indicates, two points on the radiograph can be reproduced separately if they are no farther from each other than 0.25 mm. If these points are any closer to each other, this lack of resolution results in the appearance of a single formation. This raises the question of whether such lack of resolution can be recognized by looking at a radiograph. Because of the mosaic-like structure of the retina and the lower limit of the angle of vision due to this structure (minimum separabile), the eye can distinguish from one another only those details which appear under an angle of vision of more than one arc minute.

Data on the minimum distance between two points enabling us to recognize them separately with the eye give a somewhat clearer picture than do data about the angle of vision. As a rule, radiographs are viewed from a distance of 30–35 cm. From this distance, the resolving power of the eye is so great that two points, the distance between which is 0.1 mm, can be clearly distingushed. If, as in Figure 40, the geometric lack of resolution is so large that points whose distance is 0.25 mm appear as a formation, this lack of resolution can be perceived.

It is apparent from the nomogram (Fig. 40), that for large distances between focus and plane of projection and for objects which are very close to the plane of projection, the lack of resolution is smaller than 0.1 mm and is thus no longer perceived by the eye.

It is probably impossible to avoid, especially for thick objects, a certain lack of resolution, which interferes with the recognition of details. The patient must be placed so that the organ of the body which is to be reproduced is as close as possible to the plane of projection. Moreover, the maximum possible focus-film distance should be selected.

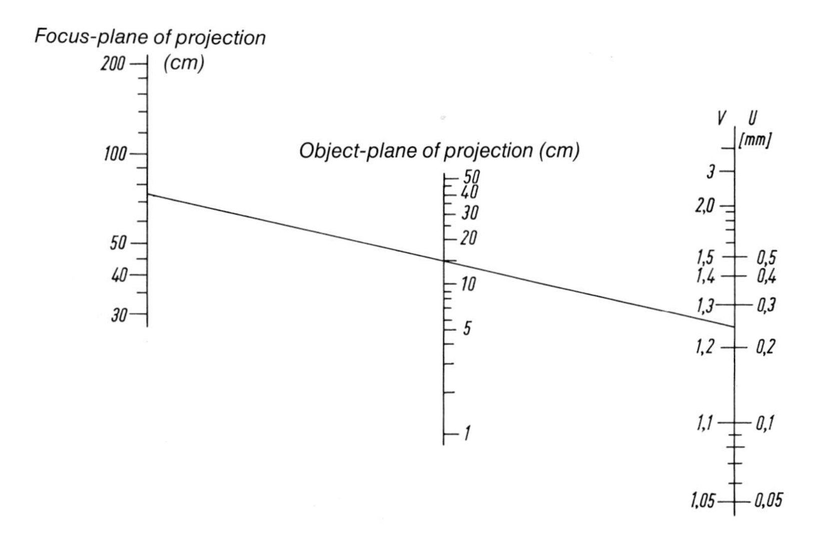

Fig. 40. Nomogram for determining the geometric lack of resolution for a focal diameter of 1 mm. U=Lack of resolution, V=Picture magnification.

A blurred radiograph can also be produced if the patient or the instrument is moved during exposure. This effect is purposively produced in body section radiography.

The representation of a certain body section is impossible under conventional conditions because, by the method of projection, all sections of the irradiated part of the body are reproduced. This cannot be prevented. By moving the instrument during the exposure, however, it is possible to reproduce in a blurred and hazy fashion all the details of objects lying outside a certain body section. Their interference with the interpretation of the details of the body section in question is minimal. The principle of this procedure is very simple. Both the X-ray tube and the film holder are moved in a vertical direction to the central ray, and care is taken that the plane of the body to be examined, independently of the instantaneous position of the tube and holder, is always projected onto the same spot of the film. This condition can be fulfilled only for a plane of the body, which alone is sharply reproduced. All other planes are projected during the movement onto various spots of the film and are therefore blurred. The stronger the blur, the more recognizable a sharply reproduced body section on the radiograph. There are many technical means of obtaining such blurred sections.

General Principles of Radiation Protection in X-Ray Diagnostics

Even without medical or technical-application ionizing radiation, man is continuously exposed to natural environmental radiation. This radiation is terrestrial on the one hand, and cosmic on the other. To this natural radiation load, the civilization radiation load is added; 80–90% of the latter is produced by medical investigations (e.g., X-ray diagnostics, nuclear medicine). Both components of radiation exposure lead to the same effects in the tissues of living organisms. These effects can be divided into those which occur in the irradiated individuum itself (somatic radiation effects) and those which lead to changes in the idioplasm (genetic radiation effects). In the somatic range, acute radiation effects occur almost exclusively in organs whose tissues show a high cell turnover. This applies to the hemapoetic system, intestinal epithelium, testicles, ovaries and the skin. The genetic effects are indicated by an increase in mutations, as can be proven by animal experiments. Although knowledge obtained in such experiments cannot be applied to man without qualification, it is expected that an increase of the potentially mutagenic physical and chemical influences will lead to an increase in genetically induced disease.

If these effects are not directly perceived, we speak of radiation load; if, on the other hand, vital functions are clearly impaired, we refer to radiation damage.

According to the above definition, X-ray investigations are included among those processes in which the organism is subjected to a radiation load. Since, such an investigation may be of fundamental importance to a patient, we cannot reduce the radiation load by altogether dispensing with such examinations. Rather, suitable protective measures are taken. For this purpose, individual countries have issued legal regulations for radiation protection, based on the recommendations of the ICRP (International Commission for Radiological Protection). The introduction to this directive gives the following essential information on radiation protection: "Radiation protection in the widest sense of the word involves good clinical judgement, correct functional design of radiation sources and protective equipment, correct application techniques and expert evaluation of diagnostic information."

The Euratom-Basic Standards (most recent version: *Official Gazette of the European Economic Community,* No. 50, 187 [1976] pp. 1–44) are not international standards. They are valid only within the European Economic Community and as a framework for national legislation on radiation protection. The World Health Organization has not issued recommendations on radiation protection. The ICRP and the ICRU are expert councils of the International Society for Radiology and, strictly speaking, as such have no official status. Another international standard worth noting is the IEC Publication 407 *Radiation Protection in Medical X-ray Equipment 10 kV to 400 kV* (1972).

Three groups of persons are identified in legislation on radiation protection: patients who, because of medical indications, are exposed to radiation; those who are exposed to radiation because of their occupations; and other persons, i.e., unconcerned third persons, who belong to the general population and have to adhere to stricter regulations than the smaller second group.

It is always recommended that an exact radiation history of the patient be obtained in order to avoid unnecessary multiple examinations. The examination record, giving data on the applied doses, must be kept for ten years, and the patient is entitled to receive a copy of his record. Those who are exposed to radiation because of their occupation are monitored for radiation load by personal dosimetry. Such persons must, at their work site, be provided with two dosimeters, and the radiation dose must always be readable on one of these instruments. As a rule, metal film-type and rod-type dosimeters are used. The maximum permissible doses differ from area to area.

Twice a year, persons occupationally exposed to radiation must take part in courses about radiation protection; moreover, once a year they must be examined for radiation damage.

Authorities also distinguish between work rooms, i.e., control areas and monitoring areas. The distinction is made according to the dose a patient receives in the area in question. The control area must be marked during operation of the X-ray equipment.

It is recommended that a table (understandable to physicians, personnel and patients) be placed in rooms where X-ray investigations are undertaken, showing the maximum doses. Also, information relating to them should be placed near the X-ray equipment for study by those involved in the control and monitoring operations.

The New Radiologic Units: *Gray* and *Becquerel*

In June 1975 the standard terms *Gray* (Gy) and *Becquerel* (Bq) were introduced on an international scale for ionizing radiation and radioactive substances, respectively. In the following table (from *Harder*), the new units are defined and their relationships to the units previously used are given.

Table 3. Radiologic Magnitudes and Units according to the ICRU Report 19 (1) and DIN 6814 (2).

Radiologic Magnitude and Symbol (DIN 6814)	*International Resignation and Symbol (ICRU)*	*Magnitude-defining Equation (DIN 6814)*	*Unit Previously Valid*	*SI Unit and Special Term*
Ion dose (J)	Exposure (X)	$J = \frac{dQ}{dm}$ (ionic charge divided by mass)	Roentgen $1\ R = 2.58 \cdot 10^{-4}\ C \cdot kg^{-1}$	Coulomb divided by kilogram $(C \cdot kg^{-1})$
Energy dose (D)	Absorbed dose (D)	$D = \frac{dE}{dm}$ (energy transferred onto matter by mass)	Rad $1\ rd = 10^{-2}\ J \cdot kg^{-1}$	Joule divided by kilogram $(J \cdot kg^{-1})$ $1\ Gy = 1\ J \cdot kg^{-1}$
Equivalent dose (D_q)	Dose equivalent (H)	$D_q = q \cdot D$ (evaluation factor times energy dose)	Rem $1\ rem = 10^{-2}\ J \cdot kg^{-1}$	Joule divided by kilogram $(J \cdot kg^{-1})$
Activity of a radioactive substance (A)	Activity of a radioactive substance (A)	$A = \frac{dN}{dt}$ (number of nuclear transformations divided by time)	Curie $1\ Ci = 3.7 \cdot 10^{10}\ s^{-1}$	Reciprocal second (s^{-1}) $1\ Bq = 1\ s^{-1}$

Table 4. The Changeover to SI Units in Radiology *(H. Lippert/H. P. Lehmann,* SI Units in Medicine, Urban & Schwarzenberg, Baltimore–Munich 1978).

	Rad (Absorbed Dose) **rd** → mGy (mJ/kg)	**Radionuclide Activity (Curie)** **Ci** → GBq **mCi** → MBq **μCi** → kBq	**Rem** (Equivalent Absorbed Dose) **rem** → mJ/kg	**Roentgen** **R** → mC/kg
Conversion	(rd)×0.01=(Gy) (Gy)×100=(rd) (rd)×10=(mGy) (mGy)×0.1=(rd) (Gy)=(J/kg)	(μCi)×37=(kBq) (kBq)×0.02703=(μCi) (mCi)×37=(MBq) (MBq)×0.02703=(mCi) (Ci)×37=(GBq) (GBq)×0.02703=(Ci)	(rem)×0.01=(J/kg) (J/kg)×100=(rem) (rem)×10=(mJ/kg) (mJ/kg)×0.1=(rem)	(R)×0.258=(mC/kg) (mC/kg)×3.876=(r)
Example	870 rd=8.7 Gy	350 μCi=12 950 kBq=13 MBq	460 rem=4.6 J/kg	4500 R=1161 mC/kg=1.161 C/kg
Names of units:	rd=rad, Gy=gray, mGy=milligray, J/kg=joule per kilogram	kBq=Kolobecquerel, MBq=Megabecquerel, GBq=Gigabecquerel, TBq=Terabecquerel	joule per kilogram	R=roentgen mC/kg=millicoulomb per kilogram
Note	Name of SI unit: the gray, symbol Gy. Resolution H2, 15 CGPM (1975) adopts "the following special name of SI unit for ionizing radiation: the gray, symbol Gy, equal to the joule per kilogram."	1 Becquerel=1 disintegration per second= 1 s^{-1} Radionuclide activity is measured in curies (Ci) (non SI unit), where 1 curie is the amount of isotope in which 3.7×10^{10} radioactive disintegrations occur per second. Resolution 7, 12 CGPM (1964) accepts "that the curie be still retained outside SI as unit of activity with the value 3.7×10^{10} s^{-1}." Resolution H 1, 15 CGPM (1975) adopts "the following special name of SI unit for activity, the becquerel, symbol Bq, equal to the second to the power minus one."		

B. Radiographic View of the Normal Adult Skeleton

I. The Skull

Radiographic Anatomy and Radiographs of the Skull, Including Exposure Techniques

The principal and most frequently applied projections are:

1. *Sagittal projections*
   a) posteroanterior (p.a.) radiographs of the facial bones and their cavities
   b) anteroposterior (a.p.) radiographs for evaluation of the occipital components of the skull
2. *Lateral projections* (frontal, bitemporal, either right or left lateral) of the facial bones and their sinuses, the lateral wall of the skull, the base of the skull with the sella turcica, the mandibular joints and the upper cervical vertebrae
3. *Axial projections,* to demonstrate
   a) the base of skull which, for anatomical reasons, can be achieved only approximately, the central ray passing in verticosubmental direction
   b) the calvarium, with submentovertical path of the central ray
4. *Inclined projections,* of unlimited variations
5. *Special projections* of the nasal bone, frontal sinuses, petrous bone, mastoid process, mandible and individual dental roots.

The *principal directions,* which correspond to the main planes of the skull, can only be applied to a small region of the head. Even with increased focus-film distance, they are, strictly speaking, not valid for the whole skull because those parts which are not focused centrally but lie more in the path of the outer branches of the cone of rays are projected axially.

For instance, the direction of the posteroanterior projection follows that of the arrows a–d (Fig. 41), moving at right angles to the forehead, which is placed parallelly to these planes, with normal posture of the head and the patient erect; but it forms a different angle with the base of the skull a–e which extends obliquely from above and anterior to below and posterior. As there is now no parallel projection, but since an infinite number of central projections is possible, the true posteroanterior projection is valid only for the central ray, e.g., arrow a in Figure 41, if the arrow corresponds to the central ray. In that case, the corresponding sagittal plane should be described more accurately. If no precise details have been given, one understands that with this projection the central ray always passes along the median plane of the body. This projection along the median plane is meant to give information about the symmetry of the body halves.

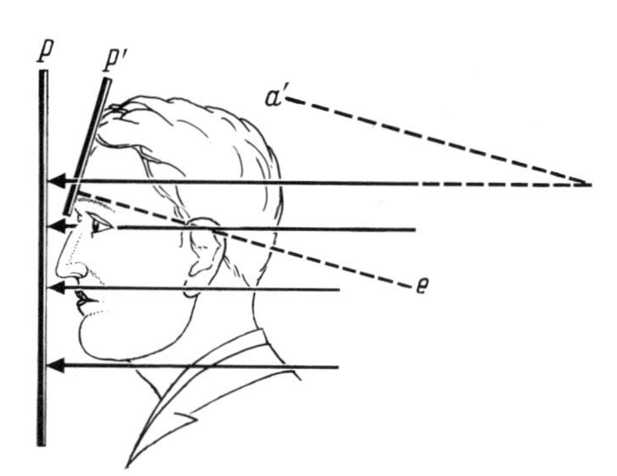

Fig. 41. Sagittal projections of the skull.

However, it must be taken into account that the skull is often asymmetrical. Therefore, if the central ray is projected along the median plane of the body, as shown by arrow a, we obtain a posteroanterior radiograph of the frontal sinuses but, at the same time, a rather poor cranio-occipitofacial view of the maxillary sinuses, and an even less distinct one of the mental region, which is crossed even more obliquely by the rays. If the tube stands in the continuation of arrow d, a view of the neck is obtained which is useless due to the long focus-film distance. But with a sufficiently large film, a caudoposteroanterior radiograph of the mandibular rami and the maxillary sinuses results. This may be valuable in some circumstances because the calvarium, which interferes greatly in projection b, will be projected away from the facial bones, which then become freely visible. If the tube is placed in such a way that film p is exposed to central ray a, and if the film is then tilted more towards the forehead (p′) in order to obtain a clearer view of the involved region here, its projection will be slightly changed, either more or less favorably, according to the incline of the forehead towards the film and the central ray.

This is also called a posteroanterior radiograph of the forehead by inclined film, although the central ray (a′) may not impinge on the film at all. It would be disadvantageous to project in the direction of e, as the active rays would have to pass a far wider diameter of the skull; in addition, the lambdoid suture could easily interfere.

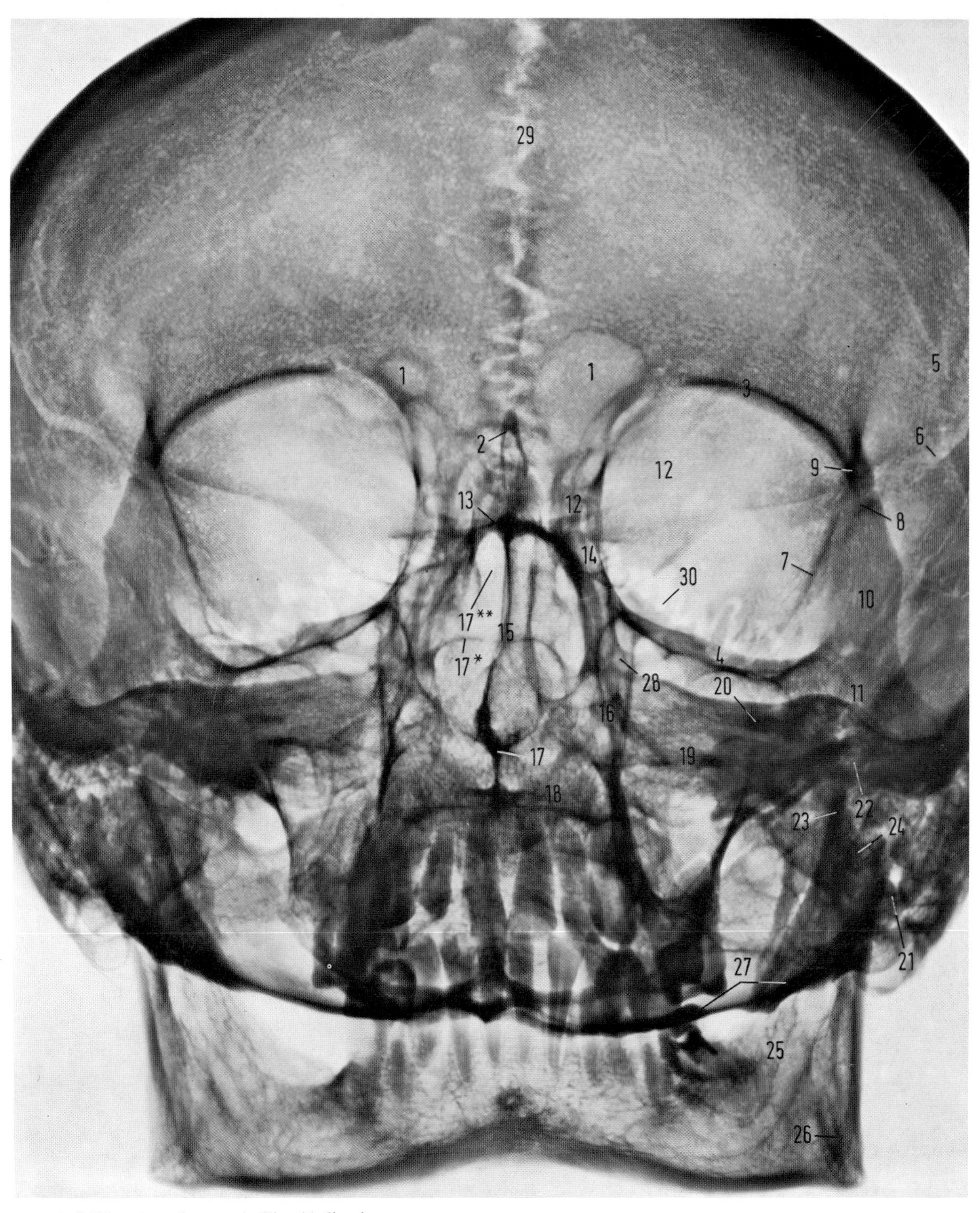

Fig. 42. Skull, macerated. Direction of ray as in Fig. 41, line b.

1 Frontal sinus, in this case rudimentary, especially on the right
2 Crista galli
3 Roof of orbita
4 Floor of orbita
5 Coronal suture
6 Sulcus for medial meningeal artery
7 Innominate line *(Mayer, Liess)*
8 Frontozygomatic suture
9 Zygomatic process of temporal bone
10 Frontal process of zygomatic bone
11 Zygomatic bone
12 Floor of anterior cranial fossa (lesser wing of sphenoid bone)
13 Cribriform plate of ethmoid bone; lateral and caudal to it: ethmoidal cells
14 Frontal process of maxilla
15 Septum of nasal cavity, showing deviation to the right
16 Lateral wall of nasal cavity
17 Vomer 17* sphenoidal sinus, 17** dorsum sellae
18 Floor of nasal cavity (projected on the incline and flattened, followed above by hard palate)
19 Maxillary sinus or antrum
20 Petrous part of temporal bone (also called pyramid)
21 Mastoid process
22 Lower margin of zygomatic arch
23 Coronoid process of mandible
24 Condyloid process of mandible
25 Mandibular canal
26 Angle of mandible
27 Floor of posterior fossa of skull
28 Foramen rotunda
29 Sagittal suture
30 Lambdoid suture

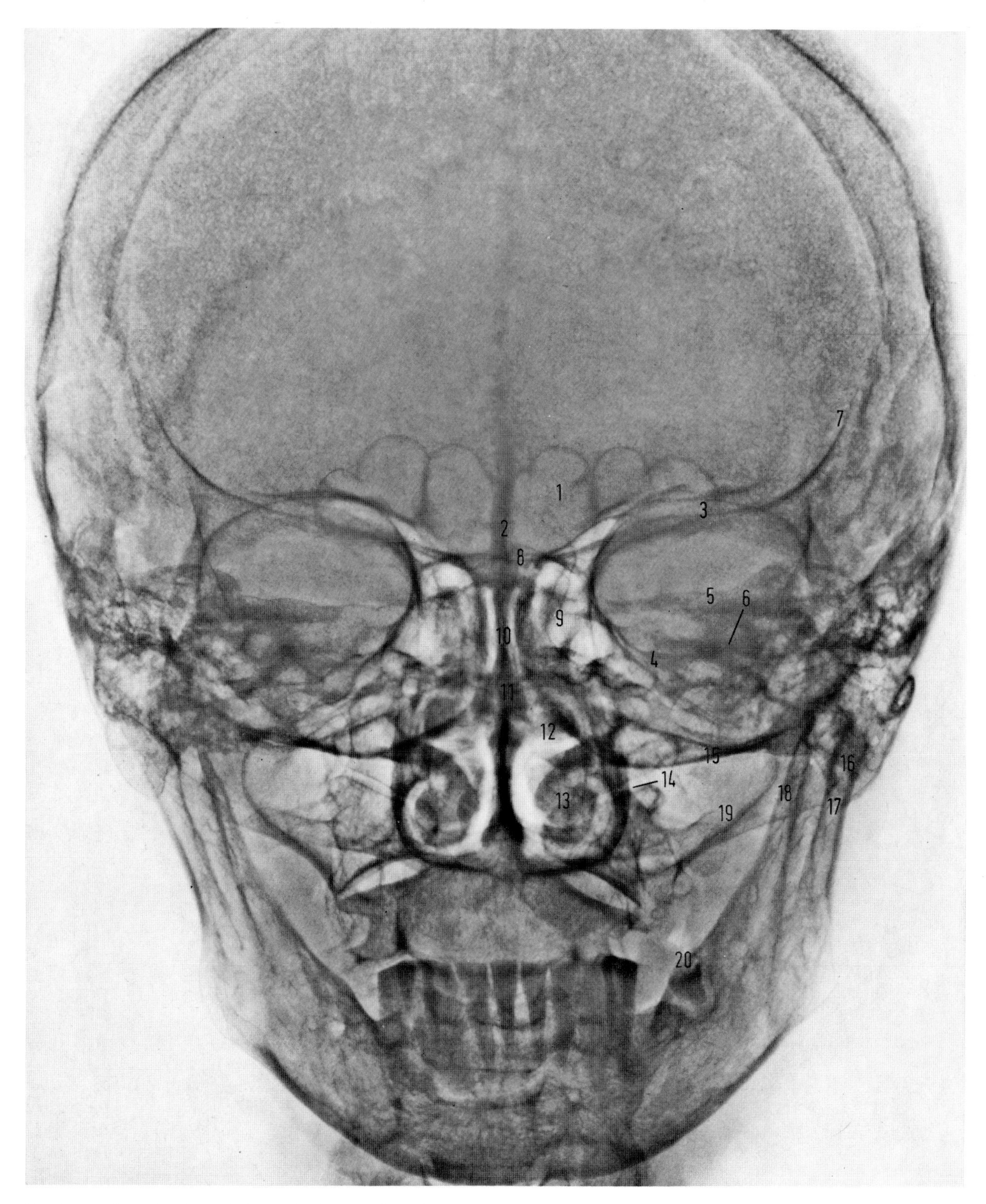

Fig. 43. Head, occipitofrontal. For projection, see Fig. 44.

1 Frontal sinus, often asymmetrical
2 Septum of frontal sinus (may be curved laterally)
3 Orbital roof
4 Orbital floor
5 Petrous bone
6 Cochlea
7 Portion of lateral wall of skull, seen from the edge
8 Base of anterior cranial fossa
9 Ethmoidal labyrinth
10 Median septum of paranasal cavities; below: bony nasal septum (frequently crooked or bent)
11 Base of skull, also forms floor of sphenoidal sinus
12 Middle nasal concha
13 Inferior nasal concha
14 Atlantooccipital joint; above: occipital condyle; below: lateral mass of atlas
15 Floor of posterior as well as middle cranial fossa; underneath: projection of maxillary sinus
16 Mastoid process
17 Condyloid process
18 Coronoid process
19 Zygomatic bone
20 Rudiment of (dental) root with periapical zone of resorption at 8

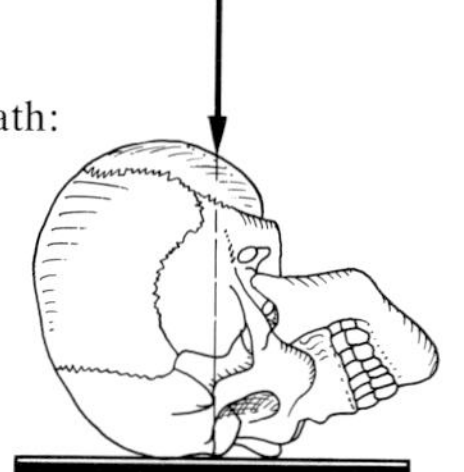

Fig. 44

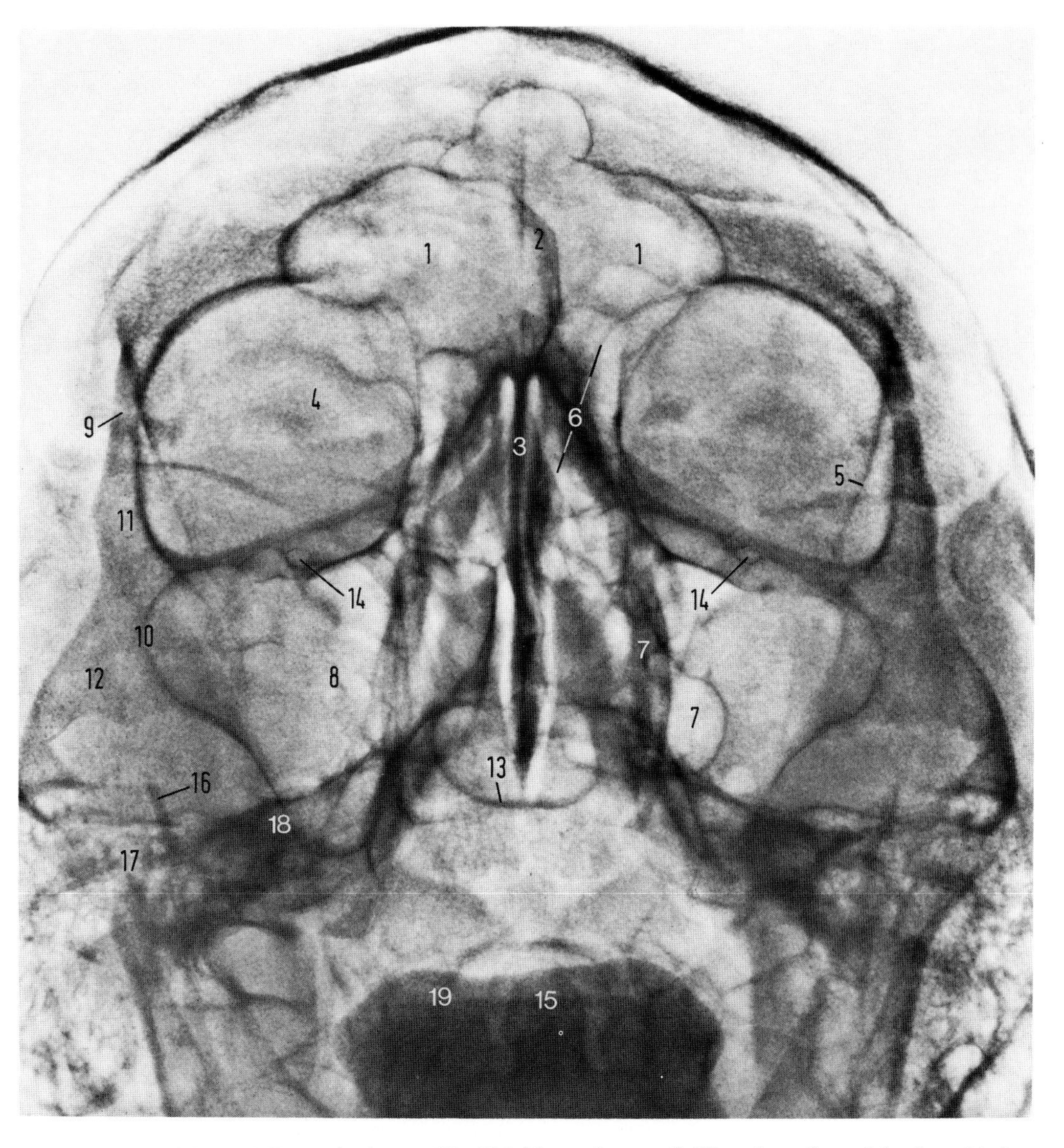

Fig. 45. Head, occipito-oral. For projection, see Fig. 46 (with mouth opened). When the radiograph is taken with the patient in an erect position, the effusion is seen as a fluid level; with the patient prone, it appears as a diffuse turbidity.

1 Frontal sinuses, variable sizes
2 Septum of frontal sinus
3 Bony nasal septum
4 Orbita
5 Innominate line (linea innominata)
6 Anterior ethmoidal cells
7 Posterior ethmoidal cells
8 Maxillary sinus
9 Frontozygomatic suture
10 Zygomatic bone
11 Frontal process
12 Temporal process (arch) of the zygomatic bone
13 Sphenoidal sinus
14 Infraorbital foramen
15 Dens (axis)
16 Coronoid process
17 Condyloid process
18 Petrous bone
19 Tongue

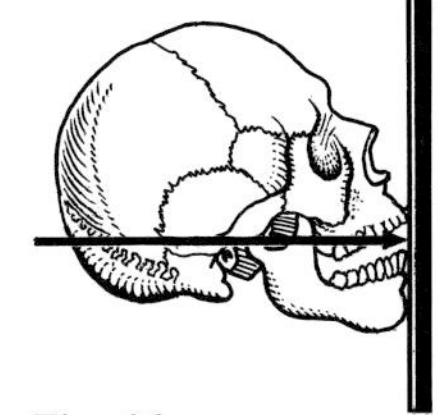

Fig. 46

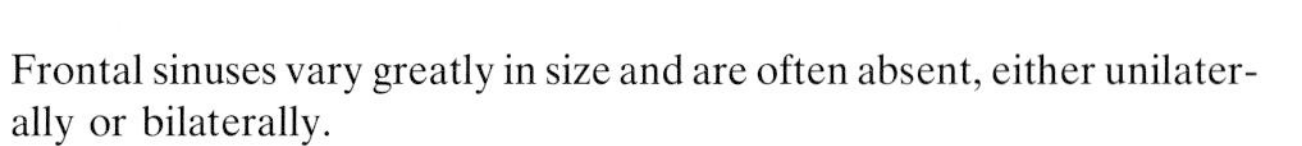

Frontal sinuses vary greatly in size and are often absent, either unilaterally or bilaterally.

Inclined posture or rotation of the head may simulate turbidities or shadows. As a sign of symmetry, observe the relation of the dens (15) to the midline. The frequently asymmetrically formed sphenoidal sinus is projected into the oral cavity.

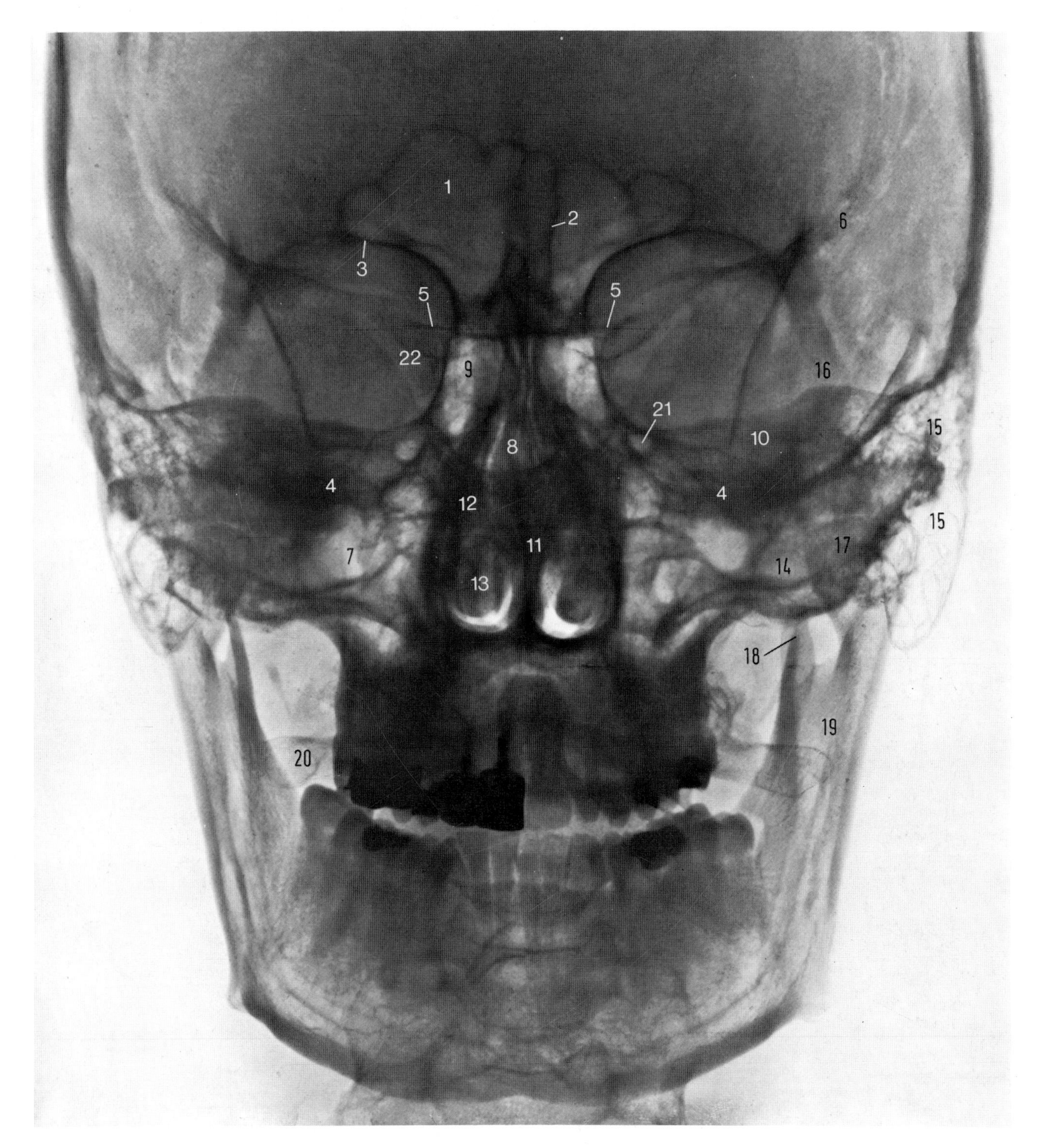

Fig. 47. Head, occipitonasal. For projection, see Fig. 48. Very suitable for a comprehensive view of all paranasal sinuses.

1 Frontal sinus
2 Septum of frontal sinus
3 Orbital roof
4 Orbital floor
5 Floor of the anterior cranial fossa (lesser wing of sphenoid bone)
6 Posterior border of anterior cranial fossa
7 Maxillary sinus
8 Floor of sphenoidal sinuses
9 Ethmoidal cells and sphenoidal sinus
10 Petrous bone
11 Bony nasal septum
12 Middle nasal concha
13 Inferior nasal concha
14 Base of posterior cranial fossa
15 Mastoid cells
16 Zygomatic process
17 Region of the mandibular condyle
18 Coronoid process
19 Ramus mandibulae
20 Transverse process of first cervical vertebra (atlas)
21 Foramen rotundum
22 Superior orbital fissure

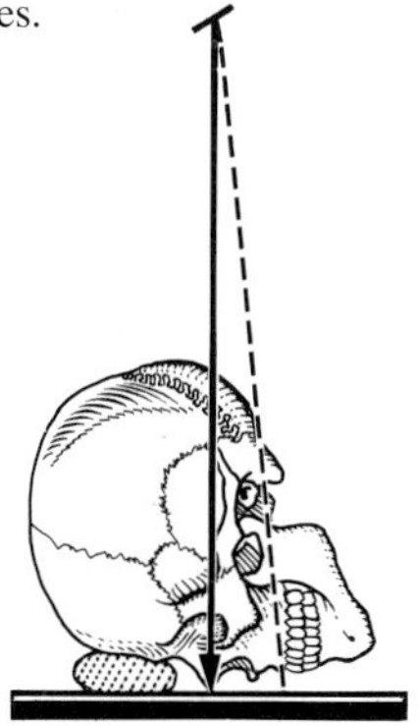

Fig. 48

Special Views of the Paranasal Sinuses

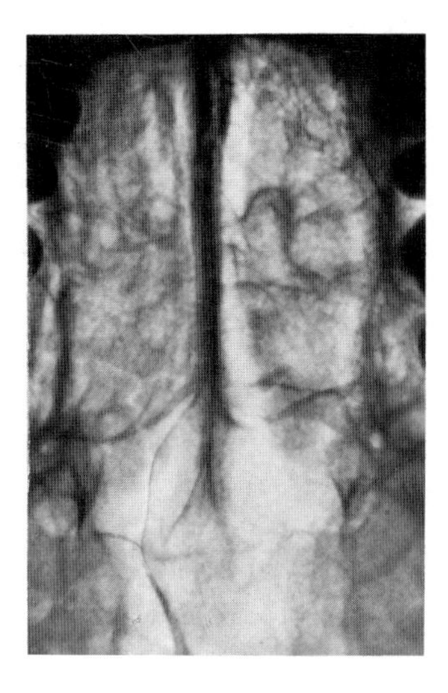

Fig. 49. Sphenoidal sinuses, axial. For projection, see Fig. 52. Superimposition upon the lumina of the sinuses by hazy posterior ethmoidal cells.

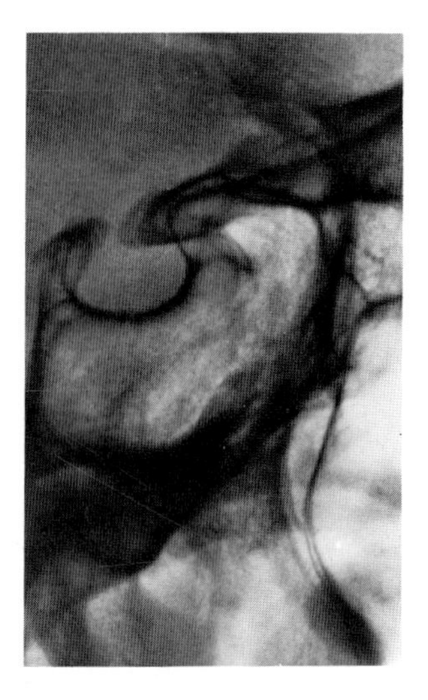

Fig. 50. Sphenoidal sinuses, lateral. For projection, see Fig. 53. This view provides information on the in depth extension of the sphenoidal sinuses.

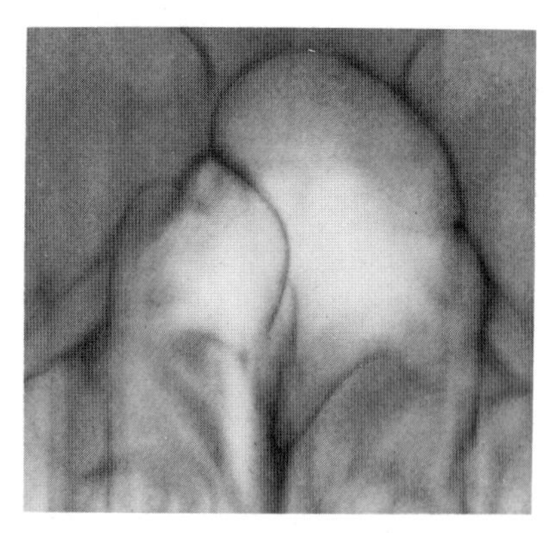

Fig. 51. Tomographic view of the sphenoidal sinuses. The tomographic examination provides a view free of superimpositions. Positioning of the patient as for axial (horizontal) tomography of the base of skull (see Figs. 54, 214 and 215).

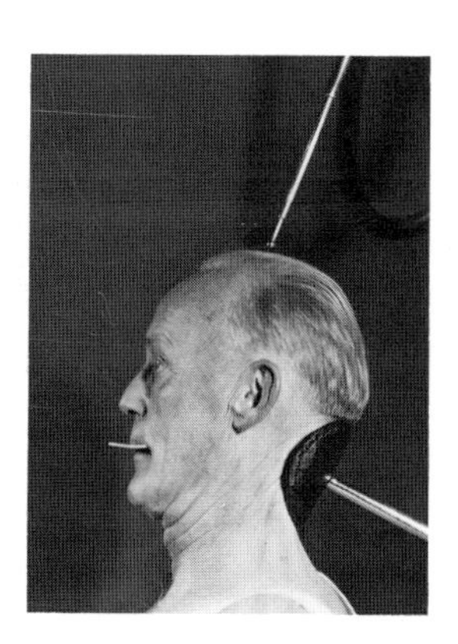

Fig. 52

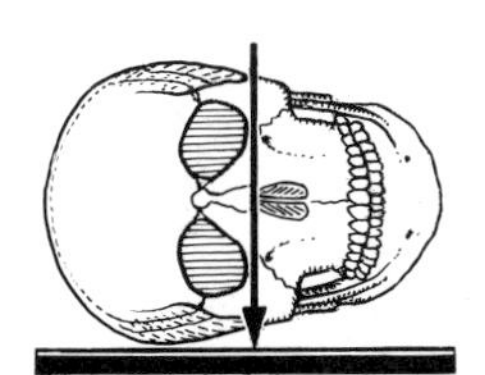

Fig. 53. The central ray is directed perpendicularly to the plane of the cassette and passes through the inferior margin of the orbitae. The sagittal plane of the head lies parallel to the film.

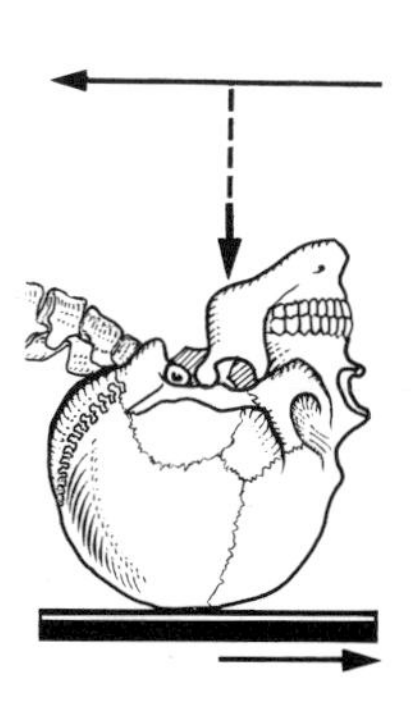

Fig. 54

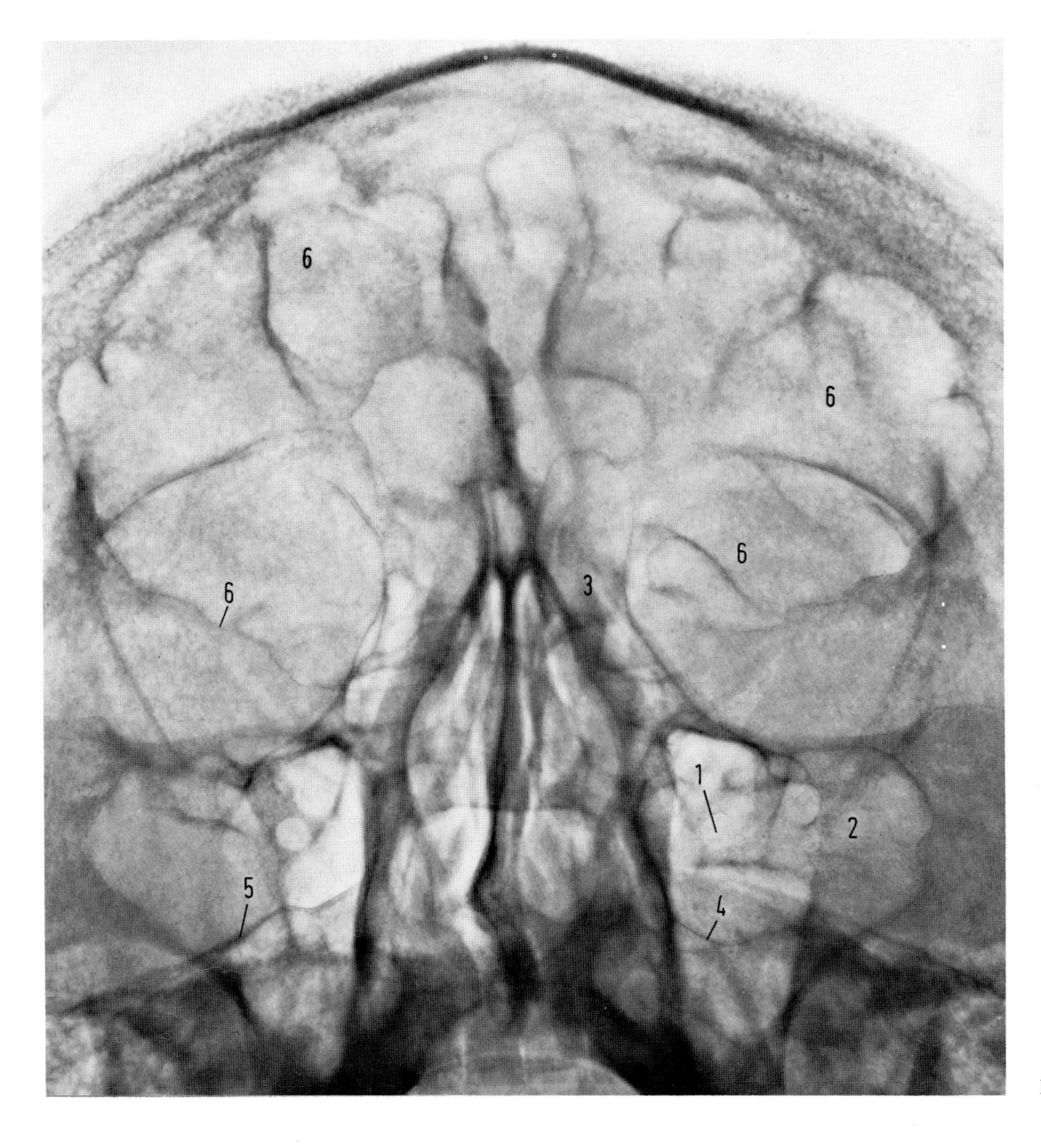

Fig. 55

Fig. 55. Hyperpneumatization of the frontal bone, with large recess above the orbita, reaching to the sphenoid bone (Pneumosinus dilatana).

1 Foramen rotundum, bilaterally well visible on this radiograph, taken according to *Schaaf's* modification
2 Maxillary sinus
3 Anterior ethmoidal cells
4 Posterior ethmoidal cells
5 Upper limit of petrous bone
6 Extensive frontal sinuses, with hyperpneumatization also in the ethmoidal cell system

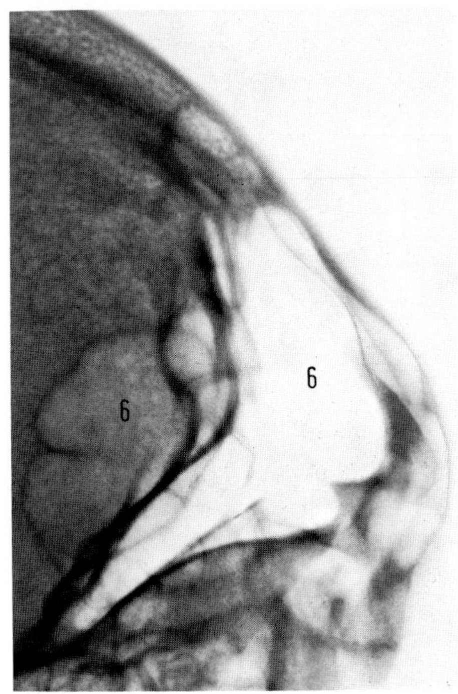

Fig. 56. The lateral view shows the actual extension of the frontal sinus.

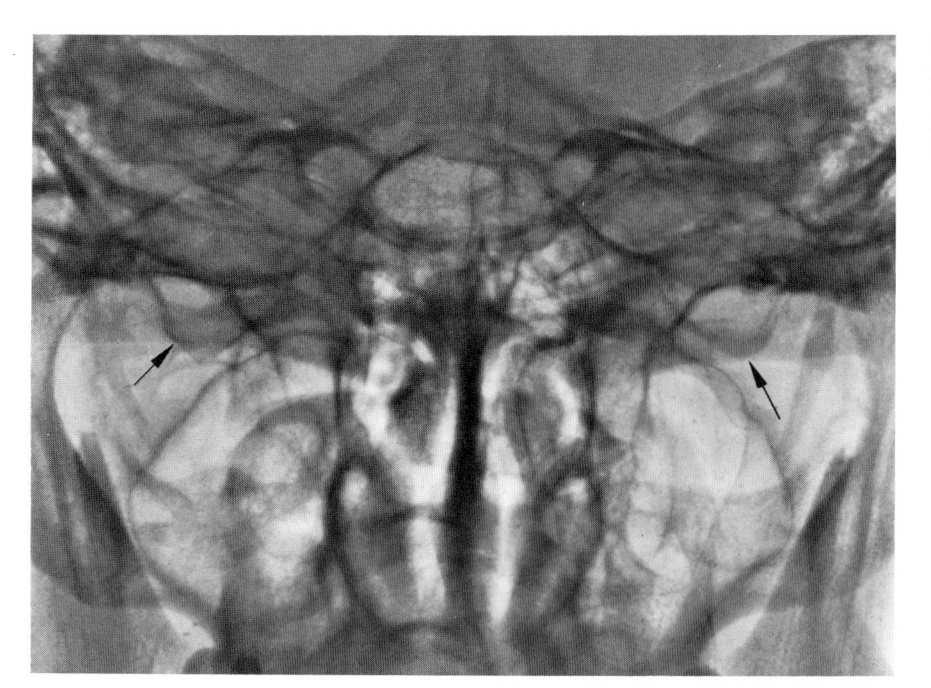

Fig. 57. Paranasal sinuses, caudo-occipito-frontal, for better demonstration of the posterior portion of the maxillary sinus *(Auer)*. For projection, see Fig. 58. Arrows are directed towards the great wing.

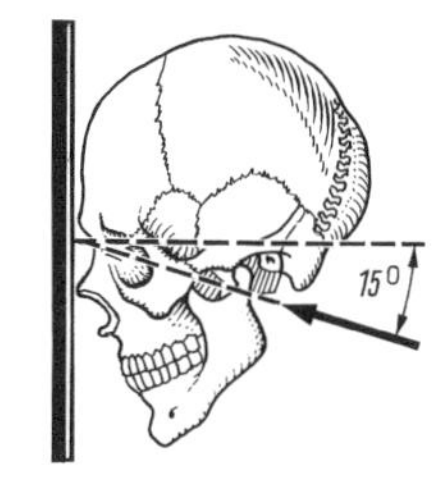

Fig. 58

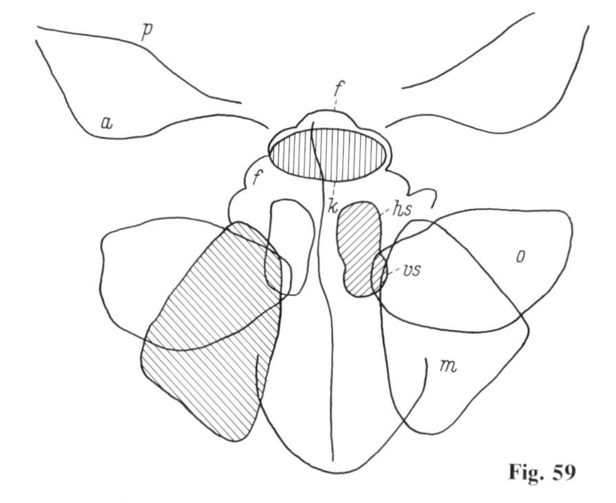

Fig. 59

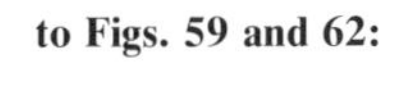

to Figs. 59 and 62:

a	Lesser wing of sphenoid bone
f	Frontal sinus
g	Auditory tube
hs	Posterior ethmoidal cells
k	Sphenoidal sinus
m	Maxillary sinus
o	Orbita
p	Petrous bone
pd	Hard palate
pm	Soft palate
t	Sella turcica
ua	Condyloid process
um	Coronoid process
vs	Anterior ethmoidal cells

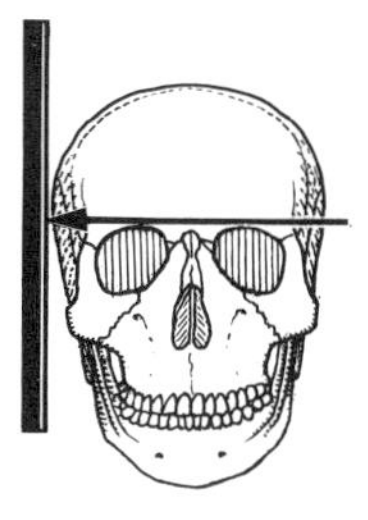

Fig. 61

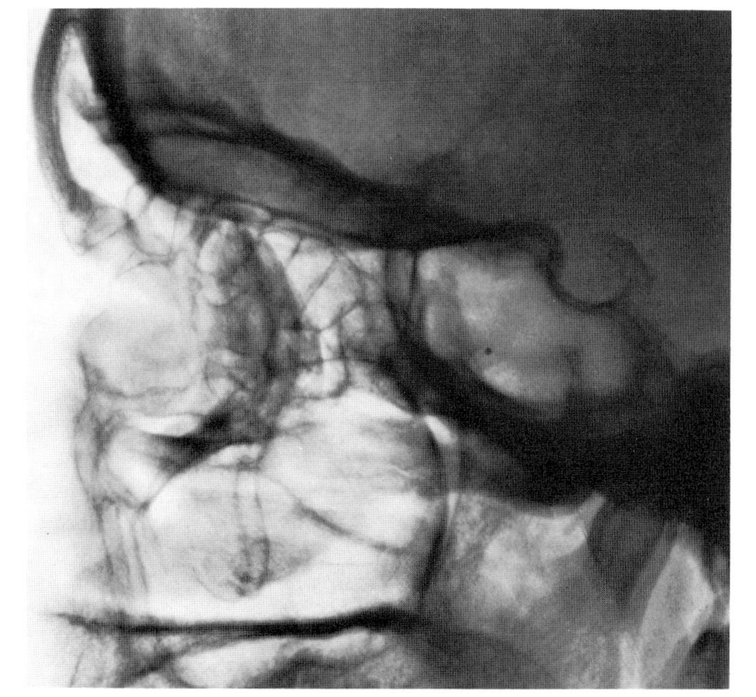

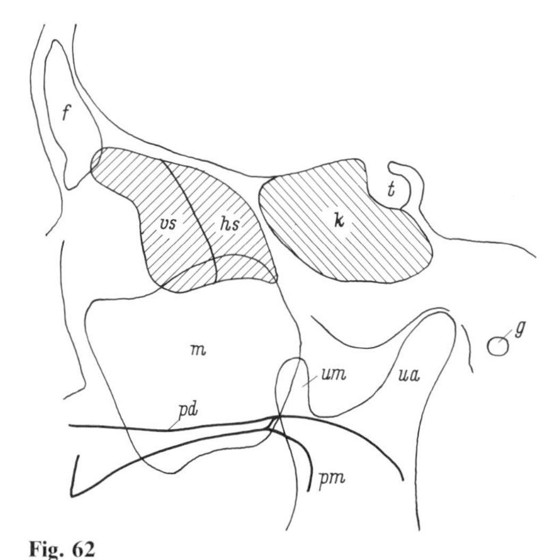

Fig. 62

Fig. 60. Paranasal sinuses, bitemporal. Good lateral survey of the paranasal sinuses. For projection, see Fig. 61.

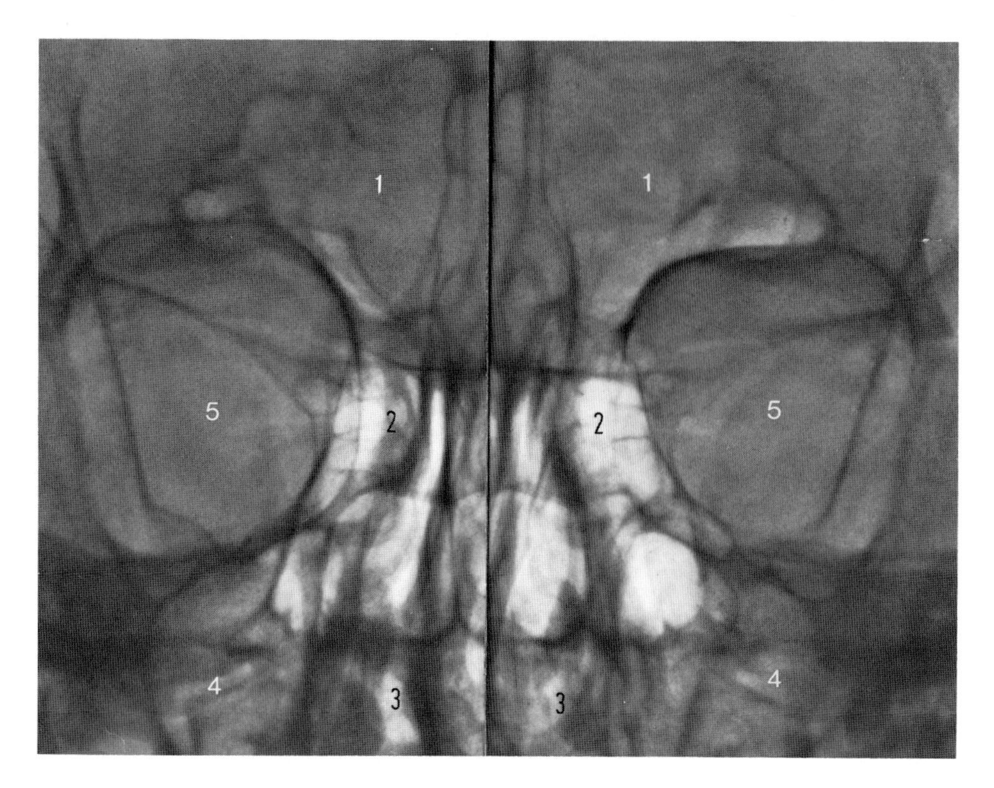

Fig. 63. Bivisual radiograph of the ethmoid bone (see *Heckmann, de Vega-Goicoechea, Dann et. al.).* Two axial radiographs are taken according to the *Rhese* technique, with an angle of about 70° between the sagittal plane of the head and the plane of the cassette.

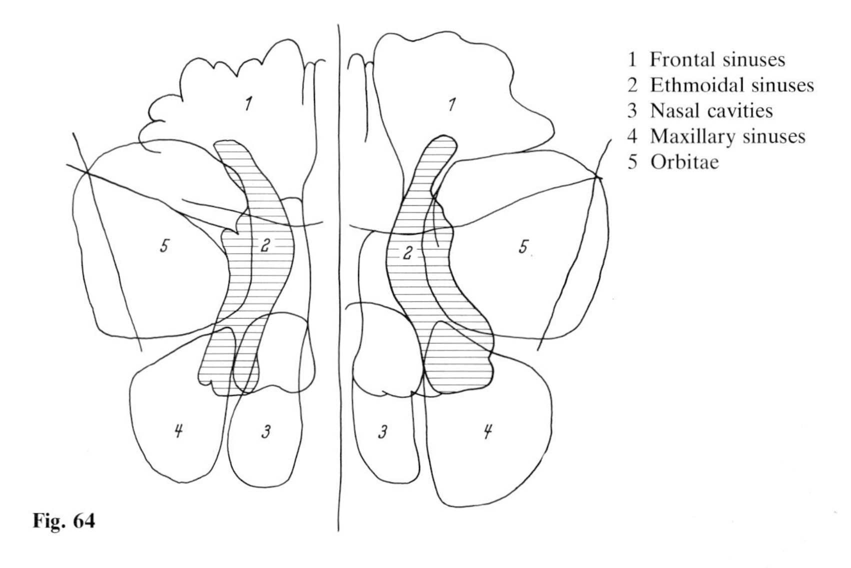

1 Frontal sinuses
2 Ethmoidal sinuses
3 Nasal cavities
4 Maxillary sinuses
5 Orbitae

Fig. 64

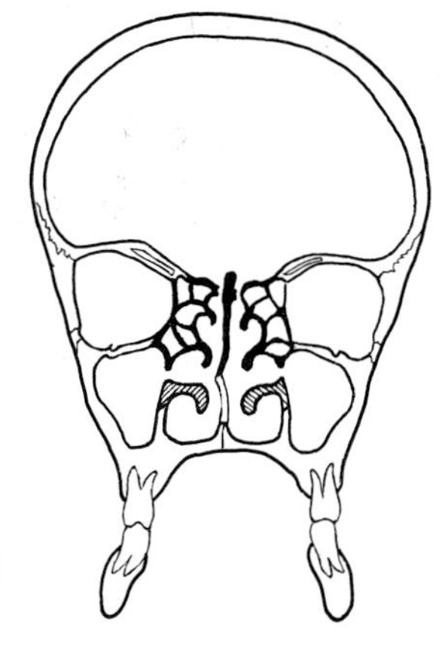

Fig. 65. Frontal section through the skull. The ethmoid bone is made prominent in black; the inferior concha is hatched. Semischematic (taken from *Corning*).

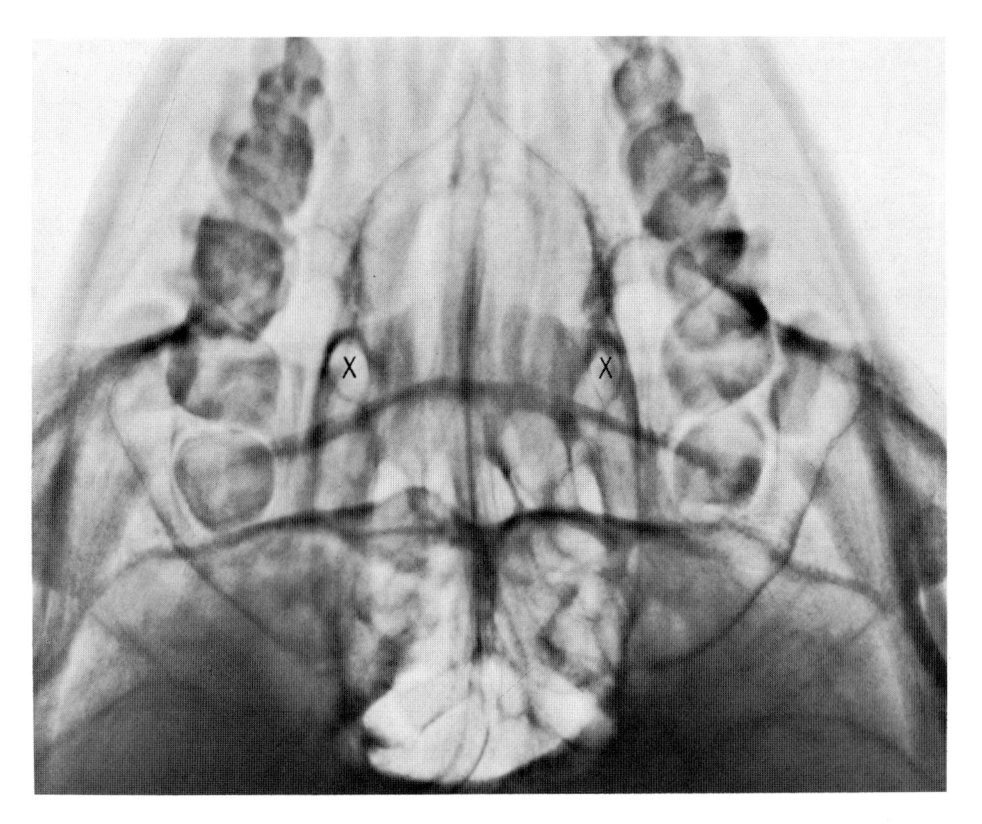

Fig. 66. Hyperextended submentovertical (axial) radiograph of the paranasal sinuses. This radiograph allows exact evaluation of the depth of the individual frontal sinuses and the thickness of their walls by means of forward projection of both rows of teeth. With this projection, the ethmoidal cells are also well demonstrated (*Mangabeira-Albernaz* and *Dasilva*). For projection, see Fig. 68.

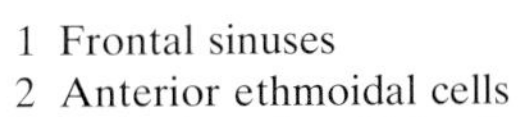

1 Frontal sinuses
2 Anterior ethmoidal cells
3 Posterior ethmoidal cells and sphenoidal sinuses
4 Maxillary sinuses
5 Nasal septum
6 Zygomatic bone
7 Maxillae with rows of teeth
** Lacrimal ducts (see also Fig. 89)

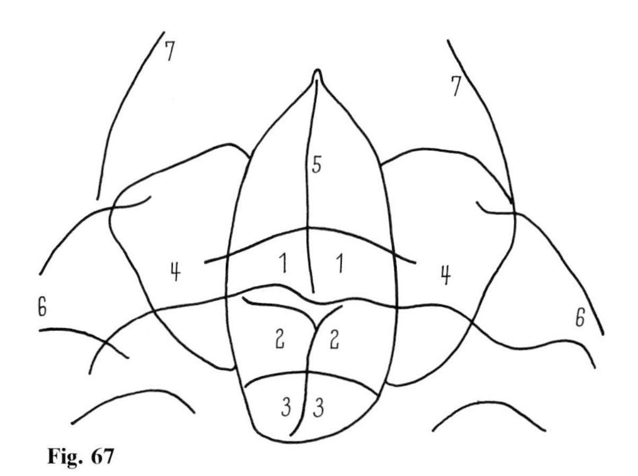

Fig. 67

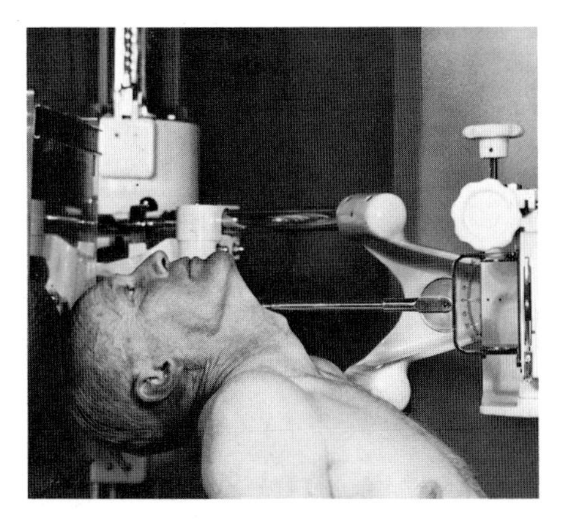

Fig. 68

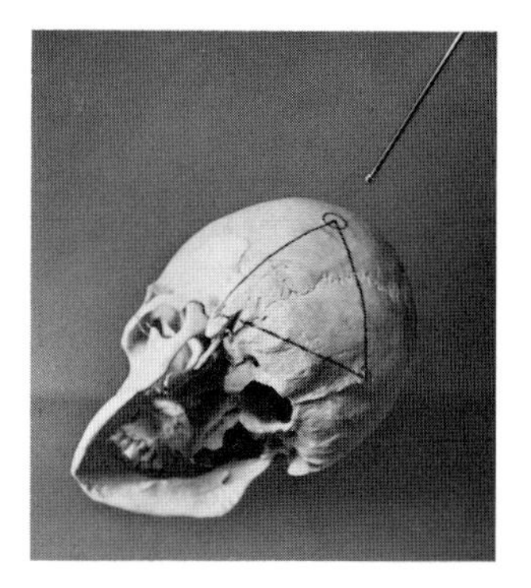

Fig. 69

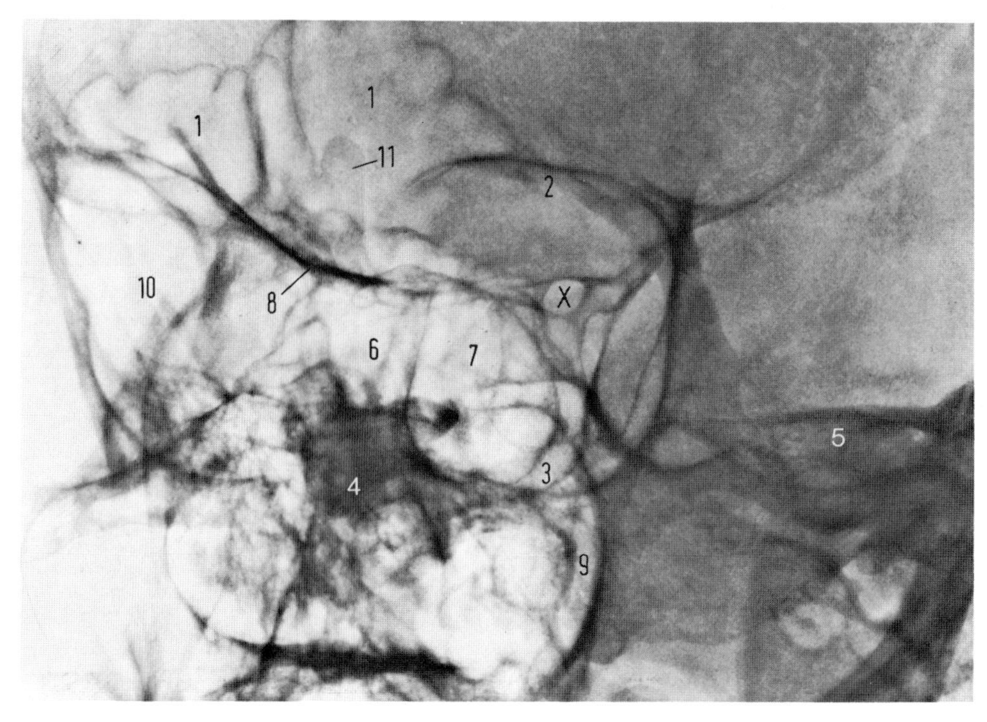

Fig. 70. Optic canal. Radiograph according to *Rhese* and *Goalwin*. For projection, see Fig. 69.

x Optic canal with ethmoidal cells
1 Frontal sinuses
2 Upper orbital margin
3 Lower orbital margin
4 Petrous bone, away from cassette
5 Petrous bone, lying near cassette
6 Ethmoidal region
7 Sphenoidal sinuses
8 Lesser wing of sphenoid bone
9 Posterior edge of maxilla, adjacent to cassette
10 Orbita, away from cassette
11 Crista galli

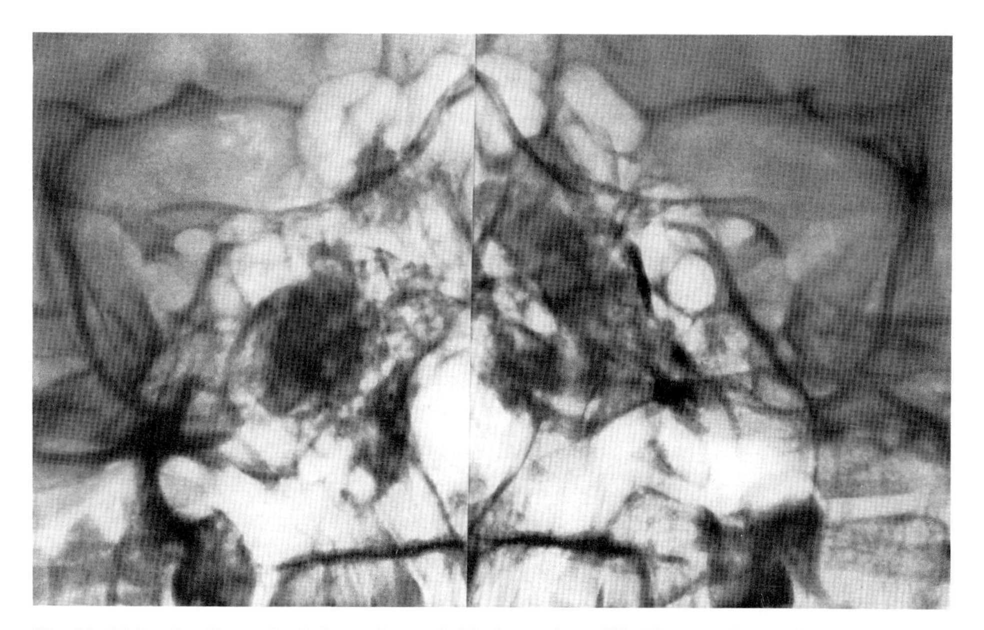

Fig. 71. Bivisual radiograph of the optic canal *(Heckmann)* modified by covering half the cassette with leaded rubber.

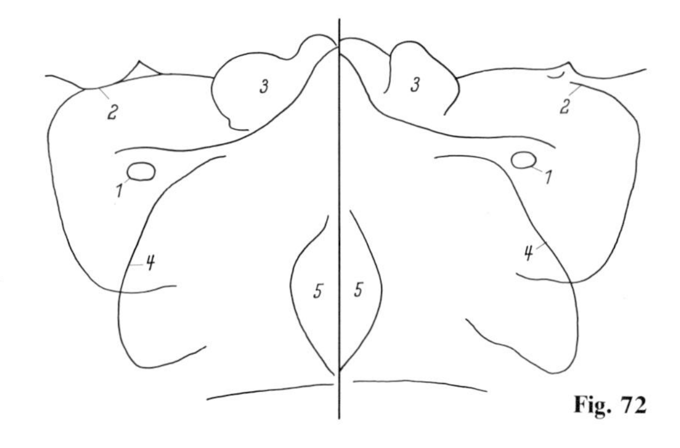

Fig. 72

This radiograph is advantageous for comparison of both sides. From the radiologic point of view, its significance is not in the absolute width of the canal but in the difference in width between the two sides and in knowledge of variants, e.g., duplications of the canal. The diameter of the optic canal, which is already fully developed by the third year of life, varies (according to *Goalwin*) between 3.5 and 5.5 mm, with an average of 4.3 to 5 mm.

1 Optic canal
2 Orbita
3 Frontal sinus
4 Maxillary sinus
5 Nasal cavity

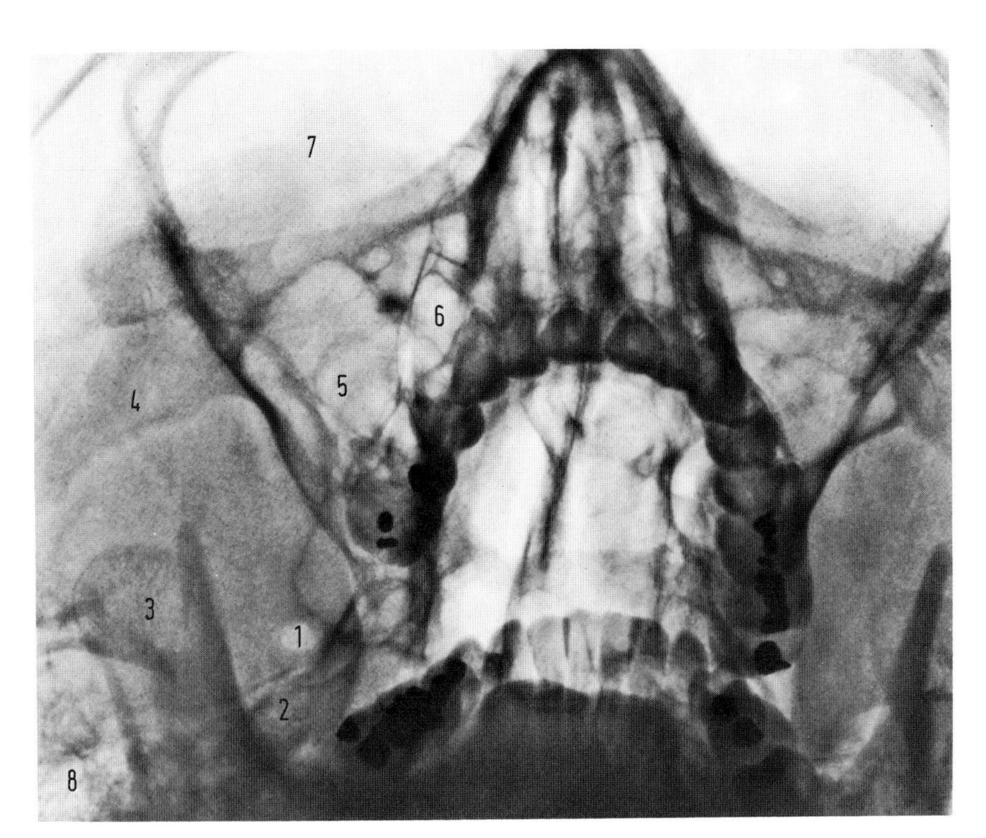

1 Foramen ovale
2 Petrous bone
3 Condyloid process of mandible
4 Zygomatic bone
5 Maxillary sinus
6 Ethmoidal cells
7 Orbita
8 Mastoid cells

Fig. 73. Foramen ovale. Radiograph is taken with the patient either prone or sitting. The head is tilted backward by 45° and rotated towards the opposite side by 10°. The projection is taken about 4 cm frontally to the tip of the lambdoid suture and about 2 cm towards the opposite side of the middle line. During the radiograph, the mouth must be wide open. The central ray impinges vertically on the cassette (see also *Clementschitsch*). By means of this radiograph, the foramen ovale is shown in its normal size (important for anesthesia of the semilunar ganglion).

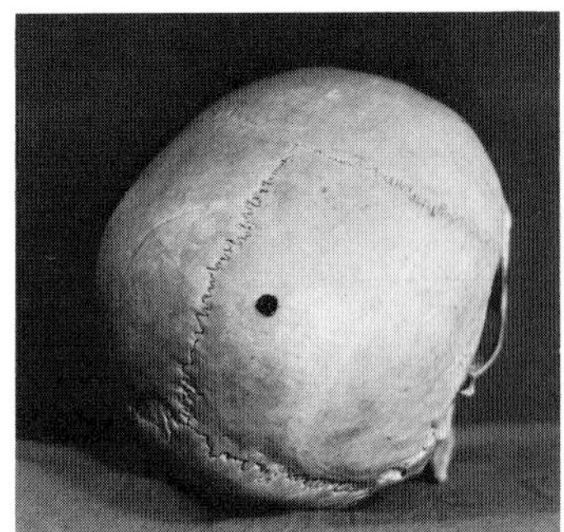

Fig. 74

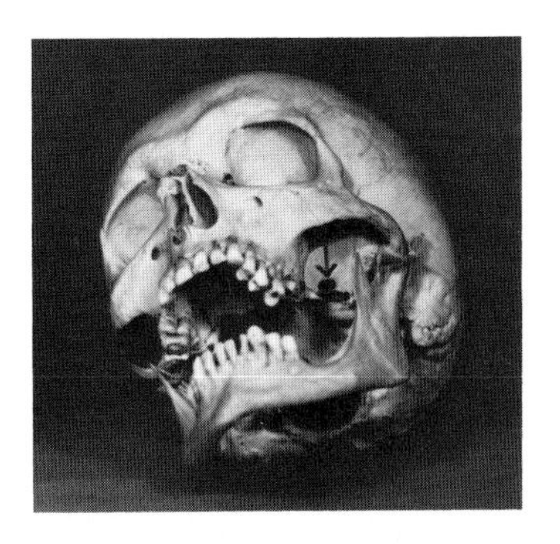

Fig. 75

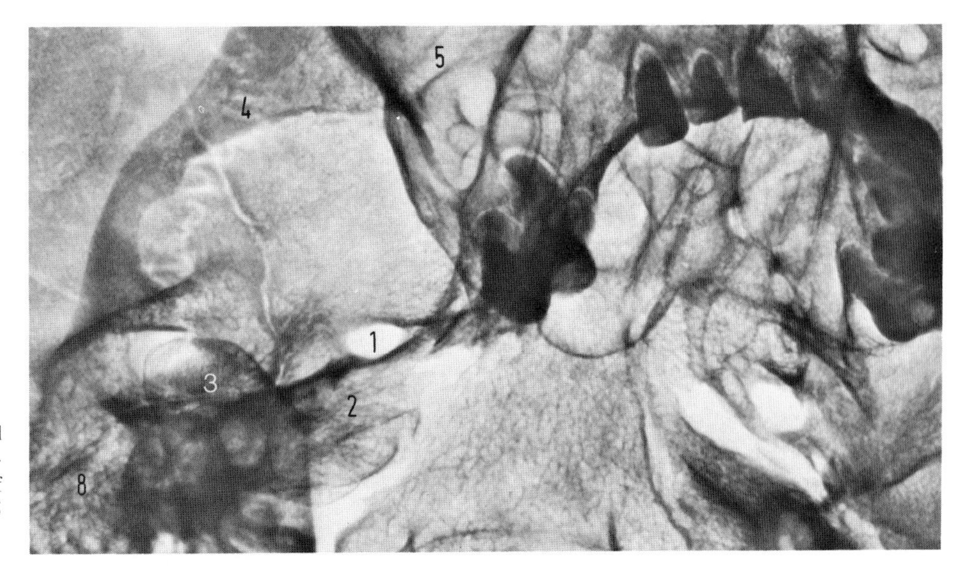

Fig. 76. Foramen ovale in macerated skull, by the same projection technique. For points of entrance and exit of the central ray, see Figs. 74 (●) and 75 (↓).

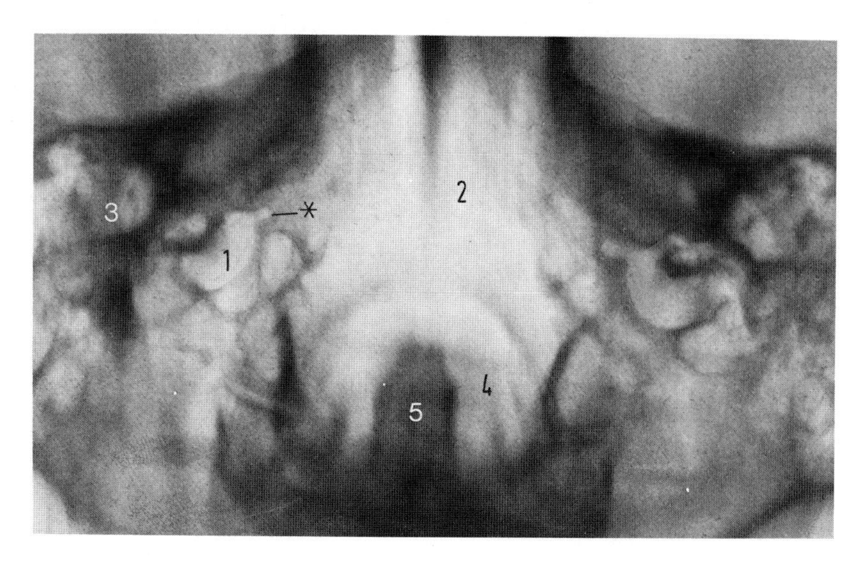

1 Jugular foramen
2 Clivus
3 Petrous bone
4 Foramen magnum
5 Dens (of axis)
* Pars nervosa

Fig. 77. Tomograph for comparative radiologic-anatomical examination of the jugular foramen on both sides, according to *Csákány* and *Donáth*. For projection, see Fig. 78. By means of the tomographic technique in half-axial projection, with the patient supine or prone, both jugular foramina are well demonstrated.

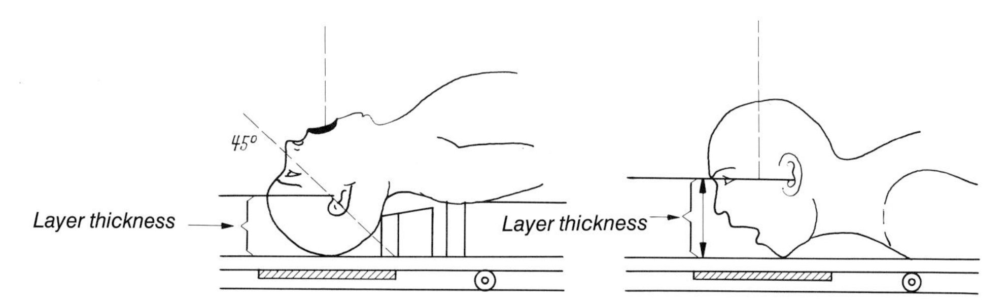

Fig. 78 (from *Csákány* and *Donáth*).

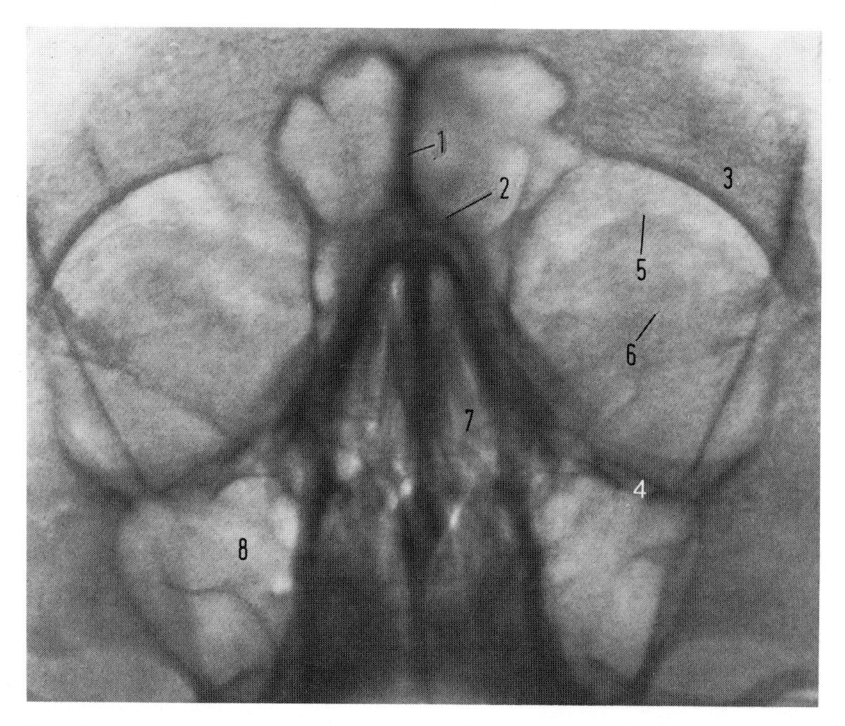

Fig. 79. Eyeball, occipito-oral radiograph. Projection as in Fig. 45. Soft rays are necessary.

1 Septum of frontal sinuses, in superimposition with crista galli
2 Contour of soft nasal tissues
3 Supraorbital margin
4 Infraorbital margin
5 Upper contour of eyeball and upper eyelid
6 Palpebral fissure (closed); the petrous bone is projected more caudally
7 Nasal cavity
8 Maxillary sinus

Fig. 80. Radiographs of the anterior portion of the eyeball, clear of bony sructures (after *Vogt*). This radiograph of the bulbus permits the demonstration of minute foreign bodies in the anterior portion of the eyeball. Figs. 80a and b in temporonasal direction of radiograph (for projection, see Fig. 81). Fig. 80c in craniocaudal direction (for projection, see Fig. 82).

1 Upper eyelid
2 Lower eyelid
3 Lateral margin of orbita
4 Frontal bone
5 Soft tissues of forehead
6 Eyeball

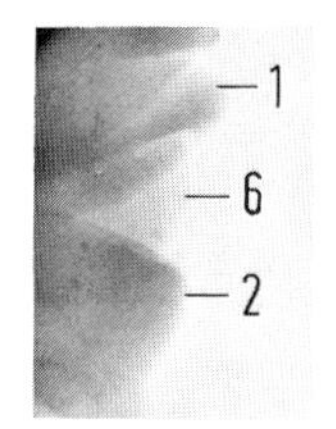

Fig. 80 a

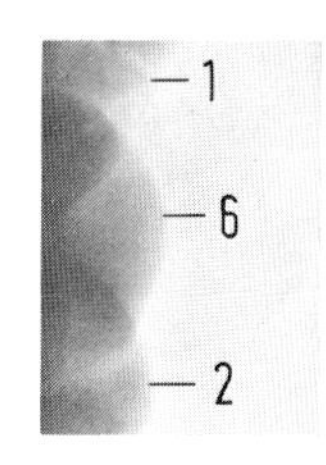

Fig. 80 b

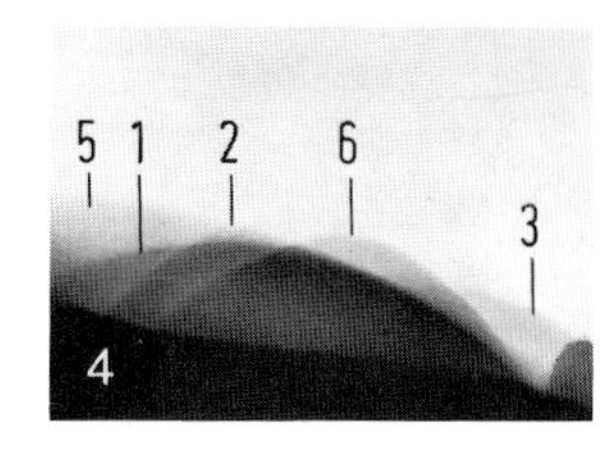

Fig. 80 c

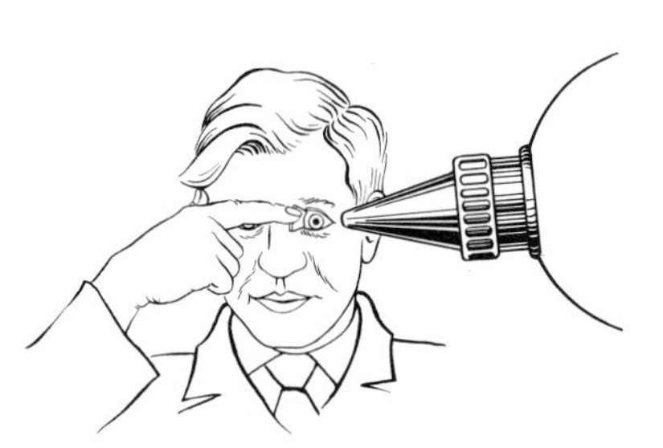

Fig. 81

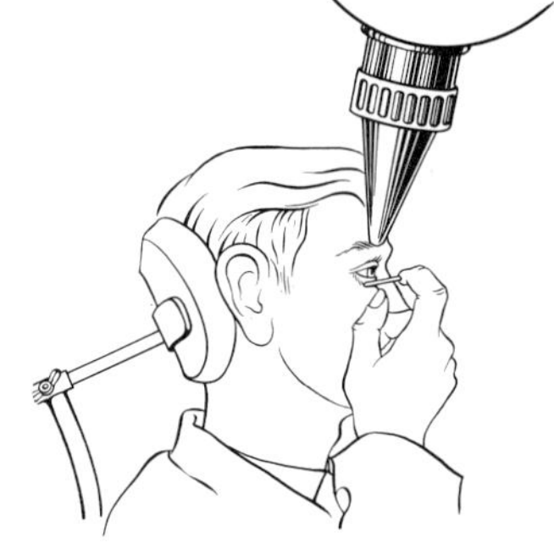

Fig. 82

Fig. 83. Nasal bone, lateral. For projection, see Fig. 84. This specialized radiograph is required only in exceptional cases (e.g., in forensic investigations). Generally, radiographs with the head lying on its right or left side, with the skull raised and the film placed at the side of the head, suffice.

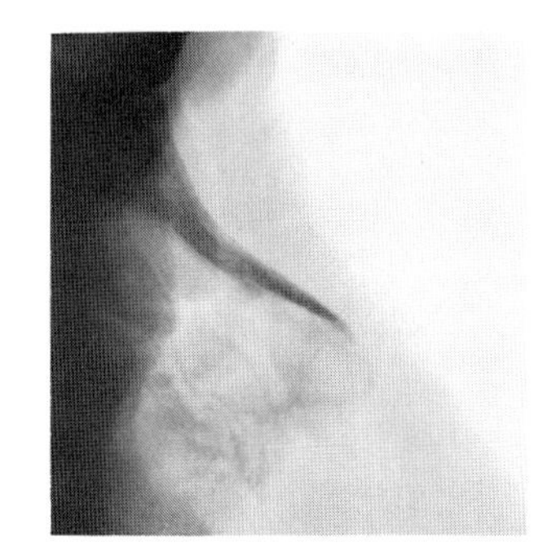

Fig. 83

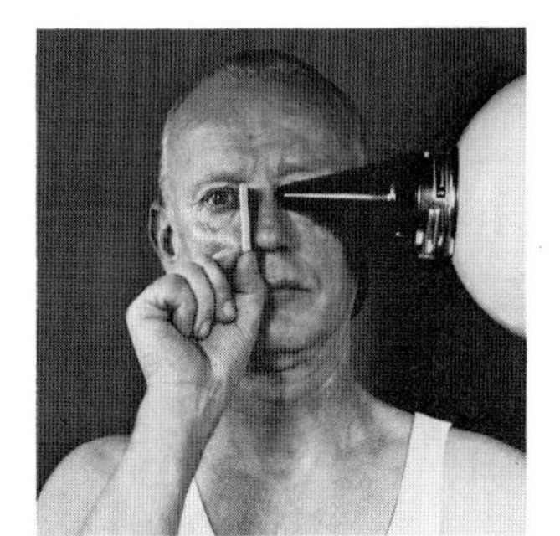

Fig. 84

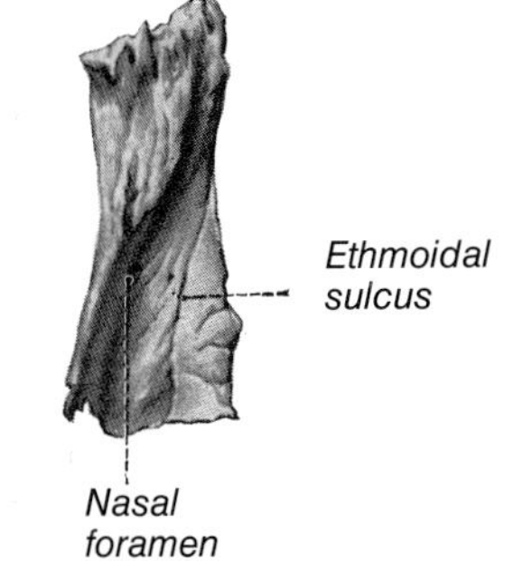

Fig. 85. Nasal bone, lateral. The distinctly recognizable furrowed structure of the nasal bone may easily simulate fissures (from *Sobotta-Becher,* 6th ed.).

Fig. 86. Nasal bone, axial. For projection, see Fig. 87. This radiograph isolates the frontal processes of the maxilla, which on both sides are directly adjacent to the nasal bones. Only the axial radiograph shows an isolated fracture of the frontal process of the maxilla; therefore, an axial radiograph of the nasal bone should also be taken *(Knetsch).*

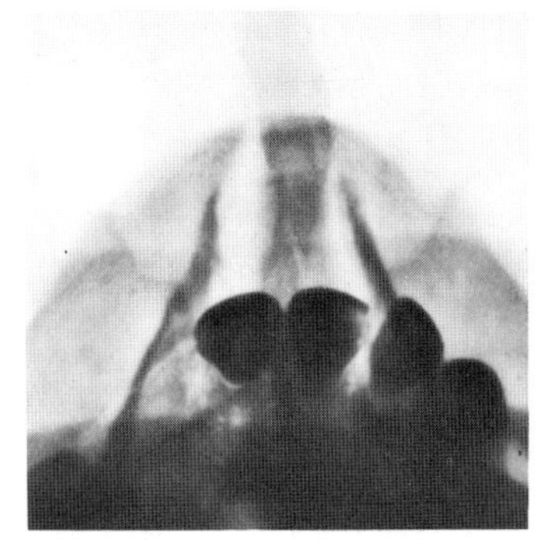

Fig. 86

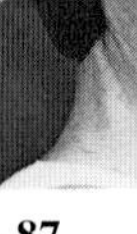

Fig. 87

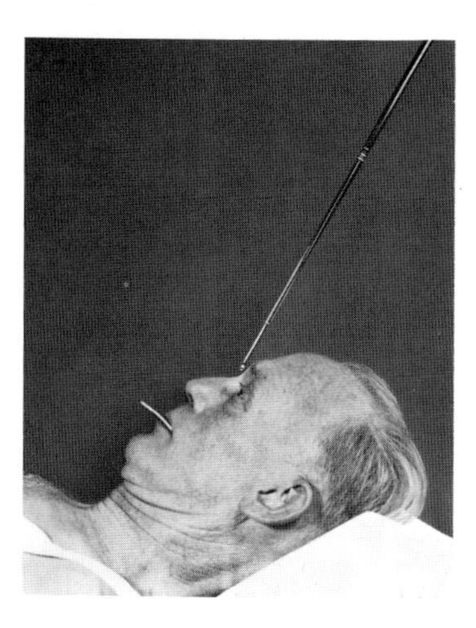

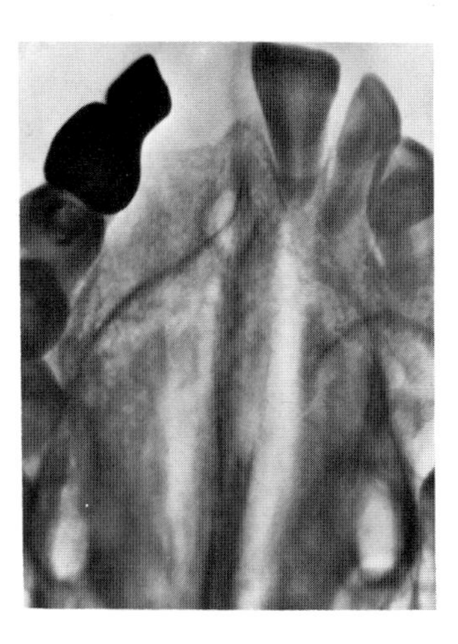

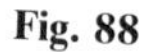

Fig. 88

Fig. 89. Bony nasolacrimal canal (after *Kopylow* and *Toth*). For projection, see Fig. 88. The central ray is focused axially in the direction of the nasolacrimal duct and impinges vertically onto the small film (4/6) placed into the oral cavity (mouth). In this connection, see Fig. 66 (axial radiograph of the paranasal sinuses in hyperextension showing the nasolacrimal canal but with the path of the beam reversed).

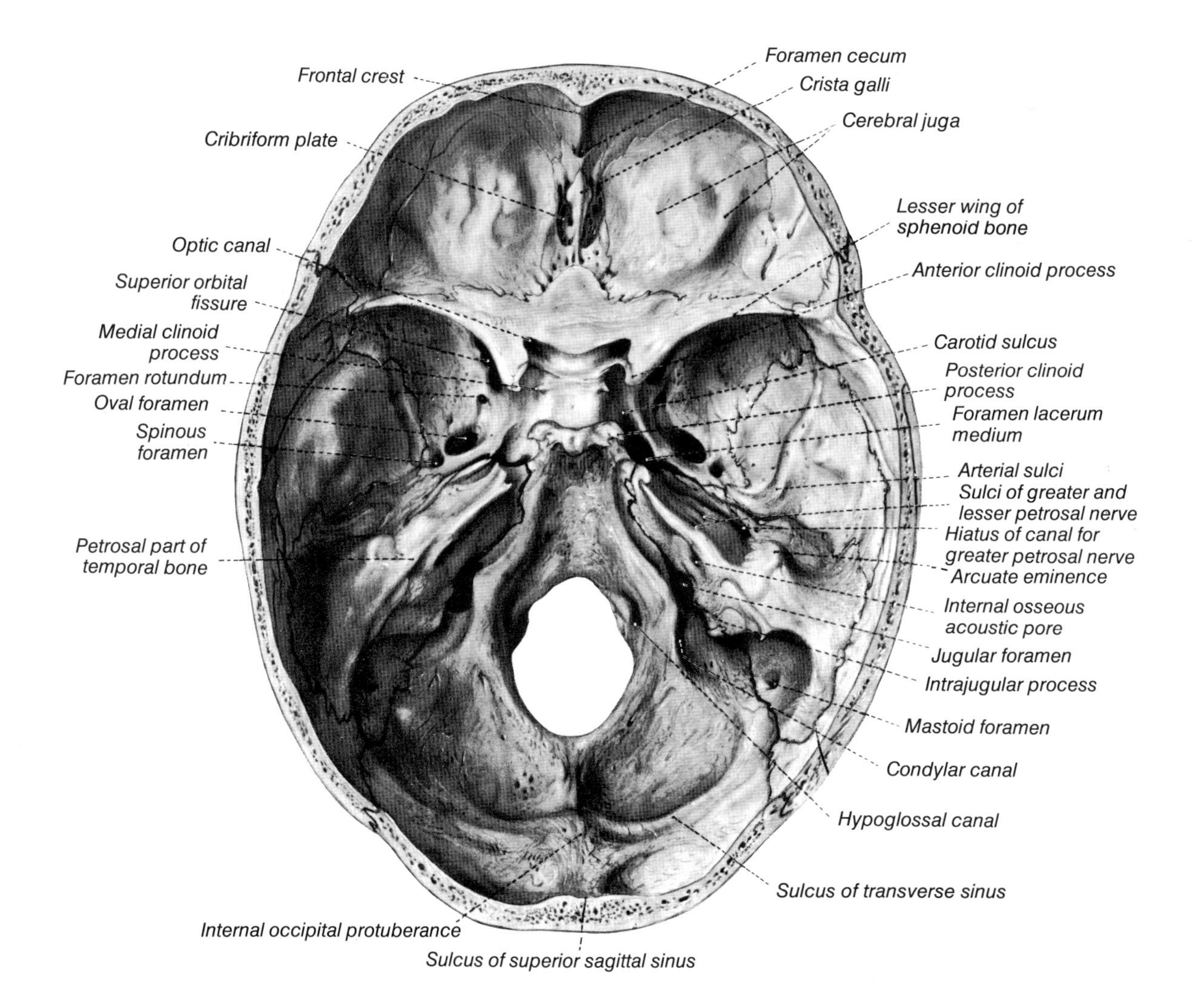

Fig. 90. Base of skull, cranial surface (from *Benninghoff/Goertler:* Lehrbuch der Anatomie des Menschen, 1. Band, 11. Aufl. Hrsg.: *H. Ferner* u. *J. Staubesand.* München-Berlin-Wien 1975).

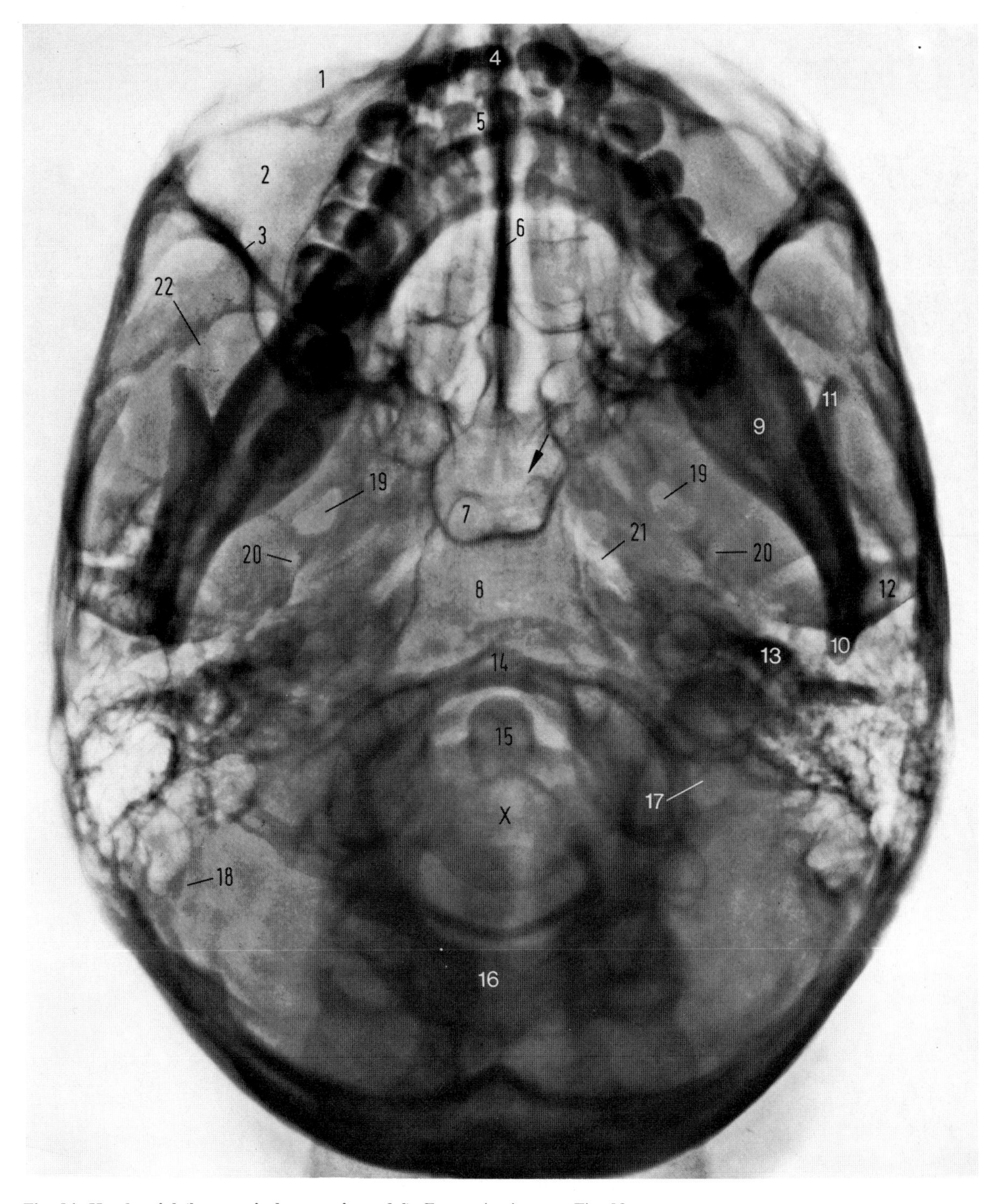

Fig. 91. Head, axial (basovertical or craniocaudal). For projection, see Fig. 92.

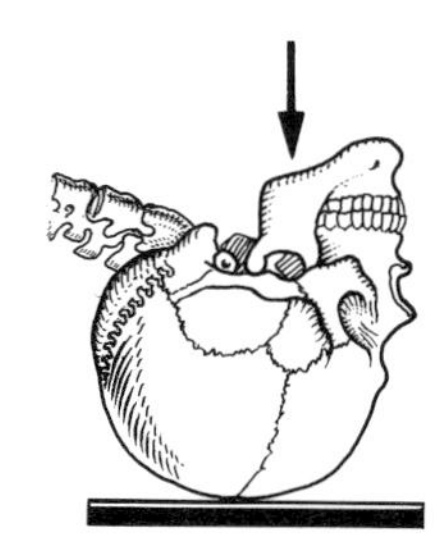

Fig. 92

1 Frontal bone
2 Orbita, projected into the maxillary sinus
3 Infratemporal surface of maxilla
4 Upper teeth
5 Lower teeth
6 Bony nasal septum
7 Dorsal portion of right sphenoidal sinus
8 Clivus
9 Mandible
10 Angle of mandible
11 Coronoid process
12 Condyloid process
13 Petrous bone
14 Anterior arch of atlas
15 Dens (axis)
16 Arch of axis
17 Foramen transversarium of atlas
18 Parietomastoid suture
19 Foramen ovale
20 Foramen spinosum
21 Foramen lacerum
22 Great wing of sphenoid bone
↙ Sagittal suture (line of pseudofracture)
X Foramen magnum

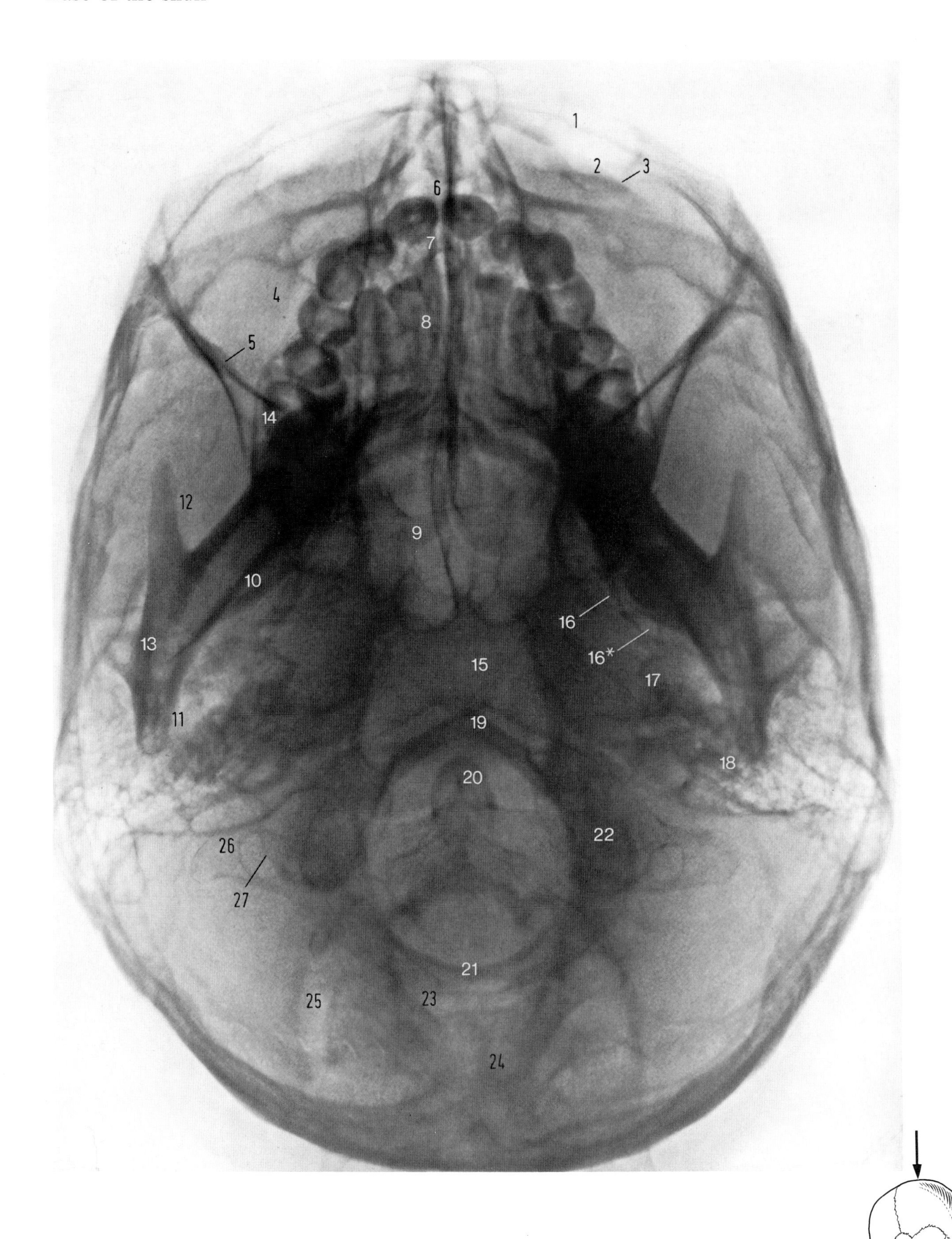

Fig. 93. Head, axial (verticobasal or craniocaudal), for demonstration of the base of the skull, paranasal sinuses and facial bones. By means of this projection, foramen magnum, dens and atlas are well demonstrated; both zygomatic arches show well with weaker exposure but are partially projected into the lateral margin of the skull (compare with Fig. 97). For projection, see Fig. 94.

Fig. 94

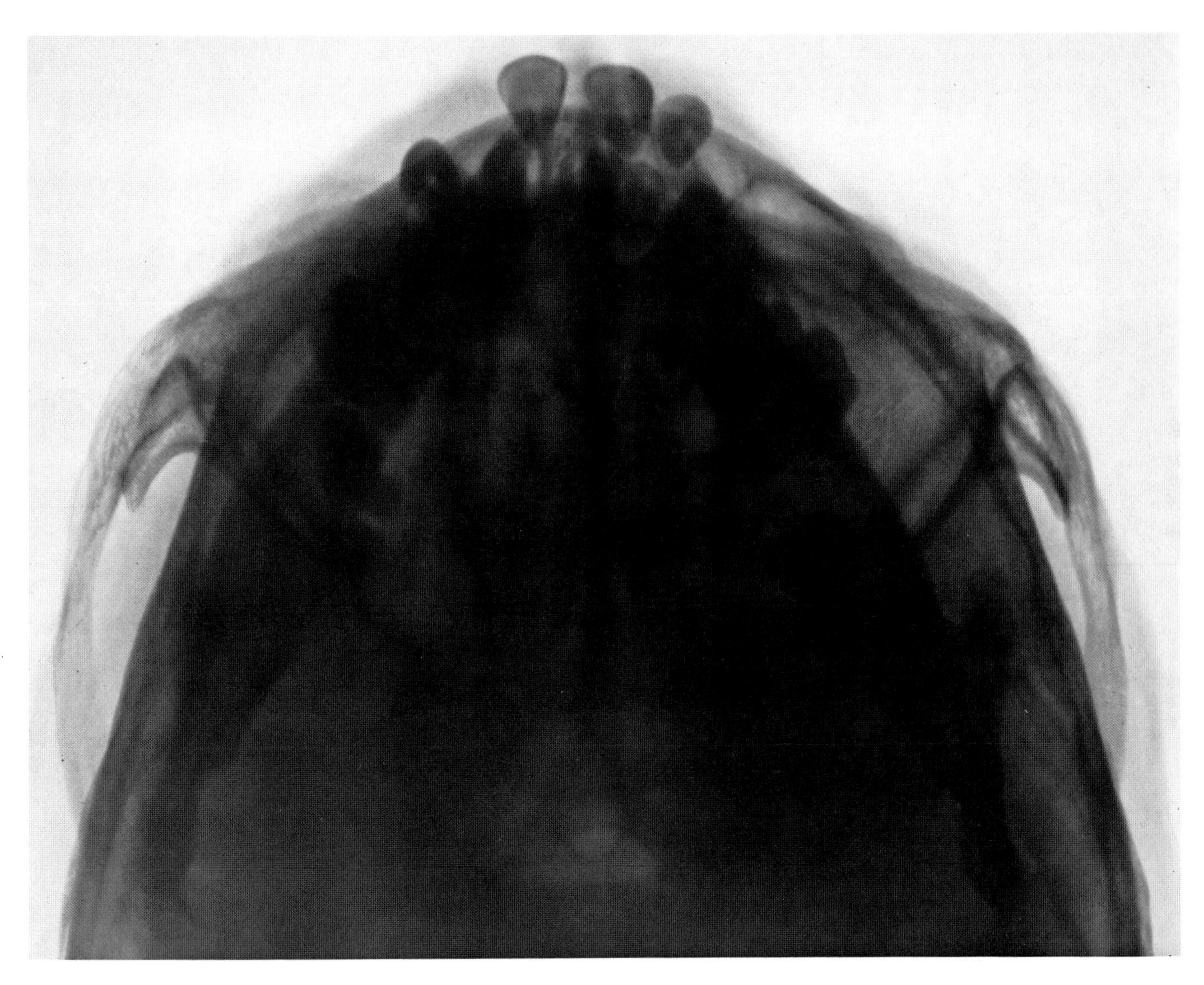

Fig. 95. Radiograph for comparison of both zygomatic arches with submentobregmatic pathway of ray *(Rösli, Pannewitz)*. Modified projection, with patient sitting (see Fig. 96). This radiograph requires soft rays in order not to overexpose the zygomatic arches. The focus-film distance is about 80 cm, to be achieved through divergence of the bundle of rays, so that the zygomatic arches are projected freely outside the skull.

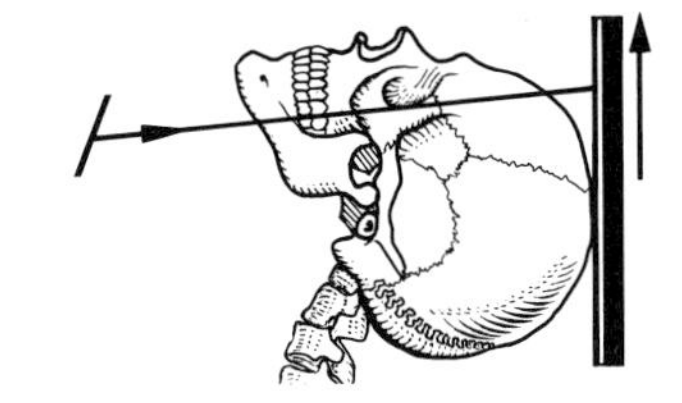

Fig. 96

◀ **to Fig. 93:**

1 Frontal bone in cross section
2 Projected horizontally
3 Contour of skin of cheek
4 Orbita, maxillary sinus
5 Infratemporal surface of maxilla
6 Nasal cavity
7 Upper teeth
8 Lower teeth
9 Right sphenoidal sinus (considerable asymmetry)
10 Mandible
11 Mandibular angle
12 Coronoid process
13 Condyloid process
14 Pterygopalatine fossa
15 Clivus
16 Foramen ovale
16* Foramen spinosum
17 Petrous bone
18 Petrous bone, pneumatic system
19 Anterior arch of atlas
20 Dens (axis)
21 Posterior arch of atlas
22 Lateral mass of atlas with joint to axis (epistropheus)
23 Arch of axis
24 Internal occipital crest
25 Occipital bone (posterior cranial fossa)
26 Transverse process of atlas
27 Foramen transversarium of atlas

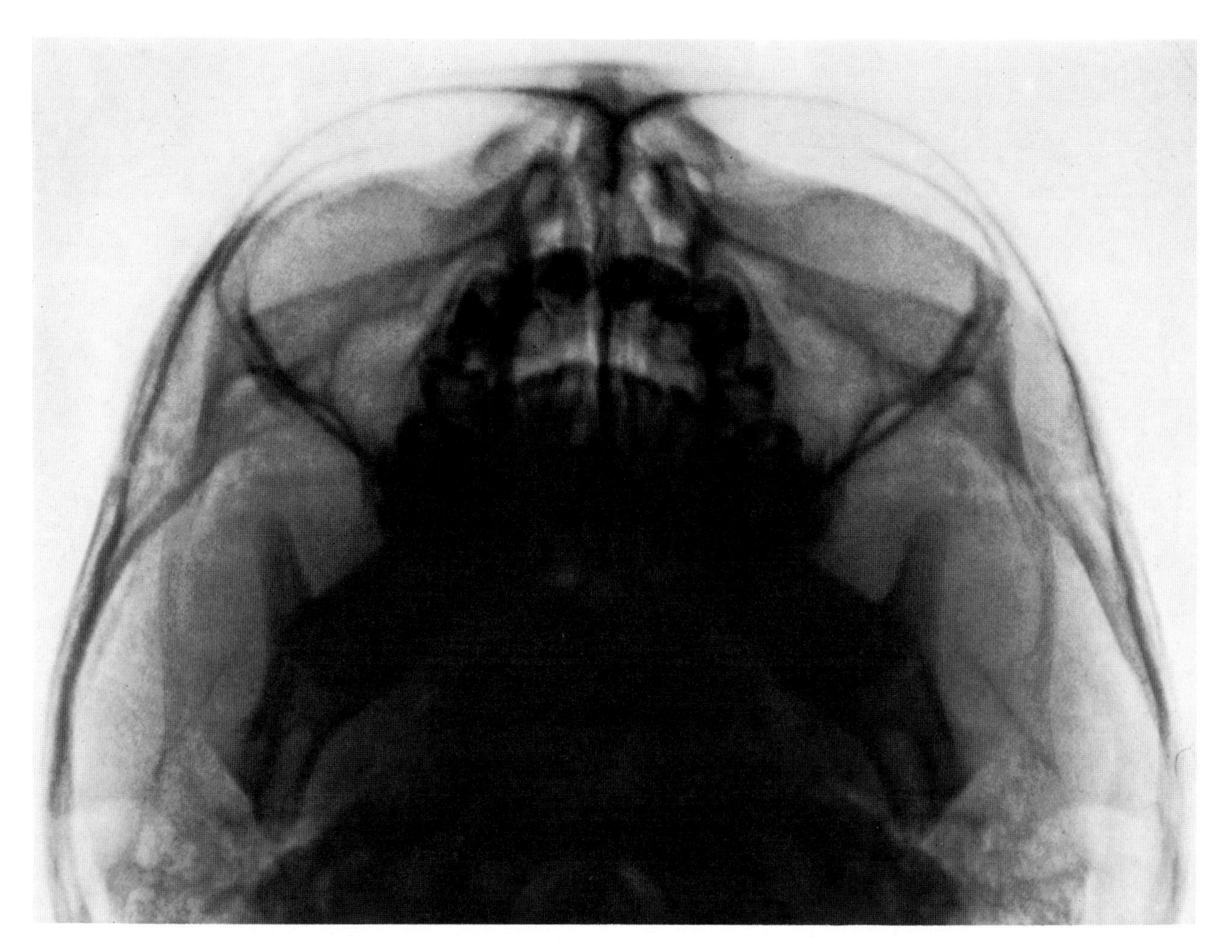

Fig. 97. Axial verticosubmental radiograph for comparison of both zygomatic arches *(Bronner* and *Koch)*. For projection, see Fig. 99.

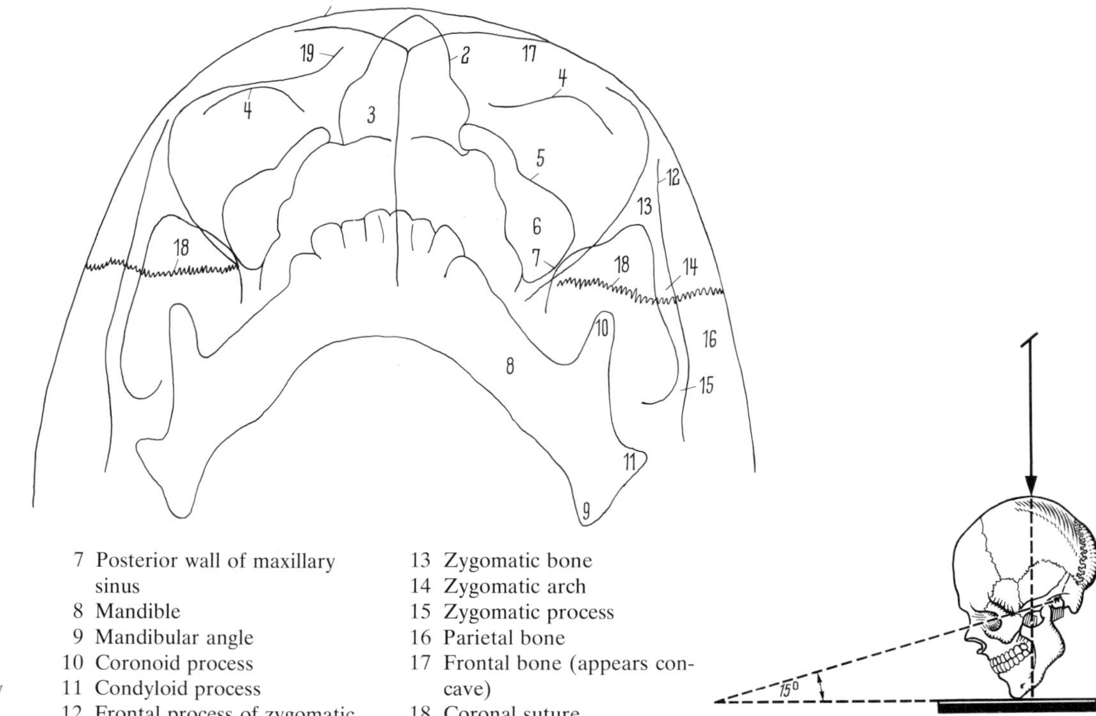

Fig. 98

1 Frontal bone
2 Lateral wall of nose
3 Nasal cavity
4 Shadow of soft tissues of eyeball
5 Anterior wall of maxillary sinus
6 Maxillary sinus
7 Posterior wall of maxillary sinus
8 Mandible
9 Mandibular angle
10 Coronoid process
11 Condyloid process
12 Frontal process of zygomatic bone
13 Zygomatic bone
14 Zygomatic arch
15 Zygomatic process
16 Parietal bone
17 Frontal bone (appears concave)
18 Coronal suture
19 Soft tissues of nose

Fig. 99

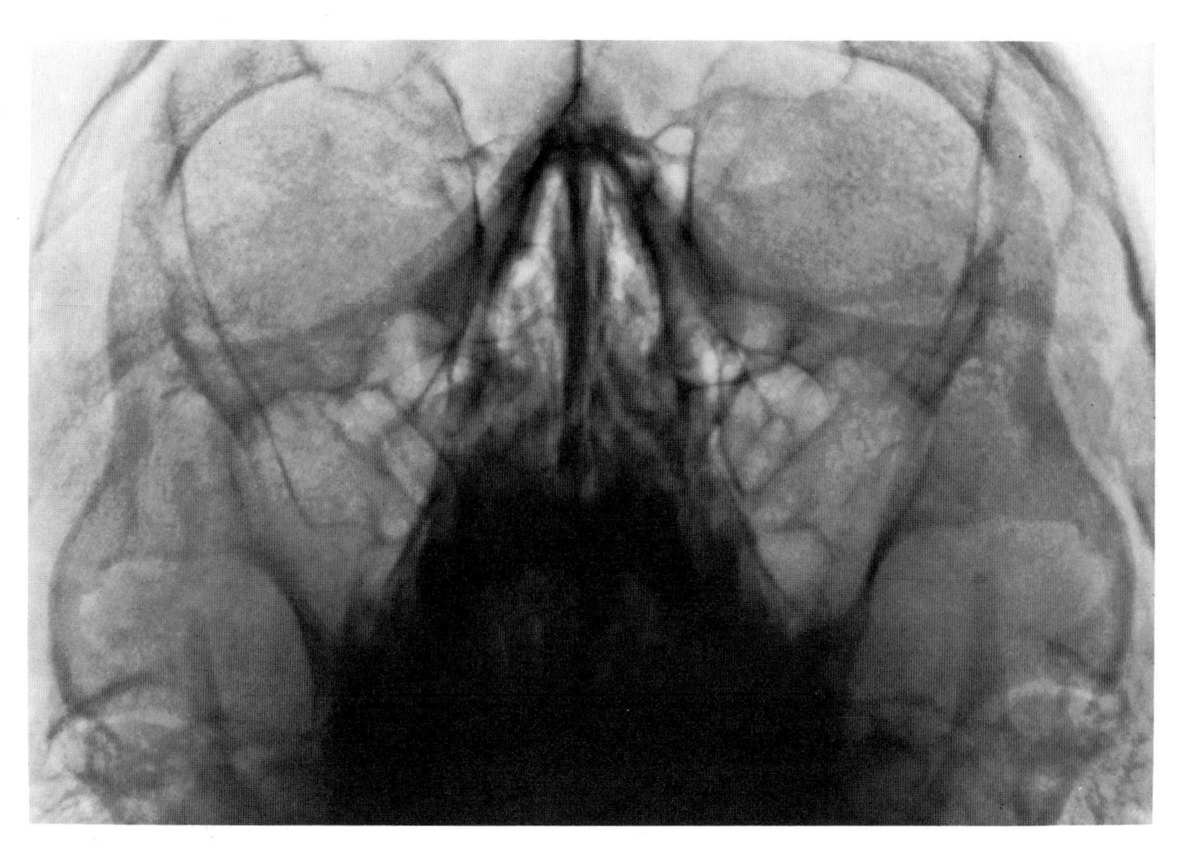

Fig. 100. Half-axial radiograph of both zygomatic arches. For projection, see Fig. 101. This radiograph is indispensable in cases of suspected fractures of facial bones. It allows the isolated presentation of maxilla, zygomatic bones and zygomatic arches.

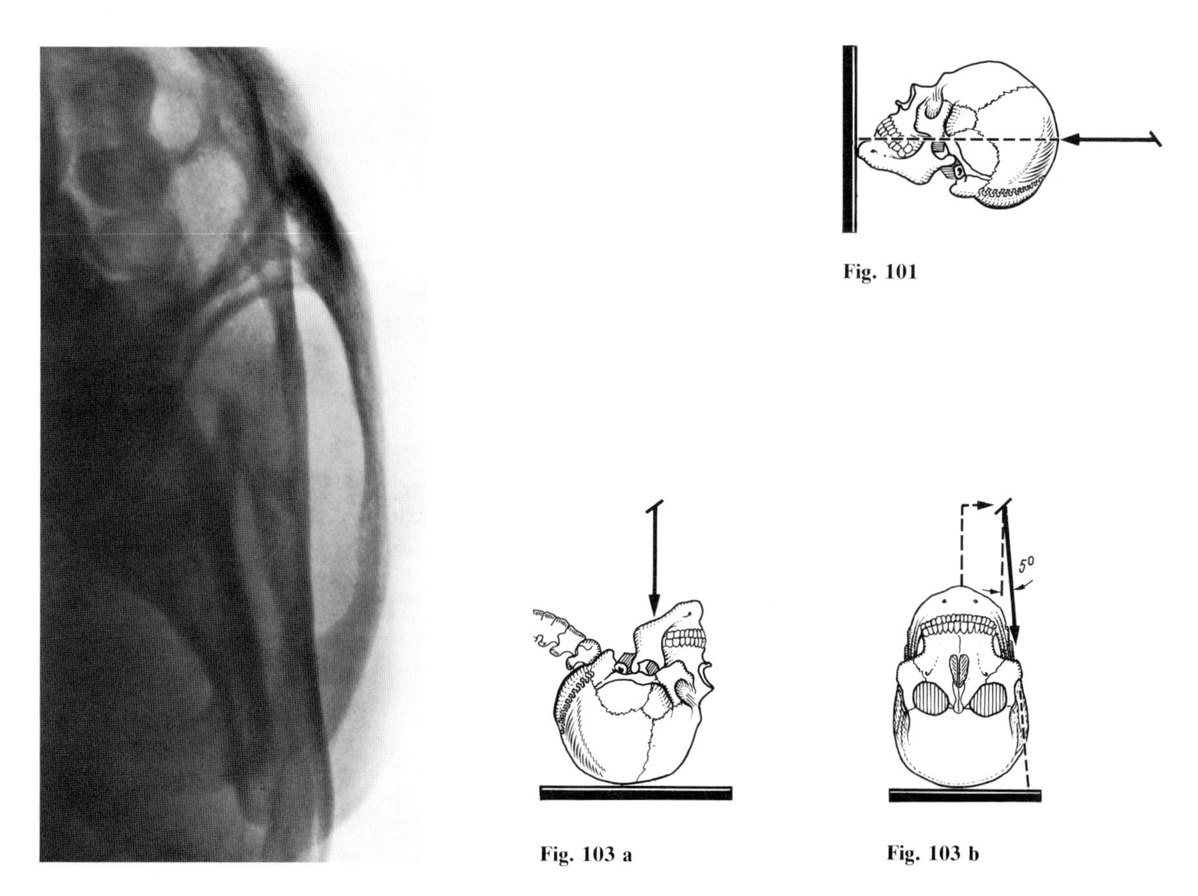

Fig. 102. Pot-handle radiograph of the zygomatic arch *(Bronner* and *Koch; Zimmer)*. For projection, see Fig. 103. By means of this radiograph, in cases of fractures of the zygomatic bones the degree of depression and the dislocation of the axes of the fragments are exceptionally well demonstrated.

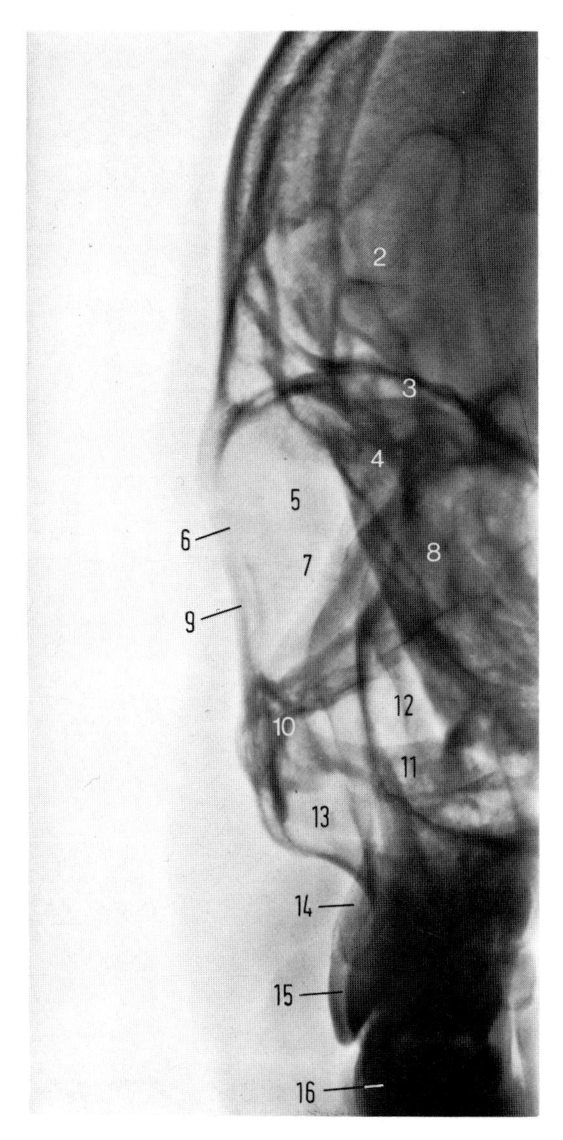

Fig. 104. Zygomatic bone, tangential, anterosinistrodextral *(Clementschitsch)*. For projection, see Fig. 106.

1 Frontal bone
2 Frontal sinus
3 Roof of orbita
4 Supraorbital margin, near nasal bone
5 Orbita of adjacent side
6 Frontozygomatic suture of adjacent side
7 Nasal bone (receding in this projection)
8 Anterior border of middle cranial fossa (adjacent)
9 Frontal process of zygomatic bone
10 Body of zygomatic bone (adjacent)
11 Zygomatic arch (adjacent)
12 Maxillary sinus (adjacent)
13 Body of maxilla
14 Alveolar process of maxilla
15 Maxillary teeth (of upper jaw)
16 Mandibular teeth (of lower jaw)

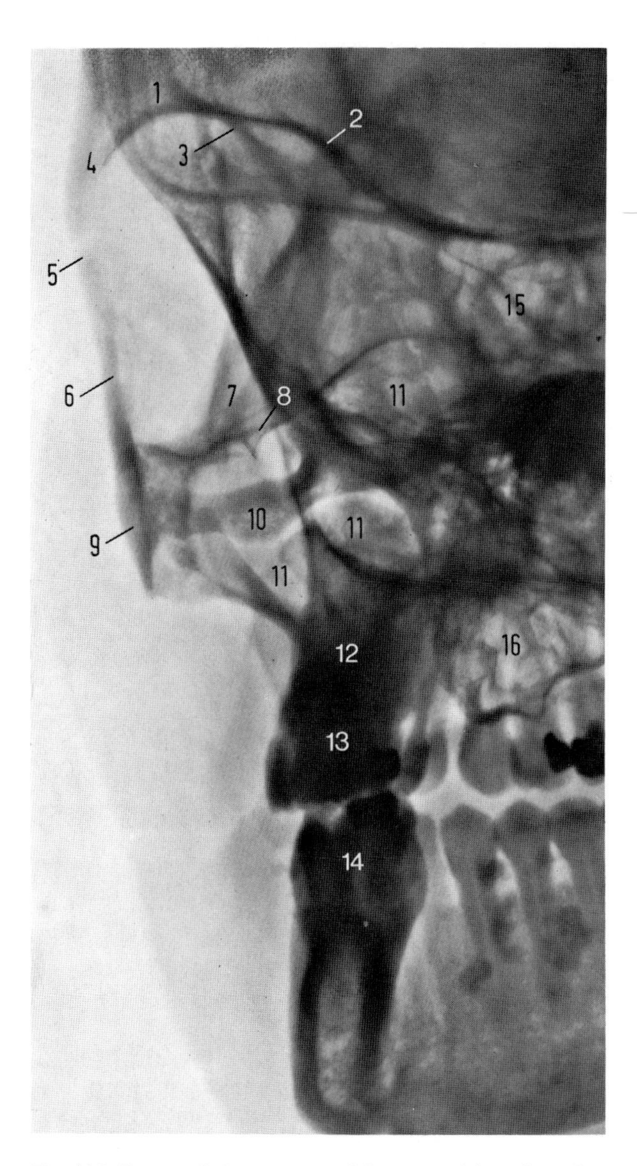

Fig. 105. Zygomatic bone, tangential, posterosinistrodextral *(Clementschitsch)*. For projection, see Fig. 107.

1 Frontal bone
2 Floor of anterior cranial fossa
3 Roof of orbita
4 Zygomatic process of frontal bone
5 Frontozygomatic suture
6 Frontal process of zygomatic bone
7 Nasal bone
8 Floor of orbita
9 Zygomatic bone
10 Zygomatic arch
11 Maxillary sinus
12 Alveolar process of maxilla
13 Maxillary teeth
14 Mandibular teeth
15 Ethmoidal cells
16 Mastoid cells

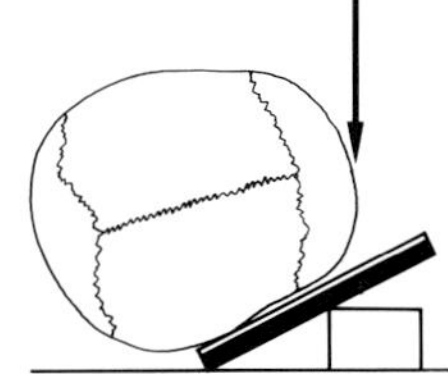

Fig. 106

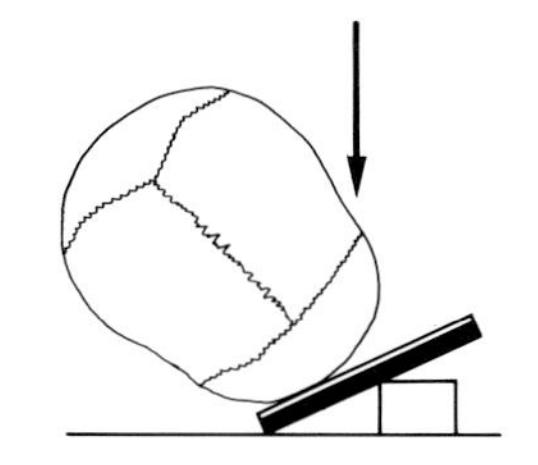

Fig. 107

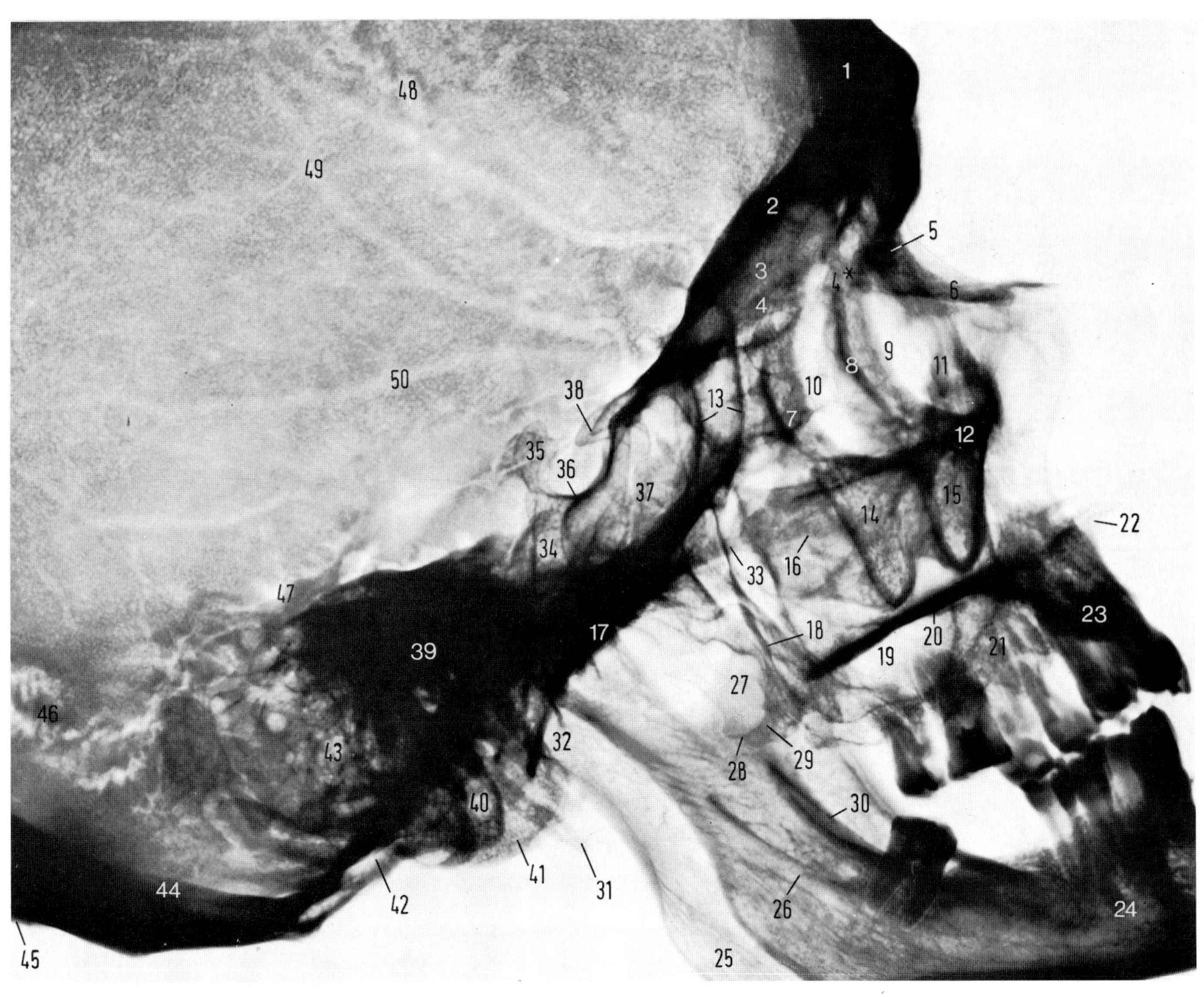

Fig. 108. Skull, macerated, bitemporal.

1 Frontal bone (frontal sinuses are not developed here)
2 Floor of anterior cranial fossa (here it also forms the orbital roof)
3 Cribriform plate
4 Zygomatic process, near to film
4* Away from film
5 Frontonasal suture
6 Nasal bones
7 Frontal process of zygomatic bone, close below the suture (adjacent)
8 Frontal process of zygomatic bone of the off-side
9 Orbita (adjacent)
10 Ethmoidal cells
11 Frontal process of maxilla
12 Infraorbital margin
13 Anterior end of middle cranial fossa
14 Zygomatic bone of adjacent side
15 Zygomatic bone of off-side
16 Lower edge of zygomatic arch adjacent to film
17 Articular tubercle of adjacent side
18 Posterior contour of maxillary body
19 Maxillary sinus
20 Palatine process of maxilla
21, 23 Alveloar process of maxilla
22 Anterior nasal spine
24 Body of mandible
25 Angle of mandible
26 Mandibular canal, terminating in the mental foramen, between the 4th and 5th teeth
27 Coronoid process of mandible (adjacent)
28 Pterygoid process
29 Pterygoid hamulus
30 Anterior edge of the adjacent ramus of the mandible; on its right, the edge of the ramus distant from film
31 Styloid process (adjacent)
32 Condyloid process of mandible (adjacent)
33 Pterygopalatine fossa (distant from film); on its left, the pterygopalatine fossa of the adjacent side
34 Clivus
35 Posterior clinoid process
36 Floor of sella turcica
37 Sphenoidal sinus
38 Anterior clinoid process
39 Petrous bone
40 Mastoid process
41 Occipital condyle
42 Foramen magnum
43 Cells of adjacent mastoid process
44 Squama of occipital bone (squama occipitalis)
45 External occipital protuberance
46 Lambdoid suture
47 Parietomastoid suture
48 Coronal suture
49 Sulcus for the anterior division of the middle meningeal artery; above and parallel to it, the corresponding sulcus of the opposite side
50 Sulcus for the posterior division of the middle meningeal artery *(Keller)*

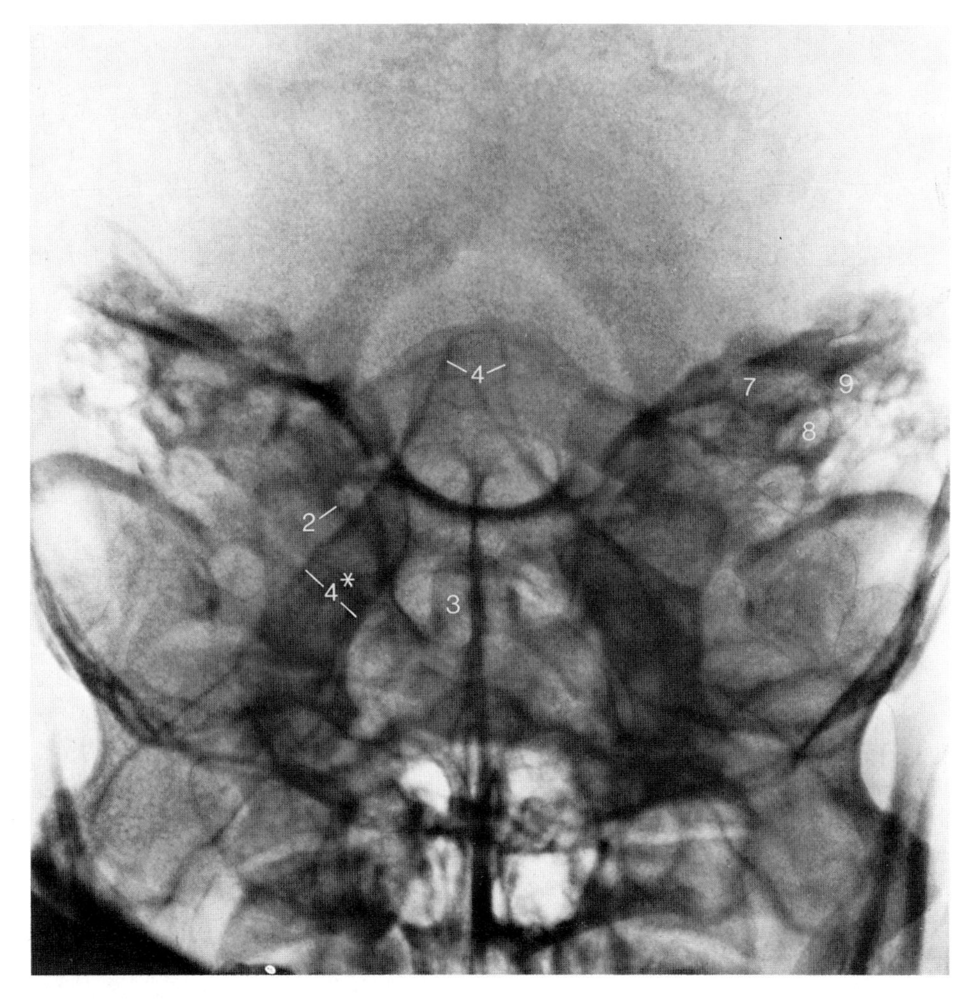

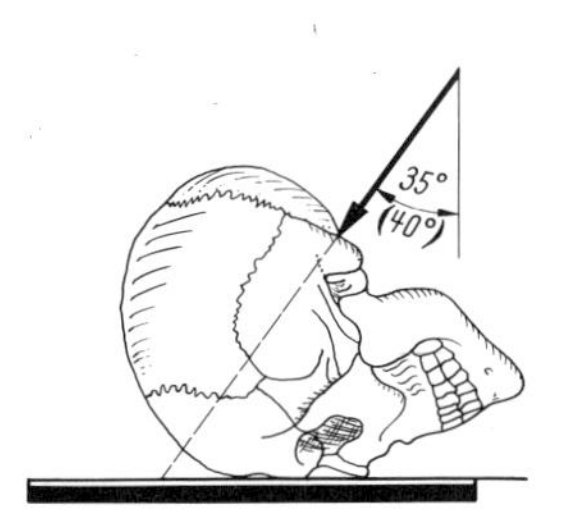

Fig. 109. Skull, nuchofrontal *(Haas)*. Both petrous bones are sagittal, with the patient prone. For projection, see Fig. 110. In this position, the posterior arch of the atlas is projected into the foramen magnum whose upper half can be visualized. The dorsum sellae itself is superimposed by the posterior arch of the atlas. In addition, one sees the squama of the occiput as well as both petrous bones in a suitable representation for comparison with one another. (See also the transcranial radiograph of the first cervical vertebra after *Kulka*.) Another good view of the arch of the atlas is provided in Fig. 117.

Fig. 110

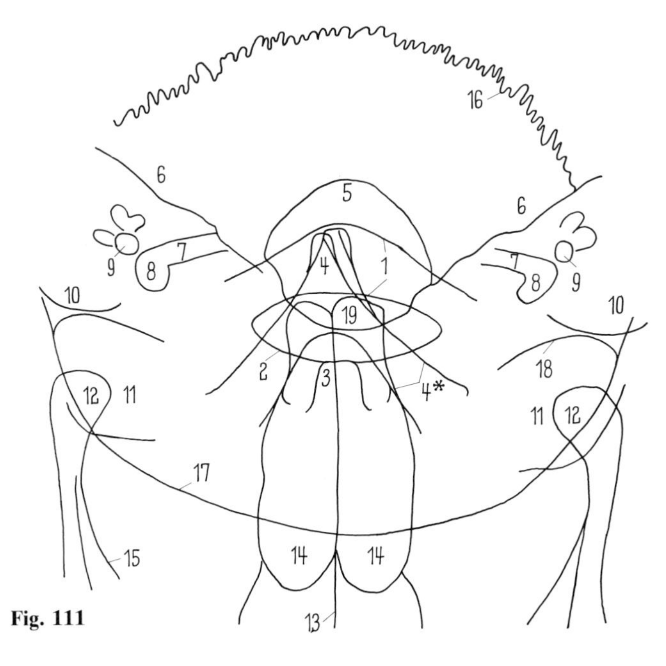

Fig. 111

To Figs. 109 and 111:

1 Posterior arch of atlas
2 Anterior arch of atlas
3 Dens (axis)
4 Spinous process of axis
4 Arch of axis (according to *Sobotta-Becher,* 16th ed.)
5 Foramen magnum
6 Petrous bone
7 Internal auditory meatus
8 Cochlea
9 Vestibule with semicircular canals
10 Mastoid cells
11 Mandibular fossa
12 Condyloid process
13 Bony nasal septum
14 Paranasal sinuses
15 Mandible
16 Lambdoid suture
17 Middle cranial fossa
18 Petrosphenoidal fissure
19 Sphenoidal sinus

To Figs. 112 and 113:

1 Foramen magnum
2 Dorsum sellae
3 Petrous bone
4 Internal auditory meatus
5 Cochlea
6 Vestibule with semicircular canals
7 Carotid canal
8 Mastoid process
9 Petrosphenoidal fissure
10 Posterior arch of atlas
11 Dens (axis)
12 Atlantooccipital articulation
13 Sphenoidal sinus
14 Nasal cavity
15 Maxillary sinus
16 Mandibular fossa
17 Zygomatic bone
18 Mandible
19 Calcified pineal body
20 Bony nasal septum
21 Middle cranial fossa
22 Orbita, posterior border

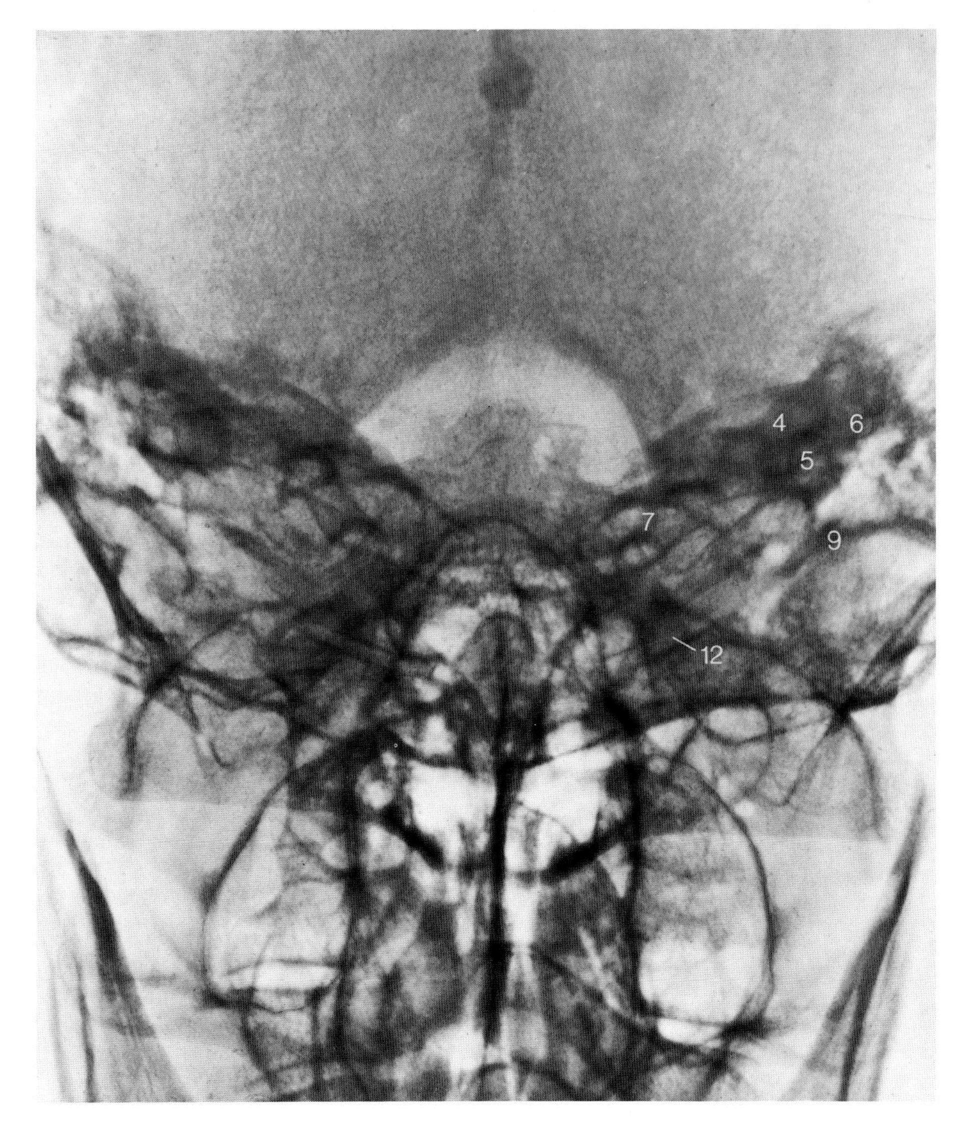

Fig. 112. Head, half-axial, nuchofrontal, after *Haas*. The projection corresponds essentially to the nuchofrontal radiograph of the skull (Fig. 108), but the central ray is directed only 30° cephalad and is aimed at the plane of the auditory canal. By projecting both petrous bones above the orbitae, one achieves an exact comparison between the apices of the petrous bones and between the internal auditory canals. At the same time, the dorsum sellae is projected into the foramen magnum, free from the arch of the atlas, which is diverted somewhat lower down through the lesser incline of the central beam.

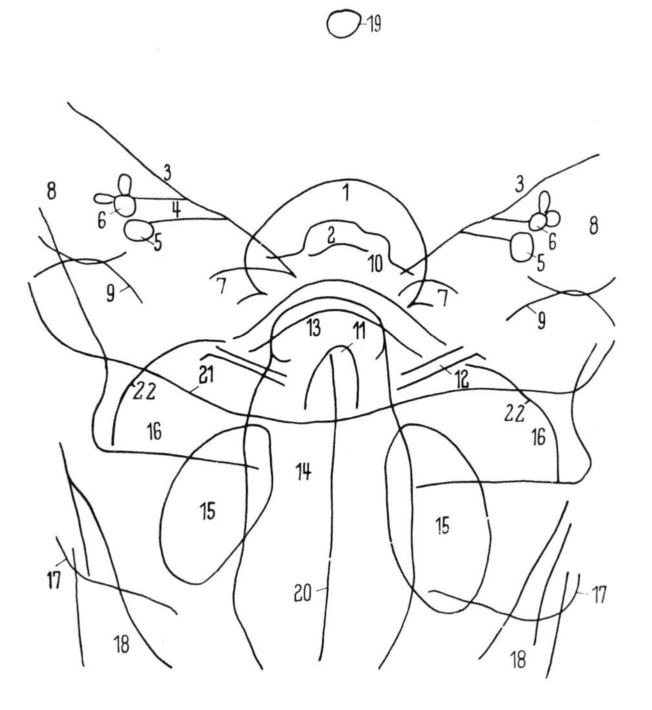

Fig. 113

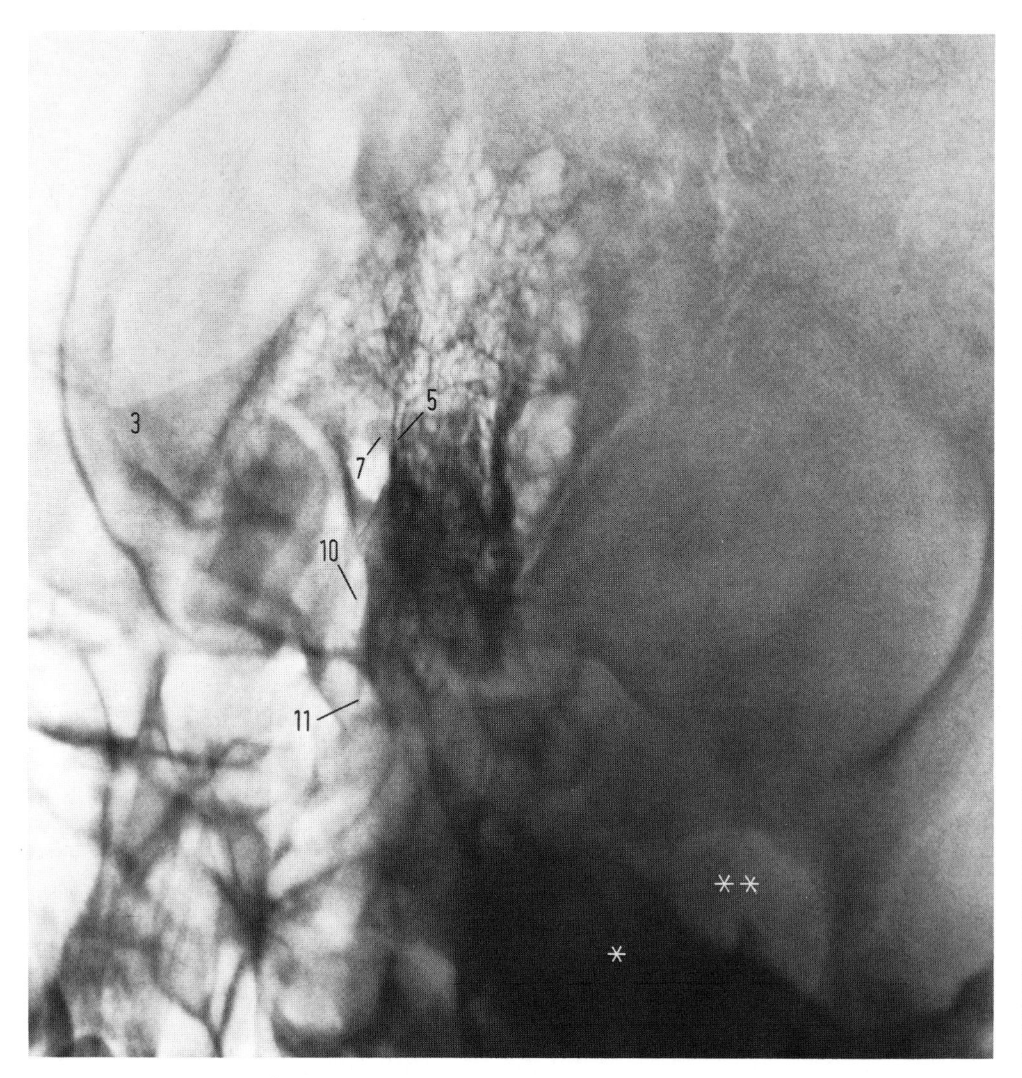

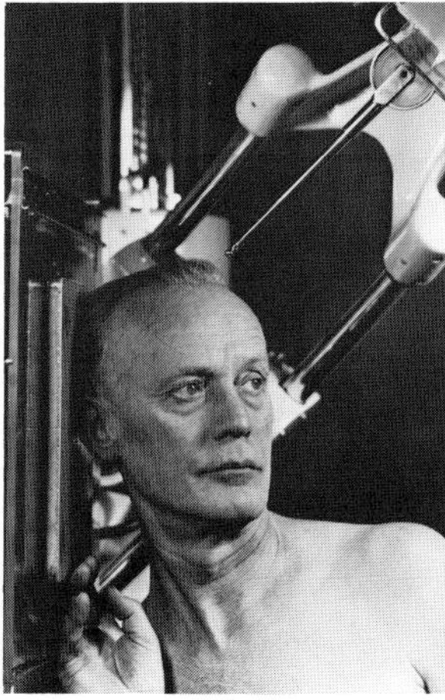

Fig. 114. Right temporal bone, axial (after *E. G. Mayer*). Central ray 45° craniocaudal, with 45° rotation of the head (see Fig. 115). By means of this technique, the petrous bone is seen at an angle of 45°. This radiograph is valuable in the search for fracture lines, defects in the wall of the tympanic antrum (cholesteatoma), as well as in distension of the antrum and the tympanic sulcus.

Fig. 115

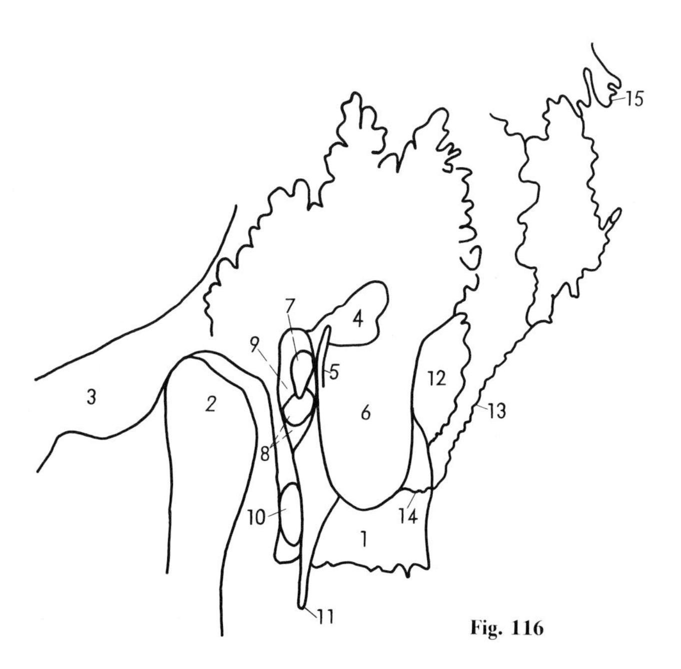

Fig. 116

To Figs. 114 and 116:

1 Petrous bone
* in X-ray, petrous bone distant from film (Fig. 114)
2 Condyloid process of mandible
3 Zygomatic arch
4 Mastoid antrum with tympanic sulcus
5 Facial canal
6 Mastoid process
7 Malleus
8 External auditory meatus
9 Tympanic cavity
10 Carotid canal
11 Styloid process
12 Incisura mastoidea
13 Parietomastoid suture
14 Occipitomastoid suture
15 Lambdoid suture
** Foramen magnum (Fig. 114)

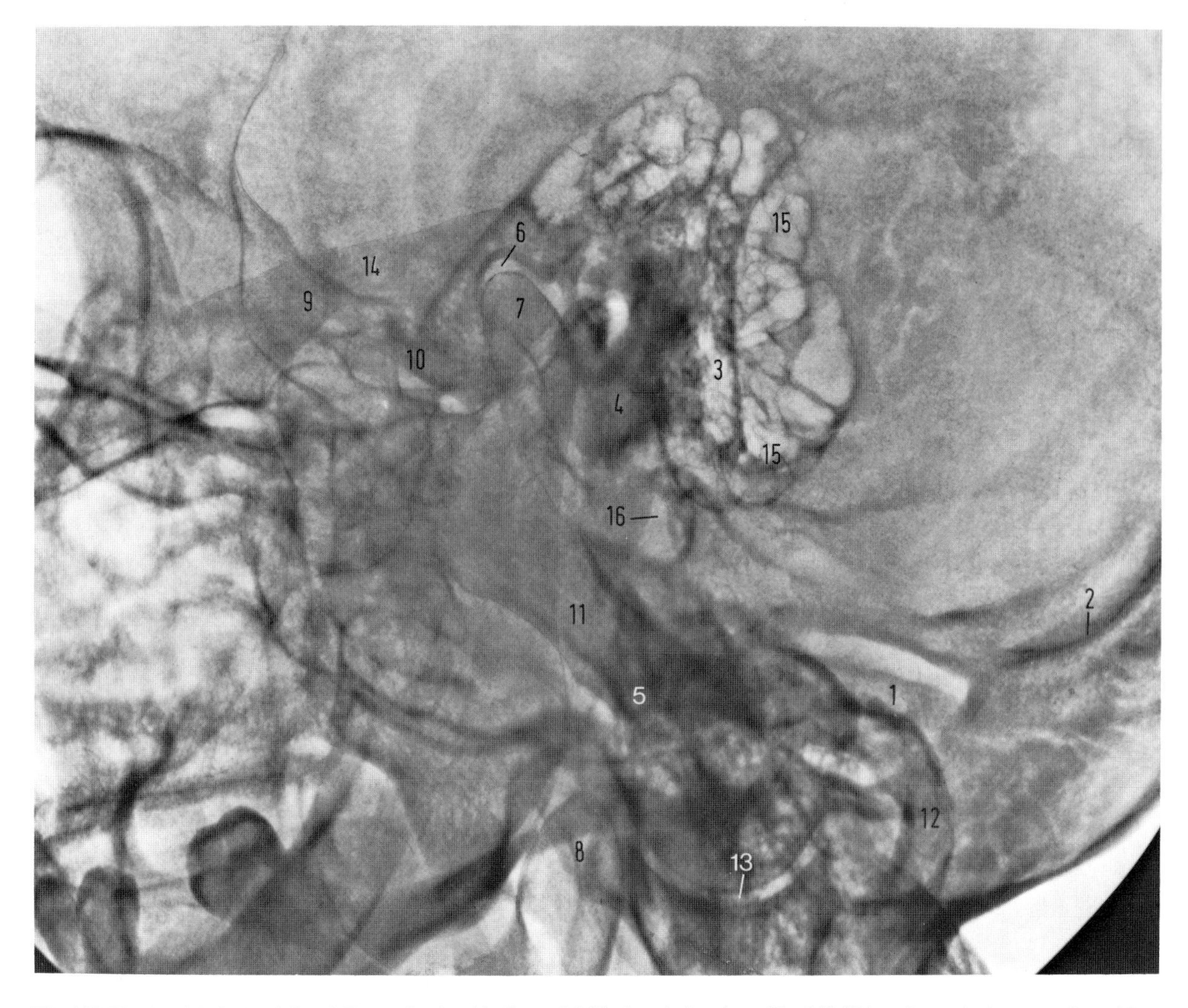

Fig. 117. Head, axial, dextrosinistral. For projection (similar to *Schüller's* technique), see Fig. 118. This radiograph gives, together with a survey of the inclined base of skull, an inclined projection of the posterior arch of the atlas (see also Fig. 109), which is partly projected into the foramen magnum. Fig. 119 demonstrates the anatomical relations by showing the inside of a skull in the direction of the central ray.

1 Foramen magnum
2 Occipital bone with internal occipital crest
3 Mastoid cells
4 Petrous bone of the adjacent side
5 Petrous bone of the off-side
6 Articular cavity of mandibular joint
7 Condyloid process of adjacent side
8 Condyloid process of off-side
9 Lesser wing of sphenoid bone
10 Sella turcica
11 Clivus
12 Posterior arch
13 Atlantooccipital articulation (distant from film)
14 Zygomatic arch (next to film)
15 Sulcus of sigmoid sinus (next to film in the upper part)
16 Jugular foramen (next to film)

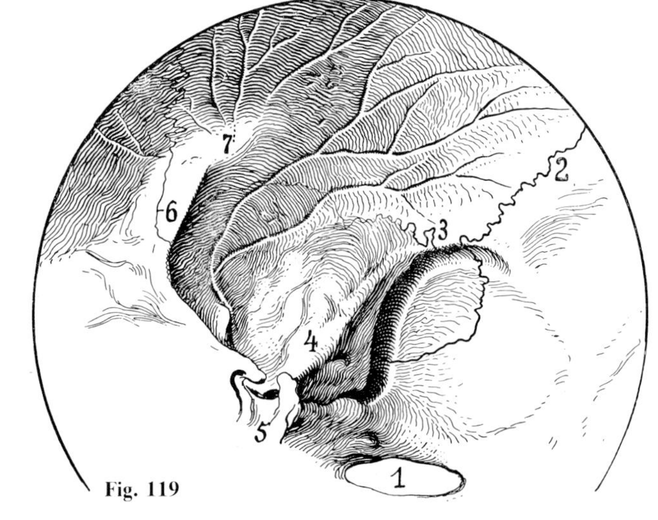

Fig. 119

1 Foramen magnum
2 Lambdoid suture
3 Parietomastoid suture; below: sulcus for the sigmoid sinus
4 Petrous bone
5 Sella turcica
6 Coronal suture
7 Lesser wing (of sphenoid bone)

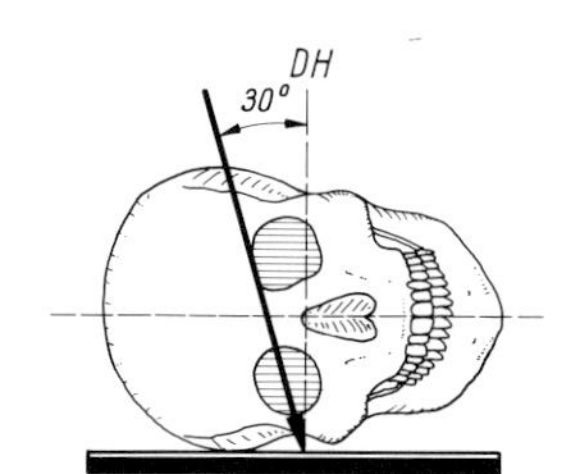

Fig. 118

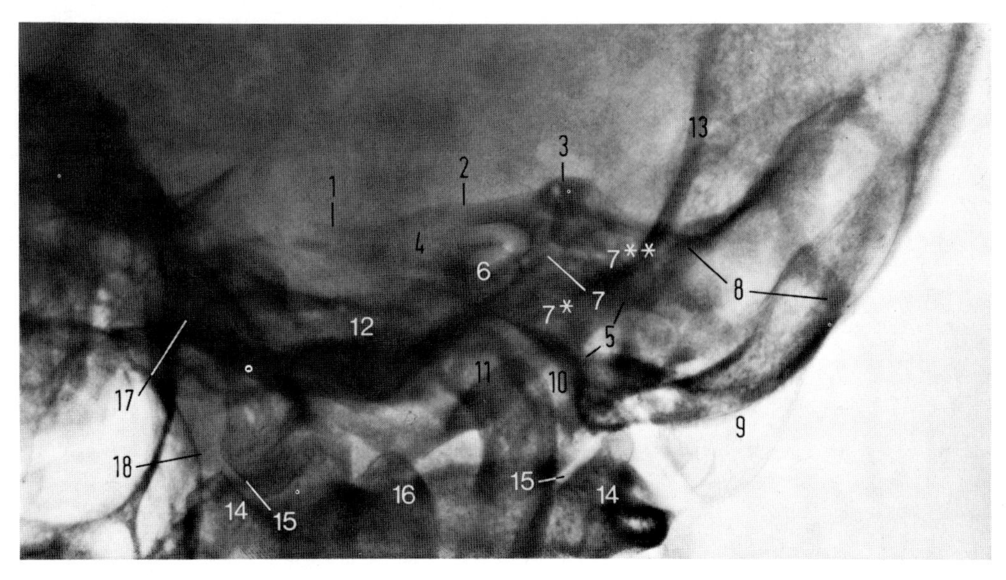

1 Apex of petrous bone
2 Upper rim of petrous bone
3 Eminentia arcuata
4 Internal auditory meatus
5 External auditory meatus
6 Cochlea
7 Vestibule with semicircular canals
7* Tympanic cavity
7** Mastoid antrum
8 Floor of posterior cranial fossa
9 Mastoid process
10 Mandibular joint
11 Condyloid process
12 Floor of middle cranial fossa
13 Occipital crest (possibly external and internal)
14 Atlas
15 Atlantooccipital joint
16 Dens (axis)
17 Orbita, lateral margin
18 Posterior margin of maxillary sinus

Fig. 120. Radiograph of petrous bone, according to *Stenvers*. For projection, see Fig. 121. With this radiograph, the petrous bone lies approximately parallel to the film. Therefore, it can be viewed well from its apex to the mastoid process. The purpose of this radiograph is to show the inner ear. The occipital crest passes laterally to the horizontal semicircular canal. The middle cranial fossa intersects the antrum.

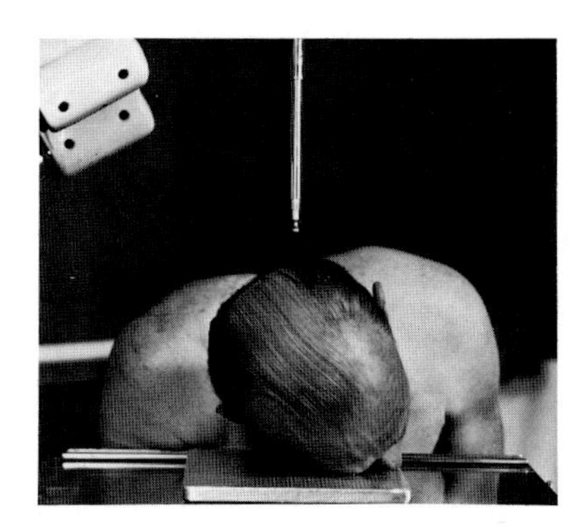

Fig. 121. Patient prone. Arms along the sides of the body, chin flexed, forehead and nose on the cassette. Rotation of the head towards the side to be examined, to make the sagittal plane form an angle of 45° with the cassette. The central ray, which is inclined 12° cephalad, meets it two fingers' breadth nasally from the occipital protuberance and is directed onto the cassette.

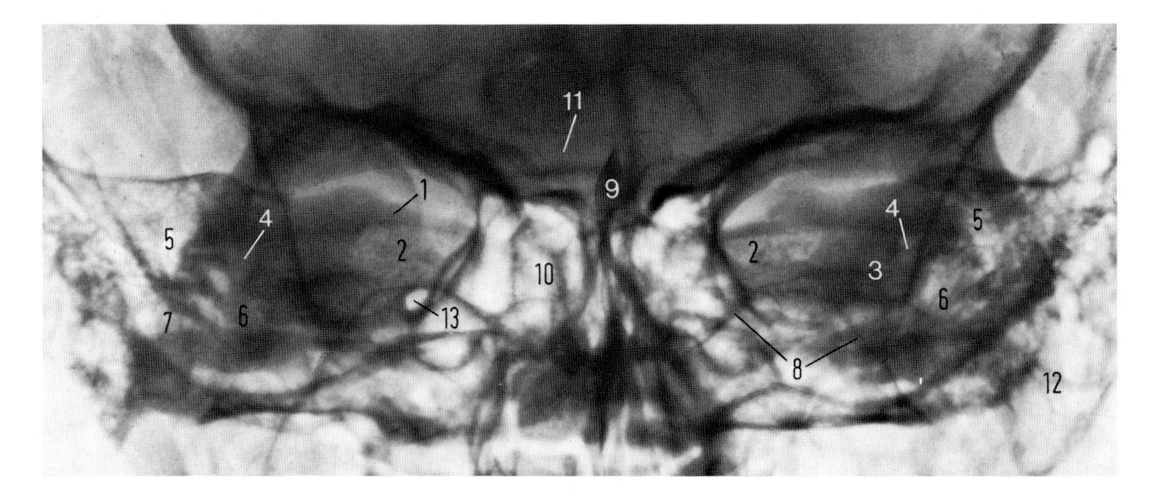

Fig. 122. Comparative orbital radiograph of the petrous bone. The projection corresponds to the occipitofrontal one of Fig. 43. With this radiograph, the auditory canals are well delineated and, therefore, an exact comparison can be made.

1 Upper edge of the petrous bone
2 Internal auditory meatus
3 Cochlea
4 Vestibule with semicircular canals
5 Antrum
6 Tympanic cavity
7 External auditory meatus
8 Posterior wall of maxillary sinus
9 Crista galli
10 Ethmoidal cells
11 Dorsum sellae
12 Mastoid process
13 Foramen rotundum

Figs. 123 and 124. Radiograph of petrous bone, after *Chaussé III.* It corresponds to the radiograph after *Stenvers,* only the central ray passes in the reverse direction. For projection, see Figs. 125 and 126. With this radiograph, one recognizes especially clearly the cochlea, vestibule and the three semicircular canals, as well as the extensive pneumatization of the petrous bone *(Lettenbauer).* Lateral to the horizontal semicircular canal the antrum is well displayed, which makes this radiograph especially suitable for diagnosis of the antrum and labyrinth. Here, the occipital crest passes medially to the semicircular canals, in contrast to the radiograph based on *Stenvers* (Fig. 120).

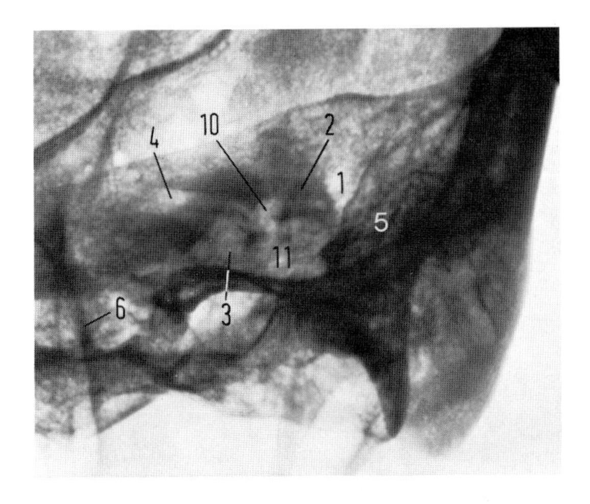

Fig. 123. Radiograph of macerated skull.
The petrous apex is superimposed by the upper outer angle of the orbita *(Reinike* and *Sprenger).*

1 Antrum
2 Crus commune
3 Cochlea
4 Internal auditory meatus
5 Floor of middle cranial fossa
6 Lateral margin of orbita
7 Condyloid process
8 Coronoid process
9 Internal occipital protuberance
10 Vestibule with semicircular canals
11 Tympanic cavity

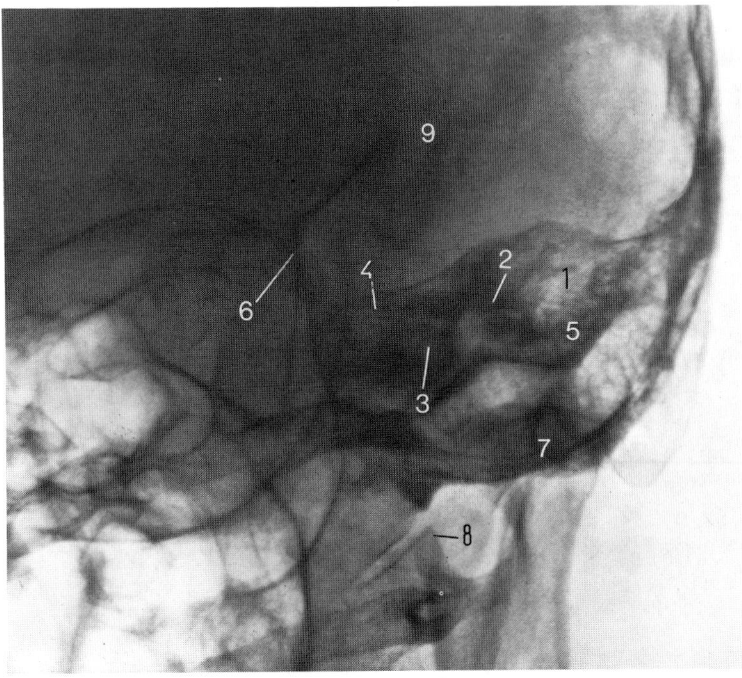

Fig. 124. Radiograph taken on patient.

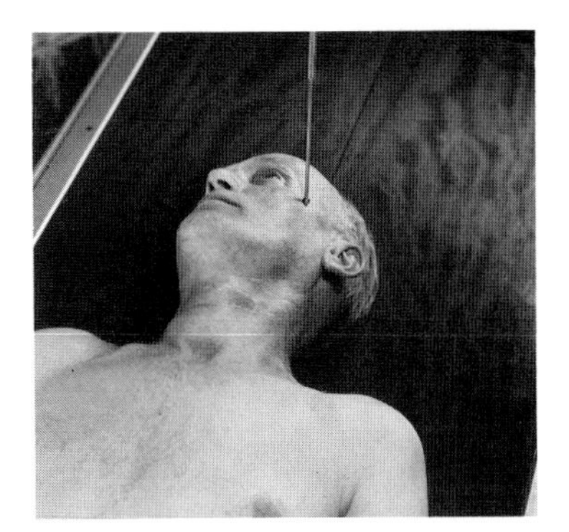

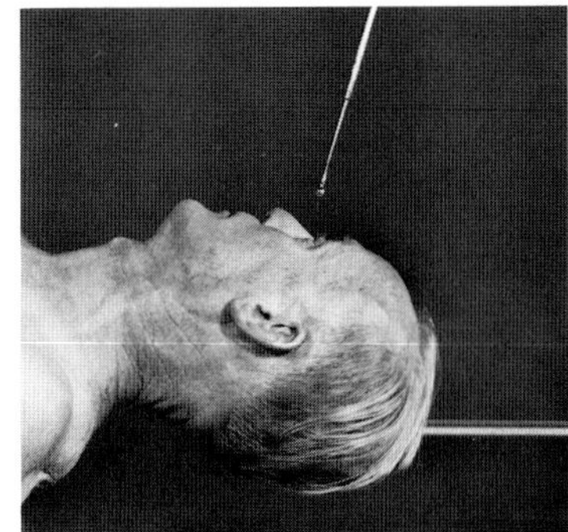

Fig. 125 **Fig. 126**

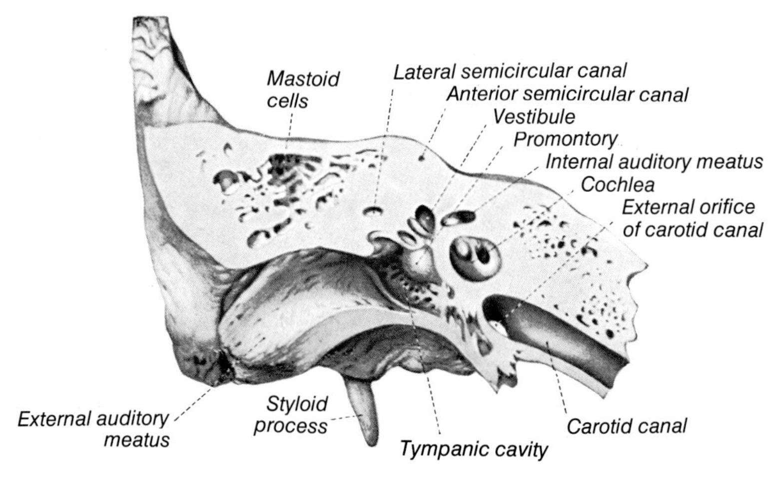

Fig. 127. Right temporal bone. The petrous part has been sawed through, parallel to its axis (from *Sobotta-Becher,* 15th ed.).

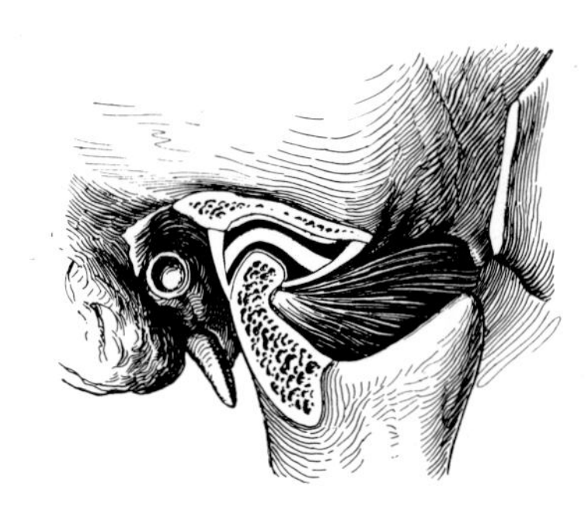

Fig. 128. Right mandibular joint, opened by sawing section. The zygomatic bone has been sawed frontally (from *Sobotta-Becher,* 15th ed.).

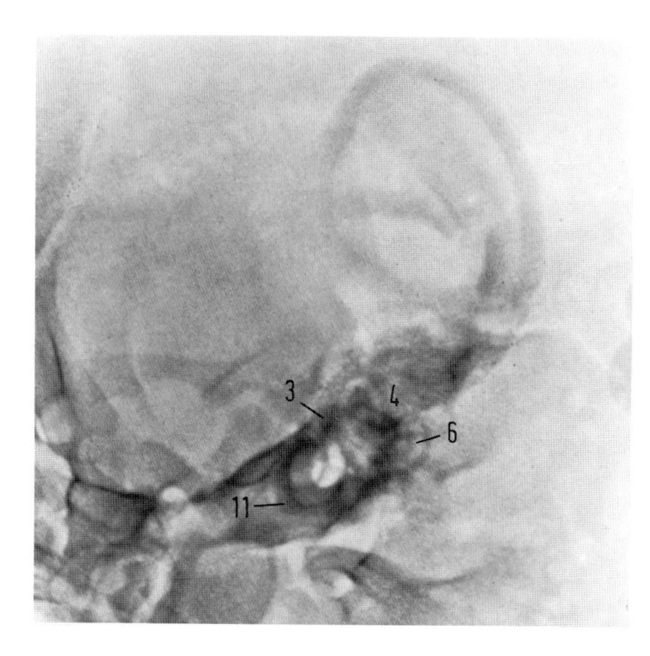

Fig. 129. **Petrous bone of an infant** (after *Rossmann*). For projection, see p. 376.

1 Carotid canal of petrous apex
2 Epitympanic recess, within the apex
3 Head of malleus and incus, projected onto one another
4 Antrum
5 Superior semicircular canal
6 Posterior semicircular canal
7 Lateral semicircular canal
8 Vestibule
9 Internal auditory canal
10 Cochlea
11 Part of the tympanic ring which later in life, shaped as a dark ring, will surround vestibule, internal auditory canal and cochlea
12 System of cells
13 Condyloid process
14 Zygomatic arch

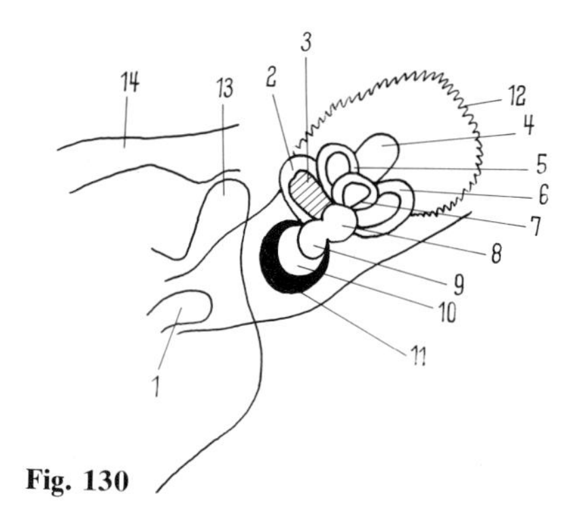

Fig. 130

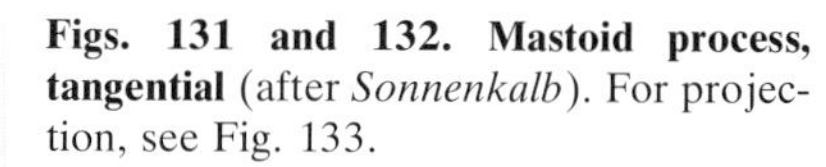
Figs. 131 and 132. Mastoid process, tangential (after *Sonnenkalb*). For projection, see Fig. 133.

Fig. 131. Good pneumatization.

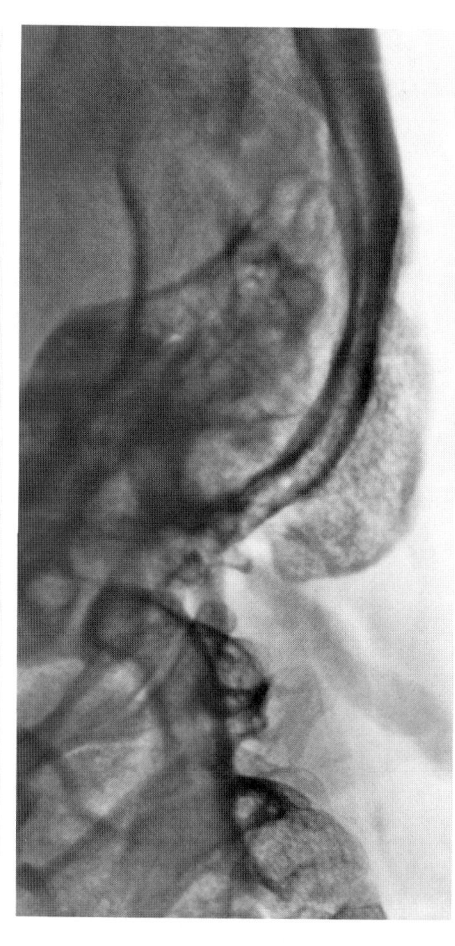

Fig. 132. Deficient pneumatization.

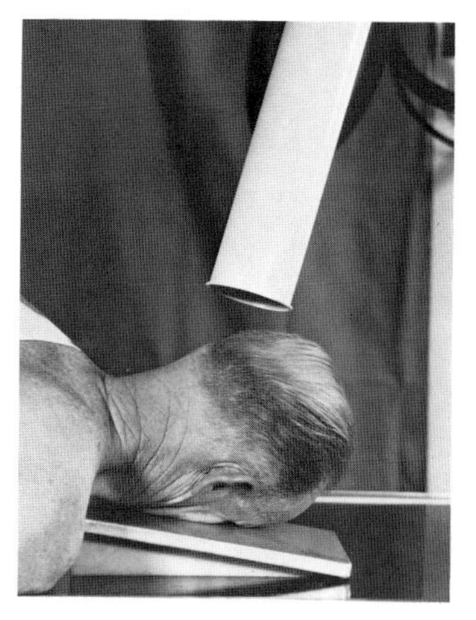

Fig. 133. Head, hanging down and forward and rotated towards the healthy side by about 45°. The central ray forms an angle of 20° with the German horizontal, open posteriorly, and with the median plane it forms an angle of 35°. The beam is aimed at the apex of the affected mastoid process, adjacent to the film.

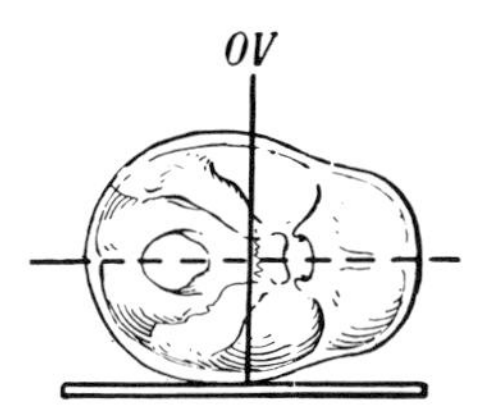

Figs. 135 and 136. Radiograph of mastoid process, according to *Schüller*. The radiograph can be taken with the mouth open or closed. If the mouth is open, the petrous apex (shown in an inclined profile) will be projected into the region of the mandibular fossa; with the mouth closed, it will be covered by the condyloid process. The radiographs are very suitable for demonstration of the mandibular joint. Fig. 134 shows the direction of the central ray in relation to the German horizontal plane (DH). This lies vertically to the median sagittal plane of the skull and connects the inferior orbital margins with the upper margins of the external auditory meatus. OV indicates the vertical plane of the ears, running at right angles to both auditory tubes.

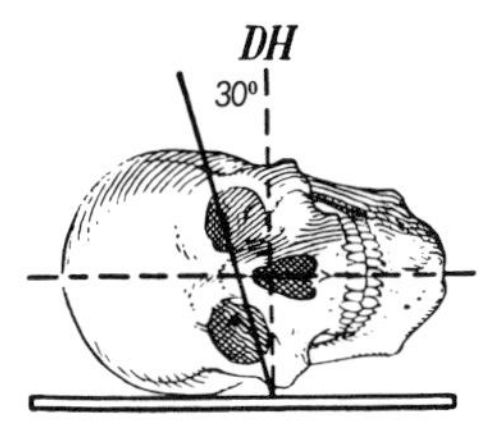

Fig. 134
(based on *E. G. Mayer*)

1 Condyloid process
2 Interstice of the mandibular joint
3 Articular tubercle
4 Sphenoidal sinuses
5 Internal auditory meatus
6 Center of labyrinth
7 Posterior contour of petrous bone
8 Posterior and inferior borders of the pneumatic system
9 Apex of mastoid process
10 Bony ledge, surrounding the foramen magnum
11 Shadow of the forward-folded pinna

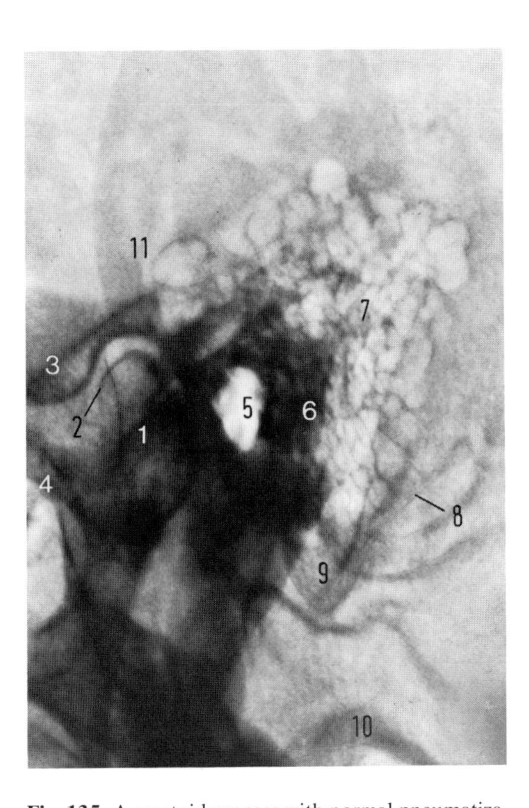

Fig. 135. A mastoid process with normal pneumatization (with mouth closed).

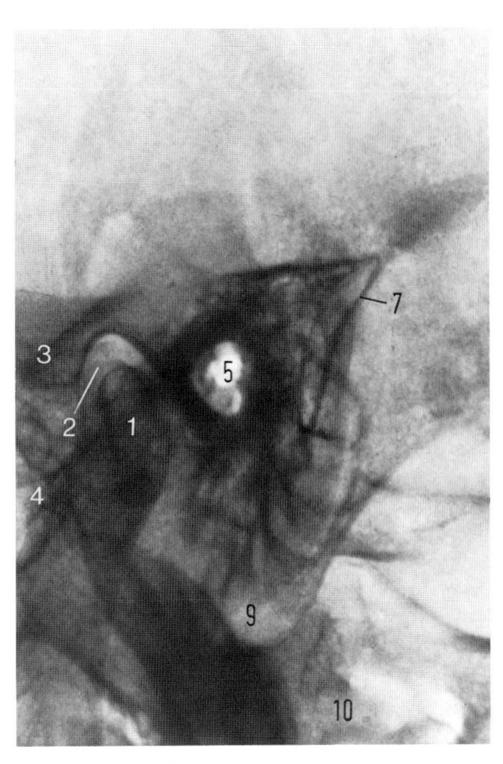

Fig. 136. A mastoid process with only slight pneumatization (with mouth open).

Fig. 139. Projection of the condyloid process into the orbita by means of the orbitoramus technique *(Grant* and *Lanting)*. The radiograph provides a clear survey of the articular tubercle and the condyloid process; laterally, the mandibular joint is enclosed by the zygomatic arch and the zygomatic bone. With this projection, the condyloid process is shown almost without foreshortening. For projection and direction of the central ray, see Figs. 137 and 138.

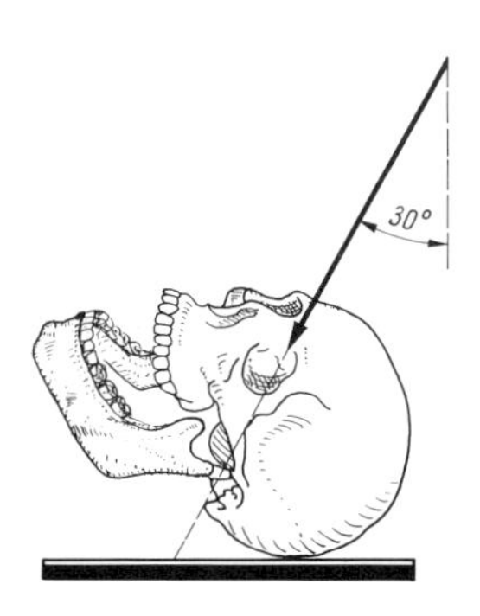

Fig. 137

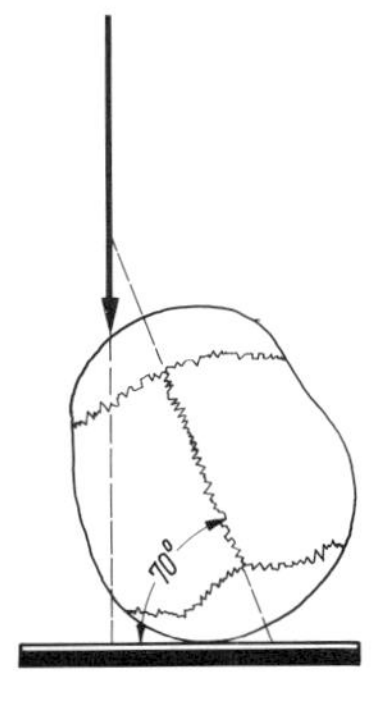

Fig. 138

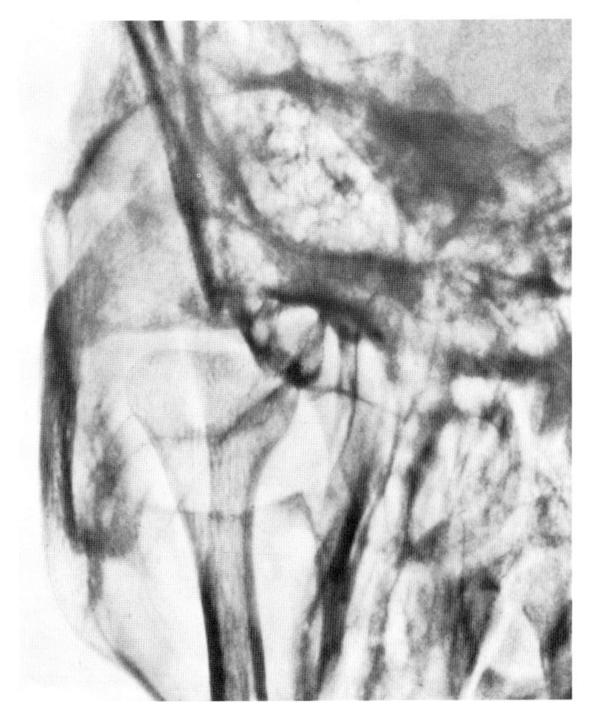

Fig. 139

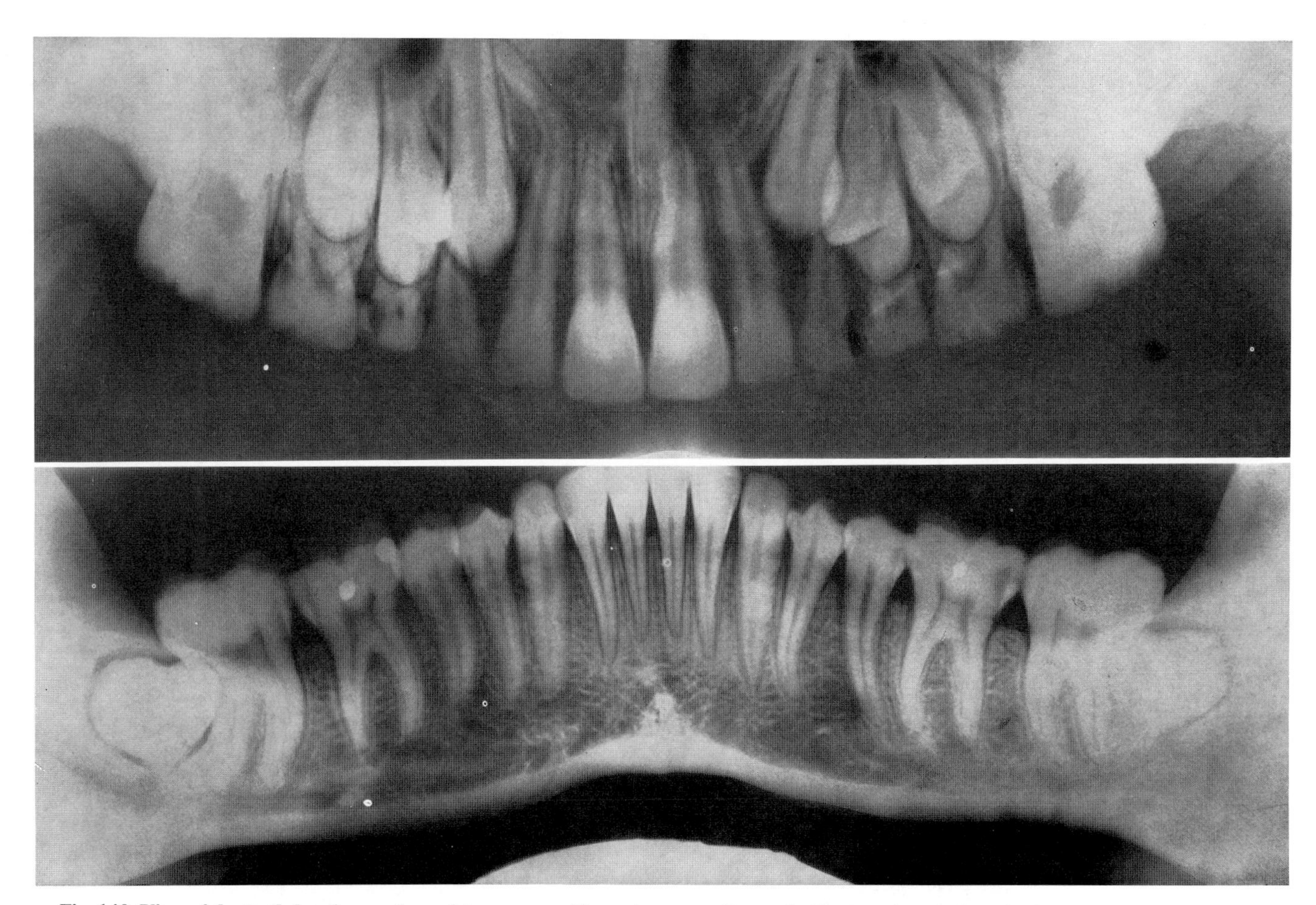

Fig. 140. View of the teeth-bearing portions of the upper and lower jaw, according to the Panoramix technique *(Lohmann, Ott)*. In contrast to the previous method of radiographs of teeth, here the cone of the X-rays is beamed from the oral cavity outwards, so that the whole set of teeth can be projected onto one film (size 10/24).

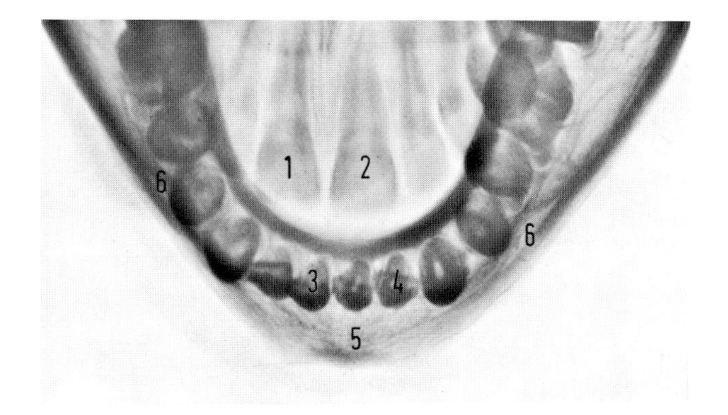

Fig. 141. Mandible, craniocaudal. For projection, see Fig. 143.

1, 2 Incisor teeth of maxilla
3, 4 Incisor teeth of mandible
5 Mental protuberance
6 Mental foramen

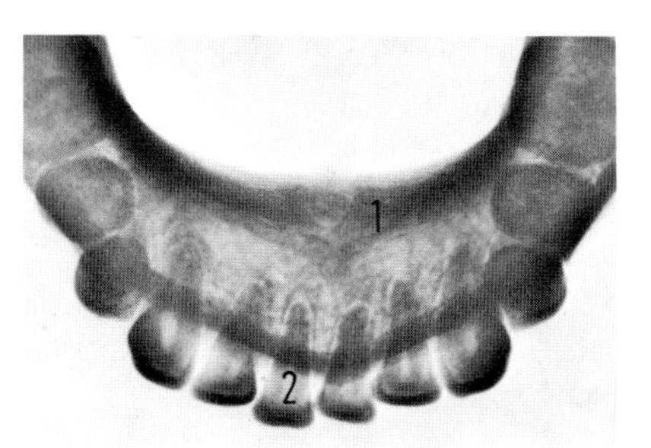

Fig. 142. Axial intrabuccal radiograph of the mandible on dental film inserted into the mouth. For projection, see Fig. 144.

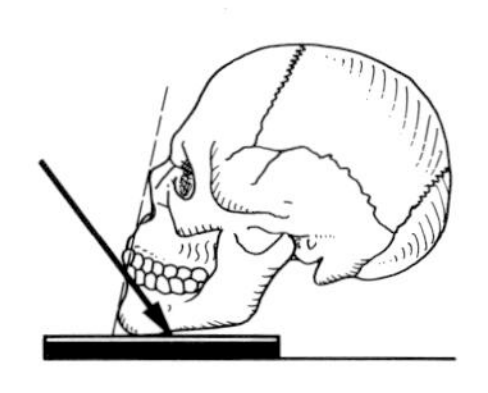

Fig. 143

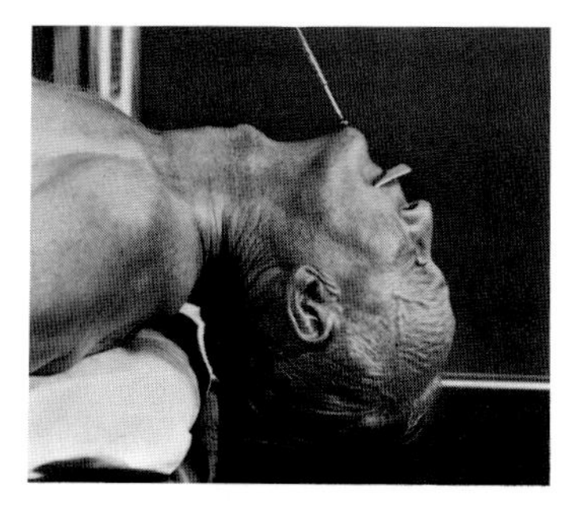

Fig. 144

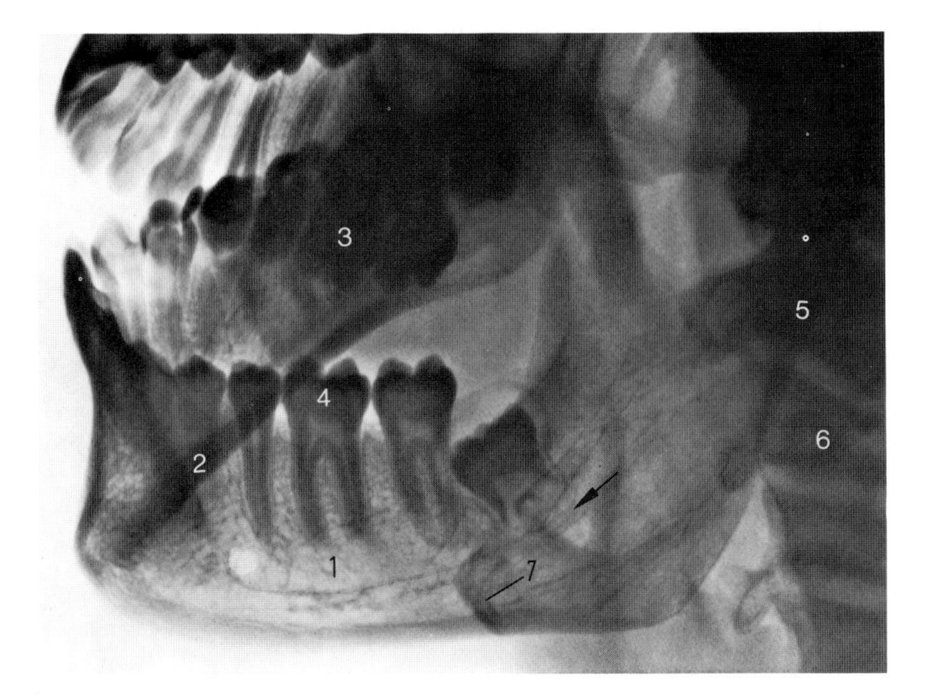

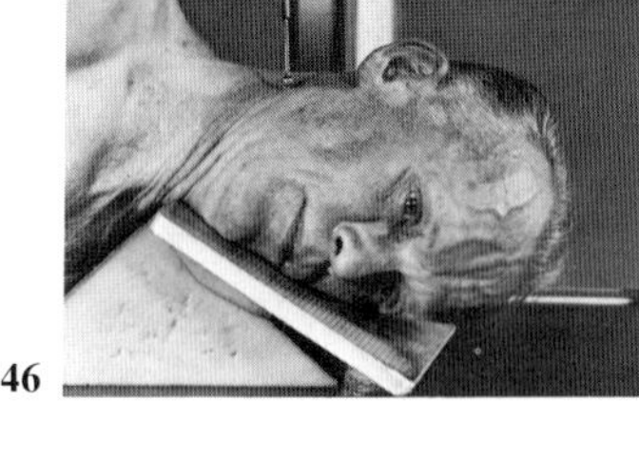

Fig. 146

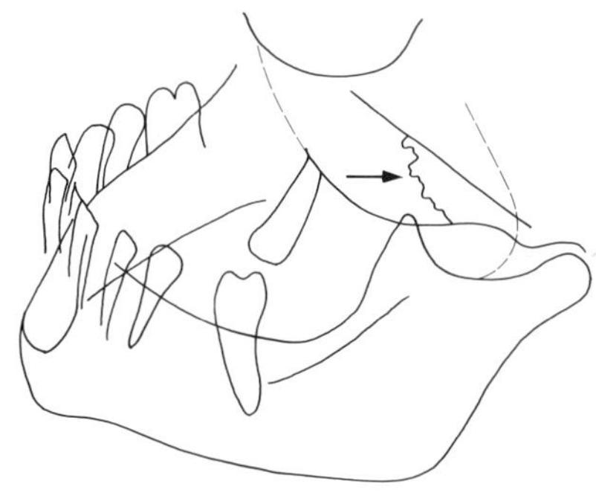

Fig. 145. "Double-axial" radiograph of mandible. Focus onto the adjacent mandibular ramus. (see Fig. 146).

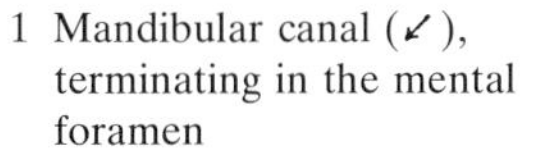

1 Mandibular canal (↙), terminating in the mental foramen
2 Mandibular body, seen from the edge
3 Upper first molar (of adjacent side)
4 Lower first molar (of adjacent side)
5 Axis
6 Body of 3rd cervical vertebra
7 Hyoid bone

Fig. 147. Shows the temporozygomatic suture (→) which can be seen only occasionally by means of clear double-axial radiographs of the mandible (female, 44 years of age).

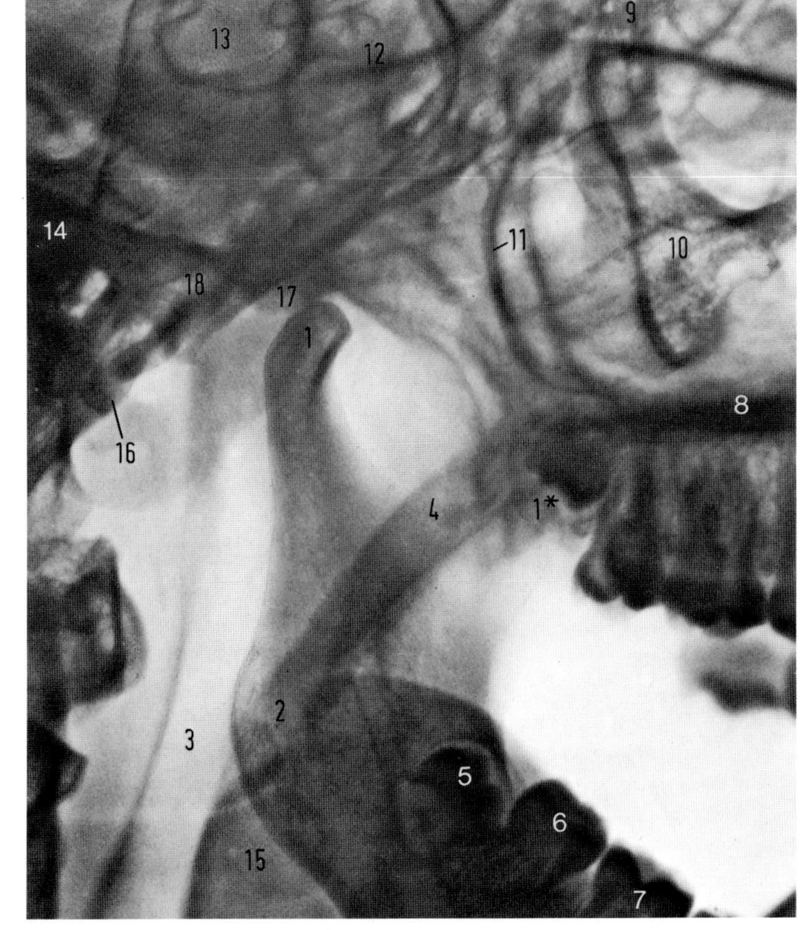

1 Condyloid process
1* Coronoid process of mandible
2 Mandibular angle
3 Weak, non-interfering shadow of the portion of the mandible away from the film
4 Soft palate
5, 6, 7 Three lower molar teeth of the adjacent side
8 Hard palate
9 Outer orbital margin
10 Zygomatic process, in cross section
11 Posterior wall of maxillary sinus
12 Sphenoidal sinuses
13 Sella
14 Petrous bone
15 Base of tongue
16 Styloid process of adjacent side
17 Articular tubercle
18 Mandibular fossa

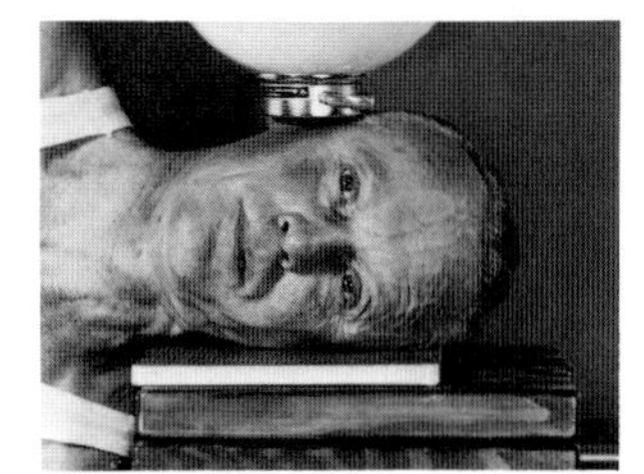

Fig. 149

Fig. 148. Mandibular joint, lateral, short-distance radiograph after *Parma* (relatively intense radiation of the skin). For projection, see Fig. 149. With this technique, only the joint adjacent to the cassette is shown; the one near the focus becomes extremely distorted and "dissolved." See *Zimmer* and *Weingraber.*

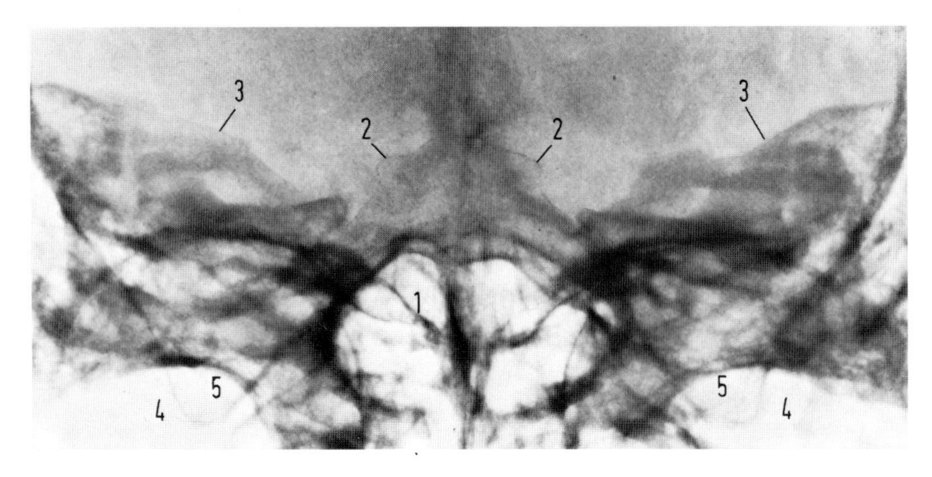

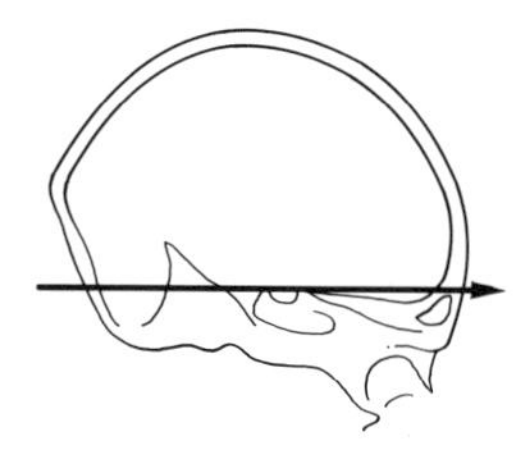

Fig. 150. Sella turcica, nuchofrontal. Fig. 151 shows the path of the rays (after *Haas*) which project the sella freely upwards into the shadow of the frontal bone.

Fig. 151

1 Ethmoid bone; on its right: crista galli
2 Lateral contour of sella, seen shaped like an anvil
3 Petrous bone (appears above the orbita)
4 Orbita
5 Great wing

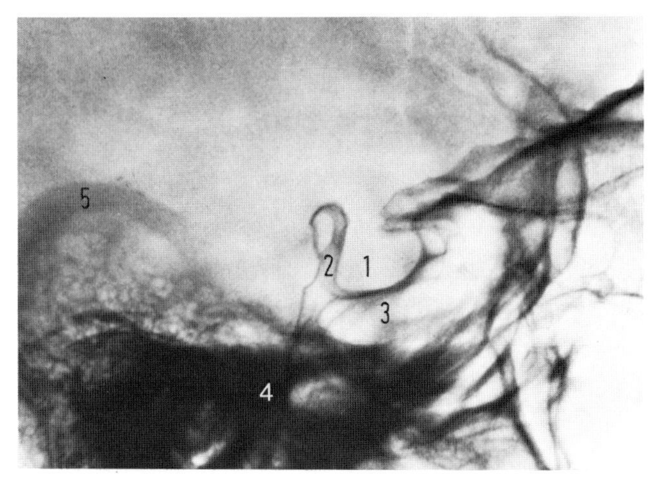

1 Sella turcica
2 Dorsum sellae
3 Sphenoidal sinus
4 Petrous bone
5 Shadow of pinna

Fig. 152. Sella turcica, bitemporal. The hyperpneumatization is due to air-containing cells in the dorsum sellae which may also continue into the clinoid processes.

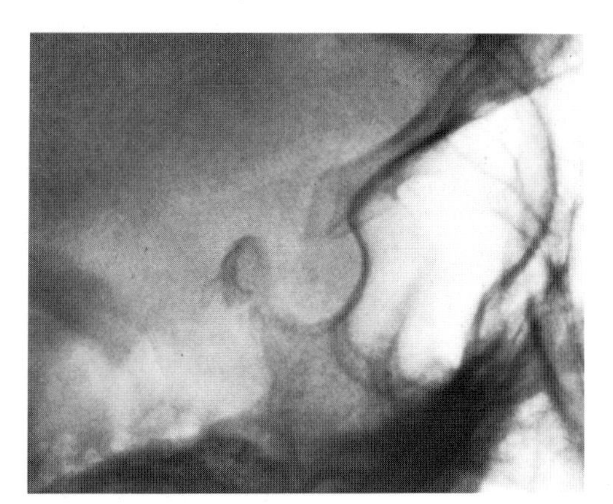

Fig. 153. Sella turcica, bitemporal. The posterior portion of the sella turcica shows a club-shaped distension directed cephalad, with a breach of contour simulated by a furrow in case of ossification of the tentorial attachment.

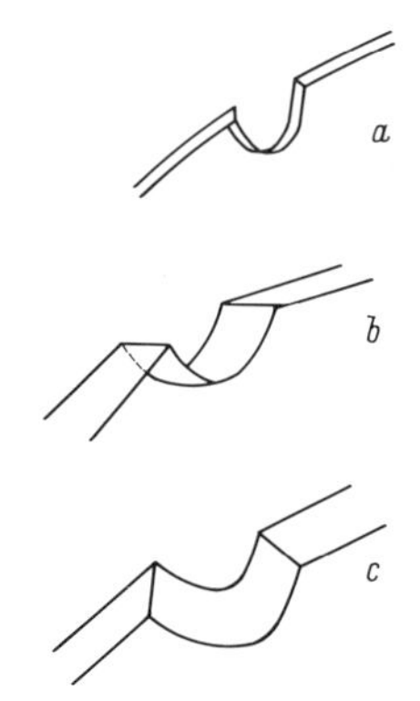

a Central projection
b Projection further from behind
c Projection further from above

Fig. 154. Projection of the sella turcica and technique for positioning. The best projection is obtained when the focus is vertically above the center point of a line which connects the outer orbital angle with the outer auditory meatus *(Takagi)*.

Figs. 155–163. Forms and variants of sella turcica.

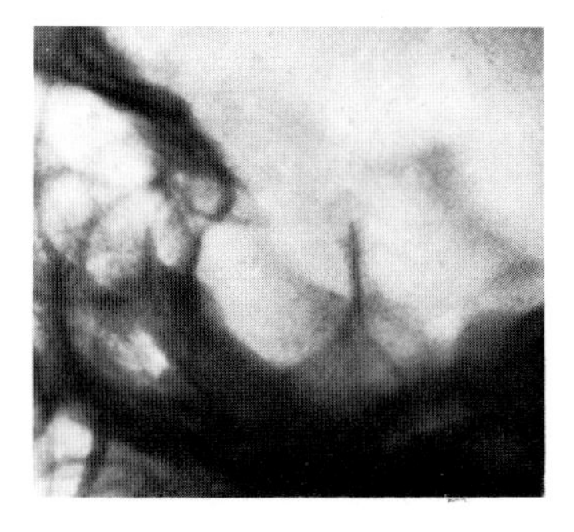

Fig. 155. Deep, round profile of sella, narrow dorsum sellae, ossification of the petrosellar or the petroclinoid ligament at the posterior rim of the dorsum sellae.

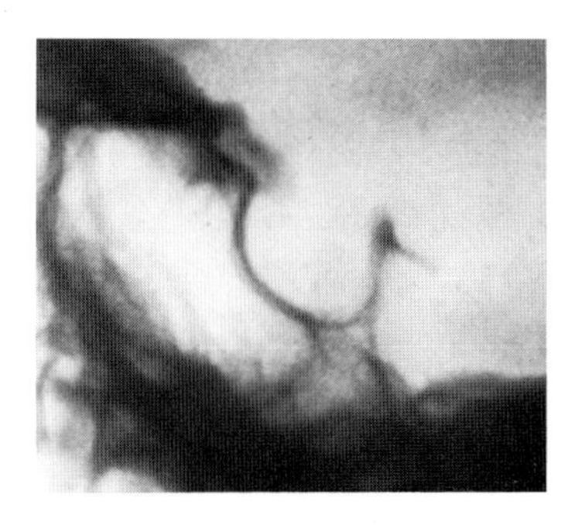

Fig. 156. Spiky ossification of the tentorial attachment at the posterior edge of the dorsum sellae, low-lying sella, high position of the sphenoid plane of the large sphenoidal sinus. Sella hanging like a knapsack. There are biological-constitutional developmental connections to pathological brain structures *(Kretschmer, Schiffer)*.

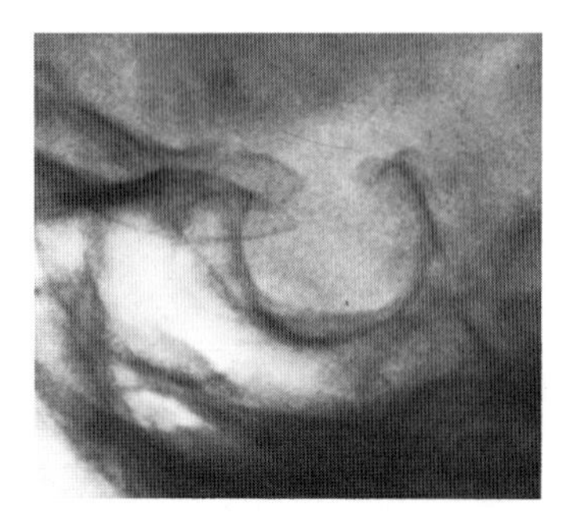

Fig. 157. Large, round profile of sella, calcification of the petrosellar ligament, reaching downwards from the posterior upper rim of the dorsum sellae (balloon-like sella, i.e., sellar excavation as in cases of intrasellar tumor).

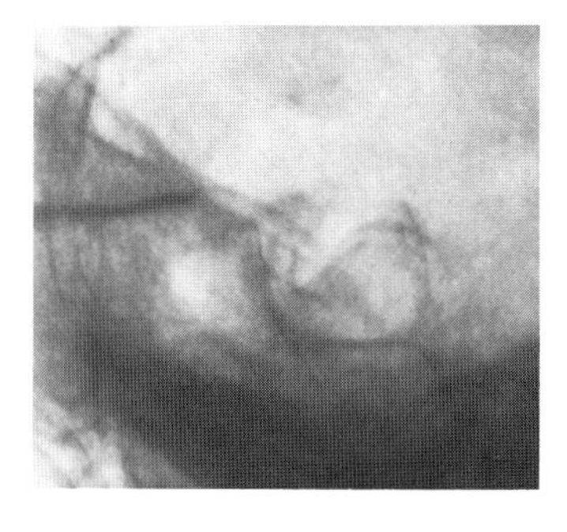

Fig. 158. Ossification in the region of the sella.

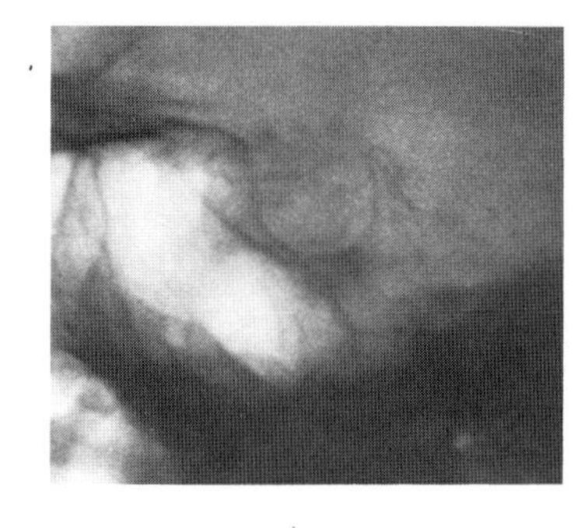

Fig. 159. Parasellar calcification.

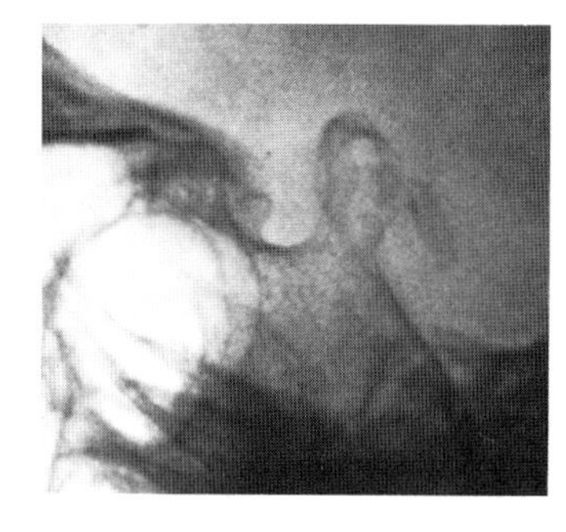

Fig. 160. Calcification of the petrosellar ligament, posterior to sella. Club-shaped, pneumatized tuberculum sellae.

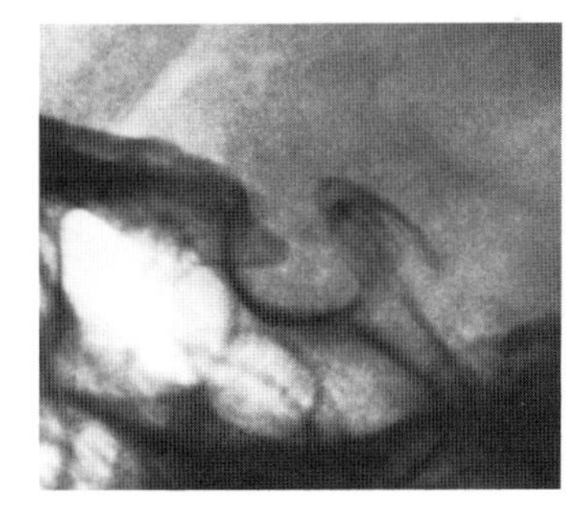

Fig. 161. Sella of normal size. Ossification of the tentorial attachment. Calcified petrosellar ligament, leading from the sellar apex downwards and posteriorly. Large anterior clinoid process.

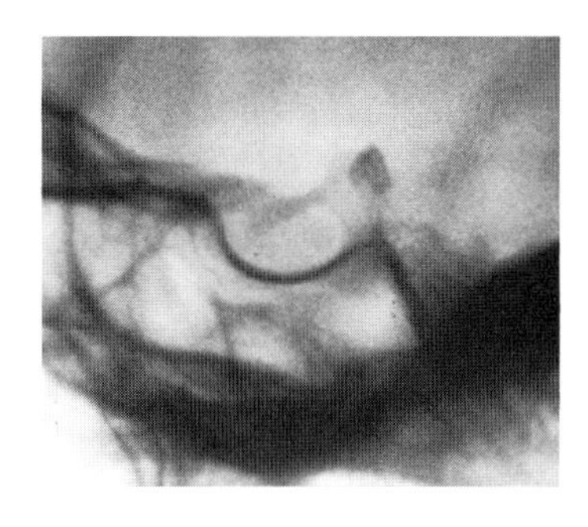

Fig. 162. Shallow shape of sella. Bony bridge across sella (probably calcified interclinoid taeniae). Low-lying sphenoidal planum in the case of a shallow sphenoidal sinus (see also Fig. 926).

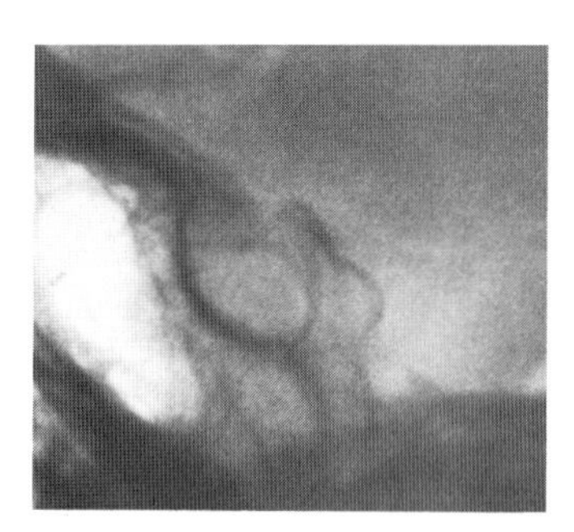

Fig. 163. Ossification of interclinoid taeniae, calcification of retrosellar ligament (petrosellar ligament). If the petrosellar ligaments are radiologically visible, they signify calcification of the dura. Ossifications in this region do not appear ribbon-like as the petrosellar ligaments, but are shaped more irregularly and look nodular.

Figs. 164–172. Forms and variants of sella turcica.

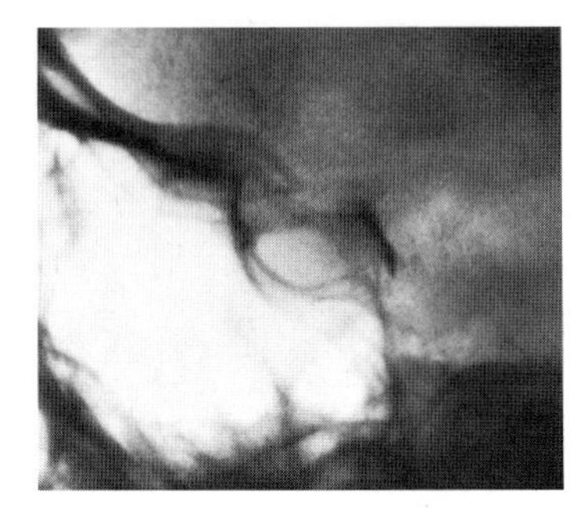

Fig. 164. Apparent narrowing of sella, caused by broad, bony sellar bridge (interclinoid ligaments, ossified interclinoid taeniae). Calcified petrosellar ligament.

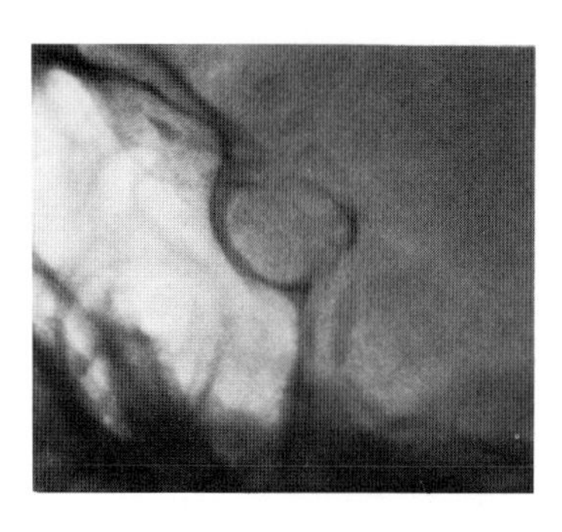

Fig. 165. Delicate bony bridge formation of the interclinoid taeniae, without reduction of the sellar space.

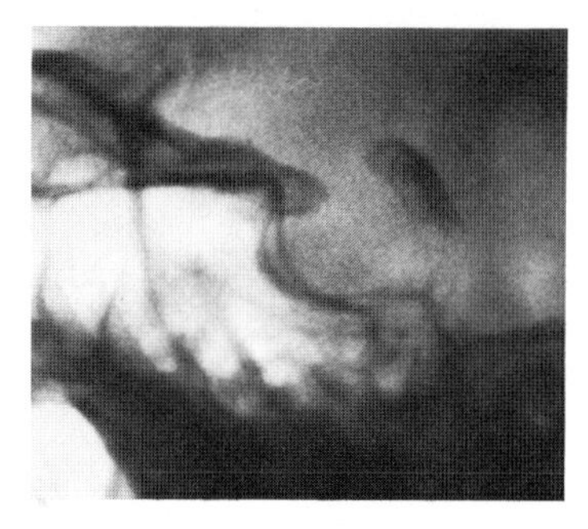

Fig. 166. Partial pneumatization of the base of the dorsum sellae.

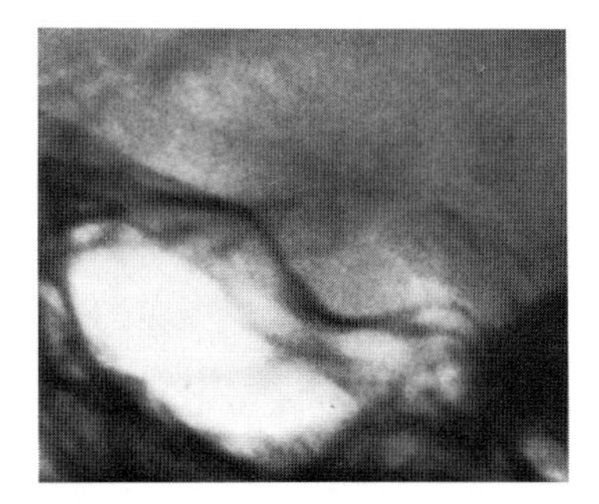

Fig. 167. Very shallow sella and very low pneumatized dorsum sellae.

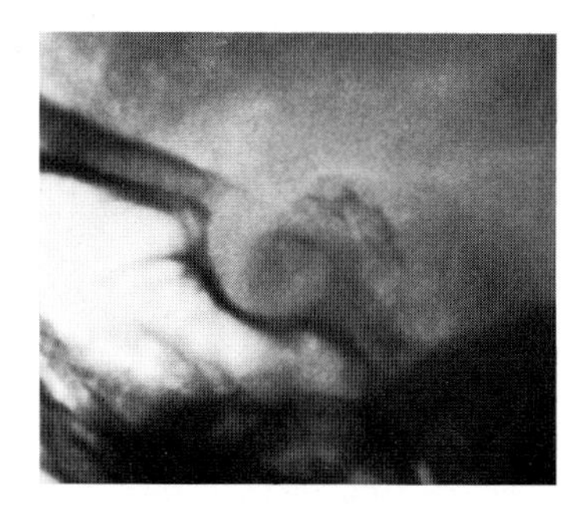

Fig. 168. Calcification of dura above the angulated dorsum sellae and within the sella (an incidental finding).

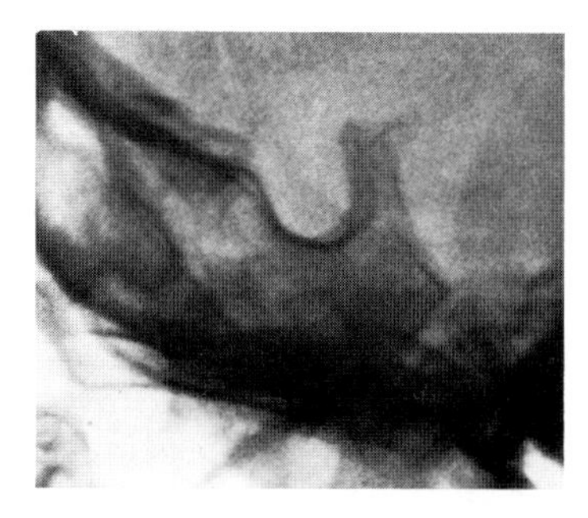

Fig. 169. Child, 3 years of age. Deep sella; thick, high and steep dorsum sellae. Developing sphenoidal sinus. Spheno-occipital synchondrosis (see also Fig. 921).

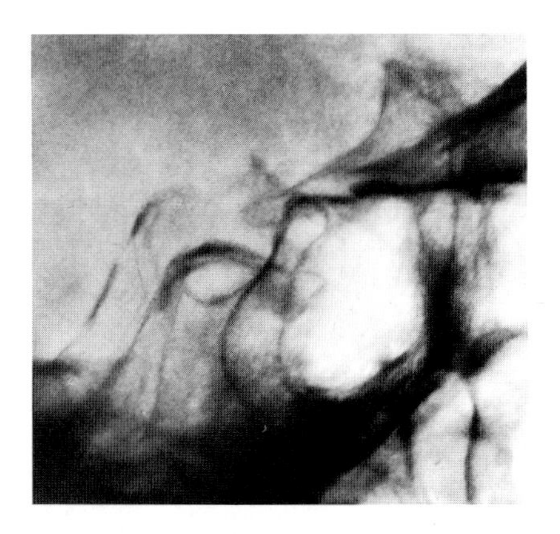

Fig. 170. Calcified double-contoured internal carotid artery. Typical twisted course within the sellar clearing. In addition, a calcified tentorial attachment visible as a dorsally directed calcified band.

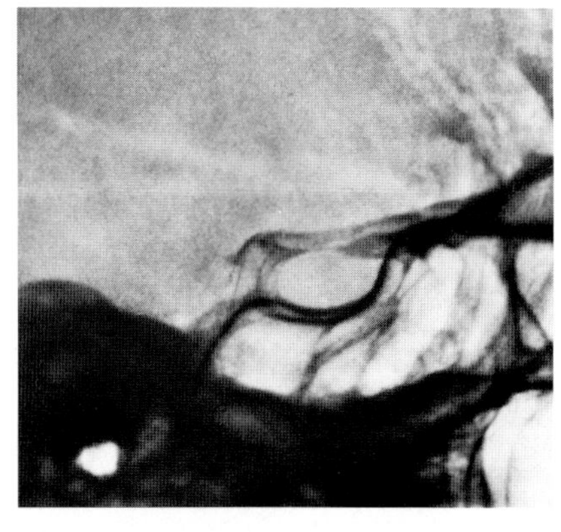

Fig. 171. Bridge formation of sella. Such malformations correspond to the type of "hypophysis-midbrain-weakling" *(Schneider, Martin, Neiss, Carstens).*

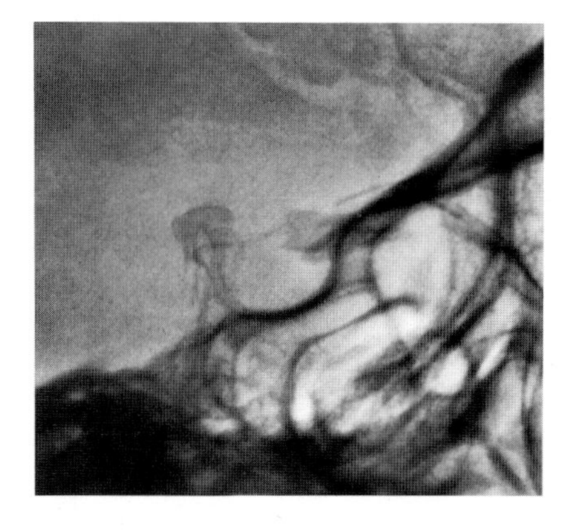

Fig. 172. Delicate bridge formation. The dorsum sella is high and club-shaped. (Hypophyseal disturbances – *Raab*'s variant, see *Carstens).* The double-contoured calcified shadow at the posterior wall of the dorsum sellae corresponds to the basilar artery.

Haas, among others, has reported details of radiologic diagnostics of the sella turcica (i.e., contours of sella, determination of its size as well as clinoid bridges). *Casazza* examined the sella turcica in different shaped skulls, finding the largest volume of the sella in excessive bradycephalic and the smallest in mesocephalic skulls. *Fischgold* and *Metzger* have reported on the normal topography of the sella turcica as well as on the radiologic view of the pathological sella, while *Haas* gives an account of the clinical evaluation of its size.

Tomography of the Head

Tomographic Examination of the Petrous Bone

The highly differentiated structures of the individual skeletal components of the skull are often difficult to analyze from an overall X-ray view. This applies especially to the petrous bone, which is extremely important clinically, its tomography was developed prior to the tomographic anatomy of the whole skull. In this volume, a fifth position (E) is added to the four standard positions (A–D) set forth by *J. Zimmer.*

Position A corresponds to the projection after *Haas* (Fig. 112), and must be carried out with the patient prone. The upper part of the body is raised by pillows to such a height that the axis of the skull forms an angle of about 30° with the plane of the table. The forehead touches the table. The central ray coincides with the median plane of the skull. This position permits a comprehensive view of the inner components of the bone.

Position B corresponds to the projection after *Schüller* (i.e., steep radiograph, with the central ray directed 35° caudally instead of 15 to 25°). The patient lies on the table on his side; the median plane is inclined towards the film to enclose, together with the table, an angle of 35°. This provides a view of the ear away from the film. At a depth of 2.5 cm (measured from the surface of the skin on the side of the focus), the antrum is found; at 2.5 to 3 cm, the distal part of the facial canal; and at 4 cm, the labyrinth.

Position C corresponds to the projection after *Stenvers* (Fig. 120). It is suitable for a view of the external auditory meatus, the antrum aditus region and the labyrinth.

In Position D, the head is placed sideways on the table; the median plane runs parallel to the film. The affected ear is adjacent to the film. This position is also suitable for the exposition of the external auditory meatus, the antrum-aditus region and the labyrinth (Figs. 225, 227, 229 and 231). Position E corresponds to the axial position of the head, with a caudocranial path of the rays (Fig. 91), the head hanging down. The tomographic horizontal section, by means of only a few layers, allows the simultaneous view of both petrous bones, as well as of the organs of the middle and inner ear.

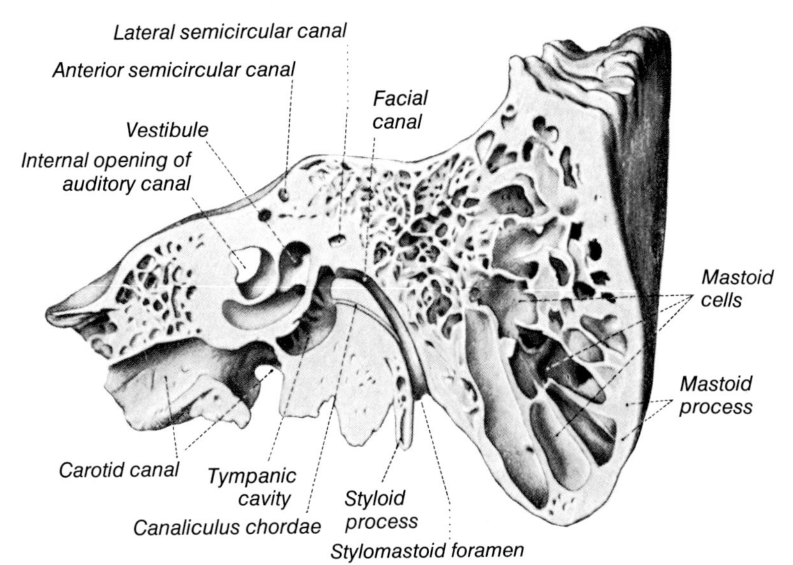

Fig. 173. Left temporal bone (from *Sobotta-Becher,* Atlas der Anatomie des Menschen, 15th edition, München – Berlin – Vienna 1957).

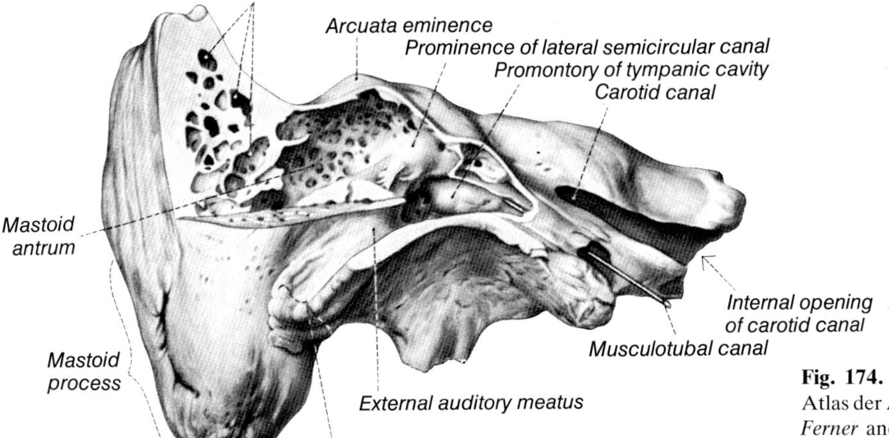

Fig. 174. Right temporal bone (from *Sobotta-Becher,* Atlas der Anatomie des Menschen, 17th edition. Ed.: *H. Ferner* and *J. Staubesand,* München – Berlin – Vienna 1972).

1. **Tomographs of both petrous bones** (Figs. 175–177) of a 62-year-old male. Standard projection as in Fig. 43, occipito-frontal. As with positions A and E (p. 67), one achieves a simultaneous view of both petrous bones, useful for comparison purposes. The difference in pneumatization is caused by a malignant process on the left side which has also invaded the antrum.

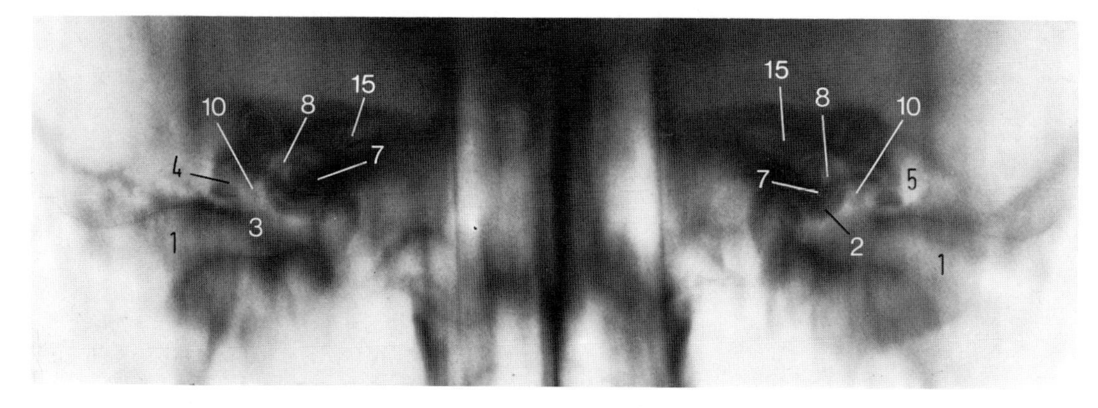

Fig. 175 (9.5 cm)

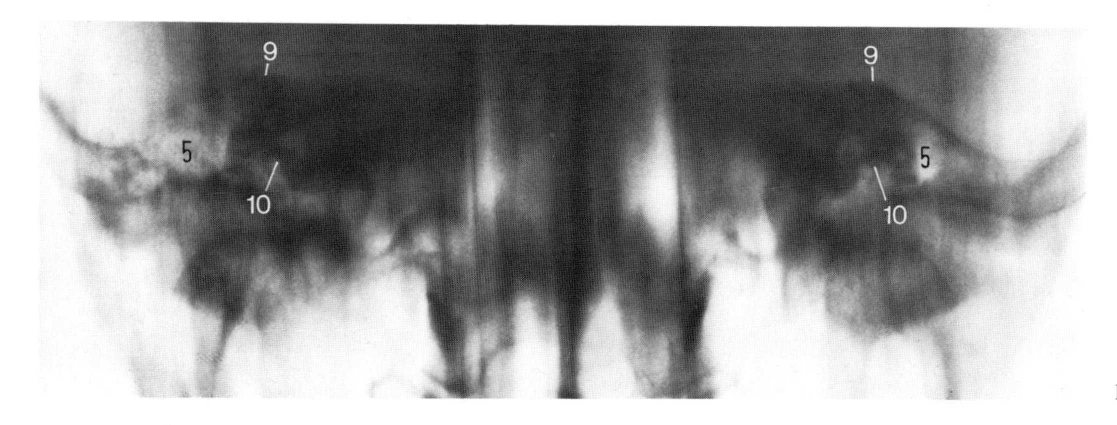

Fig. 176 (9.75 cm)

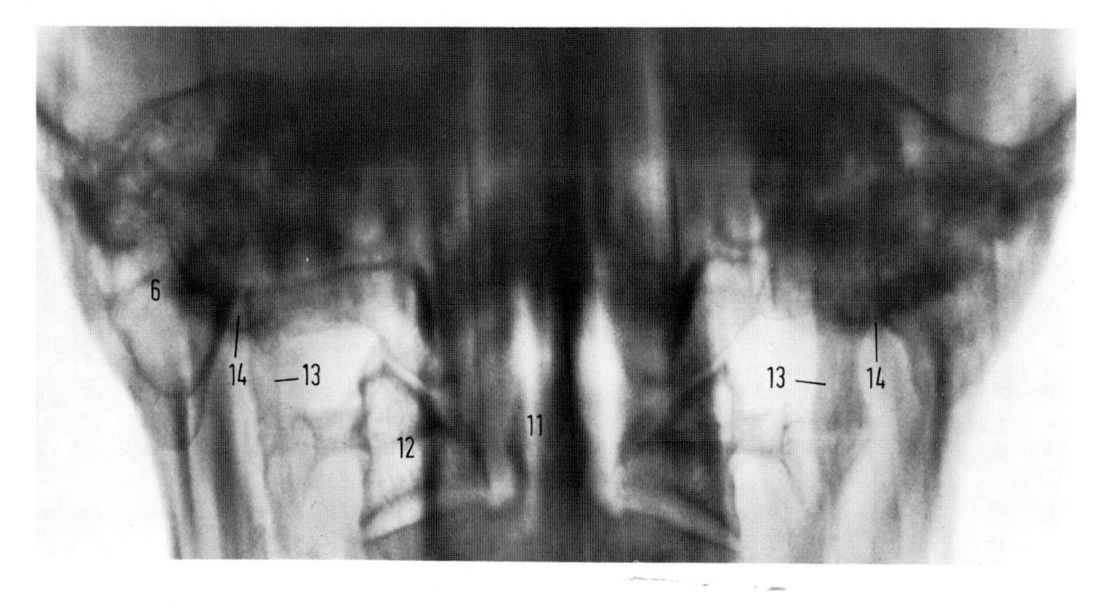

Fig. 177 (10.5 cm)

To Figs. 175, 176 and 177:

1 External auditory meatus
2 Promontory
3 Tympanic cavity
4 Aditus ad antrum
5 Mastoid antrum
6 Mastoid cells
7 Cochlea
8 Vestibule with semicircular canals
9 Arcuate eminence
10 Epitympanic recess with head of malleus
11 Dens (axis)
12 Atlas
13 Styloid process
14 Stylomastoid foramen
15 Internal auditory meatus

2. **Oriented horizontal tomography of the right petrous bone after** *Birkner* **with a linear blurring,** compared with horizontal sections on a skeleton. The advantage of this method is in the demonstration, by means of only a few layers, of the organs of the middle and inner ear. Because almost all these organs lie in one horizontal plane, this is important for otologic diagnostics. An additional benefit is the possibility of a simultaneous tomographic view of both petrous bones. The tomographs of the petrous bone, taken in the horizontal position of the head with an axial path of the rays, have an advantage over the corresponding tomographs taken occipitofrontal with a sagittal direction of the beam (Figs. 175–177), due to the separate projection of the middle and inner ear.
For comparison with skeletal sections of about 0.25 cm thickness, the tomographic layers were taken at distances of about 0.25 cm.

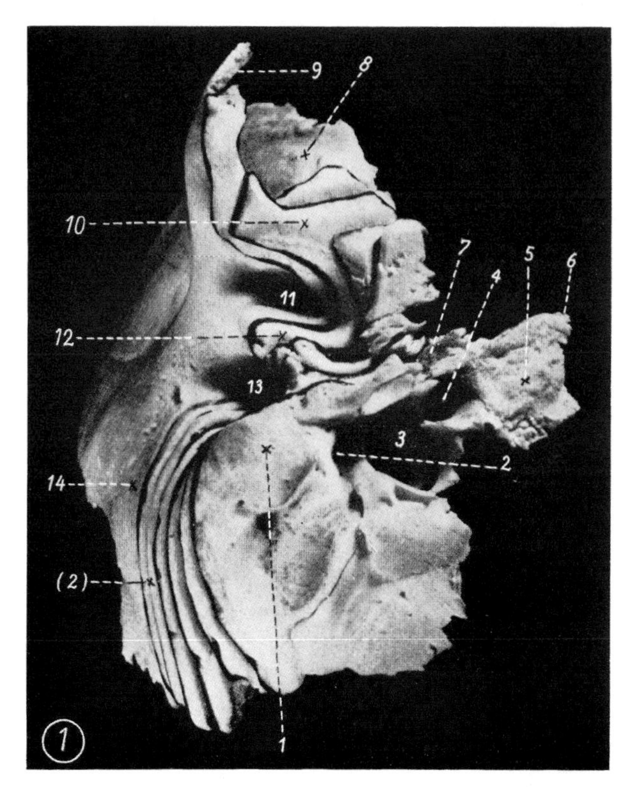

1 Mastoid process
2 Stylomastoid foramen (point of exit of the facial nerve)
3 Jugular fossa
4 External opening of carotid canal
5 Inferior surface of petrous portion
6 Apex of petrous portion
7 Termination of musculotubal canal
8 Squama
9 Zygomatic process
10 Articular tubercle
11 Mandibular fossa
12 Retromandibular process
13 External auditory meatus
14 Mastoid portion

Fig. 178. Right petrous bone with temporal squama and zygomatic process, taken from below.

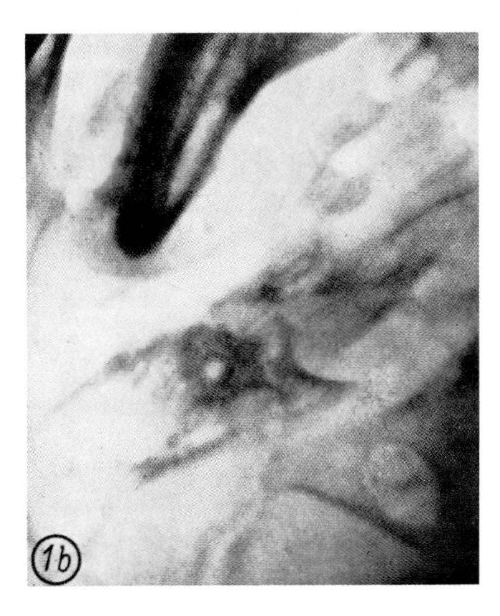

Fig. 179. General view of the right petrous bone, with patient supine.

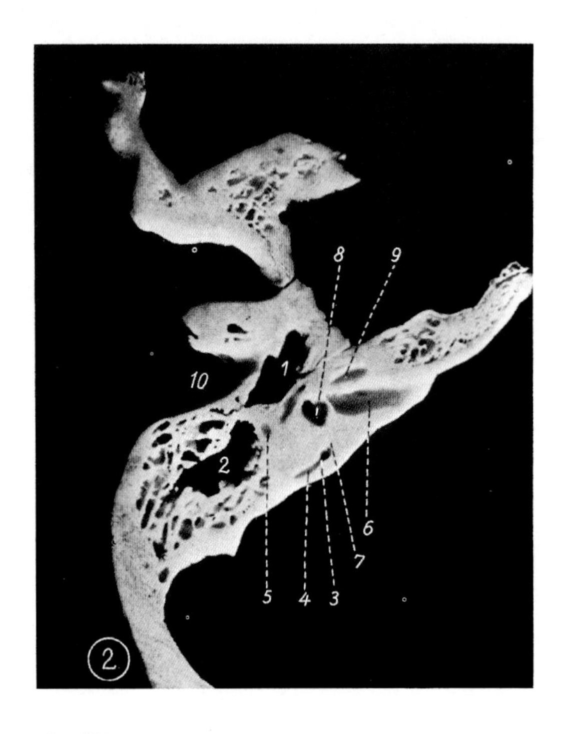

Fig. 180

The uppermost layers*, 10.75–11.5 cm (Figs. 180–186), already show an exceptional number of details. Above all, one recognizes the tympanic cavity, whose outer border is formed by the head of the malleus and its handle, which is inserted into the tympanic membrane (Fig. 186). The musculotubal canal, which contains the bony part of the auditory tube and the tensor tympanic muscle, runs forward and medially (Figs. 183 and 184). Backwards and laterally, the aditus ad antrum with the antrum itself can be distinctly recognized. The entire petrous cell system can be presented by this projection, as well as by tomographs taken in frontal and sagittal positions.

The facial canal, after separation from the inner auditory tube in vertical direction behind the tympanic cavity, becomes visible in cross section on all layers.

The component parts of the labyrinth (vestibule, cochlea and semicircular canals) are sharply outlined. The posterior and lateral semicircular canals with the crus commune appear to their full extent especially in the upper layers, while vestibulum and cochlea are best displayed in the 11.25- and 11.50-cm layers (Figs. 184 and 186).

The internal auditory meatus in its course is visible just as distinctly. Only with tomography *(Stenvers)* does one succeed in obtaining a similarly complete view of the internal auditory canal.

The groove in the occipital squama, caused by the sigmoid sinus, is shown in the 11.5- and 11.75-cm layers (Figs. 185–188). Its relation to the antrum and mastoid cells can easily be determined.

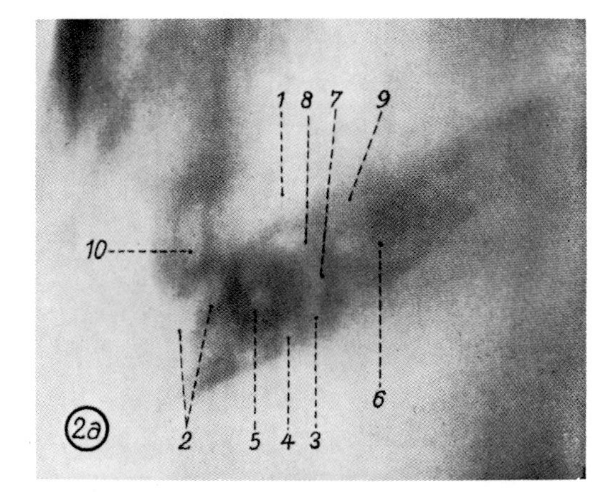

Fig. 181

To Figs. 180–182:

1 Tympanic cavity (attic)
2 Mastoid antrum
3 Crus commune of superior and posterior semicircular canal
4 Posterior semicircular canal
5 Facial canal
6 Internal auditory meatus
7 Sectioned superior semicircular canal
8 Vestibule
9 Cochlea
10 External auditory meatus

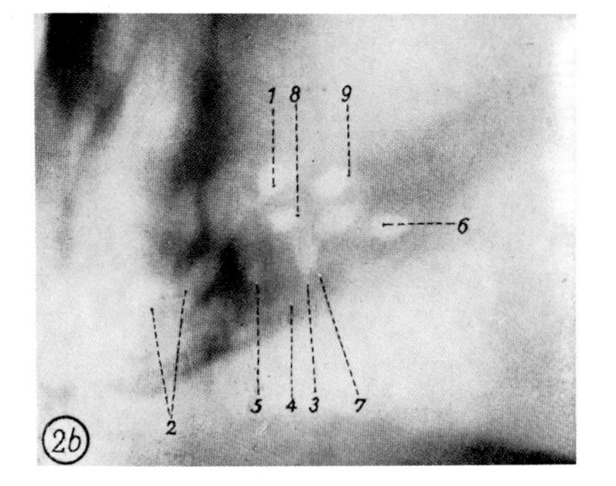

Fig. 182

* The concepts "above" and "below" refer to the normal posture of the head of a person in upright position. For example, the eminentia arcuata is "above," the foramen jugulare "below."

To Figs. 183 and 184:

1 Tympanic cavity
2 Head of malleus and manubrium
3 Musculotubal canal
4 Cochlea
5 Facial canal
6 Interior auditory canal
7 Aditus ad antrum
8 Vestibule
9 Mastoid antrum
10 Mastoid cells
11 Zygomatic process with cells

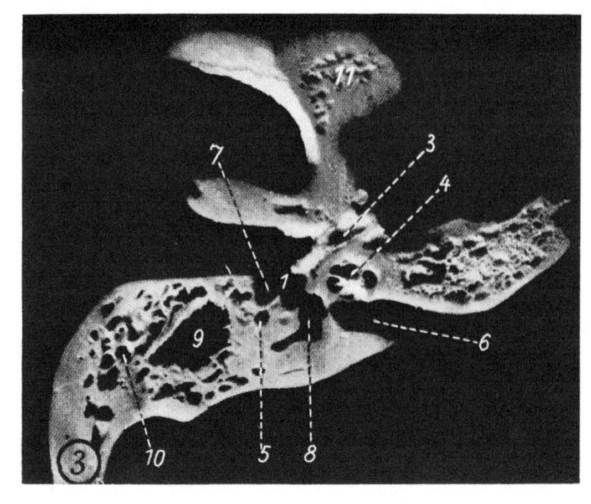

Fig. 183

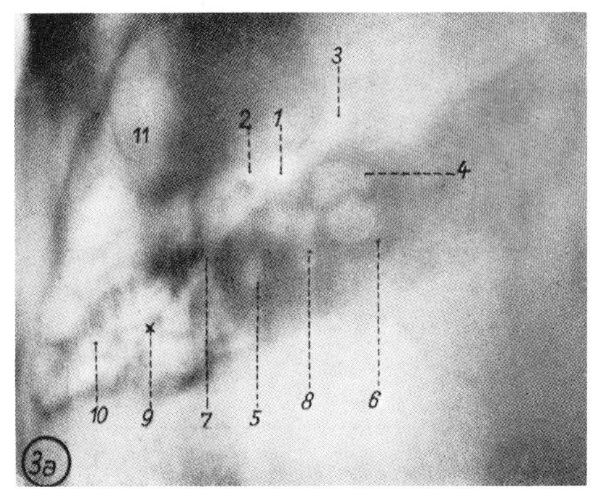

Fig. 184

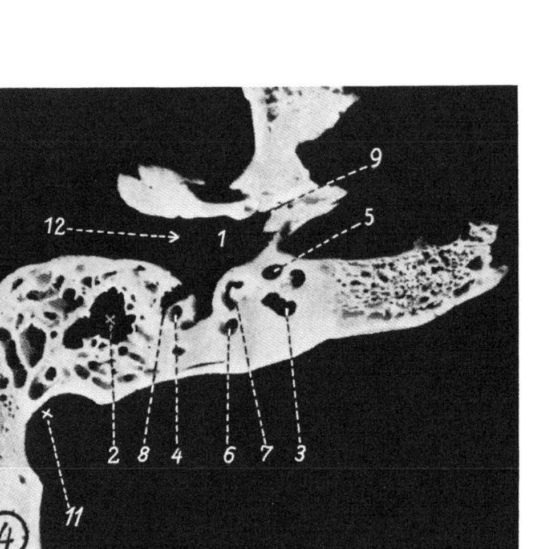

Fig. 185

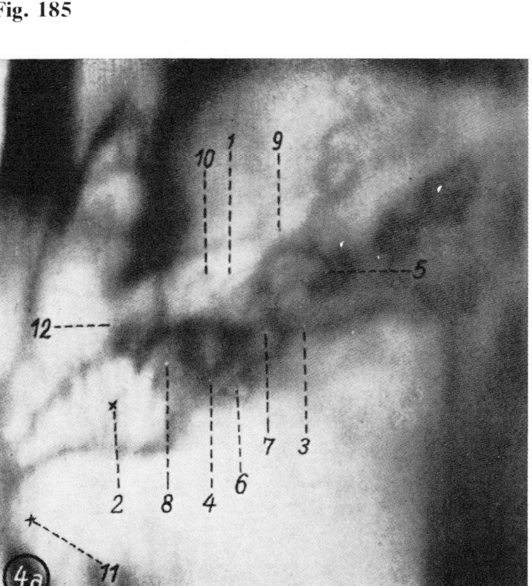

Fig. 186

To Figs. 185 and 186:

1 Tympanic cavity
2 Mastoid antrum
3 Innermost part of auditory canal
4 Facial canal
5 Convolution of cochlea
6 Cross section of superior semicircular canal and (Fig. 186) part of posterior semicircular canal
7 Vestibule
8 Aditus ad antrum
9 Musculotubal canal
10 Head of malleus with handle, inserted into tympanic membrane
11 Sigmoid sinus
12 Outer auditory canal

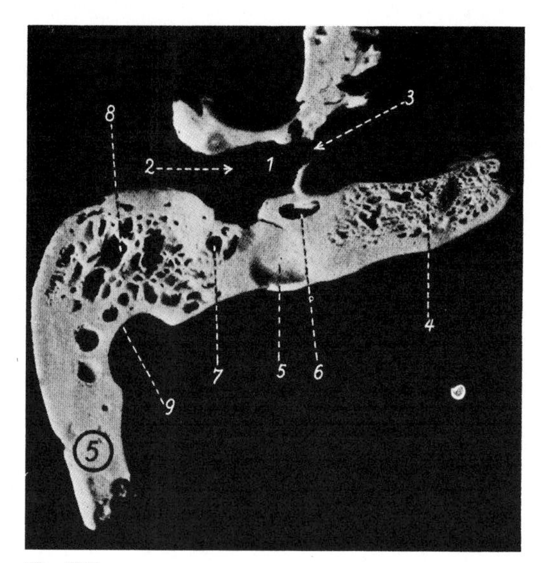

Fig. 187

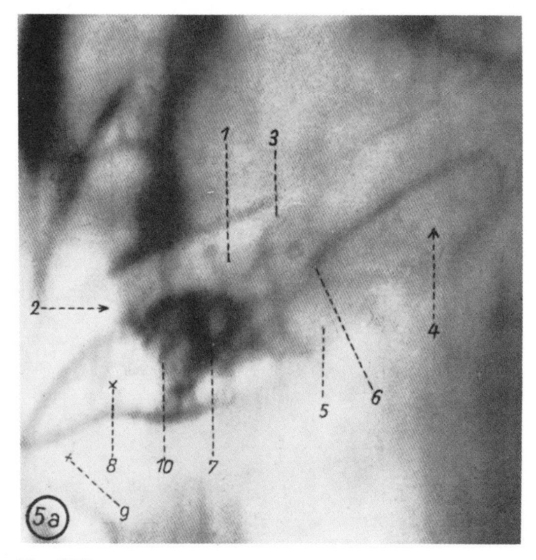

Fig. 188

Figs. 187 and 188 (11.75 cm) show the outer auditory canal, still parts of the tympanic cavity and its accessory spaces, as well as the spirals of the cochlea, the vestibule and parts of the transected semicircular canals. The roof of the jugular fossa in relation to the labyrinth is recognizable. The apex of the petrous bone contains mainly honeycombed cells. As in most of the layers, the posterior contour of the petrous bone is distinctly delineated.

1 Tympanic cavity
2 Outer auditory canal
3 Musculotubal canal
4 Base and cells of petrous bone
5 Bulb of superior jugular vein
6 Cochlea
7 Facial canal
8 Mastoid cells
9 Sigmoid sinus
10 Entrance to mastoid cells

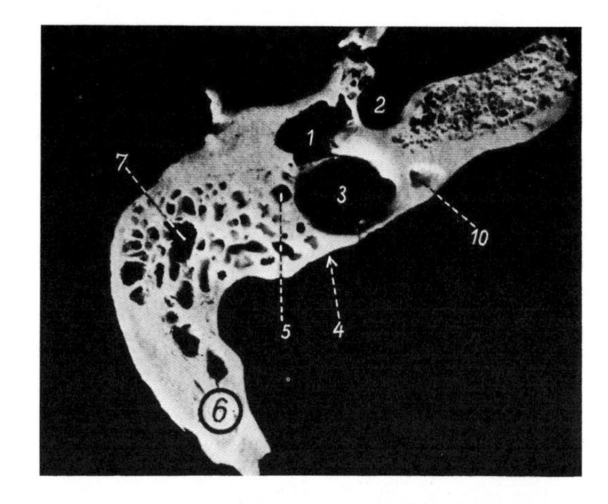

Fig. 189

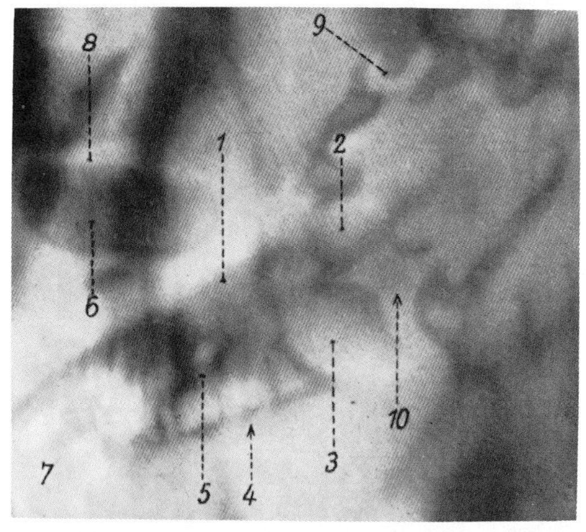

Fig. 190

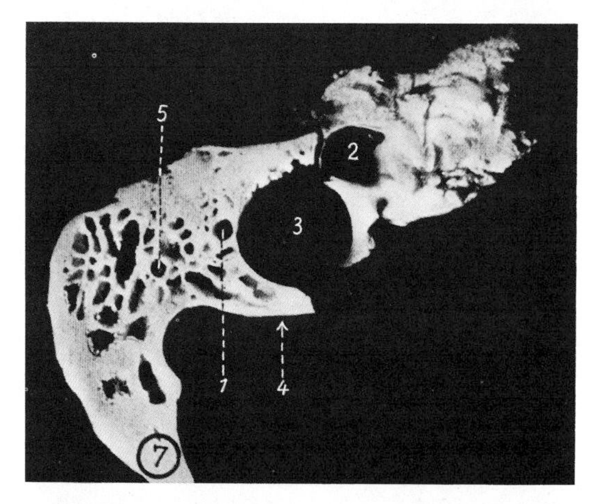

Fig. 191

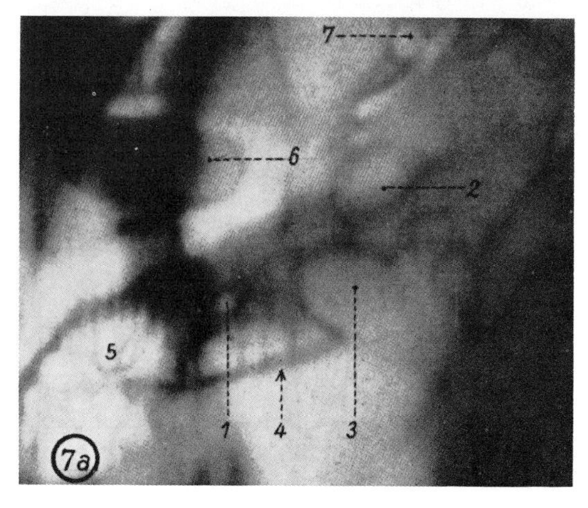

Fig. 192

◀ To Figs. 189 and 190:

1 Tympanic cavity
2 Opening of the interior carotid canal
3 Jugular fossa
4 Posterior wall of petrous bone
5 Facial canal
6 Condyloid process
7 Mastoid cells
8 Articular interstice of mandibular joint
9 Foramen ovale
10 Fossula petrosa

Figs. 189–192 (12 to 12.5 cm) show the vesicular pneumatization of the mastoid, which surrounds the massive of the facial canal. The jugular fossa and its relation to the tympanic cavity on the one hand and the carotid canal on the other can be well determined. Anteriorly, the petrosphenoidal fissure with the openings for the divisions of the trigeminal nerve (foramen ovale and foramen rotundum) can be seen. The condyloid process of the mandible and the interstice of the mandibular joint appear rather impressive here.

The diagnostically important organs of the middle and inner ear can, therefore, also be demonstrated by horizontal tomography with only three to four layers at a distance of 2.5 cm.

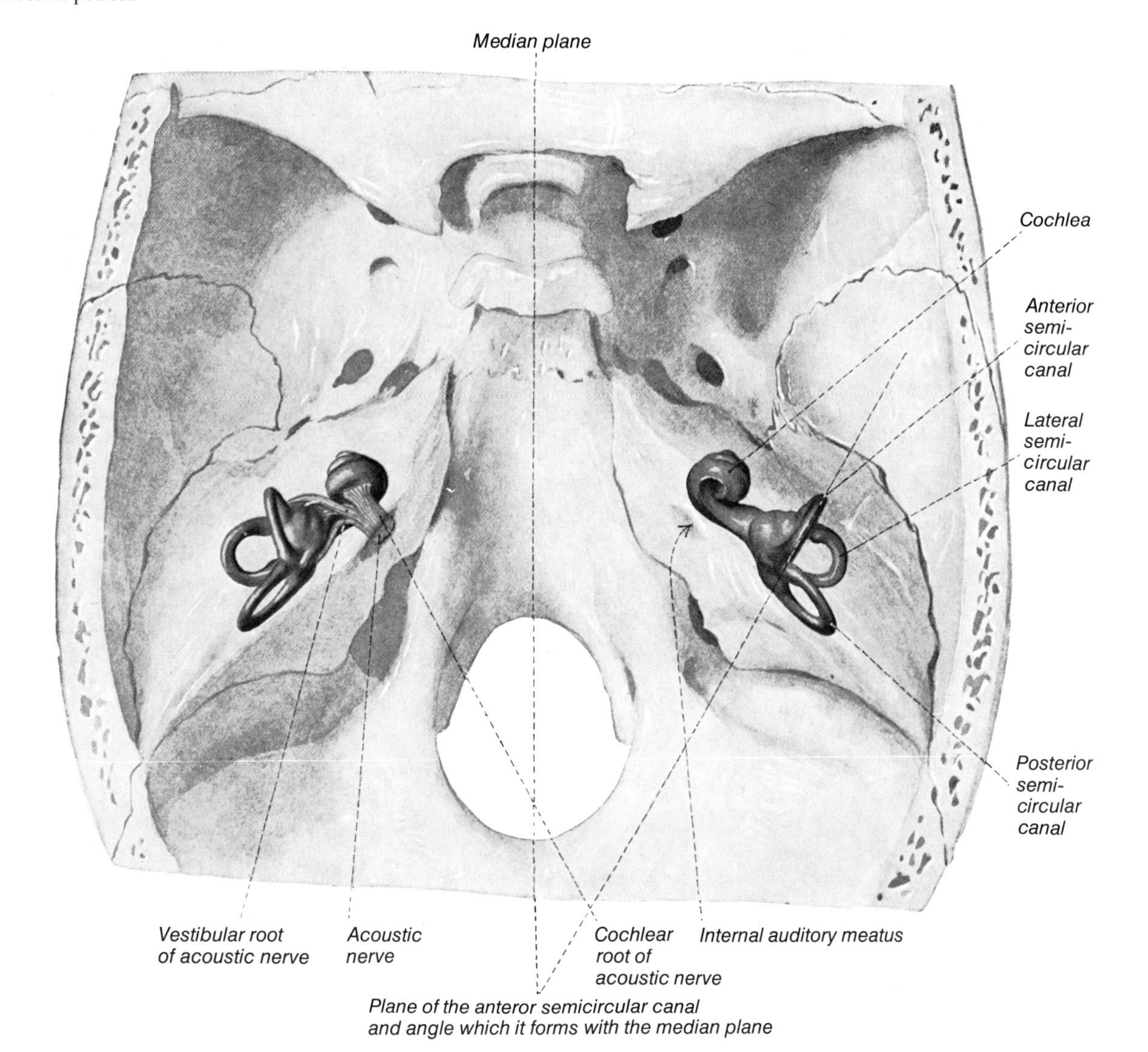

Fig. 193. The bony labyrinths in their relative position, projected onto the **internal base** of the skull. On the left side, the entering nerves are drawn schematically (from *Sobotta-Becher,* Atlas der Anatomie des Menschen, 17th edition. Ed.: *H. Ferner* and *J. Staubesand.* München – Berlin – Vienna 1972).

◀ To Figs. 191 and 192:

1 Facial canal
2 Outer opening of carotid canal
3 Jugular fossa
4 Posterior wall of petrous bone
5 Mastoid cells
6 Condyloid process
7 Foramen ovale

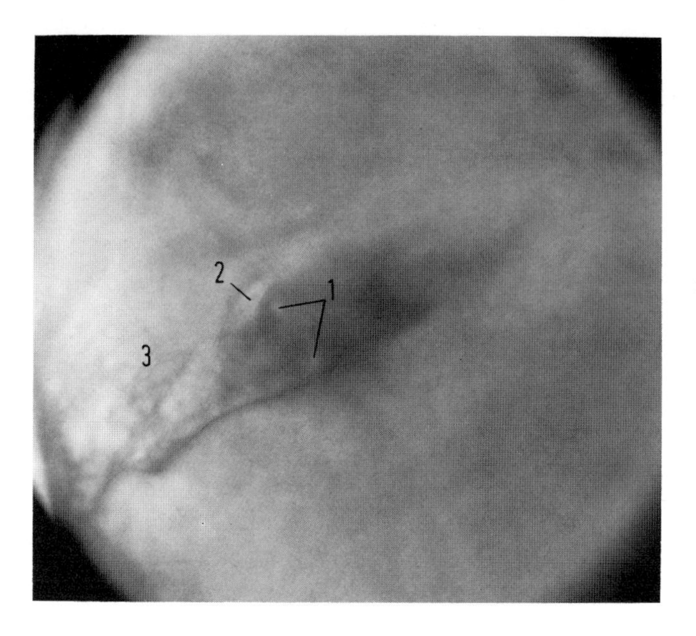

Fig. 194 (10.1 cm)

3. **Horizontal tomographic examination of the right petrous bone, after** *Birkner,* **with polycyclic blurring.** The tomographs were taken with submentovertical direction of the rays. The film is placed parallel to the German horizontal; the central ray runs vertical to it (axial position of head as in Fig. 91). The radiographs were taken with the Polytom (Tobb) of the Massiot Company, with the hypocycloid blurring moving through an angle of 45°. The distance of focus-to-film plane was kept constant at 1.45 m. The optically effective focus was 1.0 mm. To the usual circular tube grids a focus-near grid was added to shield against shaft rays (Stielstrahlen). For elimination of the scattered rays a small film-near grid was used which moved circularly in synchronization with the changing motions of the focus. (These X-ray films were placed at the author's disposal by *Frey.*)

To Figs. 194, 195 and 196:

1 Anterior (superior) semicircular canal
2 Epitympanic recess of tympanic cavity
3 Periantral cells
4 Vestibule
5 Cochlea
6 Internal auditory meatus
7 Auditory ossicles (malleus and incus)
8 Tympanic cavity
9 Antrum
10 Region of the fenestra ovalis
11 Facial canal

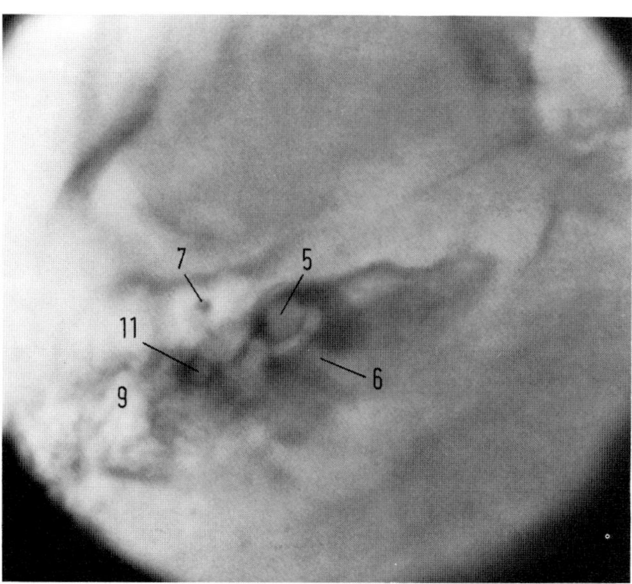

Fig. 195 (10.5 cm)

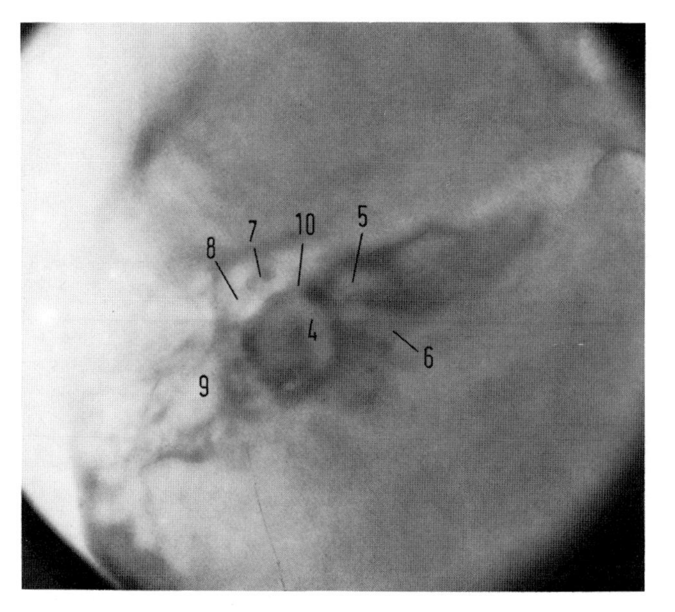

Fig. 196 (10.8 cm)

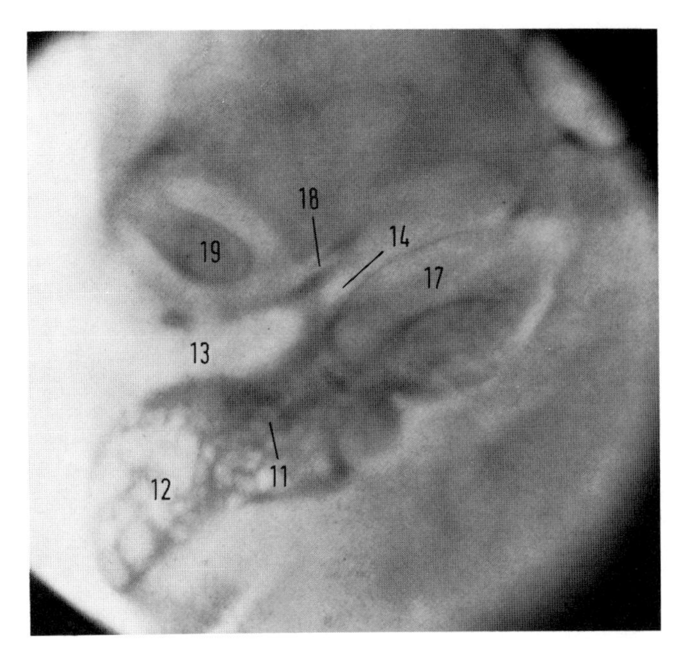

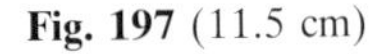
Fig. 197 (11.5 cm)

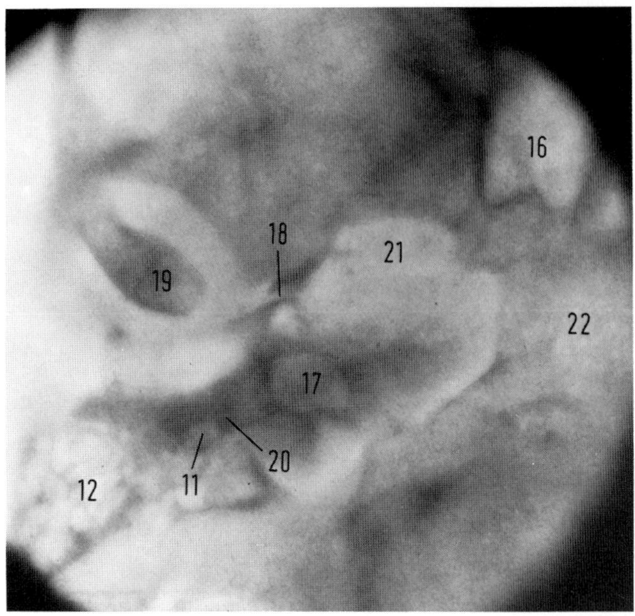

Fig. 198 (12.0 cm)

To Figs. 197 and 198:

11 Facial canal (terminating in stylomastoid foramen)
12 Mastoid cells
13 External auditory meatus
14 Musculotubal canal
16 Sphenoidal sinus
17 Carotid canal
18 Petrotympanic fissure
19 Condyloid process
20 Styloid process
21 Foramen ovale
22 Clivus

Tomographic Examination of the Skull in Comparison to Anatomical Saw-Cut Bone Sections

The systematic tomographic X-ray examination of the skull encounters certain difficulties, as is pointed out in the literature. Summary accounts have been given by *Fischgold, David* and *Brégeat; Herdner; Muntean* and others. Our method *(Birkner)* consists in contrasting tomographs of the skull of the living with corresponding saw-cut bone sections of the macerated skull. The advantages of comparison of anatomical, sawed bone sections with tomographs have already been demonstrated (Figs. 178–192) in the tomographic examination of the petrous bone in the horizontal (transverse) plane *(Birkner)*.

Here, reproduction is limited to the essential tomographs, taken in the three main planes. Only those tomographs which would conform to the bone sections and would show the most important anatomical details were selected.

The most frequent indications for tomography of the skull are diseases of the middle ear, the inner auditory organs and the paranasal sinuses. A further indication is fractures, mainly those at the base of the skull. Destruction of the skull caused by tumors can often be diagnosed more precisely by means of tomography than by a most meticulously aimed radiograph.

The standard projections in the exact frontal, transverse and sagittal planes (as reproduced on the following pages) are usually sufficient for most clinical requirements. For tomographic examination of certain regions, however, more or less extensive flexion, extension or rotation of the head frequently must be used *(Muntean)*.

4. Frontal bone section, saw-cut, and corresponding tomograph.

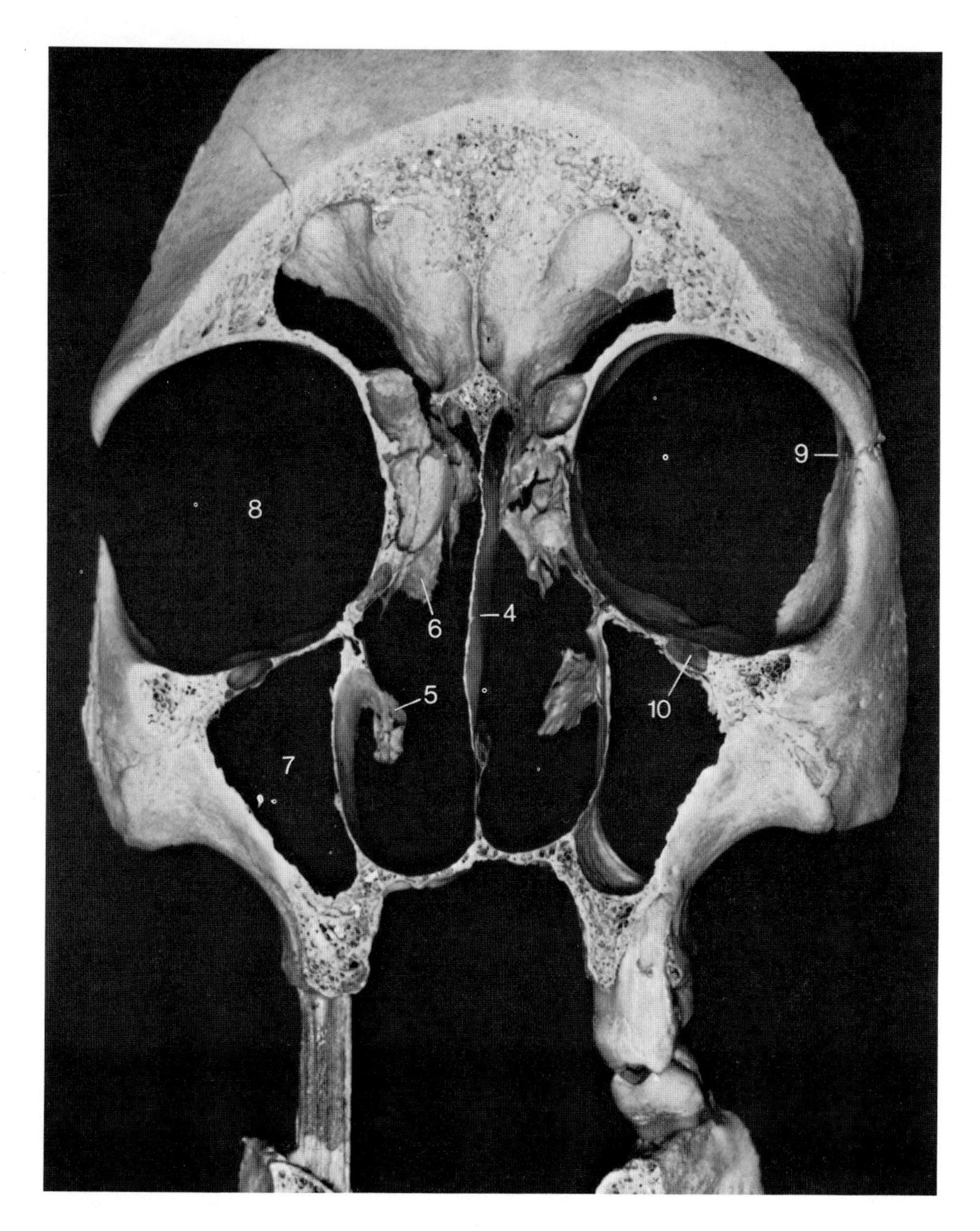

Fig. 199. Front view of section of the skeletal skull, corresponding to Fig. 200.

4 Bony nasal septum (vomer and perpendicular plate)
5 Inferior nasal concha
6 Middle nasal concha
7 Maxillary sinus
8 Orbita
9 Zygomaticofrontal suture
10 Infraorbital canal

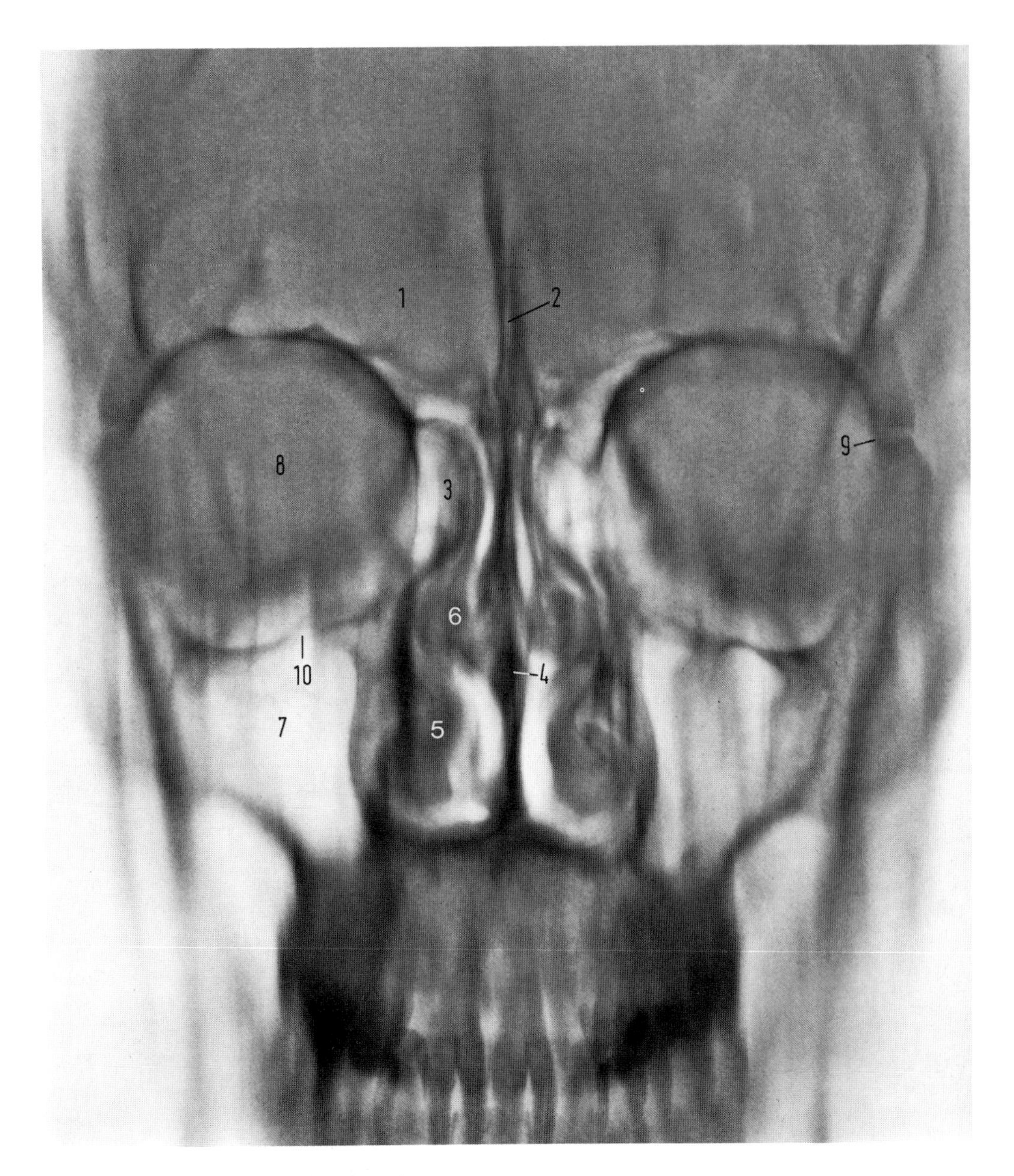

Fig. 200. Distance of layer 4.5 cm from front.

1 Frontal sinus
2 Septum, onto which the frontal crest and crista galli are projected
3 Ethmoidal cells
4 Bony nasal septum (vomer and perpendicular plate)
5 Inferior nasal concha
6 Middle nasal concha
7 Maxillary sinus
8 Orbita
9 Zygomaticofrontal suture
10 Infraorbital canal

The tomographic examination of the maxillary sinuses provides information on morphological and pathological details if it is carried out in all planes (see also Figs. 219 and 225).

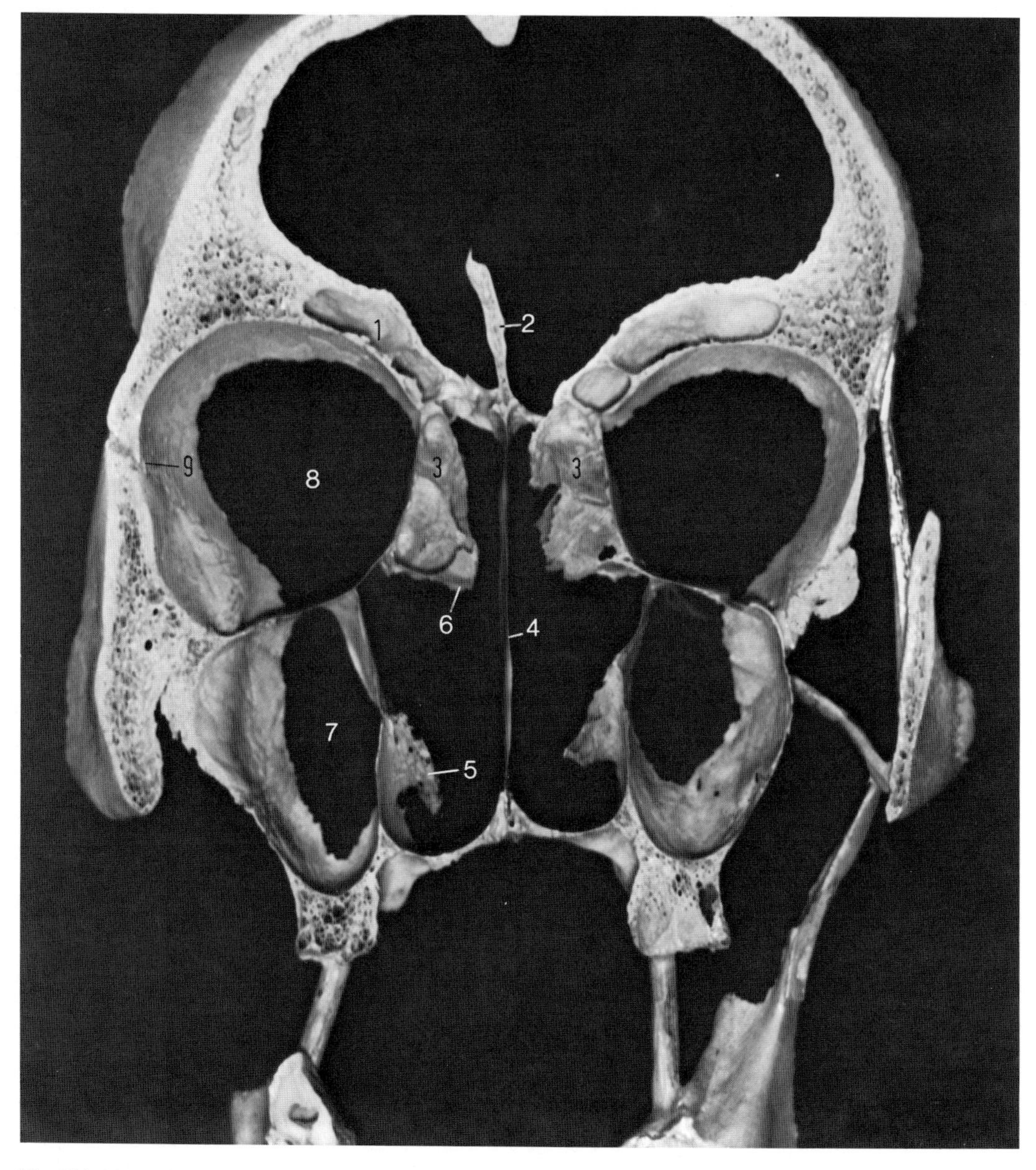

Fig. 201. Front view of section of the skeletal skull (corresponding to Fig. 202).

1 Frontal sinus
2 Crista galli
3 Ethmoidal cells
4 Bony nasal septum, cranially perpendicular plate, caudally vomer
5 Inferior nasal concha
6 Middle nasal concha
7 Maxillary sinus
8 Orbita
9 Zygomaticofrontal suture

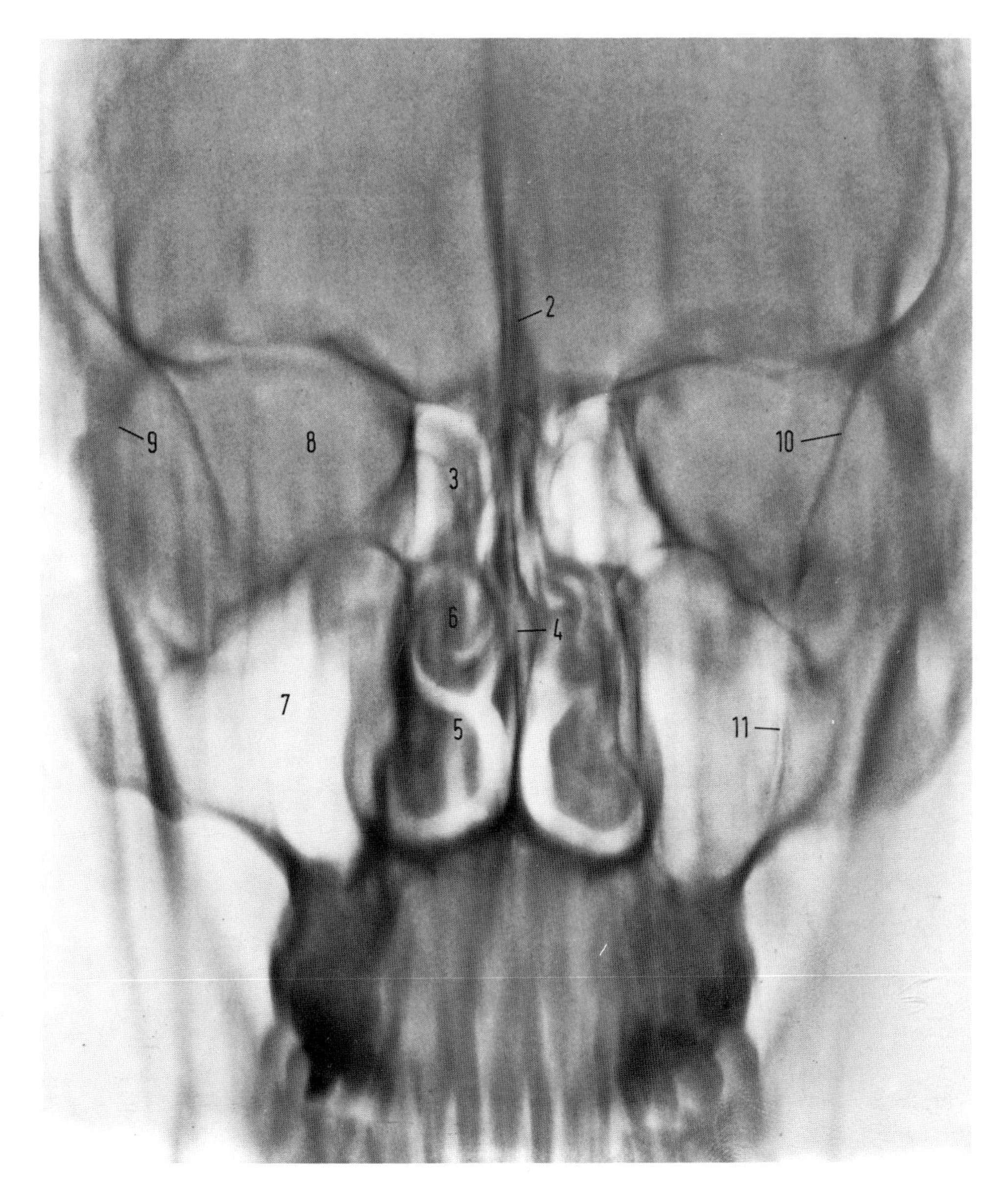

Fig. 202. Distance of layer 5.5 cm from front.

2 Crista galli
3 Ethmoidal cells
4 Bony nasal septum, cranially perpendicular plate, caudally vomer
5 Inferior nasal concha
6 Middle nasal concha
7 Maxillary sinus
8 Orbita
9 Zygomaticofrontal suture
10 Linea innominata (visible through the orbita) (see also Fig. 45, no. 5). Unilateral or bilateral absence of the linea innominata occurs as a variant in cases of a very shallow temporal fossa, as the cortical part of its floor, impinged upon tangentially, forms the anatomical substratum of the linea innominata. According to *Liess,* its loss, indistinctness or interruption provide an essential aid to the diagnosis of pathological changes of the lateral wall of the orbita (sarcomata or other tumors).
11 Pterygopalatine canal (visible through the maxillary sinus)

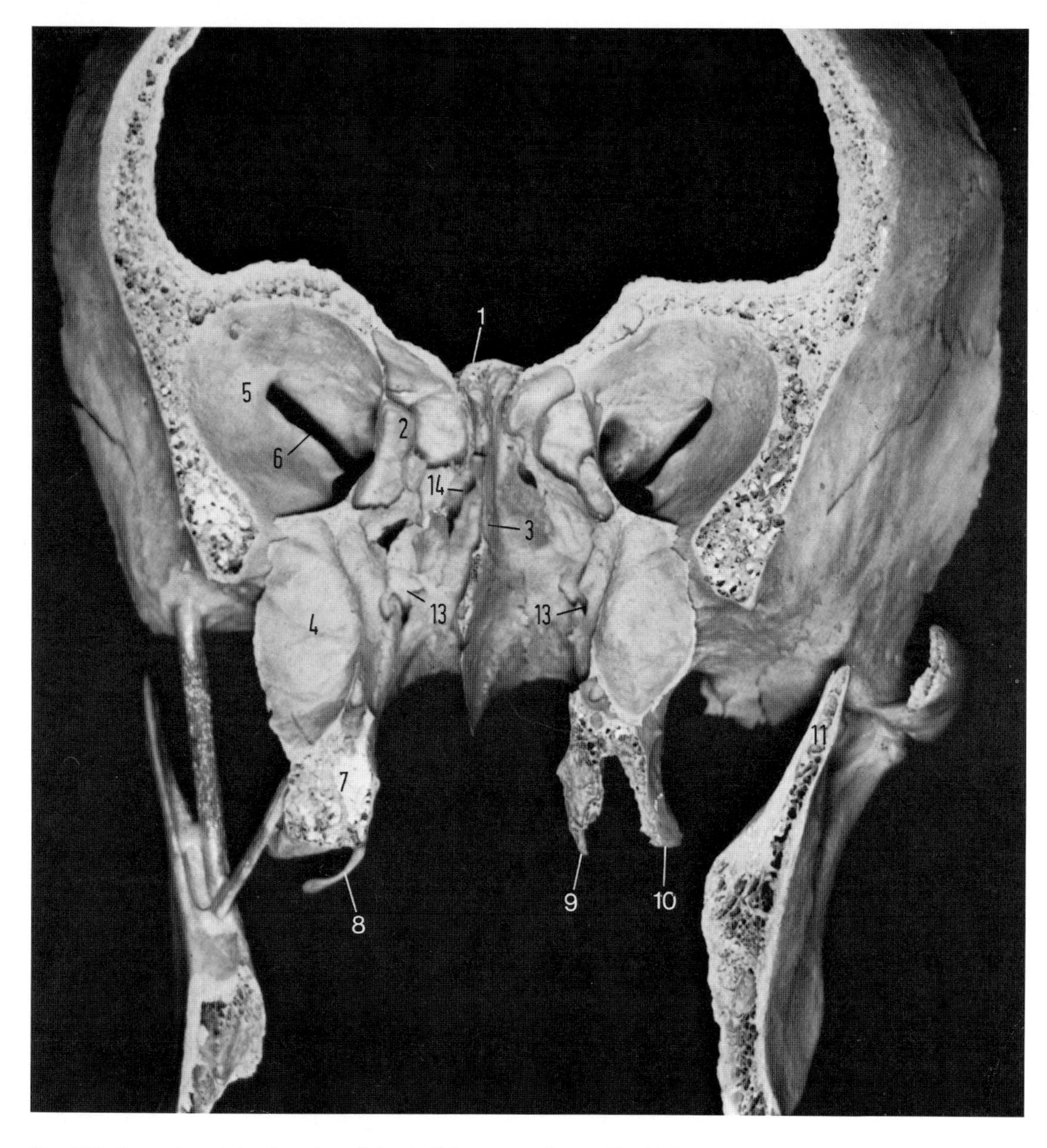

Fig. 203. Front view skeletal section of the skull (corresponding to Fig. 204).

1 Cribriform plate of ethmoid bone
2 Posterior ethmoidal cells
3 Bony nasal septum (perpendicular plate and vomer)
4 Posterior wall of maxillary sinus
5 Posterior wall of orbita; caudal portion: orbital surface of great wings
6 Superior orbital fissure; on this tomograph, distinct difference in width between the two sides. This anomaly is very rare. Narrowing, due to hyperostosis, in a case of meningioma. Distension, caused by encroachment on the small and great wings of the sphenoid bone (i.e., by tumor or metastases) or by raised intracranial pressure. This may lead to the development of a cavernous sinus syndrome (superior orbital fissure syndrome), which consists of ophthalmoplegia with loss of corneal reflex, mydriasis and ptosis. The condition may be caused by circumscribed processes around the cavernous sinus, especially near the points of exit of the 3rd to 6th cranial nerves in the region of the superior orbital fissure. If the optic chiasma or optic tract are affected, deficits in the field of vision will occur.
7 Pterygoid process
8 Pterygoid hamulus
9 Medial plate of pterygoid process
10 Lateral plate
11 Coronoid process
13 Pterygoid canal
14 Opening into sphenoidal sinus

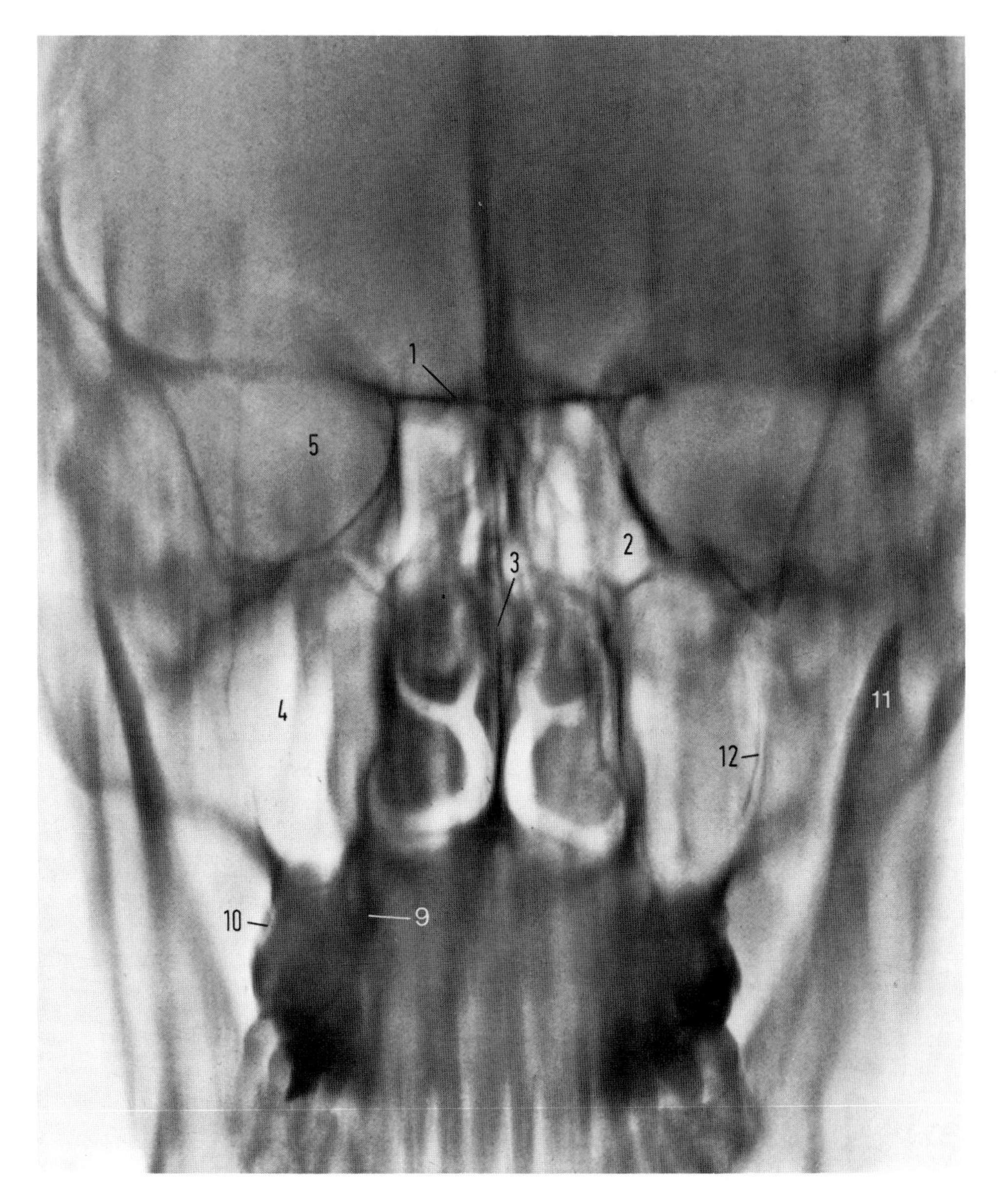

Fig. 204. Distance of layer 6.5 cm from front.

1 Cribriform plate of ethmoidal bone
2 Posterior ethmoidal cells
3 Bony nasal septum (perpendicular plate and vomer)
4 Posterior wall of maxillary sinus
5 Posterior wall of orbita; caudal portion: orbital surface of great wings of sphenoid bone
9 Medial plate of pterygoid process
10 Lateral plate of pterygoid process
11 Coronoid process
12 Pterygopalatine canal

On a tomograph, one can see only a few ethmoidal cells completely surrounded by bone when the septa are at right angles to the plane of the layer (see also Figs. 214 and 215).

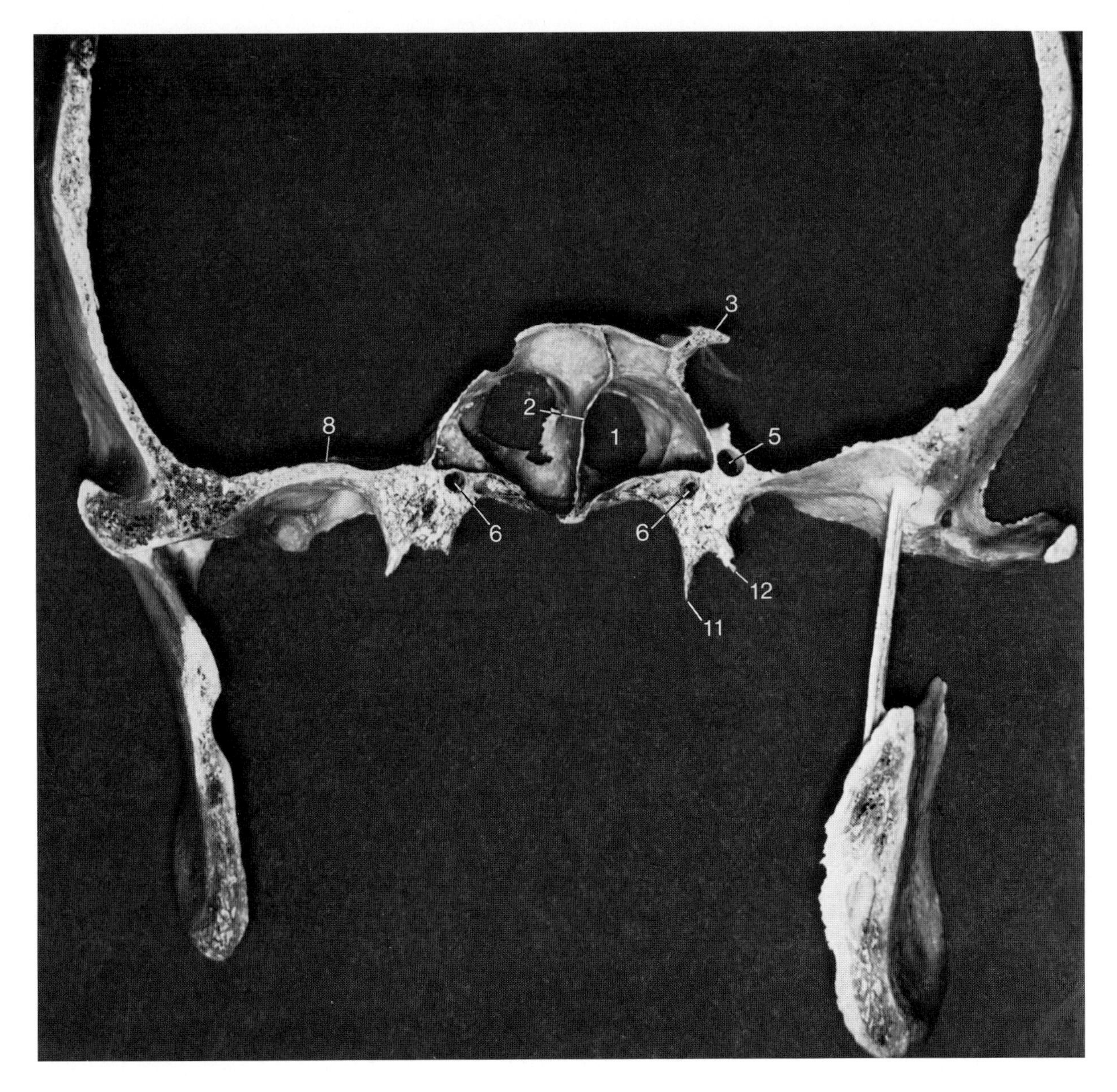

Fig. 205. Front view of the skeletal section of the skull (corresponding to Fig. 206).

1 Sphenoidal sinus
2 Septum of sphenoidal sinus
3 Anterior clinoid process
5 Foramen rotundum
6 Pterygoid canal
8 Middle cranial fossa
11 Medial plate of pterygoid process
12 Lateral plate of pterygoid process

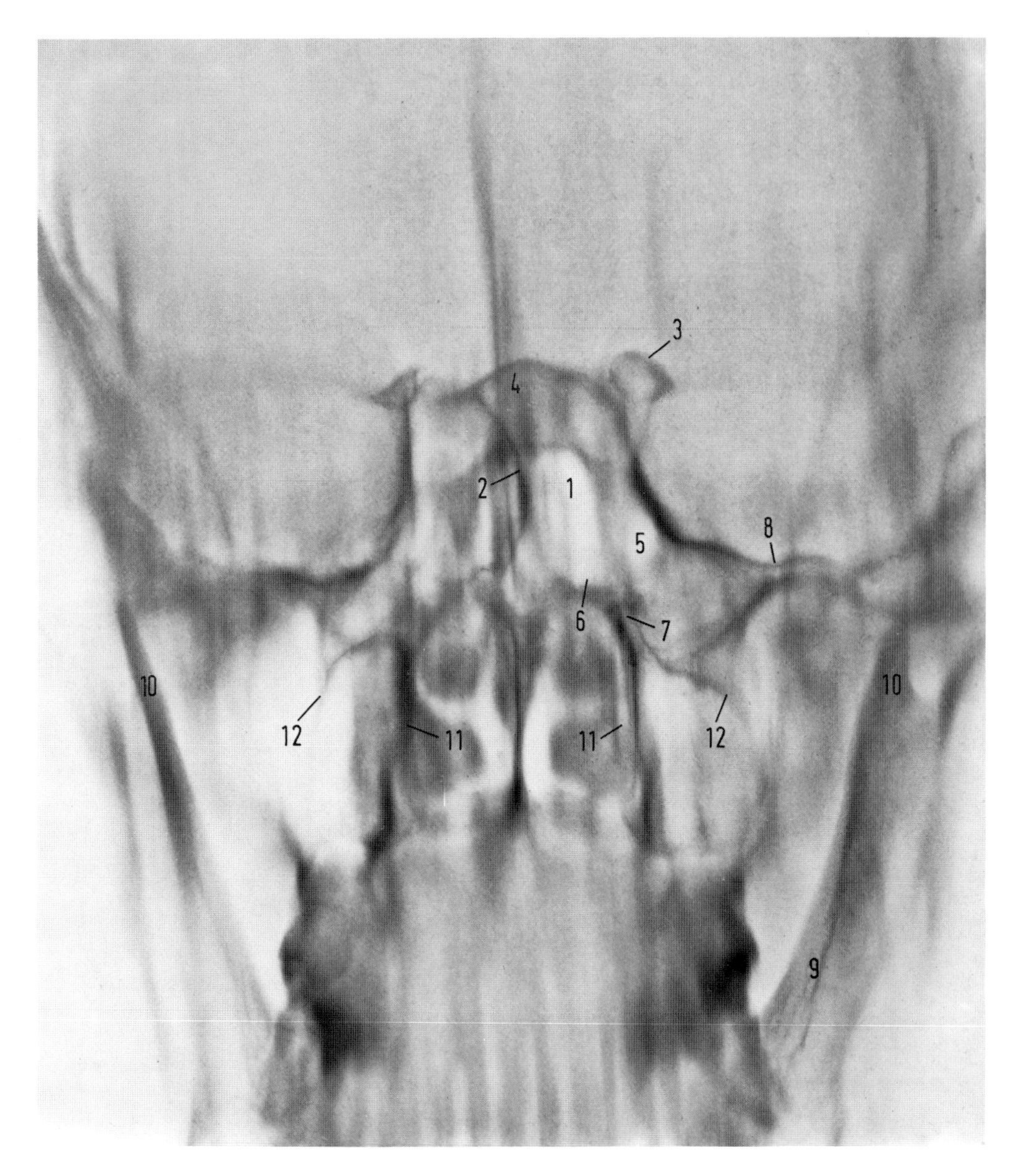

Fig. 206. Distance of layer 7.5 cm from front.

1 Sphenoidal sinus
2 Septum of sphenoidal sinus
3 Anterior clinoid process
4 Dorsum sellae (visible through sphenoidal sinus)
5 Foramen rotundum
6 Pterygoid canal
7 Major palatine sulcus
8 Medial cranial fossa
9 Mandible
10 Coronoid process
11 Medial plate of pterygoid process
12 Lateral plate of pterygoid process

The foramen rotundum may vary in size and shape between the right and left sides. Here, on both the skeletal section and the tomograph, only the left is shown. The tomographic demonstration of the foramen rotundum is important for traumatology, among other conditions, as two of three typical fracture lines of the middle and anterior cranial fossa pass here (passage of the second trigeminal division = maxillary nerve).

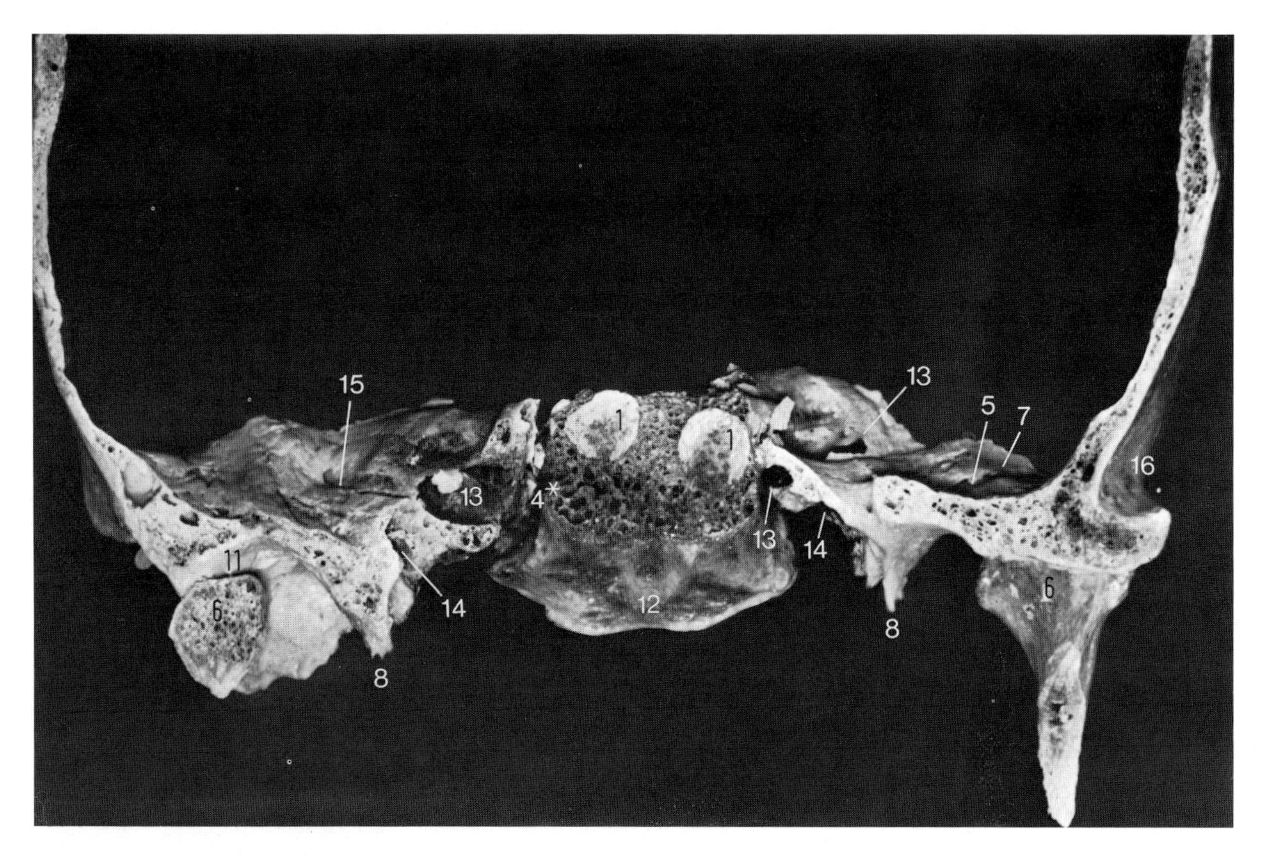

Fig. 207. Front view of skeletal section (corresponding to Fig. 208).

1 Dorsal portion of sphenoidal sinus (posterior wall)
4* Petrooccipital fissure
5 Middle cranial fossa
6 Condyloid process
7 Petrosquamous fissure
8 Sphenoidal spine
11 Mandibular fossa
12 Basilar part of occipital bone; above it: body of sphenoid bone
13 Opening of carotid canal
14 Musculotubal canal
15 Sulcus of greater superficial petrosal nerve
16 Temporal fossa

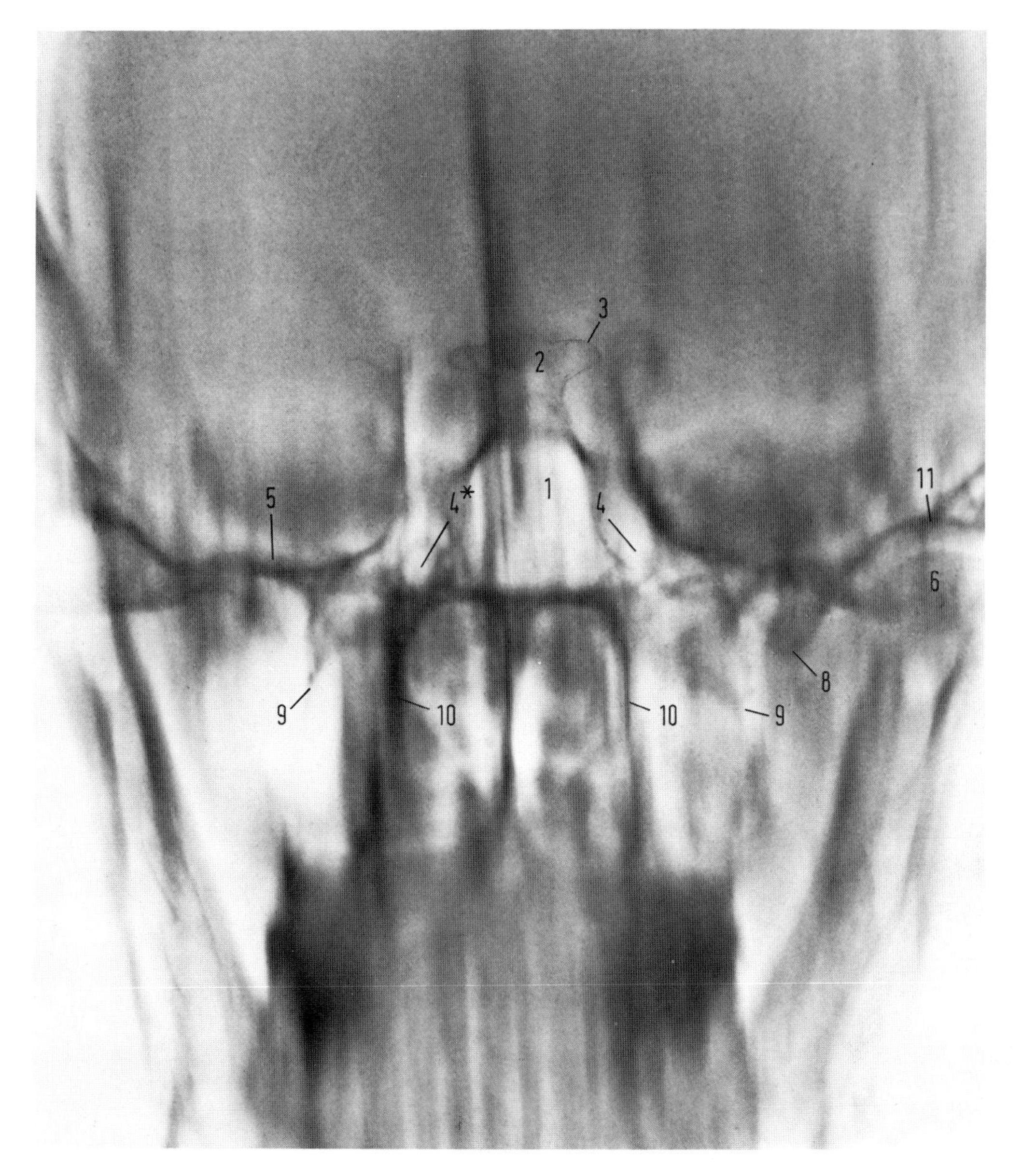

Fig. 208. Distance of layer 9.0 cm from front.

1 Dorsal portion of sphenoidal sinus (posterior wall)
2 Dorsum sellae
3 Posterior clinoid process
4 Foramen rotundum
4* Petrooccipital fissure
5 Middle cranial fossa
6 Condyloid process
8 Sphenoidal spine
9 Lateral plate of pterygoid process
10 Medial plate of pterygoid process
11 Mandibular fossa

5. Horizontal (transverse) saw-cut bone sections and corresponding axial tomographs of the living (Figs. 209 and 219).

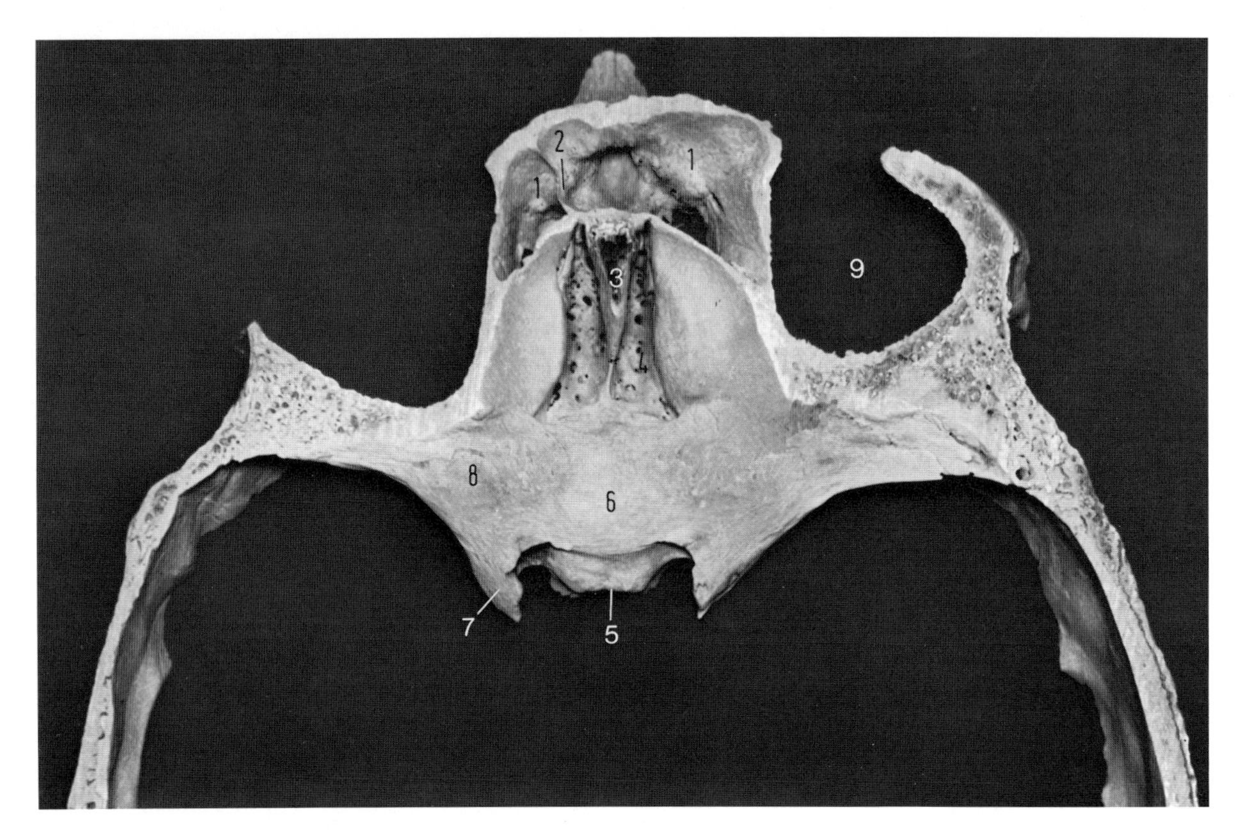

Fig. 209. Skeletal section, from cranial (to Figs. 210 and 211).

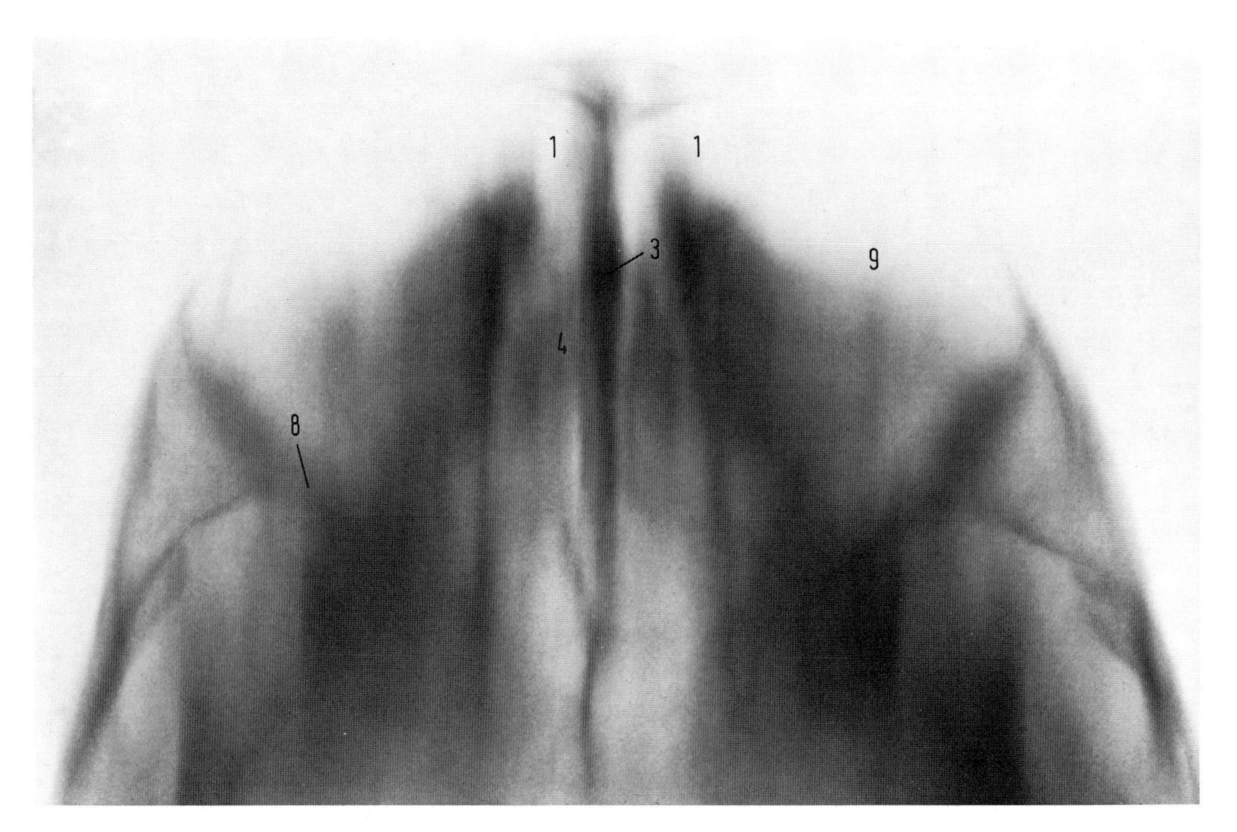

Fig. 210. Distance of layer 9.75 cm from cranial. For positioning, see Fig. 91.

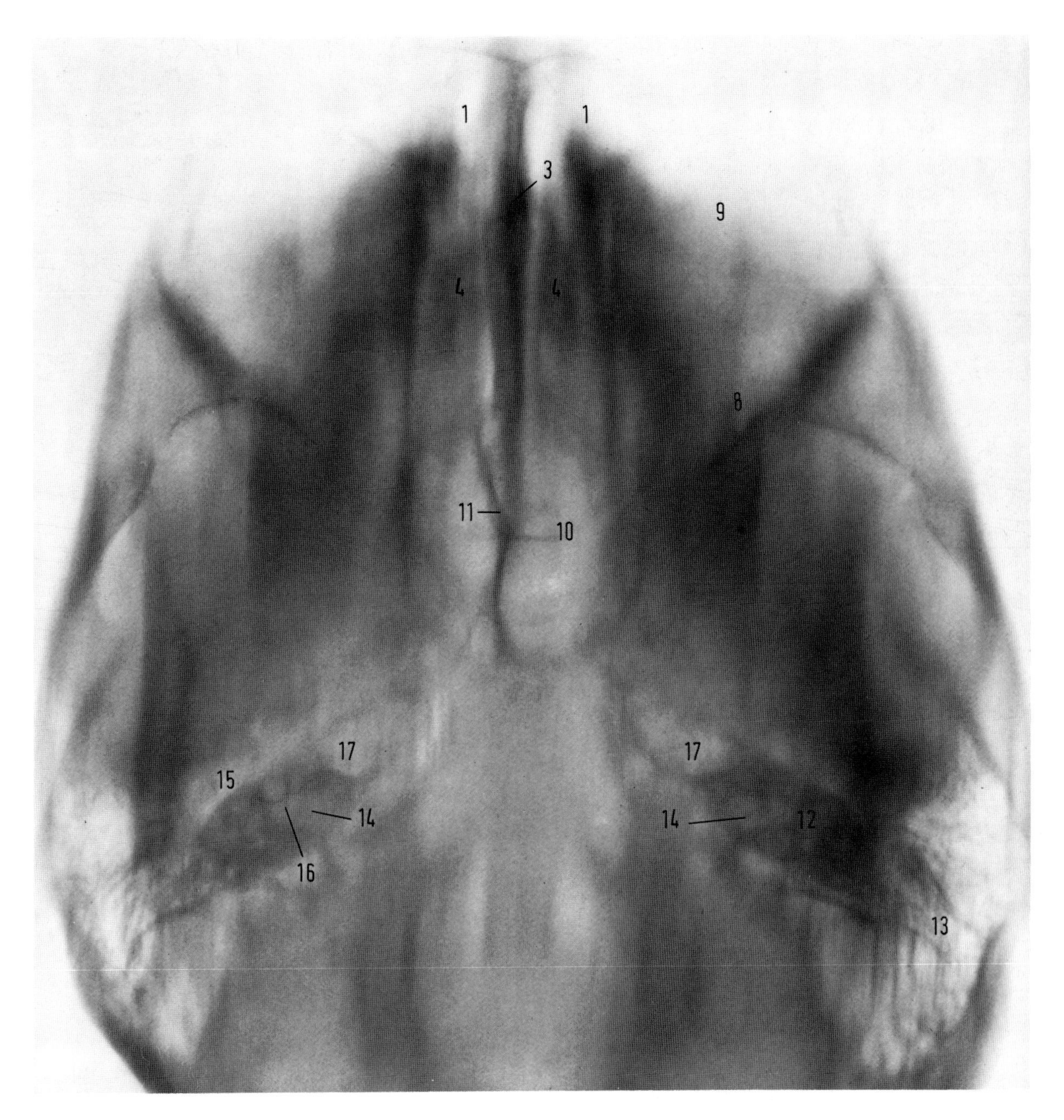

Fig. 211. Distance of layer 11.0 cm from cranial. Patient supine, with hyperextended head. Compare position to Fig. 91.

To Figs. 209, 210 and 211:

1 Frontal sinus
2 Septum of frontal sinus
3 Crista galli
4 Cribriform plate of ethmoid bone
5 Tuberculum sellae
6 Body of sphenoid bone
7 Anterior clinoid process
8 Small wing
9 Orbita
10 Sphenoidal sinus
11 Septum of sphenoidal sinus
12 Petrous bone
13 Pneumatic system of mastoid process
14 Internal auditory meatus
15 Tympanic cavity with adjoining antrum
16 Cochlea
17 Foramen lacerum

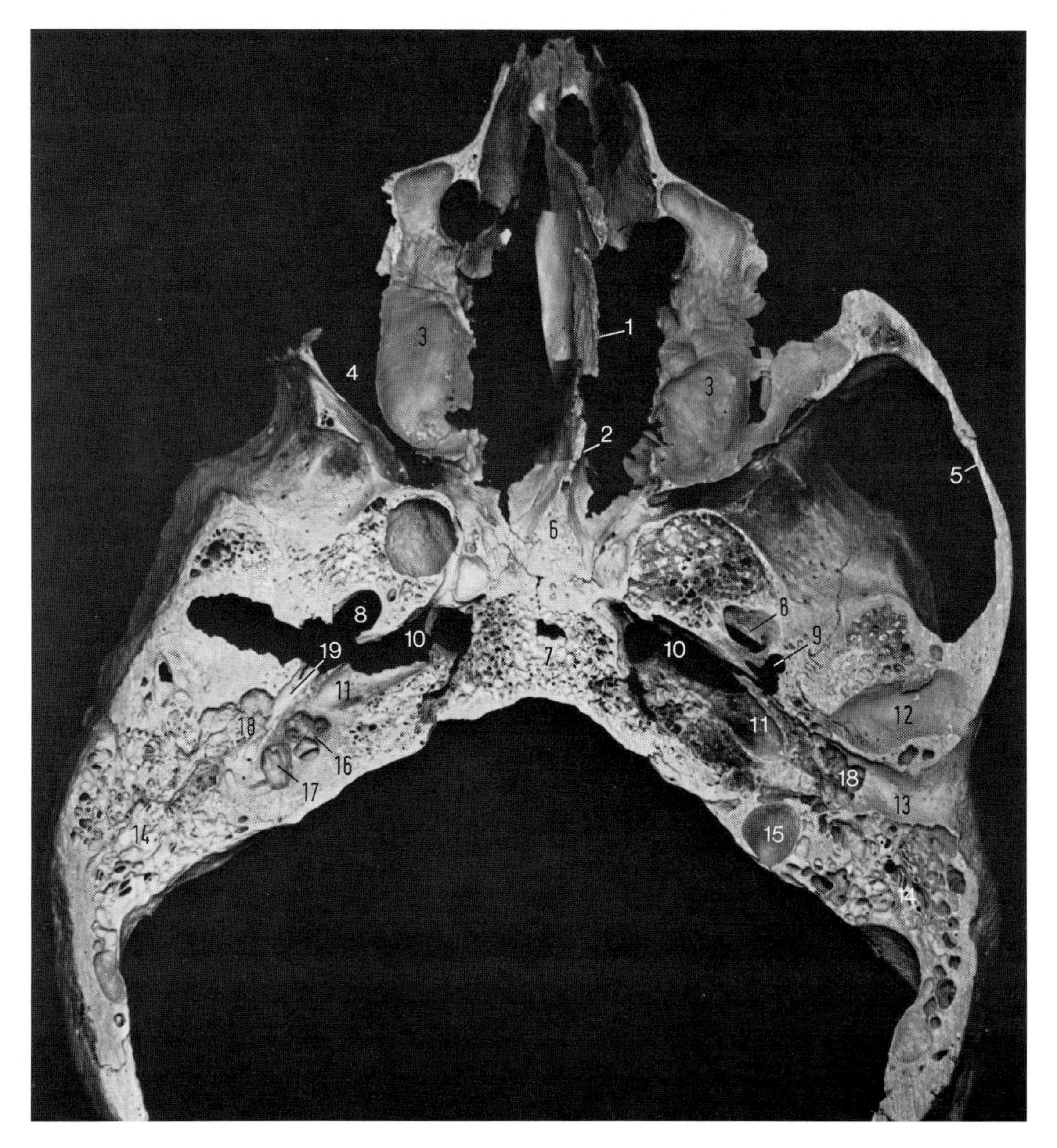

Fig. 212. Skeletal section, seen caudally, at corresponding depth (corresponding to Figs. 213 and 215).

1 Perpendicular plate
2 Sphenoidal crest
3 Roof of maxillary sinus
4 Inferior orbital fissure
5 Zygomatic arch
6 Body of sphenoid bone
7 Basilar part of occipital bone
8 Foramen ovale
9 Foramen spinosum
10 Foramen lacerum
11 Carotid canal
12 Mandibular fossa
13 External auditory meatus
14 Pneumatic system of mastoid process
15 Jugular foramen
16 Cochlea
17 Vestibule with the lateral part of the bony ampulla and of the semicircular canal
18 Tympanic cavity
19 Musculotubal canal

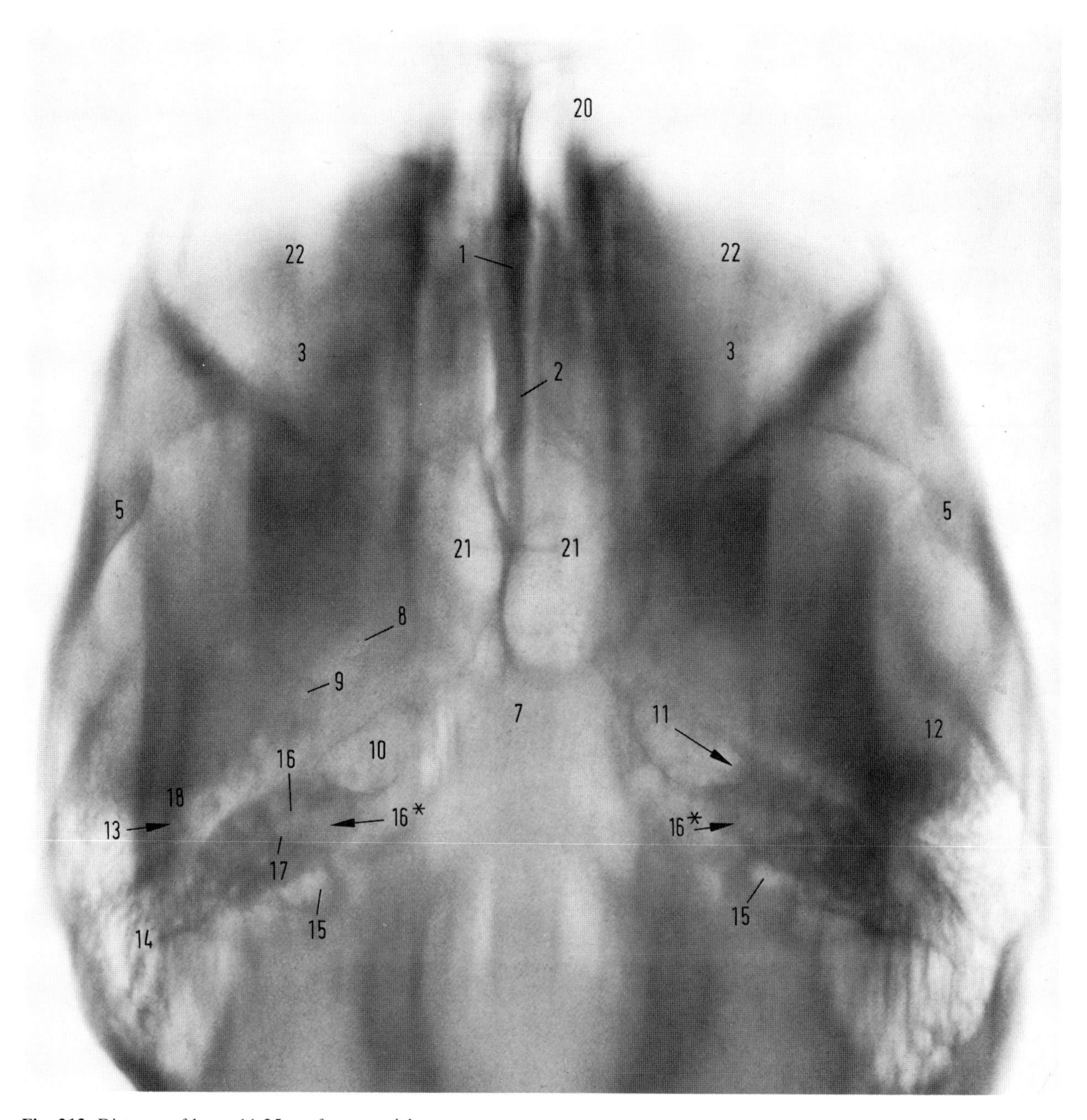

Fig. 213. Distance of layer 11.25 cm from cranial.

1 Perpendicular plate
2 Sphenoidal crest
3 Roof of maxillary sinus
5 Zygomatic arch
7 Basilar part of occipital bone
8 Foramen ovale
9 Foramen spinosum
10 Foramen lacerum
11 Carotid canal
12 Mandibular fossa
13 External auditory meatus
14 Pneumatic system of mastoid process
15 Jugular foramen
16 Cochlea
16* Internal auditory meatus
17 Vestibule with the lateral part of the bony ampulla and of the semicircular canal
18 Tympanic cavity
20 Frontal sinus
21 Sphenoidal sinus
22 Orbita

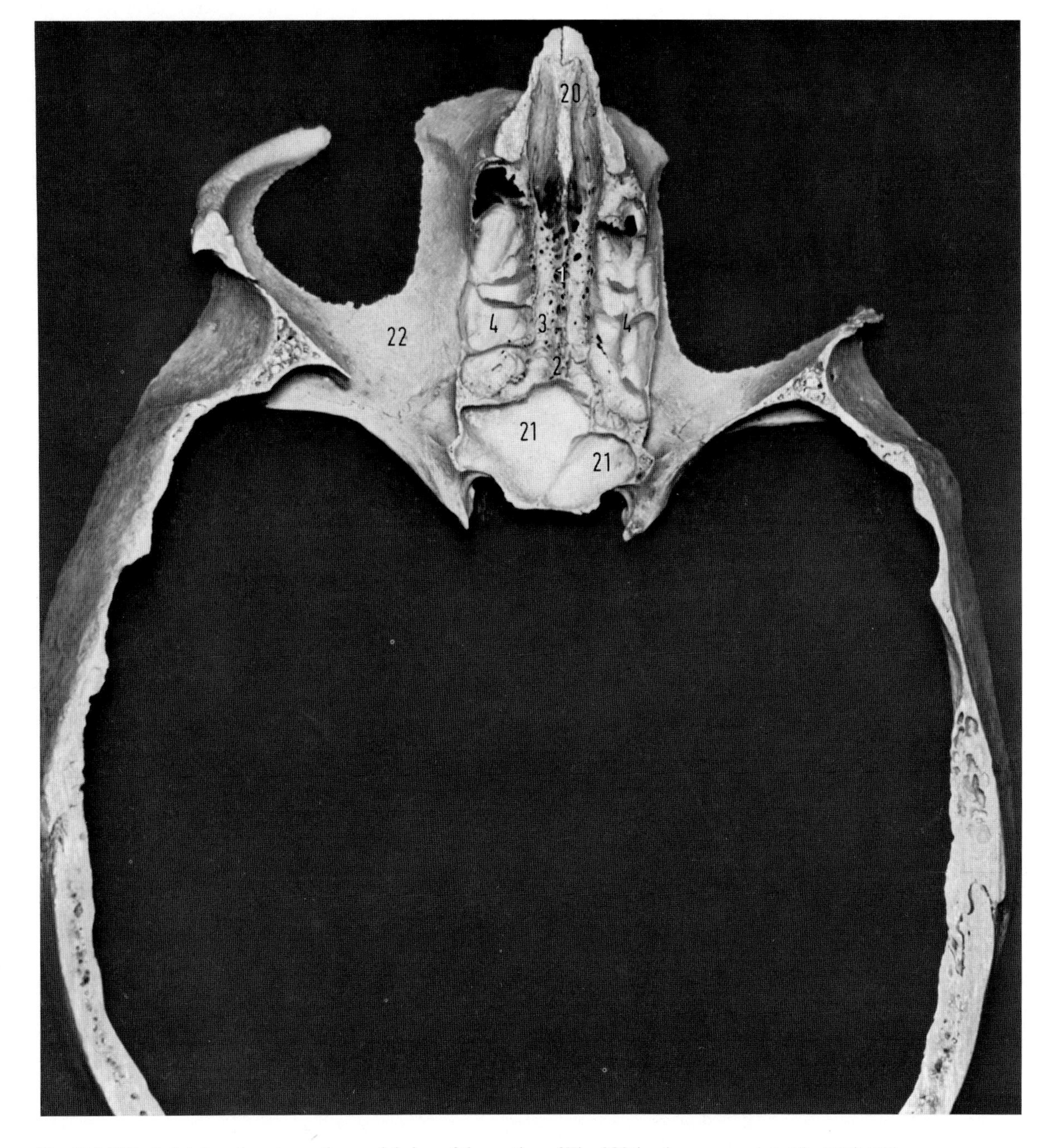

Fig. 214. This skeletal section shows the caudal view of the section of Fig. 209 (and corresponds to Fig. 215). This sequence was necessary due to a slightly different direction of the section plane, in comparison with the tomograph, in order to demonstrate the anatomical details of Fig. 215 in the anterior region of the corresponding skeletal section.

1 Perpendicular plate
2 Sphenoidal crest
3 Cribriform plate
4 Ethmoidal cells
20 Nasal bone
21 Sphenoidal sinus
22 Orbita

This skeletal layer (level, plane) shows the sphenoidal sinus and its relation to the posterior ethmoidal cells with their transverse septa. In Fig. 215 the sphenoidal sinuses are shown in complete depth. The anteriorly placed ethmoidal cells cannot be distinguished individually as their transverse septa are blurred (see also Fig. 204).

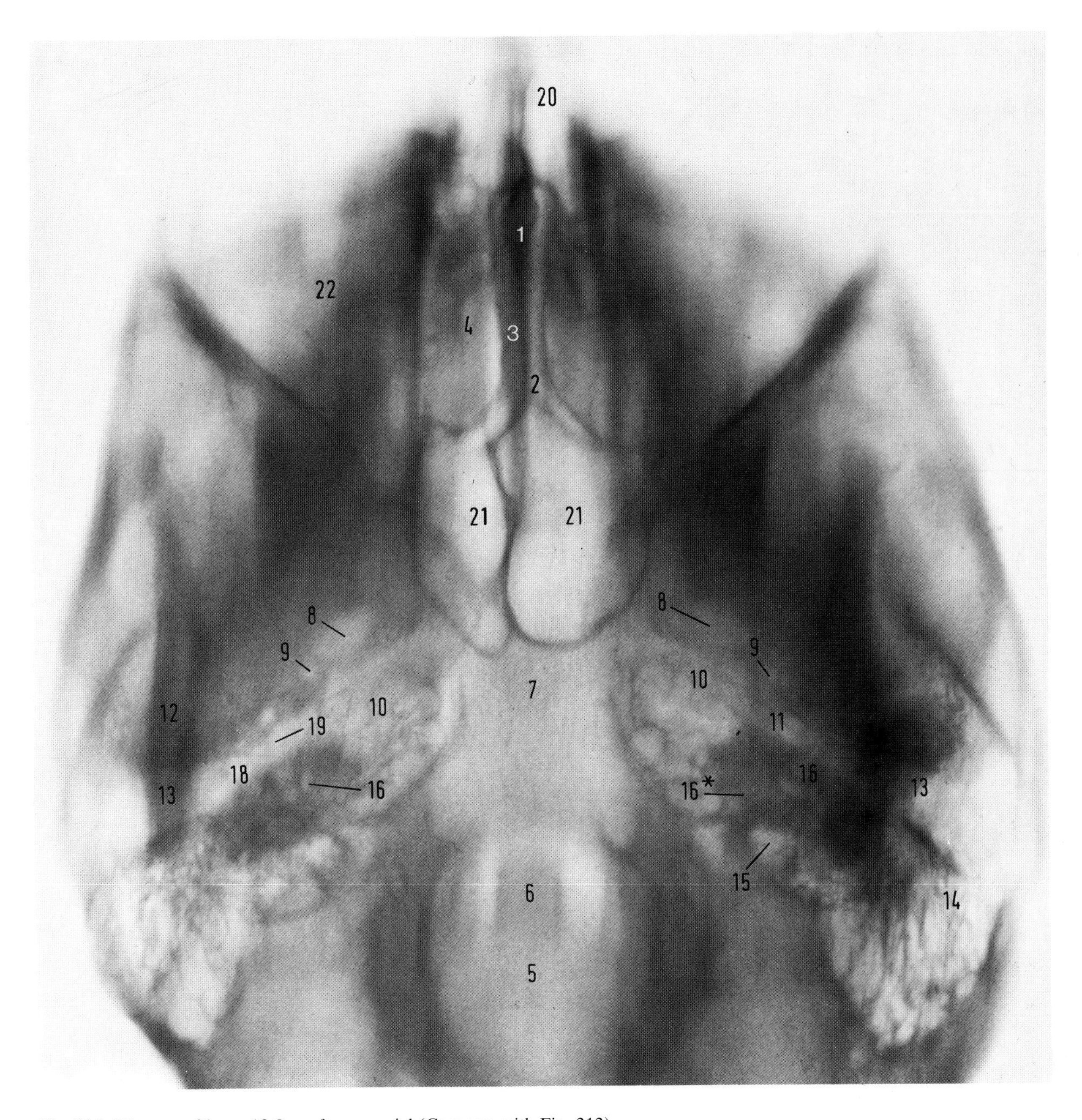

Fig. 215. Distance of layer 12.0 cm from cranial (Compare with Fig. 212).

1 Perpendicular plate
2 Sphenoidal crest
3 Cribriform plate
4 Ethmoidal cells
5 Foramen magnum
6 Dens (axis)
7 Basilar part
8 Foramen ovale
9 Foramen spinosum
10 Foramen lacerum
11 Carotid canal
12 Mandibular fossa
13 External auditory meatus
14 Pneumatic system of mastoid process
15 Jugular foramen
16 Cochlea
16* Internal auditory meatus
18 Tympanic cavity
19 Musculotubal canal
20 Nasal bone
21 Sphenoidal sinus
22 Orbita

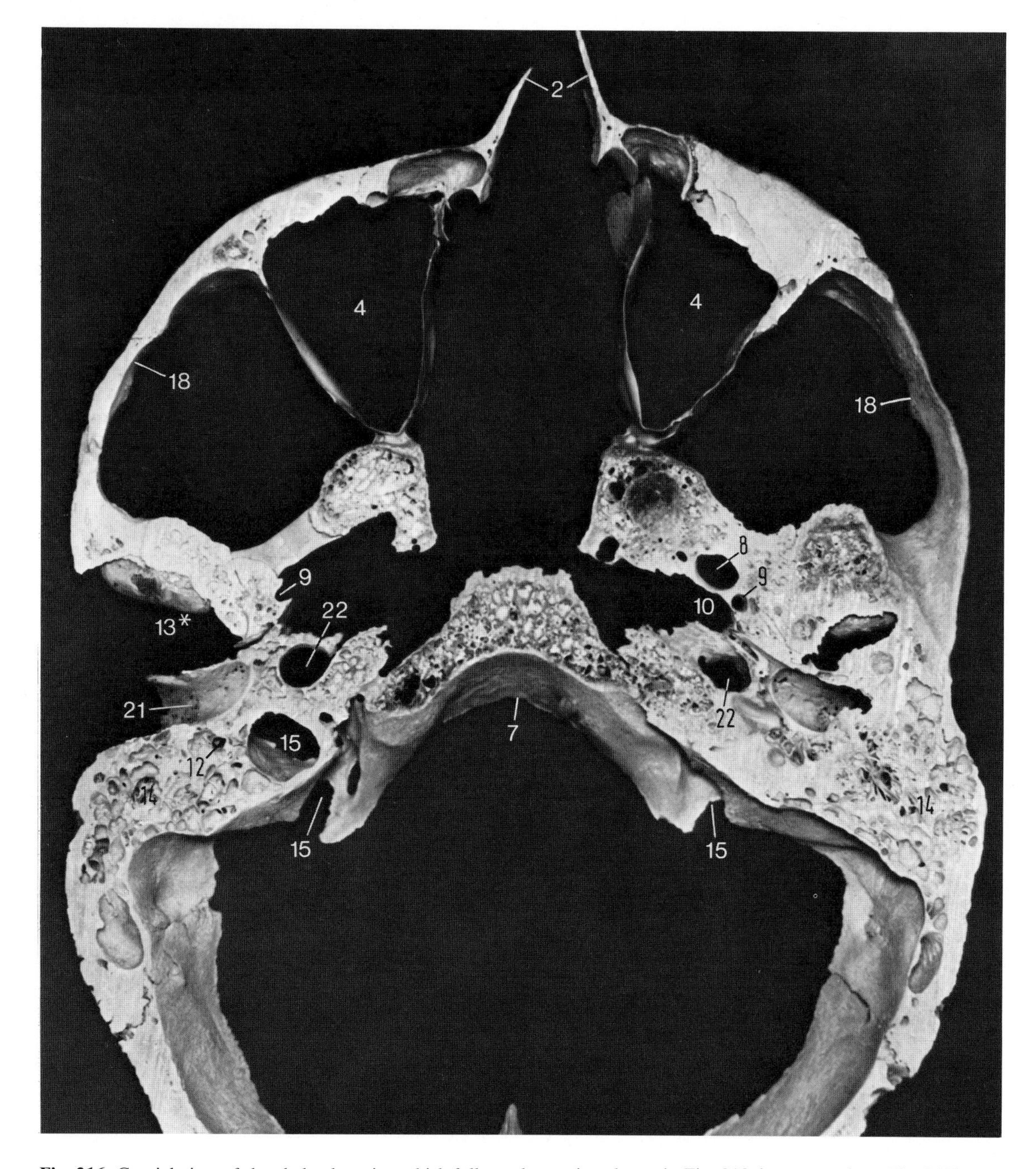

Fig. 216. Cranial view of the skeletal section which follows the section shown in Fig. 212 (corresponds to Fig. 217).

2 Nasal bone
4 Sinus maxillaris
7 Basilar part
8 Foramen ovale
9 Foramen spinosum
10 Foramen lacerum
12 Facial canal (terminating in caudal direction in the stylomastoid foramen)
13* Region of the mandibular fossa
14 Mastoid cells
15 Jugular foramen
18 Zygomatic arch
21 External auditory meatus
22 Carotid canal

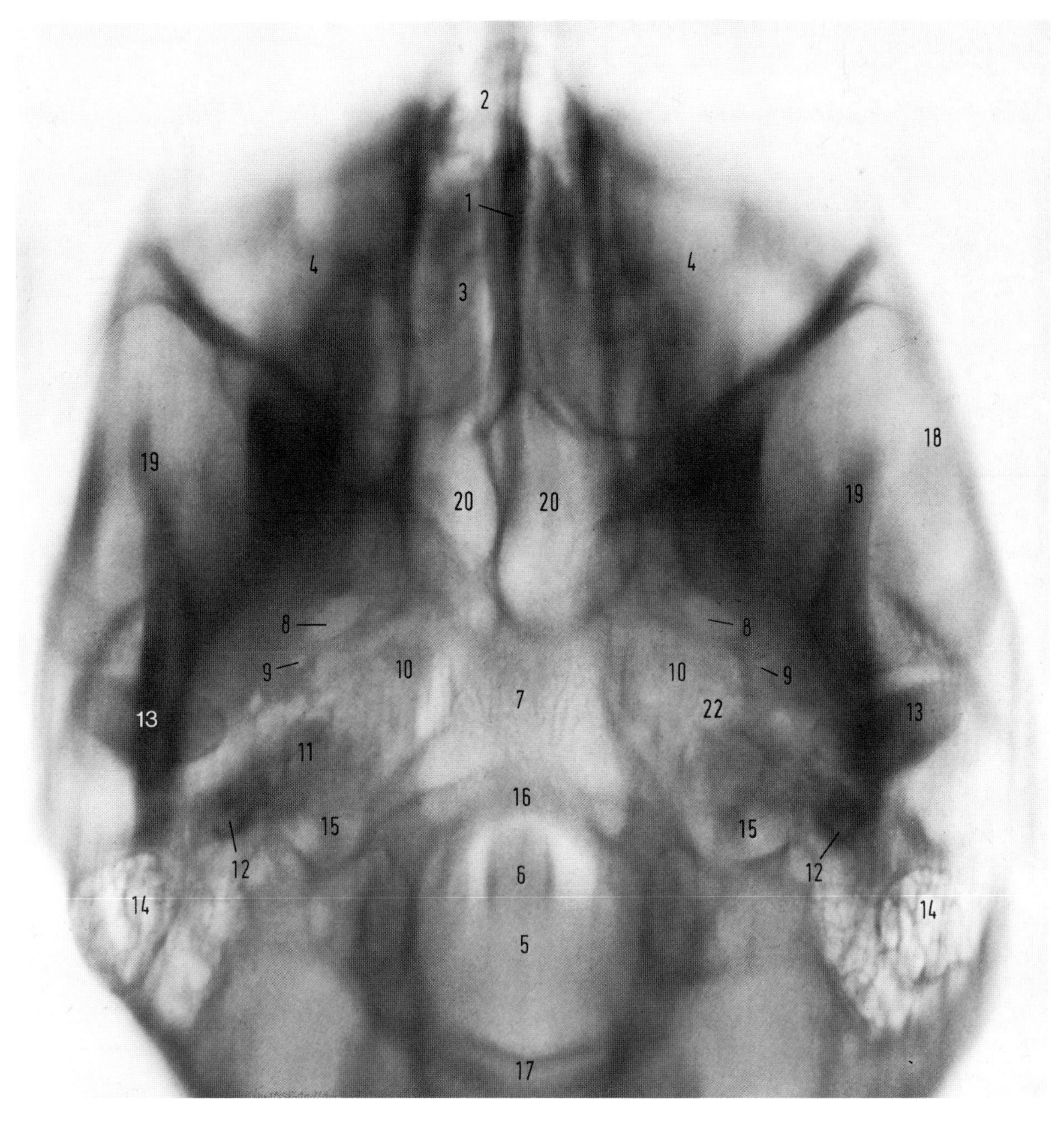

Fig. 217. Distance of layer 13.0 cm from cranial.

1 Bony nasal septum
2 Nasal bone
3 Ethmoidal cells
4 Maxillary sinus
5 Foramen magnum
6 Dens (axis)
7 Basilar part
8 Foramen ovale
9 Foramen spinosum
10 Foramen lacerum
11 Petrous bone
12 Facial canal (terminating in caudal direction in the stylomastoid foramen)
13 Condyloid process
14 Mastoid cells
15 Jugular foramen
16 Anterior arch of atlas
17 Posterior arch of atlas
18 Zygomatic arch
19 Coronoid process
20 Sphenoidal sinus with septum
22 Carotid canal

The foramina ovalia for the third division of the trigeminal nerve (mandibular nerve), and the foramina spinosa for the middle meningeal artery and for a recurrent branch of the mandibular nerve, may be of different lumen at either side. Only in cases of conspicuous difference in width should trauma or tumor be considered as its cause.

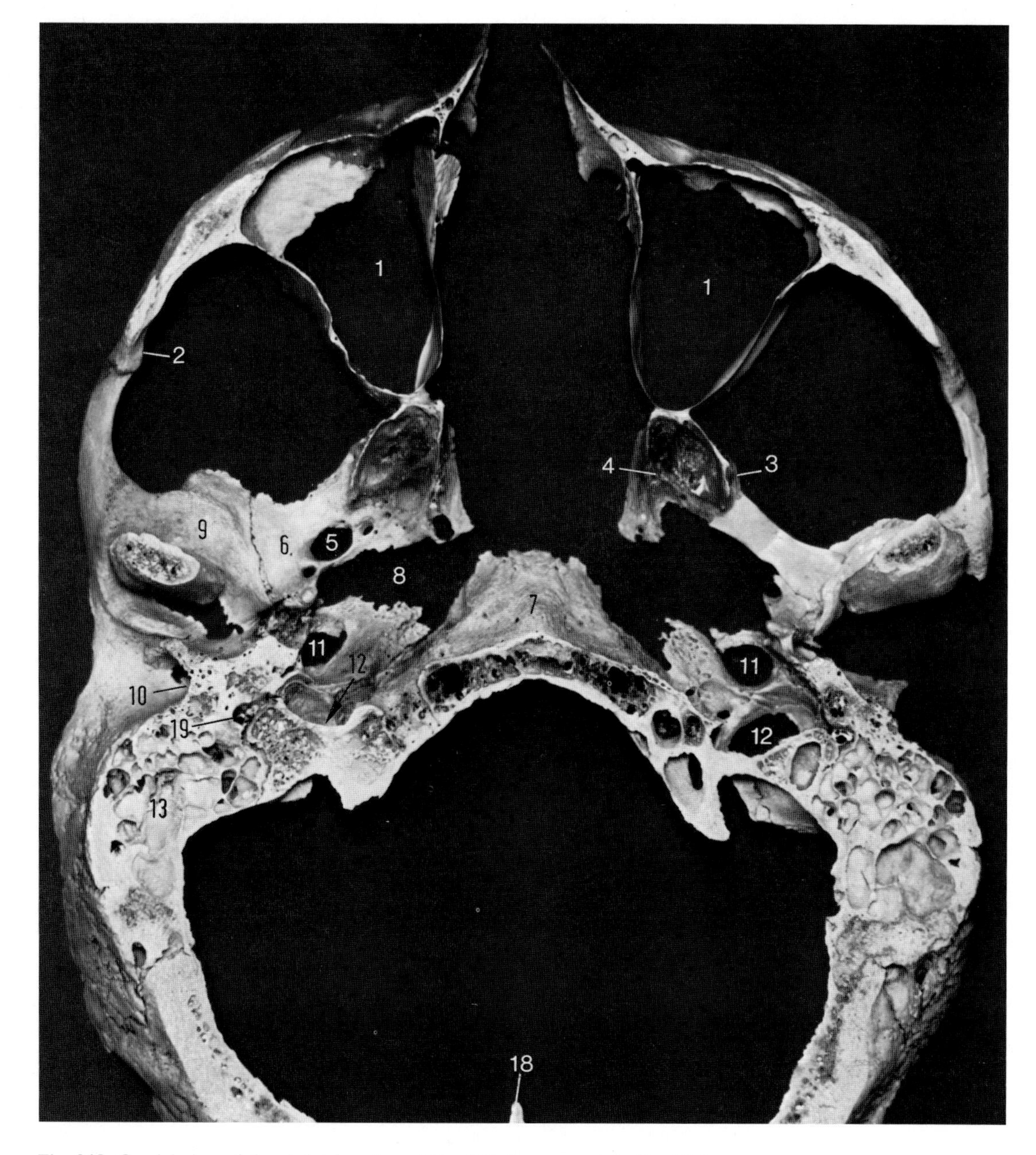

Fig. 218. Caudal view of the skeletal section of Fig. 216 (corresponds to Fig. 219).

1 Maxillary sinus
2 Zygomatic arch
3 Lateral plate of pterygoid process
4 Medial plate
5 Foramen ovale
6 Foramen spinosum
7 Basilar part
8 Foramen lacerum
9 Condyloid process
10 External orifice of auditory canal
11 Carotid canal
12 Jugular foramen
13 Mastoid cells
18 Internal occipital crest, a variable ridge on the inner surface of the occipital squama, leading from the internal occipital protuberance to the foramen magnum. It provides the line of attachment of the falx cerebri. See also Figs. 93 and 120.
19 Stylomastoid foramen (facial canal)

The vesicular cells of the pyramid, which vary in size, extend into the temporal squama, as shown on the skeletal section as well as on the tomograph.

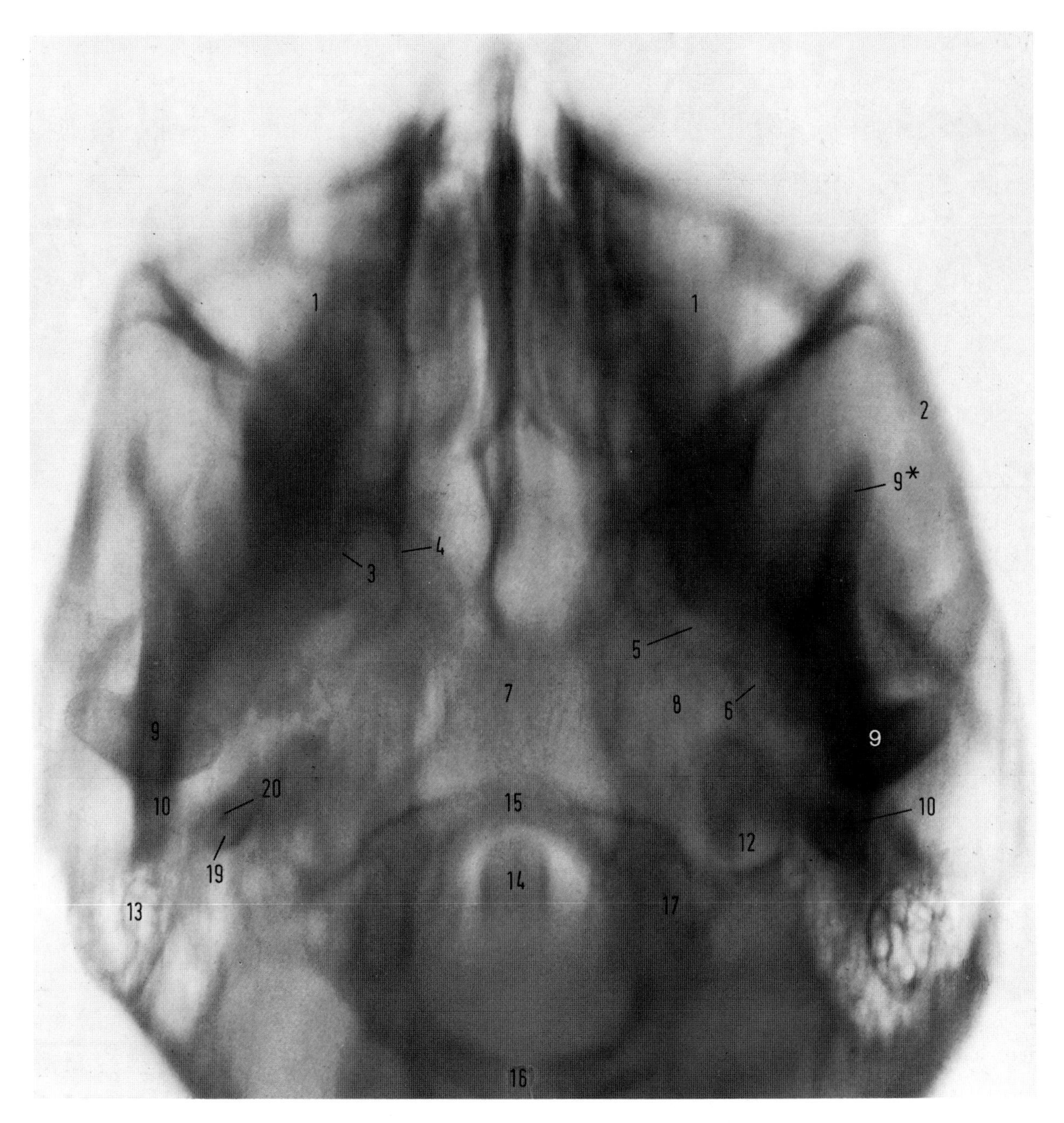

Fig. 219. Distance of layer 13.5 cm from cranial.

1 Maxillary sinus
2 Zygomatic arch
3 Lateral plate of pterygoid process
4 Medial plate
5 Foramen ovale
6 Foramen spinosum
7 Basilar part
8 Foramen lacerum
9 Condyloid process
9* Coronoid process
10 External orifice of auditory canal
12 Jugular foramen
13 Mastoid cells
14 Dens (axis)
15 Anterior arch of atlas
16 Posterior arch of atlas
17 Lateral mass of atlas
19 Stylomastoid foramen (facial canal)
20 Styloid process

6. Sagittal and parasagittal saw-cut bone sections and corresponding lateral tomographs of the living (Figs. 220–231).

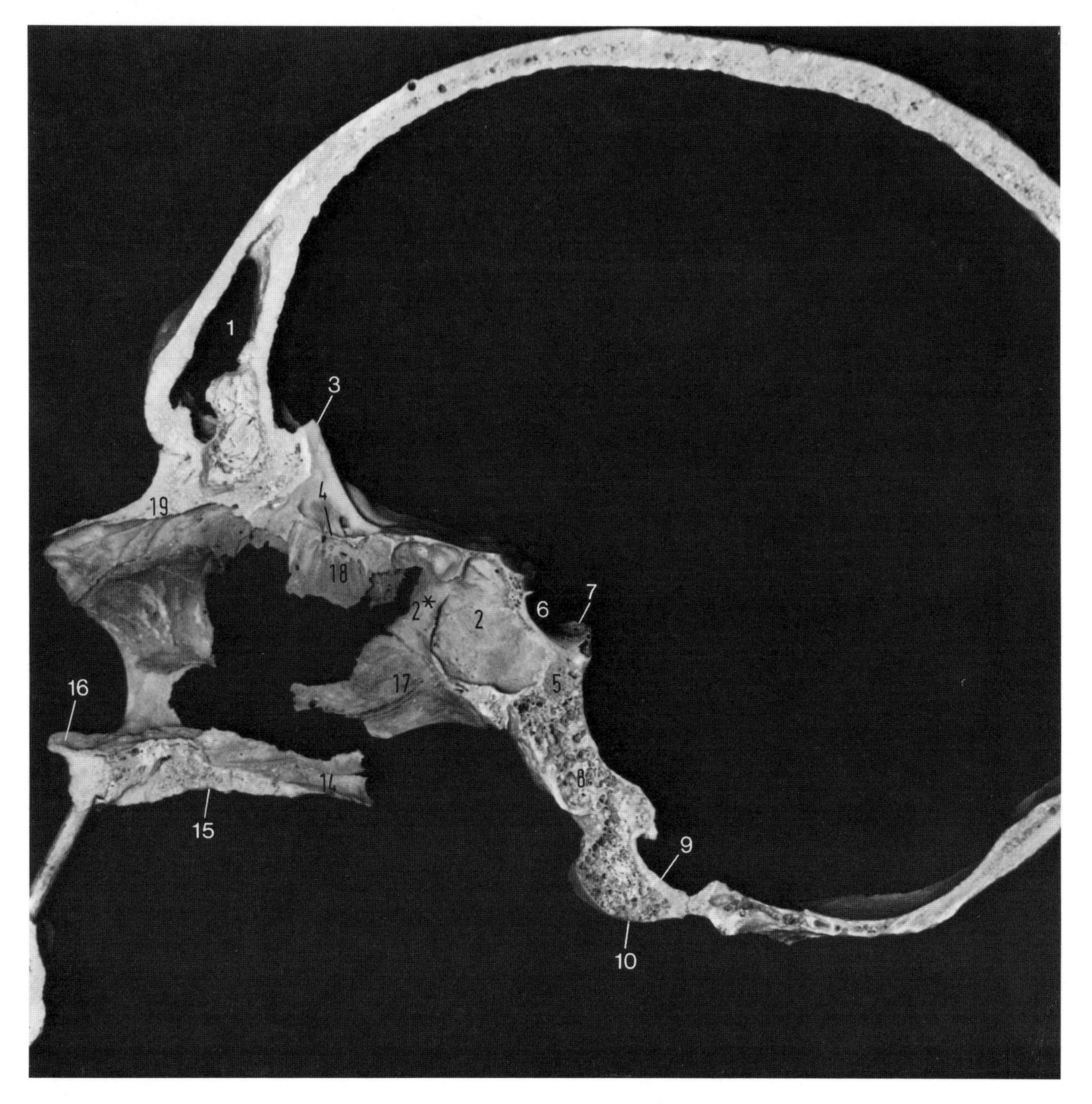

Fig. 220, corresponding to Fig. 221.

1 Frontal sinus
2 Sphenoidal sinus
2* Sphenoidal crest
3 Crista galli
4 Cribriform plate
5 Body of sphenoid bone
6 Sella turcica
7 Dorsum sellae with posterior clinoid process
8 Basilar part
9 Region of foramen magnum
10 Occipital condyle
14 Horizontal plate of palatine bone
15 Palatine process of maxilla
16 Anterior nasal spine
17 Vomer
18 Perpendicular plate of ethmoid bone bony nasal septum
19 Nasal bone

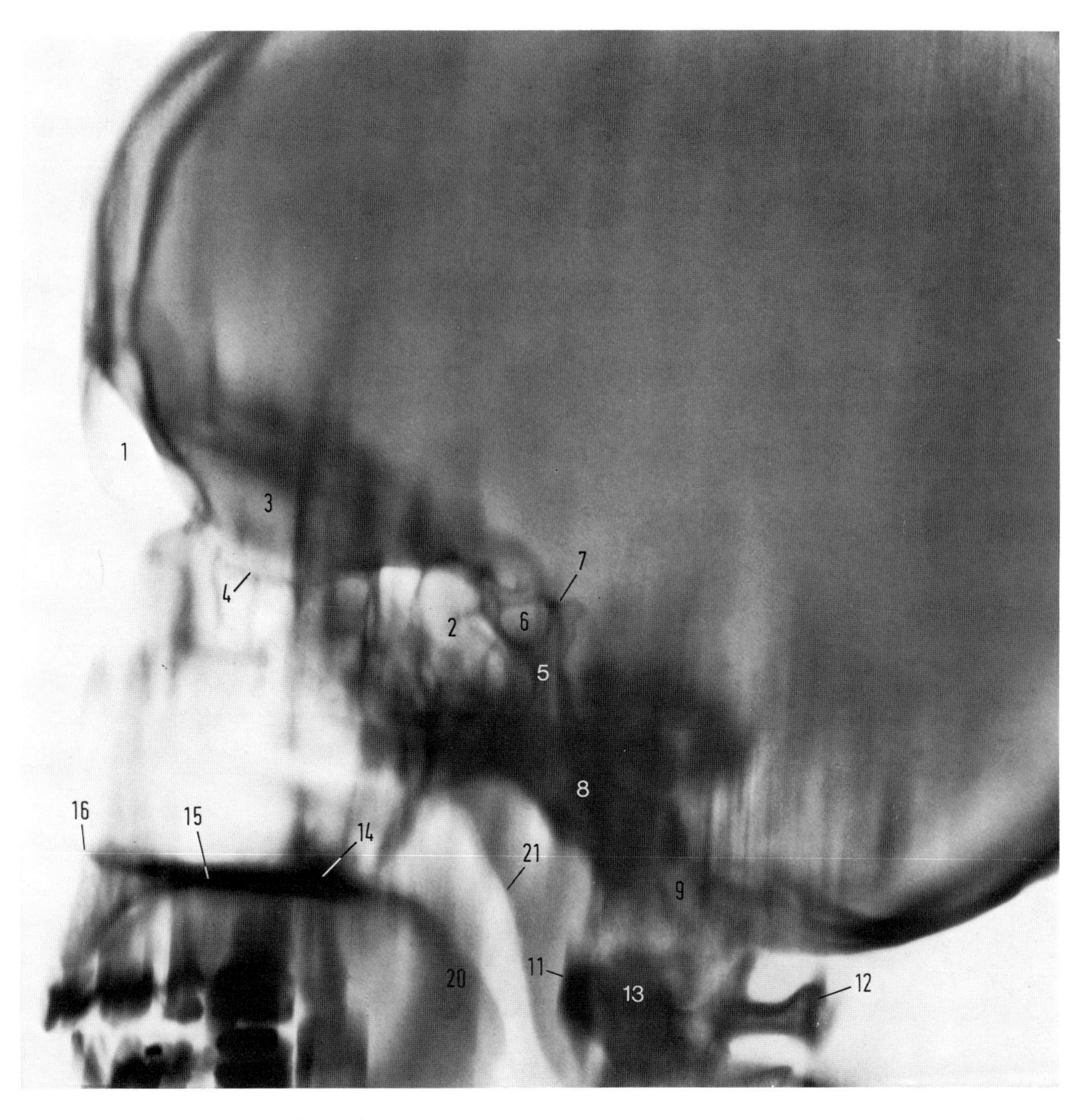

Fig. 221. Distance of layer 6.0 cm from left.

1 Frontal sinus
2 Sphenoidal sinus
3 Crista galli
4 Cribriform plate
5 Body of sphenoid bone
6 Sella turcica
7 Dorsum sellae with posterior clinoid process
8 Basilar part
9 Region of foramen magnum
11 Anterior arch of atlas with anterior tubercle
12 Posterior arch of atlas with posterior tubercle
13 Dens (axis)
14 Horizontal plate of palatine bone
15 Palatine process of maxilla
16 Anterior nasal spine
20 Soft palate
21 Posterior pharyngeal wall

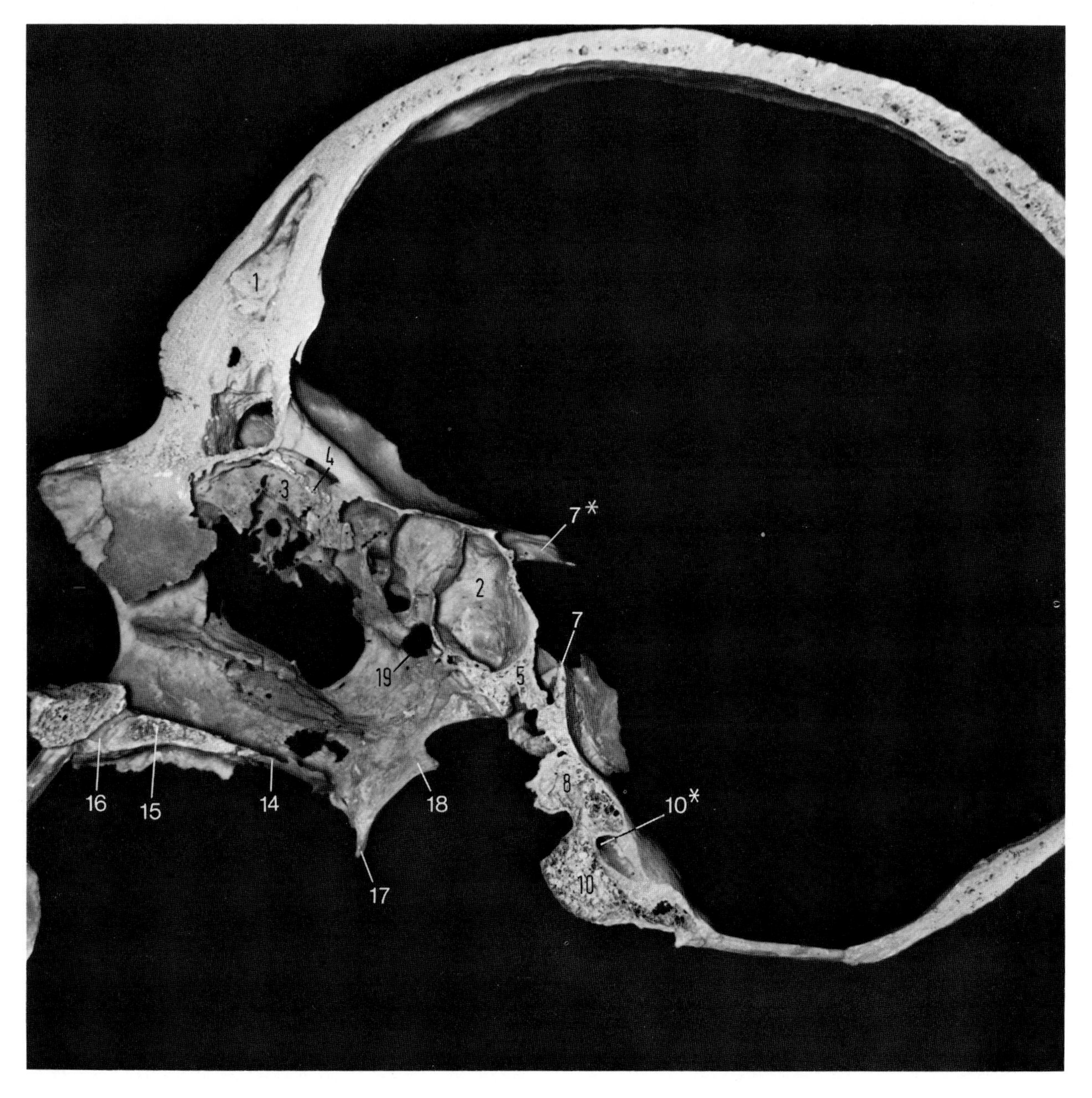

Fig. 222 (corresponding to Fig. 223).

1 Frontal sinus
2 Sphenoidal sinus
3 Ethmoidal cells
4 Cribriform plate of ethmoid bone
5 Body of sphenoid bone
7 Dorsum sellae
7* Small wing
8 Basilar part
10 Occipital condyle
10* Hypoglossal canal
14 Horizontal part of palatine bone
15 Palatine process of maxilla
16 Incisive canal
17 Pterygoid hamulus
18 Lateral plate of pterygoid process
19 Sphenopalatine foramen

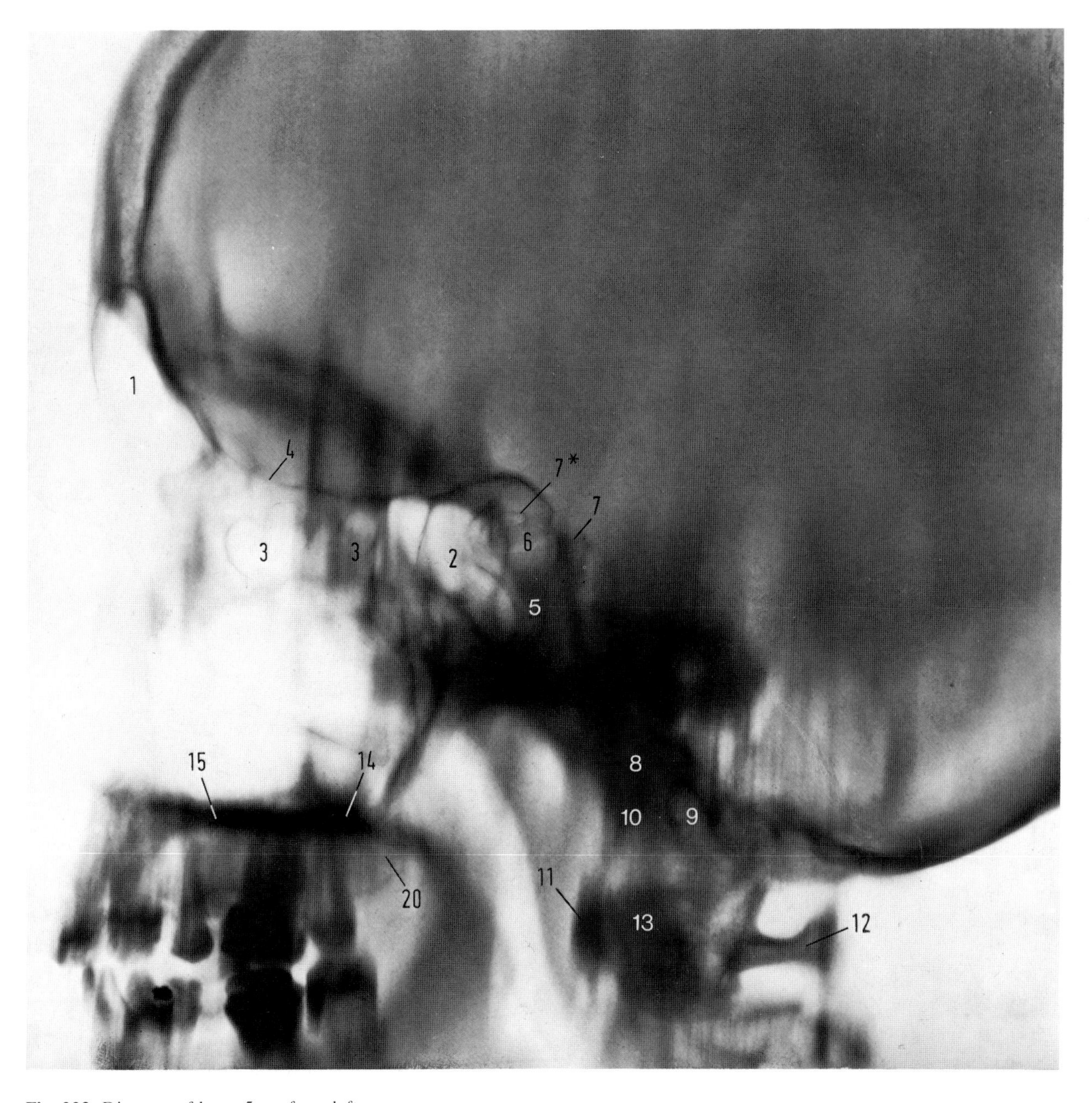

Fig. 223. Distance of layer 5 cm from left.

1 Frontal sinus
2 Sphenoidal sinus
3 Ethmoidal cells
4 Cribriform plate of ethmoid bone
5 Body of sphenoid bone
6 Sella turcica
7 Dorsum sellae
7* Small wing
8 Basilar part
9 Region of foramen magnum
10 Occipital condyle
11 Anterior arch of atlas
12 Posterior arch of atlas
13 Dens (axis)
14 Horizontal plate of palatine bone
15 Palatine process of maxilla
20 Pterygoid process

The lateral tomograph is well suited for evaluation of the extent of the paranasal cavities. In addition, fractures of the posterior wall of the frontal sinuses, severed bony splinters, or defects in the walls of the frontal and sphenoidal sinuses can be demonstrated. The paramedial lateral tomographs (Figs. 229 and 231) are indispensable for discerning the expansion of the maxillary sinus posteriorly.

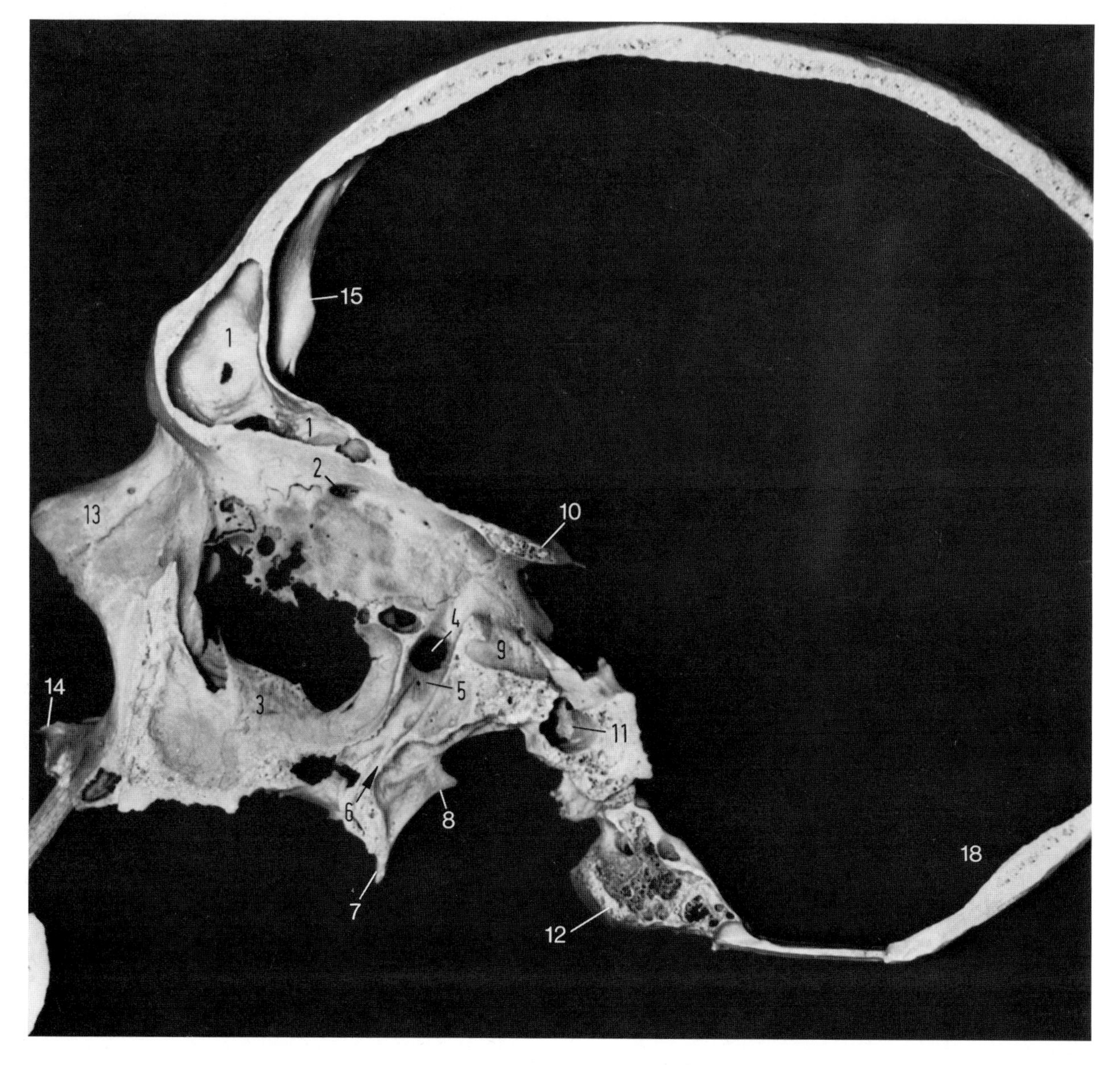

Fig. 224 (corresponding to Fig. 225).

1 Frontal sinus with recess
2 Anterior ethmoidal foramen
3 Maxillary sinus
4 Sphenopalatine foramen
5 Pterygopalatine fossa
6 Pterygopalatine canal (canalis palatinus major)
7 Pterygoid hamulus
8 Lateral plate of pterygoid process
9 Foramen rotundum
10 Small wing
11 Carotid canal
12 Occipital condyle
13 Nasal bone
14 Anterior nasal spine
15 Frontal crest
18 Posterior cranial fossa

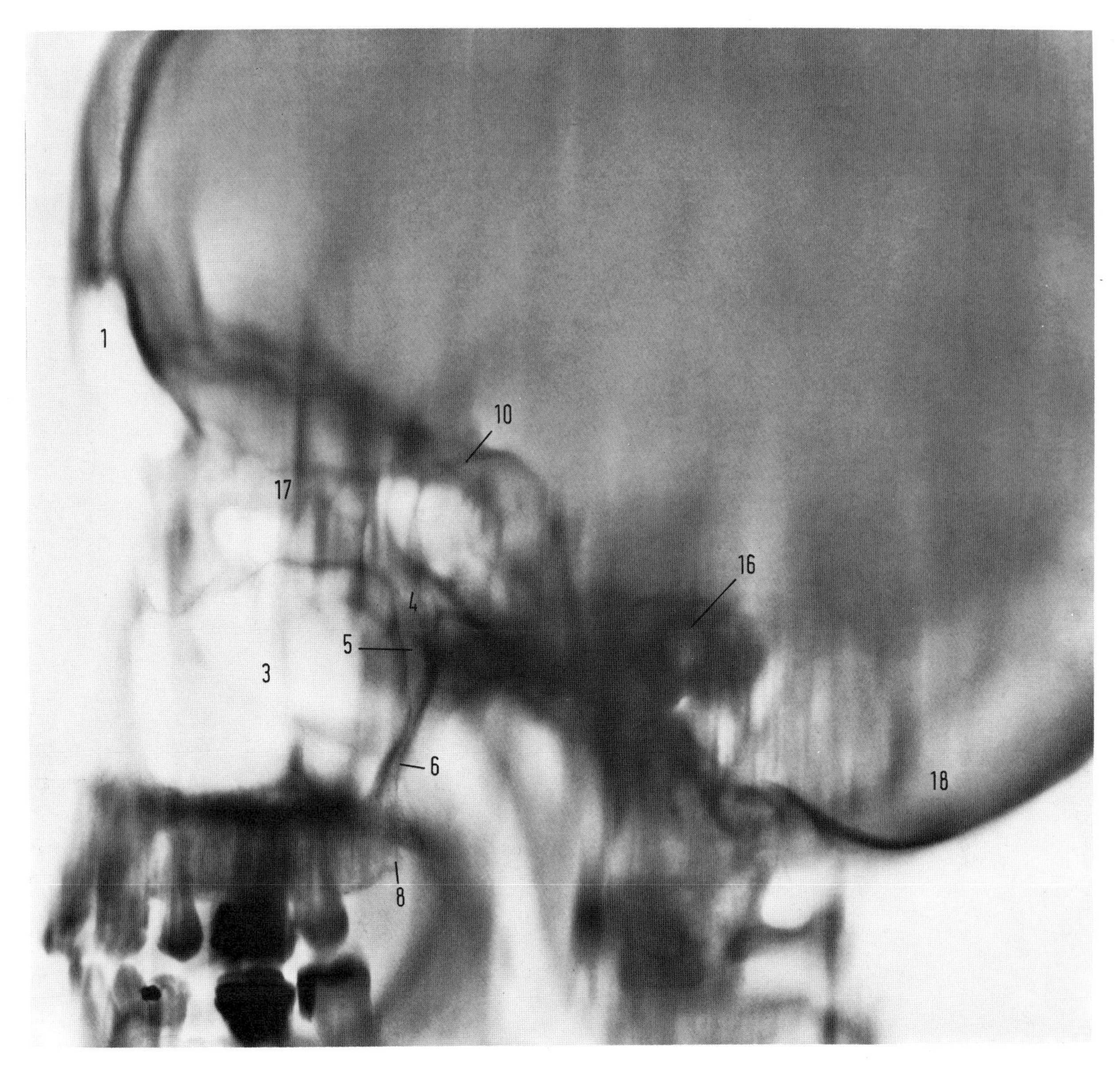

Fig. 225. Distance of layer 4.5 cm from left.

1 Frontal sinus with recess
3 Maxillary sinus
4 Sphenopalatine foramen
5 Pterygopalatine fossa
6 Pterygopalatine canal (canalis palatinus major)
8 Lateral plate of pterygoid process
10 Small wing
16 Internal orifice of auditory canal
17 Ethmoidal cells
18 Posterior cranial fossa

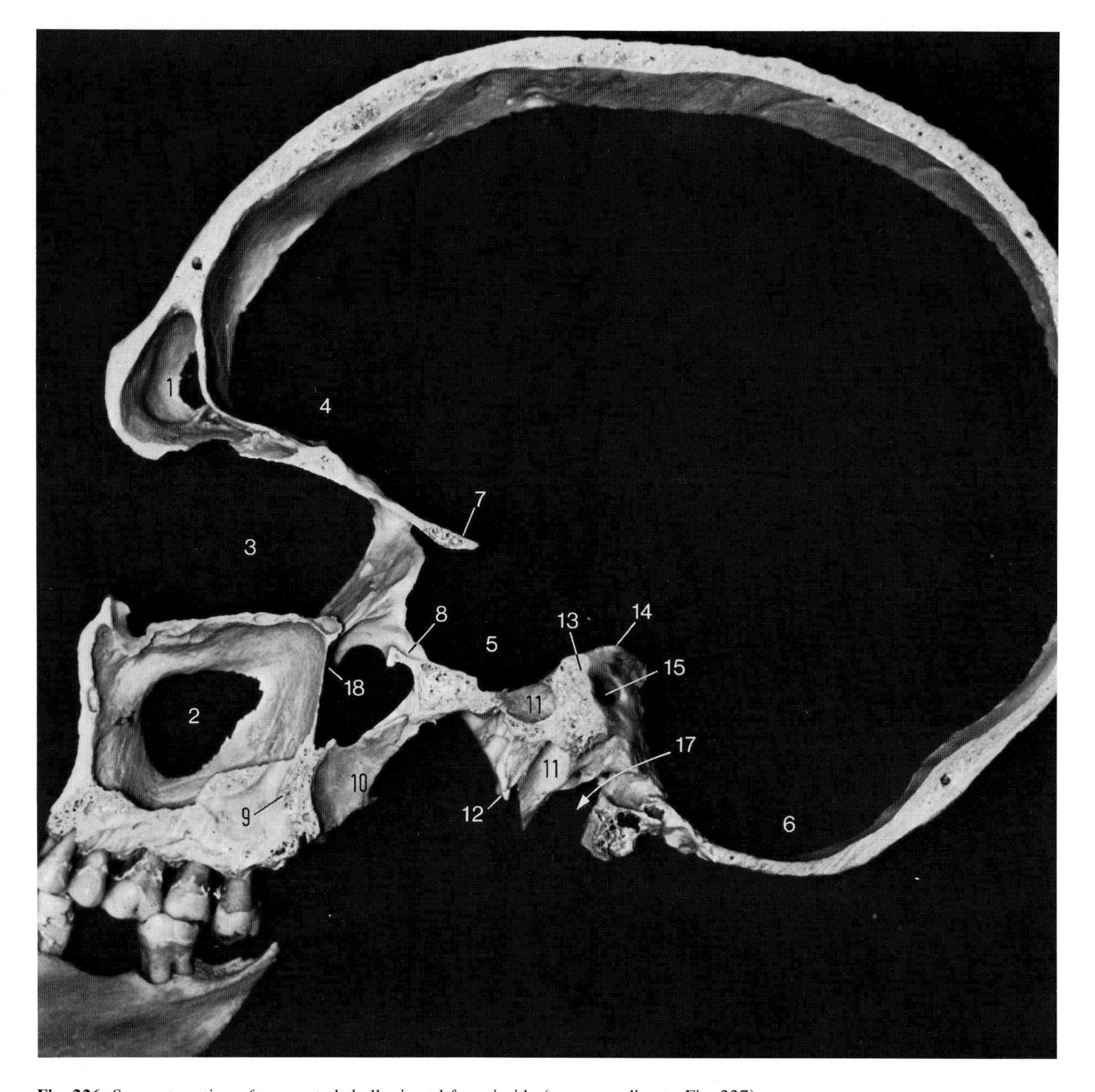

Fig. 226. Saw-cut section of macerated skull, viewed from inside (corresponding to Fig. 227).

1 Frontal sinus
2 Maxillary sinus
3 Orbita
4 Anterior cranial fossa
5 Middle cranial fossa
6 Posterior cranial fossa
7 Small wing
8 Foramen rotundum
9 Pterygopalatine canal (canalis palatinus major)
10 Lateral plate of pterygoid process
11 Carotid canal
12 Sphenoidal spine
13 Petrous bone
14 Eminentia arcuata
15 Internal orifice of auditory canal
17 Jugular foramen
18 Pterygopalatine fossa

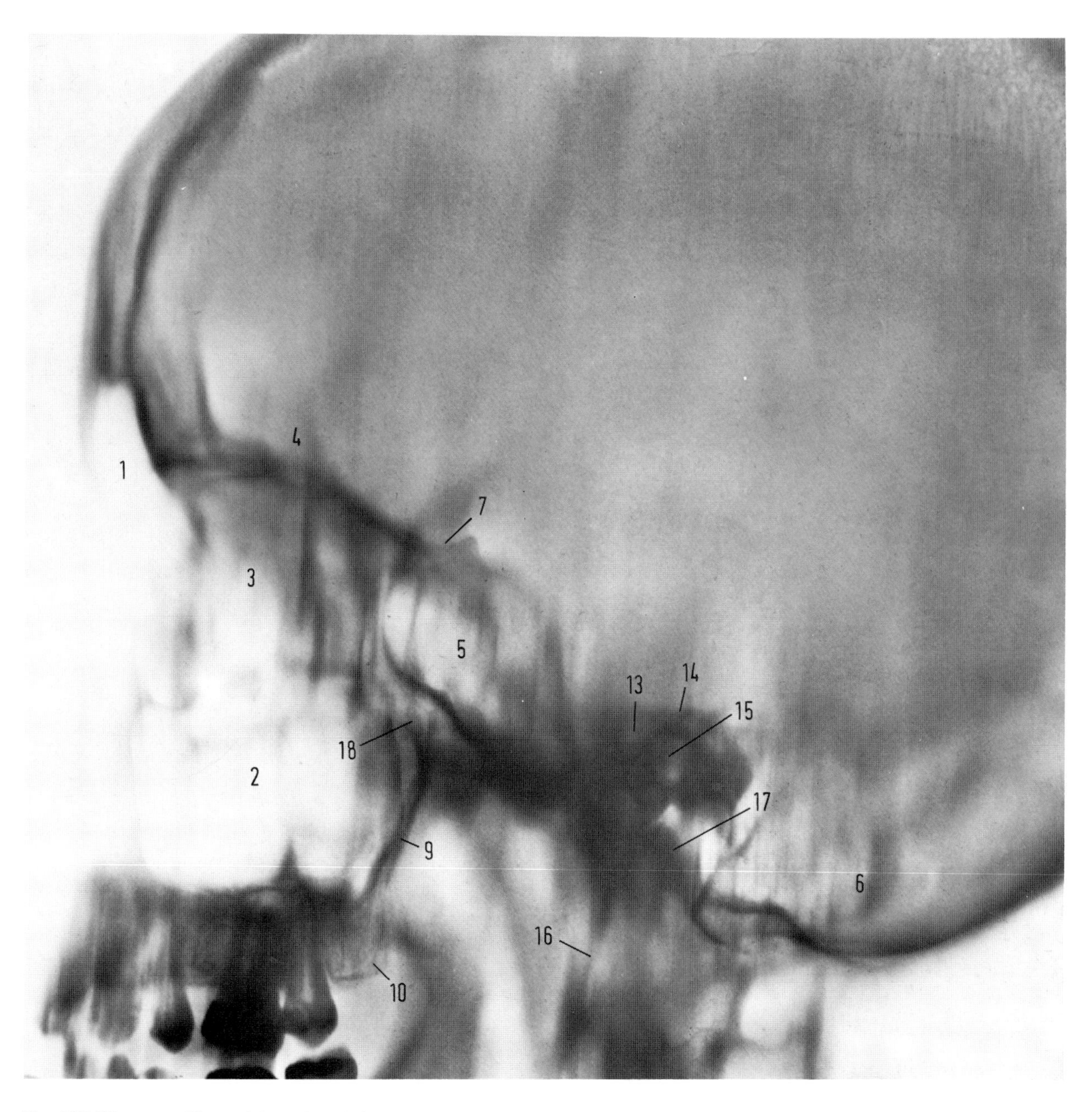

Fig. 227. Distance of layer 4.0 cm from left.

1 Frontal sinus
2 Maxillary sinus
3 Orbita
4 Anterior cranial fossa
5 Middle cranial fossa
6 Posterior cranial fossa
7 Small wing
9 Pterygopalatine canal (canalis palatinus major)
10 Lateral plate of pterygoid process
13 Petrous bone
14 Eminentia arcuata
15 Internal orifice of auditory canal
16 Styloid process
17 Jugular foramen
18 Pterygopalatine fossa

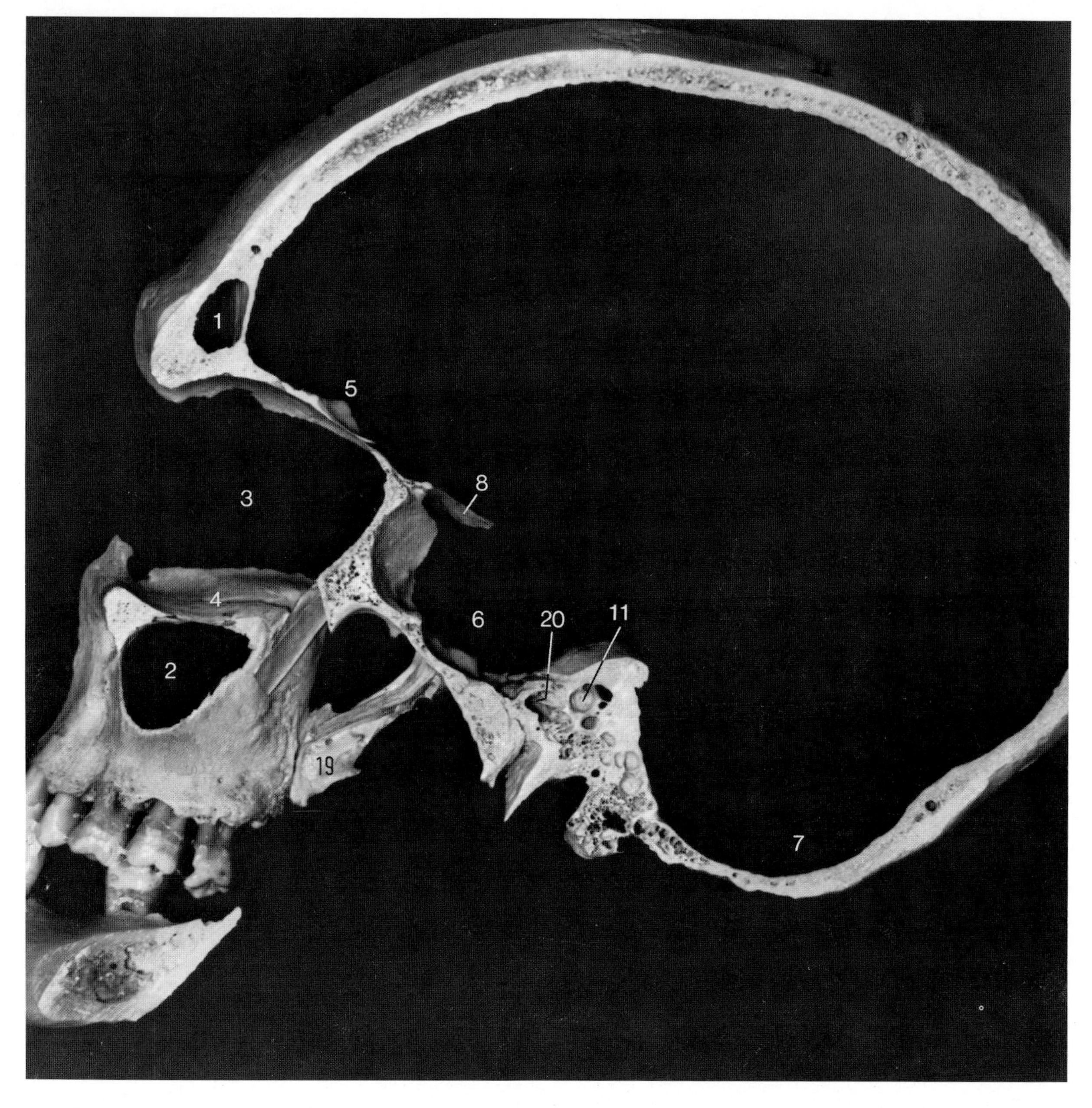

Fig. 228. Saw-cut bone section of Fig. 226, viewed from outside after turning the tomograph.

1 Frontal sinus
2 Maxillary sinus
3 Orbita
4 Floor of orbita
5 Anterior cranial fossa
6 Middle cranial fossa
7 Posterior cranial fossa
8 Small wing
11 Cochlea
19 Lateral plate of pterygoid process
20 Musculotubal canal

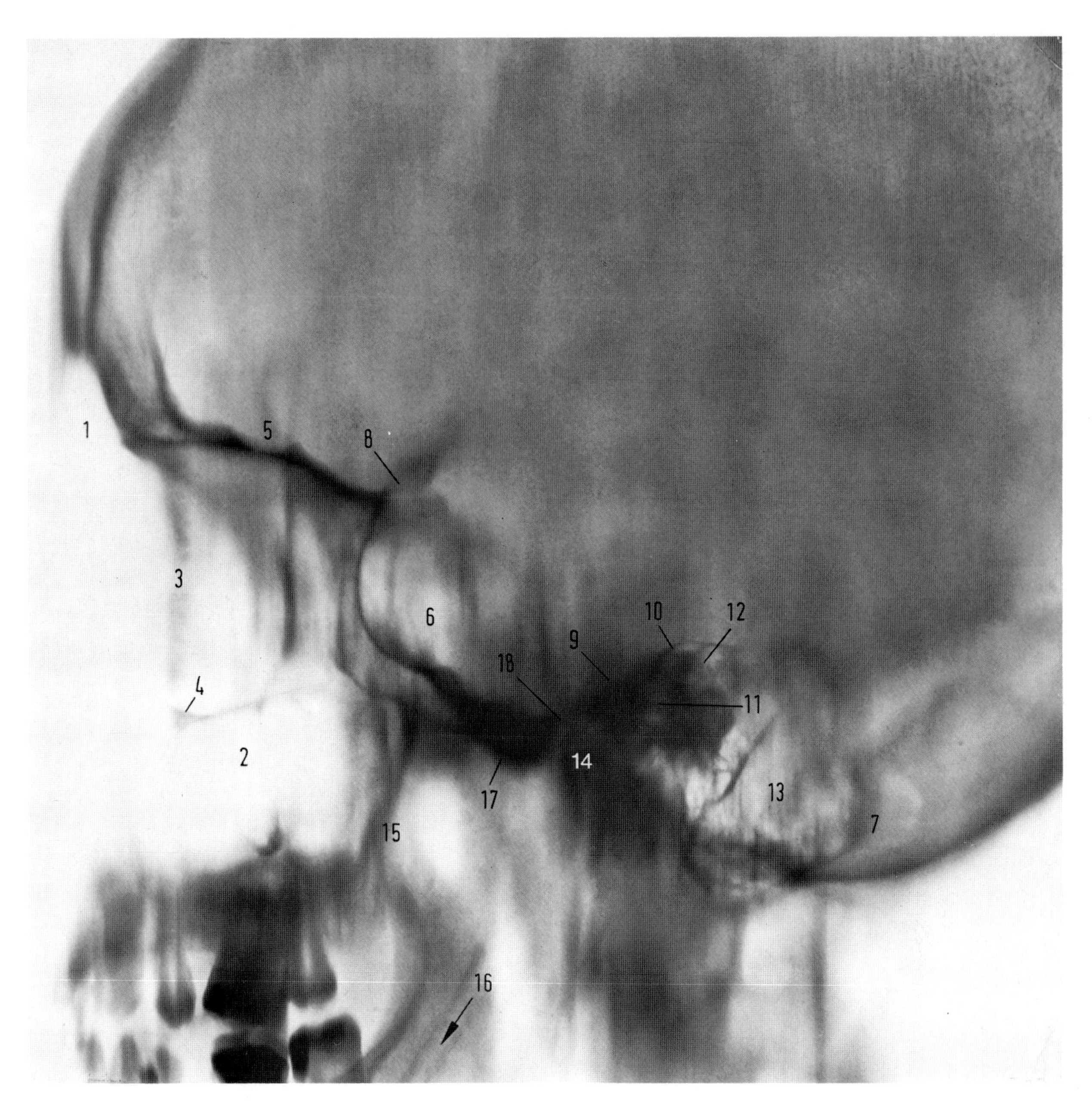

Fig. 229. Distance of layer 3,0 cm from left.

1 Frontal sinus
2 Maxillary sinus
3 Orbita
4 Floor of orbita
5 Anterior cranial fossa
6 Middle cranial fossa
7 Posterior cranial fossa
8 Small wing
9 Petrous bone
10 Eminentia arcuata with anterior semicircular canal
11 Cochlea (with vestibule)
12 Pneumatization of petrous bone
13 Mastoid cells
14 Condyloid process
15 Coronoid process
16 Mandibular canal
17 Articular tubercle
18 Mandibular fossa

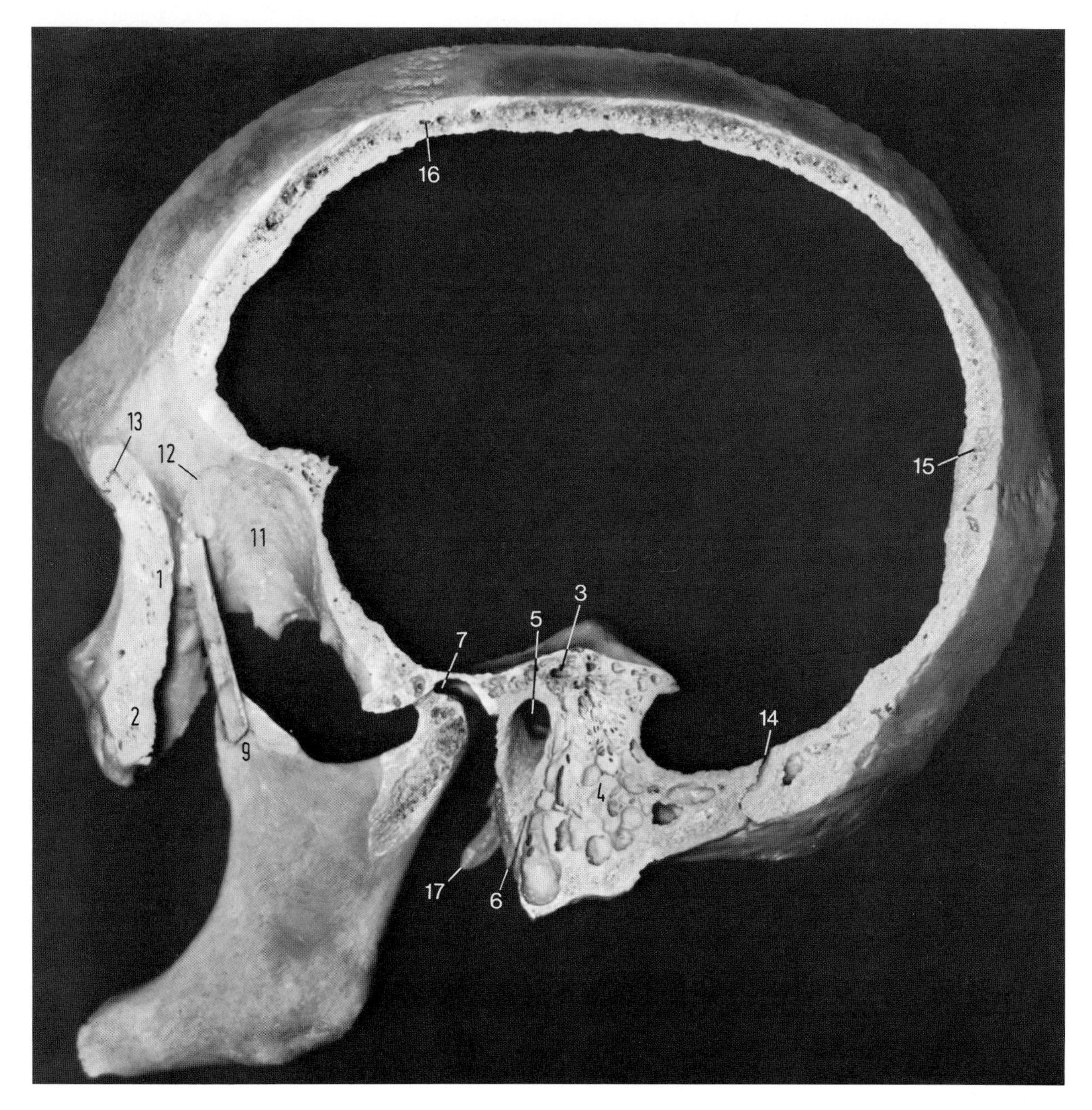

Fig. 230 (corresponding to Fig. 231).

1 Frontal process of zygomatic bone
2 Body of zygomatic bone
3 Mastoid antrum
4 Mastoid cells
5 External orifice of auditory canal
6 Tympanomastoid fissure
7 Mandibular fossa
9 Coronoid process
11 Small wing
12 Sphenofrontal suture
13 Zygomaticofrontal suture
14 Occipitomastoid suture
15 Lambdoid suture
16 Coronal suture
17 Styloid process

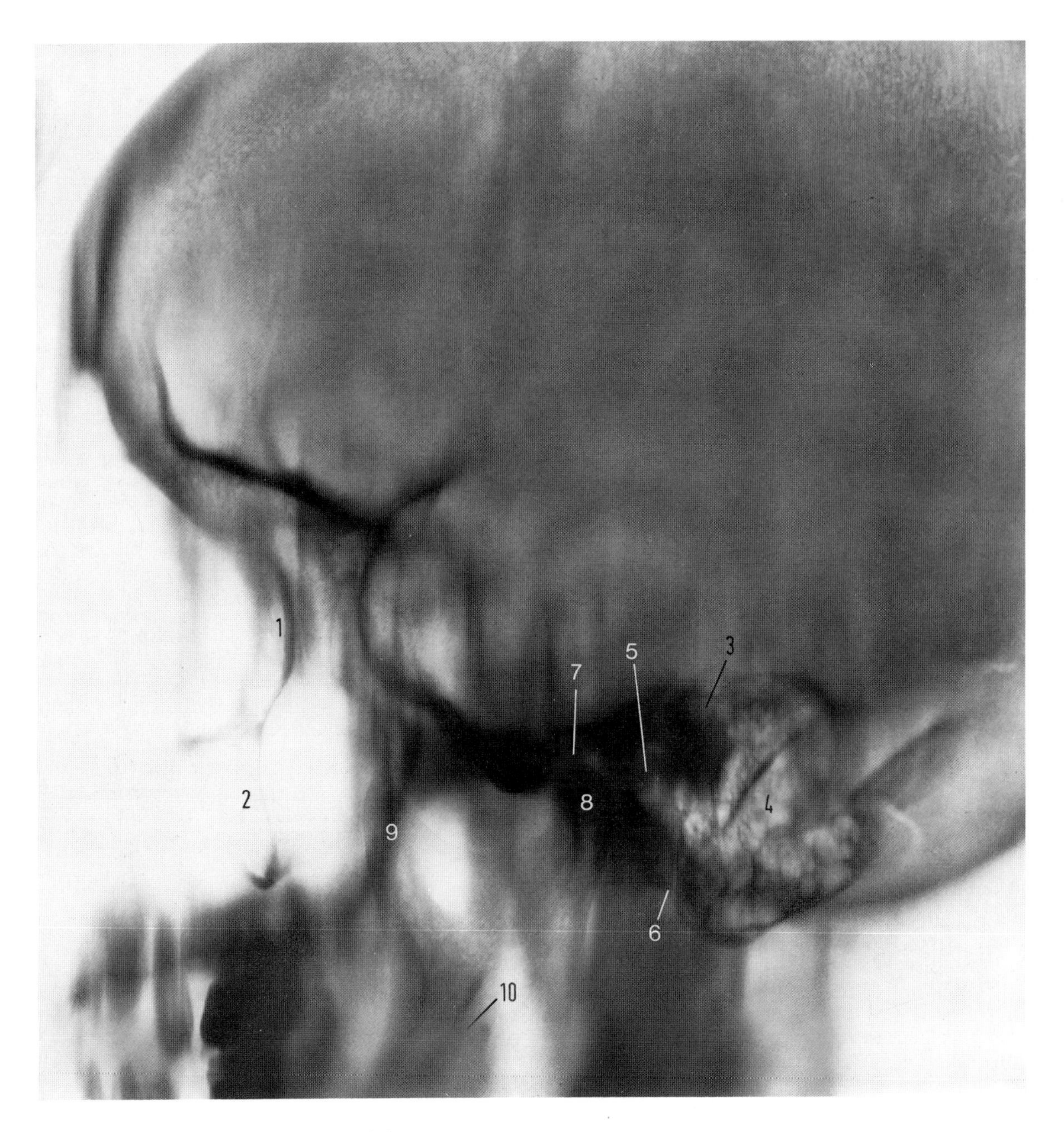

Fig. 231. Distance of layer 2.25 cm from left.

1 Frontal process of zygomatic bone
2 Body of zygomatic bone
3 Mastoid antrum
4 Mastoid cells
5 External orifice of auditory canal (with tympanic cavity)
6 Tympanomastoid fissure
7 Mandibular fossa
8 Condyloid process
9 Coronoid process
10 Mandibular canal

Variants and Sources of Diagnostic Error of the Skull and Neck

To Figs. 232 and 233:*

1 Persistent frontal (metopic) suture (see Figs. 234 and 267) occurs as a dominant hereditary factor and in relation to cretinism. It can be simulated on occipito-oral radiographs if the sagittal suture is projected into the frontal bone by steep direction of the beam. This occurs to an extent of 6.45 to 8% *(Torgersen, van Acken, Knetsch).* Occasionally, one finds in the lower third of the frontal (metopic) suture a gap (metopic fontanel) or a bone formation (metopic bone) filling this gap. *Rauber* reports on the interfrontal and supranasal bones. *Hiltemann* and *Knetsch* describe a metopic fonticulus due to failure of bony closure (inconstant persistent fontanel). The metopic fonticulus is often combined with a frontal hyperostosis (see No. 29). The failure of unification of both frontal bones is found, *inter alia,* in cases of clidocranial dysostosis, a severe disturbance of ossification of the skull, the clavicles and, frequently, of the remaining skeleton

1* Unilateral circumscribed hyperostosis, simulating defect (see Fig. 263); differential diagnosis against meningioma

2 Ossified or calcified falx cerebri (see Figs. 239, 258, 259 and 260 a), often combined with a calcified pineal gland. *Wrangel* and *Fassbender* consider it a calcifying dura (following trauma, inflammation, etc.) which also occurs in the animal kingdom and is explained by the osteoplastic tendency of the dura. Consequently, *Janker's* theory of an atavistic formation can no longer be sustained. On sagittal (Fig. 232) and axial (Fig. 259) radiographs, the bony plate is viewed from its narrow side (edge) and therefore gives a dense shadow. On lateral projection (Fig. 233), the shadow of this bony plate, seen from the side, is faintly visible at best

3 Calcified pineal body (see Fig. 112). This finding is non-pathological; it sometimes occurs in infancy and is then a possible indication of pinealoma. The calciferous shadow must be exactly in the median plane on sagittal symmetrical radiograph. Pathological processes may distort or shift it laterally. Normally, the pineal body is situated 4 cm above and 1 cm dorsal to the internal auditory opening. The structure is dot-like or granular. Frequency among the 11–20 age group is 11%, but generally 50–60%. This structure must be differentiated from calcified tubercles, which are smaller and distributed more irregularly *(Gallois)*

4 Crista galli (see Figs. 42, 90, 112 and 150). This is a process of the perpendicular lamina jutting out into the anterior cranial fossa, often superimposed upon the frontal crest and the septum between the frontal sinuses

4* Exostosis of the upper edge of the petrous pyramid *(Finze),* caused by an enlarged, usually sclerotic, bony pad at the inner auditory canal

5 Frontal diploic vein (see Figs. 234, 236 and 249), usually terminating in the supraorbital foramen

5* Frontal emissary vein (see Figs. 250–252). It runs in a bony vascular canal in the lower medial third of the frontal bone, leading from the middle line to the upper border of the orbita, usually unilateral, more rarely bilateral. It provides an anastomosis between the superior sagittal sinus and the orbital veins. Its frequency amounts to 0.2 to 0.3% of all skull radiographs *(Knetsch, Martin-Reith)*

6 Granular *(Pacchioni's)* foveolae (see Fig. 234). Not to be confused with metastases. To be differentiated from oversized parietal foramina

6* Oversized parietal foramina (see Figs. 240 and 242). This is a rare hereditary anomaly of ossification, occurring parasagittally in the dorsal third of the parietal bones, where the parietal emissary veins are also found. Should not be mistaken for pitting atrophy of the parietal bone, which mainly occurs symmetrically but may also be found unilaterally (see Figs. 239 and 241). If a foramen is circular and unilateral, it may be mistaken for a solitary metastasis. *Dahm* reported on residual skull defects after fractures. The differential diagnosis against lacunae of the vault has been extensively described by *Lièvre* and *Fischgold,* as well as by *Ghislanzoni* and *Porro. Pendergrass* and *Pepper* reported on ossification processes at persistent parietal foramina

6** Calcification of soft tissues, e.g., in epitheliomata, atheromata, scars, etc., which may simulate a fracture

7 Calcification within a foveola *Pacchioni;* if unilateral, may be confused with an osteomyelitic sequestrum

7* Pitting atrophy of the parietal bone (see Figs. 239 and 241 a,b); also occurs in younger people and is usually symmetrical

8 Sulcus of transverse sinus (see Figs. 269 and 270); there is an occasional calcification embedded in the tentorium cerebelli

9 Calcified chorioid plexus (see Fig. 265), usually occurring with advanced age but frequently the effect of chronic inflammation of the plexus, especially after toxoplasmosis (triad: hydrocephalus, chorioretinopathy and calcified foci in the brain). For differential diagnosis of intracranial calcifications, see *Tönnis* and *Friedmann*

9* Longitudinal fissure in the dens (axis); should not be confused with a simulated cleft (see Figs. 308 and 310)

10 Squamous suture between parietal and temporal bone (see Figs. 246, 946 and 947); by a scaly superimposition on an anteroposterior view, this may be mistaken for a fracture

10* Superior orbital fissure (see Fig. 47). The cranial nerves III–VI, as well as the superior and inferior ophthalmic veins, pass through it, coming from the middle cranial fossa. Pathological processes may cause the superior sagittal sinus syndrome (see Fig. 203 and Fig. 47)

11 Supernumerary bone at the tip of the lambdoid suture (Fig. 274); differential diagnosis: interparietal bone (Inka bone). The bone may be divided into several parts (see Figs. 276, 281 and 282)

11* Transverse occipital suture (developed only laterally: sutura mendosa, see Figs. 237, 274 and 275) separates the upper section of the occiput as interparietal or Inka bone (see Fig. 281)

12 Mental foramen (see Fig. 145). Avoid mistaking this exit of the mental artery, situated in the region of the roots of the lower premolars, for a cyst or granuloma

13 Angle of mandible resembling exostosis (see Figs. 47 and 108). Insertion of masseter muscle

14 Calcified internal carotid artery (orthograde projection)

14* Calcified internal carotid artery (lateral projection) (see Fig. 170). Occasionally, the artery may be projected as a double-contoured shadowy strip into the hypophyseal fossa of the sella turcica, and may be mistaken for intrasellar calcifications. This error can be eliminated by tomography (see also Figs. 170, 216, 217)

15 Dens (axis). May remain independent as odontoid bone in cases of failure of synostosis with the body of the axis, which occurs normally about the fifth year of life. The horizontal cleft should not be confused with a fracture, which is usually jagged and does not reach right to the base. Pseudofracture may appear due to *Mach* effect (see Fig. 310)

15* Unexplained apophysis-like bone shadow at the tip of the dens; most likely a terminal ossicle *(Maurer, Delvigne)*

16 Maxillary sinus (see Figs. 55, 200, 219 and 225)

16* Incisive foramen; may occur in multiples. On excentric projection, periapical destruction may be simulated

17 Eyelid, palpebral fissure; horizontal cleft on closure of eyelids (see Fig. 79)

17* Subarcuate fossa, step formation *(Psenner);* occurs in the adult sometimes as a result of raised intracranial pressure

18 Occipital diploic vein (see Figs. 234 and 236); very variable. If it occurs asymmetrically, may simulate a fracture

18* Linea innominata; may be absent; either unilateral or bilateral (see Figs. 45, 47 and 202 for a more detailed analysis)

19 Gaping wound which may simulate a fracture *(Döhner)*

---

* The numbers in heavy type are to be found either only on the lateral drawing Fig. 233, p. 109, or on both Figs. 233 and 232.

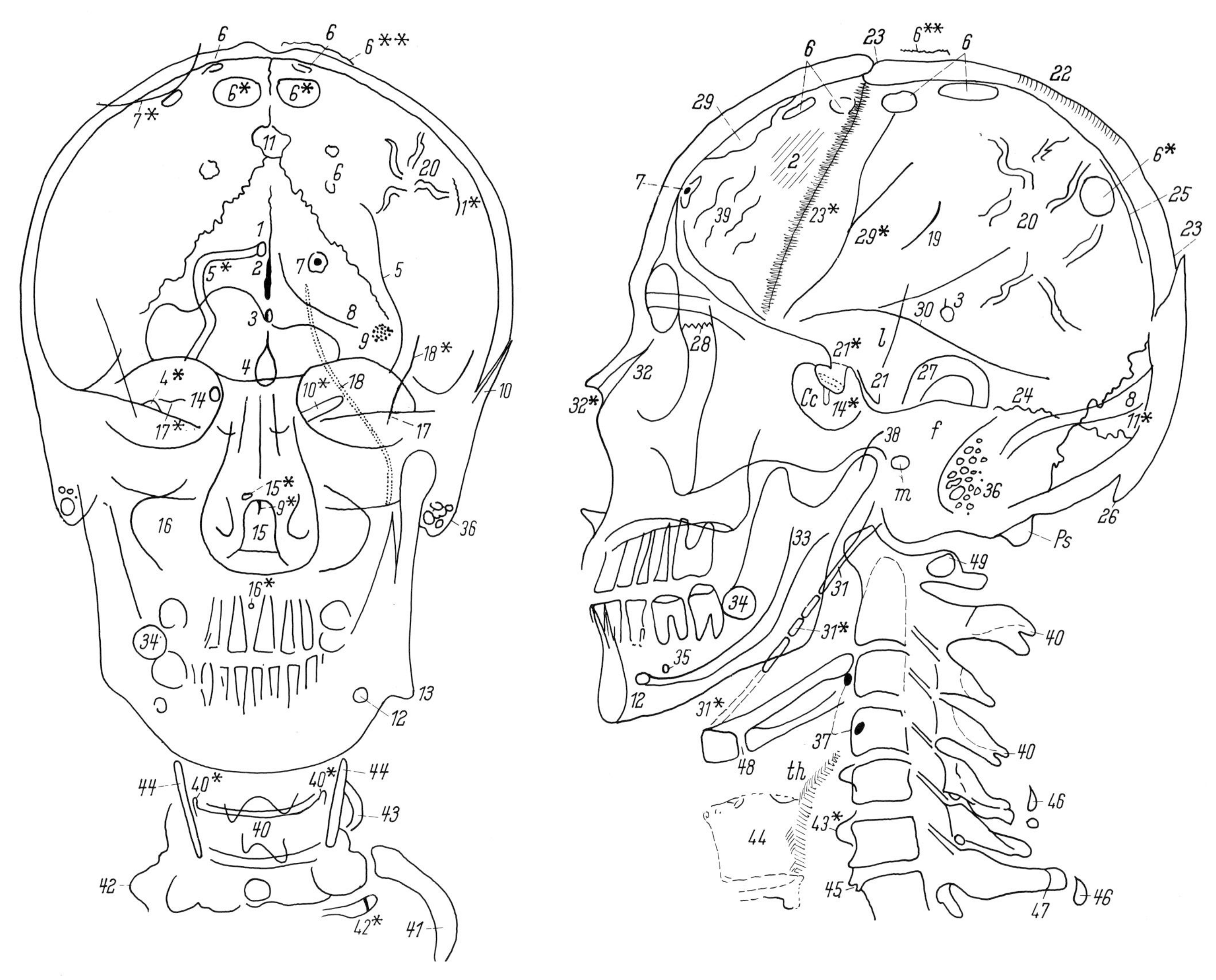

Fig. 232. Skull, neck; sagittal.

Fig. 233. Skull, neck; lateral.

20 Venous star of *Bretschet,* formed by the variable diploic veins of the parietal bone (see Fig. 234). Atypical diploic veins may either be a variation from the norm or may form an important pathognostic criterion

21 Ossified dura; calcification of the tentorial insertion; see Figs. 156, 161 and 170 *(Kresse* and *Göbbeler)*

21* Interclinoid taenia, so-called sellar bridge. According to *Platzer,* it occurs frequently in cases of an elongated course of the internal carotid artery within the cavernous sinus and therefore may be used as a diagnostic aid. The interclinoid taenia develops from a cartilagenous origin *(Carstens, Platzer). Platzer* considers it completely unlikely that an interclinoid taenia might be an ossification of the dura (see Figs. 163, 165, 171, 172)

22 Sagittal suture (velvet-like pattern). Velvet-like appearance of the sagittal suture on lateral projection is caused by its very jagged course in the external lamina; while in the internal lamina it turns wavy and almost straight *(Grashey);* see Fig. 245. Should not be confused with the pathological "brush-skull" (spicules on the thickened skull cap, e.g., in cases of sickle-cell anemia, marble disease of the bone or osteoplastic metastases)

23 Overlapping sutures (Fig. 262), pronounced step formation, called bathrocephaly. Not to be mistaken for a depressed fracture

23* Hyperostosis of the coronal suture; calcified seams, most frequent at this site (Fig. 246)

24 Parietomastoid suture (see Figs. 243 and 934), branches off ventrally from the lambdoid suture and passes into the squamous suture; may be gaping and thus simulate a fracture

25 Pseudo-depressed fracture simulated by edges of blood vessels or other ledge-shaped irregularities of the internal lamina *(Lossen);* see Fig. 955

26 Occipital spur (Fig. 266). The occipital protuberance points spur-like towards the ligamentum nuchae mainly in older people. Familial occurrence has been observed *(Psenner)*

27 Pinna (see Fig. 269). Both pinnae may be seen on a lateral radiograph; then, the one away from the film appears larger than the one against the film

28 Frontozygomatic suture (see Fig. 45); may be gaping and thus be confused with a fracture

29 Internal frontal hyperostosis (see Fig. 261 a,b). One distinguishes between the knobby (internal frontal hyperostosis) and the flower-bed-like (frontal nebula) forms. It is related to hormonal dysfunctions *(Ellegast, Bartelheimer),* with preponderance (90%) in women

29* Anterior temporal diploic vein (see Figs. 236, 255, 256 and 954); apparently terminates, in most cases, in the foveola granularis *(Lindblom)*

30 Sulcus for the posterior branch of the middle meningeal artery (see Figs. 108 and 234); may simulate a fracture

30* See on p. 110 l

31 Styloid process (see Figs. 108 and 177). Avoid confusion with a foreign body. A joint-like union with an ossified stylohyoid ligament is possible. Normal length is 2 to 3 cm, but it may reach 6 to 7 cm *(Bratt)*

31* Stylohyoid ligament (see Figs. 321, 322). May ossify in joint-like subdivisions; they could signify the remnants of a gill skeleton *(Bratt)*

32 Sulcus for blood vessel at the inner side of the nasal bones (see Fig. 83). Avoid confusion with a fracture (nasomaxillary suture and ethmoidal sulcus); see Fig. 85

32* Sulcus for anterior ethmoidal artery and nerve (see Figs. 83 and 85)

33 Mandibular canal (see Figs. 108 and 145). The mylohyoid line, which gives origin to the muscle of the same name, runs along the inner surface. Projection of this sharp line onto the mandibular canal may show a fictitious distension

34 Retained tooth (see Fig. 145); may simulate an odontoma

35 Salivary calculus; may be confused with compacta islet, exostosis or enostosis

36 Mastoid cells (see Figs. 135, 930–933 and 935–939). Above, one observes the sigmoid sinus as a continuation of the transverse sinus. In this region, emissary mastoid veins, which vary in number, position and width, are often found

37 Calcified triticeous cartilages (cartilagines triticeae) (Fig. 294a); they appear as sesamoid bones in the thyrohyoid ligament. They are projected between the greater cornua of the hyoid bone and the superior cornua of the thyroid cartilage, and should not be mistaken for ossifications in the anterior longitudinal ligament

38 Petrotympanic fissure (Fig. 198), the site of emergence of the chorda tympani nerve

39 Juga cerebralia (see Figs. 956 and 958)

40 Normally forked spinous processes (see Figs. 283a and 322); not to be confused with spina bifida (see Fig. 317)

40* Uncinate processes (Fig. 284), forming so-called half-joints with the next higher vertebra. They often show osteoarthrotic changes (so-called uncovertebral arthrosis)

41 Cervical rib (see Figs. 353 and 354). Frequency is 1%, and in up to 90% of cases it does not cause any symptoms. Is to be differentiated from an underdeveloped first rib (see Fig. 367). Both anomalies may cause a scalenus syndrome

42 Very large transverse process (see Fig. 352); fused rudimentary rib

42* Persistent apophyseal nucleus at the transverse process of the 1st thoracic vertebra (Fig. 356); must be differentiated from a fracture

43 Transverse process, protruding laterally (see Figs. 323, 996)

43* Protruding anterior tubercle of the transverse process (see Figs. 283b and 322). Differential diagnosis against ossification of the anterior longitudinal ligament (?); see also Fig. 316

44 Ossified thyroid cartilage (see Fig. 294). Ossification of the thyroid cartilage usually starts after skeletal growth has terminated

45 Deforming spondylosis (see Fig. 322)

46 Circumscribed calcinosis of the ligamentum nuchae (see Fig. 322)

47 Fatigue fracture *(Schipper* fracture). Differential diagnosis against persistent apophyseal nuclei (see also *Seibert* and *Daiker* who, in 1975, showed a persistent apophysis of the 7th cervical vertebra, together with a semilateral hyperplasia of the spinous process of the 5th)

48 Cleft in the hyoid bone; fusion of the parts of the hyoid bone may not take place at all

49 Arcuate foramen (see Fig. 311). Variant of the sulcus for the vertebral artery and vein and the suboccipital nerve. The canal is formed by a bony span which leads from the posterior rim of the superior articular surface of the atlas to its posterior arch

Cc Persistent craniopharyngeal canal, not to be confused with a persistent intersphenoidal synchondrosis *(Kullnig, Schaaf* and *Wilhelm)*

f Petrous bone

l An occasionally found clear line, which may be wrongly identified as a fissure. It is caused by the sulcus of a branch of the middle meningeal artery taking an atypical course *(Grashey).* In contrast to the sulcus for a blood vessel, a fracture usually runs in a straight line

m External auditory meatus

Ps Suboccipital process; compare also *Kerckrings'* process *(Gassmann, Caffey)*

th Thyrohyoid ligament, in process of ossification, as a continuation of the hyoid cornu

Gallois, Goldhamer, Grashey, Döhner and *Schwartz* reported on the simulation of pathological and traumatic changes in the skull caused by variants in the skeleton and by intracranial calcifications, e.g., *Pacchioni* grooves, supernumerary sutures, spheno-occipital synchondrosis, step-like skull (bathrocephaly), exaggerated development of the external occipital protuberance, shadow of the pinna, canals for blood vessels, gaping wounds and calcifications of the pineal gland and in the region of the sella turcica.

Platybasia is a designation used by anthropologists and anatomists and connotes flattening of *Welcker's* basal angle. It describes schematically the step-like relation between the anterior and posterior cranial fossa. This angle should be about 134 degrees (deviation $\pm$ 10°). For measuring the basal angle, one uses the lines from the nasion to the center of the sella, and from the basion (midpoint of the anterior margin of the foramen magnum) to this center. In most cases, the flattening of this angle is connected with an abnormal position of the basioocciput and the anterior margin of the foramen magnum. Platybasia is not infrequently combined with basilar impression.

Basilar impression or invagination denotes the changed space relation between the upper segment of the cervical vertebrae (atlas and axis) and the posterior cranial fossa. The occipital condyles, the margins of the foramen magnum and the upper segment of the cervical vertebrae are invaginated funnel-like into the interior of the posterior cranial fossa. The clivus often takes a flattened or cranioconvex course. Basilar impression may be connected with atlas assimilation, apalasia of the dens and other anomalies *(Klaus, Tobeck).*

Traumatic cephalhydrocele *(de Quervain)* connotes formation of lacunae in the skull, which may delay the healing of the fracture, presumably by a tear in the dura with keloid formation, and which may sometimes also cause a widening of the cleft *(Dahm).*

To Fig. 234:

1 *Pacchioni* grooves, varying in size and depth; very large in this case. They are especially found in the region of the original great fontanel. Lateral recesses (lateral lacunae) of the sagittal sinus are embedded in the *Pacchioni* grooves which hold, besides diploic veins, knobby bulges of the arachnoid *(Pacchionian* granulations, Fig. 235). The grooves become visible only after the 10th year of life.

2 Parietal bone

3 Sagittal suture

4 Persistent frontal suture (metopic suture); an anomaly found in 6–8% of adults, usually limited to the lower part of the frontal plate. *Torgersen* points to its dominant heredity and its relation to cretinism. Normally, the suture between the pair of frontal bones, which develop in the second embryonic month, disappears in the second to third years of life. Occasionally, a fontanel (metopic fontanel), which may be bridged by its own bony nucleus, occurs in the lower part of the suture: interfrontal or metopic bone *(van Acken, Hiltemann, Torgersen, Haas).*

5 Lambdoid suture

6 Diploic veins. These veins, which become visible only after the fifth year, are quite variable in position and course, as well as in extent. They are independent of the cranial sutures and may cross them. They anastomose among themselves as well as with the cerebral and meningeal veins, the sinuses and the lateral lacunae. On each side of the vault, one distinguishes 4 to 5 large collecting channels: the frontal, anterior, medial and posterior temporal and the occipital diploic vein (Fig. 236). Occasionally, variciform distensions, which may simulate skull defects, occur in the parietal region. Here, one also finds the venous star of *Bretschet* which on unilateral appearance may, like other diploic veins, be confused with fractures (see Figs. 232, 233). Due to the variability of the diploic veins, it is difficult to draw any conclusions to pathological processes *(Lindblom, Sorge, Santagati, Scarpa, Wanke).*

7 Sulci for the anterior branch of the middle meningeal artery

8 Sulci for the posterior branch of the middle meningeal artery

9 Coronal suture

▶

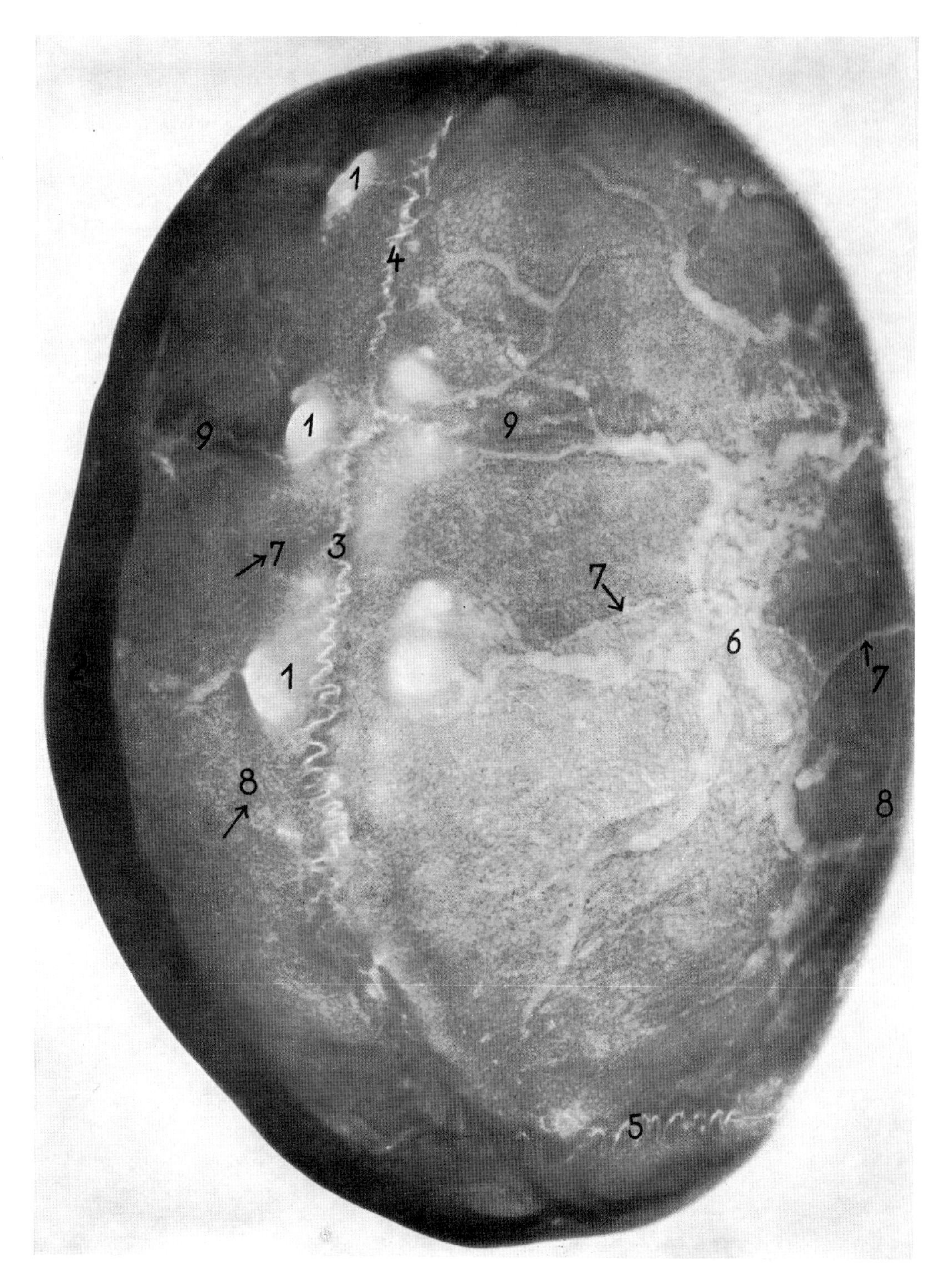

Fig. 234. Adult vault, macerated. Large *Pacchioni* grooves in the vault; also network of diploic vessels.

Ossifications of the sutures are frequent. Usually, they do not cause any discomfort. They are not different from ossifications of other soft tissues, e.g., of the larynx. The bony fusion of the most important sutures generally begins in the 25th to 40th years of life, starting in the internal lamina and proceeding later into the outer vault. If the frontal (metopic) suture (4) persists, it forms an exception and remains open when the other sutures have already been ossified. This physiological synostosis of the sutures must be delimited against the so-called craniostenoses with premature closure of the sutures. This premature closure may lead to various types of skull such as oxycephaly (steeplehead or towerhead), dolichocephaly (elongated skull), brachycephaly (short skull), plagiocephaly (oblique skull) and scaphocephaly (boat-shaped skull). Figs. 956 and 958 show a towerhead in an 11-year-old child.

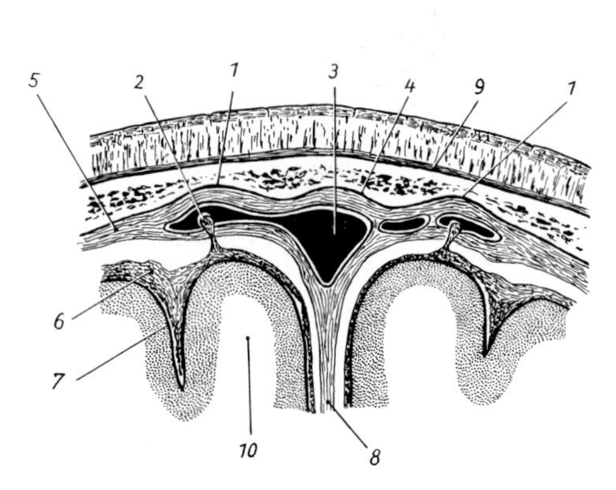

Fig. 235. Frontal section through the layers of the vault, the superior sagittal sinus and the arachnoid granulations *(Pacchioni*an granulations), from *Corning.*

1 *Pacchioni*an grooves
2 *Pacchioni*an granulations within a lateral lacuna
3 Superior sagittal sinus
4 Sagittal sulcus
5 Dura
6 Arachnoid
7 Pia mater
8 Falx cerebri
9 Galea aponeurotica
10 Cerebral gyrus

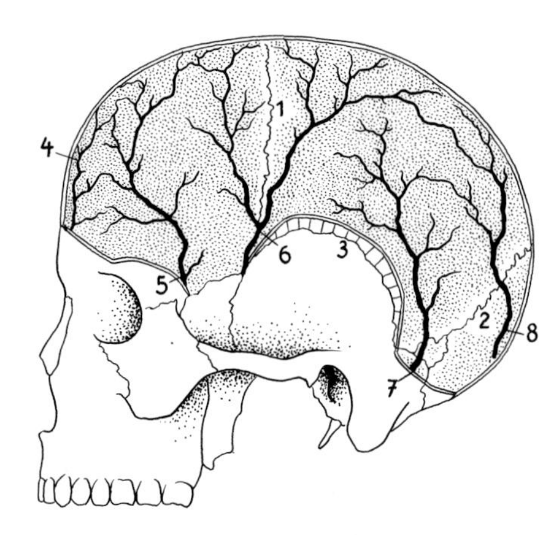

Fig. 236. Large collecting channels of the diploic veins (from *Rauber-Kopsch).*

1 Coronal suture
2 Lambdoid suture
3 Squamous suture
4 Frontal diploic vein
5 Anterior temporal diploic vein
6 Middle temporal diploic vein
7 Posterior temporal diploic vein
8 Occipital diploic vein

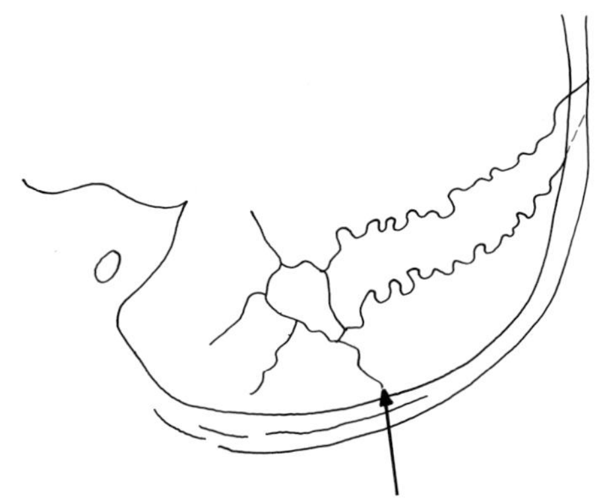

Fig. 237 shows a **sutura mendosa** (↖) in a 3-year-old child. This suture is very frequent during the first year of life, but is found more rarely from the fifth year on. According to *Pawlik,* it is present in 10% (out of 150 cases) of 16–20 year olds. The start of the sutura mendosa is found most easily at the level of the transverse sinus. Its origin is always visible at the lambdoid suture; this is important for the differential diagnosis against a fracture. Frequently, a supernumerary bone can be seen at the junction of the sutura mendosa with the lambdoid suture.

As **Figs. 237** and **238** show, the sutures of the skull of the infant are far more ramified than in the adult skull, where they partly fuse. In the thinner infantile bones of the skull the sutures appear much more distinctly, e.g., the squamous suture. Therefore, a fracture is easily suspected *(Grob).*

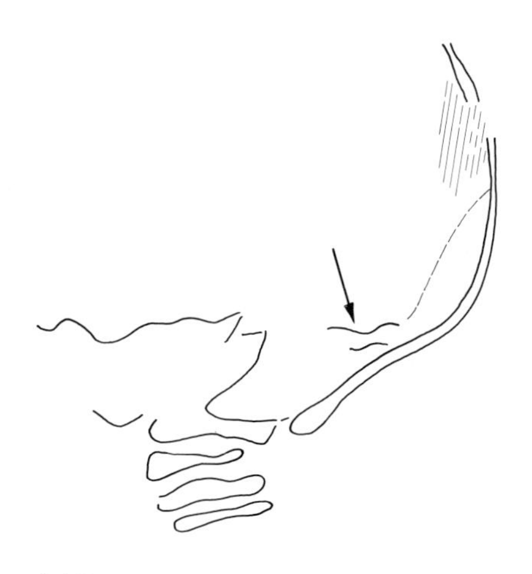

Fig. 238 shows the **posterior intraoccipital synchondrosis** (↘) in a 5-week-old infant. This may easily simulate a fracture. For digital impressions and dehiscences of the cranial sutures, see *Hünermann.*

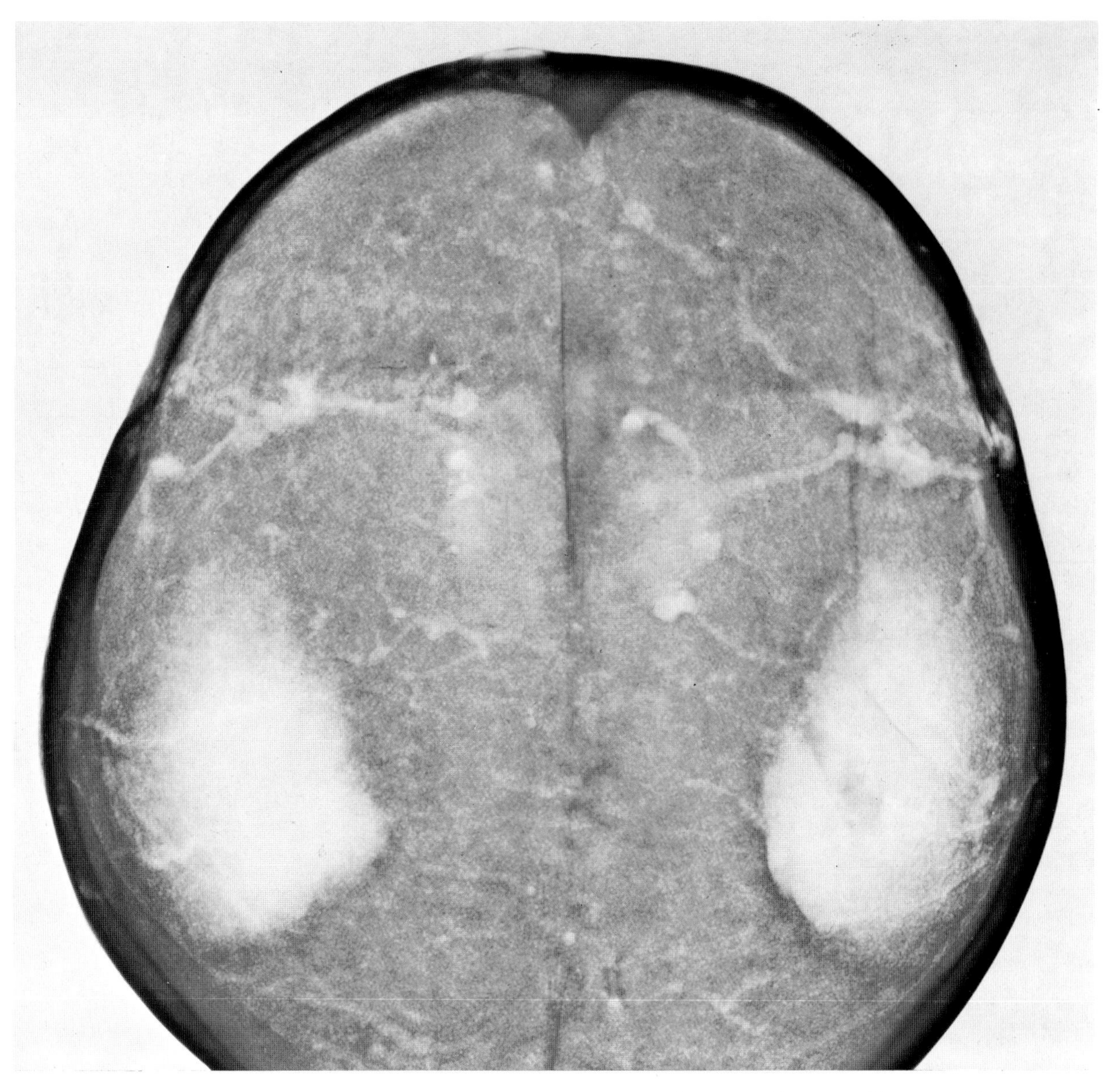

Fig. 239. Adult vault, macerated. Senile atrophy with bilateral thinning of the parietal bone *(Knetsch)*. This must be differentiated from the excessively large (permagna) parietal foramina (see below). Compare with No. 6* in Fig. 232, and Fig. 242 a and b. Ossified falx cerebri in axial projection as in Fig. 259.

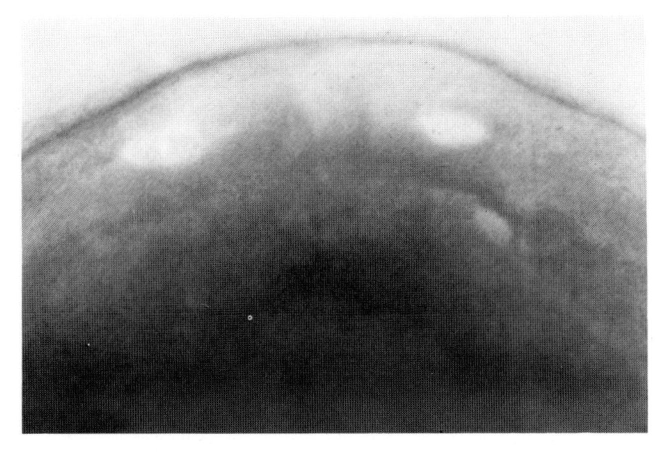

Fig. 240 a. Anteroposterior view.

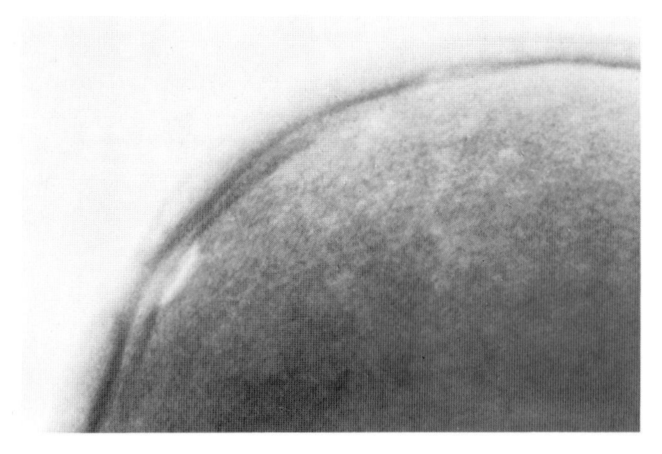

Fig. 240 b. Lateral view.

Fig. 240 a, b. Oversize parietal foramina (permagna), found parasagittal in the dorsal third of the parietal bones (see Fig. 242).

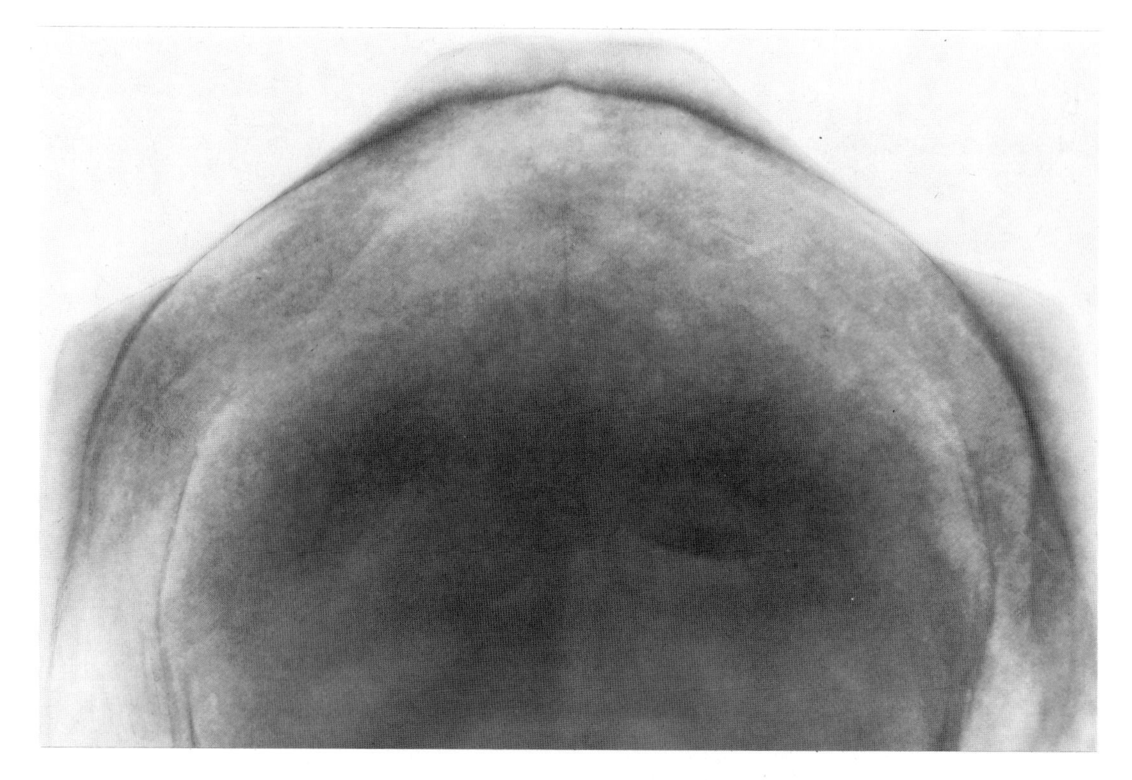

Fig. 241 a

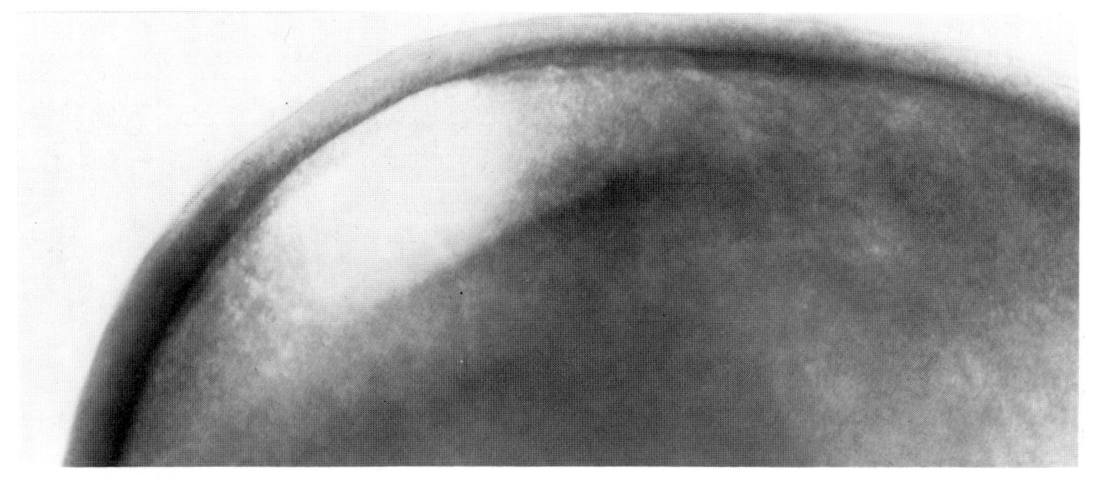

Fig. 241 b

Fig. 241 a, b. Pitting senile atrophy of both parietal bones *(Gros)*. This occurs without any additional disease. It should not be confused with the parietal foramen which, according to *O'Rahilly* and *Twohig*, is present in 60% of cases, frequently unilaterally. In 90%, the diameters of the parietal foramina do not exceed 1 mm; they serve as passages for the parietal emissary veins.

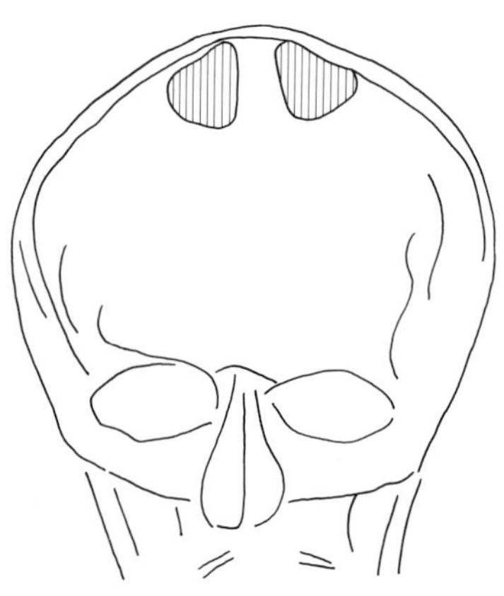

Fig. 242 a

Fig. 242 b

Fig. 242 a, b shows the described, sometimes very large, parietal foramina whose position and symmetrical arrangement are characteristic *(Wissler)*. *Pessagno* described oversized foramina, a. o., with unilateral localization. These two sketches are based on radiographs by *Travers* and *Wormley*.

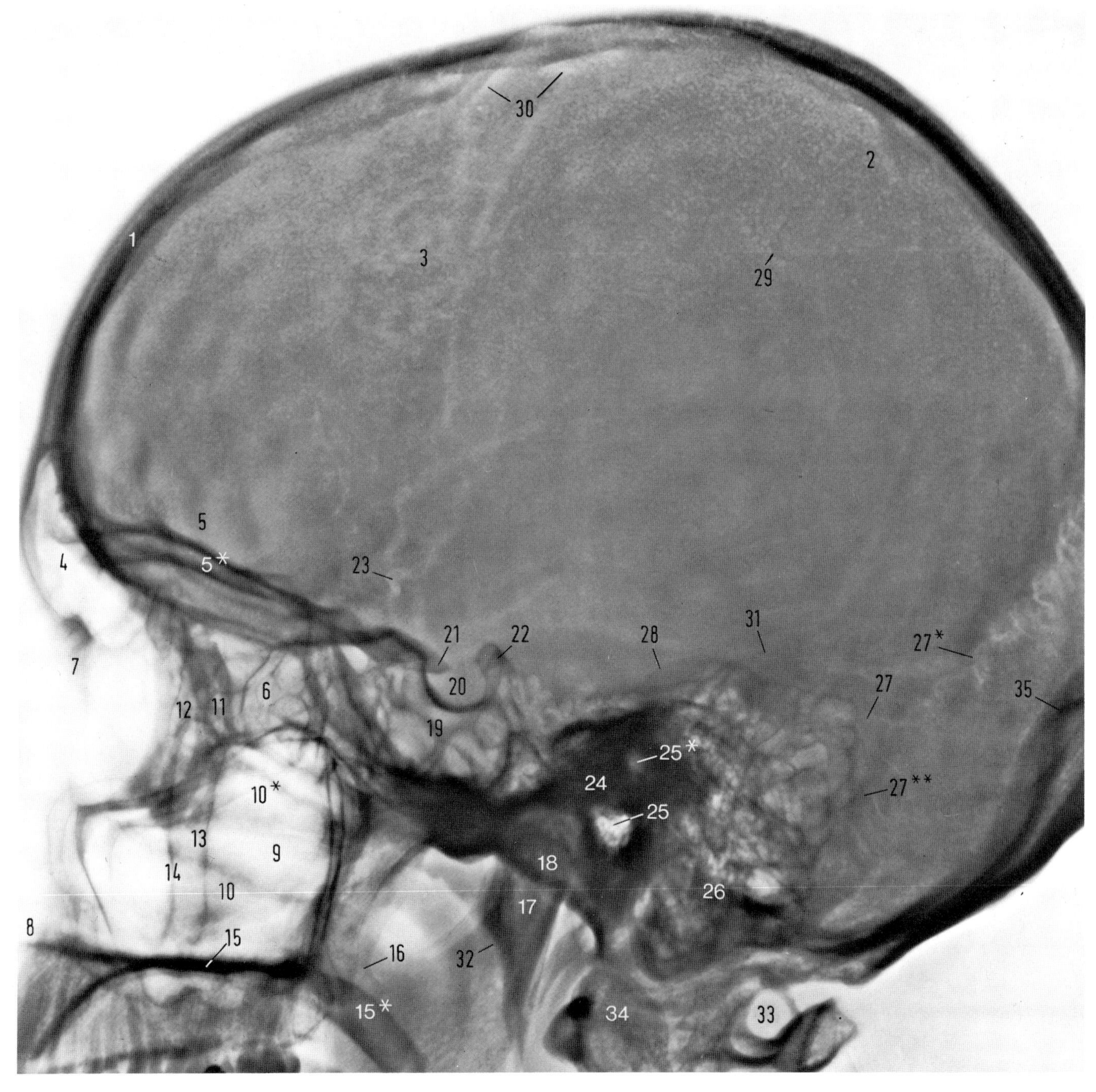

Fig. 243. Head, bitemporal. Conspicuous diploic canals and granular foveolae.

1 Frontal bone
2 Parietal bone
3 Coronal suture
4 Frontal sinus
5 Roof of the film-distant orbita
5*Roof of the adjacent orbita
6 Ethmoidal cells
7 Nasal bone
8 Anterior nasal spine
9 Maxillary sinus
10 Inferior nasal concha
10*Middle nasal concha
11 Outer margin of the adjacent orbita
12 Outer margin of the film-distant orbita
13 Zygomatic process of the adjacent side
14 Zygomatic process of the film-distant side
15 Hard palate
15*Soft palate
16 Pterygoid process
17 Condyloid process
18 Condyle of mandible
19 Sphenoidal sinus
20 Sella turcica
21 Anterior clinoid process
22 Posterior clinoid process
23 Sulcus for middle meningeal artery
24 Petrous bone
25 Opening of the external auditory canal
25*Opening of the internal auditory canal
26 Region of foramen magnum
27 Parietomastoid suture
27*Lambdoid suture
27** Occipitomastoid suture
28 Pinna
29 Diploic canals, spread net-like
30 Granular foveolae
31 Sulcus of the middle meningeal artery
32 Posterior pharyngeal wall
33 Arcuate foramen of atlas
34 Dens (axis)
35 Internal occipital protuberance

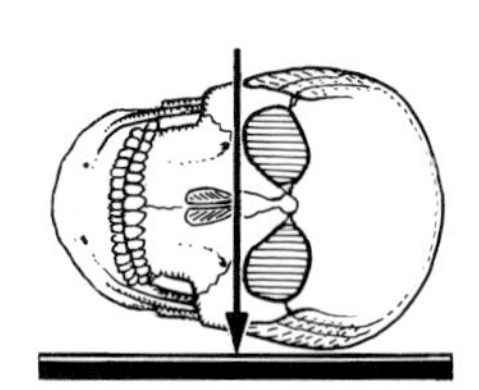

Fig. 244

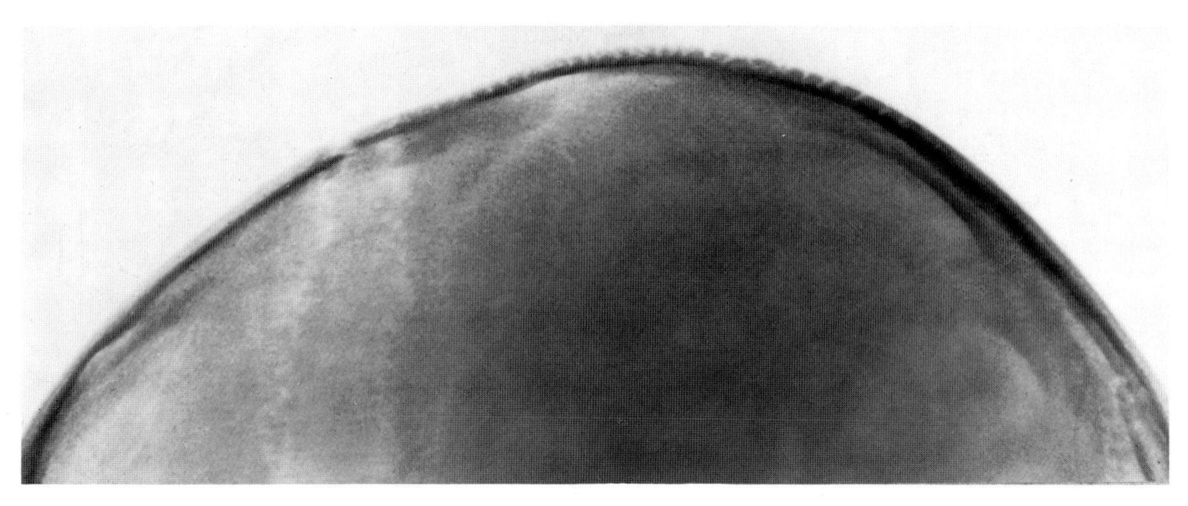

Fig. 245. Velvet-like markings on lateral view of parietal bone, caused by "indentations" which correspond to the very winding course of the sagittal suture (see Fig. 233, No. 22).

Fig. 246. Rare coincidence of massive hyperostosis of the coronal sutures with superimposed, gaping, but non-synostosed lambdoid sutures in a 70-year-old woman.

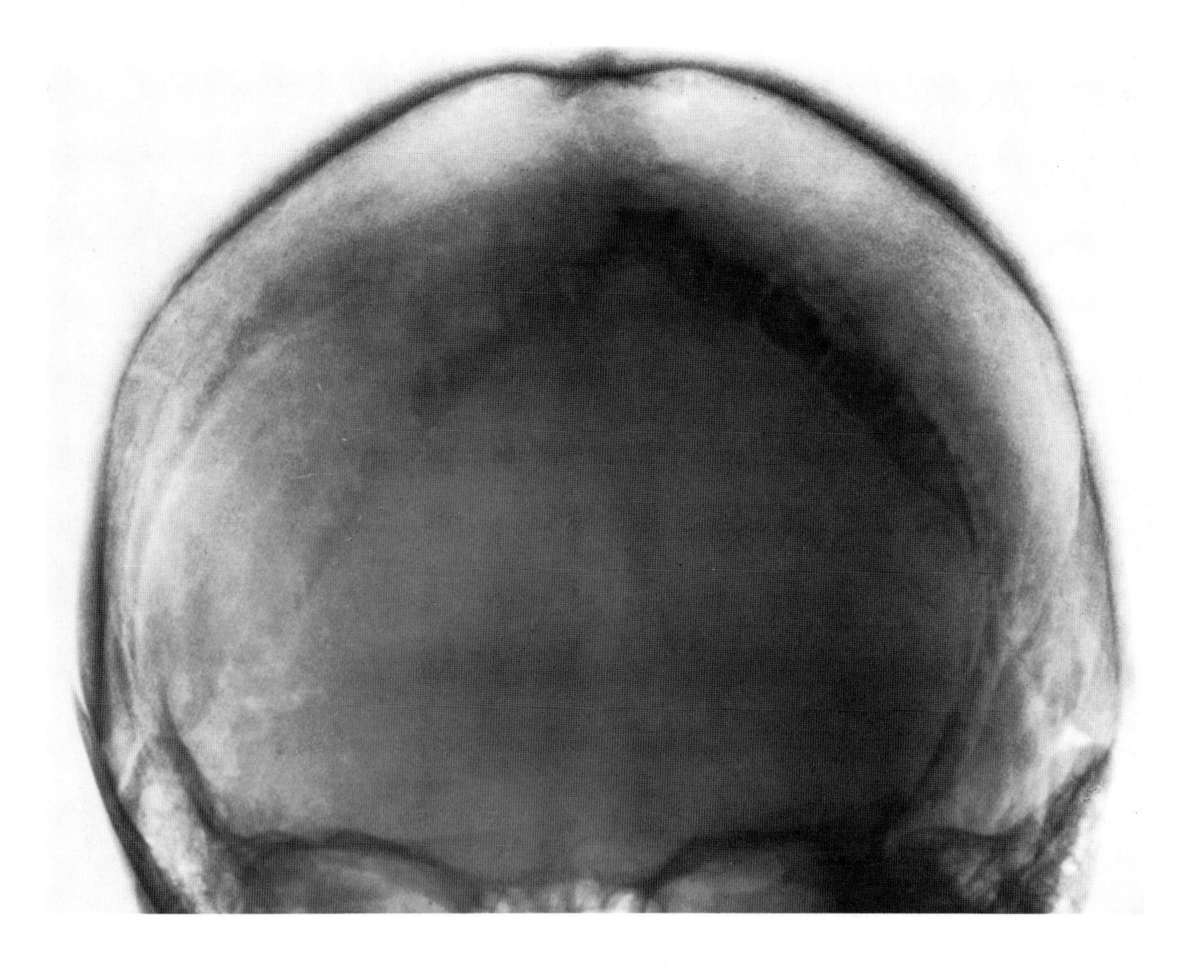

Among the main sutures, the coronal suture frequently synostoses as early as 11 to 20 years of age. The sagittal suture remains open longer, but is almost completely closed by 50 to 70 years. The lambdoid suture is still open in 60–70% of men and women aged 70–80 years. This shows that conclusions as to age cannot be drawn from the state of the cranial suture.

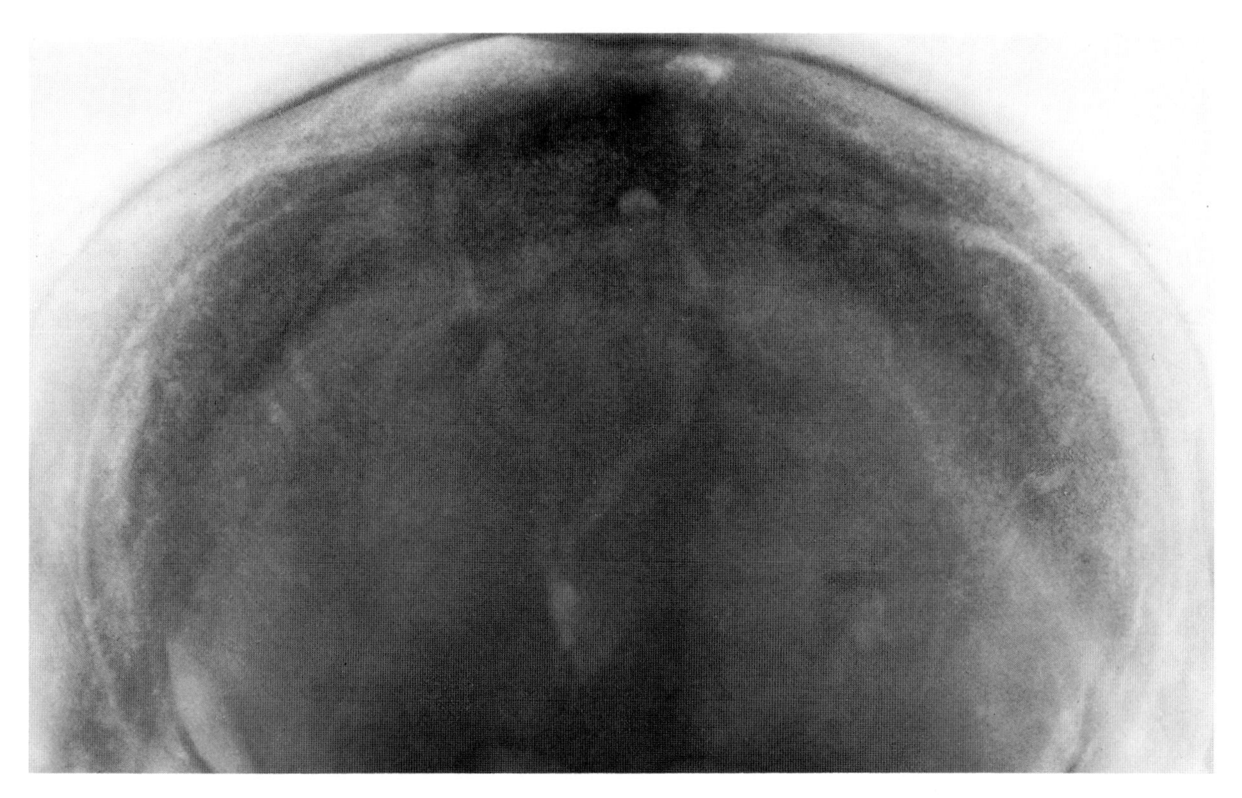

Fig. 247 a. Anteroposterior view.

The holes in the vault:
1. Granular foveolae *(Pacchioni)* are smallish grooves in the internal lamina which are caused by excrescences of the arachnoid *(Pacchioni*an granulations). These peculiar knobby formations invaginate the dura button-like, and may even perforate it *(Sobotta-Becher,* 16th ed.). They protrude into the space of the sinuses where, as a result, only a thin layer of tissue separates the blood from the cerebrospinal fluid. Lateral from the lateral lacunae of the sinuses, the arachnoid villi advance into the internal lamina of the vault towards the diploic veins and there produce the granular foveolae *(Benninghoff-Goerttler,* 9th ed.).
2. Parietal foramina, wrongly also called symmetrical parietal windows (fenestrae) *(Zarfl* and *Voigt),* are pinhead-size, bilateral paramedian holes for the passage of the parietal emissary veins.
3. Foramina permagna connote the development of the parietal foramina to larger-than-bean size. They are said to be caused by dominant hereditary derangements of ossification. Although not relevant clinically, they confer a stigma of degeneration.
4. Persistent accessory parietal fontanel, i.e., symmetrical parietal windows (fenestrae) (see also *Schmidt-Wittkamp* and *Christians; Mükke* and *Poppe).*

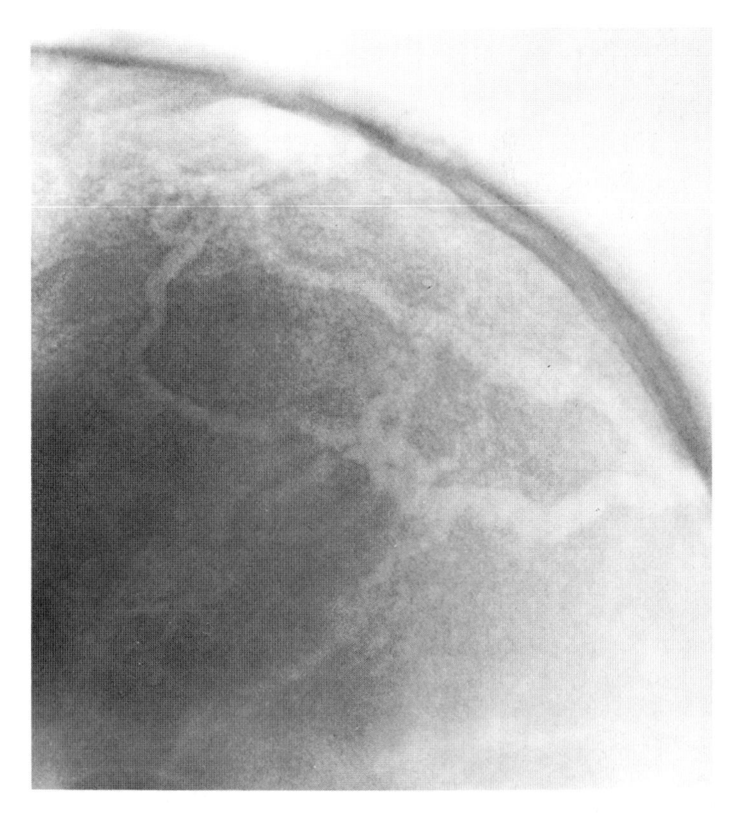

Fig. 247 b. Lateral view.

Fig. 247 a, b. Asymmetrical overside parietal foramina for the termination of deeper diploic veins which, on lateral view, form a venous star of *Breschet* as a further variant; see No. 20 on Figs. 232 and 233.

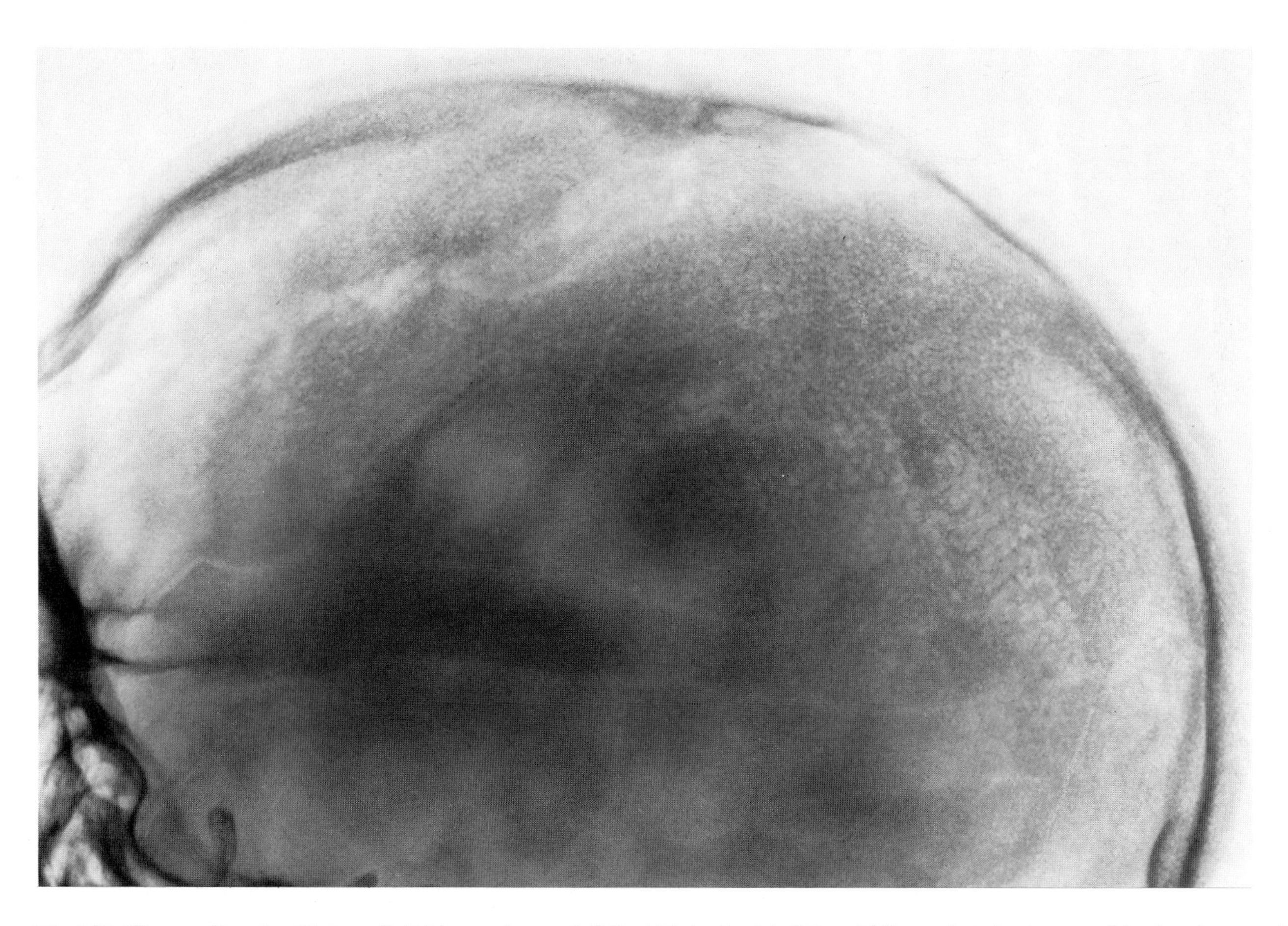

Fig. 248. 17-year-old male with deep digital impressions and distinct bilateral sulci of the middle meningeal artery, reaching into its posterior branches (the adjacent side appears smaller and more sharply outlined).

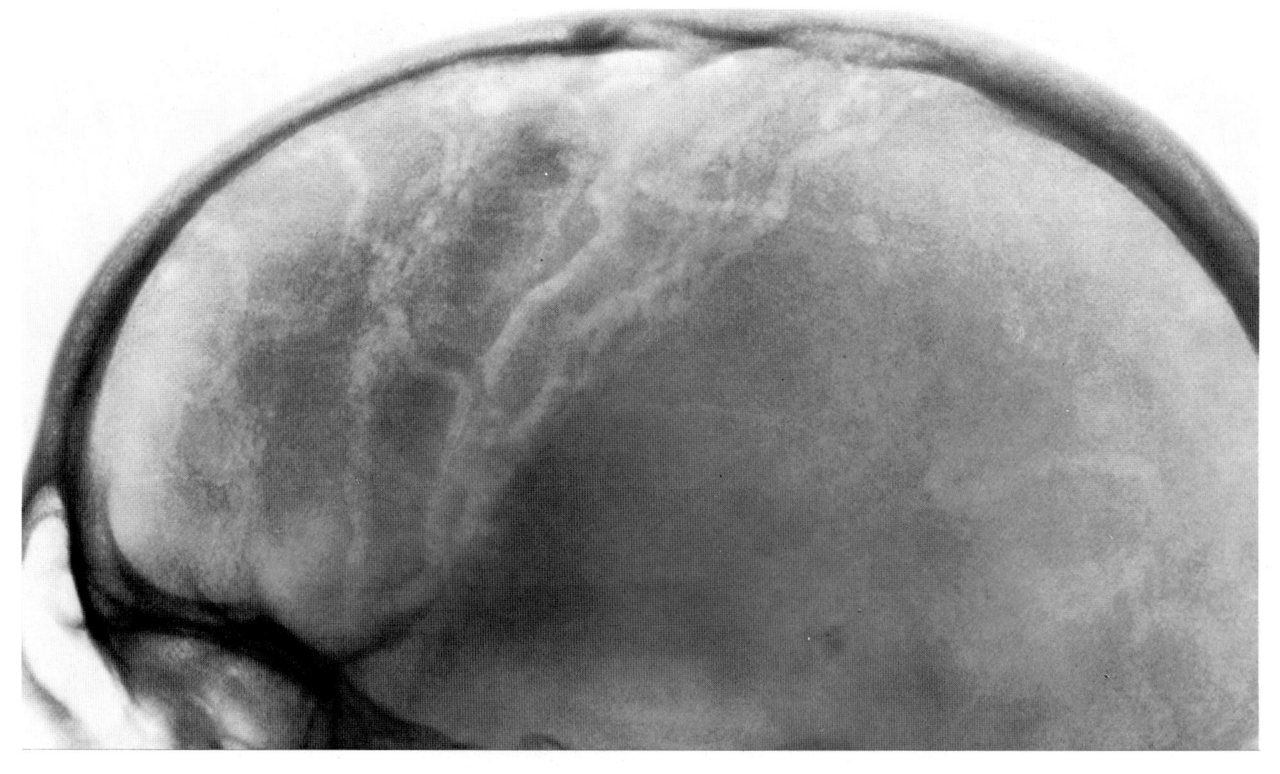

Fig. 249. Frontal and temporal, tree-like ramified diploic veins, apparently terminating in deep lacunar granular foveolae, and flowing through holes in the external lamina into the outer veins of the soft tissues or into the emissary veins.

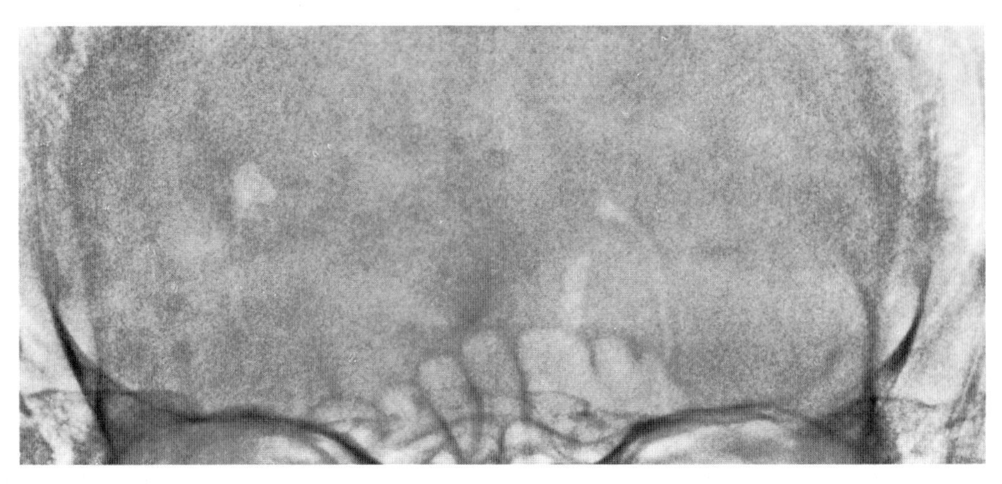

Fig. 250 (from the collection of *Knetsch*). **Left frontal emissary vein and right** *Pacchioni*an **groove.** Emissary veins connect the sinuses of the dura mater with the superficial veins of the skull. The length of the canals, which terminate in a hole-like defect, is usually 2–4 cm. In juveniles the frontal emissary vein can be demonstrated especially well. It is more frequently present unilaterally than bilaterally and is visible in 0.2 to 0.3% of all radiographs of the skull *(Knetsch)*. Confusion with fractures may occur. See also *Martin-Reith*.

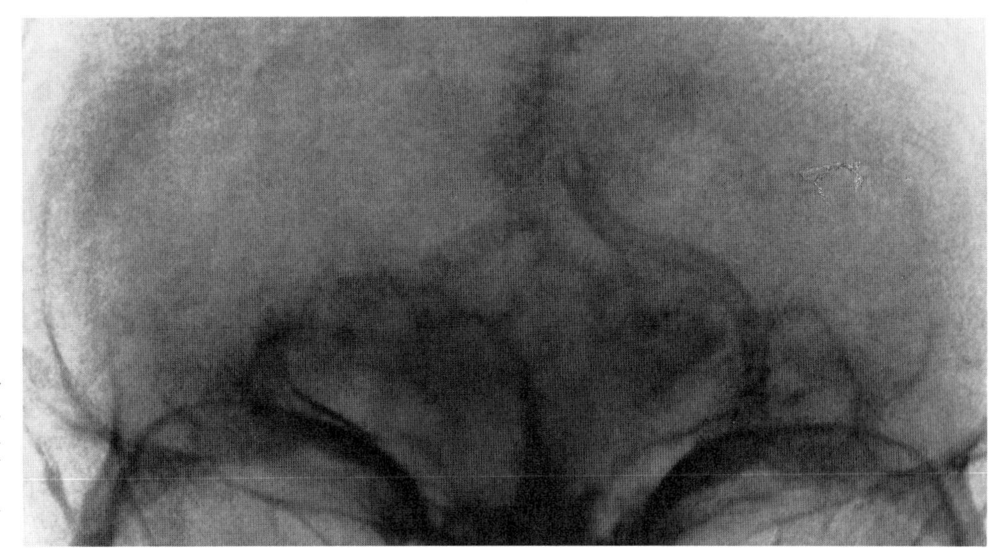

Fig. 251. Left frontal emissary vein next to sutural hyperostoses. Further emissary veins: mastoid emissary vein, parietal emissary vein, occipital emissary vein, condyloid emissary vein, emissary vein of the foramen of Vesalius.

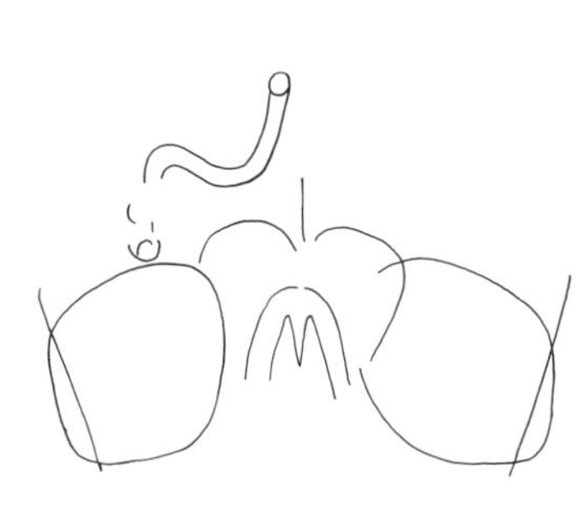

Fig. 252. The showing of the frontal emissary vein is said to signify a pathological process, e.g., increased intracranial pressure or intracranial or ophthalmic disturbances.

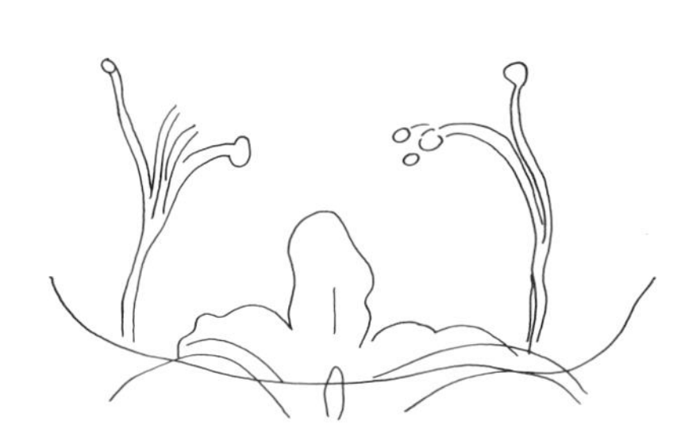

Fig. 253 shows examples of the inconstant and very variable sulci of the frontal diploic veins, which lead in an arch as bony vascular canals from the median plane to the superior orbital boundary, usually occurring unilaterally and more rarely bilaterally. They form a vascular connection of the superior sagittal sinus to the orbital veins.

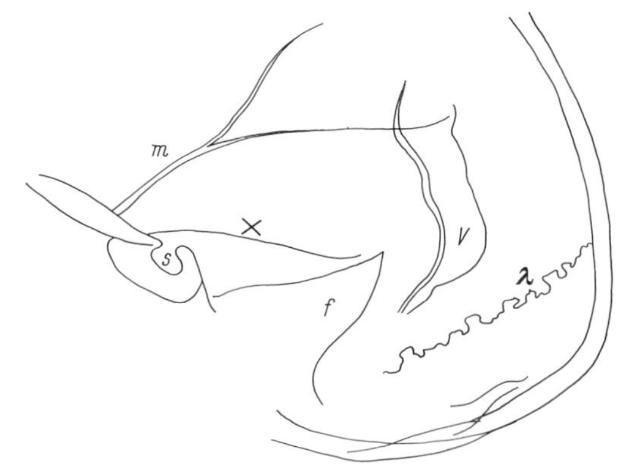

Fig. 254. Sulci for blood vessels. f=petrous bone, λ=lambdoid suture, s=sella, m=sulci of the middle meningeal artery. A lower branch (×) is often mistaken for a fracture (Fig. 233, No. 30). A radiograph taken more from the median line, verticodextrosinistral and verticosinistrodextral, can clarify the facts. V=venous sulci in the posterior region of the parietal bone, running more vertically and, in contrast to fracture lines, more arched *(Keller)*.

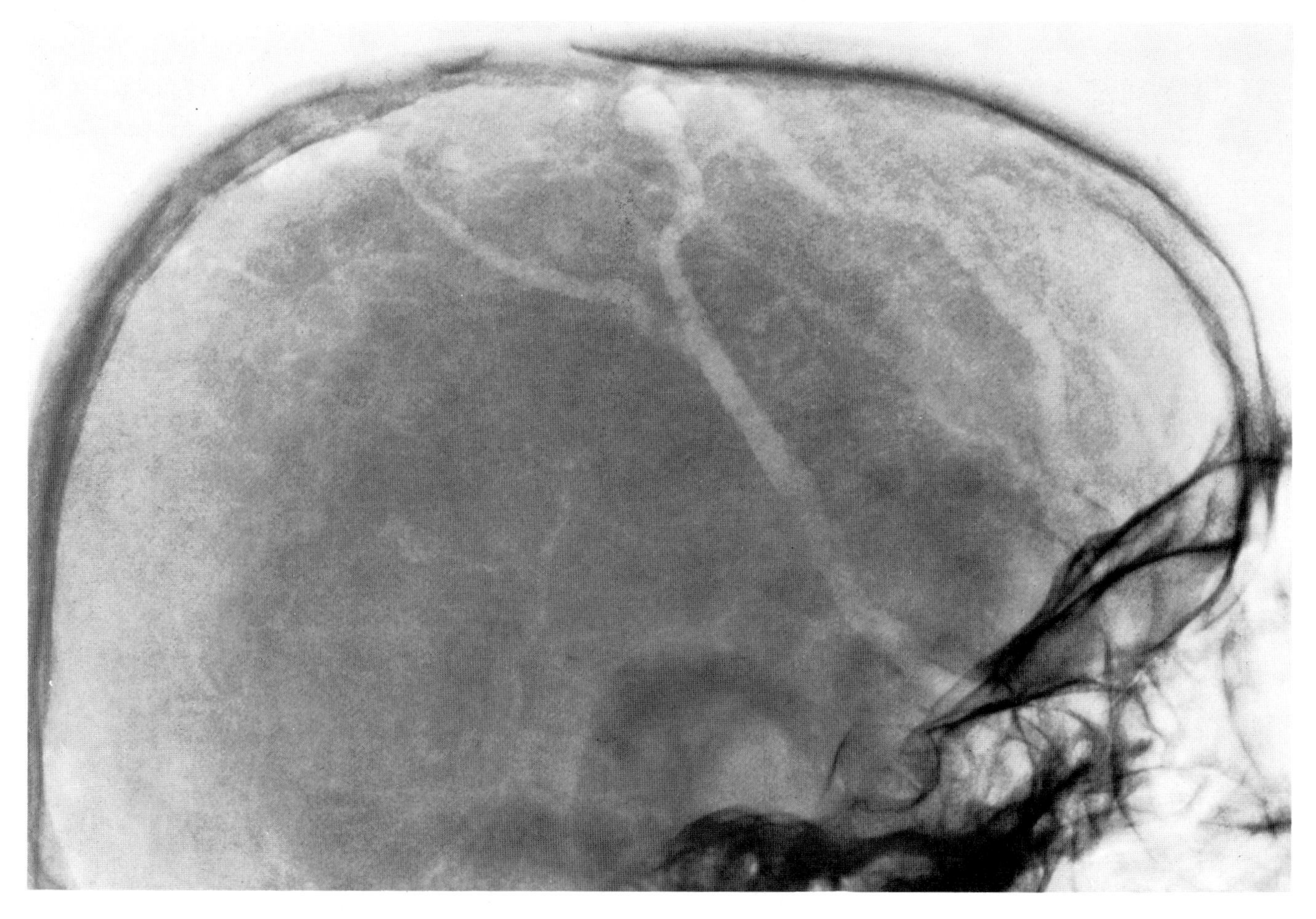

Fig. 255. Conspicuously wide diploic veins which terminate in the also widened granular foveolae, with an especially distinct view of the variable anterior temporal diploic vein. Course, shape and caliber of the diploic veins differ greatly *(Wanke, Lindblom)*. See Fig. 233, No. 29*, Fig. 236 and Fig. 257.

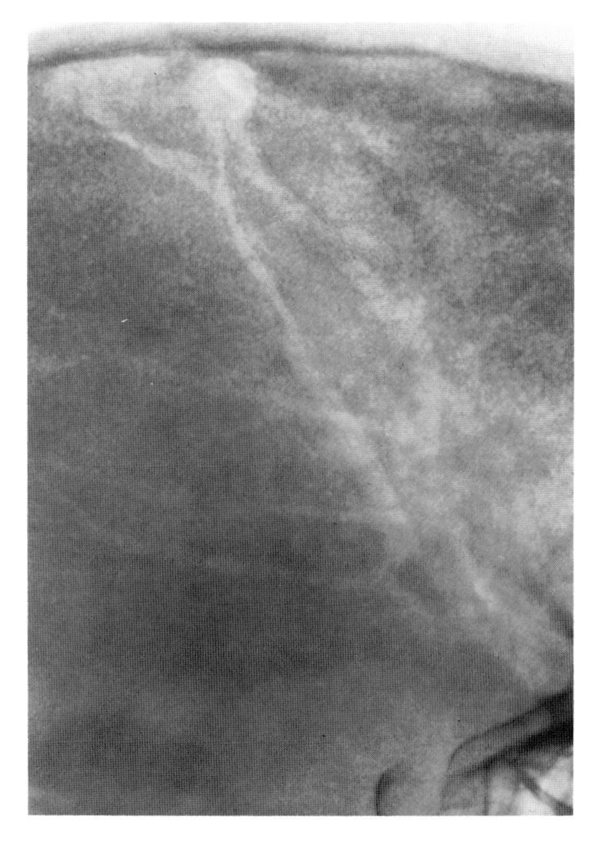

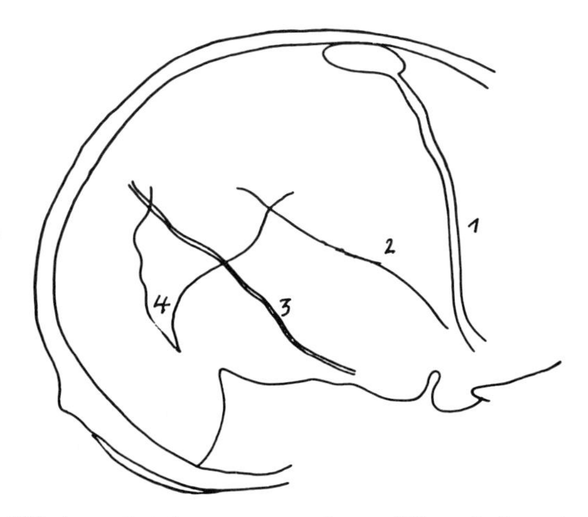

Fig. 257 shows that the venous canals run differently from the arterial sulci.

1 Anterior temporal diploic vein. Here, somewhat dilated, it seems to terminate into a granular foveola in the region of the former fontanel.
2 Sulcus of the middle meningeal artery
3 and 4 Venous canals; 4 may form ample ramifications, sometimes cobweb-like

Fig. 256. Anterior temporal diploic vein, which appears to terminate in a *Pacchioni*an groove.

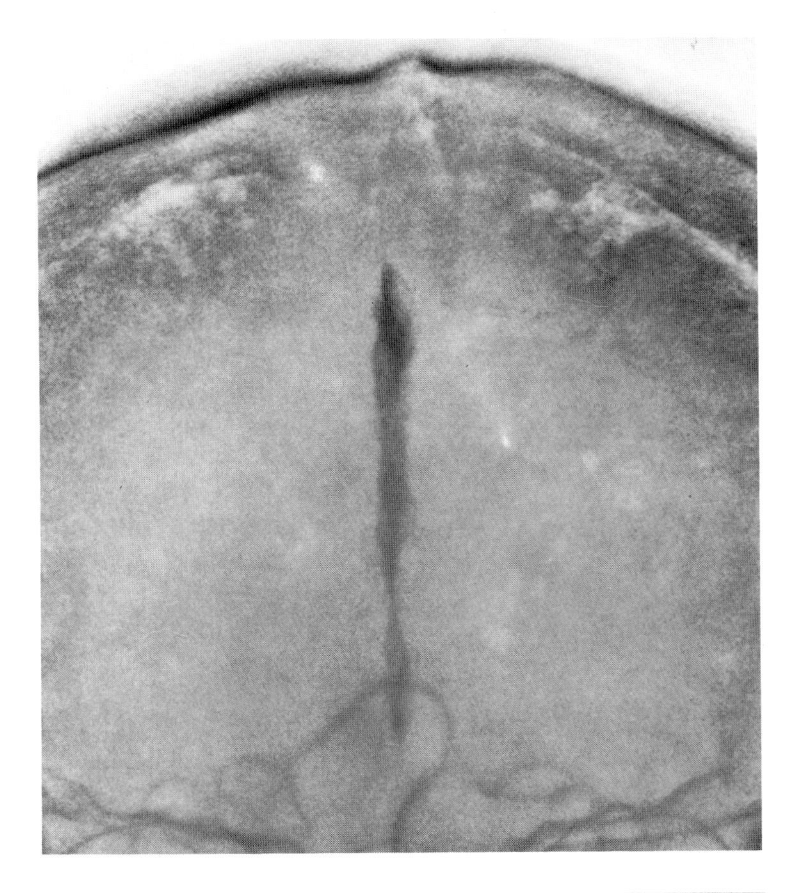

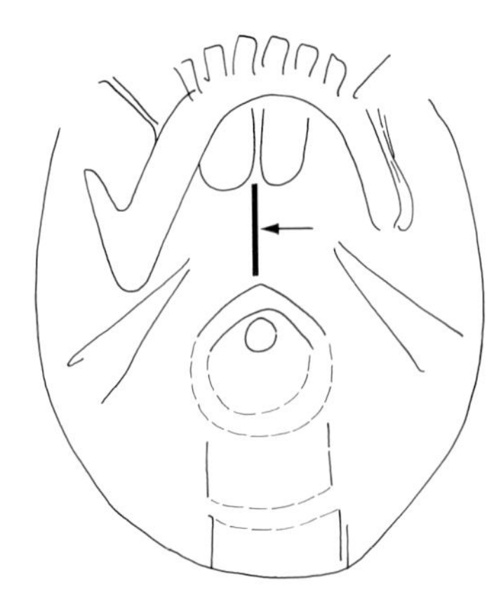

Fig. 259. Ossified falx cerebri on axial projection (←). See also Fig. 239.

Fig. 258. Ossified falx cerebri (see Fig. 232, No. 2). Distinct granular foveolae, in symmetrical arrangement (see No. 6 in Fig. 232), can be recognized.

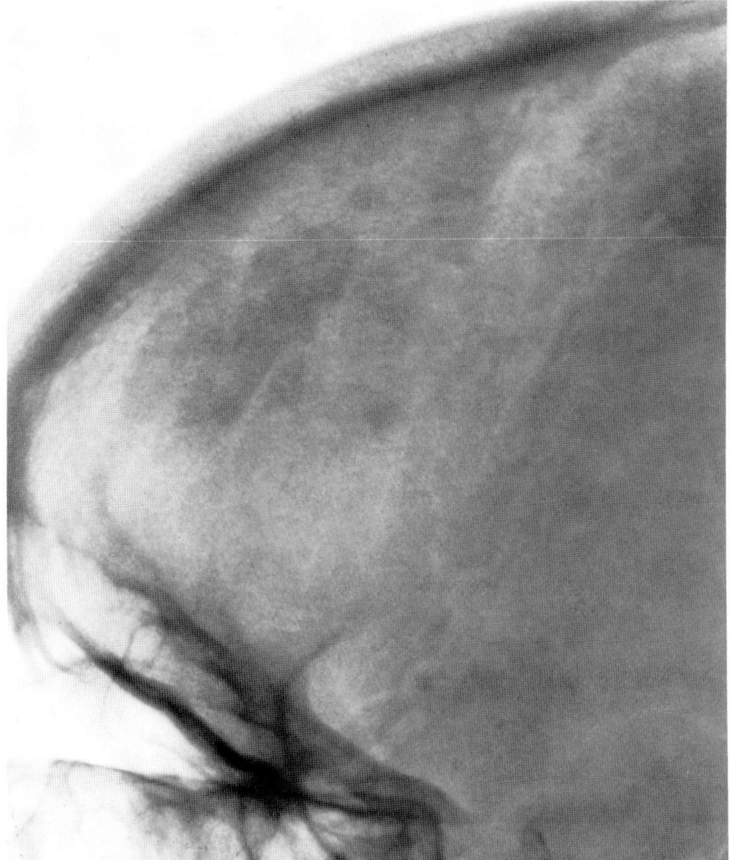

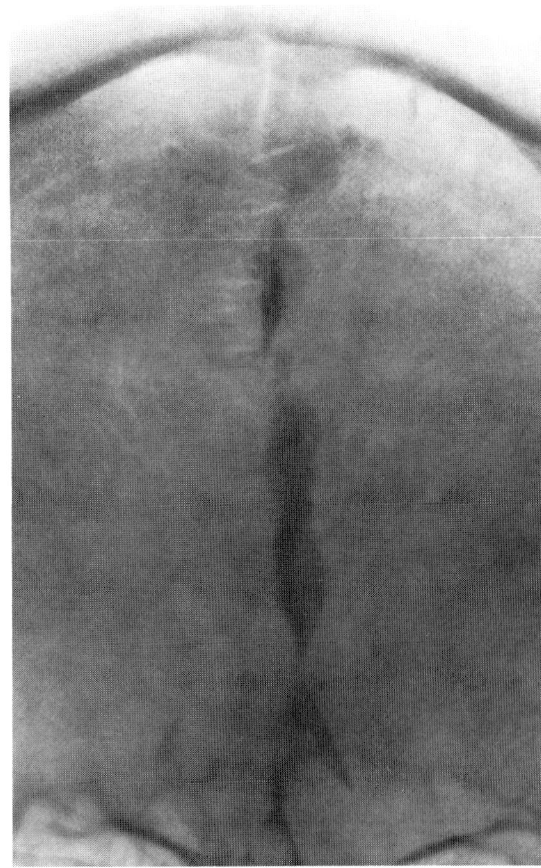

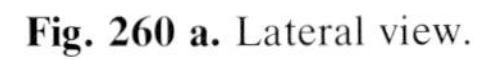

Fig. 260 a. Lateral view.

Fig. 260 b. Posteroanterior view.

Fig. 260 a, b. On the lateral view, **simulation of a frontal nebula** (a flower-bed-like shape of the frontal hyperostosis), caused by a flattened calcification of the falx (see No. 29 on Fig. 233).

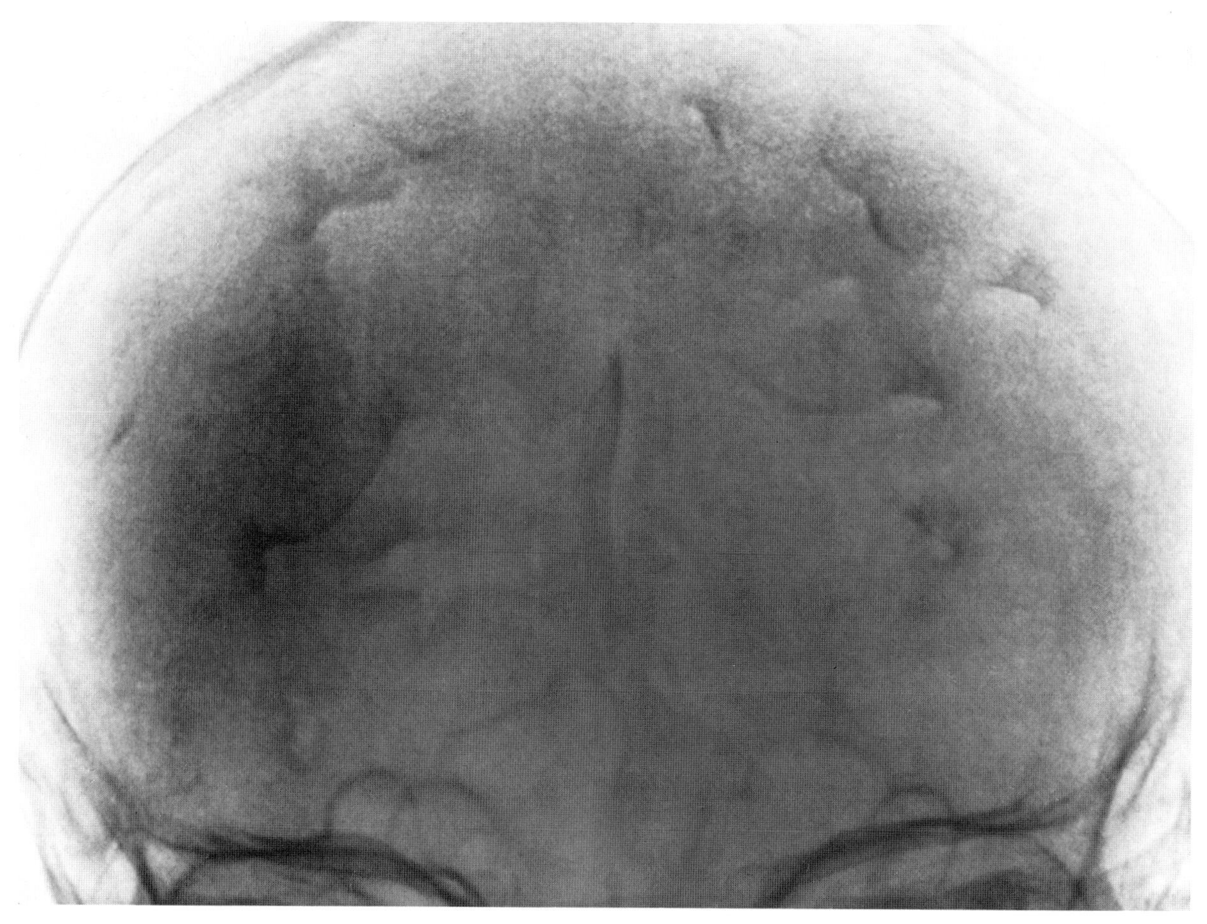

Fig. 261 a

Fig. 261 b

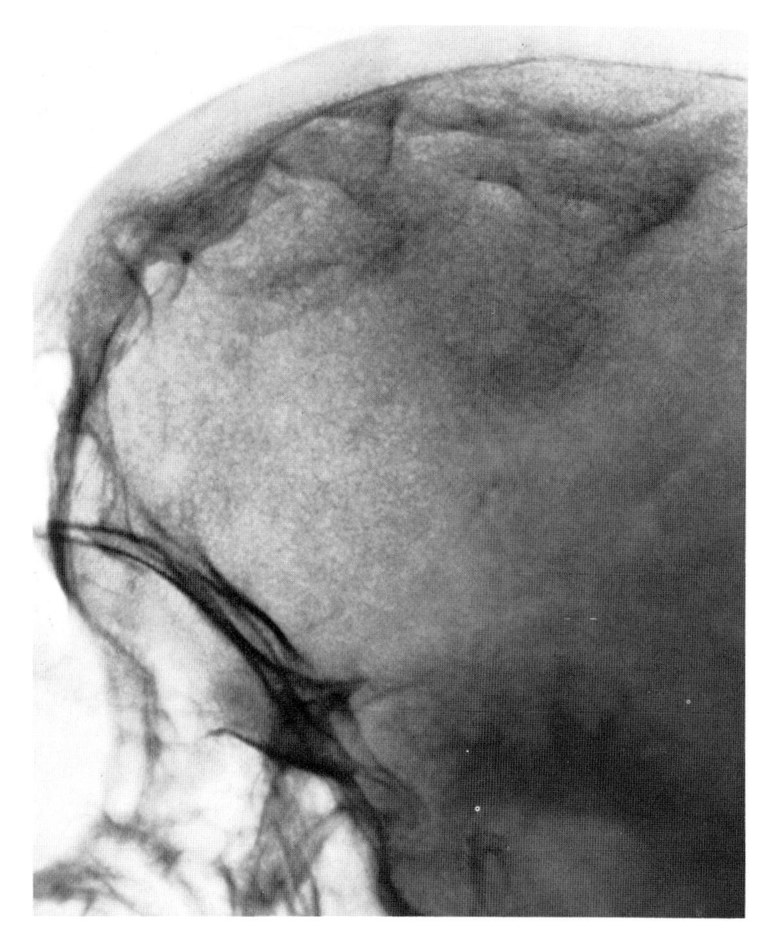

Coincidence of a hereditary developmental disposition (internal frontal hyperostosis) with calcifications of the falx and the suprasellar dural region (post-traumatic or post-inflammatory, calcified hematoma); see *Ellegast.* It sometimes occurs as part of the *Morgagni* syndrome (obesity, virilism, amenorrhea, hypertonia, internal frontal hyperostosis). The regions of the sutures, including the original frontal suture, remain free of hyperostoses. Therefore, these can easily be delimited from calcifications of the meninges. One distinguishes between knobby hyperostosis (predominantly in the frontal region), spotty hyperostosis (frontal nebula), the parietal form and diffuse calvarial hyperostosis.

Fig. 261. Frontal hyperostosis, calcification of the falx cerebri and calcified suprasellar hematoma.

Fig. 262. Step formation on the occiput (bathrocephaly).
The occipital squama may overlap the parietal bones dorsally. This causes the development of a step in the region of the lambdoid suture which, as in this case, is frequently combined with supernumerary bones (see also Fig. 233, No. 23).

1 Tip of the lambdoid suture (approximate)
2 Lambdoid suture, whose two limbs almost cover each other. The suture forms a step (visible near No. 1).
3 Supernumerary bone in the region of the lambdoid suture. This step formation, with a gaping lambdoid suture, presents an anatomical variant (bathrocephaly) which should not be mistaken for a fracture. Together with it, one usually finds numerous supernumerary bones.
4 Internal occipital protuberance, indistinct; the edge of the longitudinal sulcus for the longitudinal sinus runs upwards and downwards, protruding screen-like (inconstant); Note well, the tentorium does not produce a radiographic shadow.
5 Region of the foramen magnum

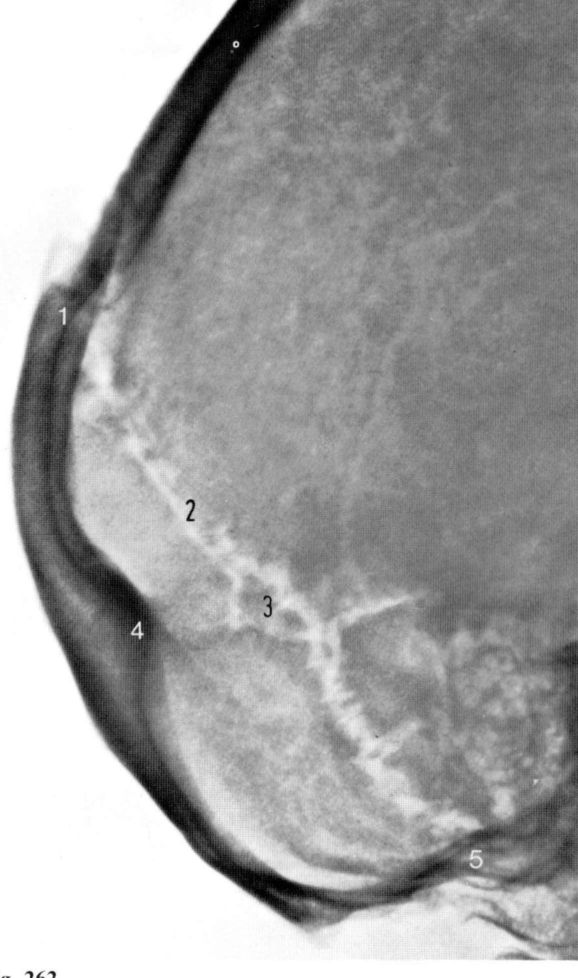

Fig. 262

Fig. 263. Unilateral sickle-shaped hypercalcinosis of the meninges. Such meningeal calcifications, which sometimes surround both hemispheres evenly (brain en cuirasse, *Birkner* and *Lagemann),* are the result of post-traumatic processes (subdural hematoma), possibly combined with the consequences of an inflammatory meningitis (internal hemorrhagic pachymeningosis).

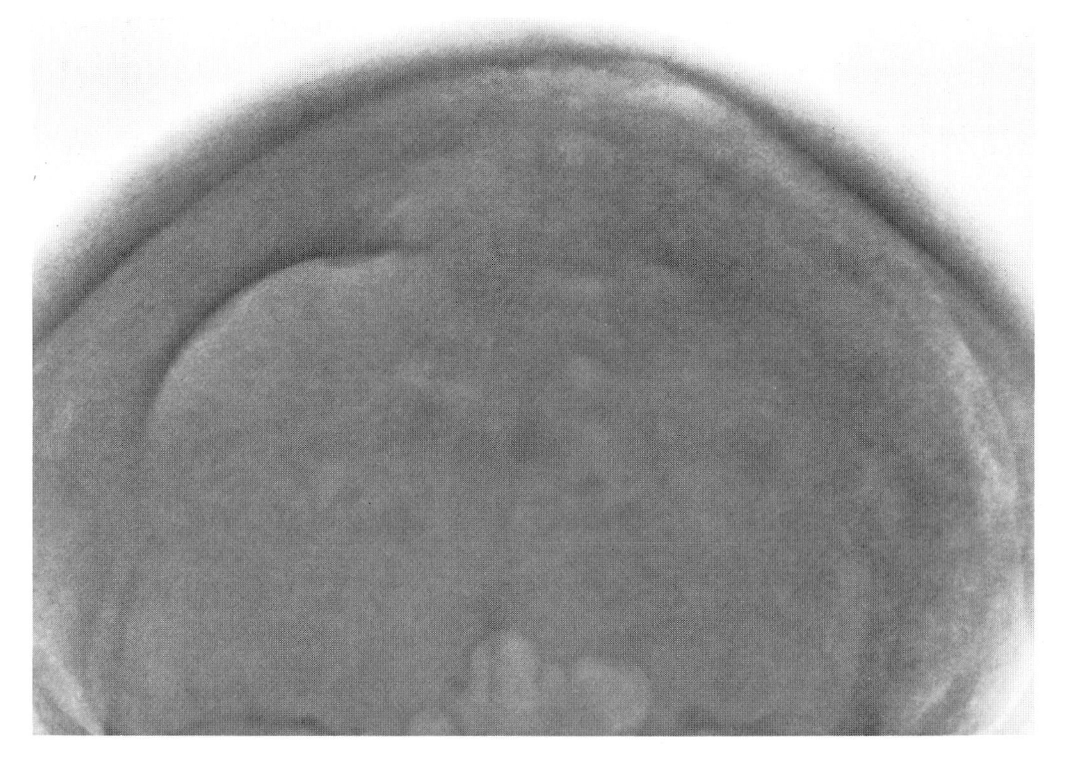

Fig. 263

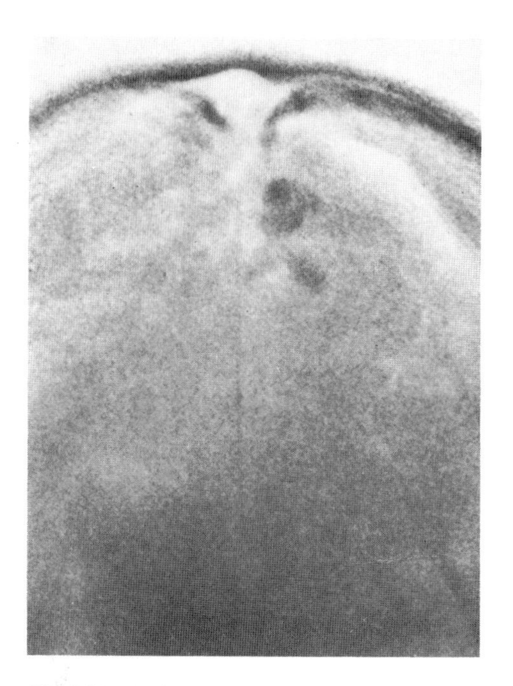

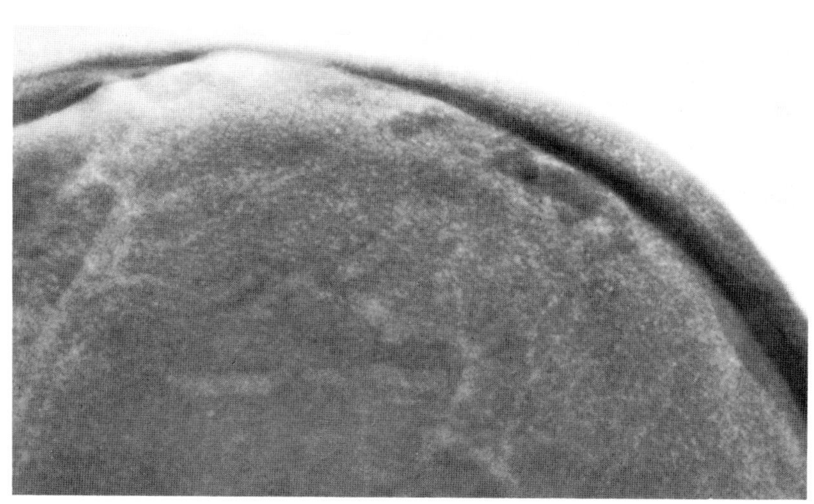

Fig. 264 a. Sagittal.

Fig. 264 b. Lateral.

Fig. 264. Male, 25 years of age; calcification of a subdural hematoma, which had not been diagnosed following trauma five years earlier, and therefore had not been operated upon. See *Tönnis* and *Friedman* for a comprehensive review of the differential diagnosis of pathological intracranial calcifications.

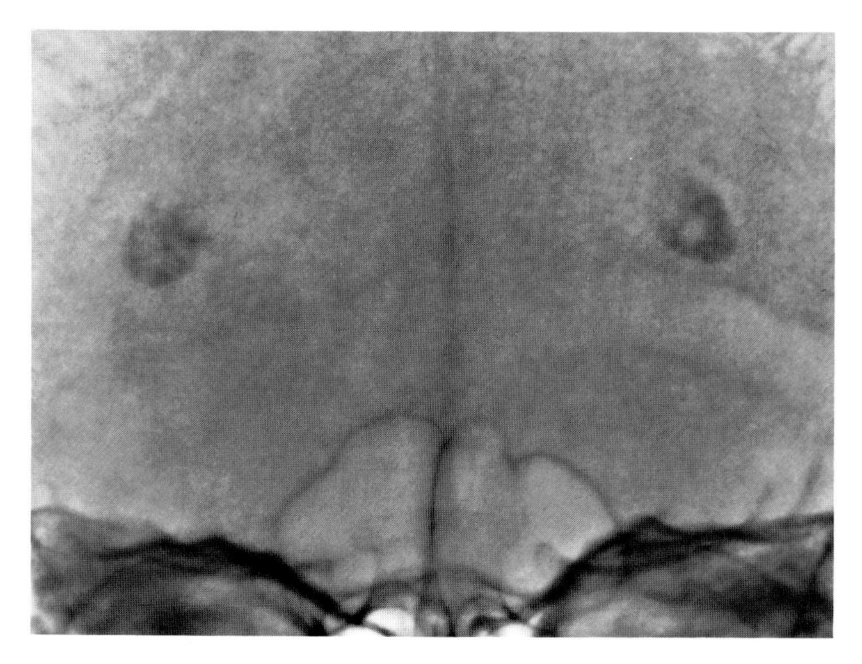

Fig. 265. Calcified chorioid plexus, usually occurring symmetrically (bilaterally up to 10%, unilaterally only 3%). For their relation to chronic inflammations of the plexus, e.g., after encephalitis due to toxoplasmosis, see Fig. 232, No. 9; see also *Schoeps, Lorenz.*

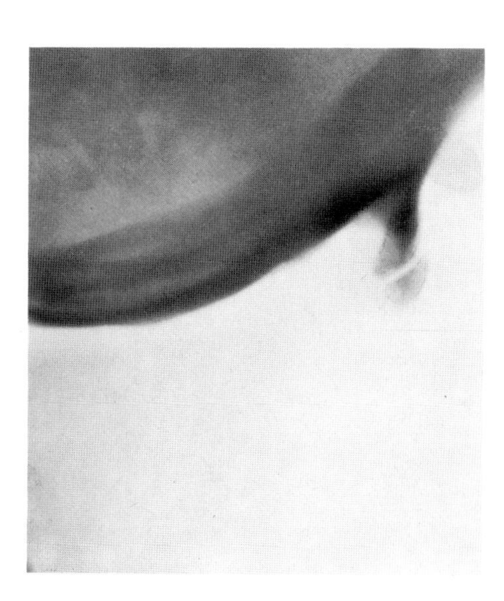

Fig. 266. So-called articulating occipital spur, a process at the external occipital protuberance *(Greineder).* This is the site of insertion for the ligamentum nuchae.

According to *Bruch, Bushe* and *Gregl,* intracranial, non-pathological calcifications (falx, sella, arachnoid, chorioid plexus, pineal body) are found in 60–75% of all radiographs of the skull of those aged 21–30 years, and in 90% of those at advanced ages or senile.

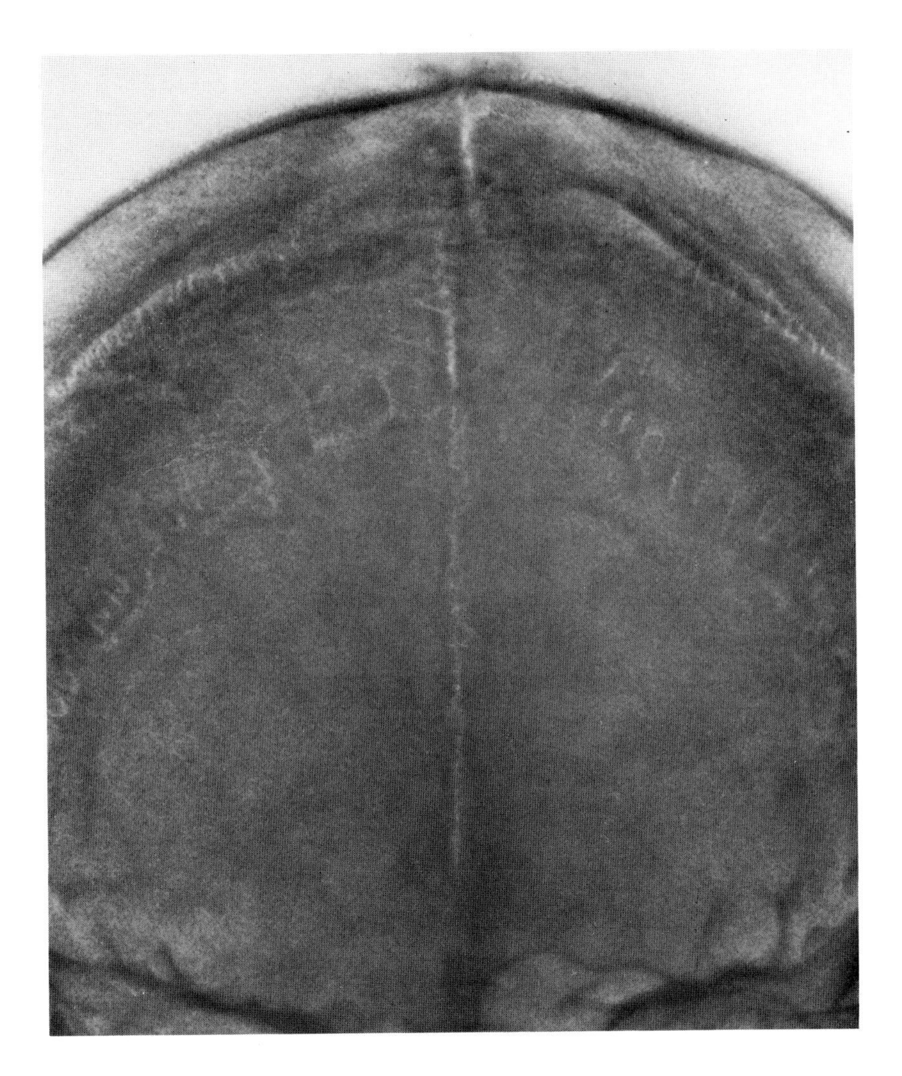

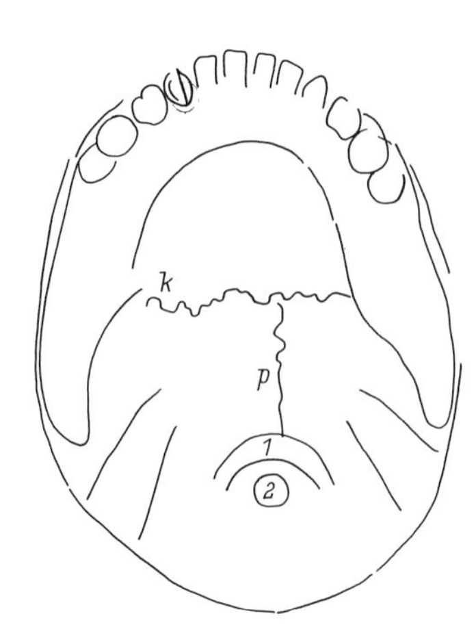

Fig. 268. On axial projection the coronal and sagittal sutures may be mistaken for fracture lines.
k Coronal suture
p Sagittal suture
1 Ventral arch of atlas
2 Dens (axis)

Fig. 267. Metopic suture (see Fig. 232, No. 1). Synostosis of the frontal suture normally starts during the second year of life. If this suture remains open beyond the third year, it is considered to be a persistent frontal suture, a metopic suture and a bifid cranium *(Terrafranca* and *Zellis); Wanke* and *Diethelm* observed this suture in 10% of those aged 10 and under and in 6% of those under 30 in their examination of a very large number of cases specifically for this condition.

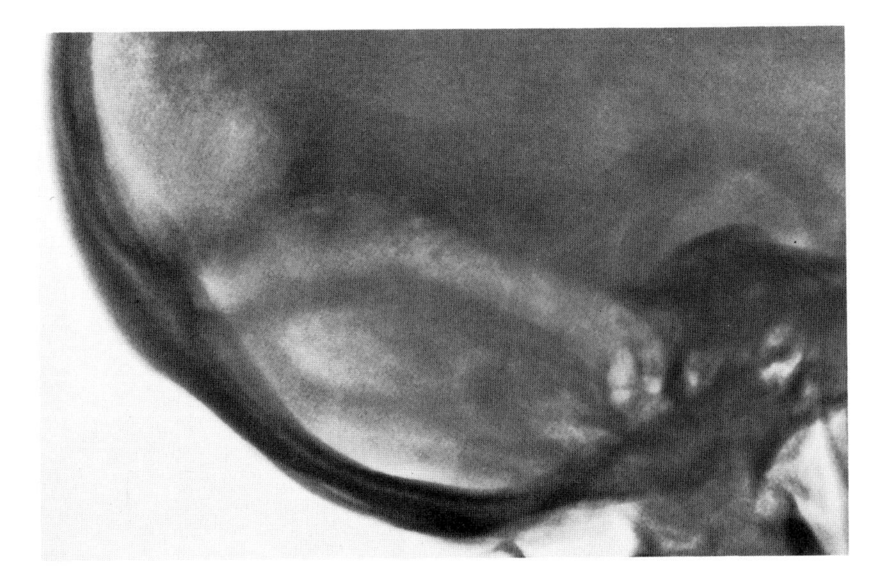

Fig. 269. Clear presentation of the sulcus for the transverse and sigmoid sinuses on a lateral radiograph of the skull. (See Fig. 233, No. 8). The pinnae are projected into the temporal squama.

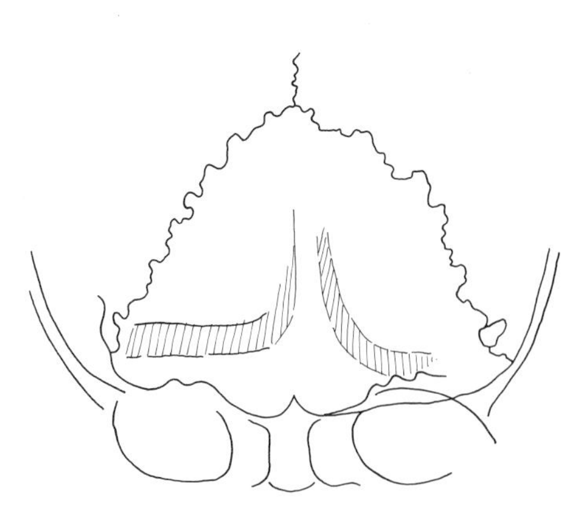

Fig. 270. Sketch of an anteroposterior radiograph. Asymmetrically developed transverse sinuses of unequal caliber are not uncommon.

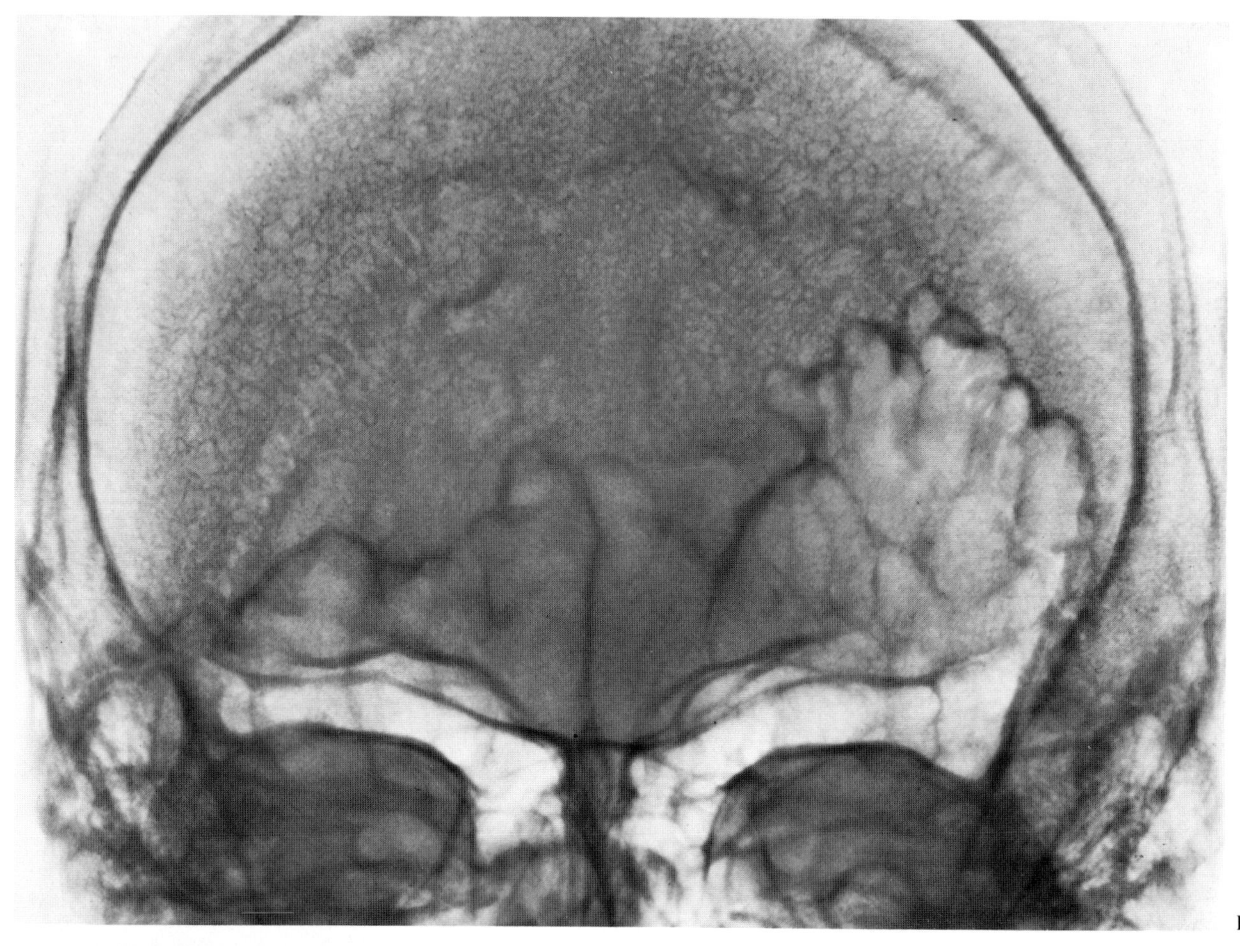

Fig. 271

Fig. 271. *Weickmann* described connections between vicarious hyperplasia of the paranasal sinuses and hypoplastic cerebral processes (perhaps an internal hydrocephalus?). Hyperplasia of the paranasal sinuses may also occur in cases of acromegaly.

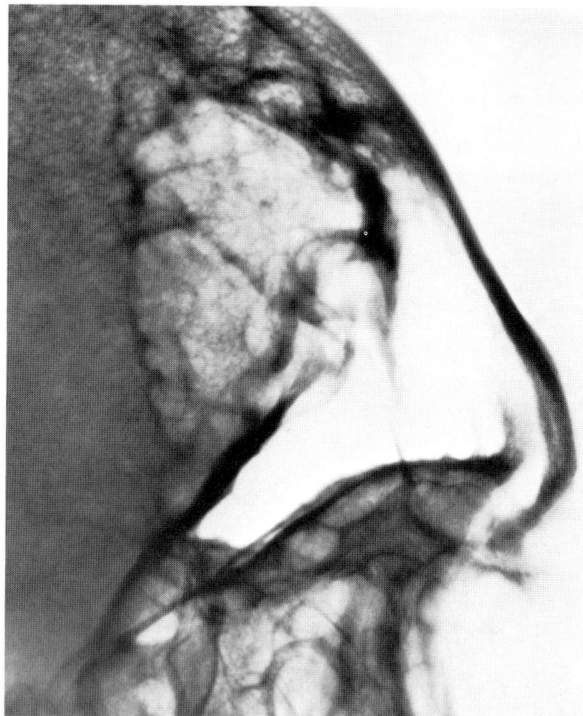

Fig. 272

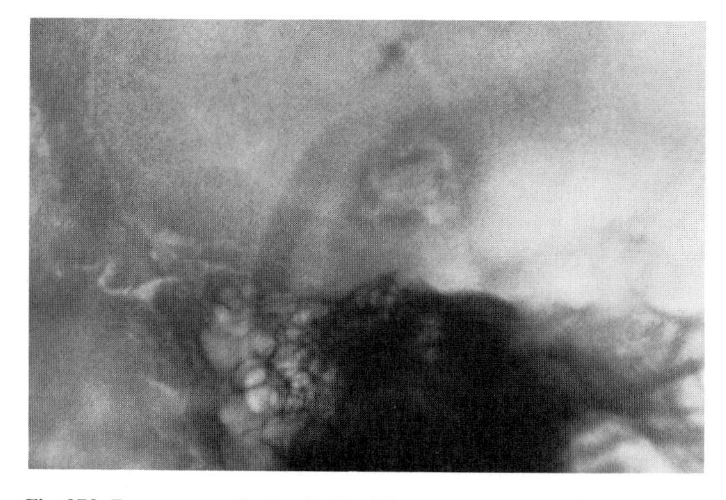

Fig. 273. Rare pneumatization in the right temporal squama in a 45-year-old female.

Figs. 271 and **272. Excessive development of the paranasal sinuses,** especially of the frontal sinuses with large recesses above both orbitae (pneumosinus dilatans); see *Weickmann.* The lateral view clearly shows the total extent of the pneumatization of the left frontal bone, as well as the recesses. In this case, the supraorbital pneumatization is mainly caused by orbital ethmoidal cells, as can be seen distinctly in Fig. 271. Especially wide extensions of the hyperpneumatization may cause difficulties in differentiating the frontal sinus from the ethmoidal cells *(Haas).*

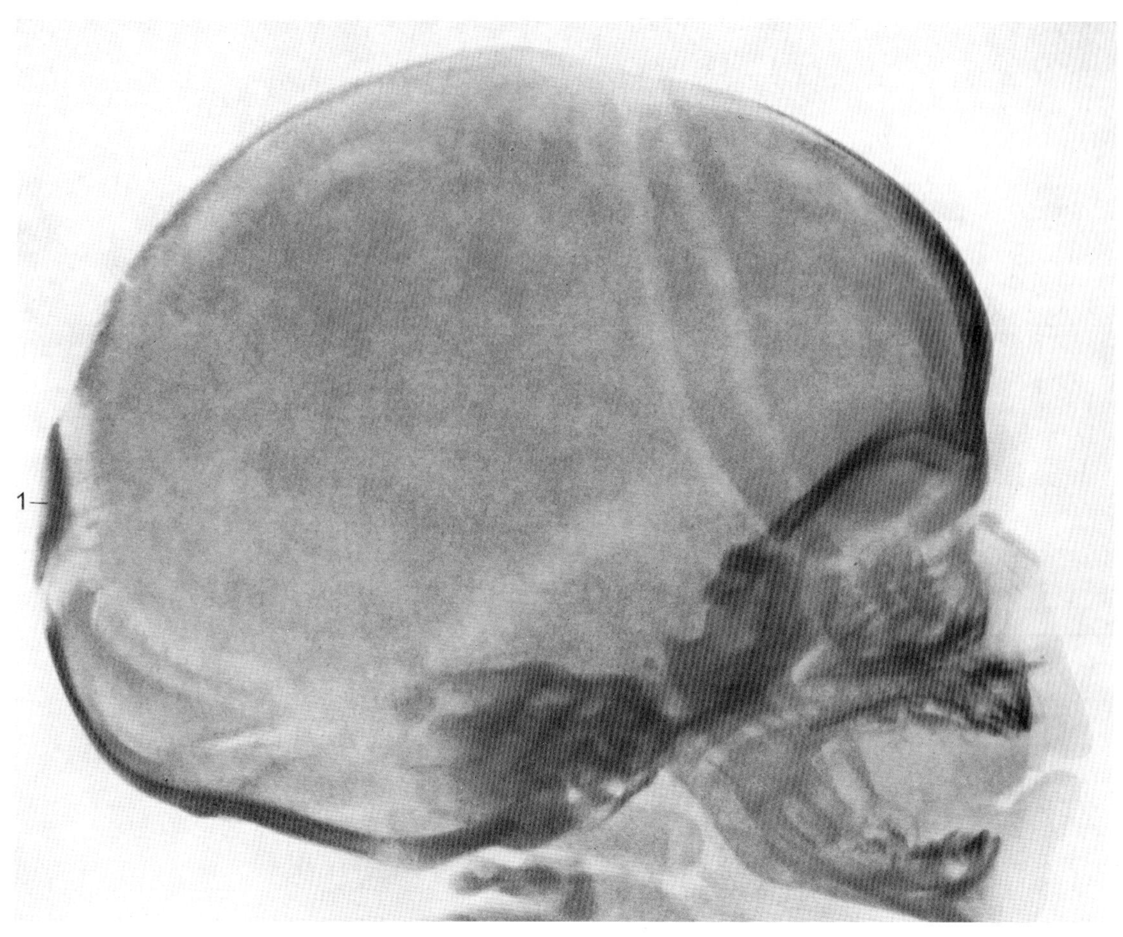

Fig. 274. Supernumerary bone, also called pointed or segmental bone, at the lambdoid suture (1) of a 3-day-old infant. The sutura mendosa, which can often still be seen during the first year of life, runs backwards and downwards.

Sutural bones (ossa suturarum), also called pointed, segmental, or fontanel bone, are bony islands surrounded by a normal cranial suture.

Fig. 275. Segmental bone at the lambdoid suture. The sutura mendosa, which starts from both lambdoid sutures, represents the remainder of a transverse occipital suture (from *Goldhamer* and *Schüller*).

Fig. 275

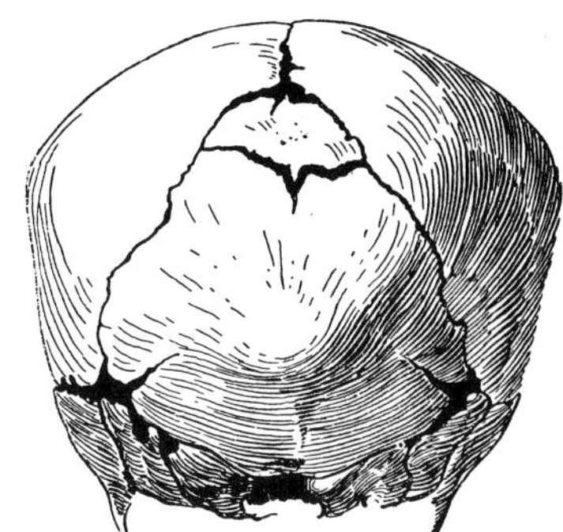

Fig. 277. Sketch to Fig. 276.

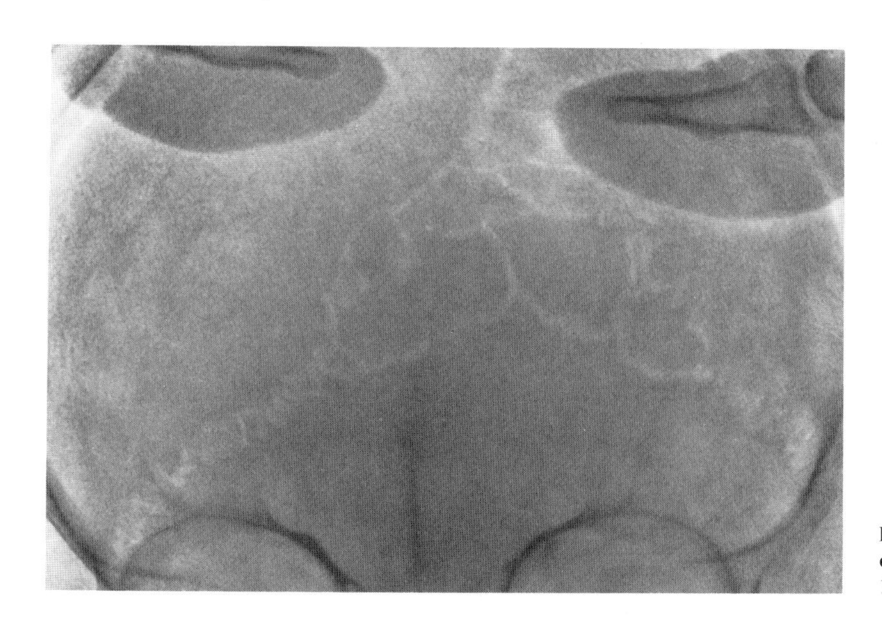

Fig. 276. Segmental bone at the juncture of the coronal and sagittal sutures (fontanel bone) in a child 1-3/4 years old.

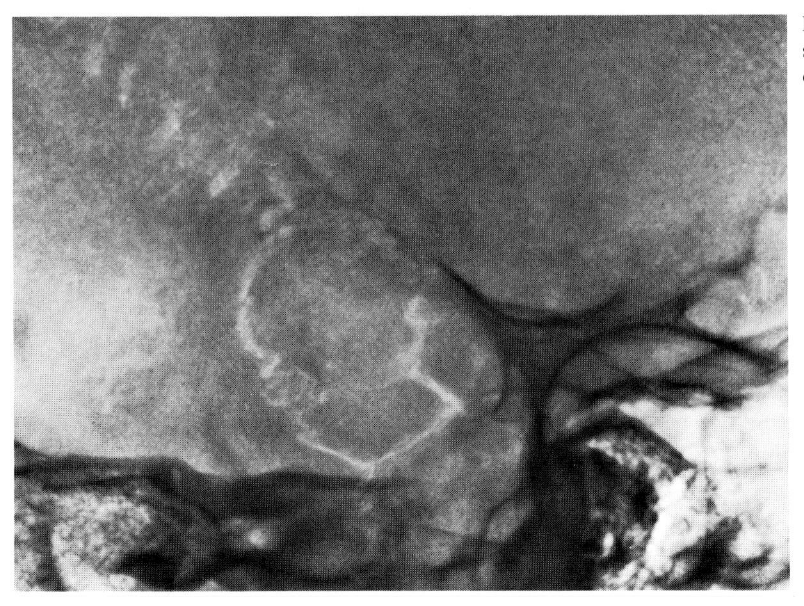

Intercalary bones (ossa intercalaria) are wholly or partly surrounded by their own suture, and therefore blow out of a larger bony squama.

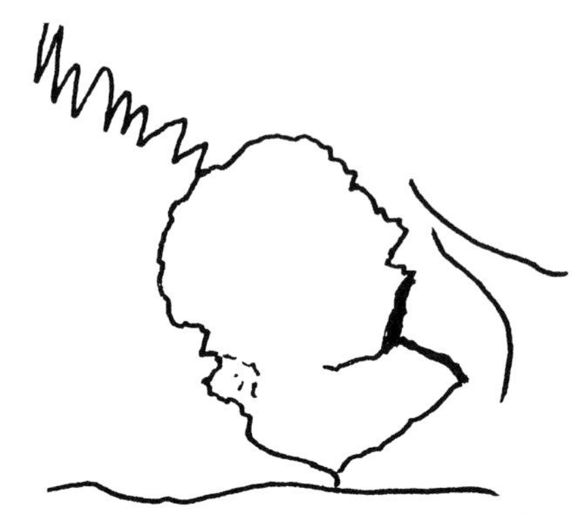

Fig. 278. Intercalary bone of the right temporal squama. Such genuine intercalary bones, which lean only partly or not at all against an ordinary suture, are obviously very rare. No similar case could be found in any of the standard references on anatomy or radiography.

Fig. 279. Sketch to Fig. 278.

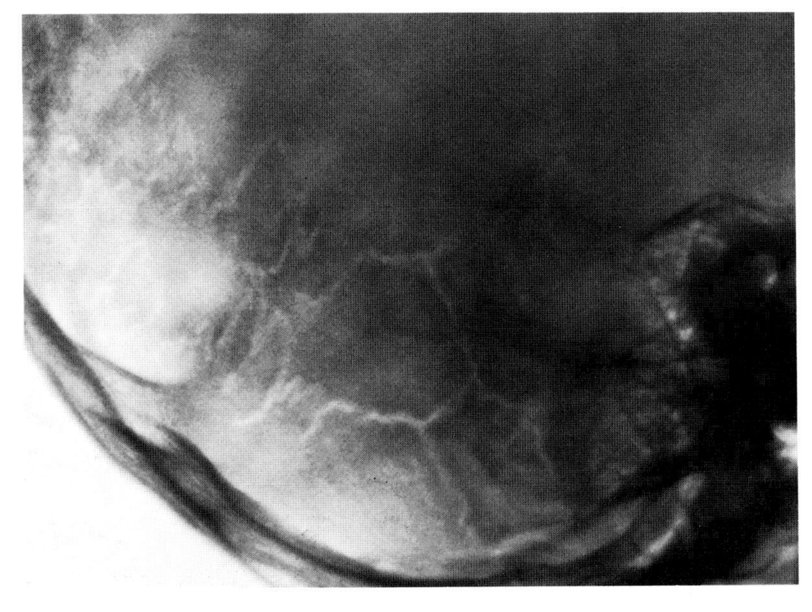

Fig. 280. A rare case of two intercalary bones, one behind the other, in the course of the lambdoid suture, which limits both of them distally. Still, such bones occur quite frequently in this region.

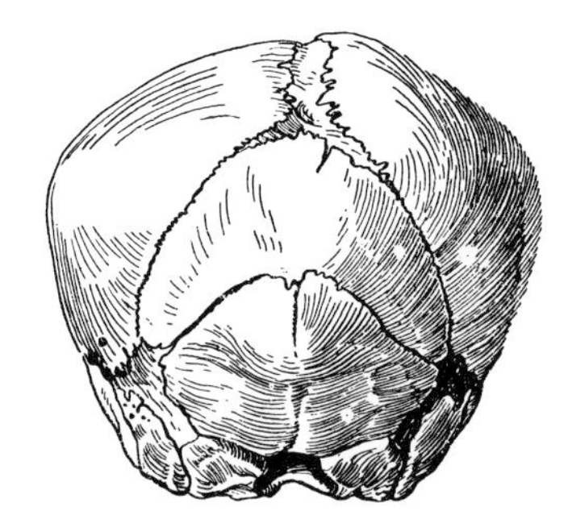

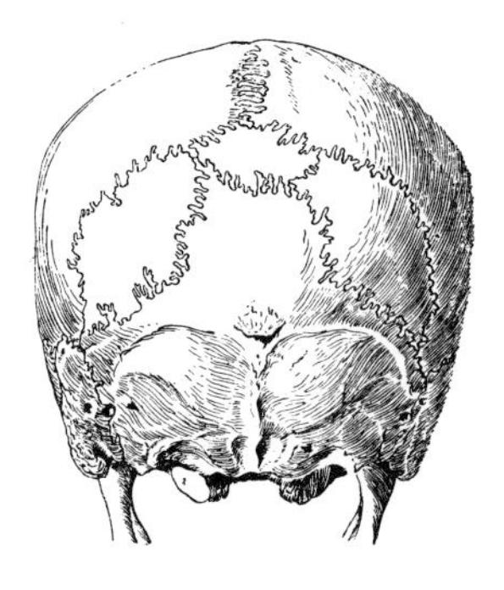

Fig. 281. Interparietal bone (Inka bone, a special form of a sutural or intercalary bone), bounded by the lambdoid suture and a persistent sutural anomaly, the transverse occipital suture (from *Goldhamer* and *Schüller*).

Fig. 282. Tripartite interparietal bone (from *Goldhamer* and *Schüller*).

Due to persistence of the transverse occipital suture, an interparietal bone (Inka bone) is formed.

II. Vertebral Column, Thoracic Cage and Pelvis

Radiographic Anatomy and Radiographs of the Cervical Spine

It is essential for the diagnosis and treatment of disorders of the spinal column to have a thorough understanding of the most important anatomical relationships of the individual vertebrae and parts of the vertebrae to each other, and to be aware of their roentgenologic appearance on radiographs taken in the usual directions of projection. For functional radiographs in the upright position of the body, exposures of the whole spinal column by *Edinger, Gajewski* and *Gepp* as well as by *Raspe* are recommended (see Figs. 884 and 885, p. 353). For the development of the spinal column during the prenatal period and during infancy, see p. 414.

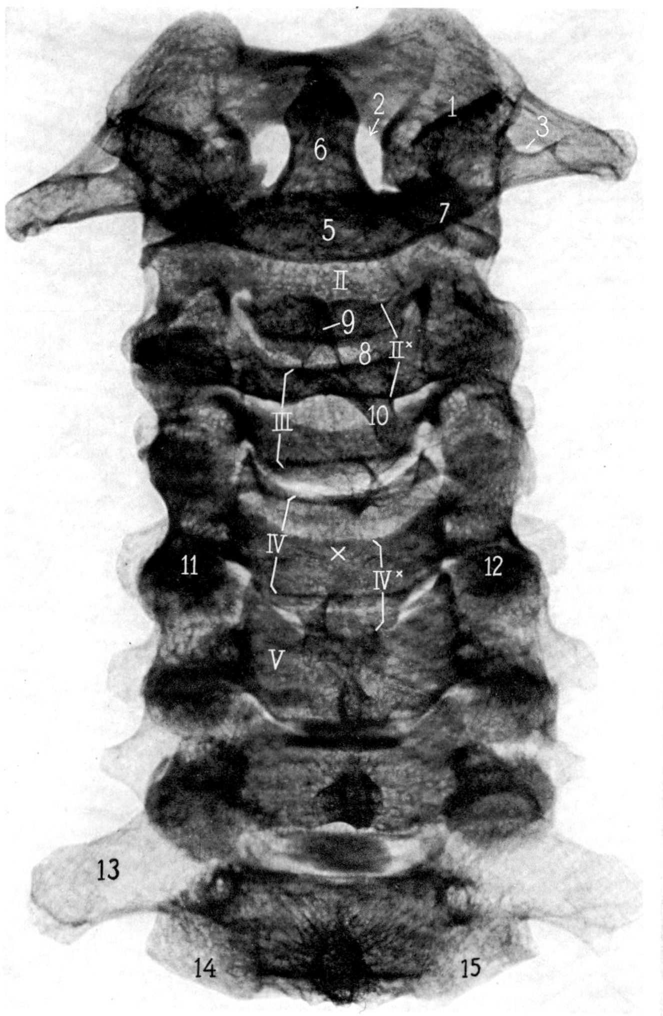

Fig. 283 a. Anteroposterior.

Fig. 283 b. Lateral.

Fig. 283. Cervical vertebral column, macerated. Centered on the body of the 4th cervical vertebra (x).

- II Body of 2nd vertebra
- II* Arch of 2nd vertebra
- III Body of 3rd vertebra
- IV Body of 4th vertebra
- IV* Arch of 4th vertebra
- V Vertebra, taken orthograde. The shadows of body and arch almost cover each other. Above, the transverse process juts out somewhat (may cause diagnostic errors).
- 1,1* Right and left superior articular facets of atlas
- 2 Vertebral foramen of atlas
- 3 Transverse process of atlas
- 4 Anterior tubercle of atlas
- 5 Posterior tubercle of atlas
- 6 Dens (axis)
- 7 Lateral atlantoaxial joint
- 8 Space for the intervertebral disk II/III
- 9, 10 "Split" spinous process (axis)
- 11, 12 Intervertebral articulations, covered because of their oblique course. At 7, the interarticular space becomes visible due to favorable direction of projection
- 13 Transverse process (cervical vertebra VII)
- 14, 15 Inferior articular processes
- 16 Superior articular process
- 17 Superior vertebral incisure } each forms half a foramen
- 18 Inferior vertebral incisure } each forms half a foramen

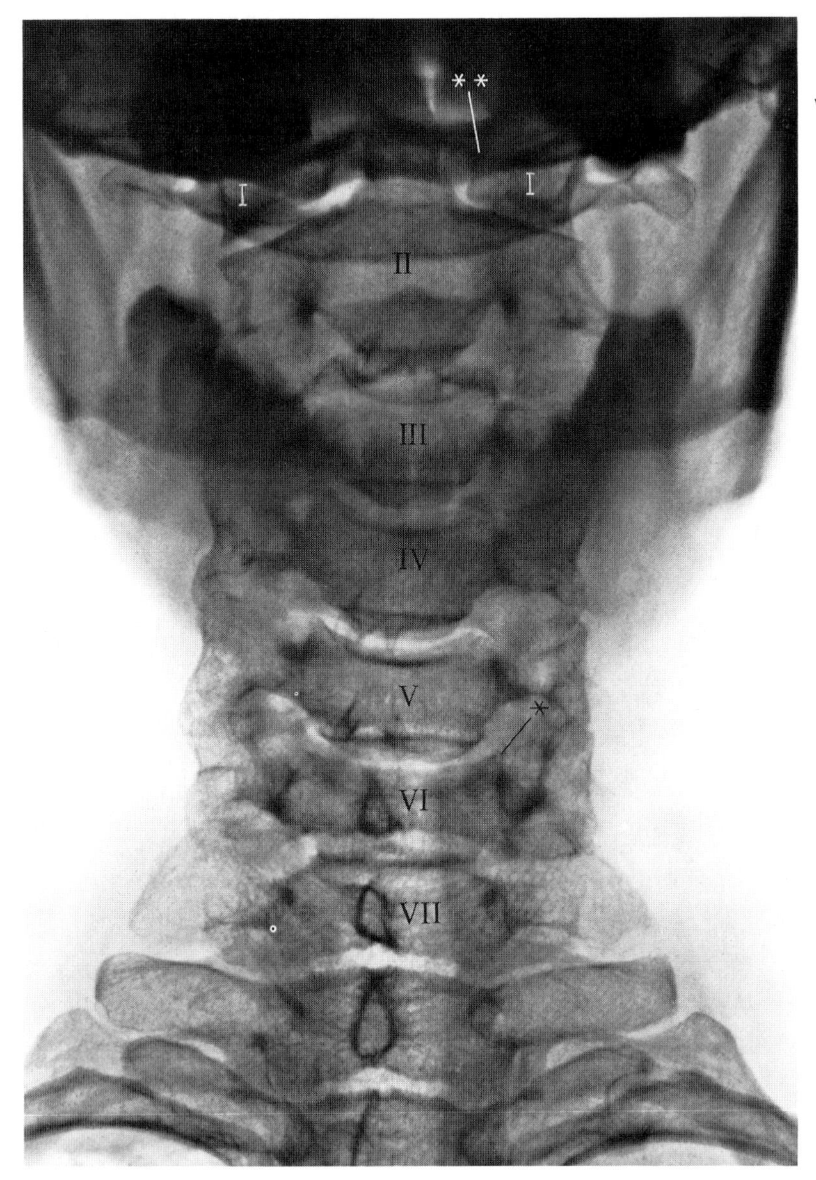

Fig. 284. Anteroposterior view of the cervical spine, with moving mandible. The atlantooccipital and atlantoaxial joints are projected into the space between maxilla and mandible. By quick opening and closure of the mouth during the entire period of exposure, the mandibular shadow becomes stretched out and blurred so much that the bodies of the upper cervical vertebrae, too, may be seen through it.

I Atlas
II Axis
III-VII Bodies of the 3rd to 7th cervical vertebrae, crossed by a band of decreased density of the trachea (subtraction effect)
* Dorsally located lateral edges of the vertebral bodies, bent in cranial direction, i.e., uncinate processes with so-called uncovertebral joint. At this location, osteochondrosis dissecans-like changes, as well as arthrotic processes may occur *(Harder).*
** View of the medial edge of the cranial articular surface of the atlas *(Viehweger)*

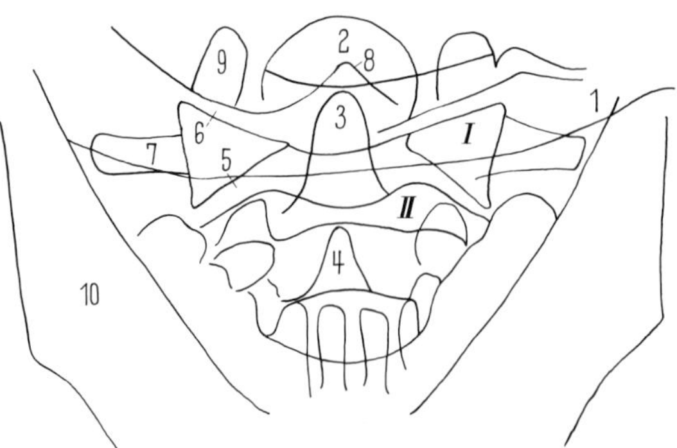

Fig. 285. Sketch of the upper vertebral joints, relating to Fig. 284.

I Atlas: lateral mass
II Axis
1 Base of the posterior cranial fossa
2 Foramen magnum
3 Dens (axis)
4 Spinous process (axis)
5 Atlantoaxial joint
6 Atlantooccipital joint
7 Transverse process of atlas
8 Internal occipital protuberance
9 Occipital condyle
10 Mandible

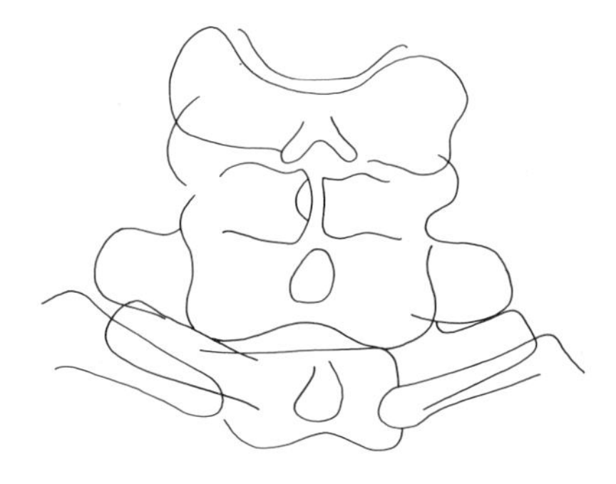

Fig. 286 a

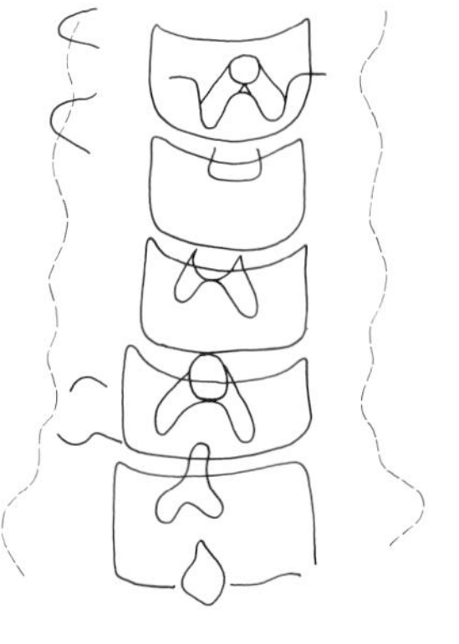

Fig. 286 b

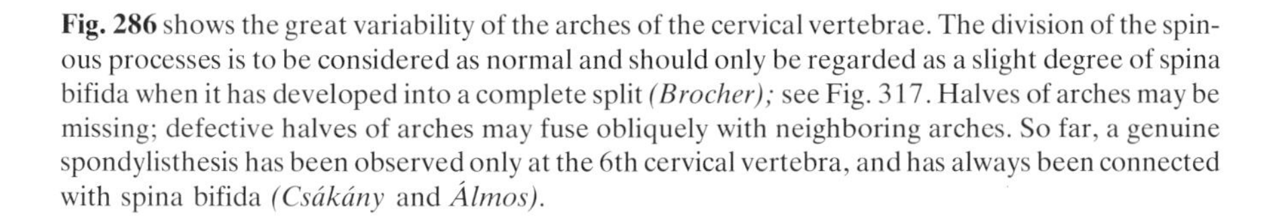

Fig. 286 shows the great variability of the arches of the cervical vertebrae. The division of the spinous processes is to be considered as normal and should only be regarded as a slight degree of spina bifida when it has developed into a complete split *(Brocher);* see Fig. 317. Halves of arches may be missing; defective halves of arches may fuse obliquely with neighboring arches. So far, a genuine spondylisthesis has been observed only at the 6th cervical vertebra, and has always been connected with spina bifida *(Csákány* and *Álmos).*

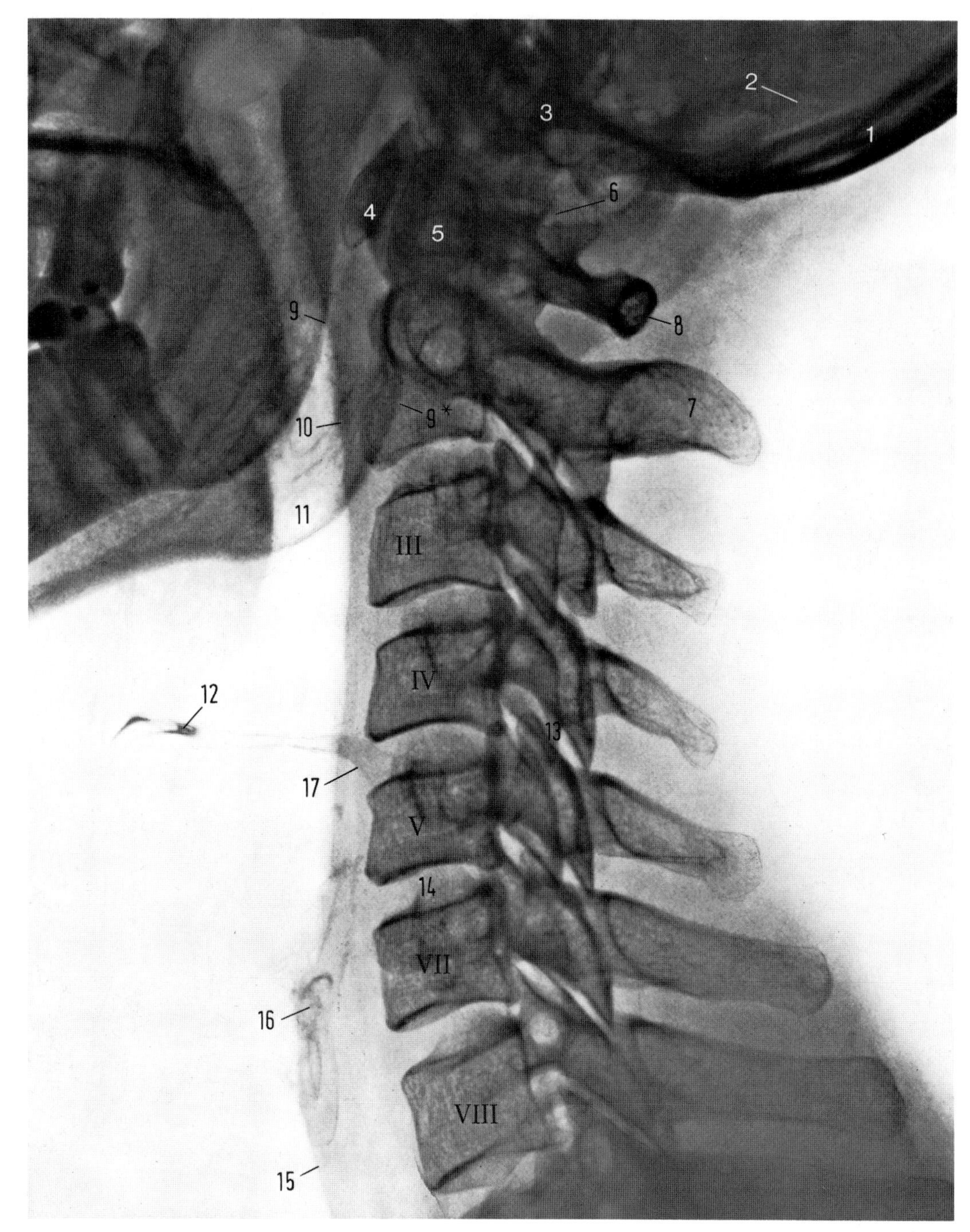

Fig. 287. Cervical spine, lateral. The strictly lateral projection of the cervical spine shows also the small joints of the vertebrae, though the joints of both sides are projected onto one another. A turn of the patient by 5° to 10° will demonstrate the isolated joints.

The healthy cervical spine exhibits a physiological lordosis, the degree of which is connected with the degree of the kyphosis in the thoracic area. With increasing thoracic kyphosis in advanced age, the cervical lordosis increases correspondingly.

III–VII 3rd to 7th bodies of the cervical vertebrae

1 Occipital squama
2 Lambdoid suture
3 Region of the foramen magnum
4 Anterior tubercle of atlas
5 Dens (axis)
6 Atlantooccipital joint (posterior part)
7 Spinous process of II (larger than the other processes)
8 Posterior tubercle of atlas
9,9* Posterior contours of both ascending rami of the mandible
10 Posterior muscle mass of the pharynx
11 Air space of the hypopharynx
12 Hyoid bone
13 Spaces of intervertebral joints
14 Intervertebral space
15 Posterior wall of trachea
16 Manifestations of ossification in the larynx
17 Greater cornu (of the hyoid bone), with decreased intensity anteriorly due to the tracheal ring

Figs. 288–290. Functional views of the atlantoaxial joints, on slight lateral tilt of the head. With lateral tilt or shift of the head, the atlas may be shifted laterally. By this process, the lateral mass slides downwards on the sloping "shoulder" and, with its lateral edge, juts out above the lateral rim of the articular surface of this shoulder. The other lateral mass is shifted in the same direction and therefore glides upwards. In this way, the edges of the lateral masses come closer to or further from the dens, so that on one side of the sliding down the distance is increased, while on the side of the gliding upwards it decreases. The coincidental finding on a radiograph of a lateral narrowing of the distance between one lateral mass of the atlas and the dens does not justify a diagnosis of a subluxation in the atlantoaxial joint. Unilateral narrowing of the distance between atlas and dens, without change of the position of the head by voluntary movements, occurs frequently due to the numerous variants of the shapes of the two upper vertebrae *(Keim, Brocher)*.

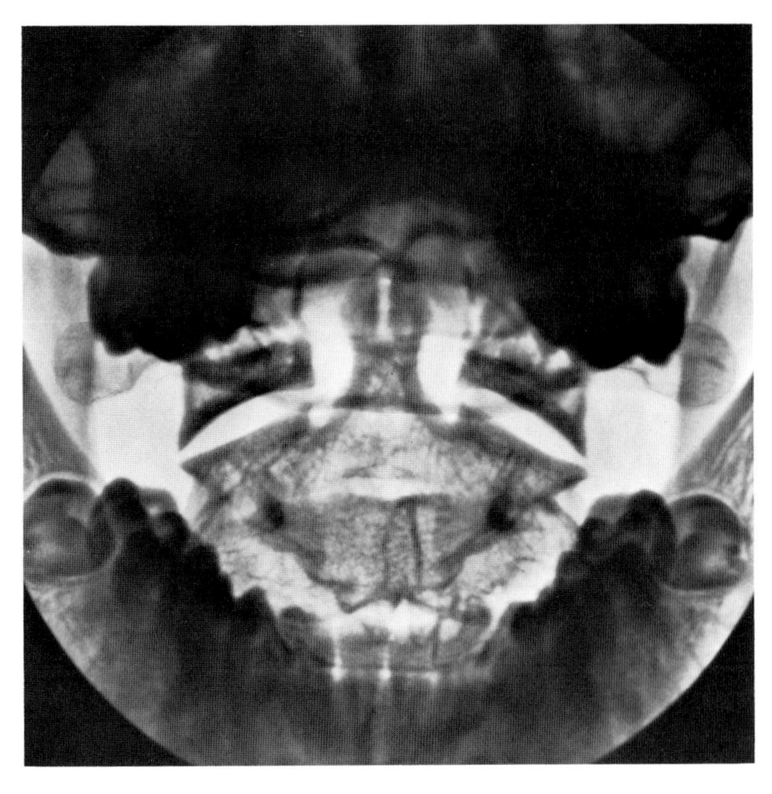

Fig. 288. Atlantoaxial articulations in normal posture, taken through the open mouth.

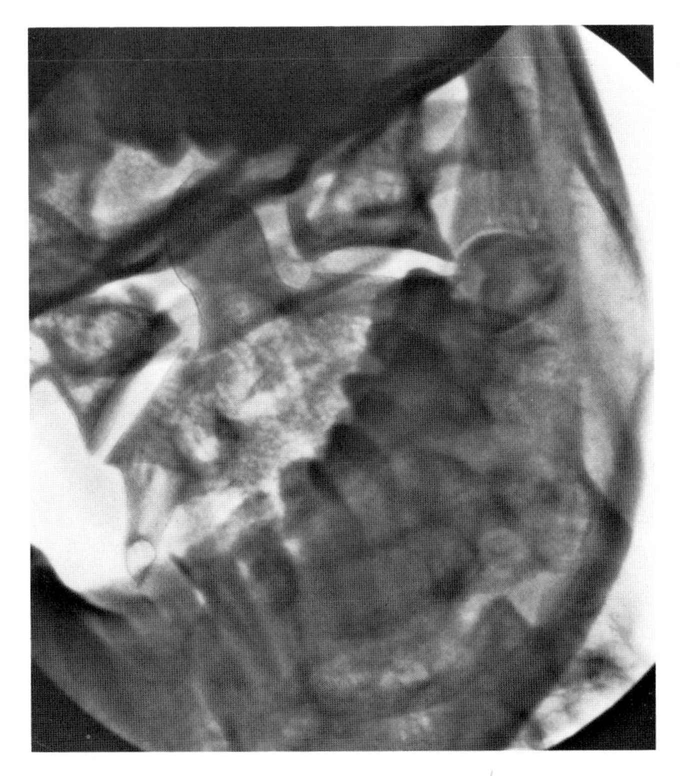

Fig. 289. Lateral inclination of the head to the right.

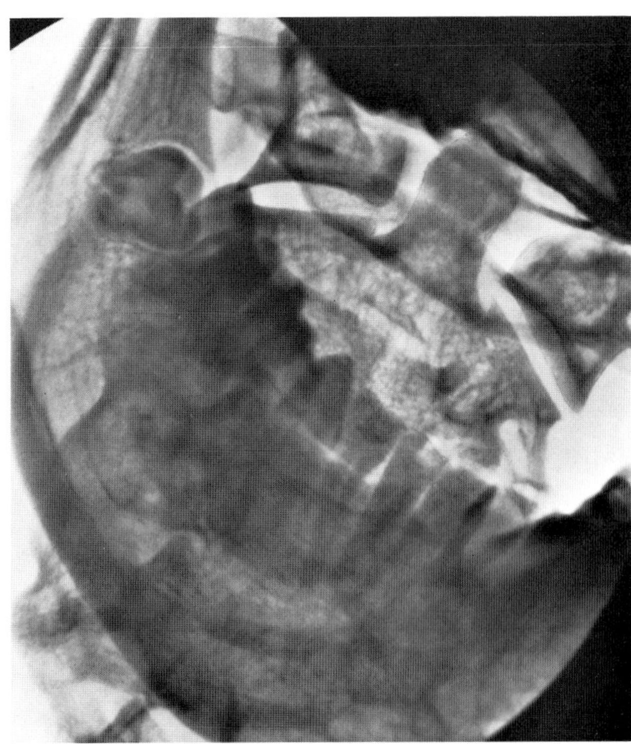

Fig. 290. Lateral inclination of the head to the left.

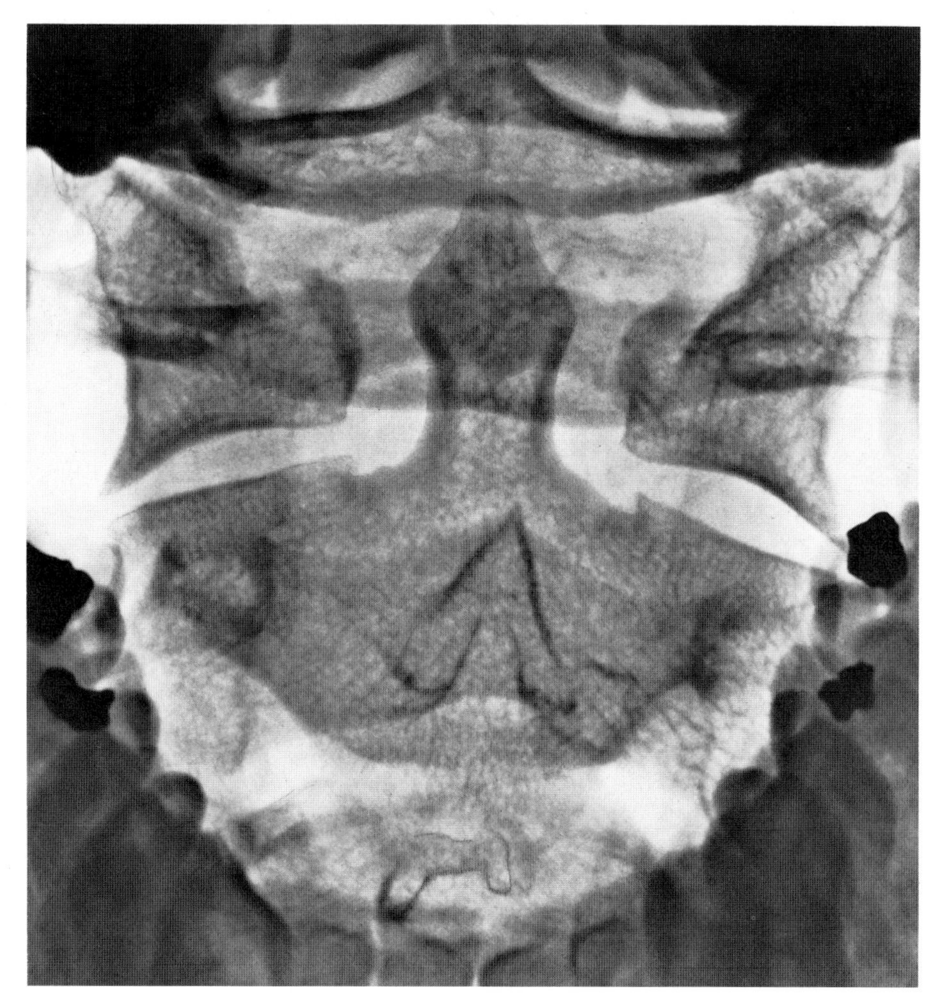

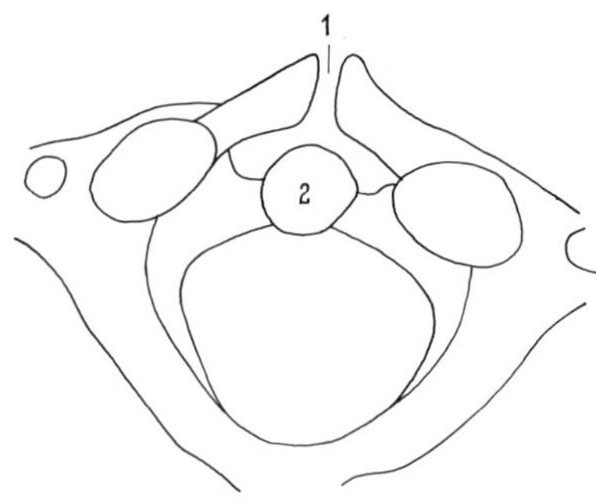

Fig. 292. Cleft formation in the anterior arch of the atlas.
1 Anterior arch of the atlas with cleft
2 Dens (axis)

Fig. 291. Enlarged view of atlas and axis; see also Figs. 109 and 219.

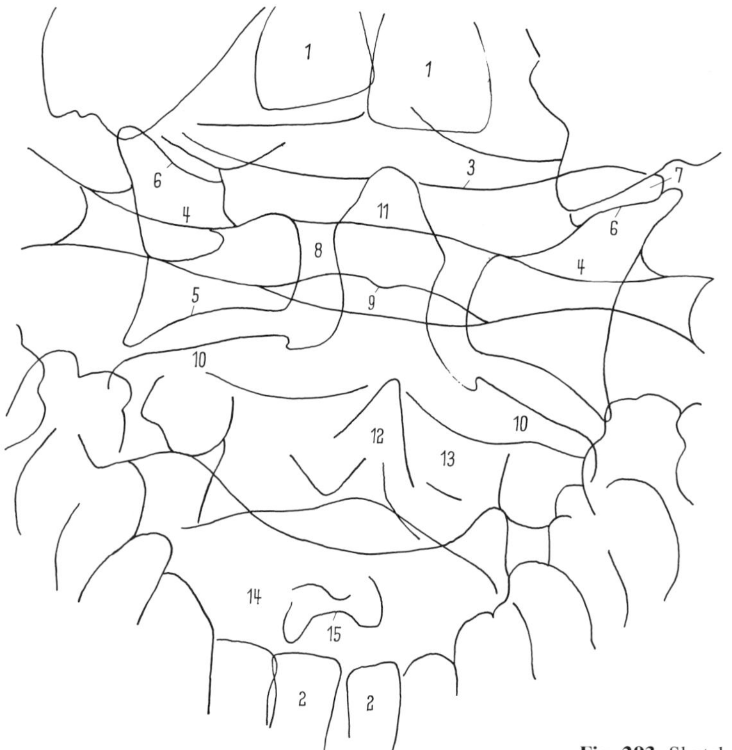

1 Upper incisors
2 Lower incisors
3 Lower limit of occiput
4 Lateral mass of atlas with transverse process
5 Inferior articular surface of atlas
6 Superior articular surface of atlas
7 Atlantooccipital articulation
8 Anterior arch of atlas
9 Anterior tubercle of atlas
10 Superior articular process of axis
11 Dens (axis)
12 Spinous process of axis
13 Arch of axis
14 Body of 3rd cervical vertebra
15 Spinous process of 3rd cervical vertebra

Fig. 293. Sketch to Fig. 291.

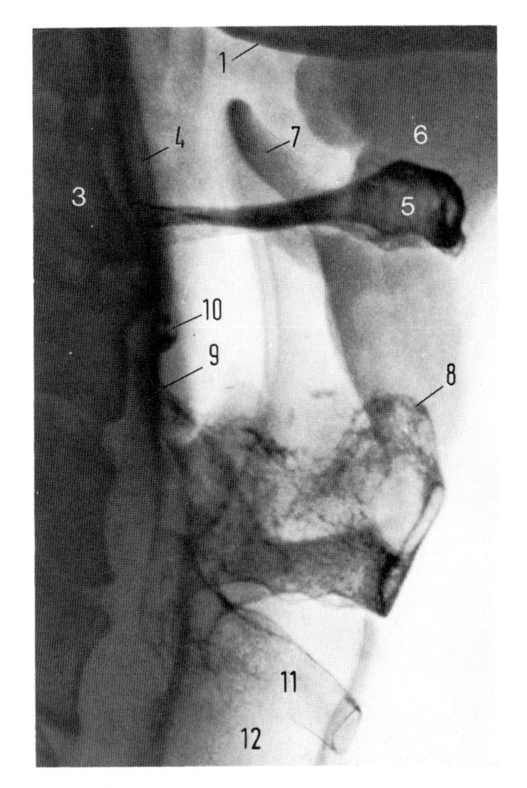

Fig. 294 a

Fig. 294 b

Fig. 294. Larynx, lateral and sagittal.

1 Angle of mandible of adjacent side
2 Calcified cervical lymph node
3 Body of 3rd cervical vertebra
4 Posterior pharyngeal wall, muscles and mucosa
5 Hyoid bone
6 Base of tongue
7 Epiglottis
8 Superior and anterior edges of thyroid cartilage
9 Superior cornu of thyroid cartilage
10 Triticeous cartilage (see No. 37, Fig. 233)
11 Cricoid cartilage
12 Trachea

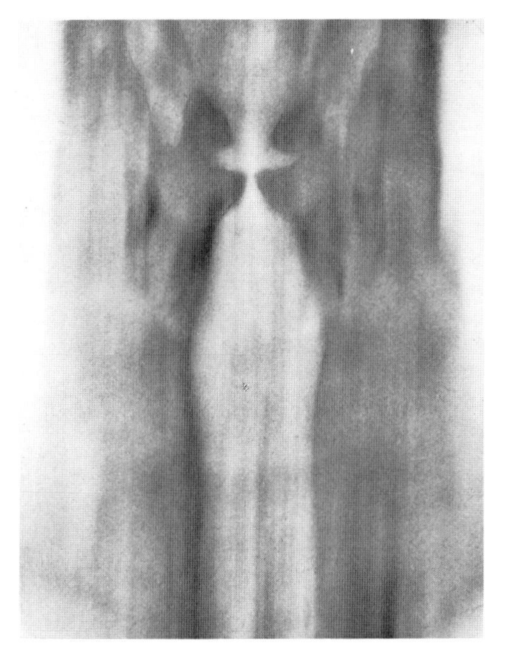

Fig. 295. Tomogram of larynx, after *Pagani.*

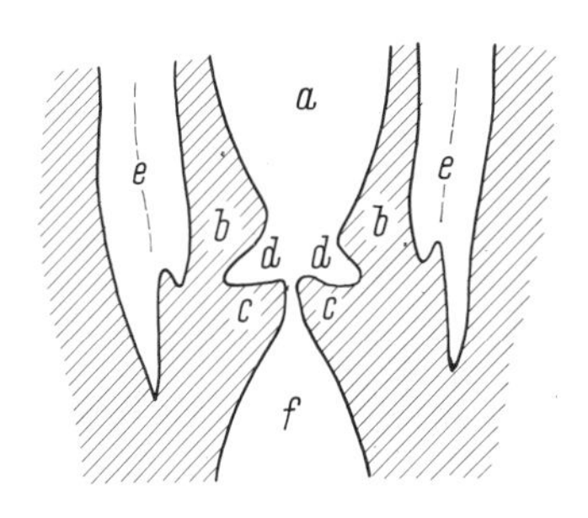

Fig. 296. Sketch to Fig. 295.

a Laryngeal vestibule
b Ventricular fold
c Vocal cord
d Ventricle of the larynx
e Piriform recess
f Subglottic space

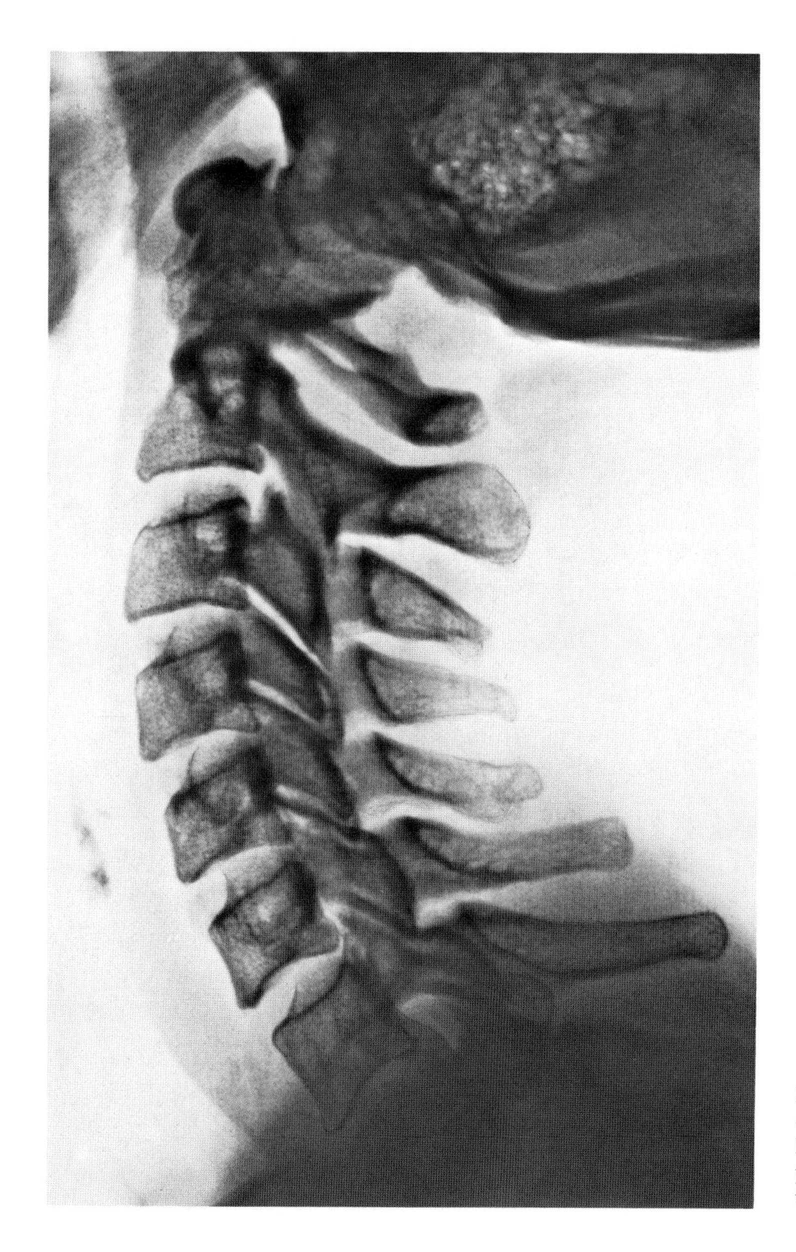

Fig. 297. Cervical spine, lateral. Well recognizable atlantooccipital joint. Is this view the lordosis is more distinct than in Fig. 287, and must be attributed to a corresponding kyphotic posture of the thoracic spine. No pathological findings in the vertebrae.

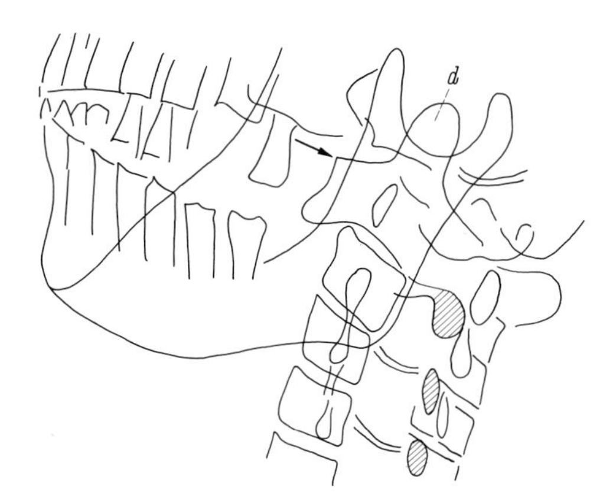

Fig. 298. On functional radiographs with slight turning of the upper cervical spine, one articular surface of the axis juts out and may give the impression of a subluxation of the 2nd cervical vertebra (→); d = Dens (axis). In cases of basilar impression or platybasia, the dens reaches into the foramen magnum, to a greater or lesser extent.

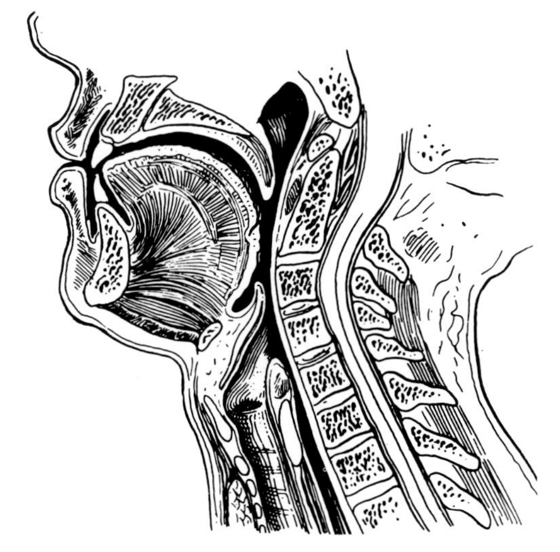

Fig. 299. Median section through the neck.

Figs. 300 and 301. Functional radiographs of the cervical spine. These views, taken with the spine overflexed or overstretched, may show changes more easily than the standard radiographs in two planes. The functional unit of the spinal column is the so-called segment of movement. It consists of the intervertebral disk, which connects two vertebrae as a so-called amphiarthrosis, the small vertebral joints and the ligaments; see also *Buetti-Bäuml, Kovács.*

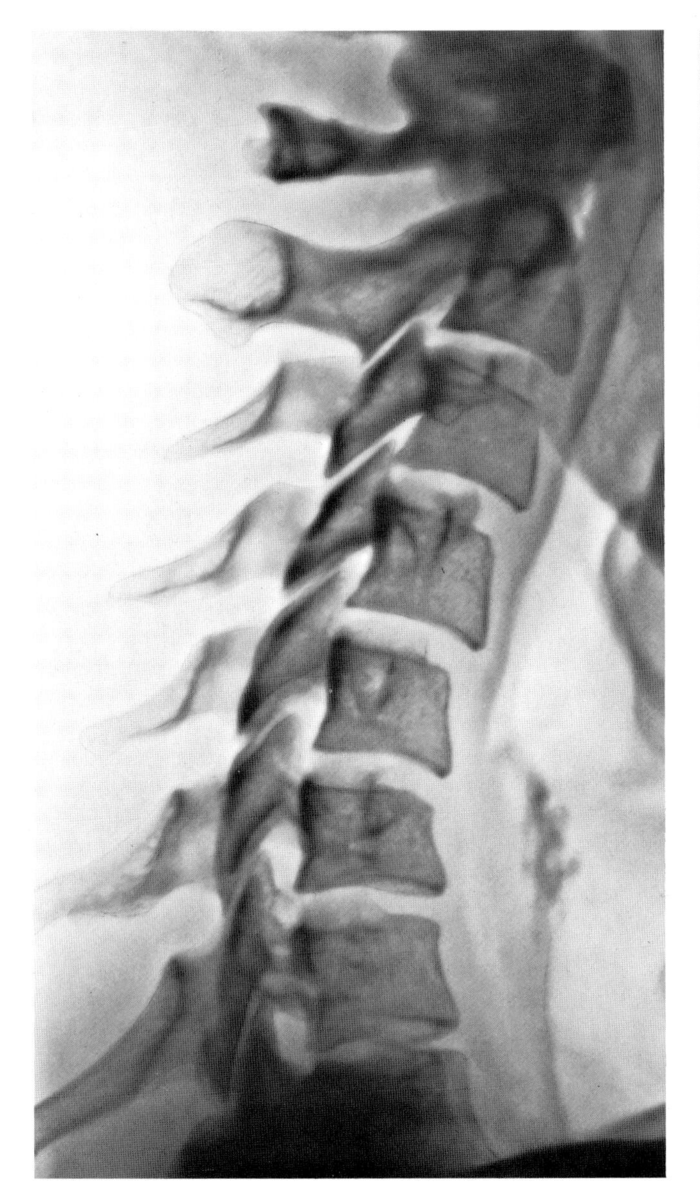

Fig. 300. Cervical spine, lateral, anteflexed. With this projection, each individual vertebra is slightly shifted and tilted forward against the next lowest one.

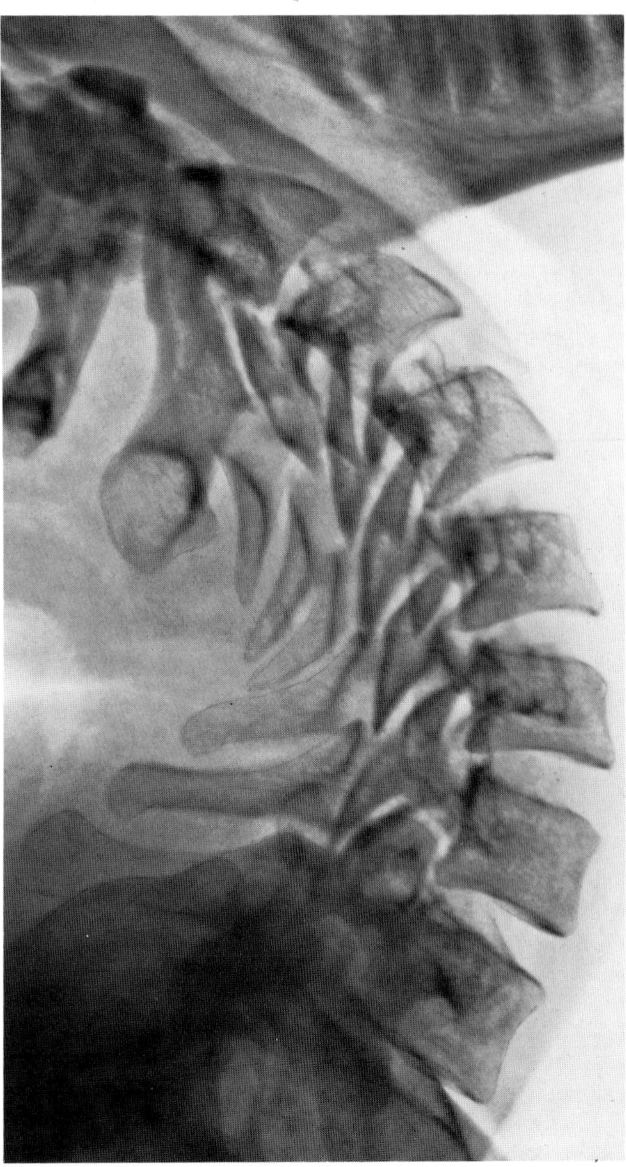

Fig. 301. Cervical spine, lateral, retroflexed. Typical for this projection is the slight dorsal shift of each vertebral body against the next lowest one. Simultaneously, the interjacent spaces for the disks are opened anteriorly, and the spinous processes are approximated to one another, especially in the middle section of the cervical spine.

These radiographs play a special role in the diagnosis of whiplash injuries and their consequences. These whiplash injuries, typically caused by car collisions, damage the cervical spine either monophasically or biphasically. The single phase form, also called hyperextension injury, is the more dangerous indirect result of the trauma. In addition to damage to muscles, intervertebral disks and the vertebral artery *(Hinz),* the following consequences of whiplash injuries may be found in the skeleton of the occiput and the cervical spine:

a) In one-phase whiplash injuries, the ligamental and muscular connections between occiput and atlas may tear, owing to rebound and hyperextension.
b) The biphasic whiplash movement may cause fracture of the axis.
c) Fracture of the base of skull in the region of the foramen magnum may occur.

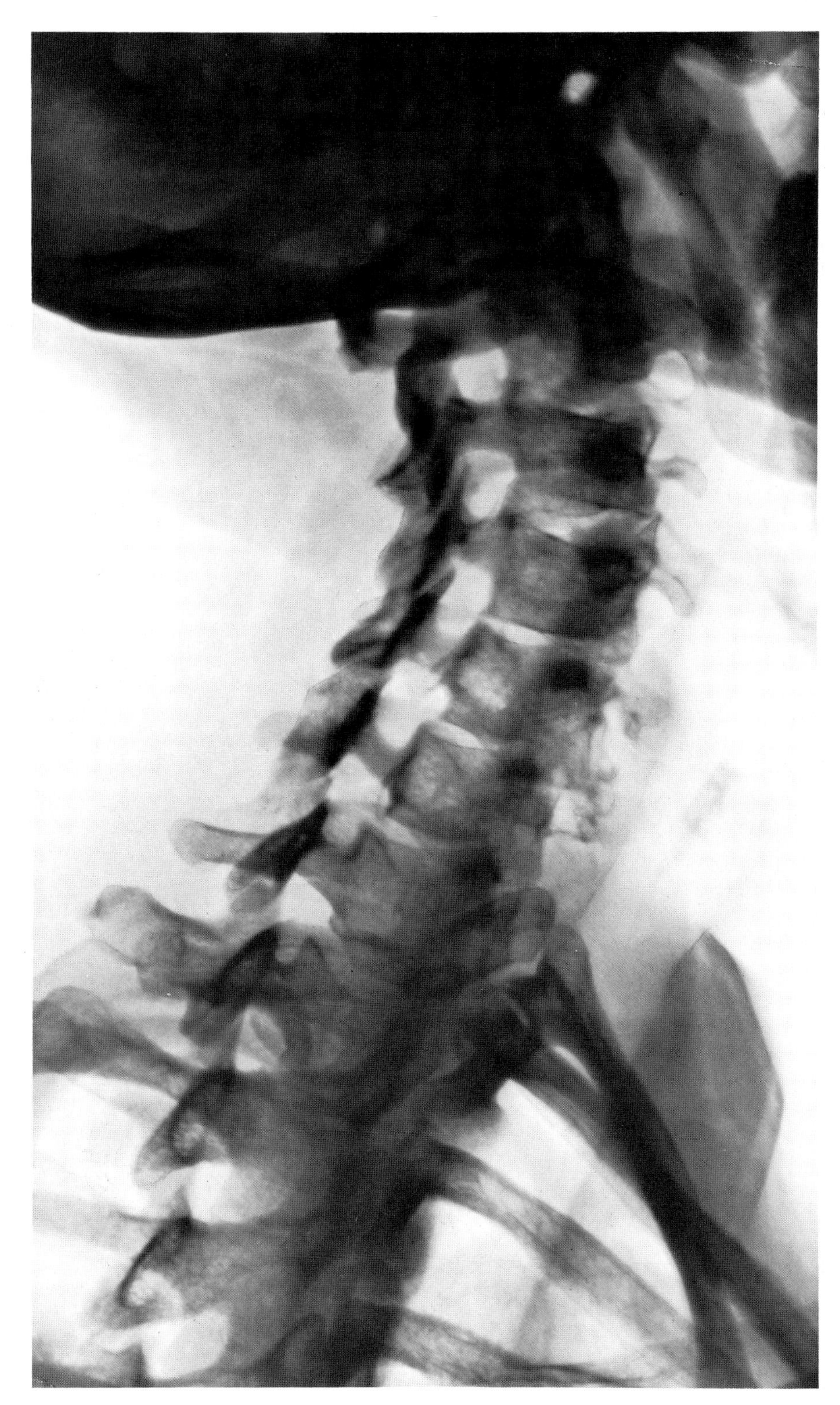

Fig. 302. **Cervical spine, oblique.** The oblique pictures show the intervertebral foramina, whose shape, size and limits are important for evaluation of cervical neuralgias. When showing the intervertebral foramina, it must be kept in mind that when the patient is turned towards the film the foramina near the film are shown, while when the patient is turned away from the film the film-distant foramina are seen.

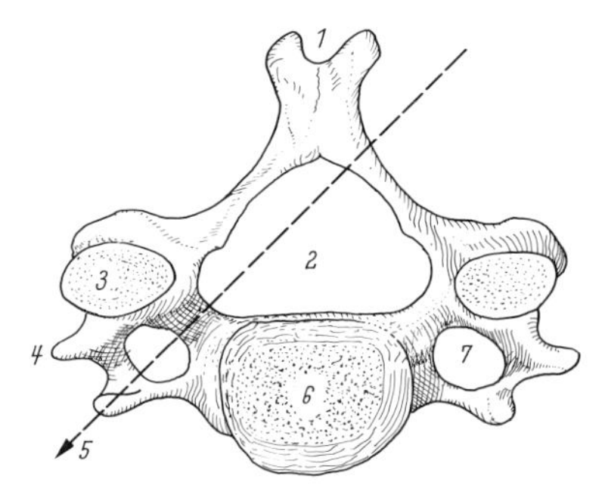

Fig. 303. Explanation of the projection for Fig. 302.

1 Cleft spinous process, normal
2 Vertebral foramen
3 Articular surface
4 Posterior tubercle
5 Anterior tubercle
6 Body of vertebra
7 Transverse foramen

The arrow passes through the intervertebral foramen; its direction corresponds to the position of the patient turned towards the film, therefore the intervertebral foramina on the film side are shown. The shape of the transverse processes of the cervical spine is characteristic. They arise in front of the articular processes from the body or the root of the arch in a lateral anterior direction. The upper sulcus between the anterior tubercle (which is the homolog of a cervical rib, i.e., the costal process) and the longer posterior tubercle (the processus transversus proper) appear most distinctly at the 4th and 5th processes.

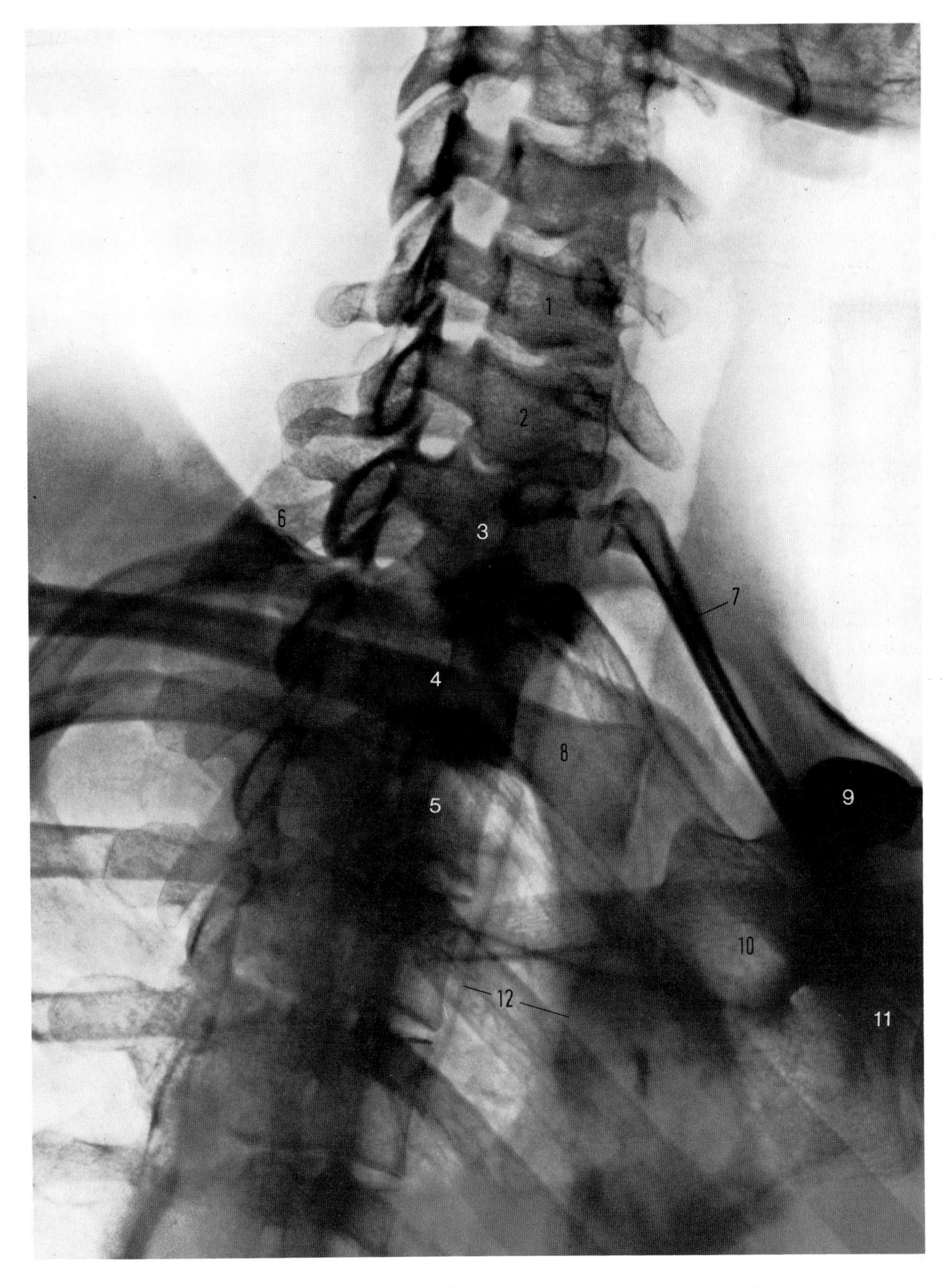

Fig. 304. Lower cervical spine and upper thoracic spine, oblique. Position: supine, with an angle of 45° towards the table. The left shoulder is directed forward, with the right shoulder so far upward and outward that the foramina will not be covered by it.

1 Body of the 6th cervical vertebra
2 Body of 7th cervical vertebra
3 Body of 1st thoracic vertebra
4 Body of 2nd thoracic vertebra
5 Body of 3rd thoracic vertebra
6 1st right rib
7 1st left rib
8 Right clavicle
9 Left clavicle
10 Manubrium sterni
11 Left scapula with glenoid cavity
12 Trachea

Variants and Sources of Diagnostic Error of the Cervical Spine

Bony abnormalities in the region of the foramen magnum:

a) Occipitalization of the atlas. It plays the greatest role among the congenital anomalies at the foramen magnum. In most cases, there is a bony connection between the anterior arch of the atlas and the anterior rim of the foramen magnum. This connection is often very narrow, up to 6 mm wide *(Climelli, McRae* and *Barnum).* Atlantooccipital articular clefts have also been observed in this region. In addition, the transverse processes of the atlas may unite with the occipital bone. Not infrequently, the following may be shown:

b) Basilar impression (see p. 100 and *H. Schmidt*). For its importance in insurance law, see *Janzen.*

c) Total absence of dens (*Miyakawa, Fullenlove, Schneider* and *Walz*) or partial aplasia of the dens (see *Hohl*). A case of fracture of the dens with maximal dorsal luxation of the atlas, without lethal consequences, has been described by *Gombert.*

d) An isolated dens *(McRae)*

e) Accessory bony elements in the area of the foramen magnum, according to *E. Fischer*, connote both manifestations of an occipital vertebra and secondary ossifications within the ligaments.

These faulty developments may be connected with a variety of disturbances of the nervous system but may also occur without recognizable impairment of the nervous substance *(Decker, Fischgold, Hacker* and *Metzger*). *McRae* found neurological changes in 30–50% of 100 cases, and *Decker et al.* found concurrent intracranial malformations in 20% of the patients examined. Luxations of the 1st and 2nd cervical vertebrae may occur e.g. in connection with anomalies of the dens.

The paratransverse process (also called epitransverse or supratransverse) has been described by *Viehweger, Brocher* and *le Double* as a rare variant at the atlas. The paratransverse process leads from the transverse process in the direction of the occipital bone or the occipital protuberance, or in a direction medial to the petrooccipital fissure. It may appear either as a delicate formation of calcified shadow or as a massively expanded ossification at the transverse process of the atlas. In modern terminology it is most commonly called the epitransverse process.

Loewenhardt described as a paracondyloid process, a bony process 13 mm wide and 10 mm long growing out laterally next to the occipital condyle. It forms a pseudojoint with a broadened transverse process of the atlas. In 1969 *Siebert* reported a similar case of formation of a pseudojoint, considered to be a manifestation of an occipital vertebra.

Gockel and *Stolze,* i.a. reported a considerable defect of the arch of the atlas; *Geipel* showed isolated centers of ossification in the posterior arch of the atlas. For demonstration of defects of the atlas arches, the following positions are recommended by *Zimmer*: the axial submentobregmatic position (Fig. 91) for evaluation of the anterior arch of the atlas, and the nuchofrontal one for the posterior arch (Fig. 109).

Budin and *Sondheimer* reported a very rare combination of an anterior and posterior spina bifida with cleft formations in the atlas.

Wackenheim tabulates the primary malformations at the passage from skull to neck in an embryologic system as malformations of:

a) the occipital squama (Inka bone, dysplasia, hypoplasia, persistence of sutures),
b) the foramen magnum (stenosis and enlargement),
c) the lateral region of the occiput (dysplasia of the condyles or their aplasia),
d) the alar and transverse ligaments,
e) the dens (dysplasia, aplasia, mobile dens),
f) the atlas (assimilation, dysplasia).

Pickhan described strikingly large transverse processes of the 2nd cervical vertebra that usually do not project beyond the wavy boundary of the lateral cervical spine.

Atypical joint formations in the region of the spinal column have been described by *Kremser* i.a. (see additional bibliography). These formations occur between the 6th and 7th cervical vertebrae. These changes are not confined only to the 6th and 7th spinous processes of the cervical vertebrae. Nor are they to be considered as secondary effects of changed statics (see pseudojoints at the spinous processes of the lumbar spine, *Baastrup*) but as genuine, congenitally preformed joint formations corresponding to the joint formations at the transverse processes of the sacrum (Fig. 476).

D. Schoen reported on the case of a line of increased radiolucency, projected onto the lower cervical vertebrae. In a male 63 years of age, with the path of the beam in frontal direction, he found in the region of the caudal half of the body of C VI a line of increased radiolucency bent convexly in the cranial direction which, sharply defined, led from the ventral edge of the body of the vertebra to the dorsal edge of the vertebral body, separated by a small line of normally structured bony tissue. Its cause had been an uncovertebral spondylosis in the region of C V to C VII which led to extensive osteophytic reactions. Therefore, what is shown here is the view of a so-called uncovertebral arthrosis that has progressed quite far. *Köhler-Zimmer* described a similar view as "simulated by the projection of the transverse processes" (Fig. 1168 in *Köhler-Zimmer*, 11th edition). But, according to *D.*

Schoen, the transverse processes of two neighboring vertebrae can only approximate to a fissure-like distance when the uncinate processes and the cranial articular processes of the caudal vertebrae are ground down to a great degree. In addition, the bodies of the vertebrae must have sunk.

Wedge-shaped cervical vertebrae may be easily confused with a fracture. They are often the cause of scolioses and frequently carry unilateral ribs; therefore, the number of ribs on the right side may differ from that on the left.

H. Schmidt reported on a rare formation of flat vertebrae. In this case, a previous trauma, as well as other illnesses, could be excluded. The entire spine had been affected, and this finding was combined with an 8th cervical vertebra and an open sacral hiatus.

The carotic tubercle of C VI, as well as that of the 7th cervical vertebra, may be very strongly developed. The latter may grow into a freely mobile cervical rib, which may even reach the sternum and cause discomfort (see Fig. 232, Nos. 41 and 42, and Figs. 355, 364, 368).

Rib-bearing cervical vertebrae arise unilaterally or bilaterally at the boundary between cervical and thoracic spine; they are known as "transitional vertebrae" and are not too rare (*Pickhan*). Out of 3650 cases examined, *Caselli* found cervical ribs in 83 women and 27 men, a frequency of 3%. Among 205 males, *Engel* found 3 cases of a bilateral cervical rib (1.46%) and 46 cases of big transverse processes (22.4%); among 95 females, cervical ribs occurred 4 times (4.2%) and enlarged transverse processes 22 times (23.2%). The appearance of cervical ribs is frequently accompanied by other anomalies of the thoracic cage. Therefore, one must not regard shadows caused by cervical ribs, and especially by calcified foci in cartilaginous cervical ribs, as pulmonary changes. Anomalies due to reduced numbers, e.g., with complete aplasia of the first rib, are very rare and may also cause diagnostic errors (see Fig. 367). According to *F. W. Schneider*, one can observe fairly frequently the formation of its own joint in a cervical rib. As during infancy, the costal processes of the 7th cervical vertebra are independent of the transverse processes; they may be mistaken on radiographic surveys for cervical ribs (*Keating* and *Amberg*). The costal and transverse processes fuse between the fourth and tenth years of life.

Embryogenetically, the costal processes are identical with cervical and thoracic ribs. Cervical ribs are already present at birth and maintain their relation in size to the thoracic ribs during the period of growth, whether rudimentary or well developed. Normally, a rudimentary rib fuses with its transverse process into a single transverse process. This then develops two tubercles: an anterior tubercle, which represents the remnant of the cervical rib, and a posterior tubercle, which forms the proper transverse process. The sulcus for the spinal nerve runs above, between the two processes, ending at the transverse foramen (see Fig. 303). Towards the lower cervical spine, the transverse foramen becomes smaller, or only fissure-like, or may even be completely absent.

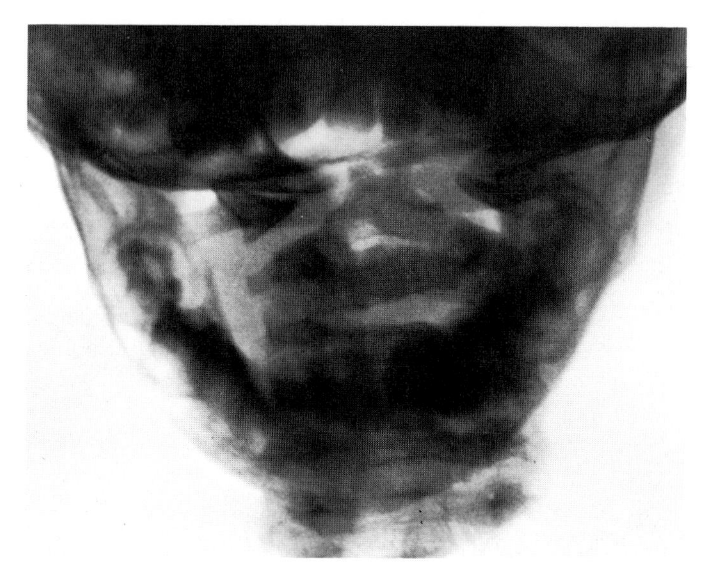

Fig. 305. **Bicornate dens** in a 6-year-old child. The bicornate dens is not a genuine anomaly but a bifurcation, sometimes still visible in infancy, representing an intermediate stage of ossification of a normal dens, which always originates from two dental processes of the axis.

The dens (axis) should not be considered embryogenetically as the body of the atlas, although this opinion is still to be found in *Schmorl-Junghans.* A body of the atlas is not projected at all in man *(Töndury);* therefore, the dens (axis) cannot arise from the body of the atlas. Rather, it originates in the shape of paired processes, the dental processes. Laterally, they are organically connected with the body of the axis. In the middle, they are separated by a septum rich in cells. In the embryo, the split in the origin of the dens is still very distinct. If care is taken to observe the lines of ossification in the dens (see Fig. 307), the V shape in the upper line of the dens is readily recognized below its tip. The secondary nucleus at the upper pole of the dens appears at about the second year of life and fuses with the dens at about the twelfth year.

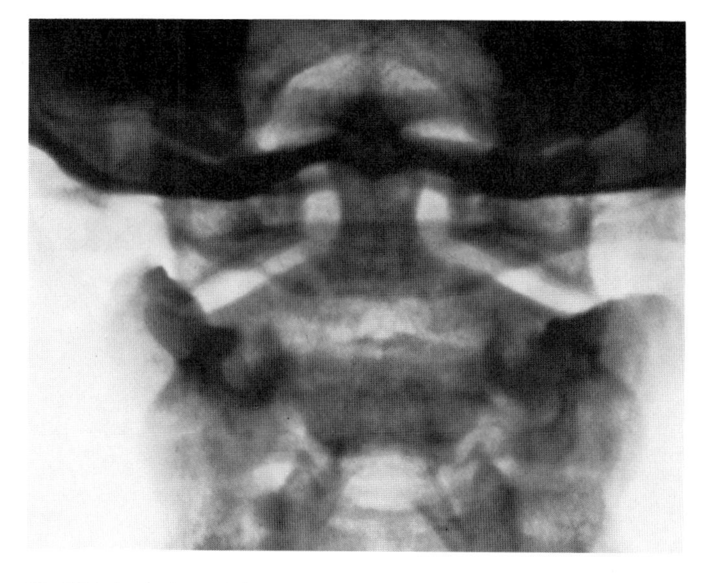

Fig. 306. At the base of the **dens,** the fusion with the body of the axis has not yet occurred in a 26-year-old male. The persistent commissures should not be mistaken for fissures because of their symmetry.

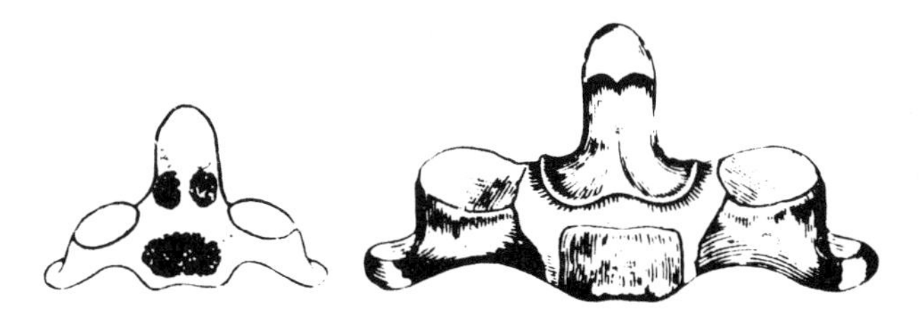

Fig. 307. Bicornate dens and commissures of fusion between dens and axis (from *Rauber-Kopsch*).

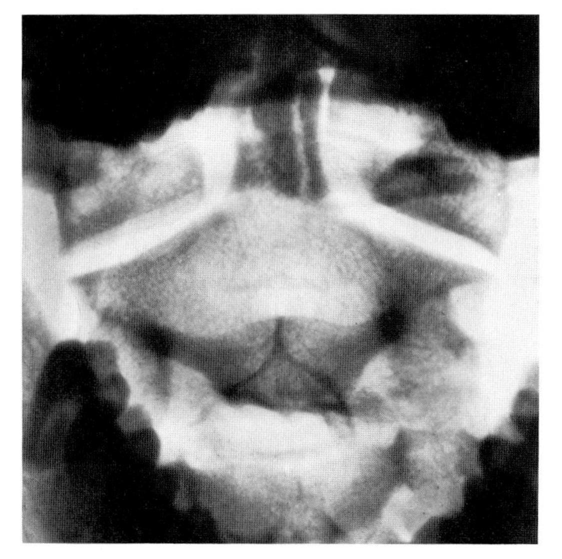

Fig. 308 a

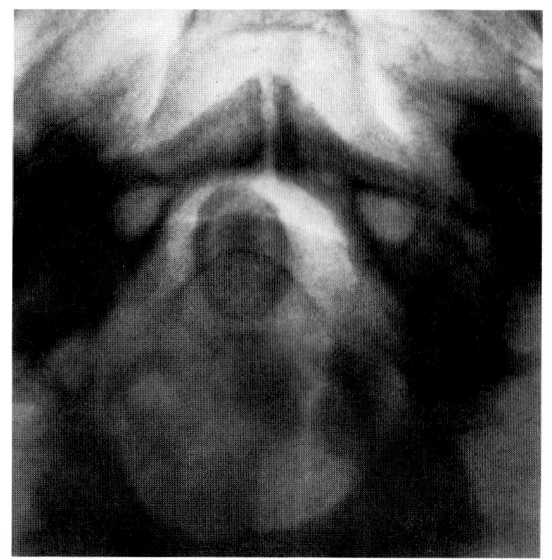

Fig. 308 b

Fig. 308. Cleft in the anterior arch of the atlas, simulating a fracture of the dens (see No. 9*, Fig. 232). Embryogenetic anomaly, i.e., persistent commissure (sometimes binuclear origin of the anterior arch of the atlas). *Sander* pointed out the importance of tomography for demonstration of changes in the uppermost cervical vertebrae (see Figs. 217 and 219 in the chapter on tomography of the skull from *Tänzer*).

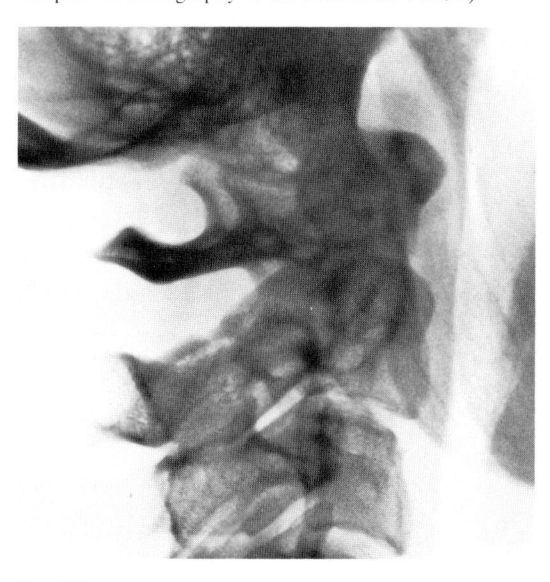

Fig. 309 a

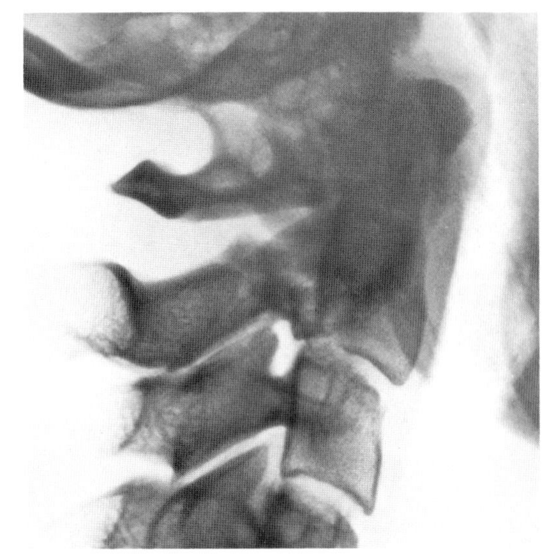

Fig. 309 b

Fig. 309 (a) A rare fracture in an arch of the axis. (b) The same patient, six weeks later; formation of callus. This was a case of luxation fracture or, more precisely, a subluxation fracture. The vertebral joint had been luxated (luxation fracture, *Böhler*) but the bodies of the vertebrae appear only subluxated against one another.

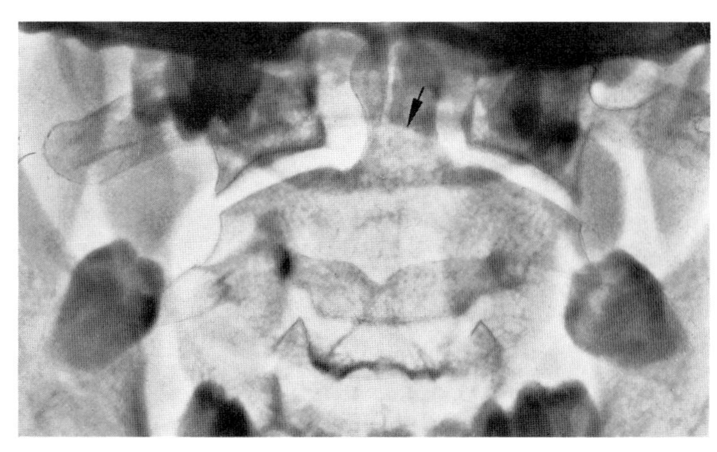

Fig. 310. Cleft between the upper-middle incisors, simulating a fracture of the dens. *Mach*-effect (↙), meaning a horizontal limitation of the shadow through the edge of an incisor. *Schneider* and *Walz* described the complete absence of the dens (axis), in whose place a tiny odontoid bone could be seen, occurring in a male 56 years of age suffering from sudden medullopathy. In this connection, the work on embryology, radiographic diagnoses and clinical findings of atlantooccipital dysplasia by *Kirschbichler* (1969) should be noted. In 1969 *Fischer* and *Schmidt* described possibilities of confusion of signs of wear in the anterior atlantodental joint with congenital malformations.

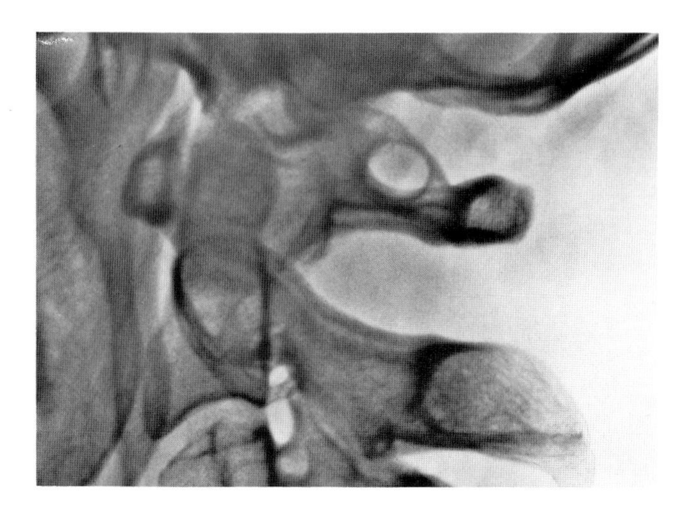

Fig. 311. Arcuate foramen of the atlas (*Kimmerle's* anomaly). A sulcus, rounded to a foramen for the vertebral artery and the suboccipital nerve (a common variant).

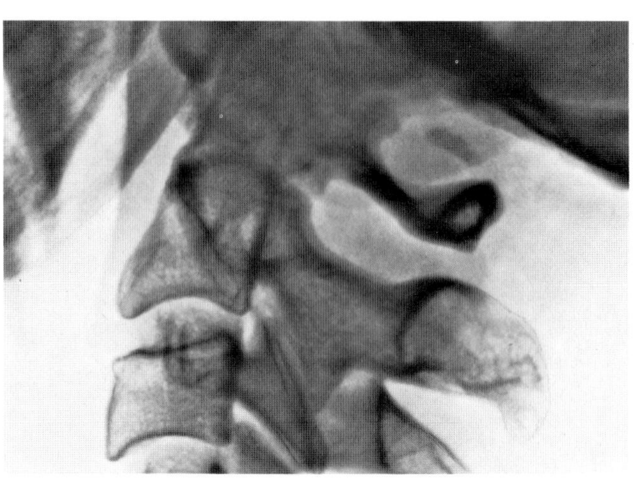

Fig. 312. Partial ossification of the atlantoocipital membrane, which bridges this sulcus. Therefore, it led only to partial formation of the arcuate foramen.

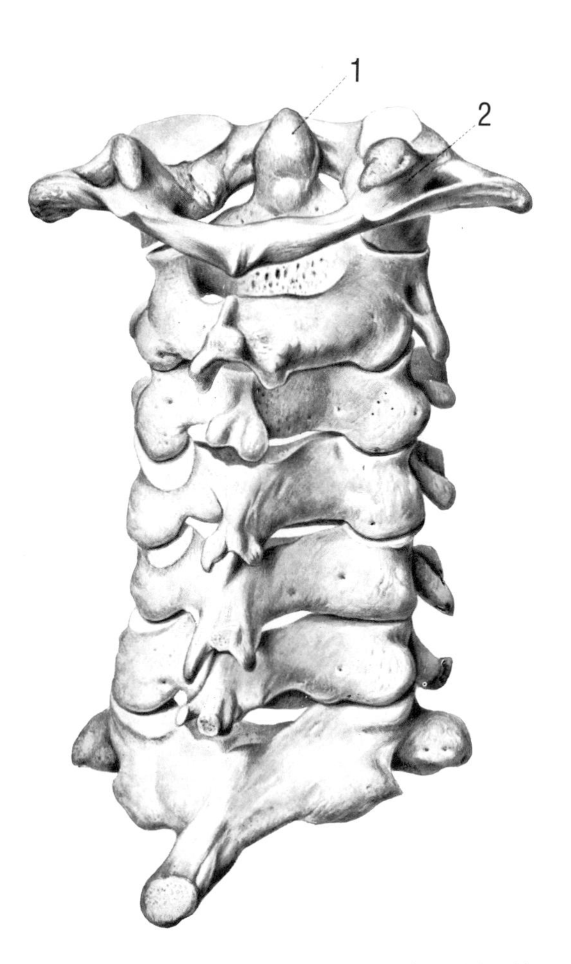

Fig. 313. Cervical spine (from *Sobotta-Becher,* 17th ed.).

1 Dens (axis)
2 Sulcus for vertebral artery and occipital nerve

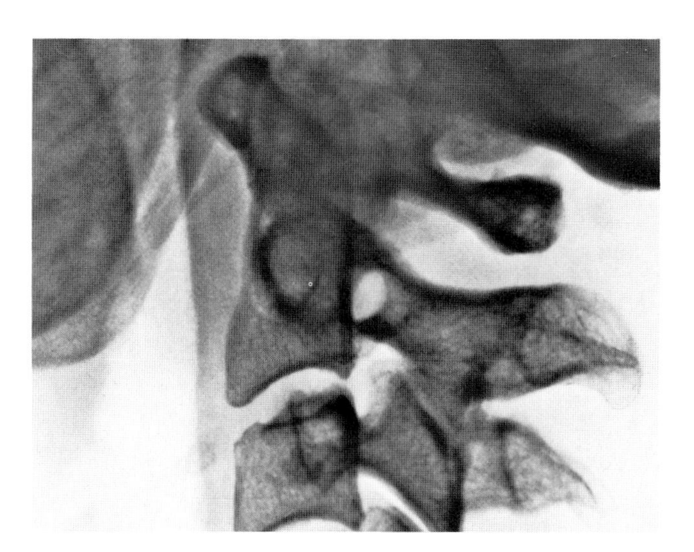

Fig. 314. Simulation of a variant foramen by a steeply placed transverse foramen of the axis. This can be observed more frequently when the rays are centered high up. *Janker* described a case of a 39-year-old patient where the transverse process of the atlas showed a peculiarity, as the greatest part of the anterior section of the transverse process had not been preformed. Therefore, part of the surrounding of the transverse foramen was missing. *Sèze* and *Djian* described a case of partial absence of the dorsal part of the transverse process of the 2nd cervical vertebra and, consequently, a gap in the transverse foramen. In 1970 *Holland* and *Stolle* reported on a case of aplasia of the root of the arch of the 5th cervical vertebra in a boy 14 years of age – an incidental finding after a severe sports accident.

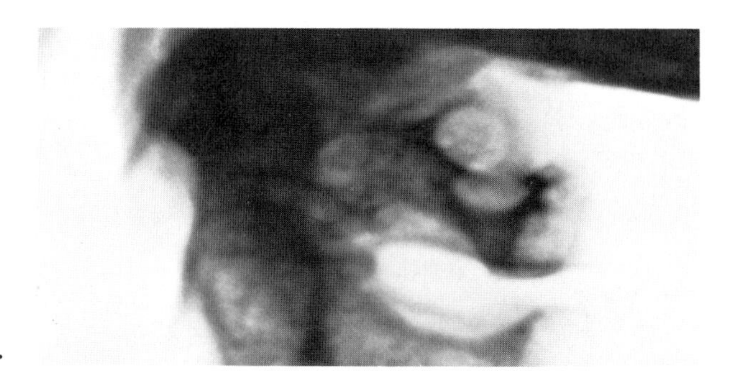

Fig. 315. Bipartite arcuate foramen.

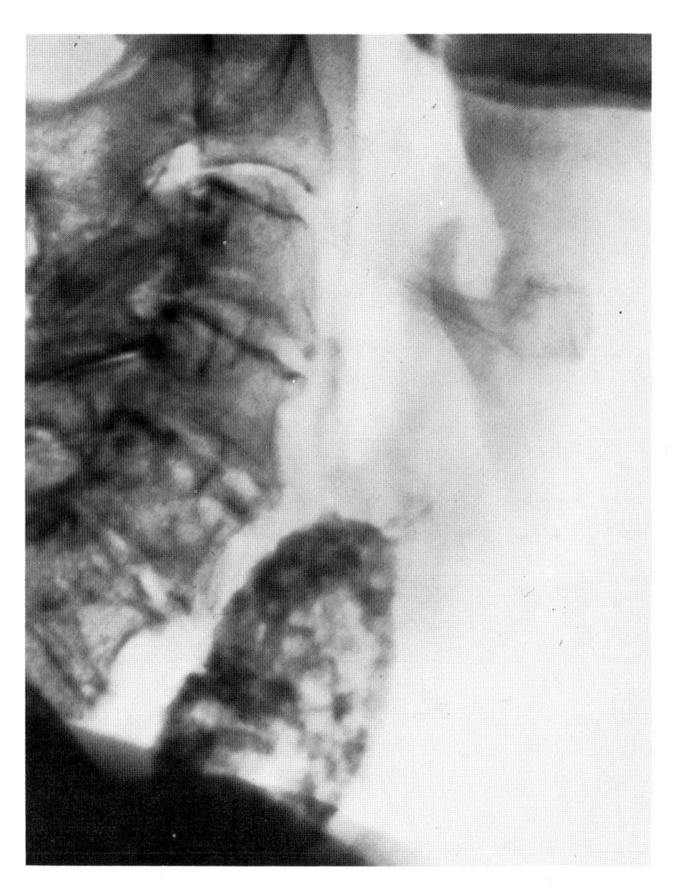

Fig. 316. Calcification of the thyroid gland. In this case, there is also a partial calcification of the anterior longitudinal ligament, as it is not infrequently found on the cervical spine in osteochondrotic changes. Calcifications of the posterior longitudinal ligament are much rarer but are then described on the cervical spine only.

Lagemann in 1972 demonstrated a case of calcification of the posterior longitudinal ligament in the region of the lumbar spine with a possible preformed excavation of the posterior body of the vertebra. But he, too, was not able to explain this single occurrence.
In 1975 *Op den Orth* demonstrated three cases of calcification of the posterior longitudinal ligament of the cervical spine and ascertained the frequency according to geographical locations in Japan. "The practical significance of these changes lies in the possibility that they may cause myelopathy by narrowing of the spinal canal."

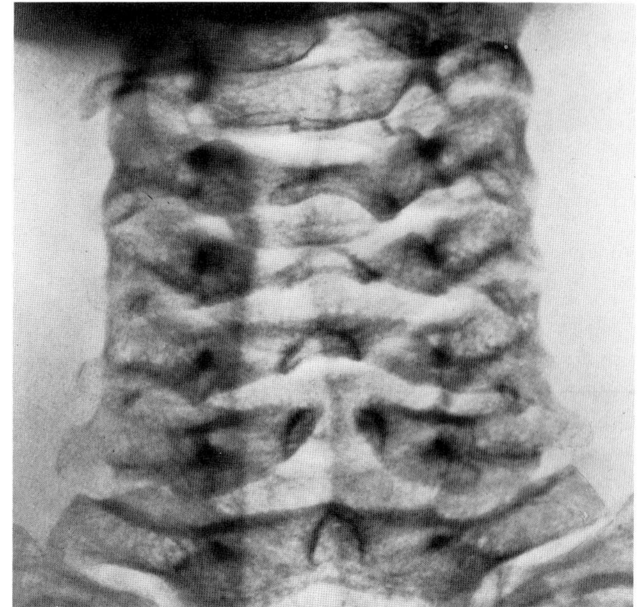

Fig. 317. Spina bifida at the 7th cervical vertebra in an 8-year-old boy. See text to Fig. 286a.

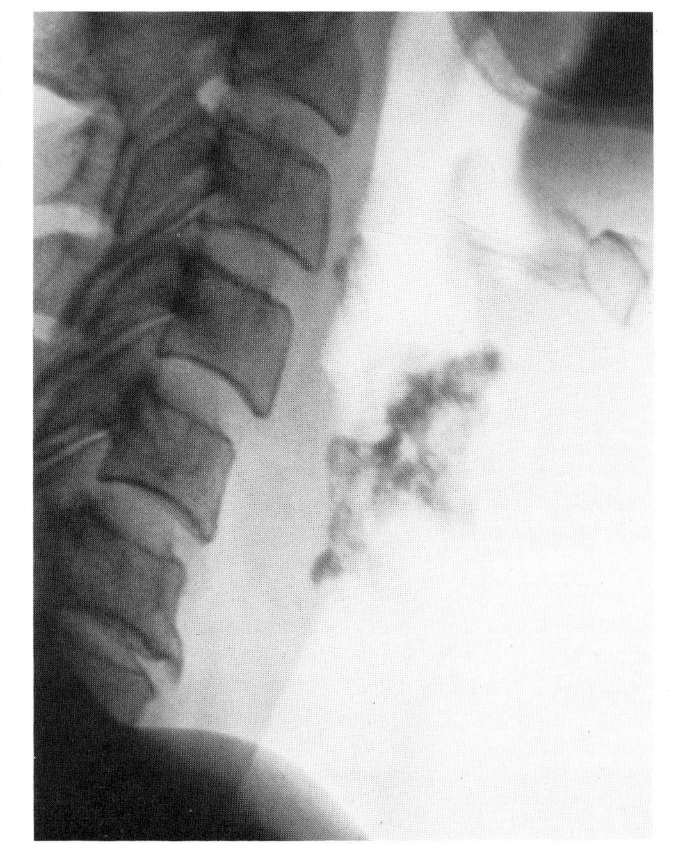

Fig. 318. Calcification of the thyroid cartilage. The ossification of the larynx starts at the end of the second decade, beginning at the posterior margin of the lamina of the thyroid cartilage *(Fraenkel)*. Viewed from the front, the shadows of the ossified thyroid cartilage appear as two ledges, converging downwards (Fig. 232, No. 44), which can easily be taken for a callus after fracture or for arthrotic hooks. On the lateral view, foci of ossification are sometimes misinterpreted when they appear as very irregularly dispersed spots.

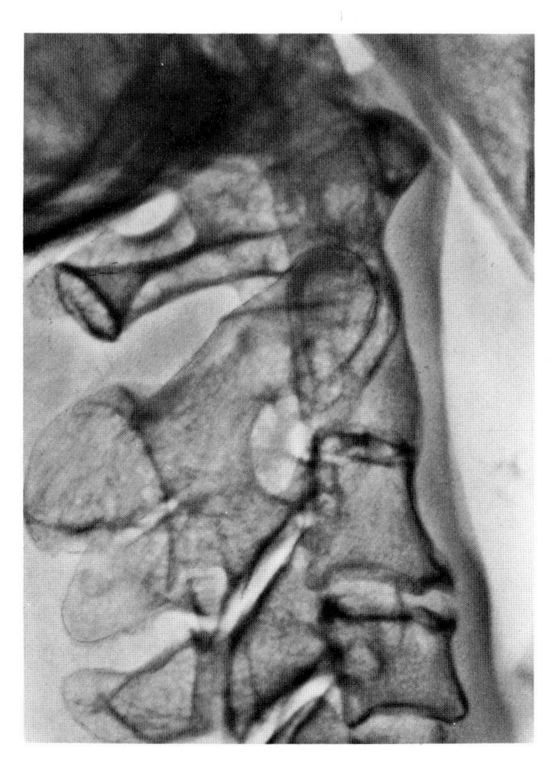

Congenital block formation in the cervical spine is not rare. Concurrent fusion of the arches speaks against inflammatory synostoses. Fusion of the two vertebrae (apart from the 1st and 2nd), synostosis of the atlas with the occiput or fissures in the atlas need not cause any disturbances, in contrast to extensive, more or less typical synostotic complexes (*Klippel-Feil's* disease, clidocranical dysostosis). The significance of these variants increases with any additional trauma. Errors in diagnosis are expecially common when radiographs are taken only some time after an accident. *Wuensch* considers the fusion of the anterior sections of the vertebral bodies in the region of the lower cervical spine (IV–VI) a "rarity" and, with *Brocher,* calls it a coalitio vertebrae.

Wackenheim reported a functional atlantooccipital block.
Oblak showed, in a 68-year-old female patient, the following combination of occipitocervical malformations:

1 Basilar impression, based on an asymmetrical medial occipital hypoplasia, condylar hypoplasia and platybasia,
2 Manifestation of an occipital vertebra, through persistence of a hypochordal clasp of the pro-atlas in the shape of a pre-basiooccipital arch and a tertiary condyle,
3 Odontoid bone,
4 Persistence of the hypochordal clasp of C II, and
5 Incomplete formation of a block vertebra between C II and C III.

Ebermaier reported on rare effects of the formation of block vertebrae of the cervical spine. Through insufficient excursions of the cervical spine, due to partial block formation of two cervical vertebrae, kinking of and pressure on the cervical medulla may be caused by extensive movements of the head. Such incidents may manifest themselves as passing spinal cord symptoms, e.g., increased reflexes, pyramidal symptoms, paresthesias and muscular weakness.

Fig. 319. Congenital formation of block vertebrae between the 2nd and 3rd cervical vertebrae, with fusion of vertebral arches and bodies. The intervertebral space has been preserved, though much reduced in height. Secondary deforming spondylosis can be seen at the neighboring vertebrae.

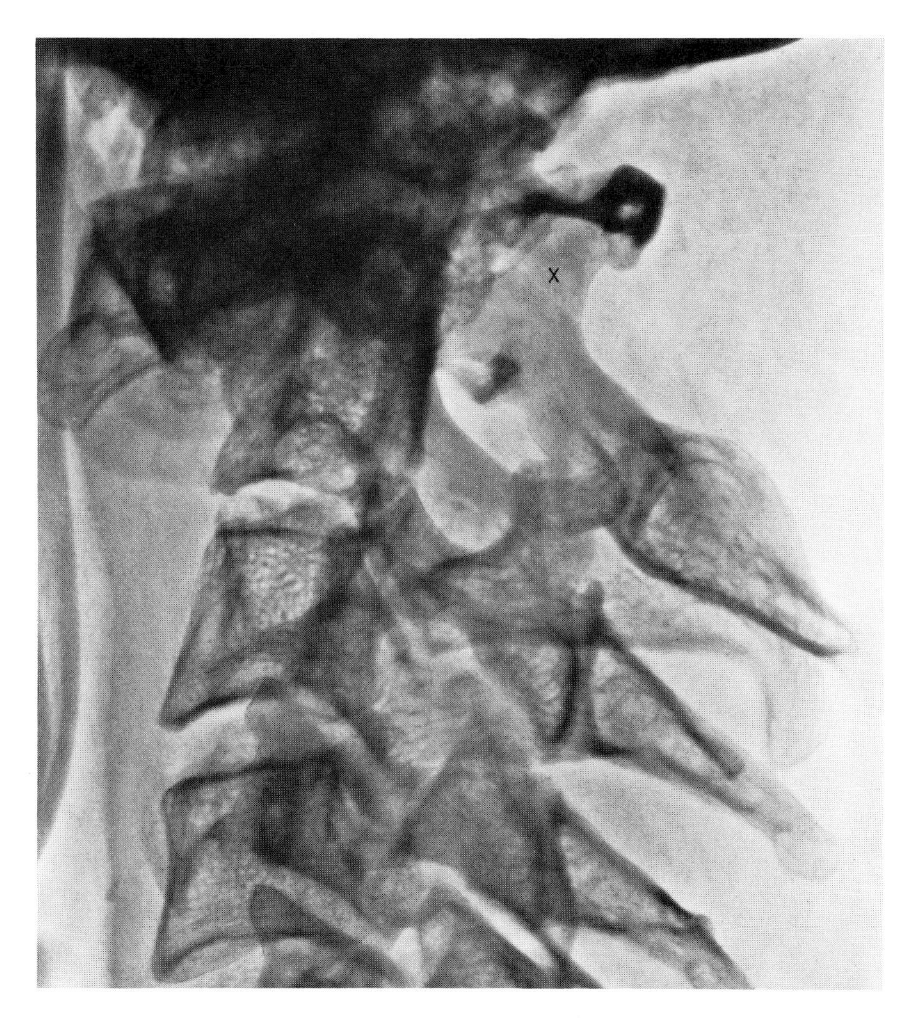

Fig. 320 (from the collection of *W. Werner,* Berlin). **Radiograph with meticulous focus of partial fusion of the vertebral arches of atlas and axis.** This partial fusion (×) of the arches belongs in the realm of block vertebrae formations, which may be partially of congenital origin and partially the result of inflammatory bone necrosis. Without doubt, this case presents a congenital anomaly which occurs very rarely in atlas and axis alone *(Köhler-Zimmer).* On causes of formation of block vertebrae, see p. 173.

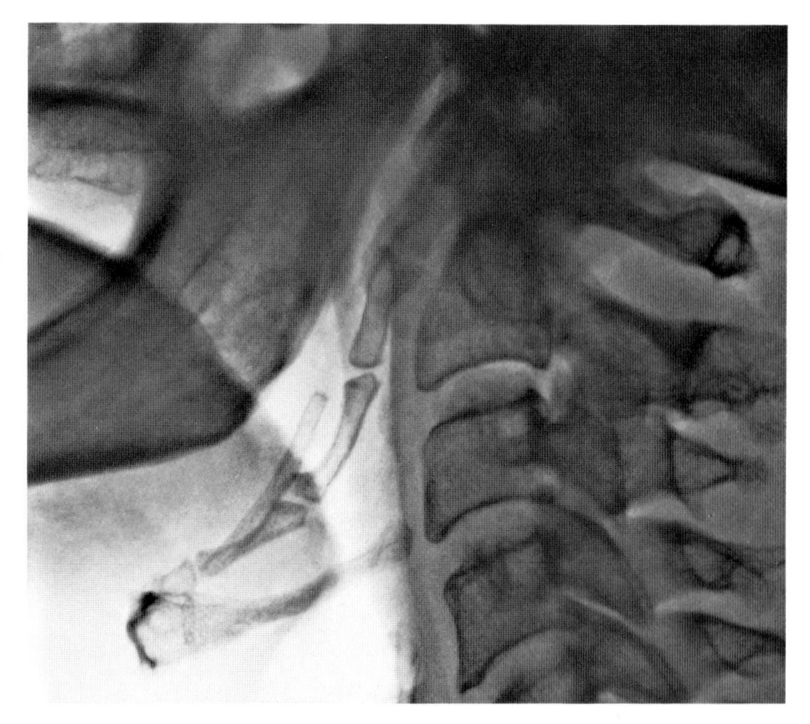

Fig. 321 (from the collection of *W. Werner,* Berlin). **Ossification of the stylohyoid ligament with joint-like subdivisions.** In a great number of vertebrates the hyoid apparartus consists of a bony chain that, on both sides of the neck, connects the hyoid bone with the base of the skull. In man, only its outer parts remain, i.e., the styloid apophysis and the lesser cornu of the hyoid bone, while the middle part has been replaced by the stylohyoid ligament. There are several types of anomalies of the hyoid apparatus:

a) A long styloid process,
b) Cartilaginous and bony nuclei in the stylohyoid ligament (a regression to a gill arch),
c) Replacement of the entire ligament by bone.

The styloid process is connected ontogenetically with the 2nd arch of gills; the ossification of the stylohyoid ligament is, so to speak, a retained arch of gills and, according to *H. A. Simon,* a genuine regression, constituting a rare anomaly. Elongation of the cornua of the hyoid bone without ligamental ossifications is also to be found *(Carones).*

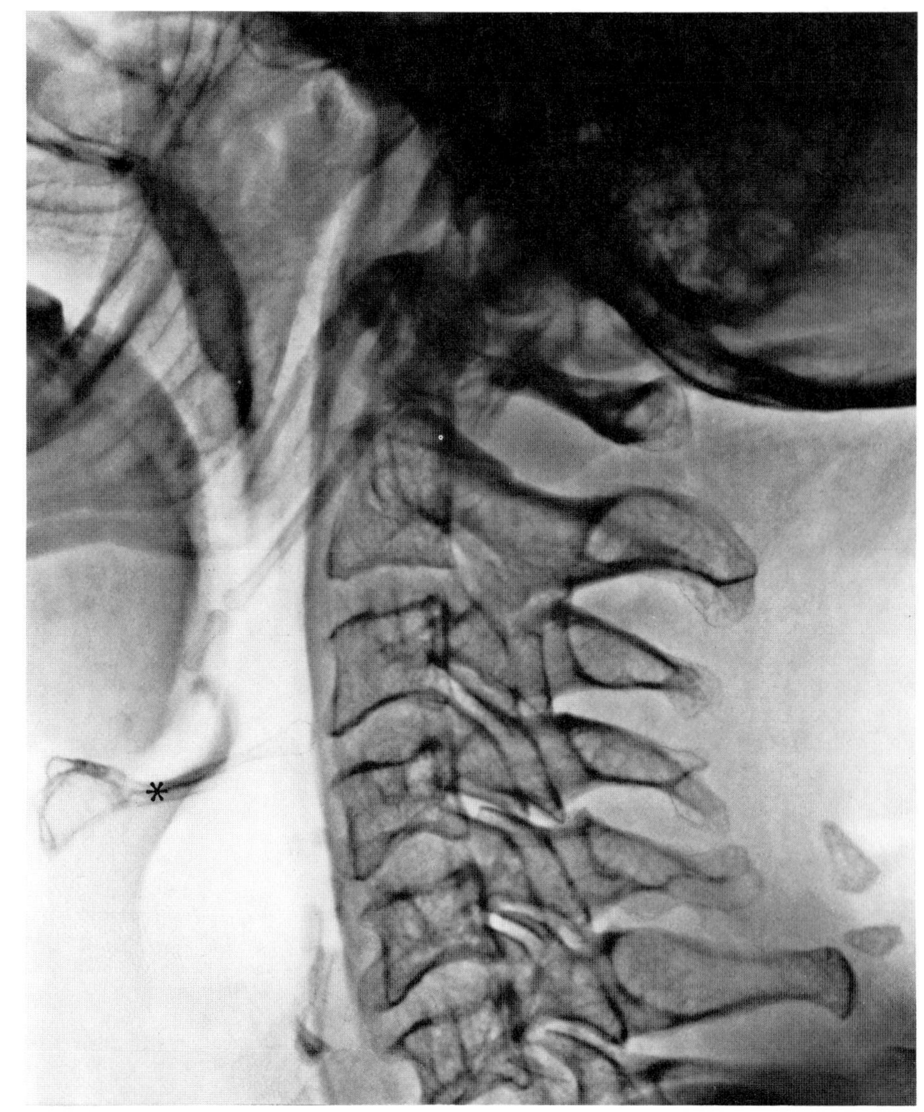

Fig. 322. Circumscribed calcinosis of the ligamentum nuchae (see Nos. 46 and 47 in Fig. 233). The differential diagnosis is for fractures with tearing-off of the spinous processes, partial ossification of the stylohyoid ligament (see No. 31* in Fig. 233), beginning of embedded calcifications in the thyroid cartilage (see No. 44 in Fig. 233), deforming spondylosis (see No. 45 in Fig. 233). The palatine velum (soft palate) and the epiglottis show up well on this view. *= hyoid bone.
Normal bifurcation of the spinous processes C II–C V.

Radiographic Anatomy and Radiographs of the Thoracic Spine, Ribs and Sternum

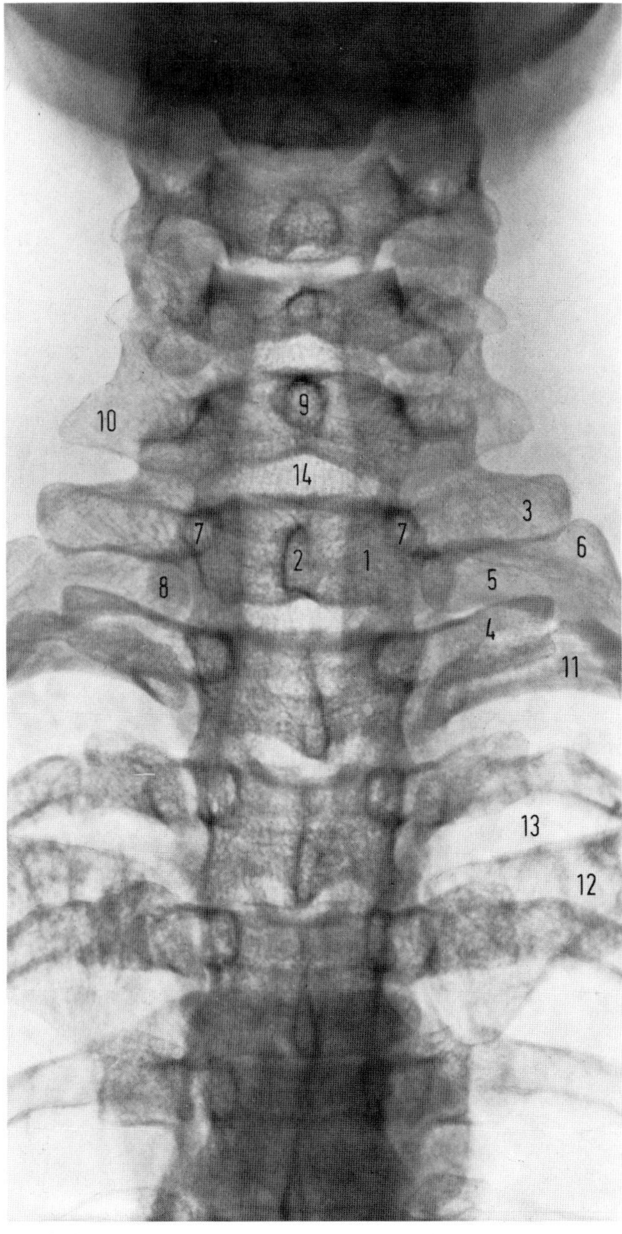

Fig. 323. Lower cervical and upper thoracic spine, ventrodorsal.

1 Body of 1st thoracic vertebra
2 Spinous process of 1st thoracic vertebra
3 Transverse process of 1st thoracic vertebra
4 Transverse process of 2nd thoracic vertebra
5 Neck of 1st rib
6 Tubercle of 1st rib
7 Root of the arch of the 1st thoracic vertebra
8 Head of the 1st rib; on its left, the articular space
9 Spinous process of the 7th cervical vertebra
10 Transverse process of the 7th cervical vertebra, sometimes, as on this view, misshapen in height or length (as rudiments of a cervical rib are fused into it)
11 2nd rib
12 Clavicle, enlarged because film-distant; lateral from the number: shadow of the 1st rib, at its transition into cartilage which becomes visible only with the start of ossification
13 Outline of lung
14 Tracheal ring

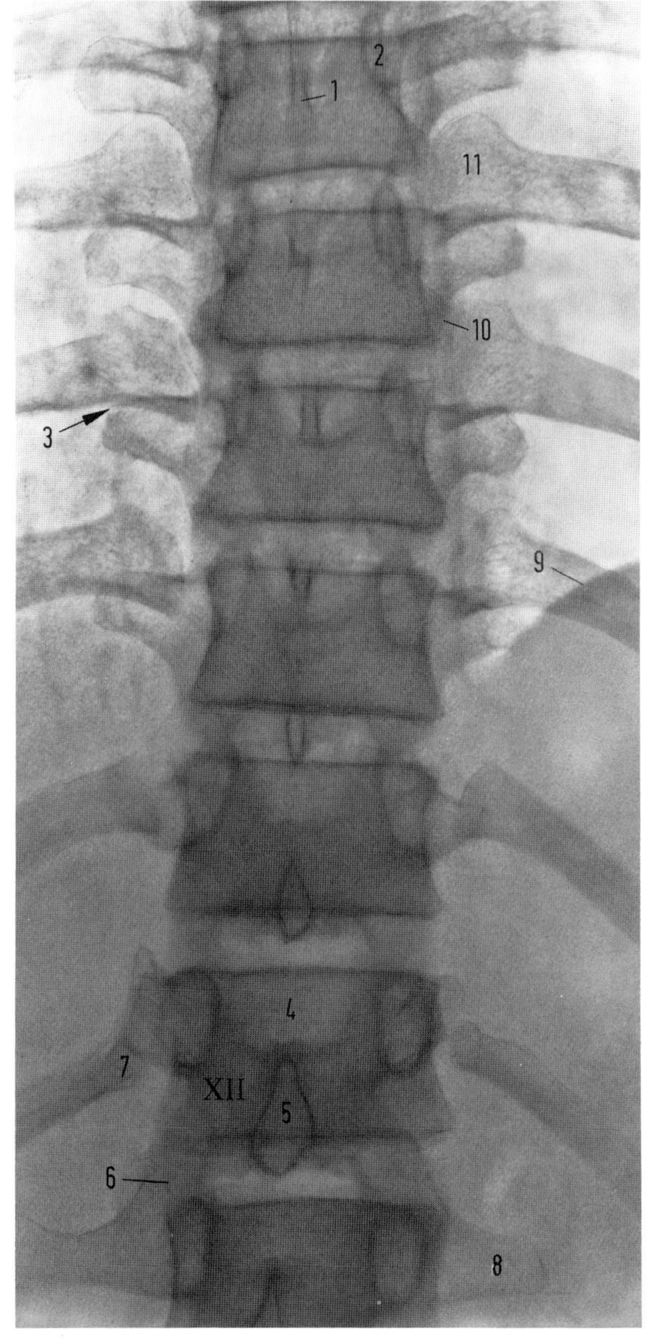

Fig. 324. Lower thoracic spine, ventrodorsal.

1 Spinous process of the 6th thoracic vertebra (the 6th and 7th thoracic vertebrae cover one another)
2 Root of arch of 7th thoracic vertebra
3 Costotransverse articulation
4 Radiolucent field, which the costal arch leaves free in an upward direction
5 Spinous process of the 12th thoracic vertebra
6 Intervertebral articulation Th 12/L I. From here on, the articular spaces are directed caudally and sagittally
7 Neck of rib
8 Costal process
9 Shadow of diaphragm
10 Costovertebral articulation (the rib articulates with two vertebrae)
11 Head of rib

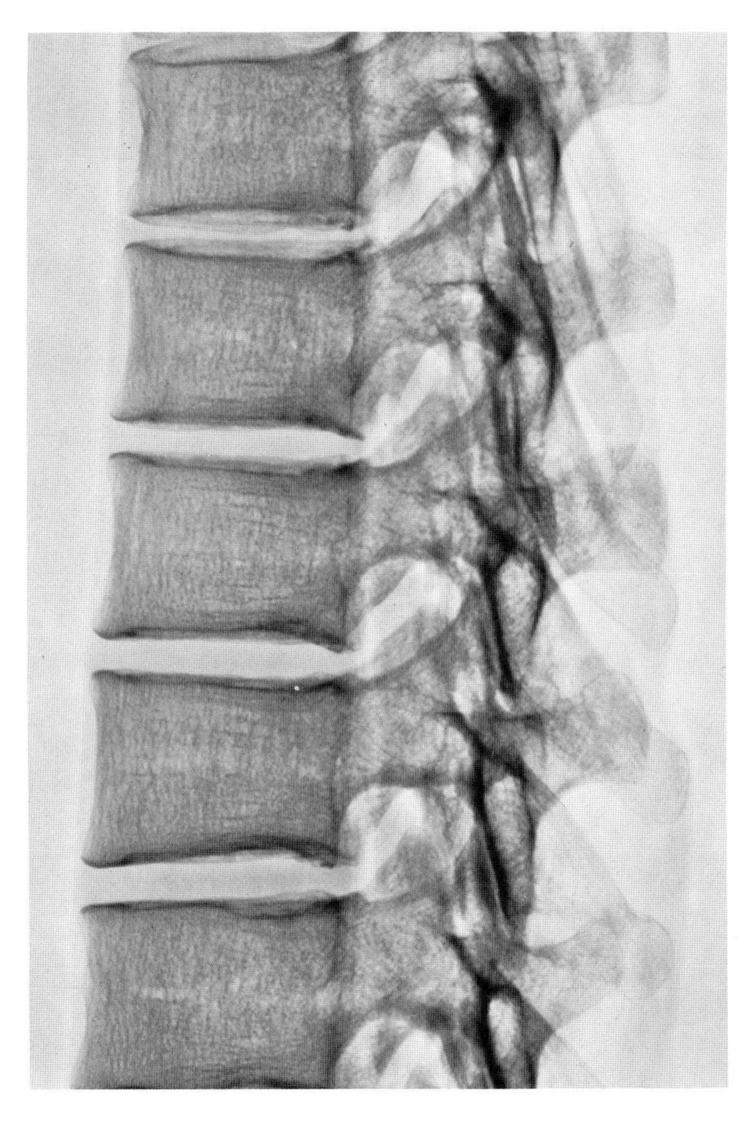

Fig. 325. Lower thoracic spine, preparation of the skeleton including ligaments, position $^3/_4$ oblique. The preparation with ligaments shows the normal relationships in the region of the intervertebral spaces, the small vertebral joints and the processes. By removal of the ribs, the position of the spinous processes is easily recognizable, while up to the spinous process of the 10th thoracic vertebra, they overlap like roof tiles; caudally from then on, they straighten up more and more and, in the region of the lumbar spine, they are directed almost straight dorsally. *Lutz* has reported on the development of the small vertebral joints.

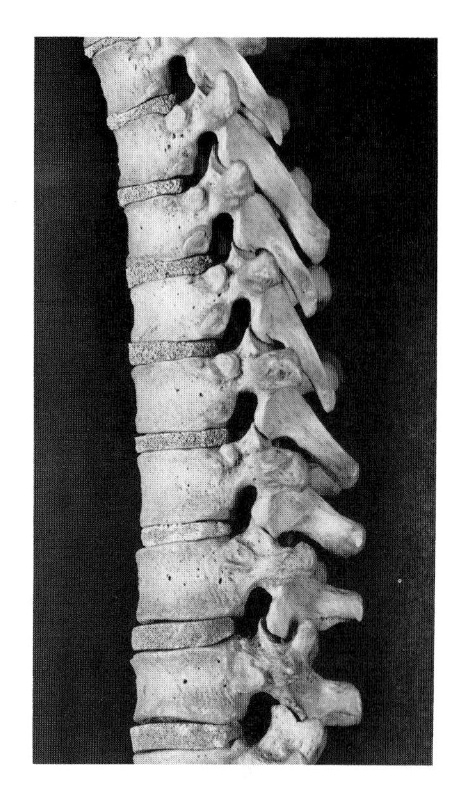

Fig. 326 demonstrates the various directions of the course of the spinous processes.

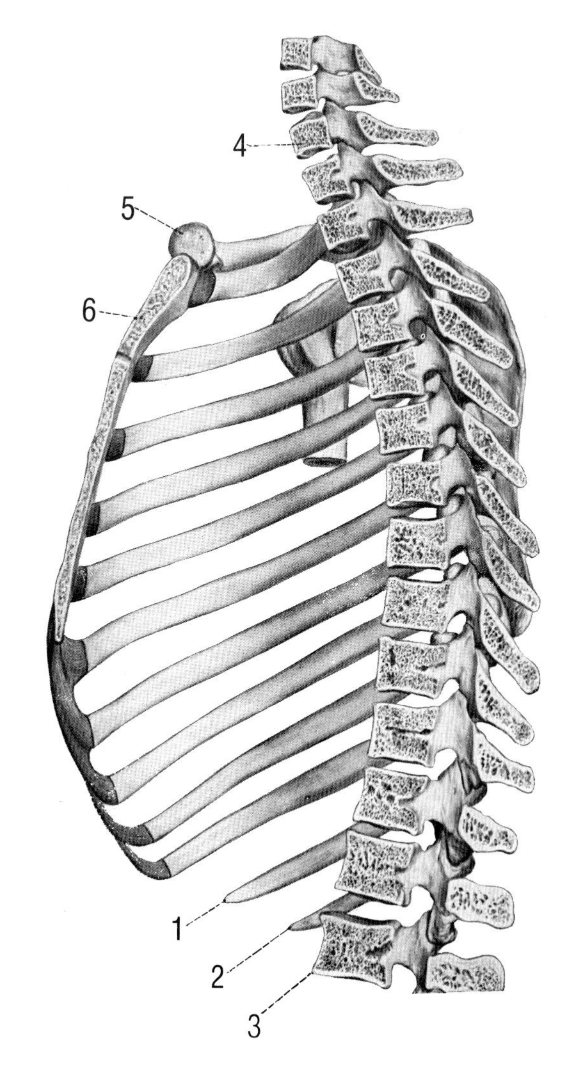

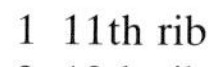

1 11th rib
2 12th rib
3 1st lumbar vertebra
4 6th cervical vertebra
5 Clavicle
6 Manubrium sterni

Fig. 327 (From *Sobotta-Becher*) shows a median sagittal section through the bony chest.

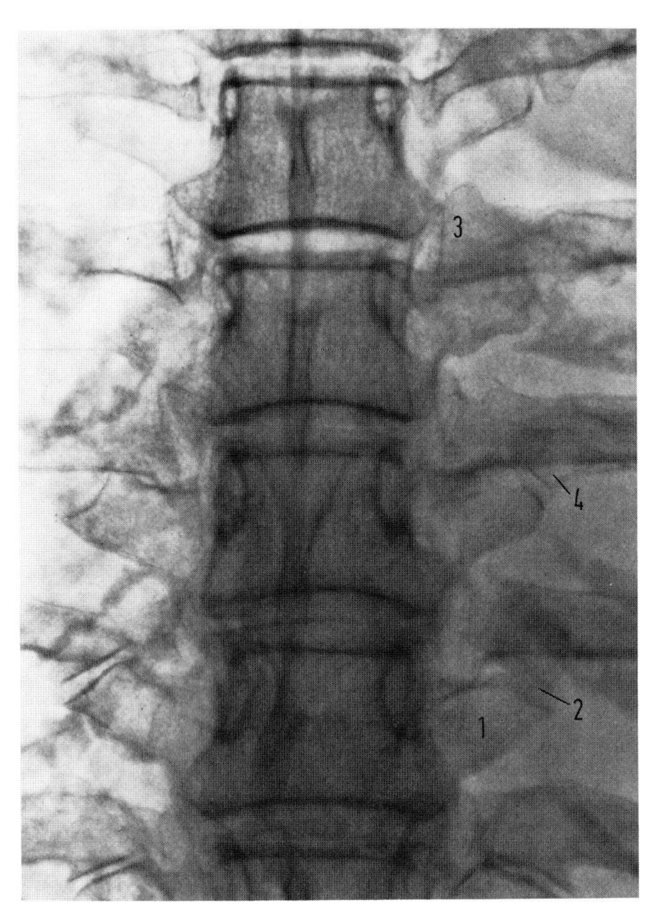

Fig. 328. Demonstration of the costotransverse joints. The central ray is beamed onto the body of the 6th thoracic vertebra at an angle of 20° in caudocranial direction.

1 Transverse process
2 Costotransverse articulation
3 Head of rib
4 Costal tubercle

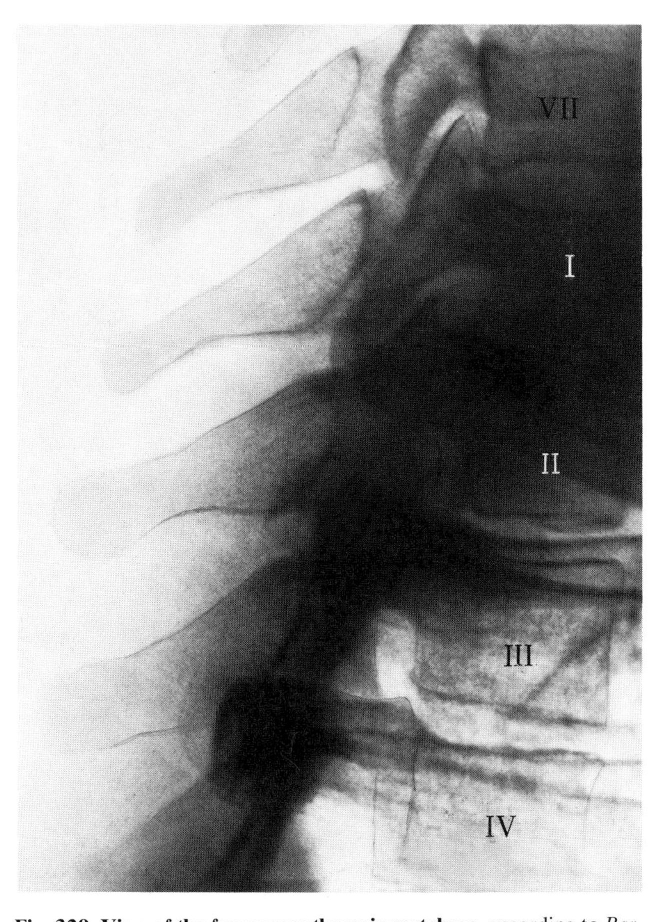

Fig. 329. View of the four upper thoracic vertebrae, according to *Barsony*. For position see Fig. 331.

VII Body of 7th cervical vertebra
I–IV Bodies of the 1st to 4th thoracic vertebrae

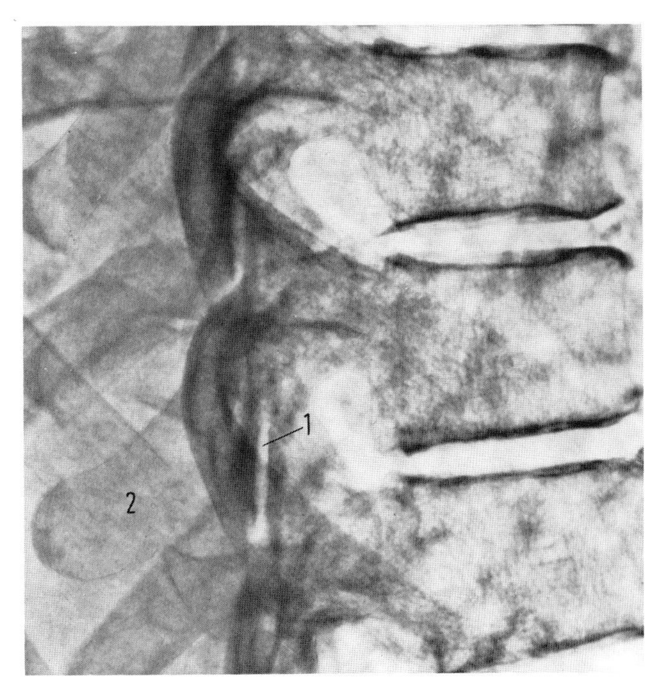

Fig. 330. Thoracic spine, oblique, patient standing, for demonstration of the film-near intervertebral joints.

1 Intervertebral joint
2 Spinous process

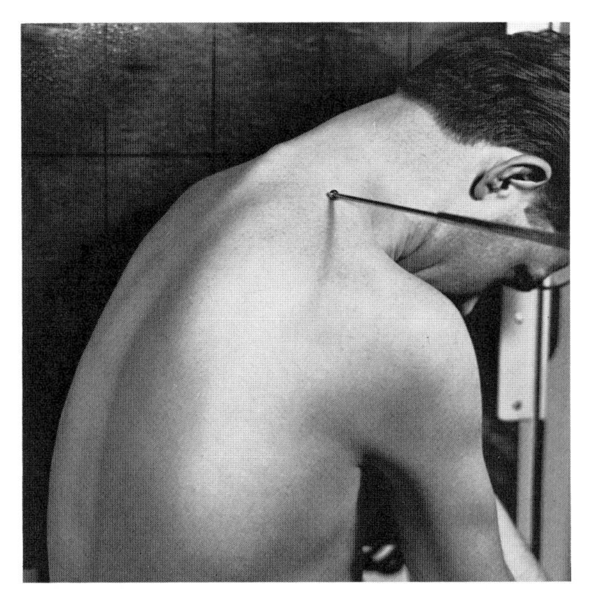

Fig. 331. Position for Fig. 329. The patient sits exactly laterally and leans with his shoulder against the *Bucky* wall-stand. The head is bent forward; the shoulders are pulled forward and downward by the hands, which are either crossed forward or pressed between the knees. In this way, a free projection of the upper thoracic vertebrae is achieved. The central ray is directed at the 1st and 2nd thoracic vertebrae and beams vertically onto the cassette.

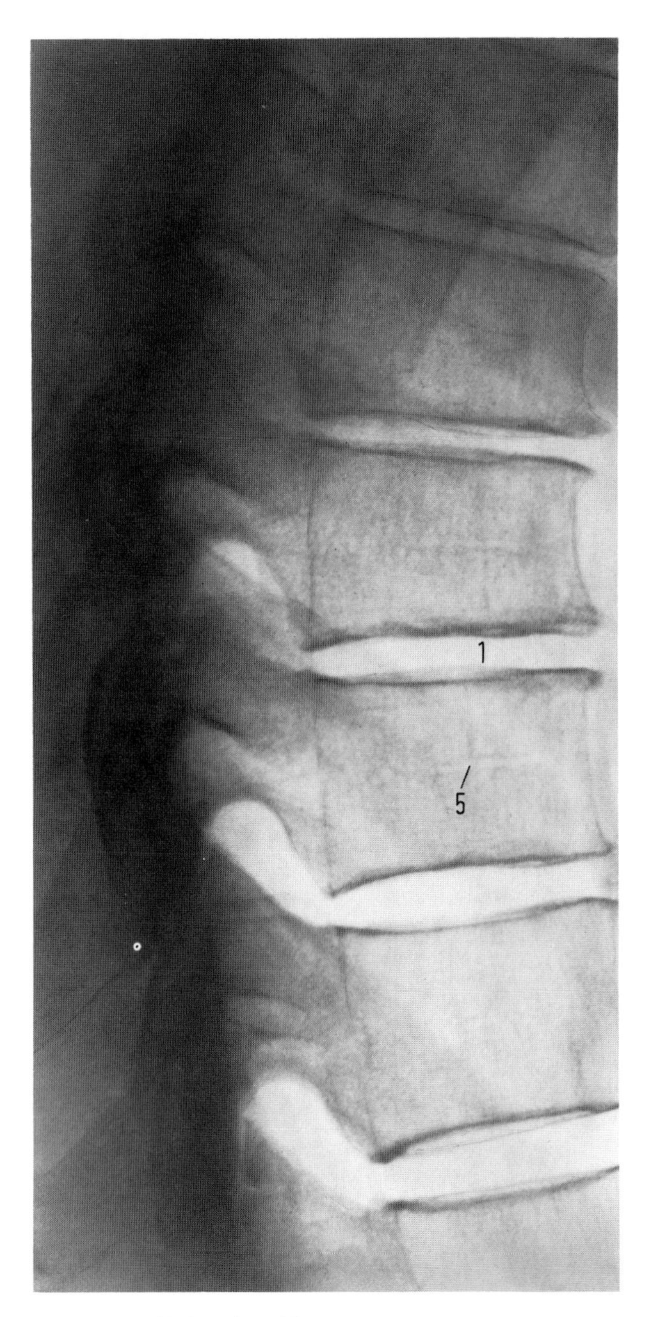

Fig. 332a. With lung breathing.

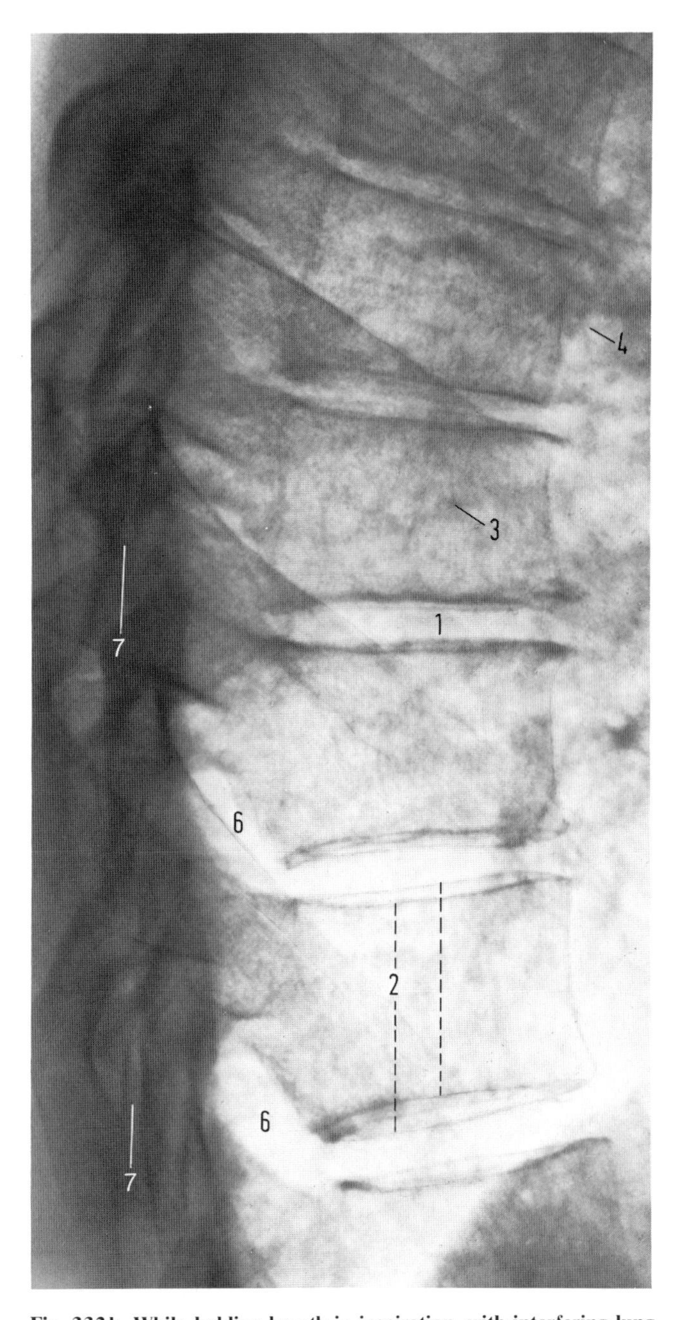

Fig. 332b. While holding breath in inspiration, with interfering lung shadow.

Fig. 332. Thoracic spine, lateral, while holding breath and while breathing. The intervertebral spaces are seen obliquely in the upper and lower thirds of the radiographs. Two contours, bent in the same direction, belong together, one pair of which corresponds to the film-near space between the margins of the two vertebral bodies, the other pair to the film-distant space.

1 Intervertebral space VII/IX, taken orthograde; therefore, it appears distinct and of simple construction
2 Height of the body of the 10th thoracic vertebra (film-distant side; on its right, the film-near side); see also Fig. 398
3 Lower angle of scapula
4 Medial margin of scapula
5 Canal of *Hahn* (see also Fig. 443, No. 107)
6 Intervertebral foramina
7 Intervertebral articulation

The indication of a rounded back, the wedge-shaped narrowing anteriorly of the upper vertebrae and the displacement of the covering laminae are reminiscent of the late stage of *Scheuermann's* disease, occurring in later infancy. He still includes the juvenile deforming osteochondritis, as well as the flat osteonecrotic vertebra *(Calvé),* among the aseptic bone necroses (see also Figs. 385 and 393). Just as constitutional-hereditary causes, combined with endocrine disturbances, are now accepted for *Scheuermann*'s disease, the flat vertebra is also attributed to a multiple genesis. It occurs as a congenital malformation, as an acquired osteonecrotic flat vertebra, manifesting itself in early infancy *(Calvé)*, and as an acquired traumatic flat vertebra. The flat vertebra in cases of eosinophile granuloma probably should be considered purely as a symptom, as in systemic diseases (rickets, osteofibrosis of *Recklinghausen*). On further aseptic bone necroses, see p. 536.

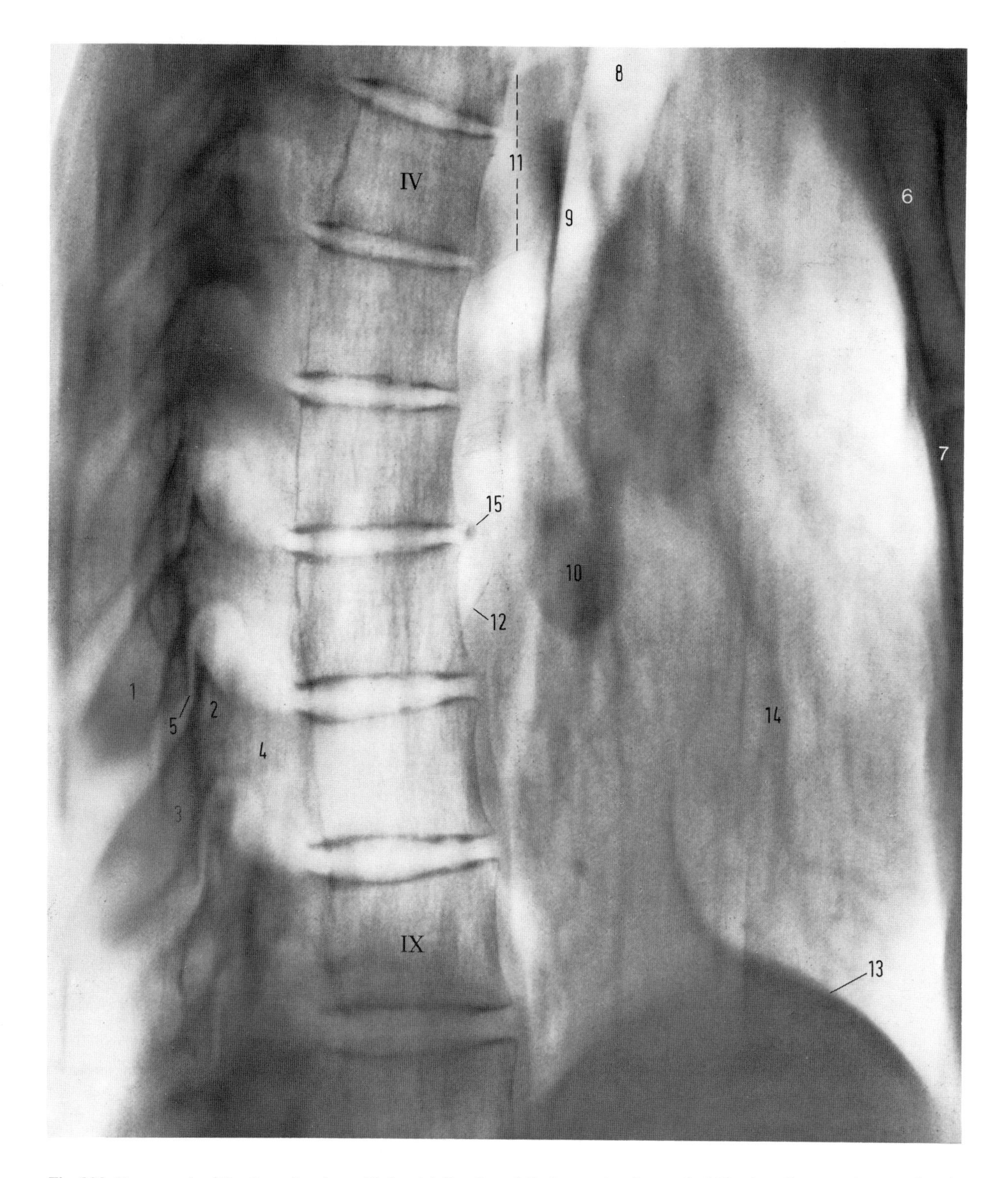

Fig. 333. Tomograph of the thoracic spine, with frontal direction of the beam, showing vertical blurring. On normal comprehensive views, foci of destruction become visible only from a diameter of 1.0 to 1.5 cm and up. Much smaller osteolytic processes or defects in the cancellous tissue can be observed with tomograms, but the structure of the vertebral bodies is shown better on comprehensive views as the patient continues normal breathing.

1 Spinous process
2 Superior articular process
3 Inferior articular process
4 Vertebral arch
5 Intervertebral joint
6 Manubrium sterni
7 Body of sternum
8 Trachea
9 Bifurcation
10 Shadow of a calcified lymphoma of hilum
11 Aortic arch, descending portion
12 Dorsal contour of heart (left ventricle)
13 Diaphragm
14 Blood vessels of the lung
15 Embedded calcification in the anterior longitudinal ligament

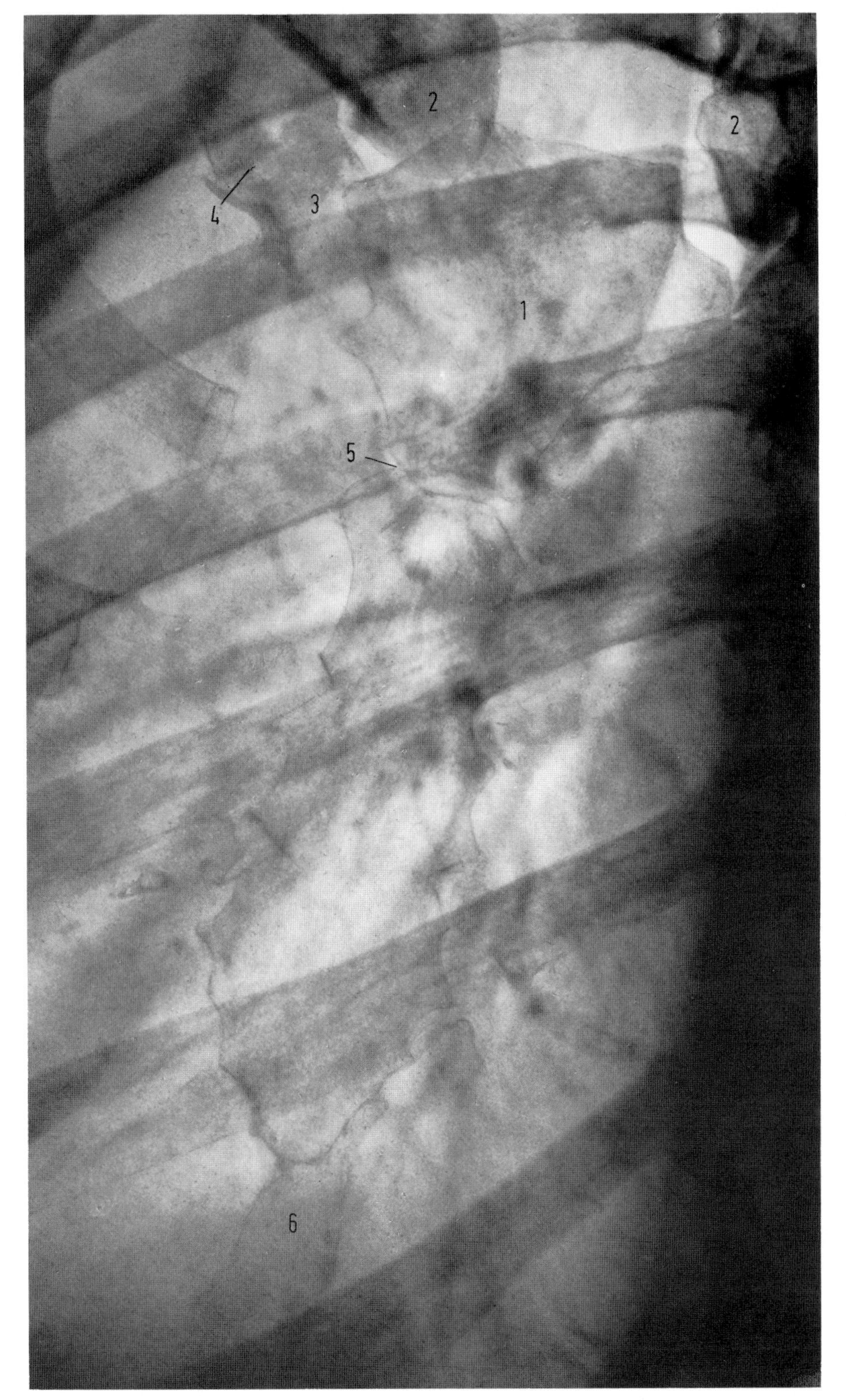

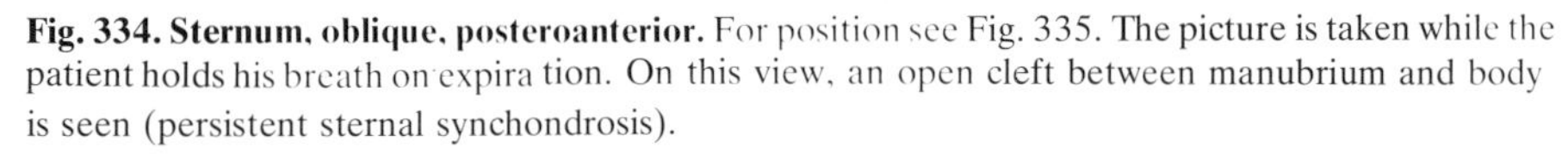
Fig. 334. Sternum, oblique, posteroanterior. For position see Fig. 335. The picture is taken while the patient holds his breath on expira tion. On this view, an open cleft between manubrium and body is seen (persistent sternal synchondrosis).

1 Manubrium sterni
2 Clavicle
3 Calcified cartilage of 1st rib
4 Cleft, free of calcification, which separates the calcified costal cartilage from the bony rib; such clefts may also remain within the calcified cartilage. According to *Stehr,* they fulfill the function of joint-like formations, providing retention of mobility of the thorax during respiration
5 Superior sternal synchondrosis (fibrocartilage)
6 Xyphoid process

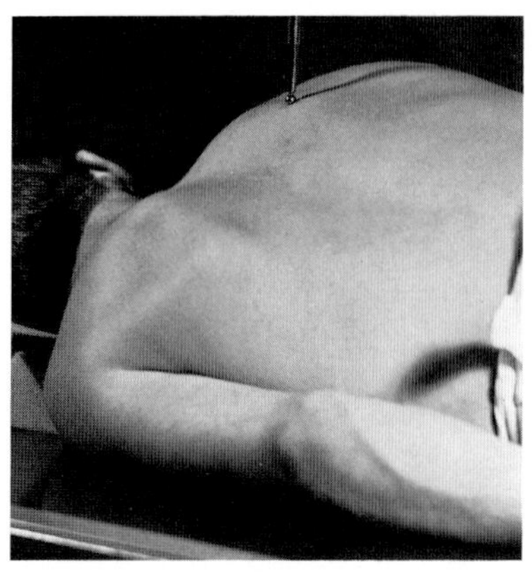

Fig. 335. Prone position, turned 45°, left side toward film, so that the shadows of heart and spine do not cover the sternum. The left arm lies close to the body, the right supports the semi-oblique position. The central ray is beamed from a point three fingers wide right of the spine to the center of the sternum, vertical to the cassette.

The persistent superior sternal synchondrosis forms a site of diminished resistance for post-traumatic and inflammatory (e.g., tuberculosis-like) diseases. Here, *Bechterew*'s disease produces early changes, as in cases of osteochondrosis and of osteochondrosis dissecans with necrosis of cartilage.

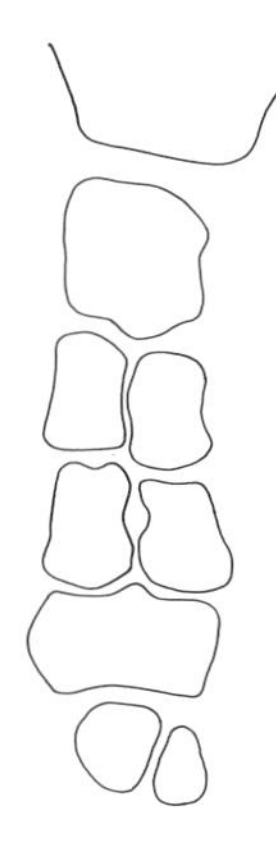

Fig. 336. Sketch according to a radiograph by *Thews.*
Fusion of the bony nuclei at the sternum has failed; therefore, apart from the normal horizontal cleft between manubrium and body, further horizontal as well as vertical clefts remain.
In addition, congenital complete sternal fissure is a recognized malformation, which is often discovered only in the adult; see *Zimmer.*

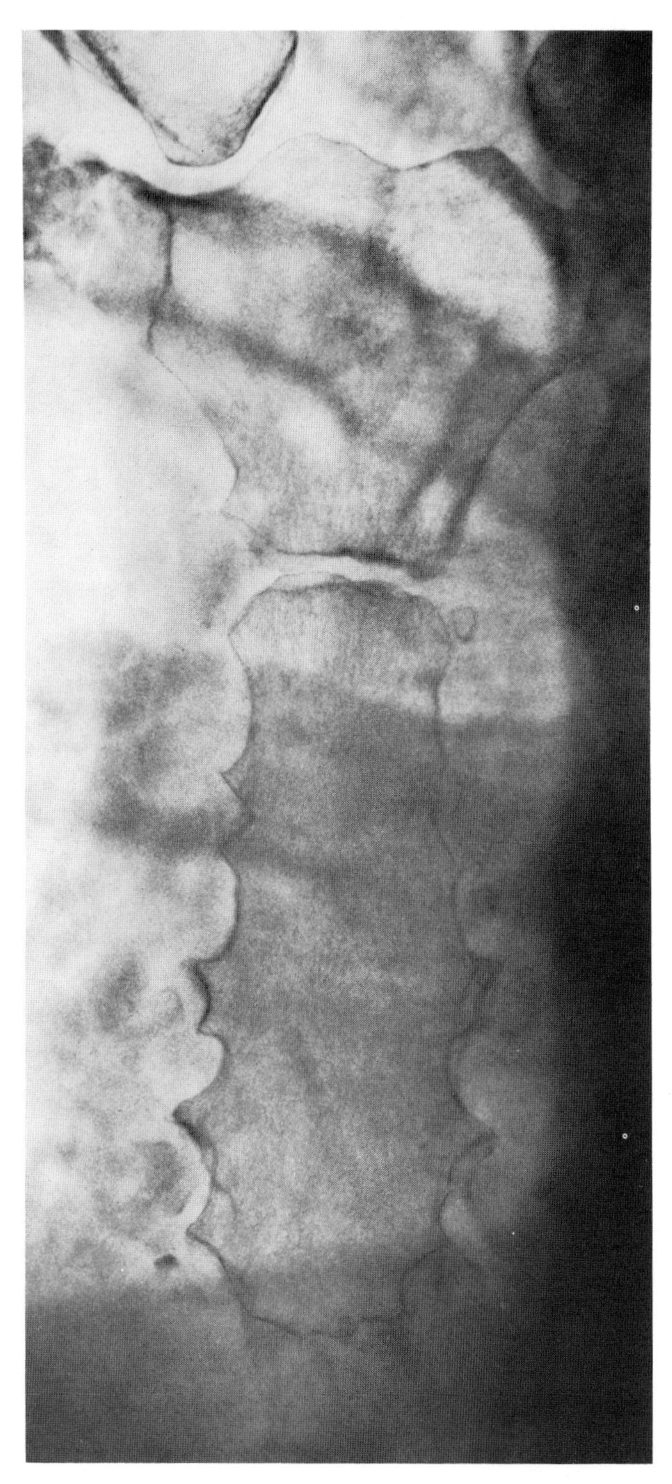

Fig. 337. Contact radiograph of the sternum, after *Lauven,* with patient prone. Because of the high load of irradiation, contact radiographs are permissible only in exceptional cases, after the most intense consideration that they are indicated. With the cylindrical tube placed close dorsally, the central ray is directed onto the sternum. One obtains a view rich in contrast, with the sternoclavicular joints showing well, without the interfering cover of the vascular system of the lung. On this view, the calcification of the cartilage of the 1st rib is still distinctly visible, while at the remaining costal cartilages the beginning of ossification can be seen faintly (see No. 3, Fig. 334). At the anterior end of the rib, the non-calcified cleft (described in Fig. 334) can just be recognized.

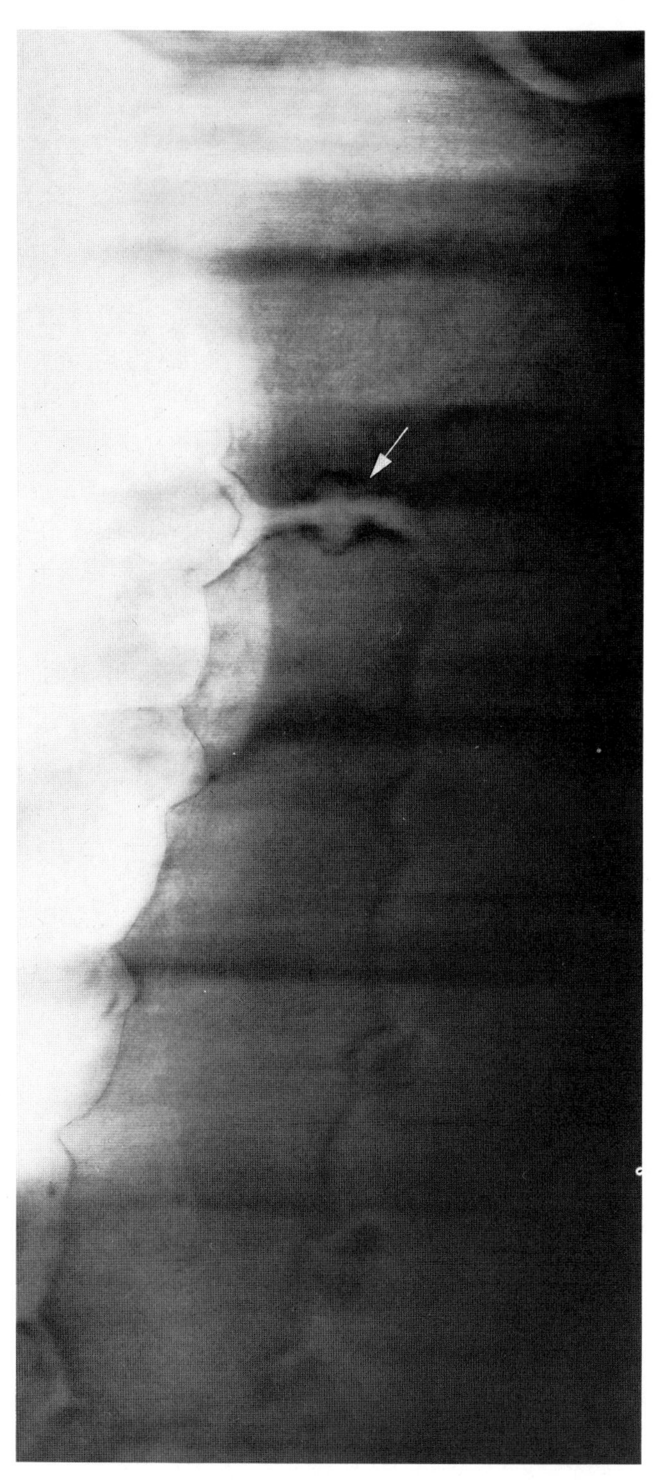

Fig. 338. The tomographic examination of the sternum and the sternoclavicular joints; horizontal blurring. With this method, even minor pathological processes at the sternum, sternoclavicular joints and clavicles can be recognized exactly and in detail. Due to its similarity to the intervertebral disks, the sternal synchondrosis sometimes produces similar views, as in cases of *Schmorl*'s cartilaginous nodules (↙) *(Pässler)*.

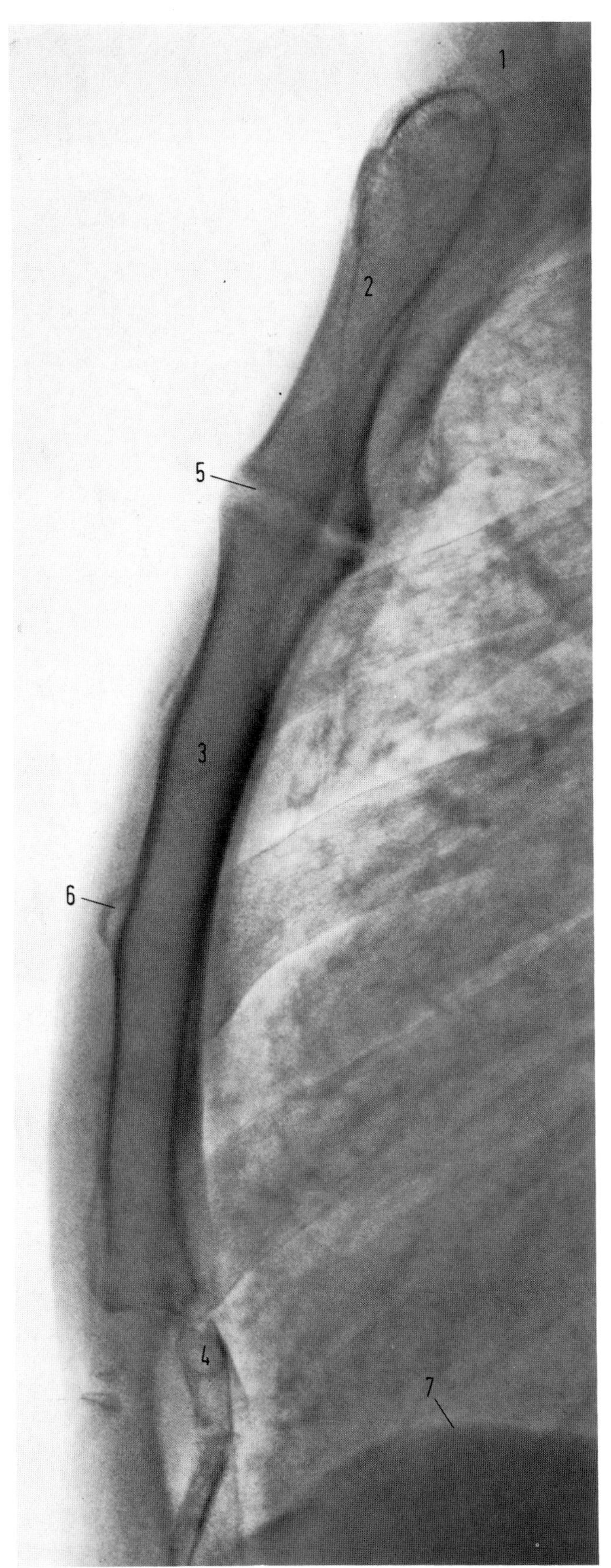

Fig. 339. **Sternum, lateral.** For position see Fig. 342.

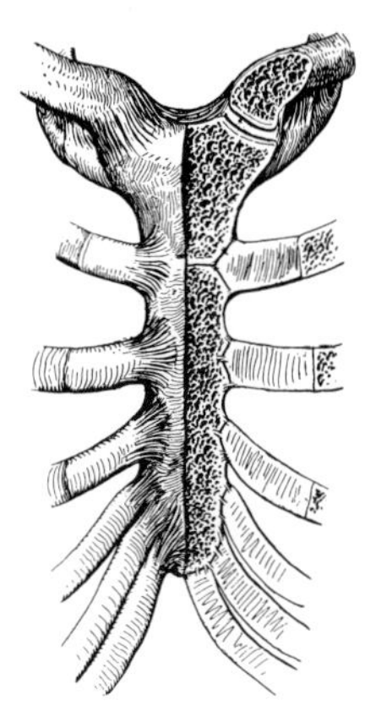

Fig. 340. Sternum, with the articulations for the clavicle and with the 2nd to 7th costal cartilages (from *Sobotta-Becher,* 15th ed.).

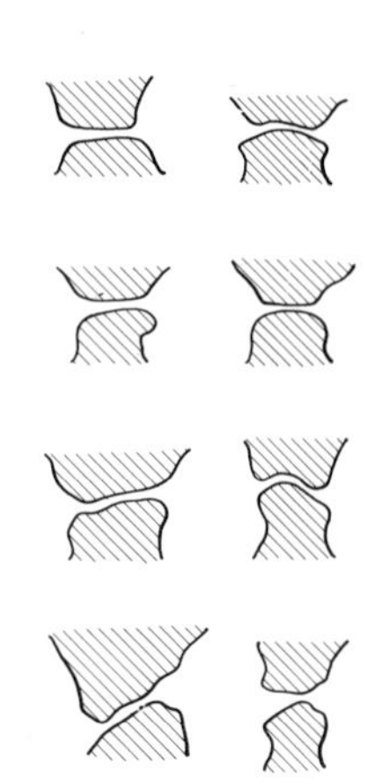

Fig. 341. Different types of superior sternal synchondrosis, viewed from the front (after *Zimmer*).

1 Both clavicular shadows, by projection fused into one pointed arch
2 Manubrium sterni
3 Body of sternum
4 Xyphoid process, not fused with the sternal body
5 Sternal synchondrosis, which may show increased formation of osteophytes *(Gassmann)*
6 Calcified costal cartilage
7 Diaphragm

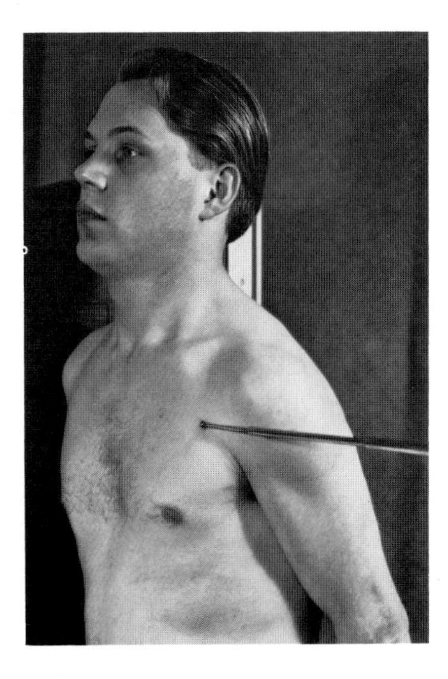

Fig. 342. Position for Fig. 339. The patient stands exactly laterally at the *Bucky* wall-stand, with both arms placed behind the back and the shoulders pulled down. The central ray is beamed vertically onto the cassette and impinges tangentially onto the middle of the sternum.

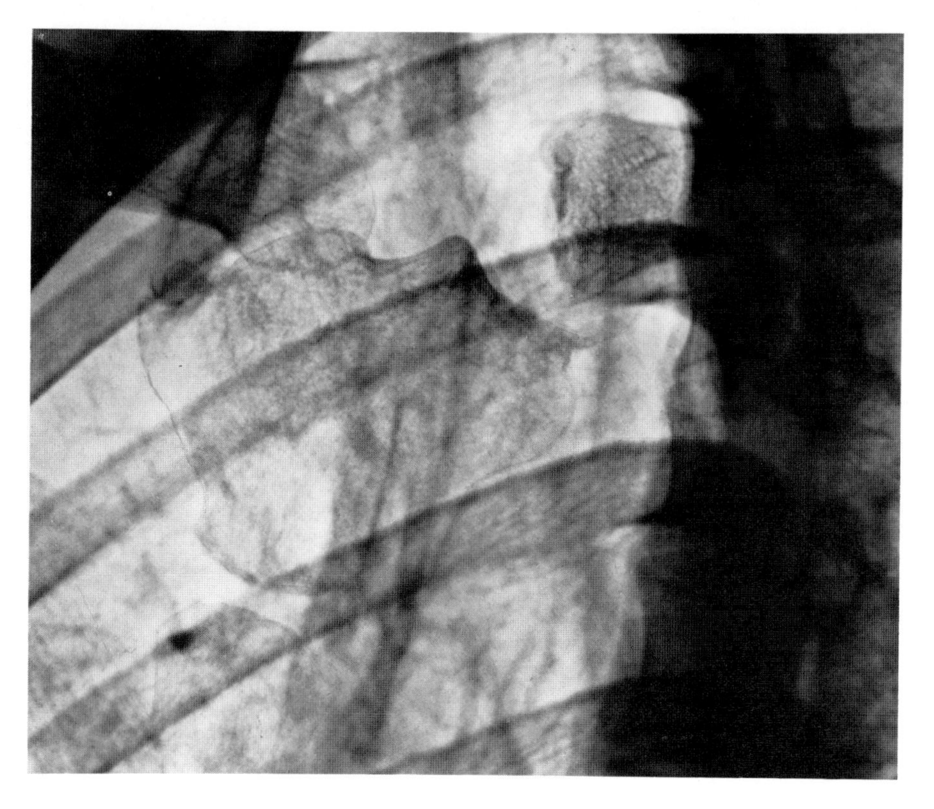

Fig. 343. Manubrium sterni. Position as for the oblique posteroanterior radiograph. The central ray is beamed onto the film-near sternoclavicular joint. A second large, bony nucleus, situated caudally to the main nucleus, led to the formation of an extremely long manubrium sterni (*Schmid* and *Weber*).

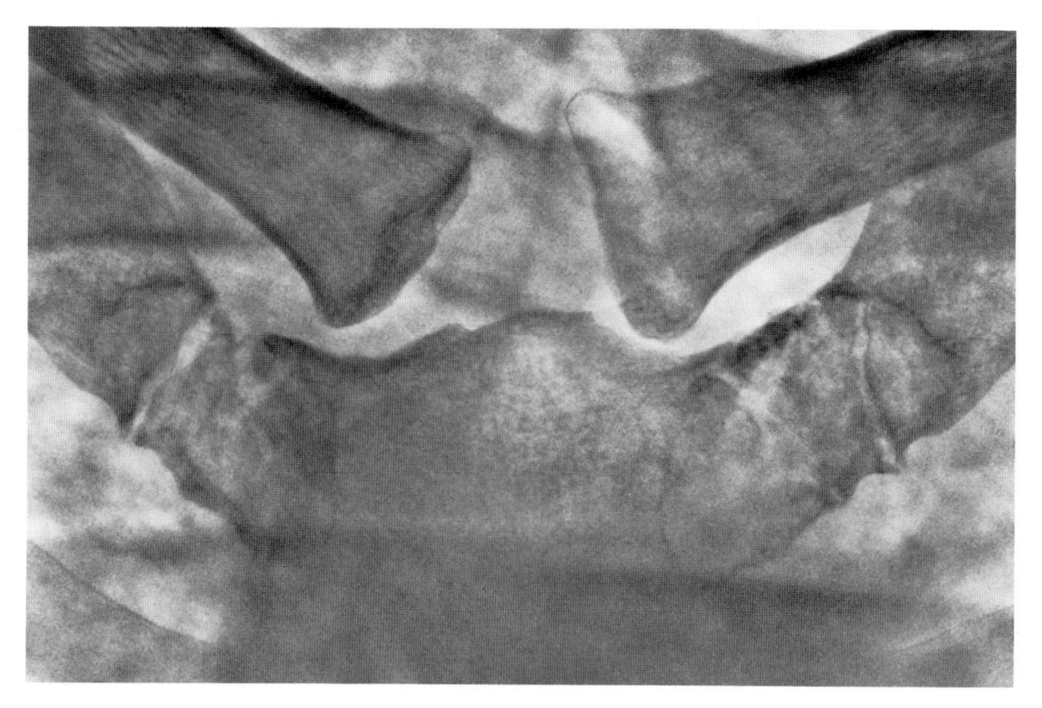

Fig. 344. Double-contact radiograph, for precise comparison of both sternoclavicular joints *(Zimmer)*. Position: prone. The shoulders are pulled forward as far as possible. The tube is centered on a "vertebral point" at the height of the sternoclavicular joints. The central beam is directed slightly cranially in order to pass the clavicular fossa. Then the tube must be shifted parallelly, once 6 cm to the right and once 6 cm to the left, and the shot is taken on the same film, each time with less exposure time than is used for an ordinary contact radiograph. The patient's position remains unchanged. The advantage of a contact radiograph compared to a tomogram lies especially in the presentation of the details of the bony structure. A serious disadvantage of contact radiographs is in the high load on the skin, especially when soft rays are applied, but this is unavoidable because of the short distance.

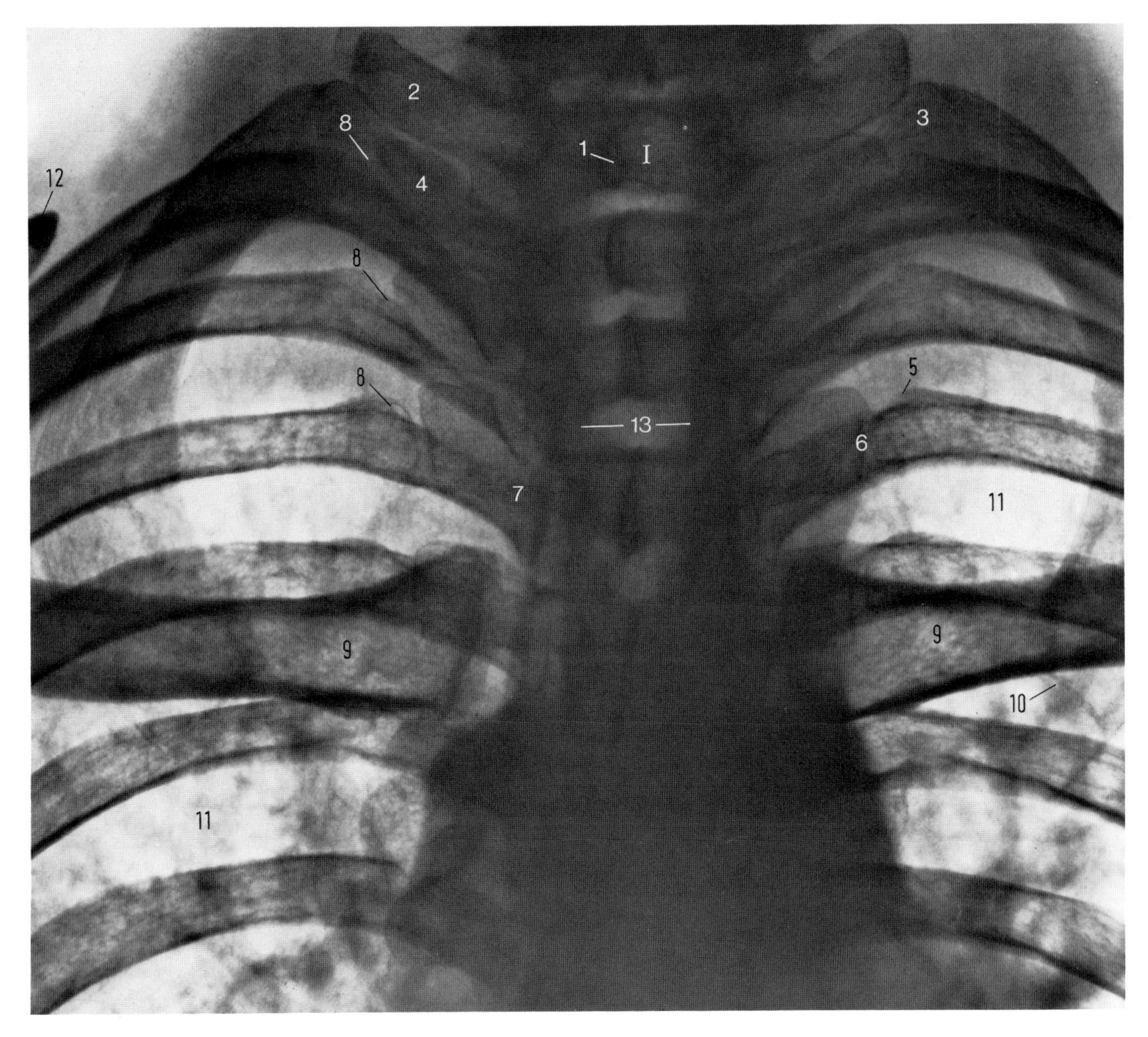

Fig. 345. Pulmonary apices, ventrodorsal, with obliquely craniocaudal-directed central ray. For position see Fig. 346. By means of this direction of the radiograph, the otherwise interfering clavicular shadow moves caudally out of the area of the pulmonary apices. In addition, the upper costovertebral joints are more clearly visible with this position.

I 1st thoracic vertebra
1 Spinous process of 1st thoracic vertebra
2 Transverse process of 1st thoracic vertebra
3 Tubercle of 1st rib
4 Neck of 1st rib
5 Tubercle of 4th rib
6 Neck of 4th rib
7 Head of 4th rib
8 Costotransverse articulations II–IV, on right side
9 Clavicle, film-distant therefore enlarged
10 Border between bone and cartilage, 1st rib
11 Lung field
12 Superior angle of scapula
13 Radiolucent band of trachea

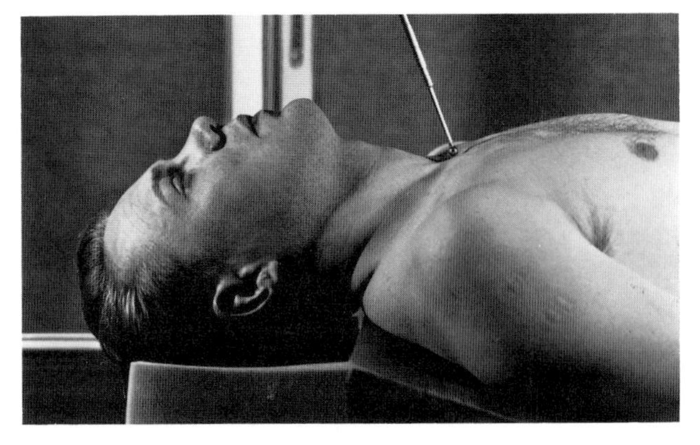

Fig. 346. Direction of beam obliquely onto collar bone, shoulders pulled forward.

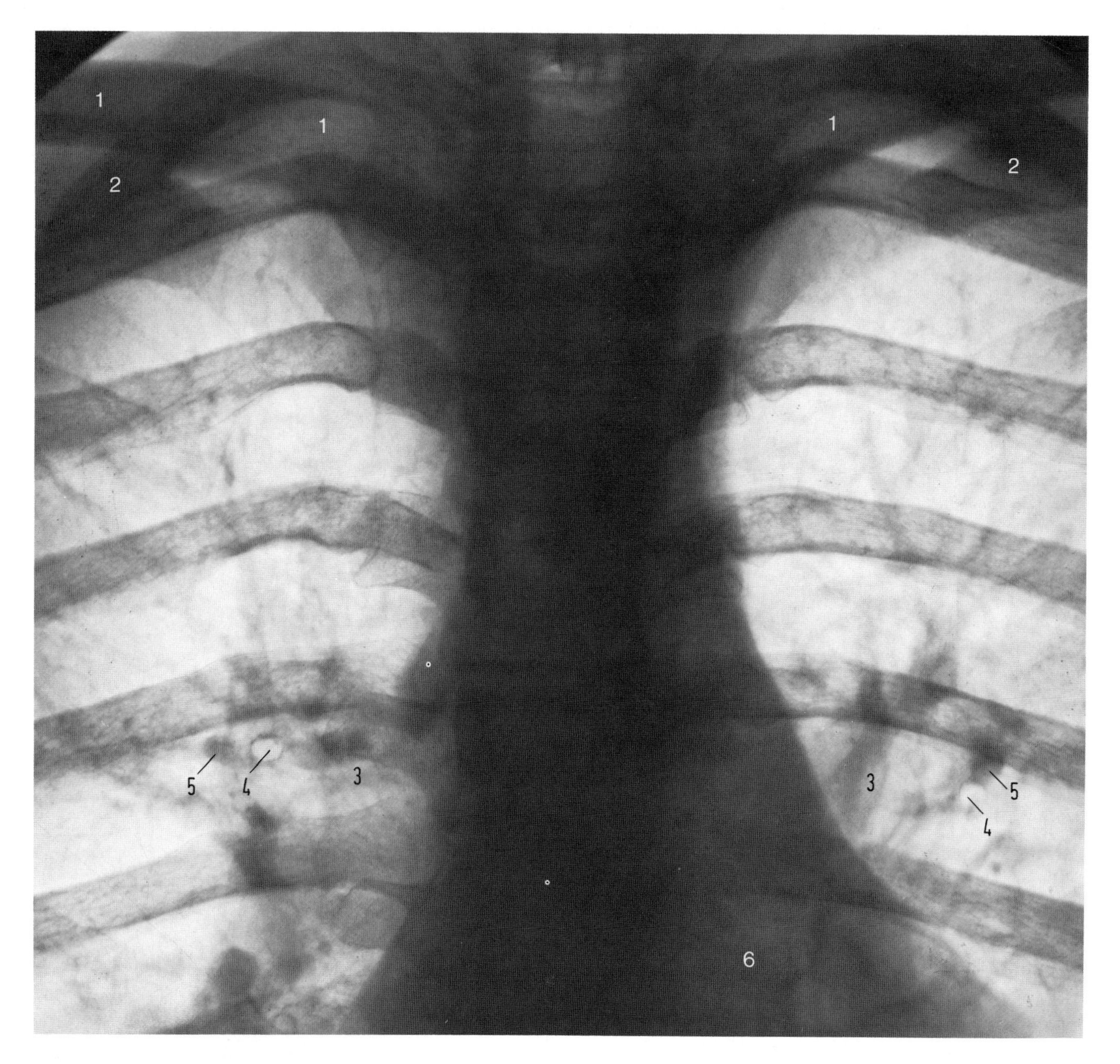

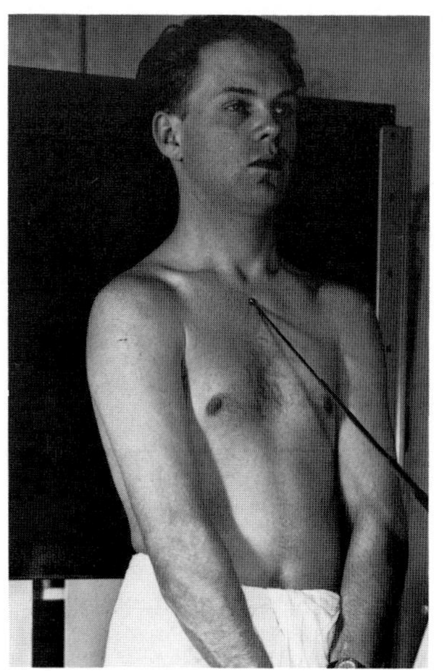

Fig. 347. View of pulmonary apices, in lordotic position, ventrodorsal, with obliquely entering craniocaudal central ray. For position see Fig. 348. With this position the central ray runs parallel to the posterior intercostal spaces and the clavicles are projected in the cranial direction away from the pulmonary apices. In addition, the shadow of the hilum is thrown upwards and rises from the shadow of the heart.

1 Clavicle
2 1st rib
3 Pulmonary hilum
4 Bronchus, taken axially
5 Pulmonary blood vessel running parallel; this is also taken axially and therefore gives a dense shadow. It should not be mistaken for a "shadow of calcification" of calcified pulmonary foci or of hilum lymphomata
6 Shadow of heart

Fig. 348. The standing patient leans his back against the *Bucky* wall-stand, obliquely in lordotic position. The arms are maximally rotated inward. The central ray is aimed caudocranially at an angle of 30° at the lower clavicular margin. Picture taken after inspiration.

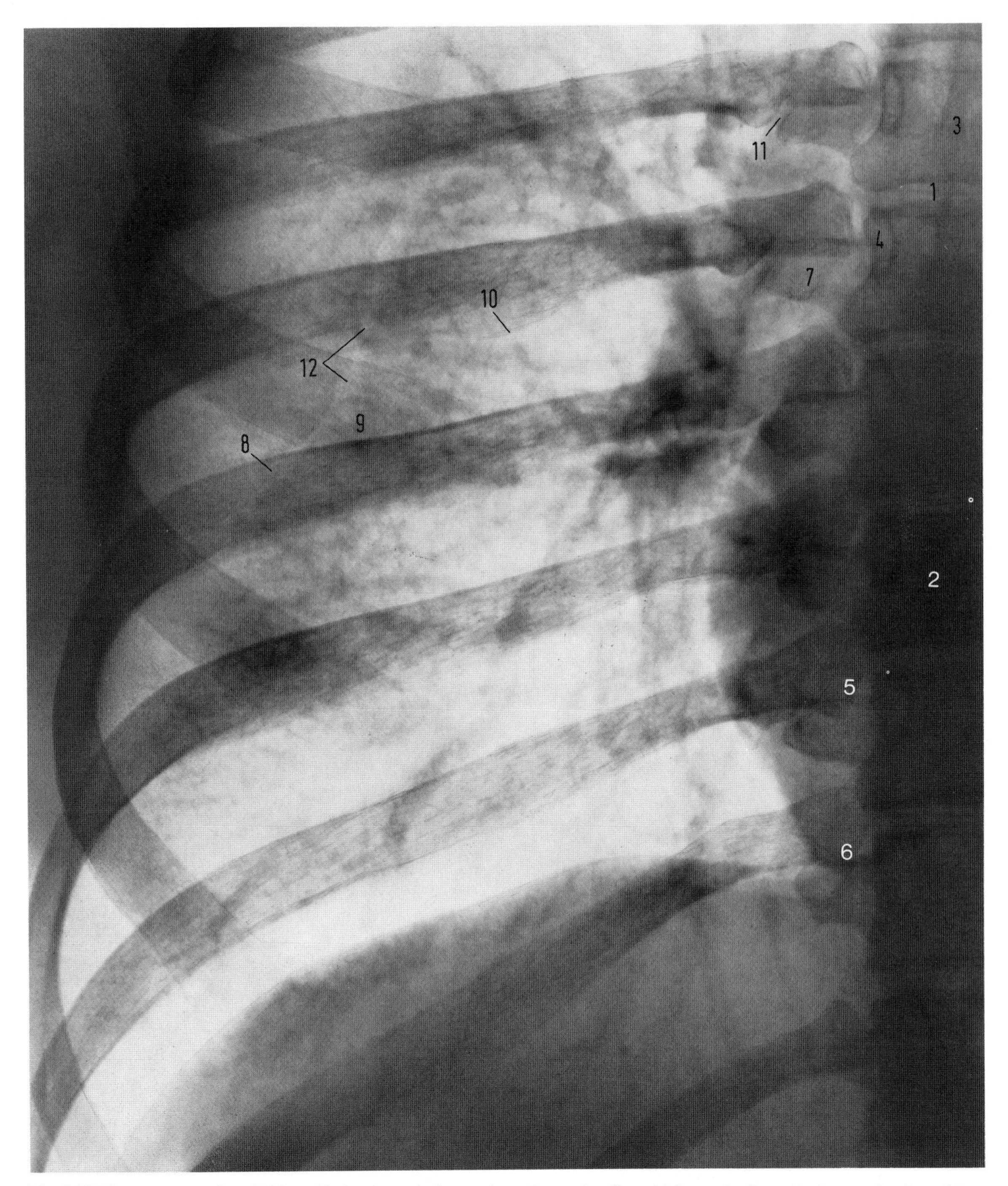

Fig. 349. Thorax, ventrodorsal. More distinct lung design projected onto the ribs, which may lead to mistaken evaluation of the structure of the ribs. Confusion with osteolytic metastases is possible. Because of motion (breathing), ribs may appear double. The lower angle of the scapula is important for orientation in case the upper and lower ribs are not visible. The 7th or 8th rib is to be found below the scapular angle.

1 Intervertebral disk
2 Body of 8th thoracic vertebra
3 Spinous process of the vertebra above it
4 Root of the arch
5,6 Heads of ribs (two articulations with the neighboring vertebrae
7 Transverse process
8 Inferior angle of scapula, projected into the dorsal sections of the 8th rib
9 5th rib, ventral
10 Rough ledge for the costal sulcus (reminiscent of pathological formations, e.g., ossifying periostitis, callus)
11 Costotransverse articulation
12 Simulated fracture of rib, caused by *Mach* effect at the medial margin of the scapula, near C V ventral and C VII dorsal.

The costal sulcus should not be confused with erosions of costal tissue, which occur more laterally from the costal tubercle. Costal erosions arise not only through collateral circulations in stenosis of the aortic isthmus but also in a multiplicity of other forms of insufficient blood supply to the lung, through neurinomata of the intercostal nerves and also from unexplained causes (*Boone, Swenson* and *Felson; Drexler, Stewart* and *Kinkaid*).

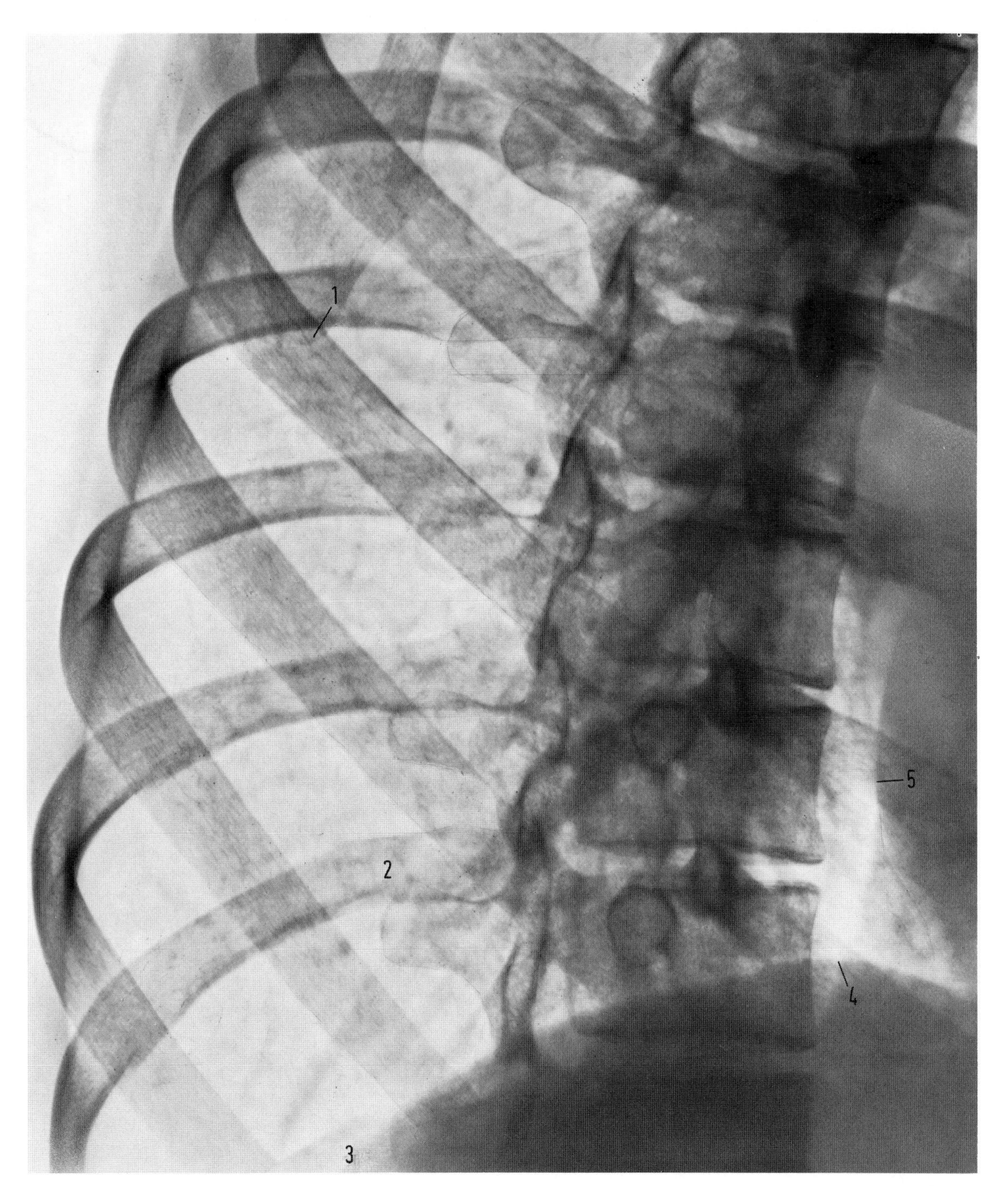

Fig. 350. Lower half of the thorax, dorsoventral (may also be taken in reverse, according to the position of the greatest pressure sensitivity). For position see Fig. 351. By bending towards the healthy side and through inspiratory fixation of the diaphragm at the moment of exposure, a large part of the lower ribs outside the diaphragmatic dome is successfully projected.

1 Inferior angle of clavicle
2 11th rib
3 12th rib
4 Diaphragmatic dome
5 Right cardiac margin

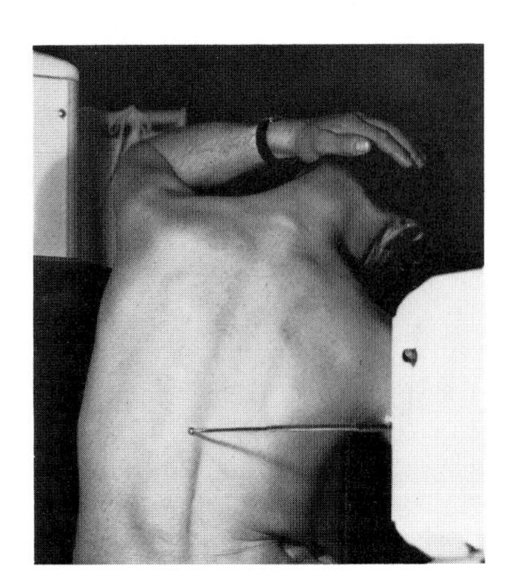

Fig. 351. The patient stands with the front of the hemithorax to be examined either obliquely or semiobliquely at the *Bucky* wall-stand. He rests the hand of the healthy side on the hip, while the arm of the diseased side is placed over the head.

Variants and Sources of Diagnostic Error of the Thoracic Spine, Ribs and Sternum

(As a supplement, see Fig. 525)

Variants are most frequent at the transition from one section of the spine to the other. Therefore, variants are especially numerous at the 7th cervical and the 1st thoracic vertebrae. They also extend to the ribs: cervical ribs on one side, defects on the 1st rib on the other, which sometimes makes it difficult to assign a vertebra to the cervical section or – as "rib-carrying" – to the thorax (transition vertebra). The correct procedure is to enumerate the vertebrae from the top downwards and to name their particulars. That the overall number of vertebrae may vary must also be taken into account.

Of 153 human spines examined, *Krmpotič* found in about 80% of the cases a tubercle on the body of the 2nd thoracic vertebra, which might serve as a mark of recognition of this vertebra. It has been proven that it is produced by the lower, regularly tendinous insertion of the medial part of the musculus longus colli. Therefore, it is called tuberculum musculus longi.

The vascular canals, called "*Hahn's* clefts" after the author who described them first, can be demonstrated distinctly only occasionally on radiographs in profile of the adult thoracic spine, and then only on isolated vertebral bodies. When they appear on repeated radiographs, they are judged clinically again and again as symptoms of vertebral osteoporosis. In fact, demonstration of these nutritive canals in a vertebra is without any clinical significance. They appear as bands of increased radiolucency in the center of the vertebral bodies and take a horizontal course.

Schmitt pointed out that on lateral radiographs of the thoracic spine, the actual upper margin of the upper thoracic vertebral body may be covered near the shoulder joint in such a way that a wedge-shaped vertebra may be simulated.

Probst described a congenital, solitary unilateral cleft formation in the interarticular part of a 7th thoracic vertebra. Bridge formations and additional intervertebral joints in most of the ribs are not rare. (See also Fig. 525, No. 58 and 58*.) *Wilhelm* showed a bony intermediary fragment in the 2nd rib. *Langeland* was able to observe the extraordinary rare luxation of the 12th rib in the costovertebral joint.

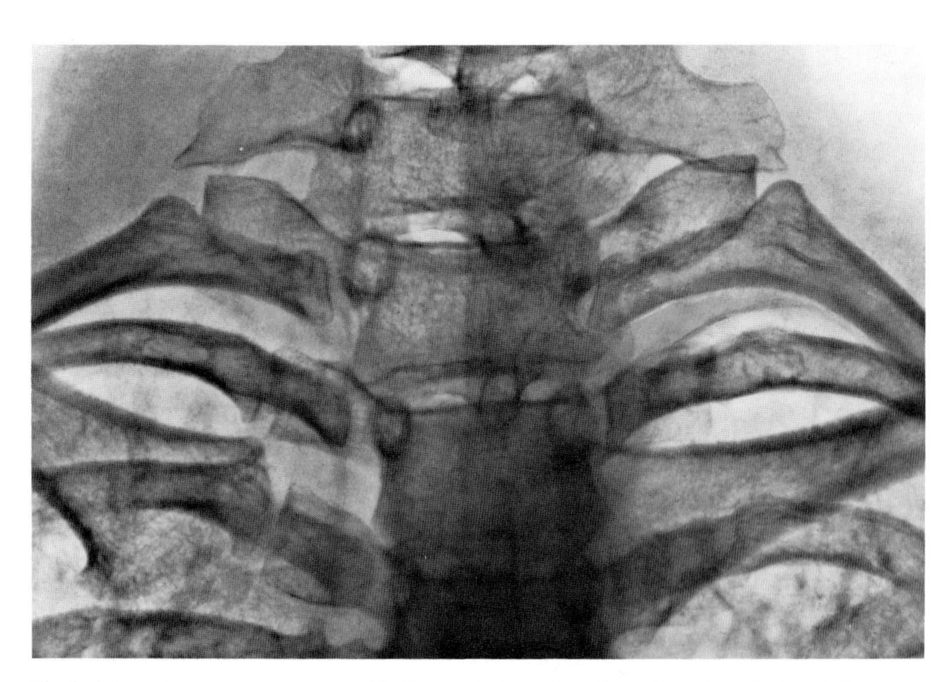

Fig. 352. Long transverse processes of the 7th cervical vertebra with rudimentary ribs. In addition, one is given the impression of the formation of a right pseudojoint, but this is only simulated by the course of the central ray. One can find any transition from these elongated transverse processes to completely formed cervical ribs (see Fig. 353 a,b). These rudimentary ribs may cause the so-called scalenus syndrome (from the collection of *J. Probst*).

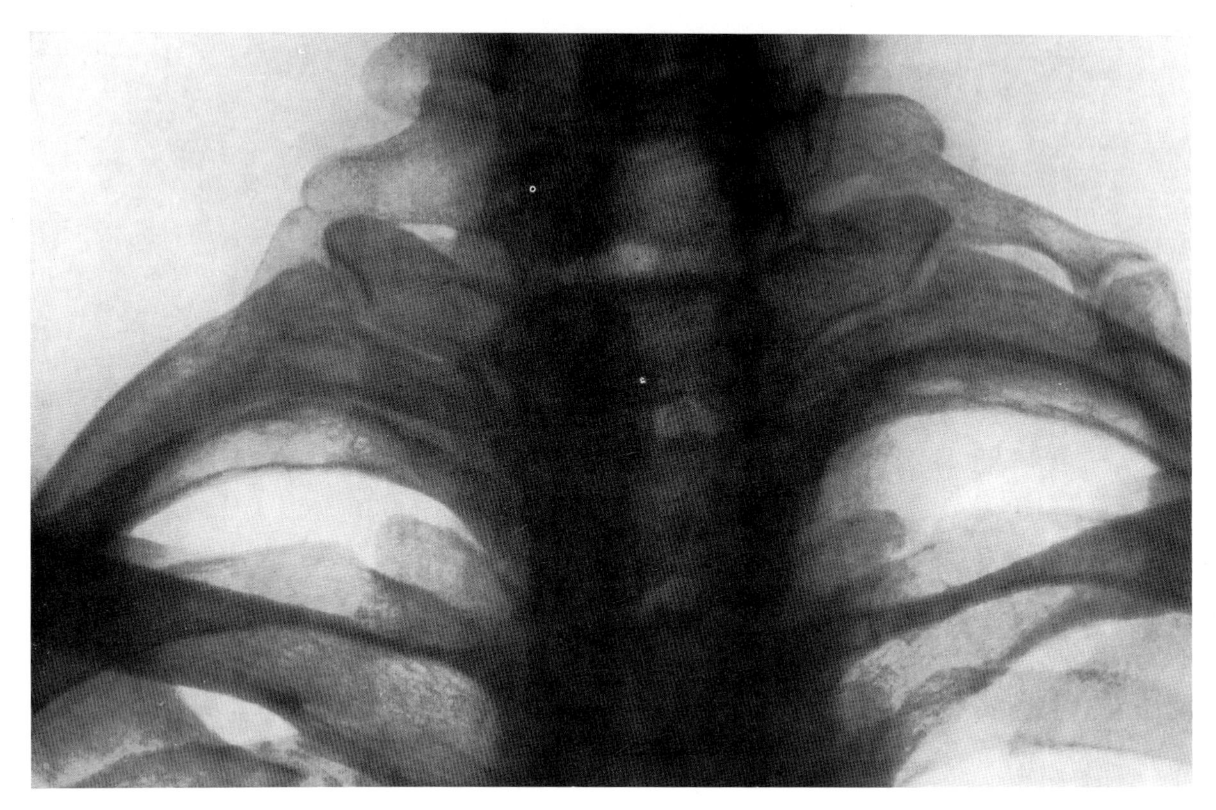

Fig. 353 a

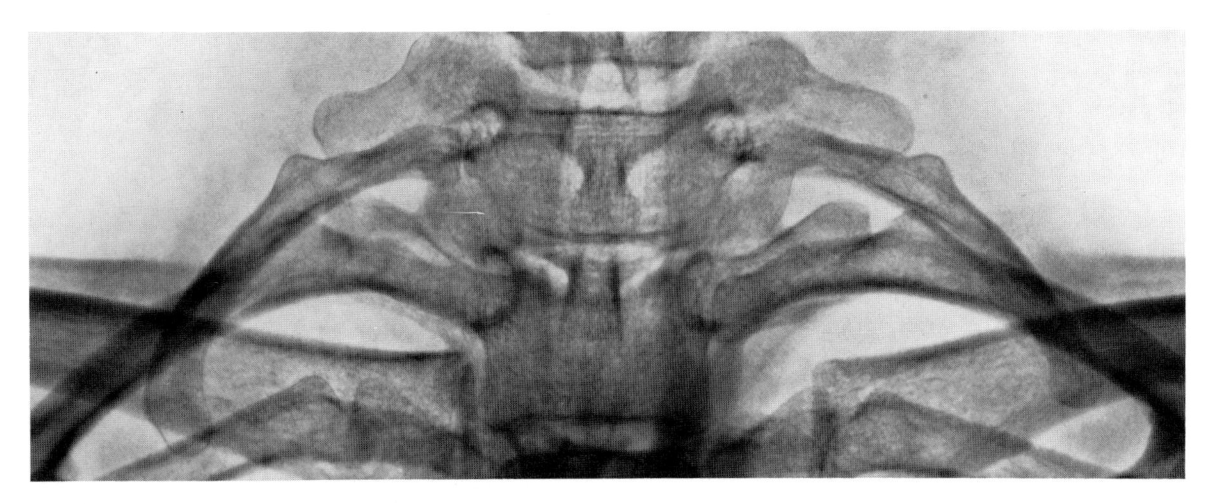

Fig. 353 b

Fig. 353. Bilateral cervical ribs on the 7th cervical vertebra. Fig. 353 a shows a special variant of a left cervical rib, i.e., with a joint-like interruption, resembling interruption in the region of the 1st rib in Fig. 362 (see also Figs. 355, 364 and 368). As to possibilities of error, see *Keating* and *Amberg*. *Pickhan* designated rib-bearing cervical vertebrae as transitional vertebrae; *Cascelli* established their frequency at about 3%.

Cervical ribs occur predominantly bilaterally, one often longer than the other. Not infrequently, they are associated with hypertrophy of the spinous process. *Overhof* reported an unusual form of two small cervical ribs at the 5th and 6th cervical vertebrae, which were in articular connection, with interposition of a small bone or cartilage. *Fleischner,* as well as *Keating* and *Amberg,* described anomalies of ribs, especially cervical ribs, as a source of diagnostic error and incorrect therapeutic indications. In addition, development of cervical ribs is often the cause of unilateral shadows in the pulmonary apices.

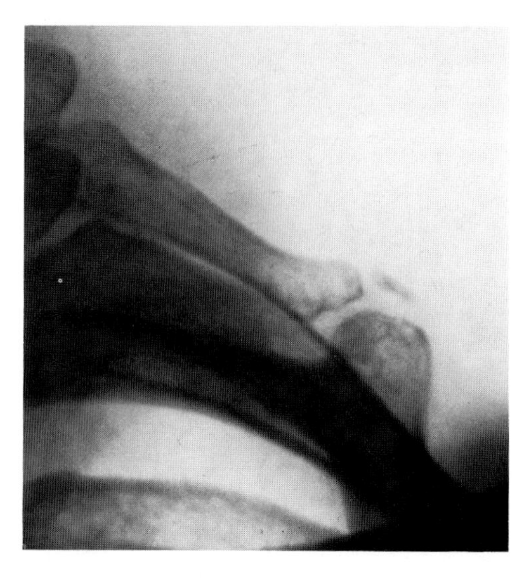

Fig. 354. A similar case of a joint-like, subdivided cervical rib with an interposed fragment, resembling an apophyseal nucleus.

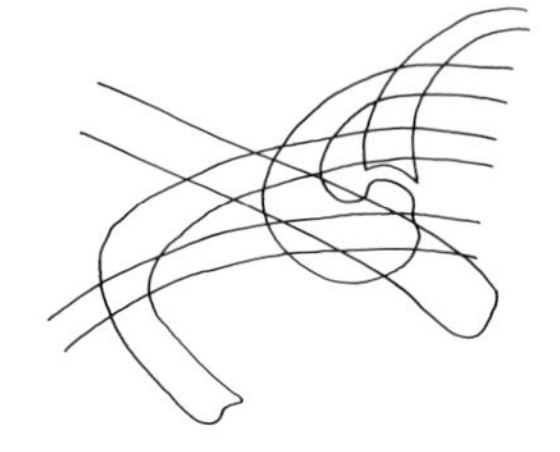

Fig. 355. Strong cervical rib, forming an articulation with the 1st rib.

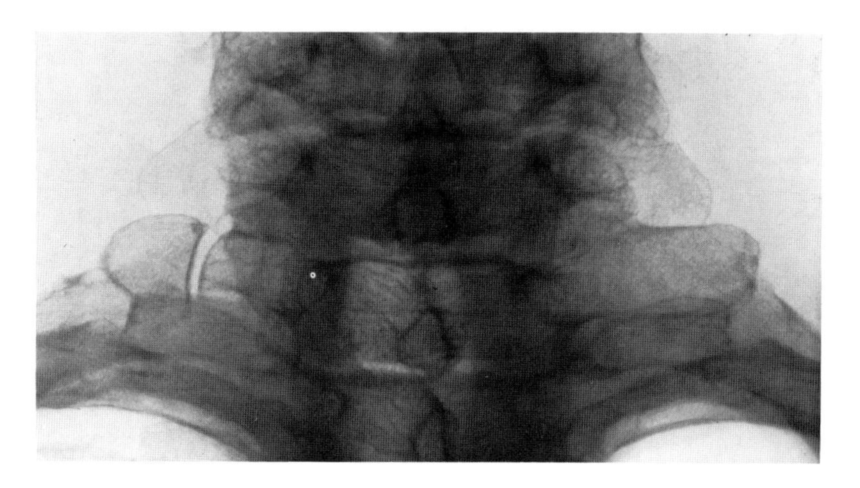

Fig. 356. Isolated transverse process at the right 1st thoracic vertebra, in an adult. No previous trauma. The X–ray findings essentially conform with those shown in Fig. 357.

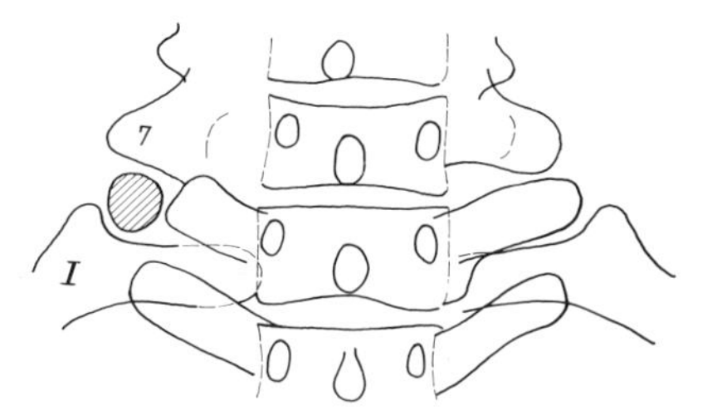

Fig. 357. At 7, there is an enlarged transverse process of C VII and, hatched, between the transverse process of the 1st thoracic vertebra and the tubercle of the 1st rib (unilateral), an independent tiny bone which articulates with the tubercle. No previous trauma.

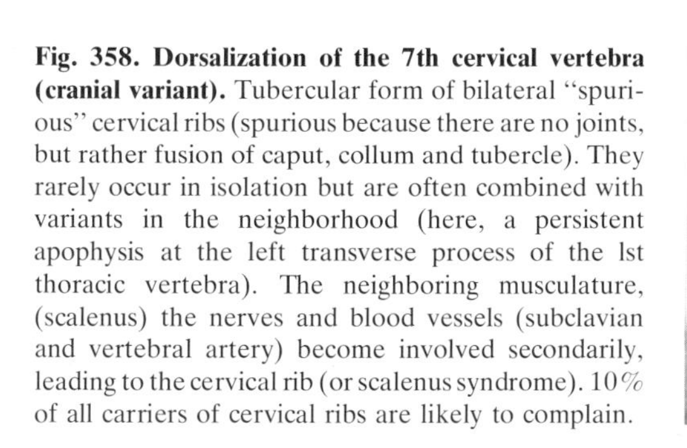

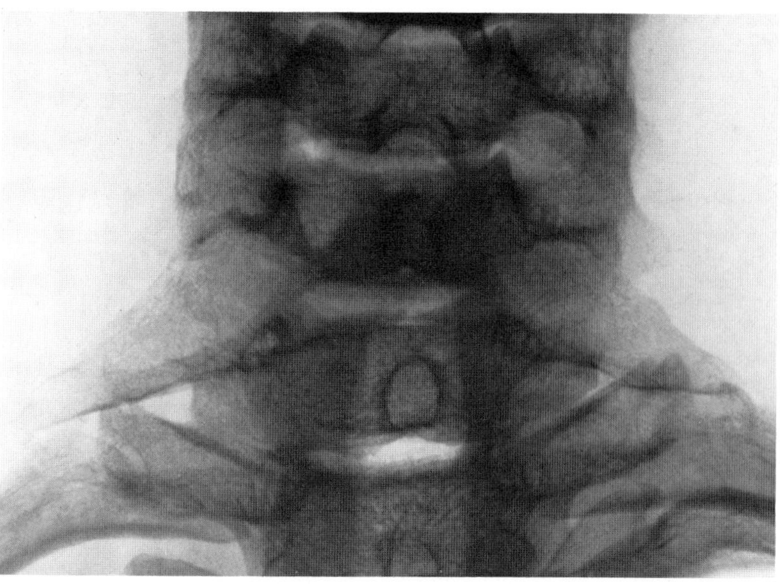

Fig. 358. Dorsalization of the 7th cervical vertebra (cranial variant). Tubercular form of bilateral "spurious" cervical ribs (spurious because there are no joints, but rather fusion of caput, collum and tubercle). They rarely occur in isolation but are often combined with variants in the neighborhood (here, a persistent apophysis at the left transverse process of the 1st thoracic vertebra). The neighboring musculature, (scalenus) the nerves and blood vessels (subclavian and vertebral artery) become involved secondarily, leading to the cervical rib (or scalenus syndrome). 10% of all carriers of cervical ribs are likely to complain.

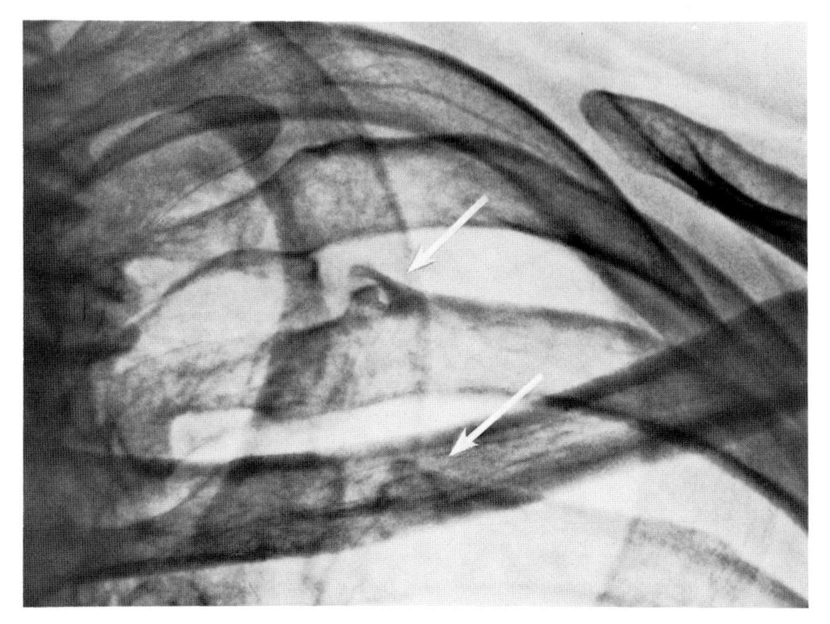

Fig. 359. Costotransverse deforming arthrosis (↙). Costovertebral joints with jagged swellings at the margin. *Kraus* demonstrated, in a radiologic-morphological and histological study, the inflammatory-degenerative character of these changes and their relation to chronic pulmonary diseases (emphysema).

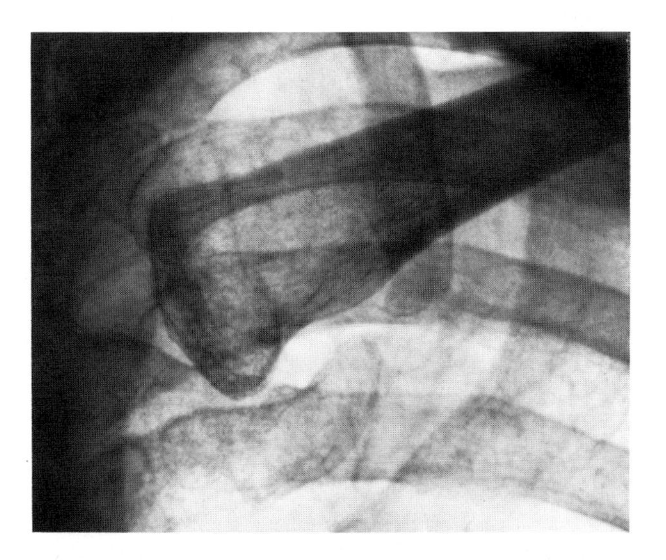

Fig. 360. Hypoplastic 1st rib. The cartilage is ossified boomerang-like and separated by an apparent cleft from the bony part of the rib. Hypoplasiae of the 1st or of the 1st and 2nd ribs are designated as Srb anomaly, especially if the regression of both ribs is connected with a bony, laminar fusion (see also *Wenz* and *Geipert*).

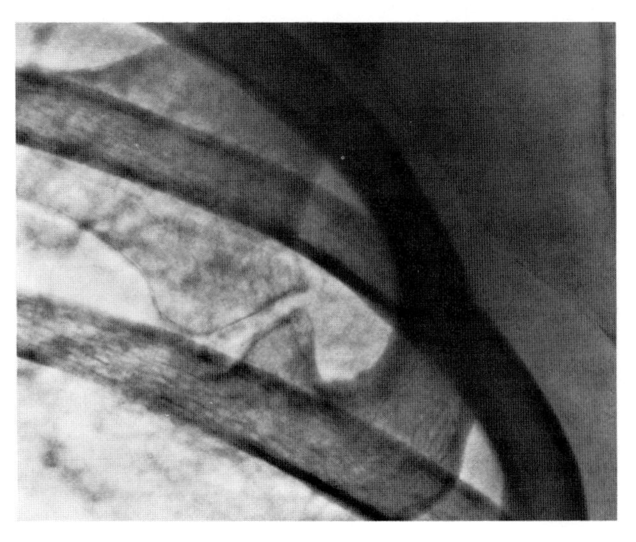

Fig. 361. Rare costal anomaly in the shape of an anterior costal bridge with formation of a pseudoarticulation. Usually it occurs unilaterally.

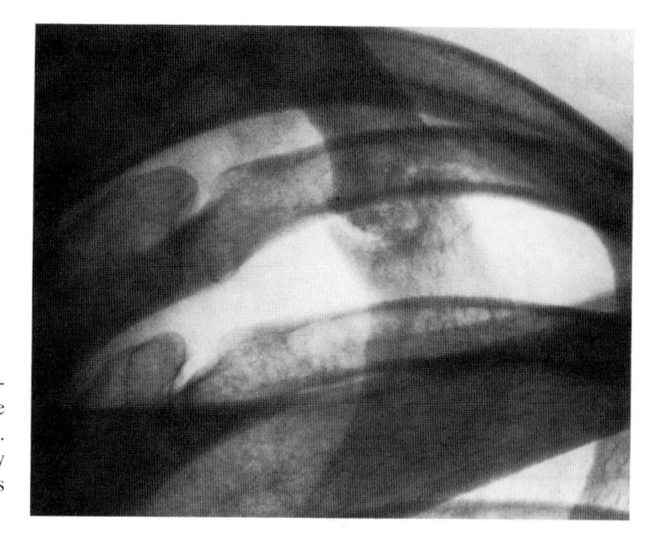

Fig. 362. Pseudoarthrosis within the 1st rib, an anomaly that is found occasionally in the region of the 1st or 2nd rib. In this case, there is a joint-like interruption in the bony part of the 1st rib whose genesis is not quite clear. This "discontinuity" is considered to be a stress fracture, even in its very rare bilateral occurrence (*Dietzel* and *Schirmer*), and there is doubt that it is a congenital developmental disturbance.

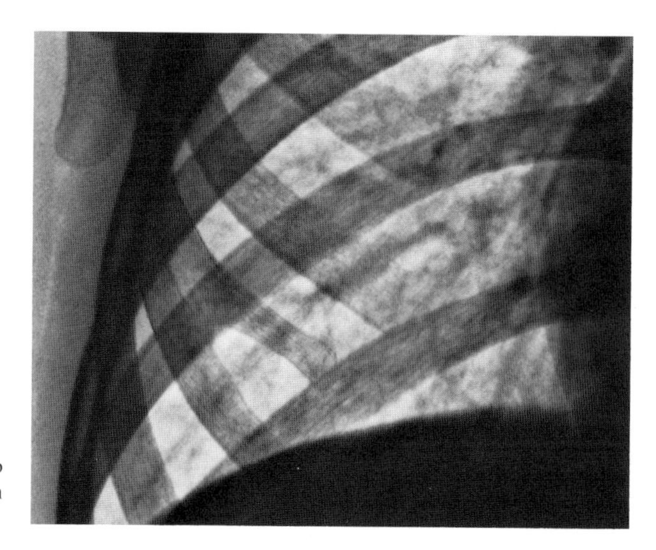

Fig. 363. *Luschka*'s **forked rib,** C VI, in a 7-year-old girl. Forked ribs, also called shovel ribs if the bifurcation is incomplete, are often shorter than normal ribs.

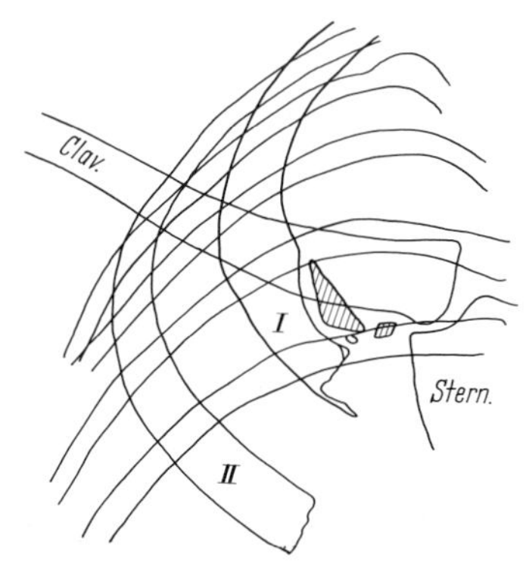

Fig. 364

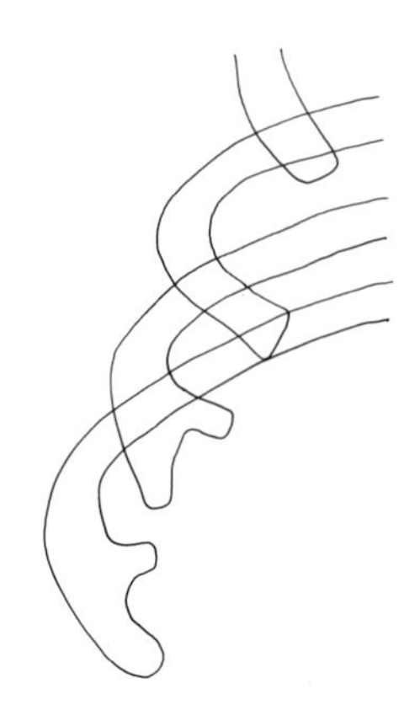

Fig. 365

Fig. 364. Peculiar cleft at the upper margin of the 1st rib, near the ossifying cartilage. Such anomalies may simulate sequestra. Joint-like connections between the first rib and clavicle are possible.

Fig. 365. Two forked ribs in a 4-year-old girl (sketch of a roentgenogram from *St. Simon*).

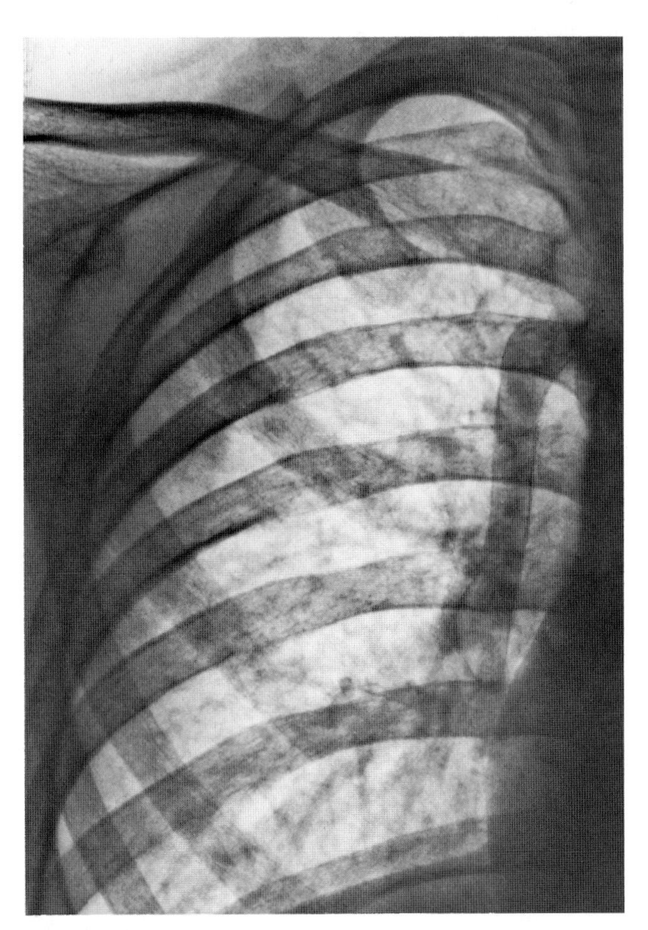

Fig. 366 a

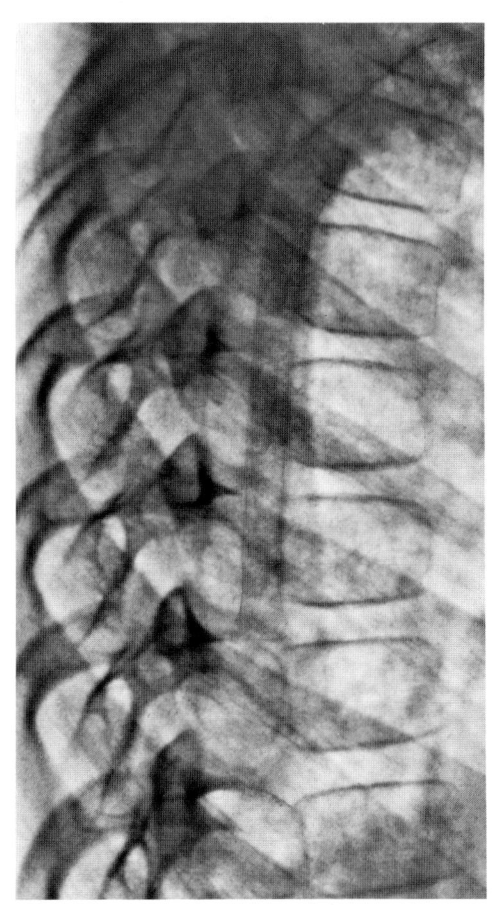

Fig. 366 b

Fig. 366. Forked rib (from the *W. Werner* collection, Berlin). The bifurcation starts immediately paravertebrally. The caudal prong runs steeply downwards, almost parallel paravertebrally.

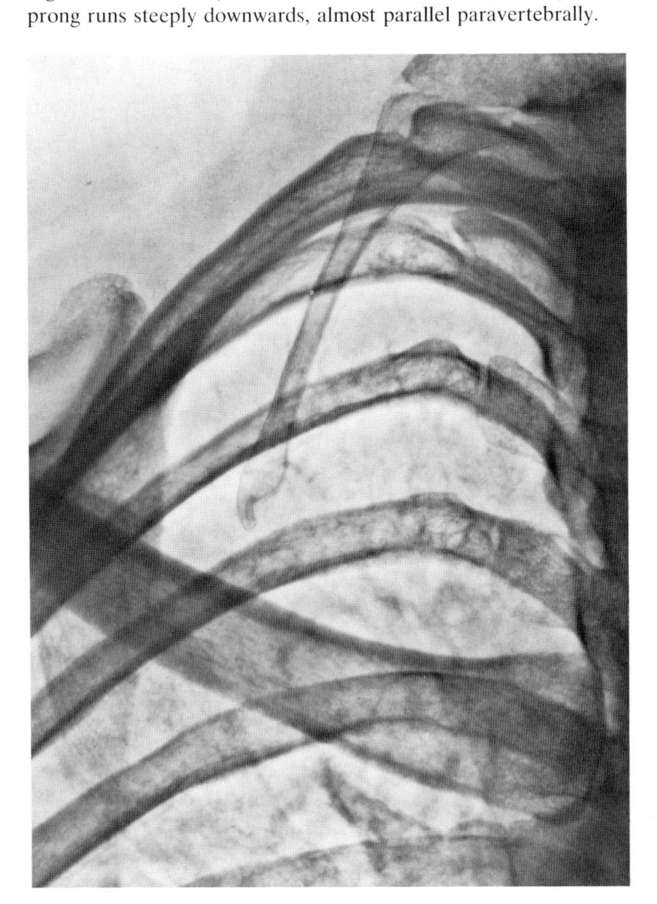

Fig. 367. Underdeveloped right 1st rib, with calcified, band-like insertion at the sternum (a form of Srb anomaly). Underdeveloped 1st ribs, as well as supernumerary cervical ribs, may cause the scalenus anticus syndrome. This is a neuralgic-neurovascular complex of symptoms caused by mechanical compression of the nerve vessel bundle in the region of the scalenus muscle; this complex belongs to the conception of the cervicobranchial syndrome. Confusion of an underdeveloped 1st rib with a cervical rib is possible. The missing support by the 1st rib causes a lowering of the clavicle, the sterno-clavicular joints and the sternum. This changed static and mechanical load at the upper thoracic cage may cause severe discomfort.

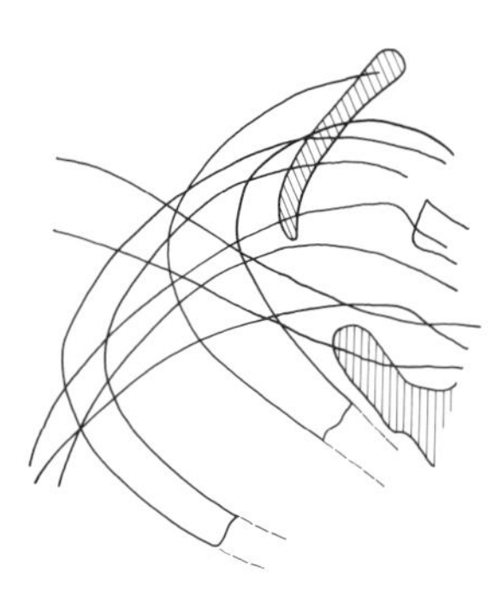

Fig. 368. *Grashey* explained a similar hypoplasia of the 1st rib as a "defect of the 1st rib whose central portion, reduced like a cervical rib, has been stunted".

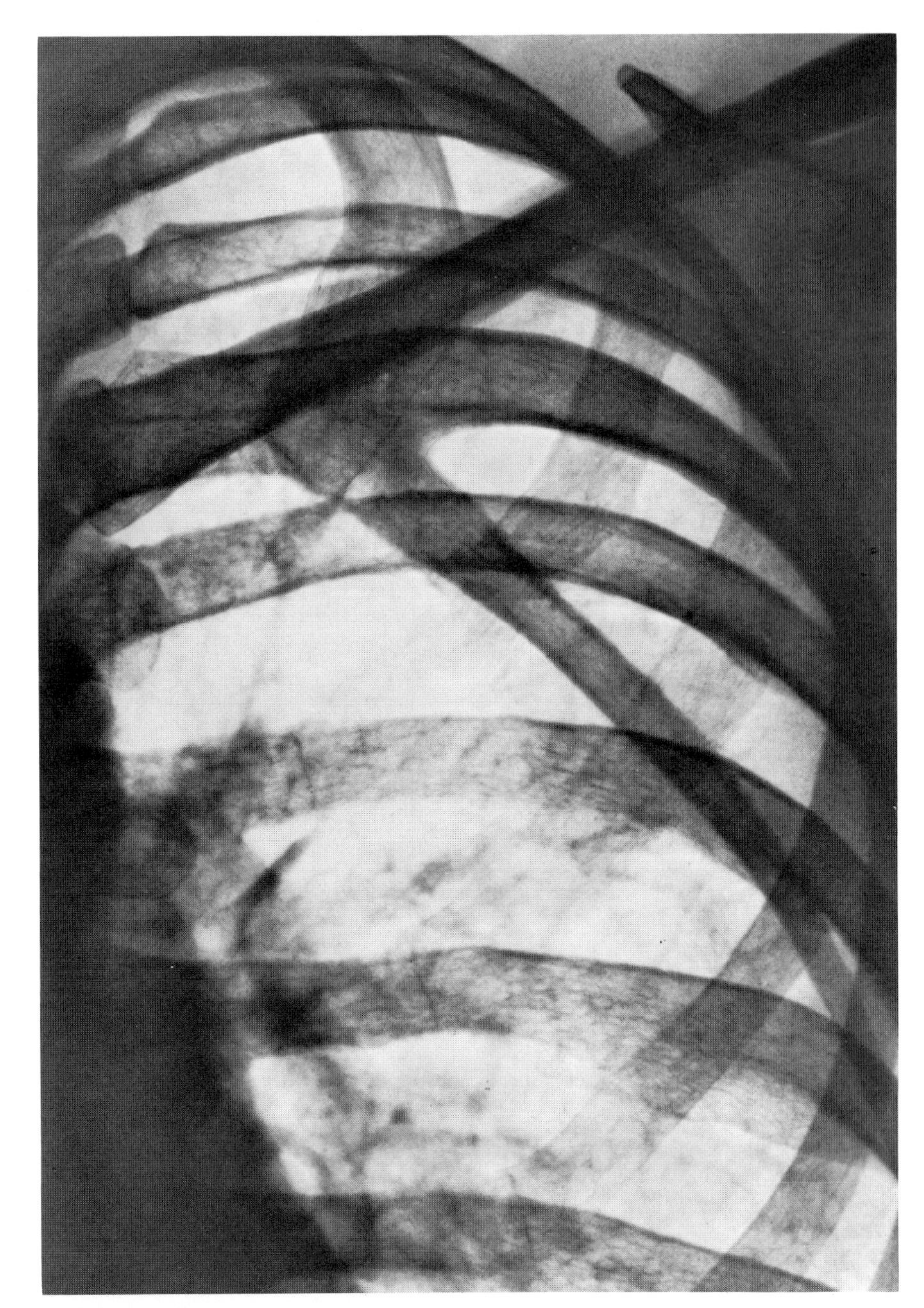

Fig. 369. Rare bifurcation of the left 5th rib dorsally, next to the costotransversal articulation (from the *W. Werner* collection). Both clasps surround the lung but do not penetrate into the lower parts of the lung, as did the caudal prong in a similar case described by *Wilk* and *Hülshoff.* The scaly, early calcifications of the parasternal costal cartilages 1 and 2, but also of 3 and 4, point to the late stage of a *Tietze* syndrome. Parasternal inflammatory swelling and reddening on the basis of osteochondritis or osteochondrosis of the cartilaginous bony sternocostal regions occur. The disease may start at any age. Often, this illness can only be diagnosed from its long and frequently painful course and its favorable reaction to weak X-ray irradiation, as typical radiographic symptoms are absent.

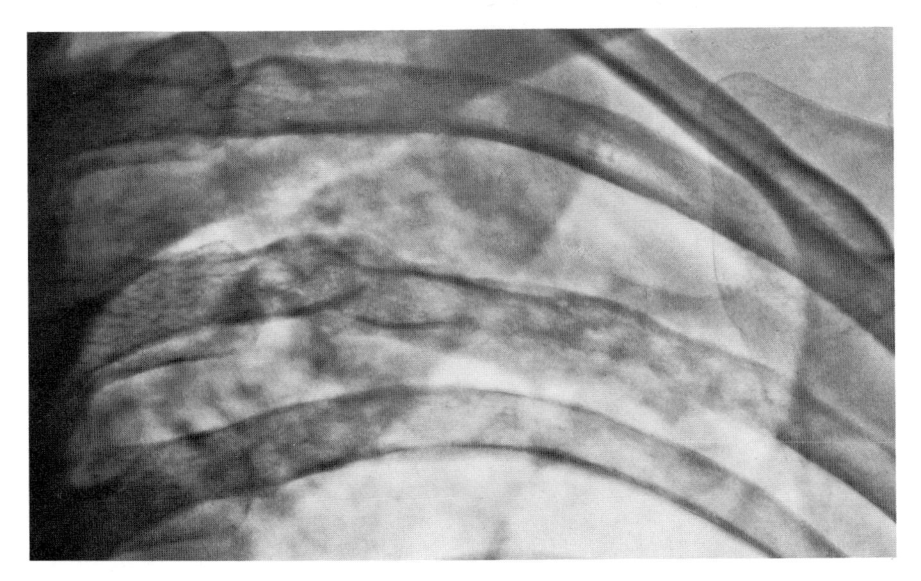

Fig. 370. Contact radiograph. **Regeneration of rib after partial paravertebral resection of the 4th left rib.**

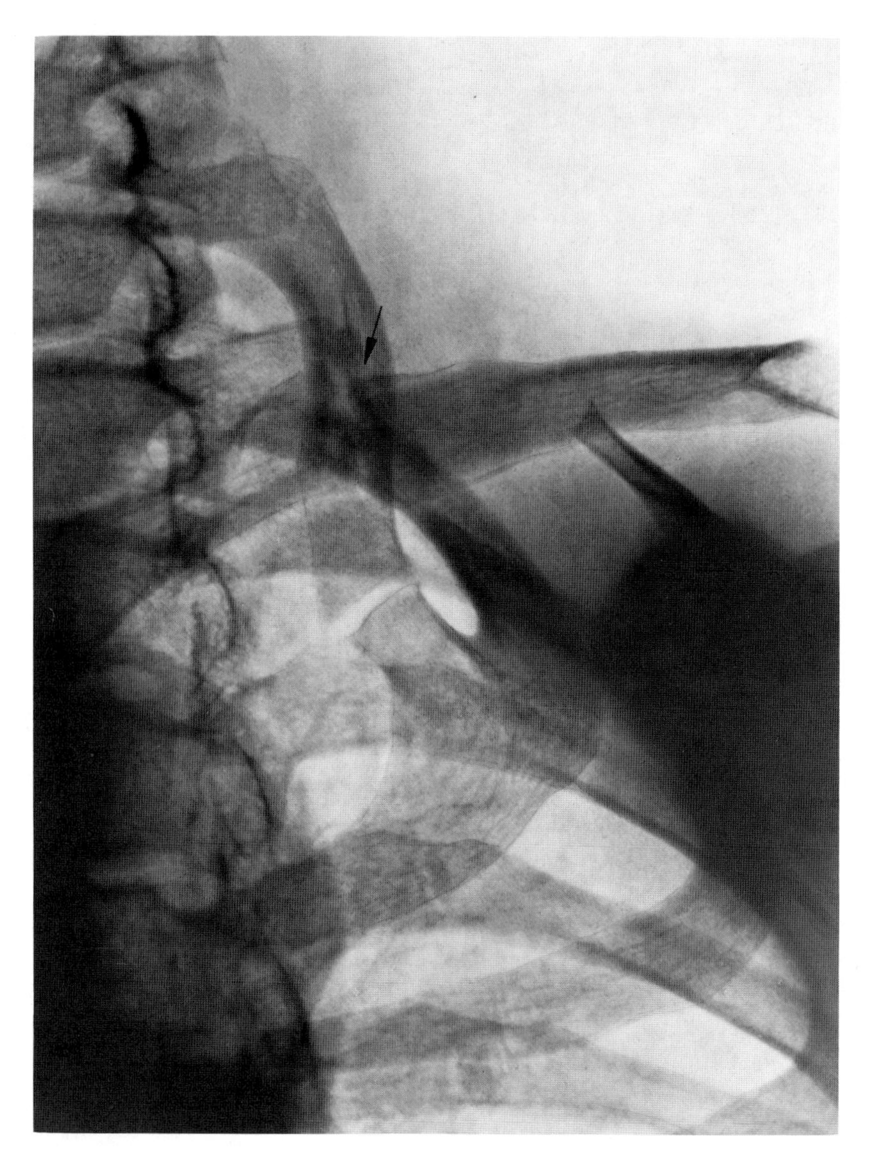

Fig. 371. Cervical rib at the 7th cervical vertebra (from the *W. Werner* collection), which is connected, via a pseudojoint in the anterior axillary line, to the slightly lowered 1st rib. In addition, there is a fracture in the shaft of the clavicle (↙), with formation of a pseudoarthrosis and a triangular bone defect at the lateral end of the clavicle. The latter denotes a clavicular osteolysis, which may also occur after a blunt trauma.

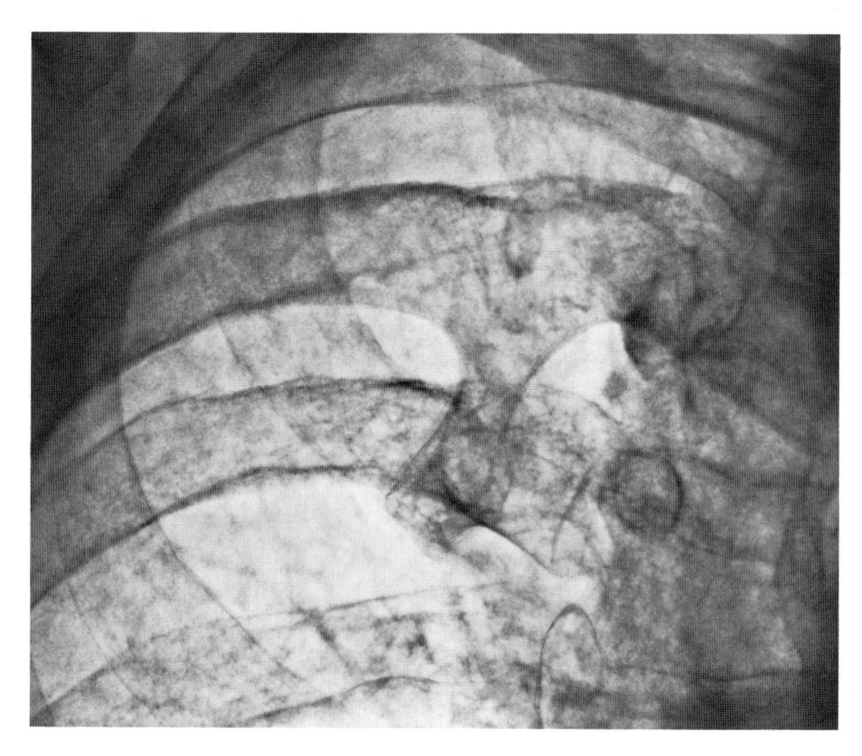

Fig. 372. Rare costal anomaly with paravertebral rudimentary costal branching off from the lower margin of the 5th rib, corresponding to a forked rib. This simulates a paravertebral bony bridge formation between the 5th and 6th ribs. But in fact, the lower contour of the 6th rib is superimposed in the caudal direction by the rudiment. *Hülshoff,* too, describes an anomaly of the right 5th rib. But in his case, it is a spur, 5–6 cm long, which developed from a medial to lateral direction into the pulmonary tissue, ending there in the shape of a button.

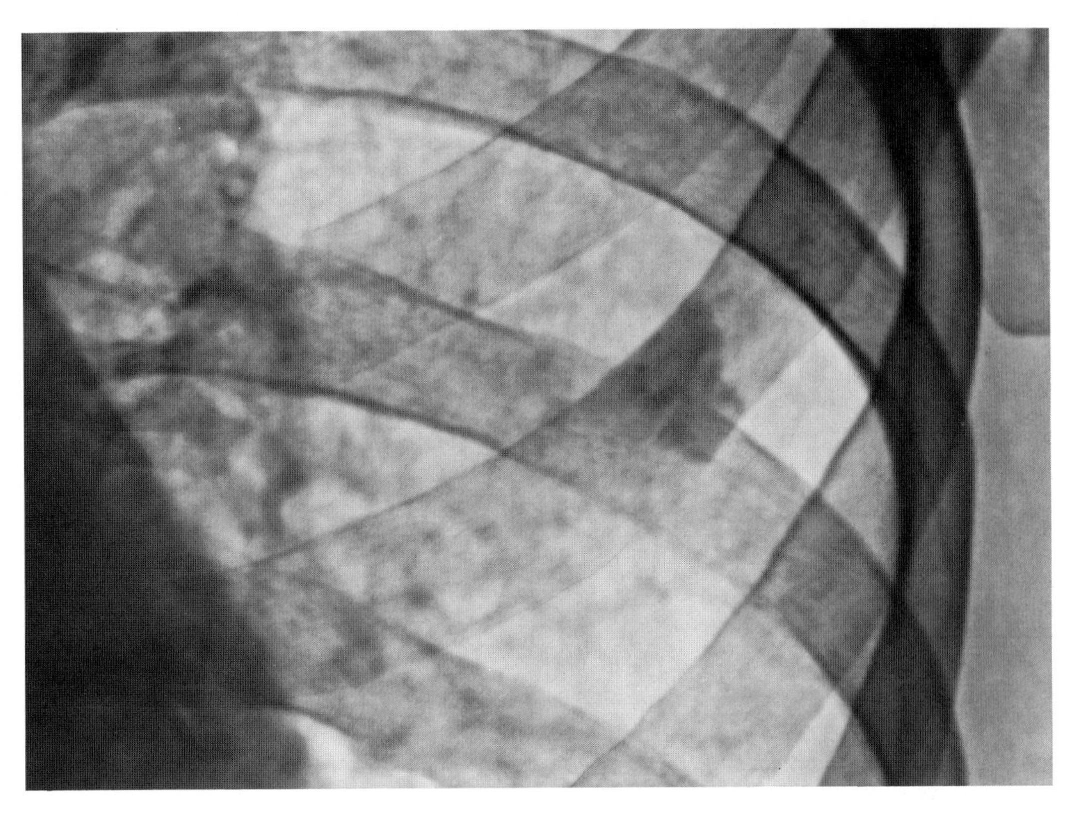

Fig. 373. "Ostéopathie condensante et hypertrophiante" in the anterior axillary line of the left 4th rib (from the *W. Werner* collection). This rib is very often involved. Such circumscribed osteosclerotic parts within the bone are also called enostoses. In these cases either a delicately reticulated thickening of the cancellous tissue develops or this is replaced by the compact tissue. When such band-shaped zones of increased density are seen, *Léri*'s melorrheostosis, a recessive hereditary disease, must also be considered. The thickened calcified strips occurring in this condition are predominantly localized in the bones of the extremities, but may also be found isolated in the ribs (*Schinz, Baensch, Friedl* and *Uehlinger*).

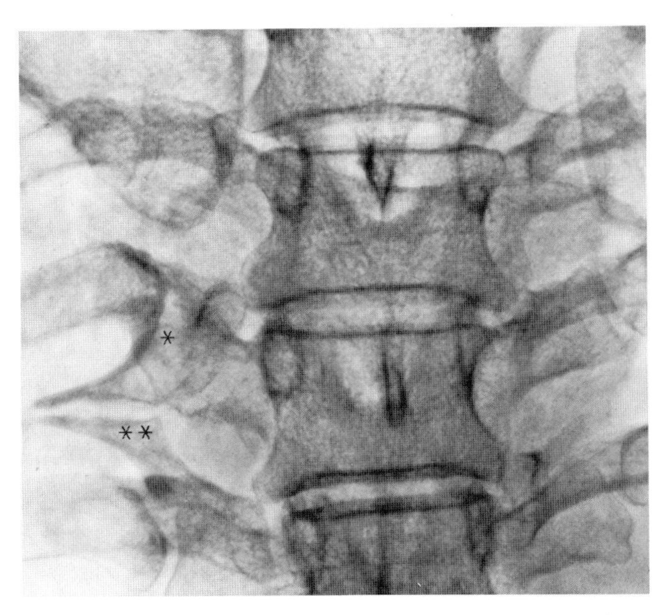

Fig. 374. Rare anomaly on the right 4th rib with deformed head (*) and a supernumerary bone (**) towards the 5th thoracic vertebra, with formation of a pseudoarticulation.

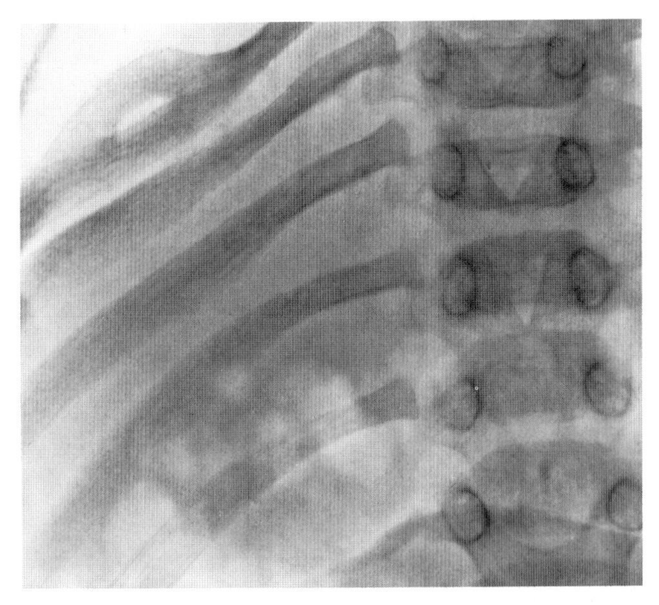

Fig. 375. Hole in the right 7th rib, in a 10-month-old infant. Concurrently, this case presented a vertebral malformation (spina bifida with meningocele). Holes are often found in the region of the chondrocostal boundary. This partial bifurcation is a malformation of arrested development, as a result of genetic or early damage. Such rounded shadows may be confused with cavities if the lungs are examined only by fluoroscopy.

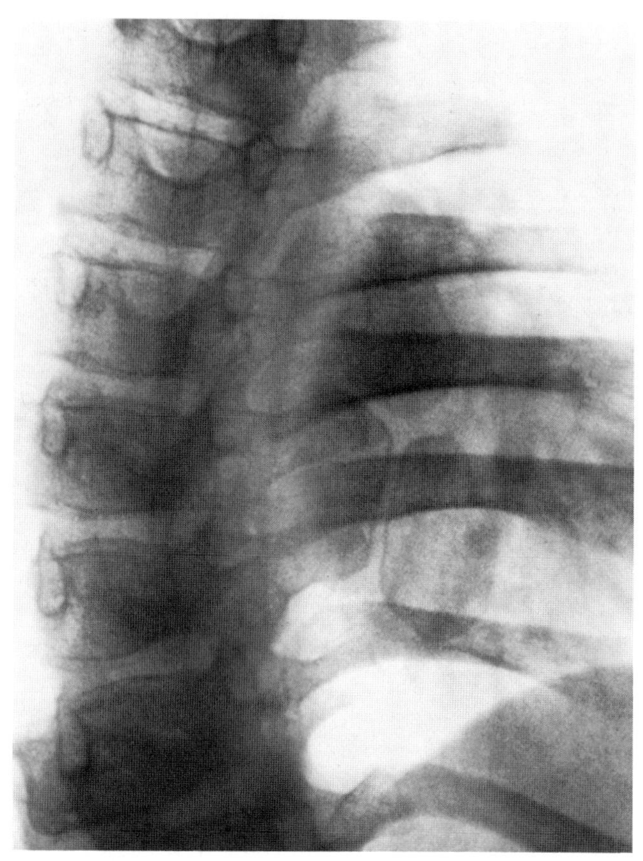

Fig. 376. Double origin of the lower sternal segment in a youth (normal, until 20 years). See also Fig. 336.

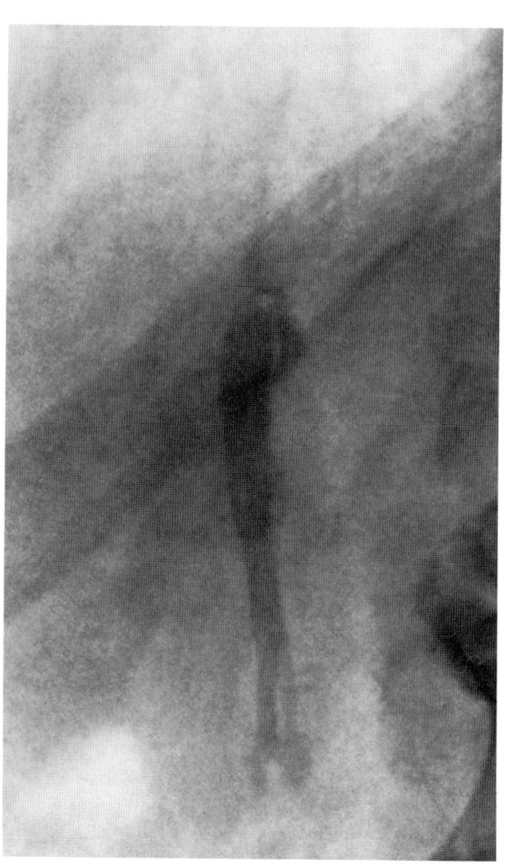

Fig. 377. Extremely long xyphoid process, split at the end (see also *Colosimo*). It is found more frequently in the male; combinations with malformations of the heart, pericardium and diaphragm are said to occur as a syndrome of congenital defects.

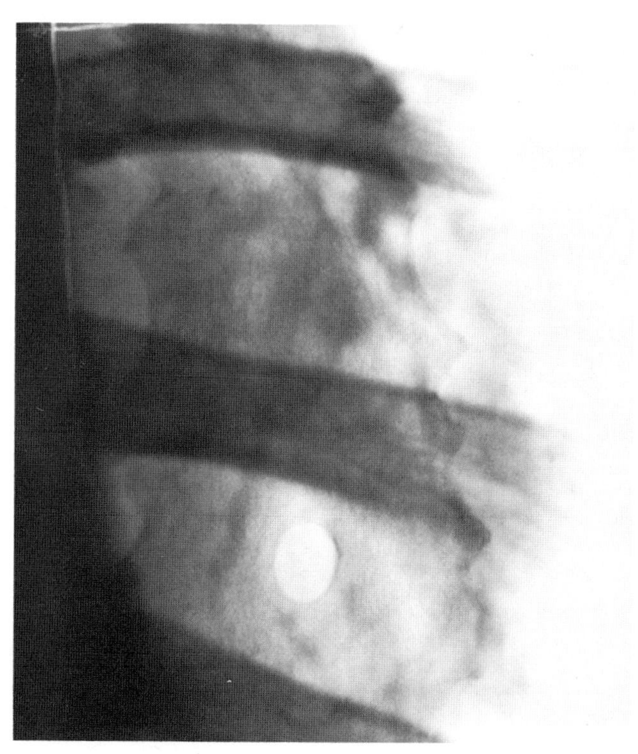

Fig. 378. Hole in the lower sternum (variant). According to *Pässler*, ossification failed due to the passage of a broad bundle of blood vessels through the cartilaginous nucleus during the embryonal period (see also costal theory, p. 433).

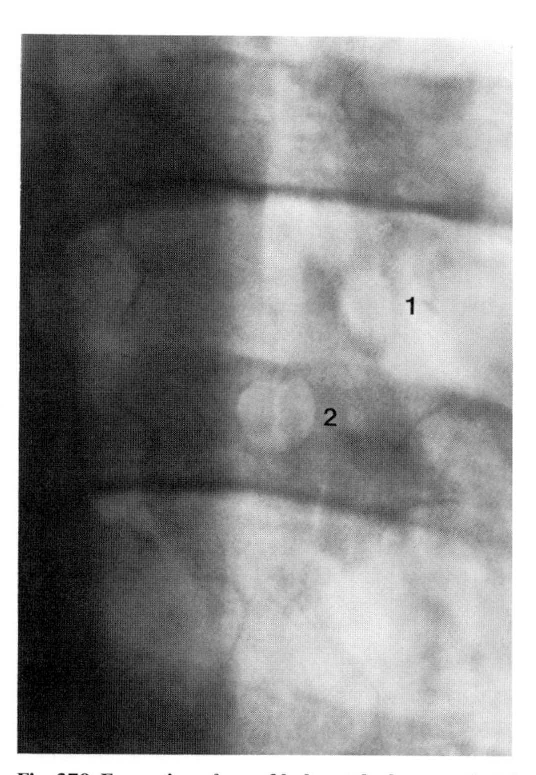

Fig. 379. Formation of round holes at the lower end of the sternum (2). Simulated hole (1) at a deep notch of the sternal margin.

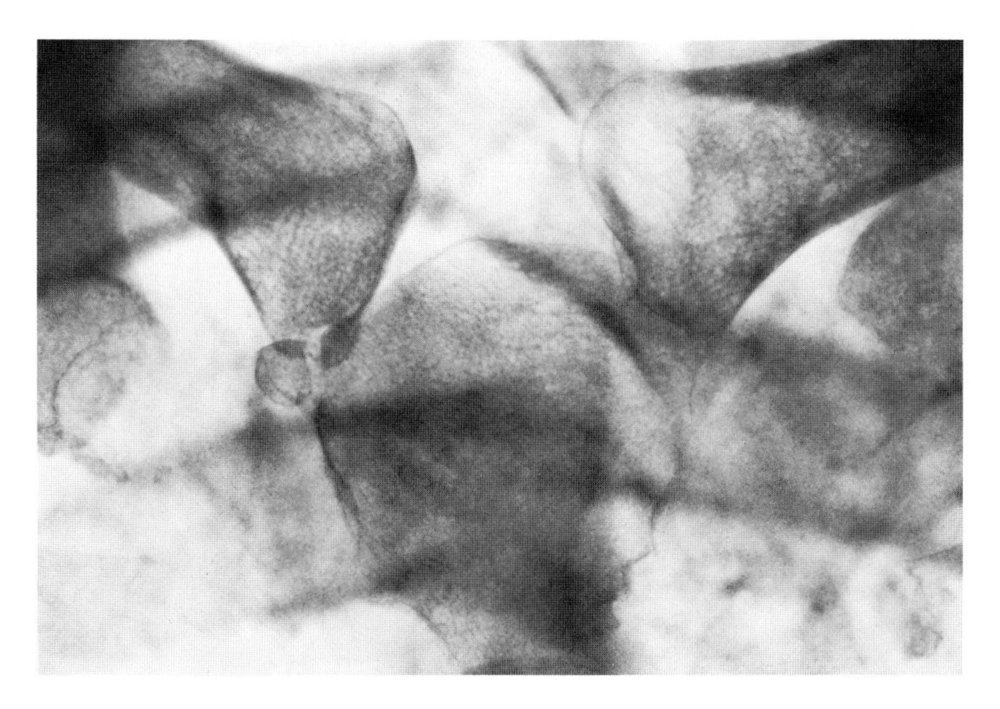

Fig. 380. Free parasternal bone, right; fusion of such an ossicle on the left. A triangular bony shadow is seen near the manubrium sterni in the cartilage of the 1st rib. The ossicle may also be fused with the manubrium sterni on one side, and may persist only unilaterally *(Ravelli)*. A thorough examination of these cases originates from *Zimmer*. According to *Stehr,* this ossicle has no connection with a cervical vertebra. When it fuses with the manubrium, it causes the latter to develop a peaked elongation. According to *Ravelli,* the parasternal ossicle should be regarded as a sternal rudiment of the coracoid which, in the monotremata, reaches to the sternum.

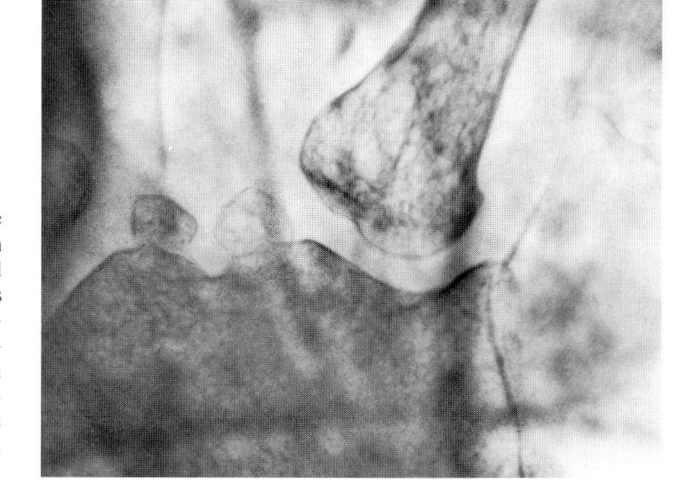

Fig. 381. Suprasternal bones on the upper edge of the sternum, a rare variant. It is possible that this represents the rudiments of an episternum of the saurians and monotremata. Usually, one finds two symmetrical ossicles about the size of the pisiform bone. Ligamentous connections lead from these ossicles e.g. to the articular disk (sternoclavicular articulation). In cases of fusion of the episternal bones with the manubrium, the former appear as strongly developed sternal tubercles which are embedded in the interclavicular ligament. The interclavicular ligament often passes over the episternal bones. Important and extensive analytic descriptions are to be found in *Lossen* and *Hofer,* as well as in *Kipshoven.*

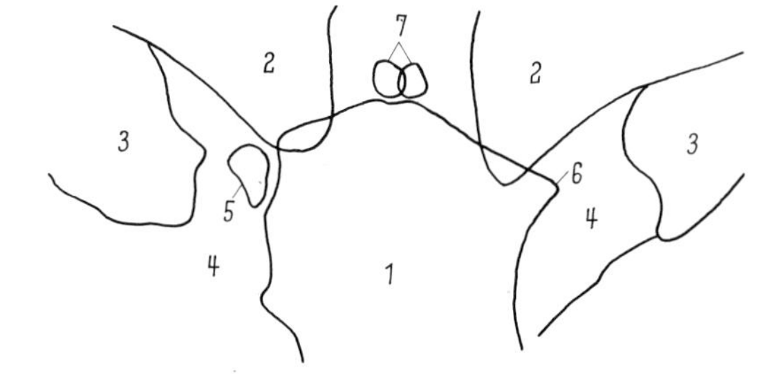

1 Manubrium sterni
2 Clavicle, sternal end
3 1st rib
4 Costal cartilage, left, partly calcified
5 Right parasternal ossicle
6 Left parasternal ossicle, fused with the manubrium
7 Two suprasternal ossicles

Fig. 382. Supra- and parasternal ossicles (sketch from a radiograph by *Ravelli*).

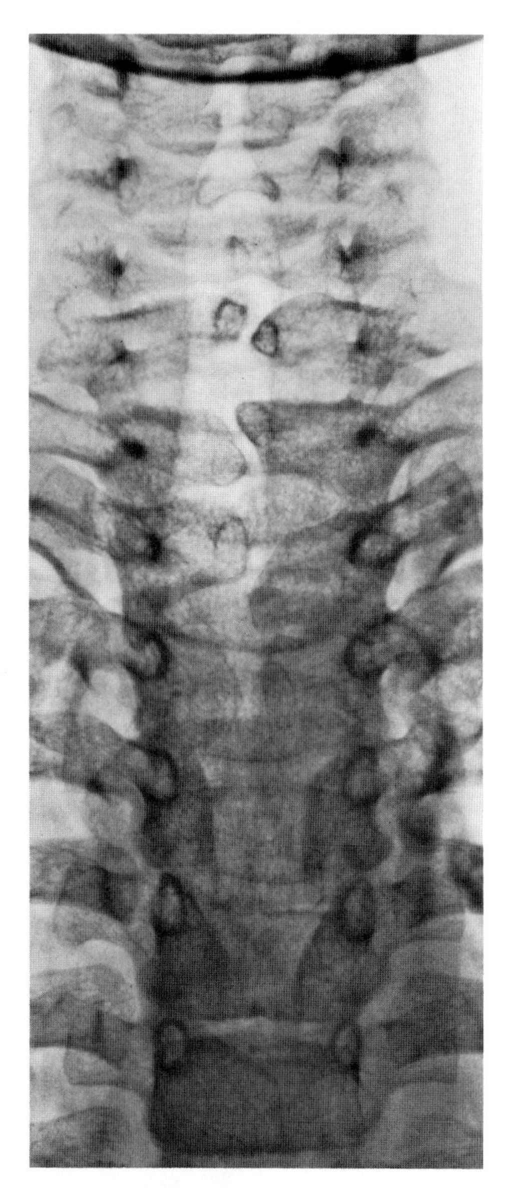

Fig. 383 a

Fig. 383 b shows the soft tissue shadow of the meningocele in profile; it can be seen and felt from outside.

Fig. 383. Extensive spina bifida, from the 6th cervical to the 6th thoracic vertebrae, with meningocele, in a 3-year-old child. The clefts in the arches may appear in the midline (spinous processes), where they can be demonstrated most frequently, further in the interarticular part of the lamina of the arch and, very rarely, at the roots of the arch. Clefts of the arches are counted among the most frequent malformations of the vertebral arches and result from failure of the fusion of both limbs of the arch. They can be demonstrated more often at the transition from the lumbar spine to the sacrum than at the remaining spinal column. At the cervical spine a spina bifida may sometimes be simulated by superimposed projection of the glottis. This finding would occur at the level of the 4th cervical vertebra.

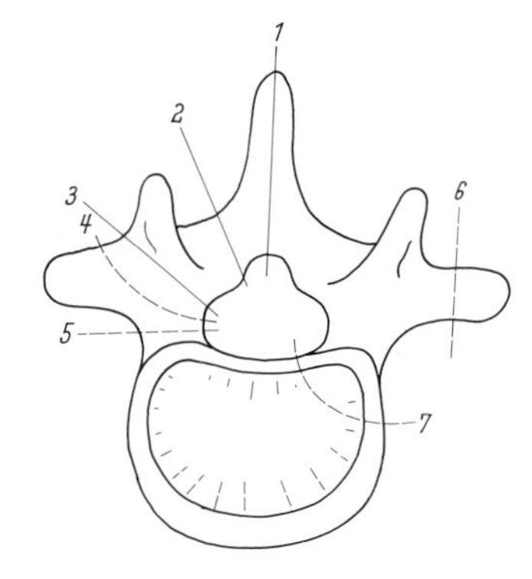

1 Split spinous process
2 Lateral cleft in a case of asymmetrical development of the halves of the arch
3 Split interarticular portion, i.e., interarticular spondylolysis
4, 5, 6 Rare cleft formations (see *Probst*)
7 Approximately the spot where the root of the arch and the vertebral body meet

Fig. 384. Cleft formation in the vertebral arch (from *Schmorl* and *Junghanns*). See also Fig. 463. The cleft-like anomalies in the region of the arches and the spinous processes are so numerous (e.g., in children, up to 60–70%) that one should only give a radiographic description of cleft formations in the various sections, without pronouncing a diagnosis. One should speak of an occult spina bifida only in cases of clinical-neurological relevance. If a meningocele is present, an open spina bifida is involved.

Scheurmann's disease leaves the following radiographic indications:
1. Torn top and bottom plates with thread fibers
2. *Schmorl*'s cartilaginous nodules of the covering plates
3. Irregularities of the marginal ledges
4. Enlargement of the anteroposterior diameter of the vertebrae
5. Box vertebrae
6. Reduction in thickness of the intervertebral disks
7. Vertebrae, wedge formed
8. Block vertebrae

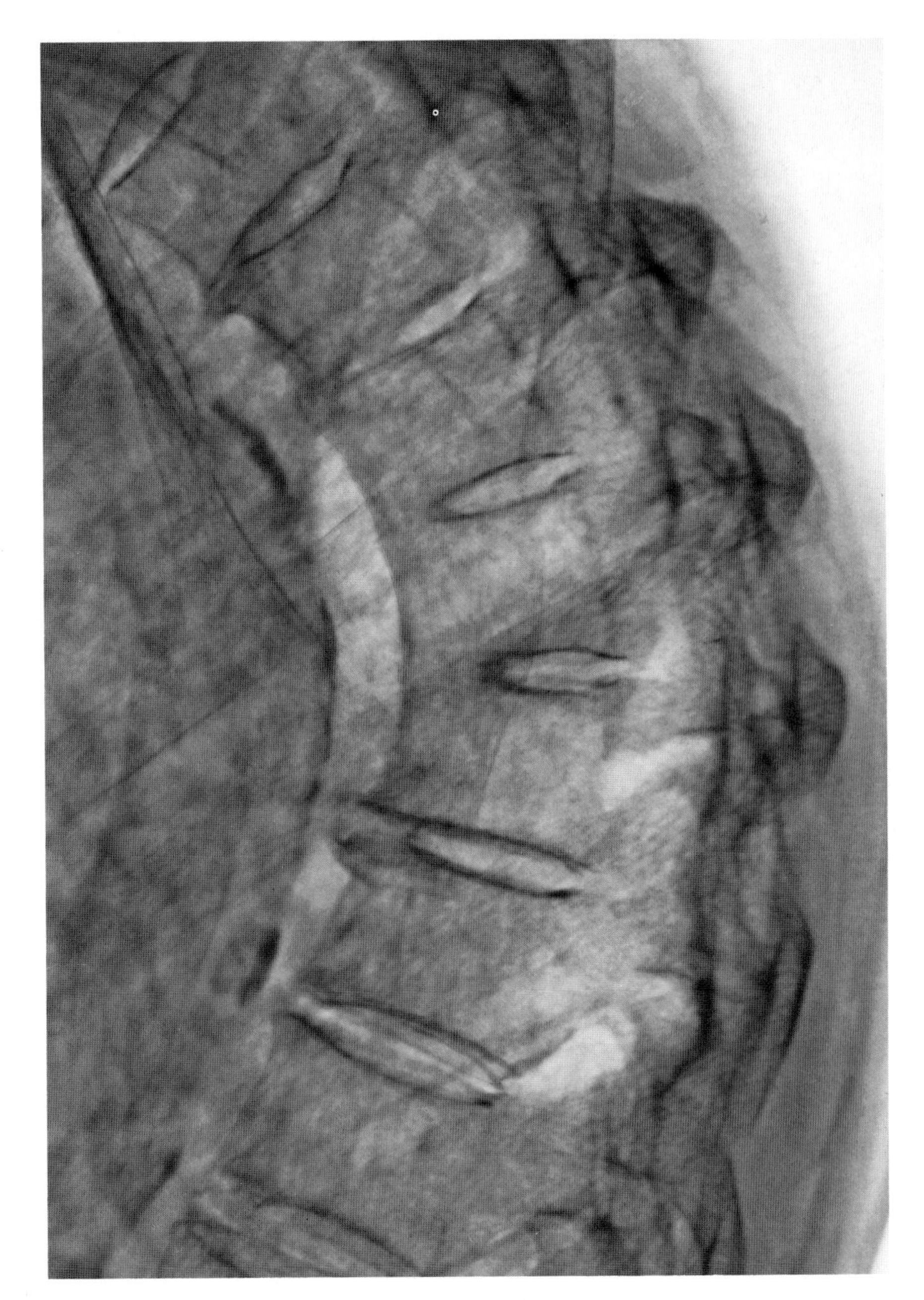

Fig. 385. Late stage, after *Scheuermann*'s disease in an 80-year-old female (on *Scheuermann*'s disease, see also Fig. 332). At the height of the most pronounced curvature, the thoracic vertebrae are fused only in their anterior parts, which causes the partial formation of block vertebrae. Apart from degenerative changes in the disks due to old age, with partly recognizable deforming spondylosis, a distinct calcification of the aorta is also shown. *Clandriello* proposed three types of synostosis in the formation of block vertebrae: formation of block vertebrae on a congenital basis, secondary block formation due to inflammatory processes of the spine, and, more rarely, after injuries (resorption of a necrotic intervertebral disk).

Causes of formation of block vertebrae (abridged according to *Langhof*):

1. Congenital formation of block vertebrae, with lack of differentiation, often at the lumbar spine, without gross malformations
2. *Kippel-Feil*'s disease; when, they occur together with malformations such as cleft vertebrae, cervical vertebrae and similar anomalies
3. After tuberculous spondylitis; generally with kinking of the axis and lateral shift, sometimes with calcification of hypostatic abscesses
4. Following infectious spondylitis, e.g., after typhoid
5. Ankylosing spondyl arthritis (*Bechterew-Pierre-Marie-Strümpell* disease); see also *Aufdermaur, Davies*
6. *Paget*'s disease
7. After traumata with fractures and compressions
8. Senile kyphosis sometimes leads to the formation of wedging and block vertebrae, mostly at the level of the middle thoracic spine
9. Deforming spondylosis; formation of block vertebrae is caused by bony lateral steps (ossified longitudinal ligaments) or by bony marginal bulge formation from vertebra to vertebra
10. Juvenile deforming osteochondrosis *(Scheuermann)*

Figs. 386–388. Separation of vertebral margins by disk tissue. This condition must be differentiated from the so-called supernumerary bones of the intervertebral disks. The following three figures are sketches from radiographs done by *Teichert*.

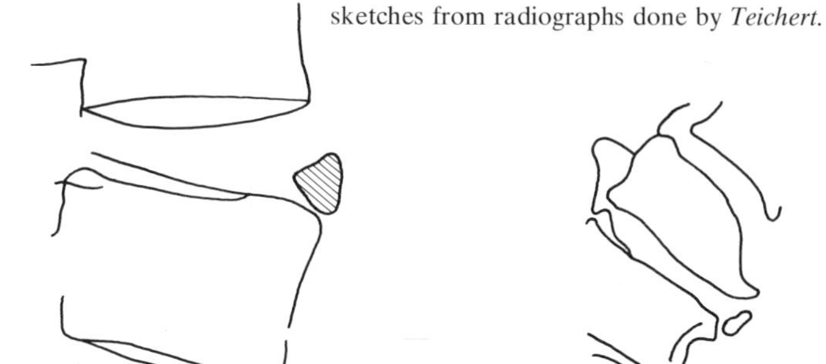

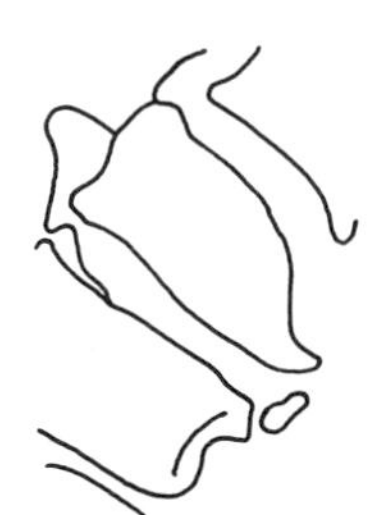

Fig. 386. Separated margins of the vertebra complement the vertebral body to a normal shape.

Fig. 387. Supernumerary bones seated upon normal vertebral margins.

Fig. 388. Supernumerary bone of the cervical spine, with spondylosis.

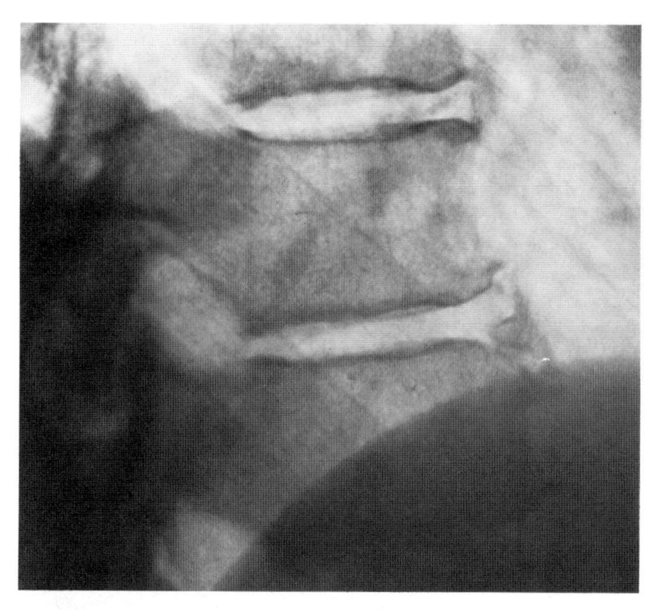

Fig. 389

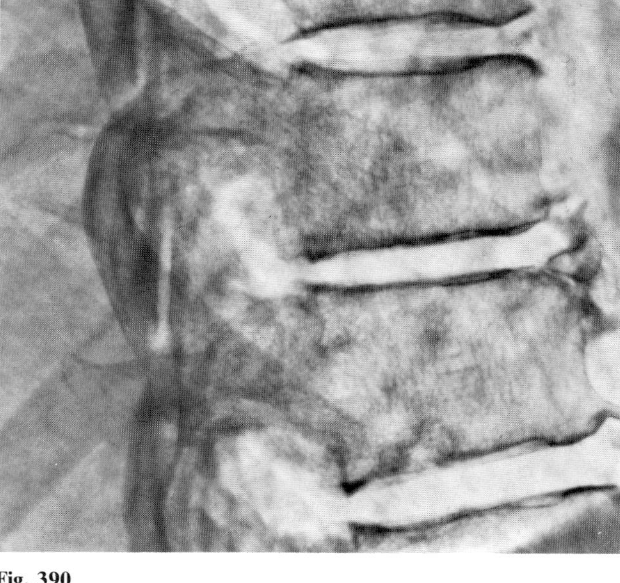

Fig. 390

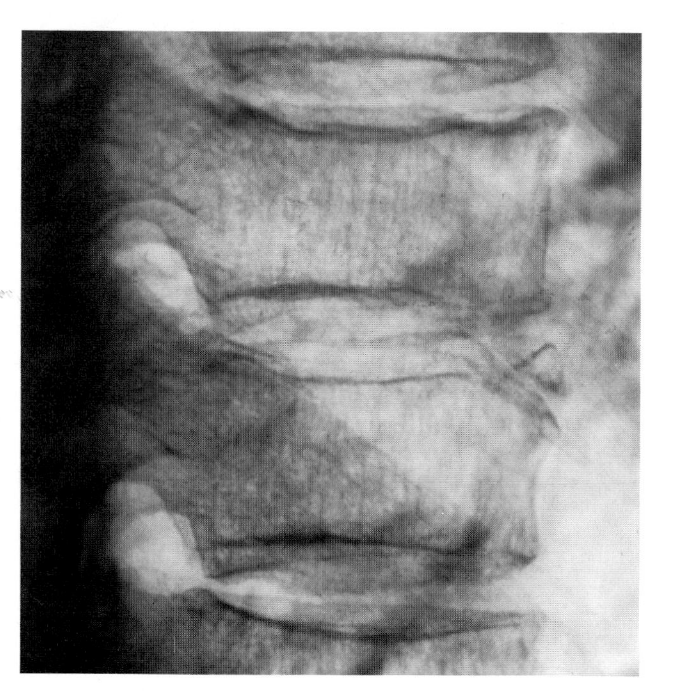

Figs. 389–391. Separation of vertebral margins in deforming spondylosis (see *Junghanns*).

For the connection between heavy work and degenerative changes in the vertebrae, which may be important when an expert opinion is required, see *Th. Becker*.

Fig. 391. Classical structure in osteoporosis. In ordinary radiographs osteoporosis becomes apparent only when the degree of demineralization is greater than 30%. In this view, apart from a separation of the margins in the body of a thoracic vertebra, an osteoporosis that has progressed to such an extent, the following can be seen: increased radiolucency, due to distinctly reduced bony structure, which has led to a skeined appearance of the structure, and a relatively augmented outline of the covering plates. Effects of this osteoporosis are infractions of the covering plates with formation of fish vertebrae, as well as collapse, with formation of wedging vertebrae (senile kyphosis) and spontaneous fractures.

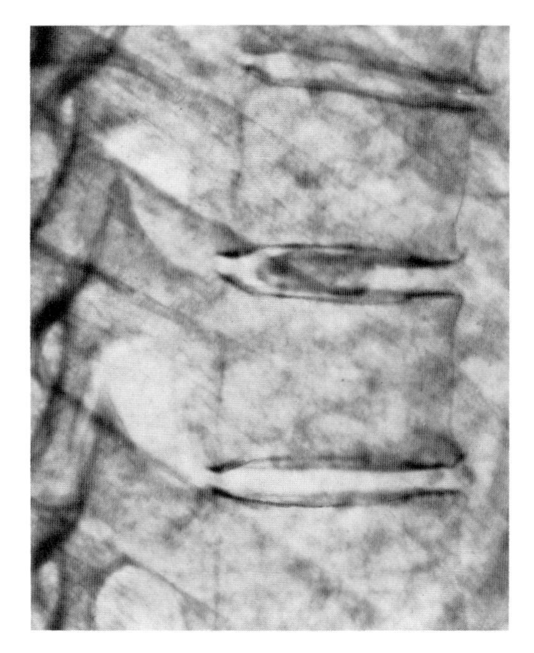

Fig. 392. Calcification of a nucleus pulposus of the thoracic spine. Calcifications of the annulus fibrosus are more frequent, and increase greatly after the 30th year of life, according to *Rathcke*. On the precise structure of the juvenile nucleus pulposus in this connection, see *Meachim* and *Cornah*.

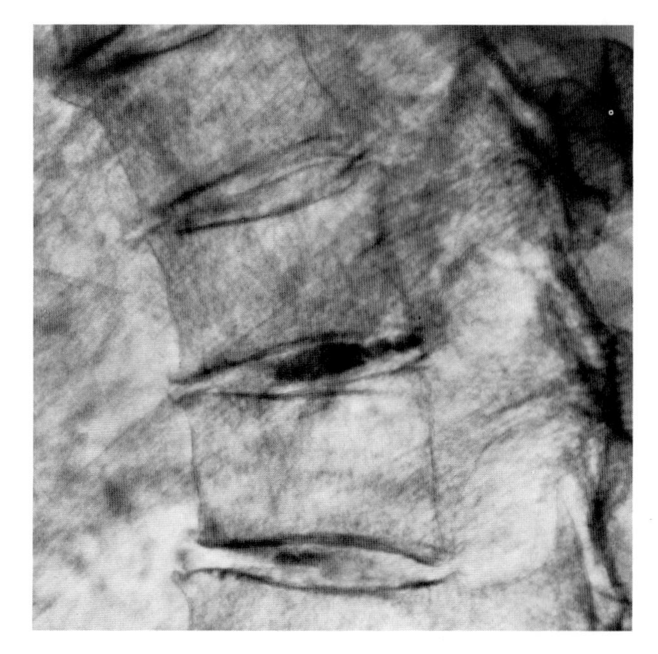

Fig. 393. Calcification of nucleus pulposus and annulus fibrosus. This finding is not rare in *Scheuermann*'s disease or after traumata. *Priessnitz* reported on the connection of intervertebral calcinosis to *Scheuermann*'s disease.

The rare, but frequently described calcifications in infancy of nucleus and disk are noteworthy. *Hayem et al.* described calcifications of nucleus and annulus fibrosus in 1- to 7-year-old children, decreasing in frequency in the cervicosacral direction. *Mainzer* and *Harzheim* also described this rare complication in infancy. Its causes include traumata, infections, metabolic anomalies and vitamin D hypervitaminosis.

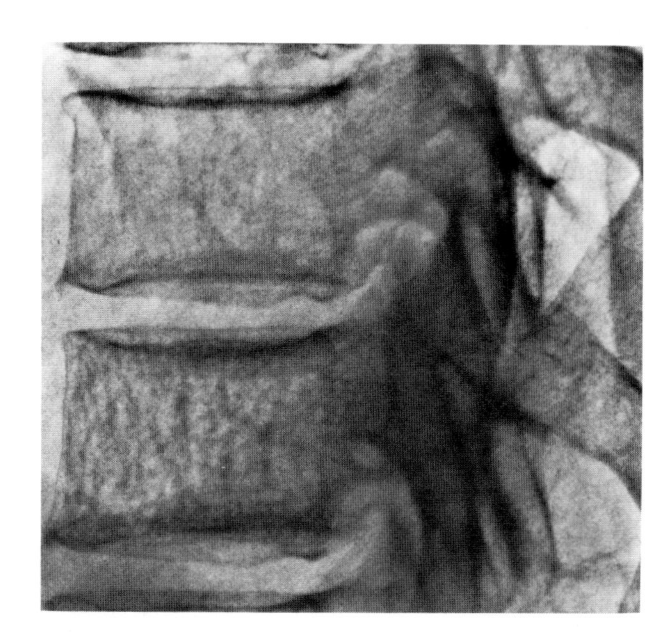

Fig. 394. Radiograph of a vertebral cavernous hemangioma, in its most frequent axial type with skeined sclerosis, in a 59-year-old male. The shape is unchanged. In contrast to the image of osteoporosis with its skeined vertebral structure (see Fig. 391), in this case the sclerosis as well as its limitation to a single or a few vertebrae are characteristic. The vertebral hemangioma of the so-called woolly type with wide-meshed, honeycomb-like structure of the cancellous tissue is rarer *(Schinz, Baensch, Friedl and Ühlinger)*. The vertebral hemangiomata are of clinical significance, e.g., compression of the spinal cord. With advancing age its frequency increases. Its favored localization is the middle thoracic spine.

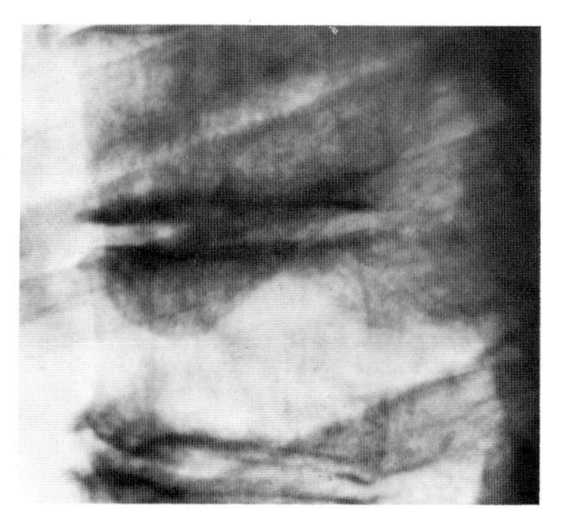

Fig. 395 a

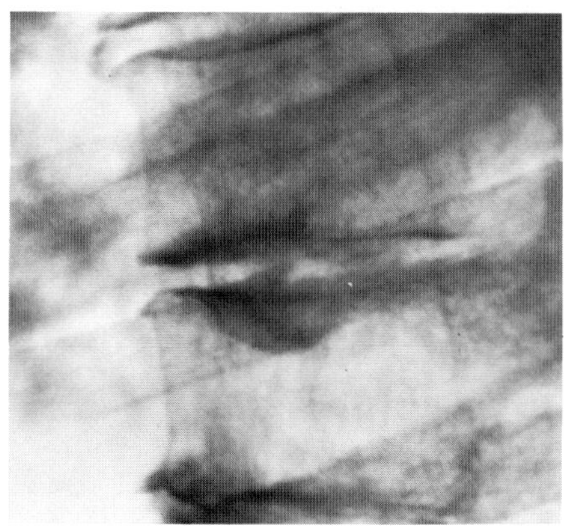

Fig. 395 b

Fig. 395. Osteoma-like increased density of the spongy tissue, with sharply curved demarcation caudally, apparently arising from the upper covering plate; actually, it is the inferior angle of a scapula, varying in size during breathing.

Radiographic Anatomy and Radiographs of the Lumbar Spine, Pelvis and Hip Joint, Including Exposure Techniques

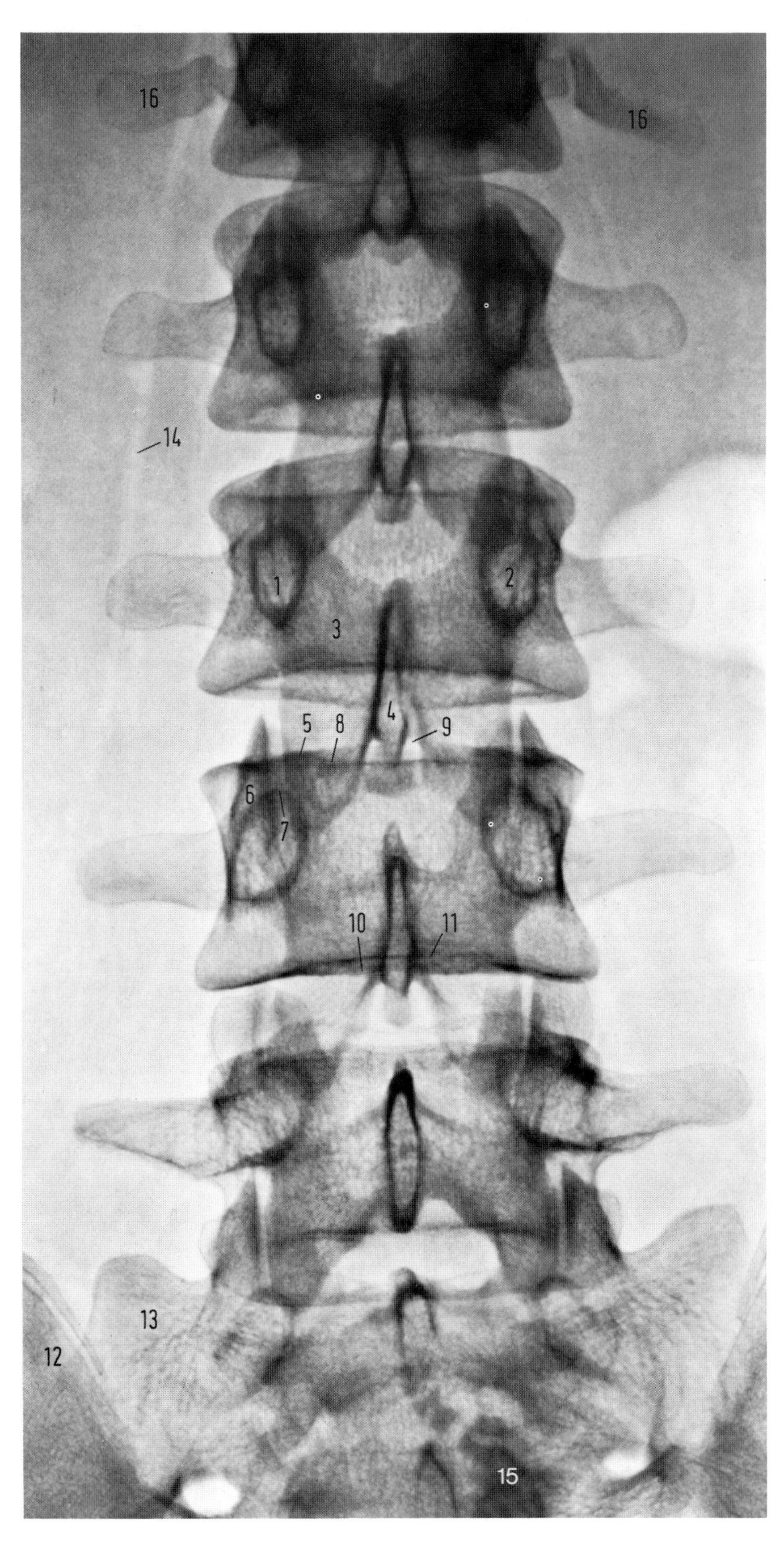

Fig. 396. Lumbar spine, ventrodorsal. Position: supine. The knees are pulled up to slightly reduce the curvature of the lumbar spine. One can also bend the hip joints maximally in order to further "straighten up" the 5th lumbar vertebra (lithotomy position). The central ray is directed to the level of the 3rd lumbar vertebra.

- 1,2 Roots of the arch (3) of the 2nd lumbar vertebra, terminating in the spinous process (4)
- 5 Lower articular process of the 2nd lumbar vertebra which forms, with the upper one (6) of the 3rd lumbar vertebra, the intervertebral articulation (7)
- 8 Dorsal upper, 10 dorsal lower, 9 ventral upper, 11 ventral lower contours of the 3rd lumbar vertebral body
- 12 Iliac crest (the apophysis is visible; juvenile patient; see also Fig. 442, No. 113)
- 13 Transverse process of 5th lumbar vertebra, fused on both sides with the sacrum; the 5th lumbar vertebra is sacralized (transition vertebra)
- 14 Lateral margin of the musculus psoas major
- 15 Calcified mesenteric lymph node
- 16 Rudimentary ribs, joint-like contiguous to the rudiment of the transverse process of the 12th thoracic vertebra

The cranially convex, curved lines belong to the ventral margin of the vertebral body and those convex caudally to the dorsal margin, when the focus was directed below the transverse surface (cover- or ground-plate, respectively), and vice versa. In our case, the cranially convex margins of the vertebral bodies of the 1st and 2nd lumbar vertebrae correspond to the ventral margin of the vertebral body, and those convex caudally to the dorsal margin (see Nos. 8–11).

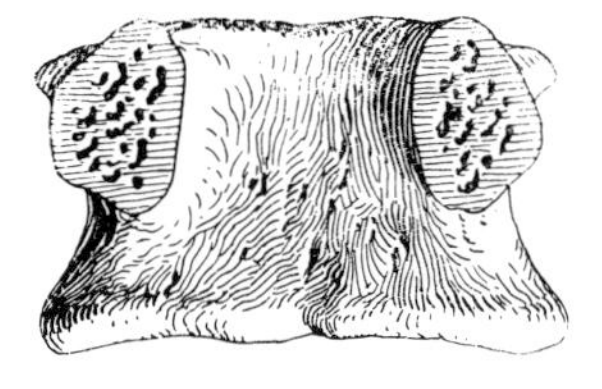

Fig. 397 shows a vertebra whose arches had been sawed off at their roots. This view of a transverse section of the roots of the arch appears on the normal radiograph (according to *Heitzmann*).

Fig. 398. Pathway of rays upon ventrodorsal picture of the lumbar spine. Only the intervertebral space IV/V is projected free and appears translucent on the radiograph. Each vertebral body gives two shadow lines of the upper and the lower margins. One corresponds to the ventral, the other to the dorsal half of the vertebral body. The more obliquely the rays impinge, the more the ventral and dorsal contours of the margin move away from one another. Where they almost cover each other, the rays have travelled in the plane of the transverse section of the intervertebral disk (in Fig. 396 between the 3rd and 4th lumbar vertebrae) whose interspace, therefore, appears as the brightest. The visible spinous processes in this section belong to the next higher vertebra. Only the spinous processes of the last two lumbar vertebrae are standing straight, i.e., in the dorsal continuation of the vertebra, the 5th is directed slightly upwards.

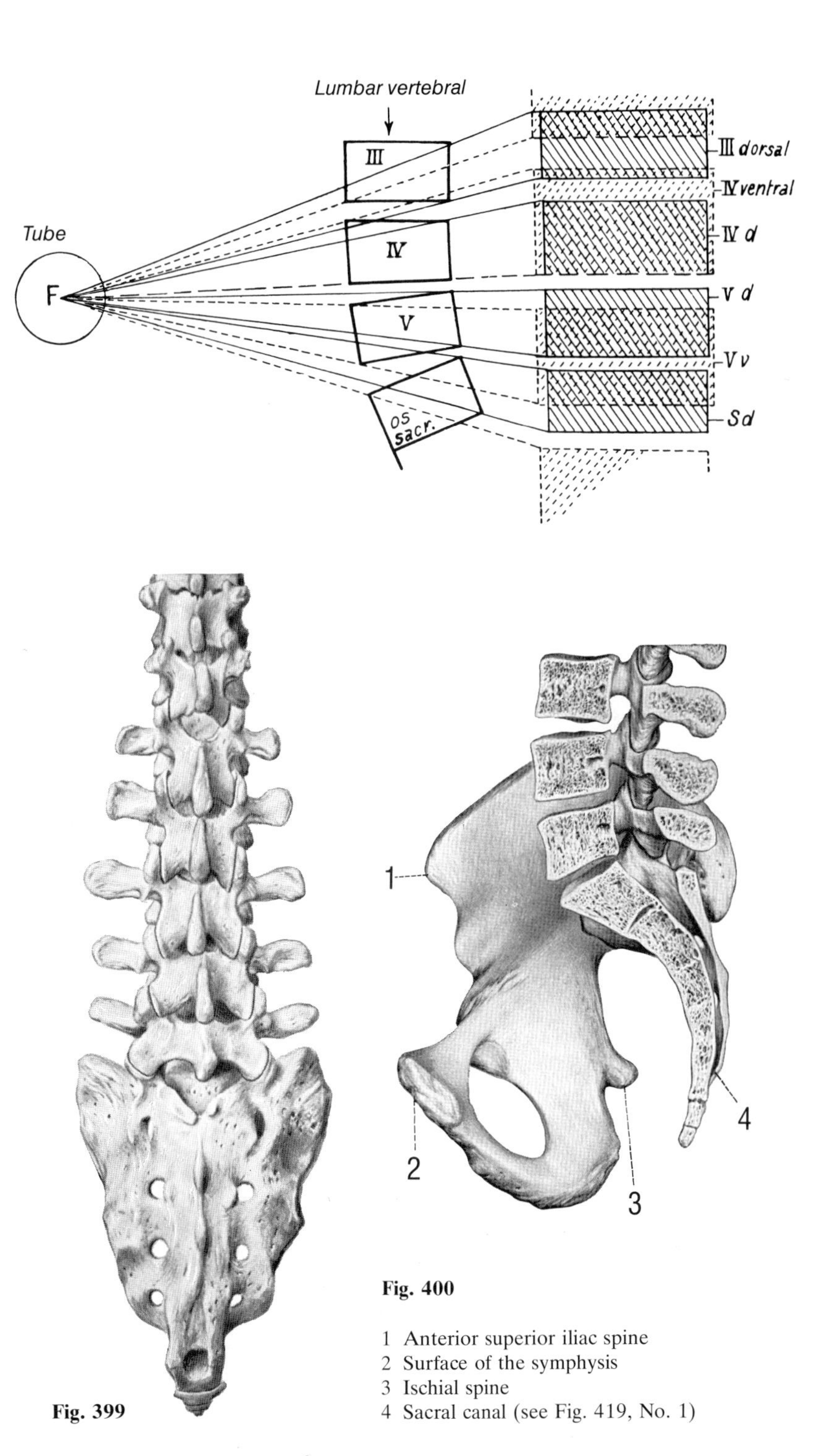

Figs. 399 and 400. Articular processes of the lumbar spine. The intervertebral articulations between the 5th lumbar vertebra and the sacrum take a direction different from the upper ones. Fig. 400 is important for the understanding of the projection of vertebrae; it shows that the lower half of the inclined and wedge-shaped 5th lumbar vertebra is bound to be projected into the shadow of the sacrum. For the importance of the overall radiograph of the lumbar spine in cases of prolapse of lumbar disks, see *Stoessel et al.* (from *Sobotta-Becher,* 17th Edition).

Fig. 399

Fig. 400

1 Anterior superior iliac spine
2 Surface of the symphysis
3 Ischial spine
4 Sacral canal (see Fig. 419, No. 1)

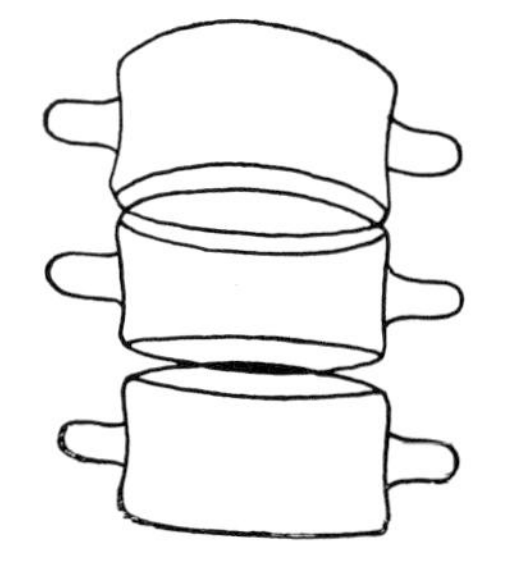

Fig. 401. Schematic sketch of the spine, illustrating:

1. It is possible to get the impression of an ossification within the intervertebral disk (nucleus pulposus), in the lower intervertebral space, in cases of a narrow overlap.
2. Oblique projection, like that on comprehensive radiographs, especially at the upper vertebrae visible on the radiograph, may easily simulate a lateral union or fusion of two vertebrae. Therefore, care should be taken that those vertebrae whose examination is essential are exposed to vertical rays as far as is possible.

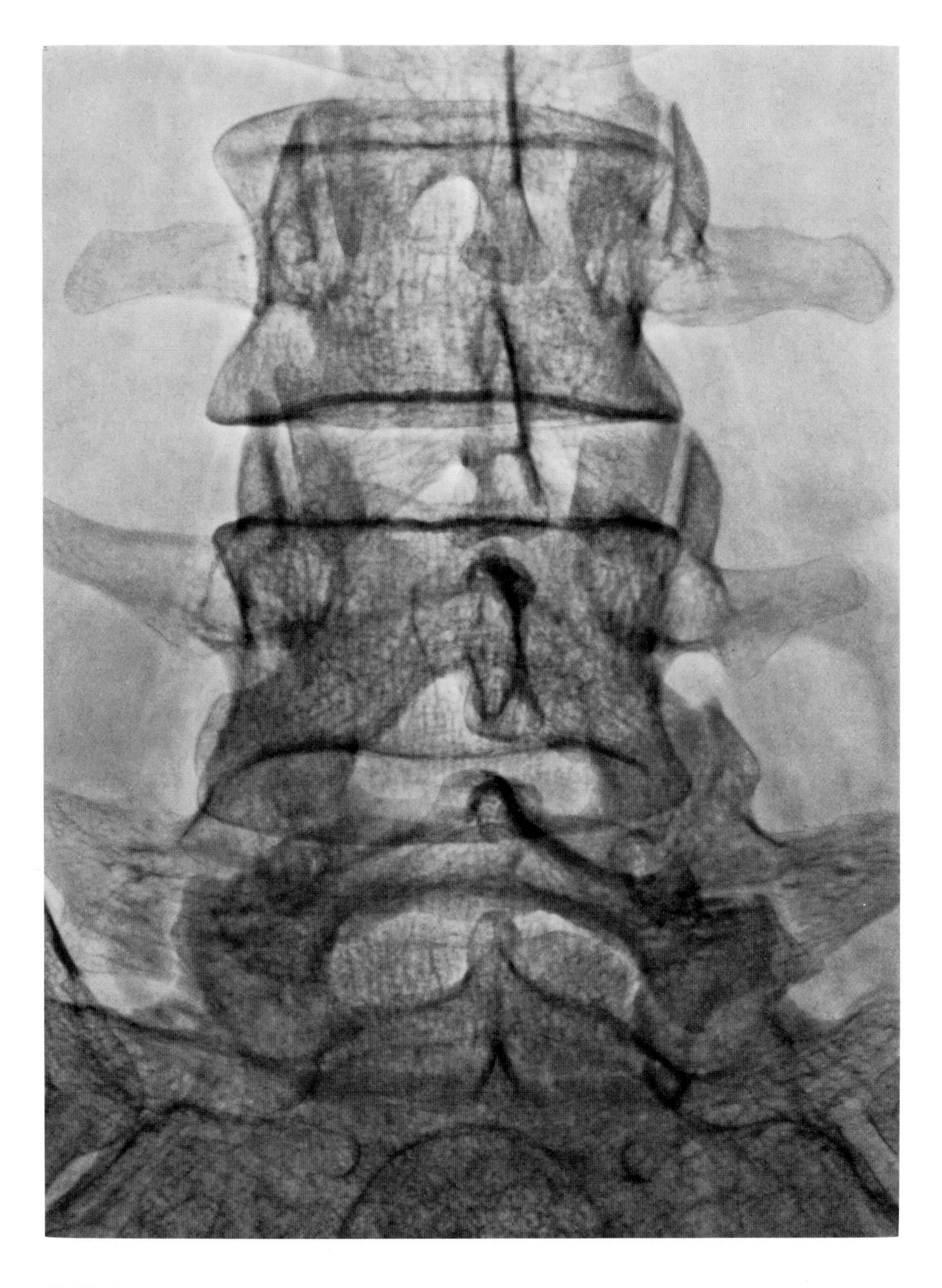

Fig. 402. Meticulously focused radiograph of the lower lumbar spine, with transition into the sacrum. The lumbar spine has been slightly turned; therefore, the spinous processes do not appear exactly median. They are shown a little to the left, corresponding to a barely observable turn towards the right of the supine patient.

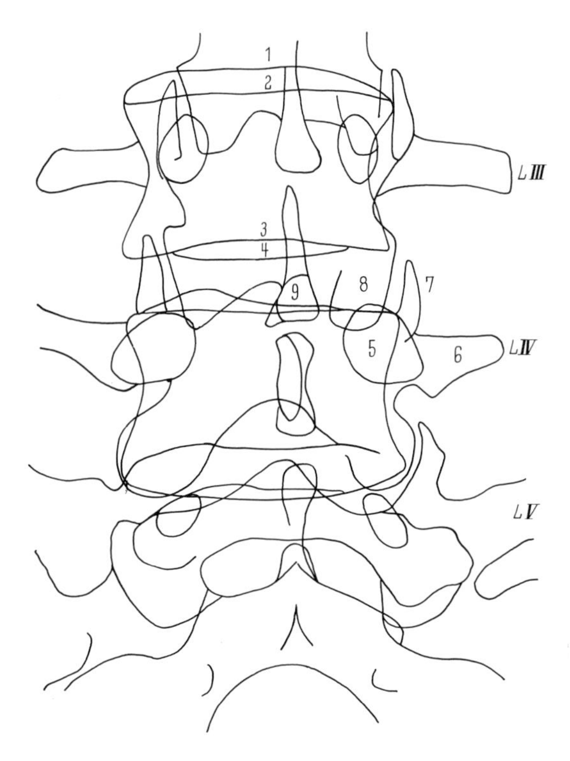

◄
Fig. 403. Sketch to Fig. 402.

1 Anterior upper border of the vertebral body (see Fig. 398)
2 Posterior upper border of the vertebral body
3 Anterior lower border of the vertebral body
4 Posterior lower border of the vertebral body
5 Insertion of arch
6 Transverse process
7 Upper articular process of the intervertebral articulation (= joint of the articular process)
8 Lower articular process of the intervertebral articulation (= joint of the articular process)
9 Spinous process

The anatomy and pathology of the small vertebral joints have been described by *Reinhardt.*

The lumbosacral skeletal region shows numerous variations. Therefore, one generally speaks of lumbosacral transition vertebrae. It is often difficult, apart from views of the entire spinal column, to enumerate the lumbar and sacral vertebrae with certainty; though on this partial view, the long, thin, slightly rising transverse processes, with their bulge at the lower medial margin, are typical for the 4th lumbar vertebra. At the lumbosacral transition vertebrae, one can find any imaginable partial or total fusion or other deformities. Here, the right club-shaped transverse process of the 5th lumbar vertebra must be mentioned as a transitional form towards partial sacralization. Further variants are possible, up to complete symmetrical lumbalizations or sacralizations, with widely different formations of pseudoarticulations.

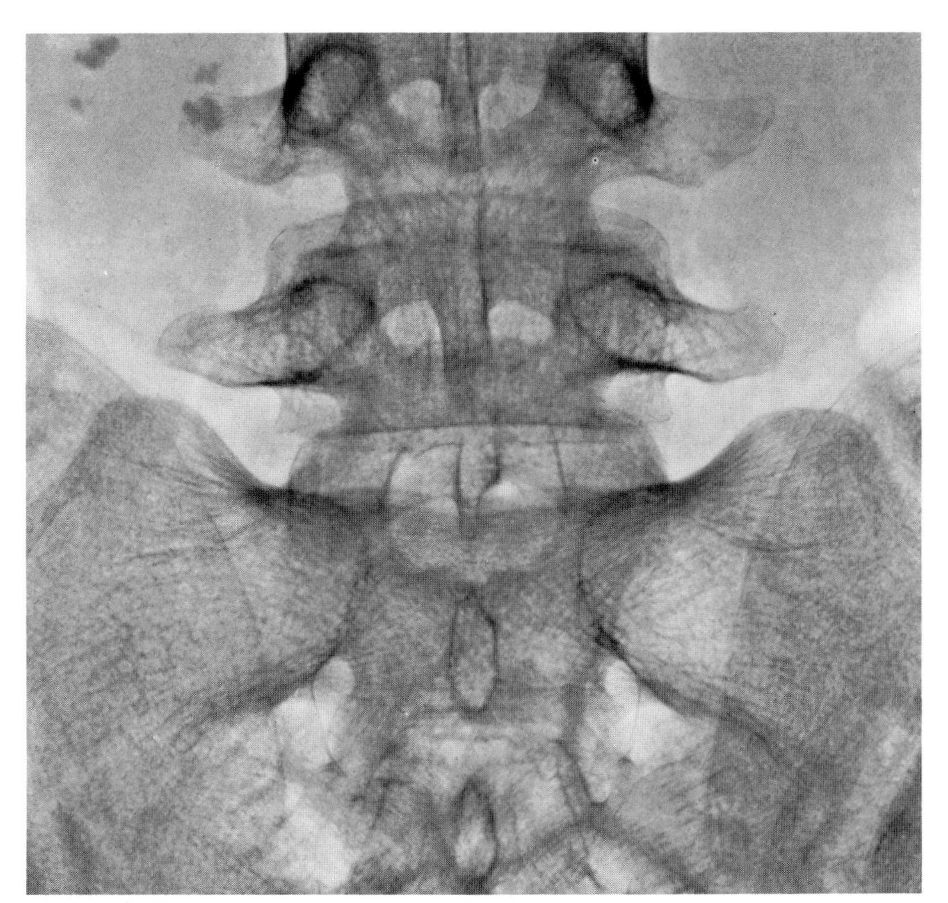

Fig. 404. Region of lumbosacral transition, inside view. For position see Fig. 405. With the path of rays inclined caudocranially by 30°, the central ray is aimed at a point just above the symphysis.

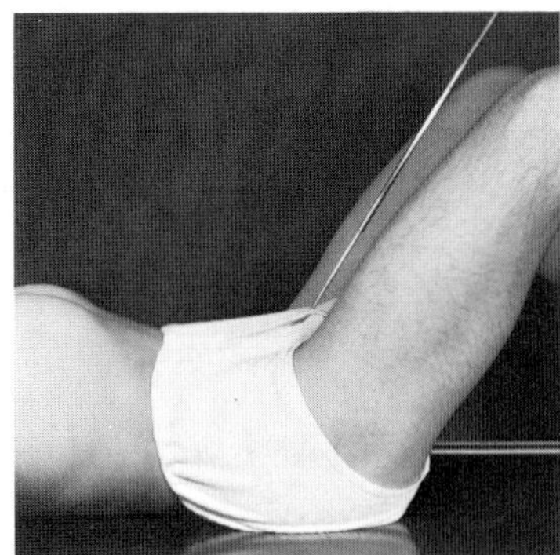

Fig. 405. Patient is supine, with knees slightly raised and thighs in abduction. With a caudocranial pathway of rays inclined by 30°, the central ray is beamed slightly above the rim of the symphysis onto the lumbosacral transition.

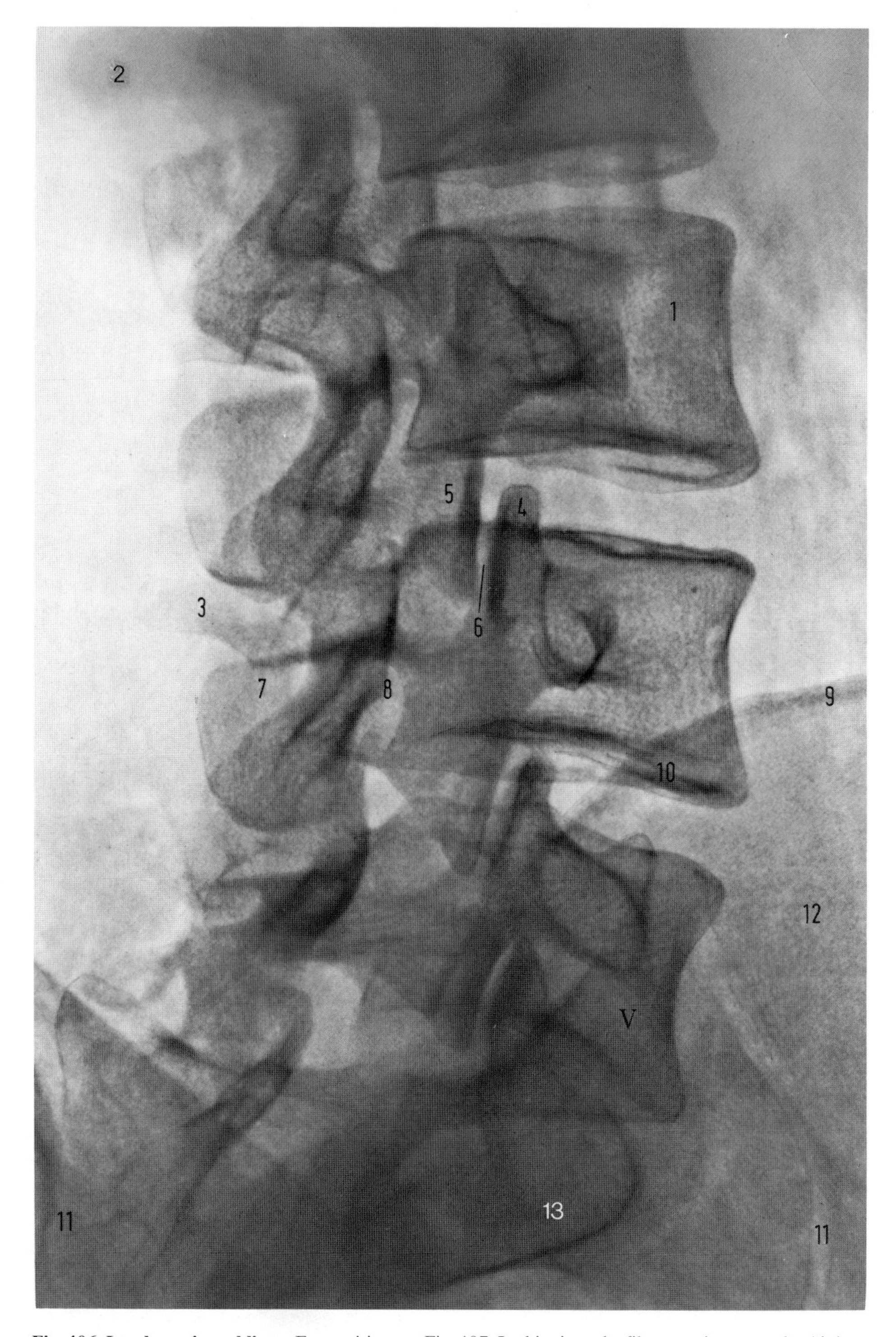

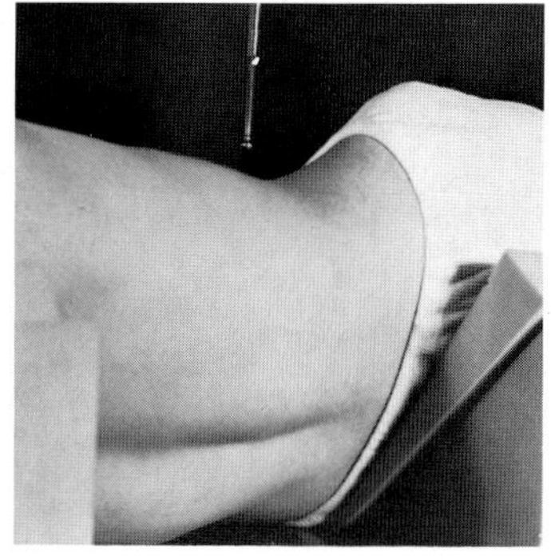

Fig. 407. Pads are placed under the shoulder and pelvis of the supine patient for an oblique position of 35–45°. The knees are slightly drawn up.

Fig. 406. Lumbar spine, oblique. For position see Fig. 407. In this view, the film-near intervertebral joints are demonstrated, and simultaneously, with slightly less rotation (20–30°), the film-distant sacroiliac joint (see Fig. 423). For an accurate diagnosis, comparative radiographs of both sides must be made.

1 Body of the 3rd lumbar vertebra
2 Costal process of the 2nd lumbar vertebra *
3 Costal process of the 4th lumbar vertebra
4 Superior articular process
5 Inferior articular process
6 Articular space of the joint of the articular process
7 Spinous process, shortened by perspective
8 Intervertebral foramen
9 Iliac crest
10 Lower contour (adjacent and distant side) of the body of L IV
11 Sacroiliac joint
12 Ilium
13 Sacrum
V Body of L V

* The transverse process at the lumbar spine fuses with a costal remnant to the costal process.

The symmetrical lumbalization of the 1st sacral vertebra (= 6 lumbar vertebrae), as well as the sacralization of the 5th lumbar vertebra (which leaves 4 lumbar vertebrae), are usually findings that do not cause complaints. Incomplete unilateral lumbalization or sacralization, with their acquired formations of pseudoarticulations, ground-off bone and oblique weight-bearing, may explain some painful states. In any case, an exact roentgenologic analysis of this statically complicated region is of the greatest importance, e.g., in insurance medicine. The surgeon or orthopedic surgeon urgently needs all the details of deviation from the norm for his final diagnosis.

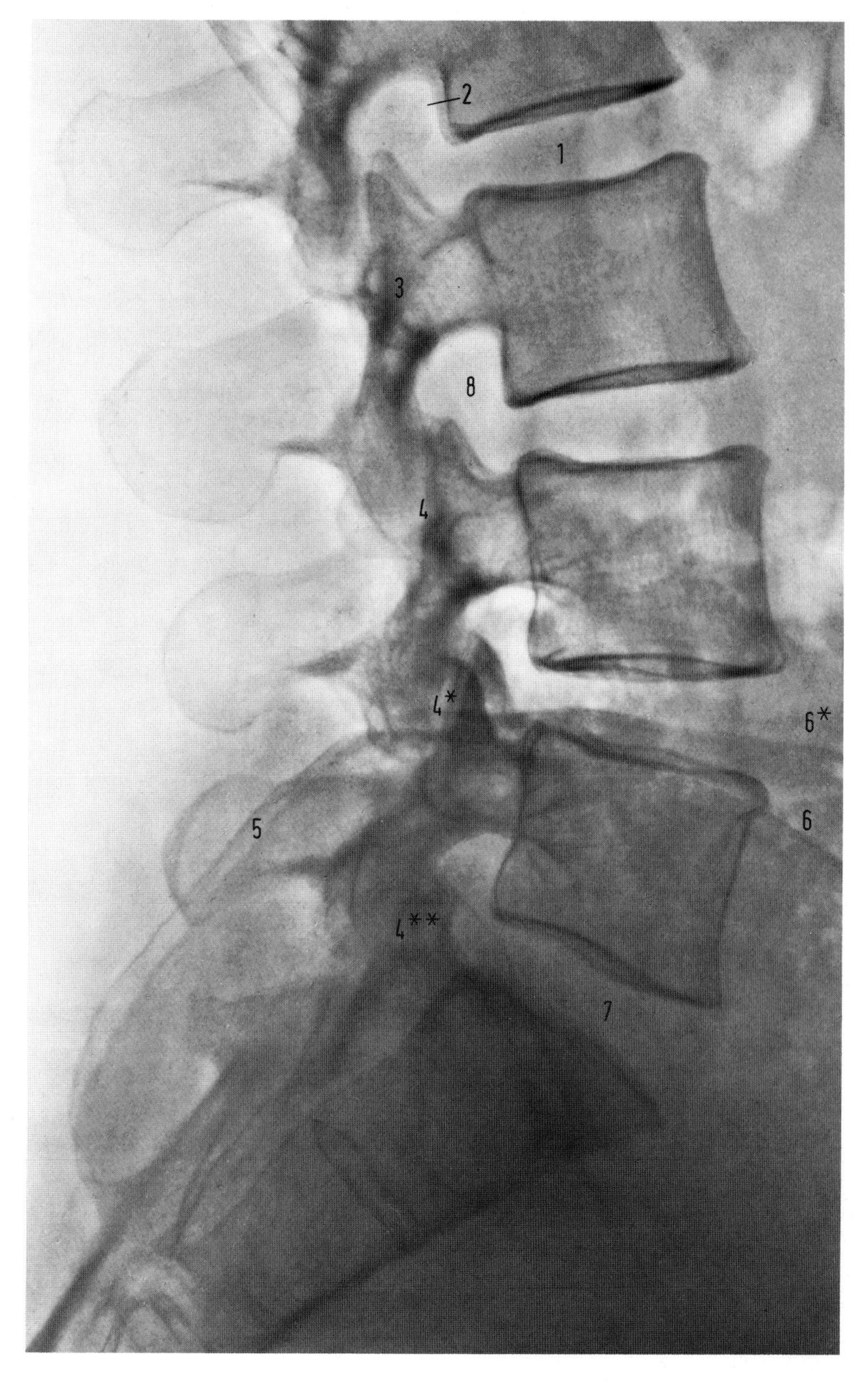

Fig. 408. Lumbar spine, lateral. Projection: the central ray is beamed vertically onto the 5th lumbar vertebra (above the iliac crest).

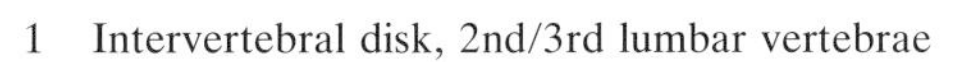

1 Intervertebral disk, 2nd/3rd lumbar vertebrae
2 Dorsal surface of the vertebral body (furnishes two contours)
3 Costal process, seen in transverse section
4 4*, 4** Articular spaces of the intervertebral joints (= spaces of the articular processes)
5 Spinous process
6 Film-near pelvic crest
6* Film-distant pelvic crest
7 Intervertebral disk between L V and sacrum
8 Intervertebral foramen, boot-shaped

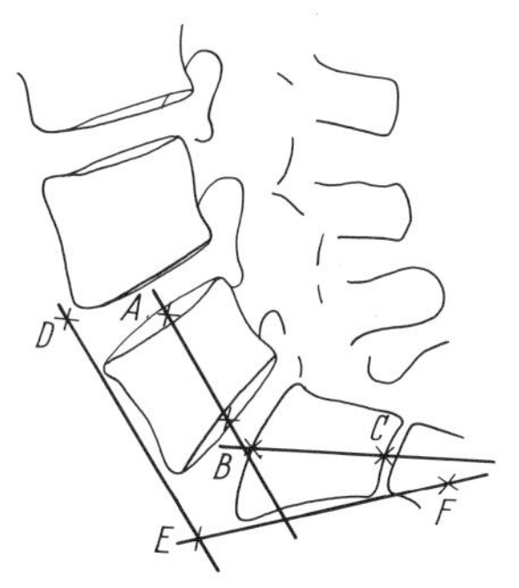

Fig. 409 (from *Schmorl-Junghanns*). **Lumbosacral angle** (ABC), amounting to 135°, with a deviation from 115 to 160°. DEF is the angle of the promontory (120–135°).

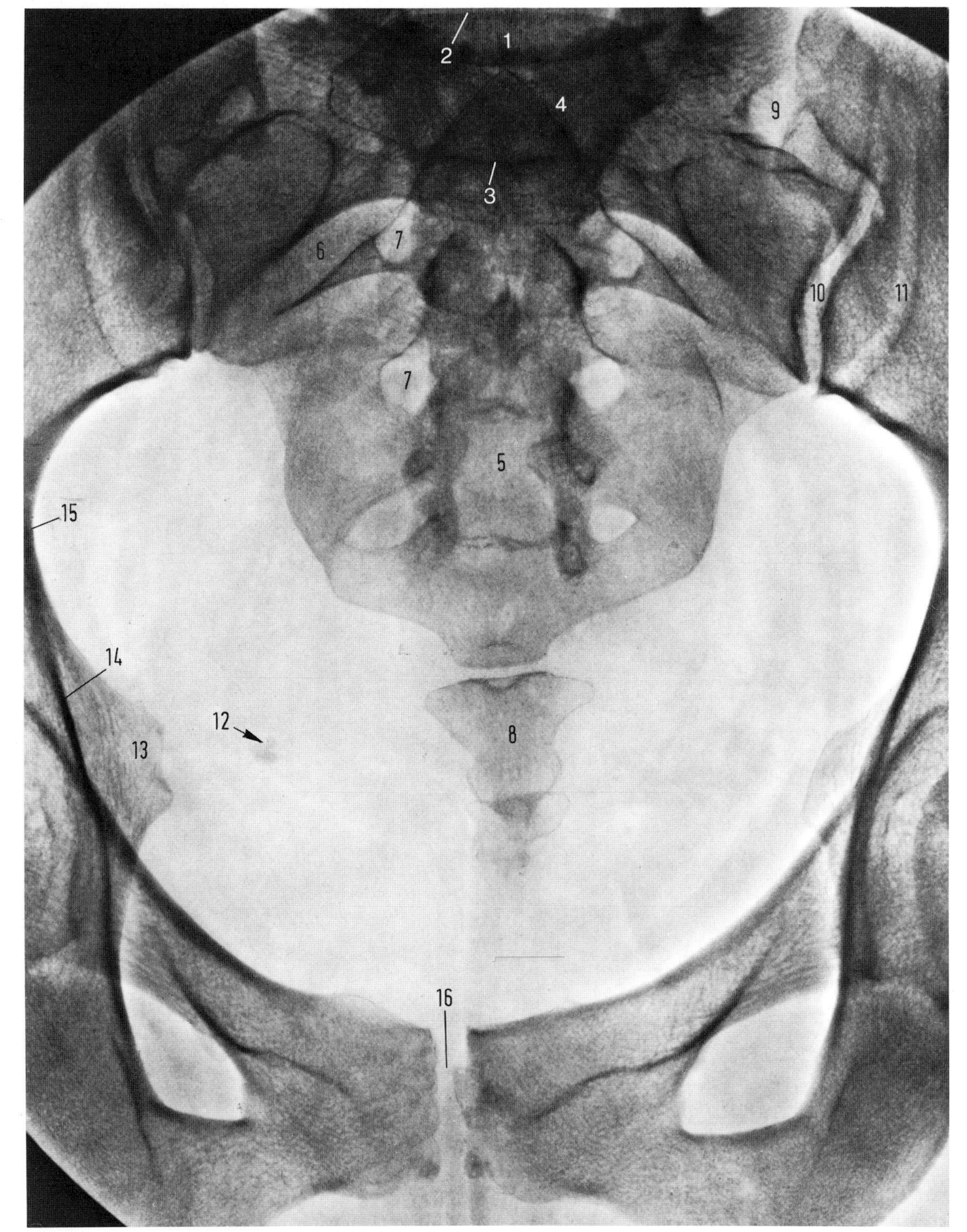

Fig. 410. Sacrum and coccyx, ventrodorsal.

1 Anterior inferior margin of LV
2 Posterior superior margin of base of sacrum
3 Anterior superior margin of S I
4 Promontory
5 Sacral hiatus
6 Lateral sacral crest
7 Sacral foramina
8 1st vertebra of coccyx, here not fused with the sacrum; the remaining coccygeal vertebrae are arranged in scoliotic fashion
9 Shape due to projection, formed by the sacral part of the ilium and the dorsal surface of the sacrum
10, 11 Spaces of the sacroiliac articulation
12 (↘) Ureteral calculi or phleboliths because of their round shape; rigth in front of the bladder
13 Ischial spine
14 Lateral pelvic wall, transverse section, due to projection
15 Linea terminalis
16 Symphysis (enlarged, being film-distant)

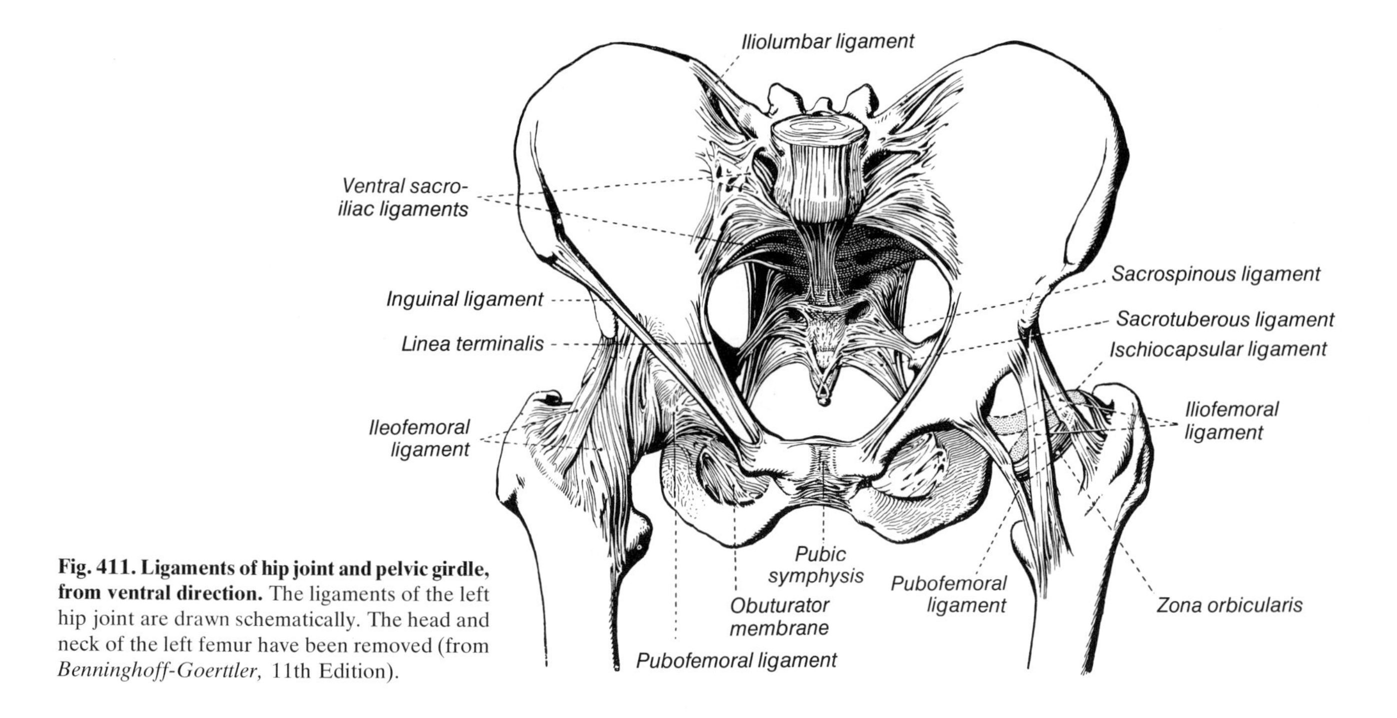

Fig. 411. Ligaments of hip joint and pelvic girdle, from ventral direction. The ligaments of the left hip joint are drawn schematically. The head and neck of the left femur have been removed (from *Benninghoff-Goerttler,* 11th Edition).

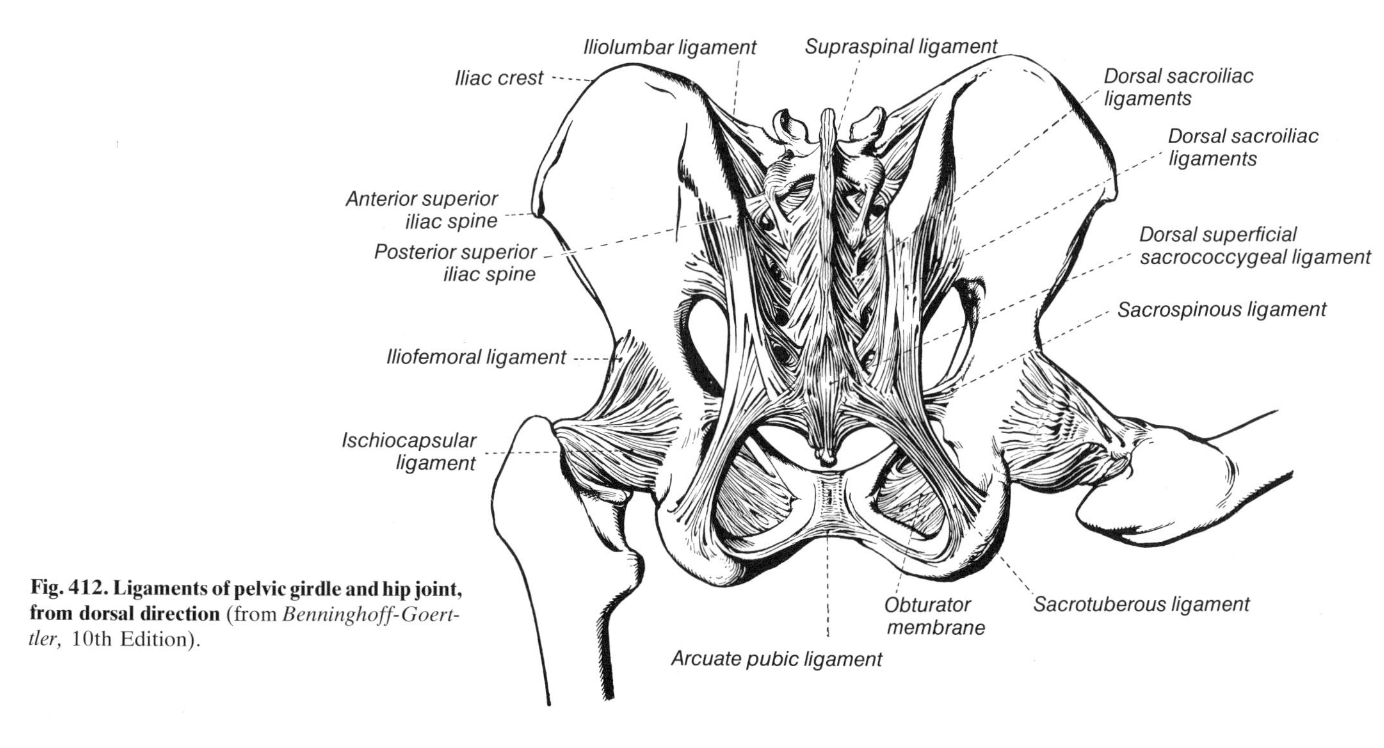

Fig. 412. Ligaments of pelvic girdle and hip joint, from dorsal direction (from *Benninghoff-Goerttler,* 10th Edition).

Average schema of the cranial and caudal variants of the spinal column (see also *Illchmann-Christ* and *Diethelm*).

Cranial variant (often dominantly hereditary)
C VII with long transverse process or cervical ribs
12th rib, very short or absent

L IV with short rudimentary transverse processes
L V sacralized
Clefts in vertebral bodies
Clefts in vertebral arches

Caudal variant (often recessively hereditary)
C VII with short transverse process
Well-formed 12th ribs
L I with lumbar ribs
L IV with fully developed transverse processes
S I lumbalized
Clefts in vertebral bodies
Clefts in vertebral arches

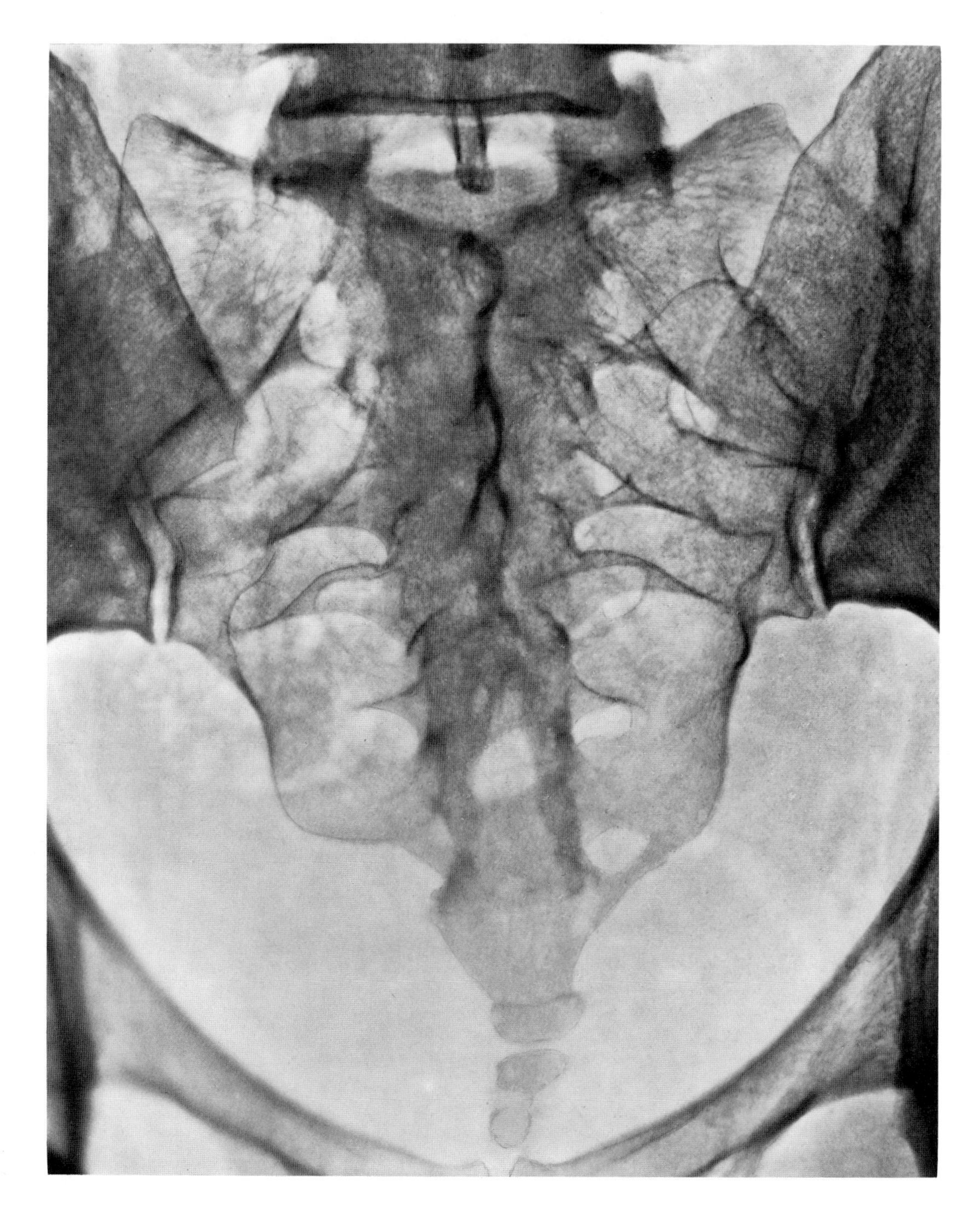

Fig. 413. View of sacrum and coccyx in "lithotomy position." In principle, it corresponds to the "inside-view" (Fig. 404). Position: supine, knee and hip joints are strongly bent, thighs are maximally abducted. The central ray is directed onto the midpoint between navel and symphysis at an angle of 10° craniocaudal. This radiograph is suitable for better demonstration of sacrum and coccyx and, concurrently, of the lumbosacral transition.

The sacral foramina, especially those of the lower sacral vertebrae, are often only partially closed or completely open. These cleft formations must be differentiated from fractures, as the fracture lines in the sacrum usually lead to the foramina too. The lower end of the spine shows great variability and asymmetry.

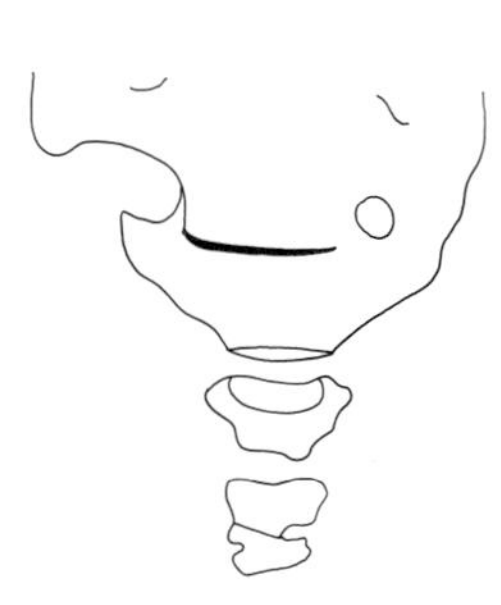

Fig. 414. A so-called **sacrocaudal transition vertebra.** The last coccygeal vertebra may present very strange shapes. Sacral curvatures are caused by asymmetrical development. The 1st sacral vertebra may articulate unilaterally or bilaterally with the ileum. Pains arising from the coccygeal or pericoccygeal region are called coccygodynia.

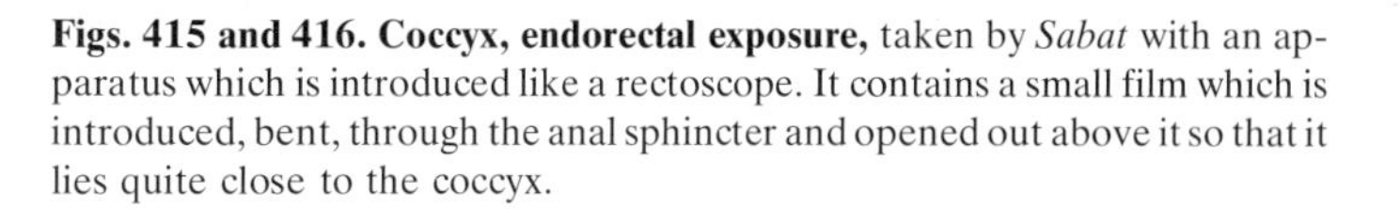

Figs. 415 and 416. Coccyx, endorectal exposure, taken by *Sabat* with an apparatus which is introduced like a rectoscope. It contains a small film which is introduced, bent, through the anal sphincter and opened out above it so that it lies quite close to the coccyx.

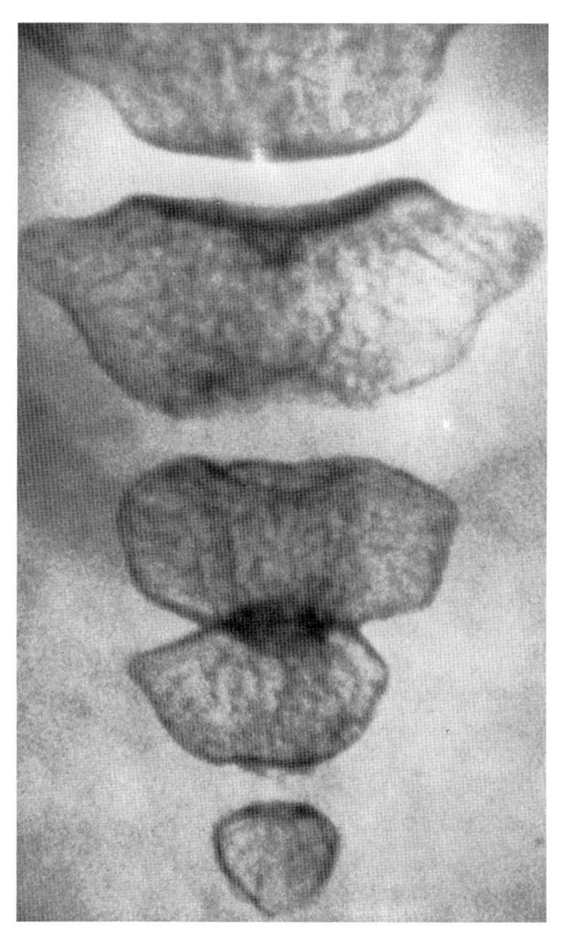

Fig. 415. Only four coccygeal vertebrae have developed (a frequent finding). Bilateral, rudimentary transverse process at the 1st coccygeal vertebra.

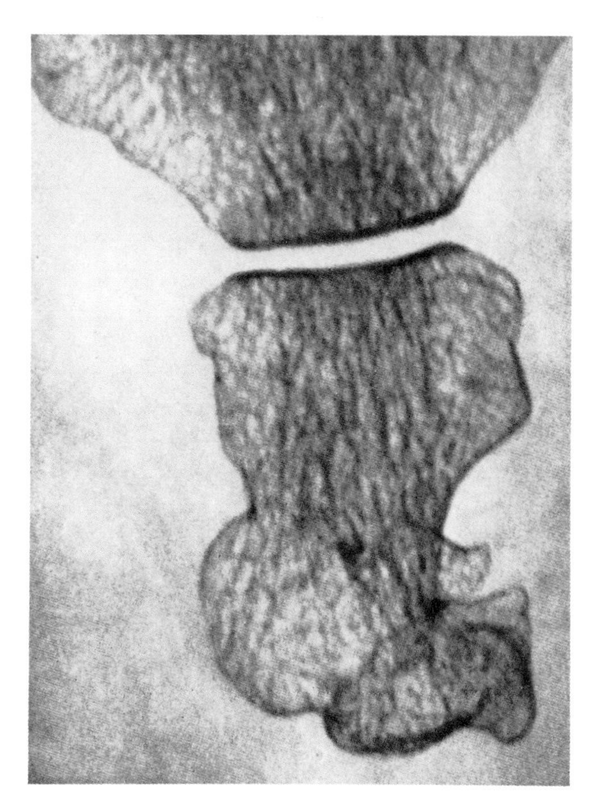

Fig. 416. This is one of the variable rudimentary forms (fusion). These fusions, which usually decrease from the caudal to cranial direction, are congenital block vertebrae. Because of the rigidity of the coccyx, which is often bent inwards, these block vertebrae may be an impediment to delivery.

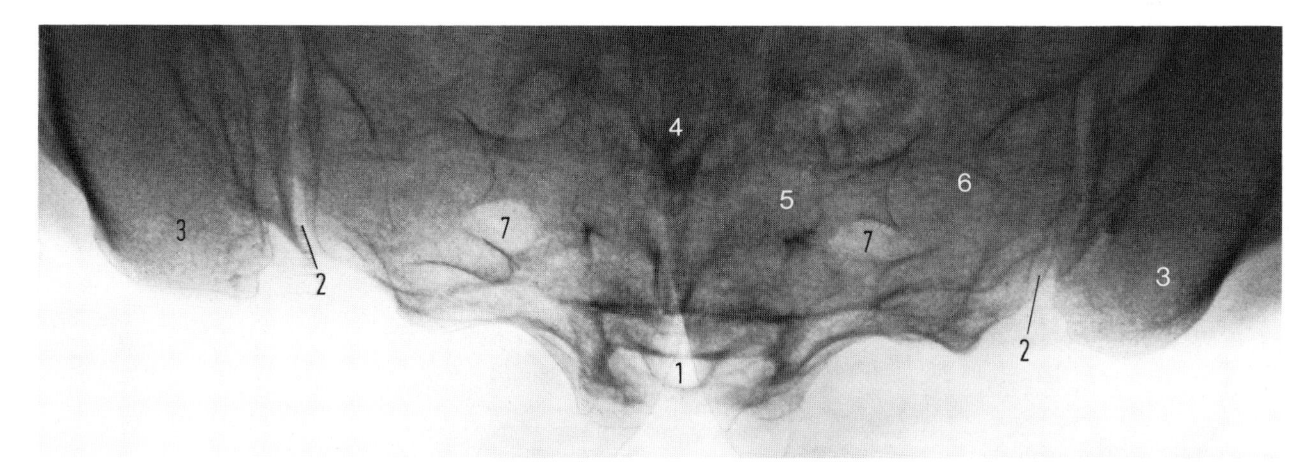

Fig. 417. Axial picture of the sacral canal. For position see Fig. 418.

1 Crescent-shaped sacral canal
2 Articular space of the sacroiliac joint
3 Ilium
4 Medial sacral crest
5 Intermediate sacral crest
6 Lateral sacral crest
7 Sacral foramina

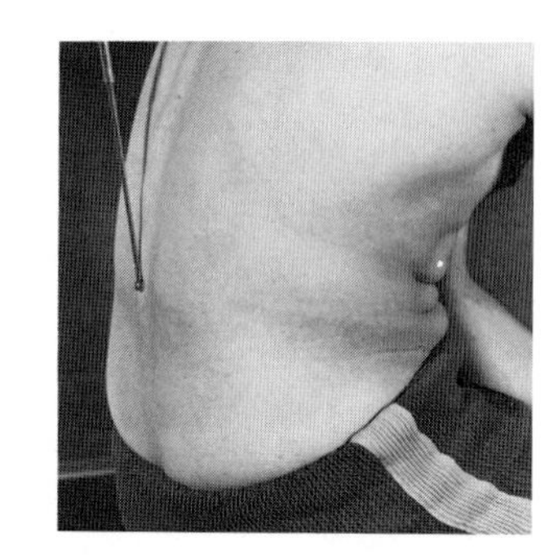

Fig. 418. This radiograph is especially important for clarification of the causes of refractory coccygodynias. These may be caused not only by the coccyx itself or by the pericoccygeal soft tissues but also by the nerves passing through the sacral canal. For instance, after jodipin myelographies, neurofunctional disturbances are not rare.

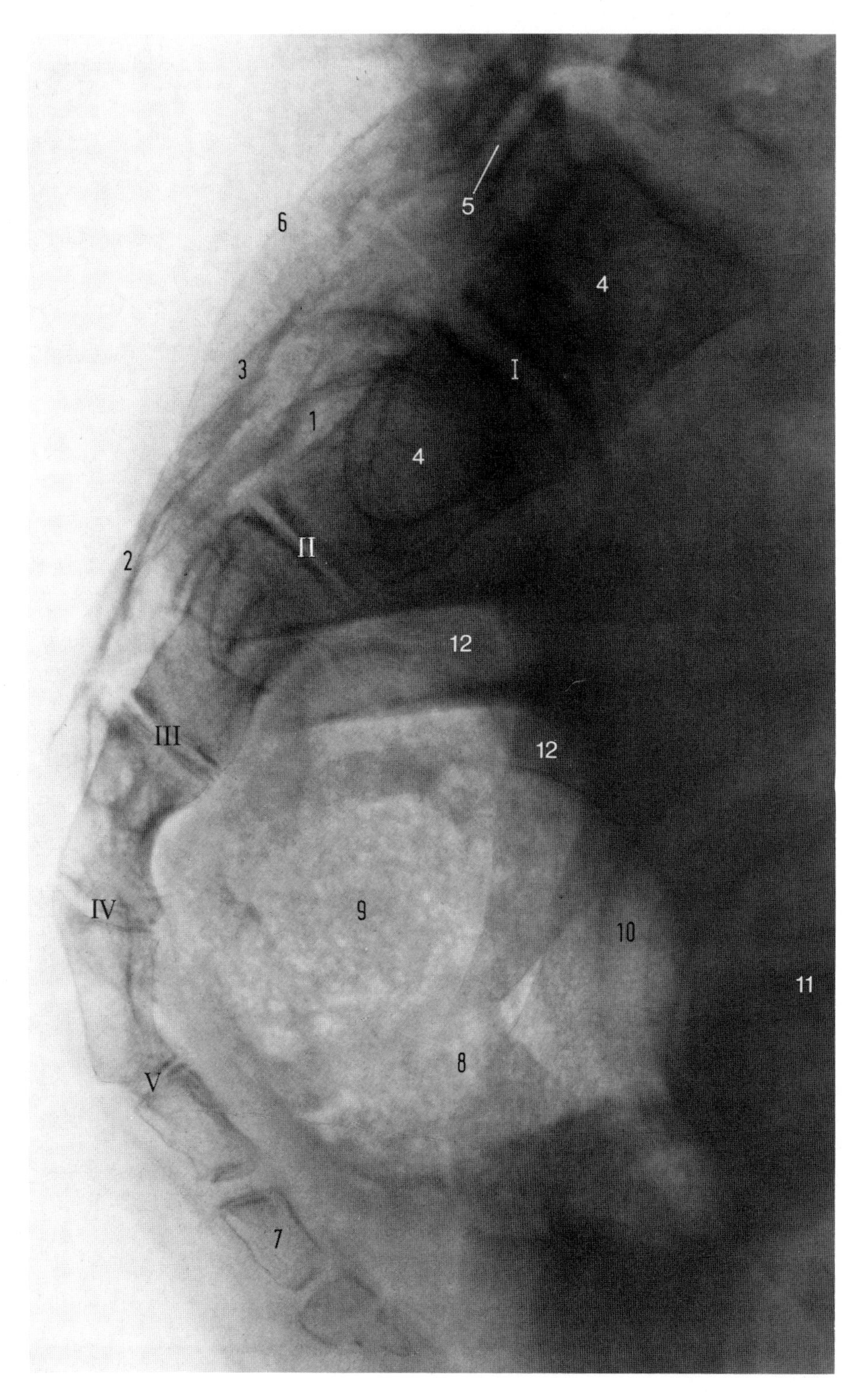

1 Sacral canal
2 Posterior sacral wall
3 Medial sacral crest
4 Auricular surface of the sacroiliac articulation, seen frontally (may simulate a cyst)
5 Articulation between 5th lumbar and 1st sacral vertebrae
6 Iliac crest
7 Coccygeal vertebra
8 Ischial spine
9 Gas-filled rectal ampoule
10 Space of hip joint
11 Femoral head, both sides projected onto each other
12 Greater sciatic notch, both sides projected slightly shifted against each other

I Border between 1st and 2nd sacral vertebrae
II Border between 2nd and 3rd sacral vertebrae
III Border between 3rd and 4th sacral vertebrae
IV Border between 4th and 5th sacral vertebrae
V Border between 5th sacral and 1st coccygeal vertebrae

Fig. 419. Sacrum, lateral. The central beam is directed onto the center of the sacrum, frontal. A sharply angled kink from the sacrum to the coccyx is observed. This kink in the sacrococcygeal joint may also become an impediment to delivery. Today, such malformations are especially important with regard to sedentary occupations or functions (e.g., long car drives, horseriding, cycling). Coccygodynia is a very frequent result.

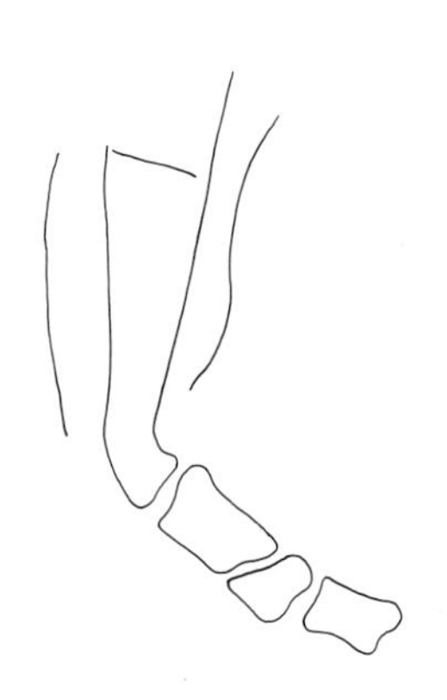

Fig. 420 shows one of the most frequent unusual shapes of the coccyx. Kinks, deformities of individual coccygeal vertebrae and lateral deviation of the end of the coccyx are frequent variants. See Fig. 443, No. 139.

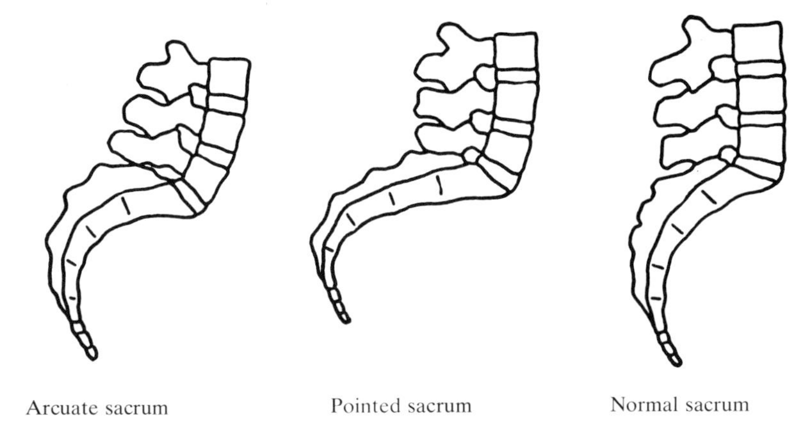

Fig. 421. Shapes of the sacrum
(according to *Scherb).*

The pointed and the arcuate sacrum are especially frequent with faulty posture. Early arthrotic changes of the small vertebral joints in the lower lumbar region are characteristic of the pointed sacrum. For measuring the lumbosacral angle, see Fig. 409.

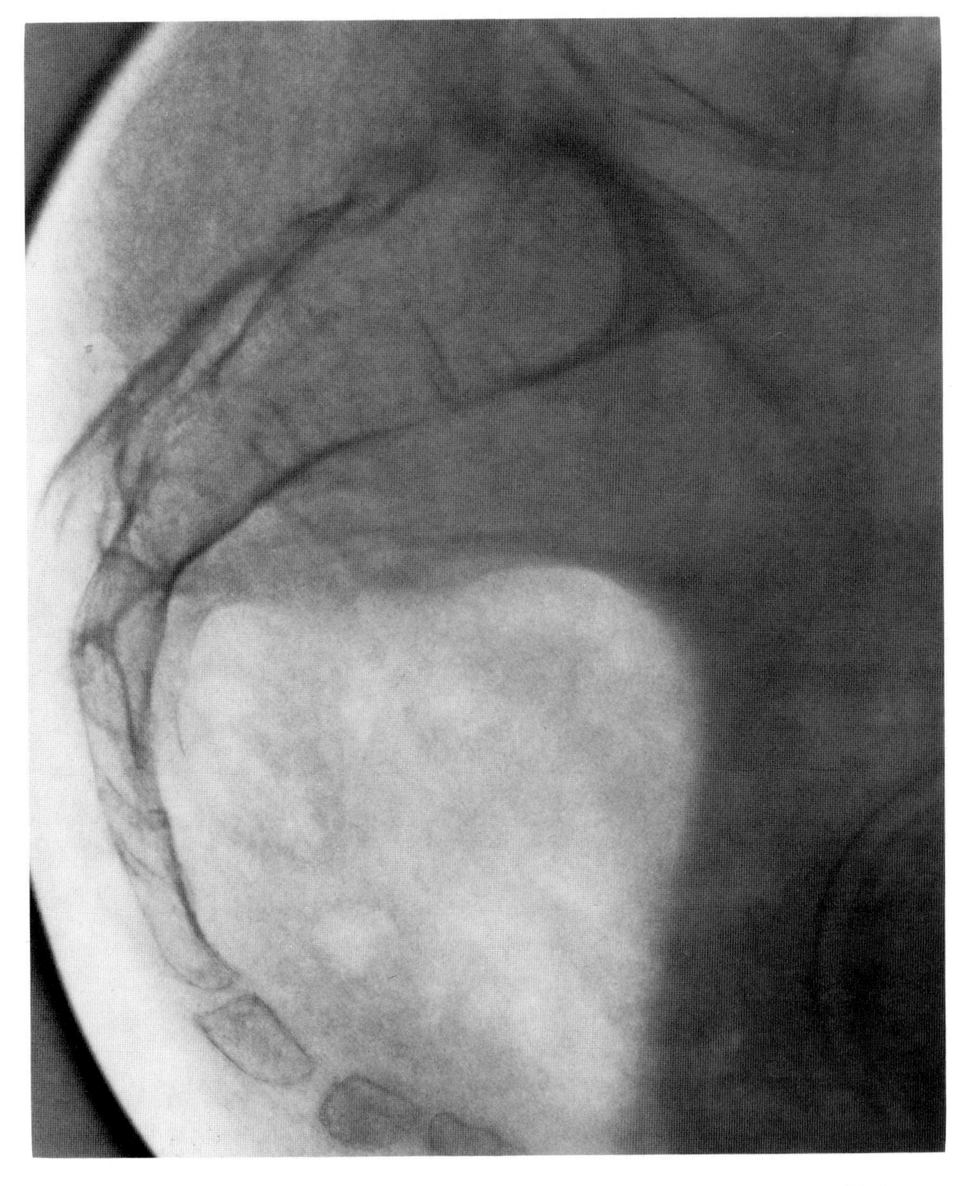

Fig. 422. "Cyst-like" appearance of the auricular surface of the sacrum. Arcuate sacrum with fracture-like kink.

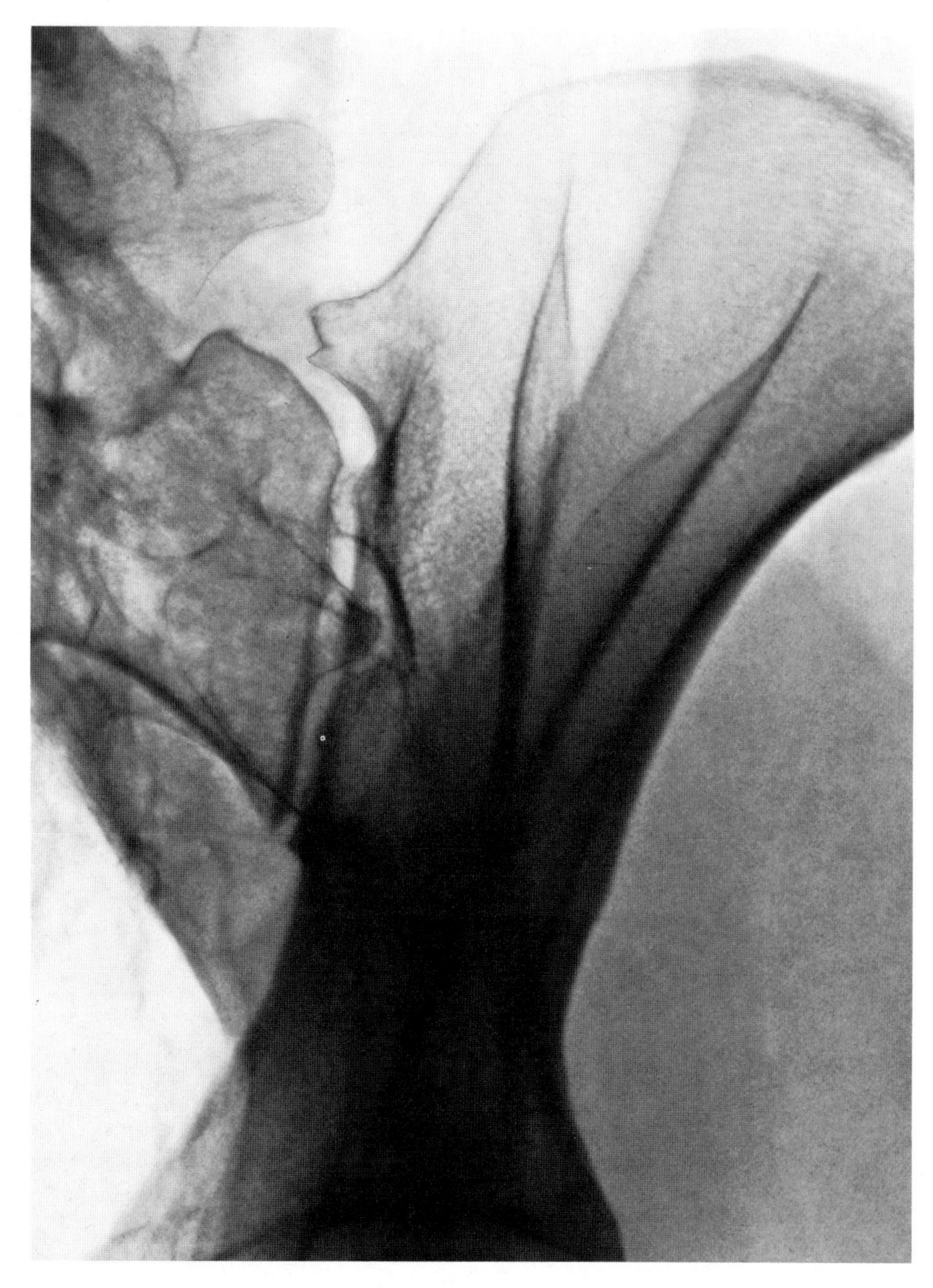

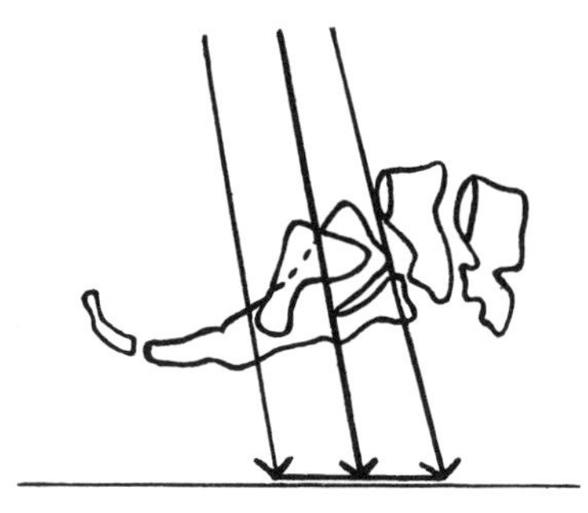

Fig. 424 a

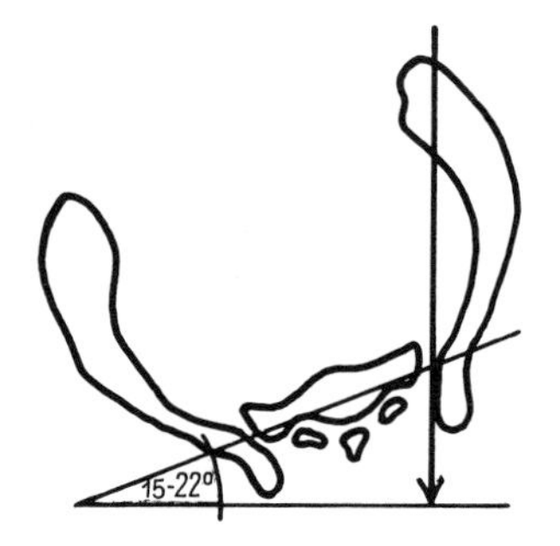

Fig. 424 b

Fig. 424. The central ray is directed cranially by 10–12°, and the patient is lifted by 15–22° off the side to be examined.

Fig. 423. Demonstration of the sacroiliac joint, according to *von Kovács*. For projection see Fig. 242. The sacroiliac articulation consists of three unequal parts, lying in different planes *(Cohen)*. The cranial parts of both sides are parallel to the axis of the sacrum but diverge forward. The larger middle parts always converge caudally, and often also forward. The caudal parts are almost always parallel to the sagittal plane. Depending on the direction of the projection and the extent of the lumbar lordosis, different views of the articular spaces are obtained. Tomography of the sacroiliac joints is very suitable as a supplement to the usual summary radiographs. By this method, the topical relations of zones of increased and reduced density to the articular space can be defined more exactly. The essential indications for this method are consequences of weight bearing (kyphoscoliosis, *Pauwels*) at the sacroiliac joints, condensing iliac osteitis, *Bechterew's* disease and sacroiliac tuberculosis *(Frik* and *Hesse)*.

The roentgenologic conception of sacroiliac arthritis denotes the results of chronic inflammatory processes in that joint. It occurs most frequently in *Bechterew's* disease. As this joint possesses only limited mobility and takes a very variable course, the early roentgenologic changes (about 70% of the juvenile *Bechterew* cases start with sacroiliac arthritis) are of special importance. On the other hand, there are no characteristic X-ray symptoms for *Bechterew's* disease. Sacroiliac arthritis takes a course similar to chronic polyarthritis, with beginning para-articular osteoporosis and inflammatory destruction and, finally, proliferative reaction. The degeneration of the joint, the sacroiliac arthrosis, with often much widened articular space, is more frequent; it often arises unilaterally and is always accompanied by band-like marginal sclerosis and debris cysts.

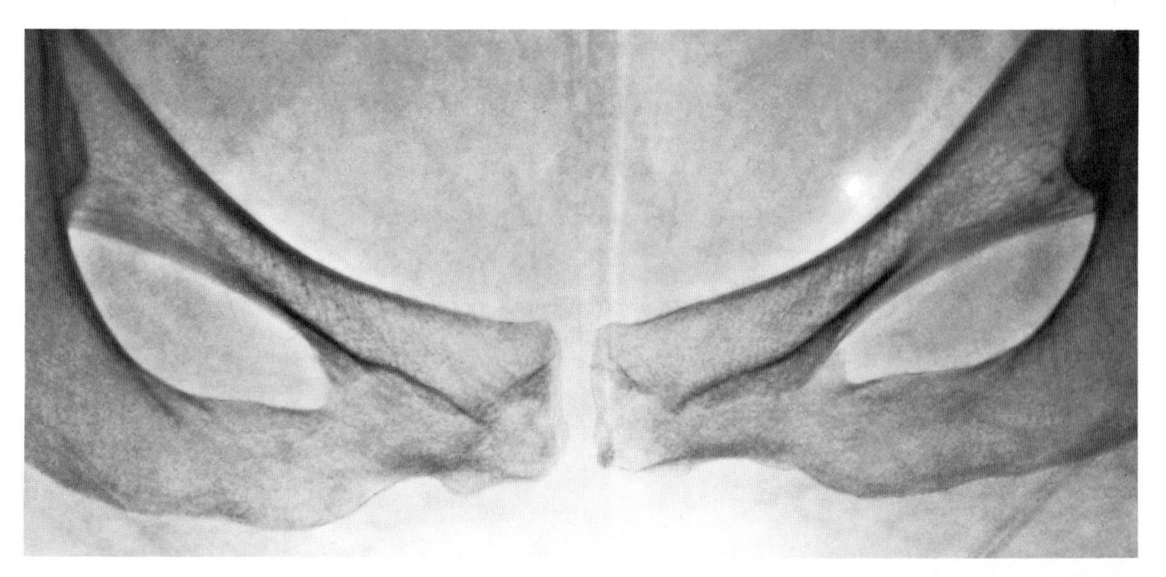

Fig. 425. Pubis, posteroanterior. Position: prone, the central ray aimed in the median plane at the symphysis at an angle of 10° caudocranial (see Fig. 426). The thickening of the medial lower rim on the right is a sign of sclerosis of the spongy substance with pseudocystic increased radiolucency. In addition, there is a widening of the symphyseal cleft. Such degenerative changes occur most frequently after traumata during confinement or after fractures of the pelvic girdle.

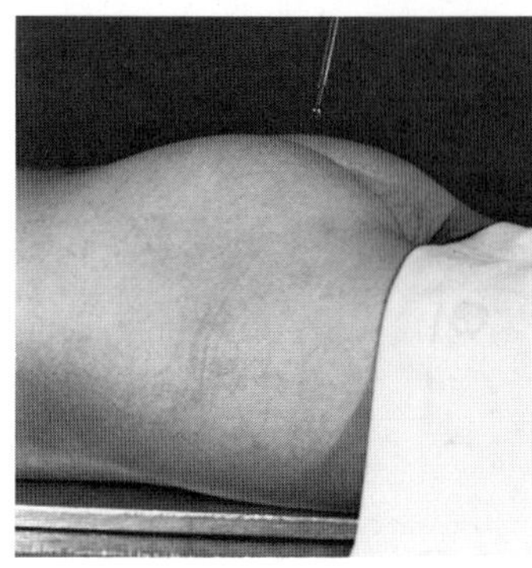

Fig. 426

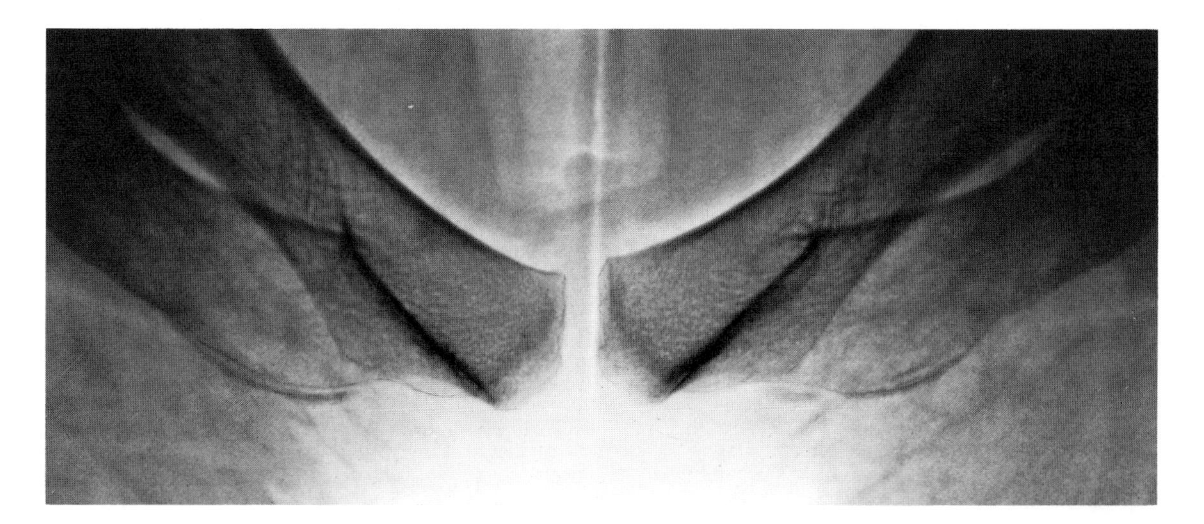

Fig. 427. Symphysis, axial. The central ray is aimed in the median plane vertically onto the symphysis. For position see Fig. 428. Irregular contours and variants of shape are normal. The width of the symphyseal cleft is about 5–6 mm, 10 mm still being normal. Comparatively frequently (about 20%), there is an uneven height of the symphysis; it occurs mainly with loosening of the pelvic girdle (*Kamieth* and *Reinhardt*). In accordance with the laws of central projection, the symphyseal cleft appears wider here as it is film-distant. The slight step formation at the upper edge suggests a real widening of the cleft (symphysiolysis) in this case.

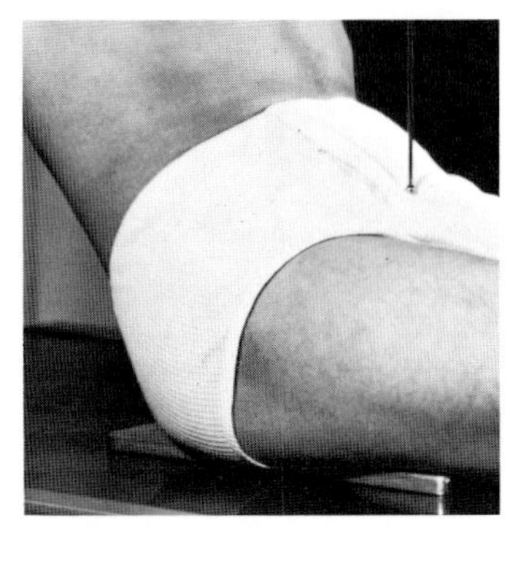

Fig. 428

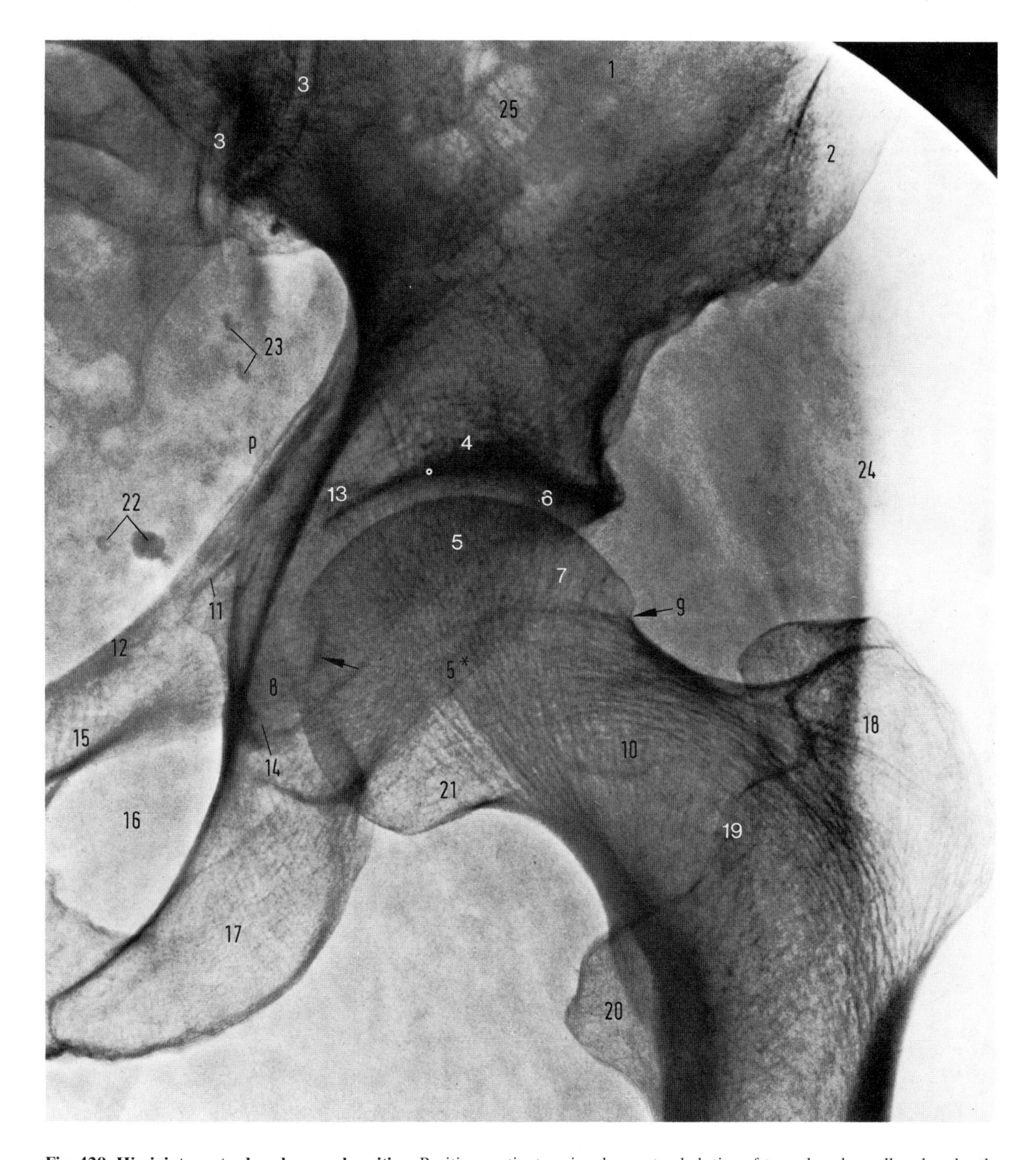

Fig. 429. Hip joint, ventrodorsal, normal position. Position: patient supine, legs extended, tips of toes closed, small pad under the knees. The central ray is beamed vertically, slightly lateral from the middle of the inguinal ligament. With extreme outward rotation with bent hip *(Lauensteins*'s position), the phenomenon of vacuum may be produced due to the incongruity of the articular surfaces, described by the anatomist *R. Fick* in 1898. *Butt* and *Samuel* have dealt with the radiographic anatomy of the proximal end of the femur.

1 Ilium
2 Anterior superior iliac spine
3 Sacroiliac joint
4 Roof of acetabulum
5 Anterior rim of acetabulum
5* Posterior rim of acetabulum
6 "Articular space" – two layers of articular cartilage
7 Femoral head
8 Apparent widening of articular space
← Fovea of the head of the femur
9 Border between head and neck
10 Neck of femur
11 Ischial spine
12 Pecten pubis
13 Lateral line of pelvic wall (seen from the edge), passes into
14 *Koehler*'s teardrop sign
15 Pubis
16 Obturator foramen
17 Ischium
18 Greater trochanter
19 Intertrochanteric crest
20 Lesser trochanter
21 Brighter zone at the border between head and neck (normal)
22 Phleboliths
23 Calcification within the arterial pelvic blood vessels
24 Lateral edge of the gluteal musculature
25 Intestinal gases, not to be mistaken for osteolytic metastases
P Pseudoperiostitis

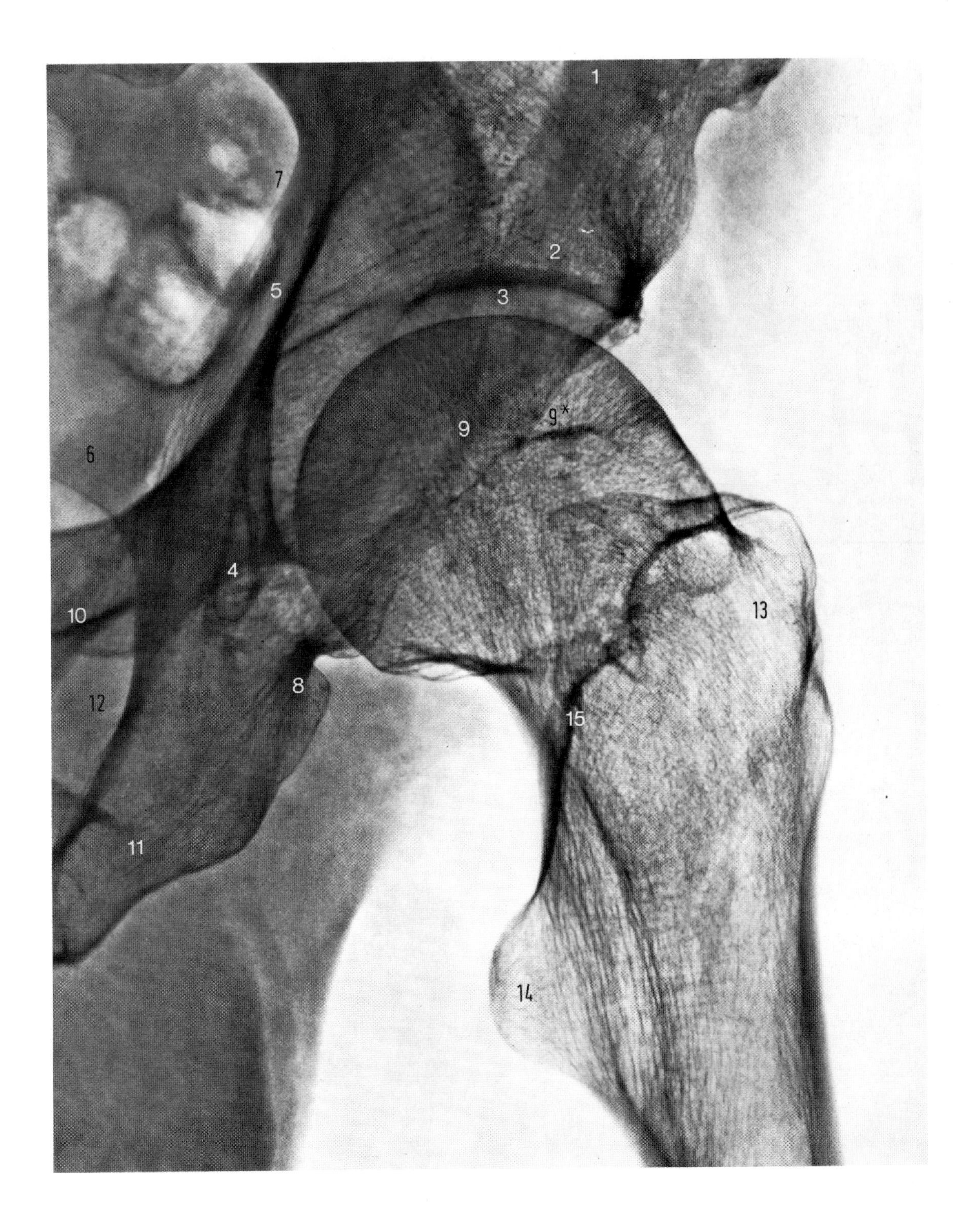

Fig. 430. Hip joint, ventrodorsal, in outward rotation. The outward rotation by the perspective shortening of the femoral neck and the heavy jutting out of the lesser trochanter are seen. See also Fig. 434.

1 Ilium
2 Upper rim of acetabulum, jutting out somewhat so that the head is well covered
3 "Articular space"; the line of the floor of the acetabulum is interrupted and its distance from the head is greater in the lower half
4 *Koehler*'s teardrop sign
5 Lateral pelvic wall
6 Ischial spine
7 Linea terminalis
8 Region of the ischial tuberosity
9 Anterior rim of acetabulum
9* Posterior rim of acetabulum (usually straighter)
10 Pubis
11 Superior ischial ramus
12 Obturator foramen
13 Greater trochanter
14 Lesser trochanter
15 Intertrochanteric line

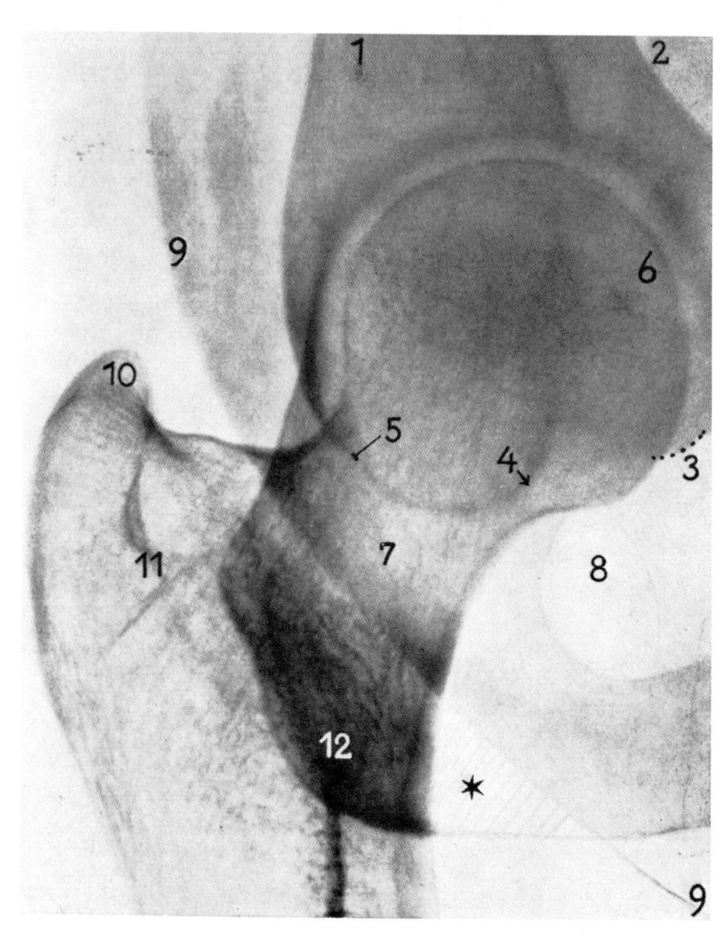

1 Ilium
2 Linea terminalis of pelvis
3 Anterior, 4 posterior rim of the acetabular notch
5 Posterior superior rim of acetabulum
6 Fovea capitis femoris
7 Neck of femur, acetabular part of the ischial rami and bulge of soft tissue
8 Obturator foramen
9 Contour of the gluteal region
10 Tip of greater trochanter
11 Intertrochanteric line
12 Ischial tuberosity; its shadow adds to the shadow of the femoral neck. A bright field (hatched) that lies outside the shadows of femur and gluteal regions follows.

Fig. 431. Right acetabulum shown in top view (plane of entrance into acetabulum runs parallel to the plane of the film); 35-year-old female.

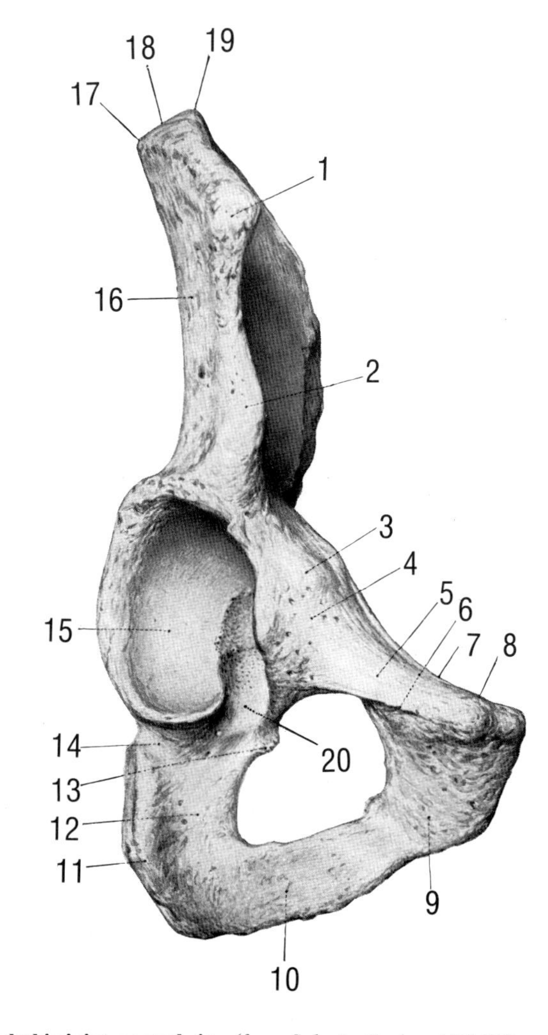

Fig. 433. Right hip joint, ventral view (from *Sobotta-Becher,* 15th Edition).

1 Anterior superior iliac spine
2 Anterior inferior iliac spine
3 Iliopectineal eminence
4 Body of pubis
5 Superior ramus of pubis
6 Obturator crest
7 Pecten of pubis
8 Pubic tubercle
9 Inferior ramus of pubis
10 Ramus of ischium
11 Ischial tuberosity
12 Body of ischium
13 Posterior obturator tubercle
14 Body of ischium
15 Acetabulum (lunate surface)
16 Iliac ala
17 Labium externum
18 Intermediate line
19 Labium internum
17–19 Iliac crest
20 Acetabular notch

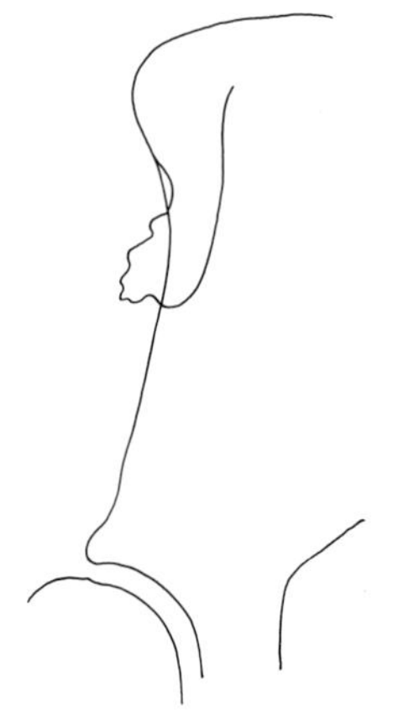

Fig. 432. Spiky exostoses at the anterior superior iliac spine. This sometimes forms a partial symptom of a generally "spiky pelvis." See Fig. 442, Nos. 122, 124, p. 198, 199.

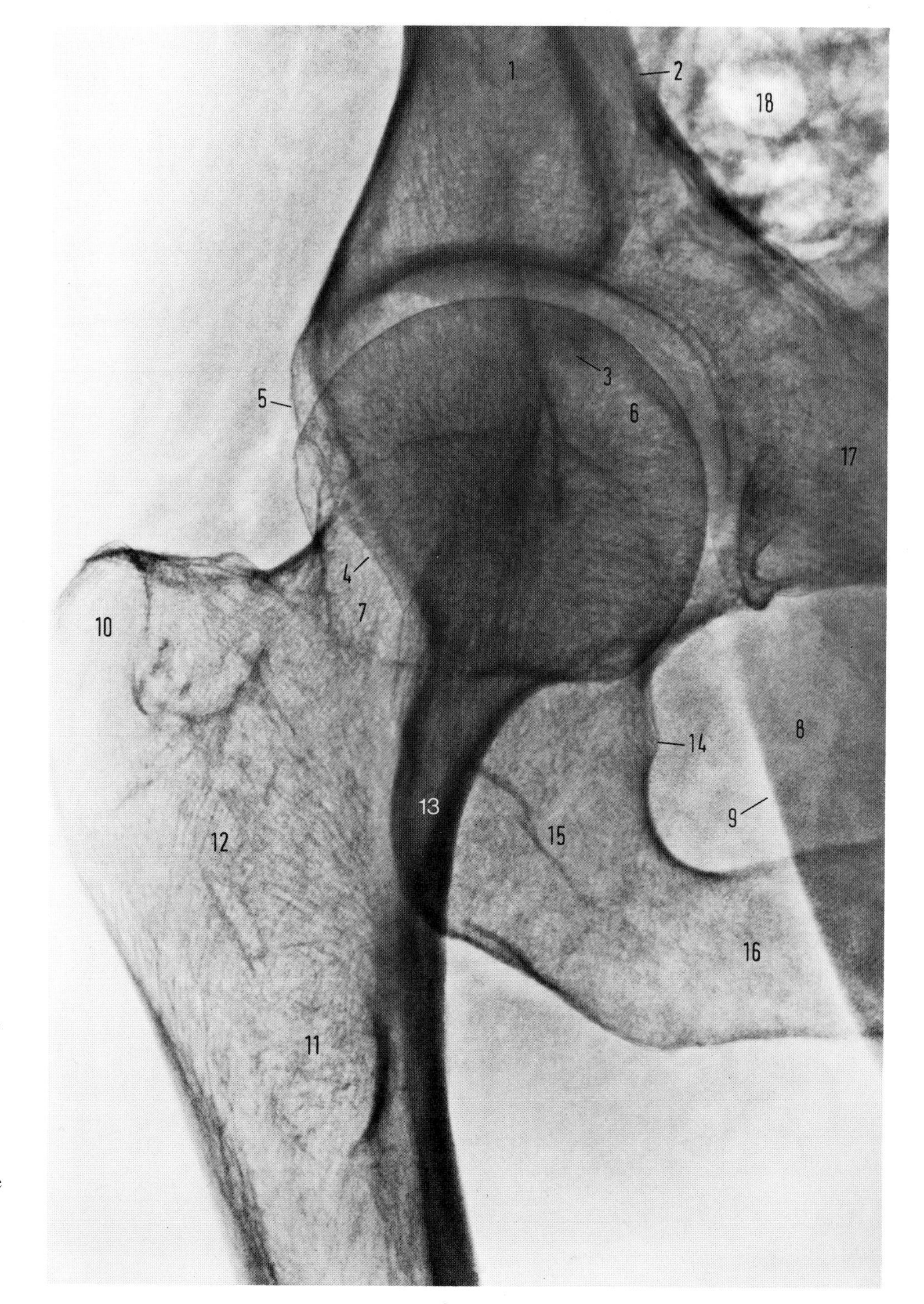

1 Ilium
2 Linea terminalis
3 Anterior margin of acetabulum
4 Posterior margin of acetabulum
5 Posterior superior margin of acetabulum
6 Fovea capitis fermoris
7 Neck of femur
8 Obturator foramen
9 Gluteal fold, contour of the opposite gluteus
10 Greater trochanter
11 Lesser trochanter, turned dorsally
12 Intertrochanteric crest
13 Tuberosity of ischium
14 Posterior obturator tubercle
15 Body of ischium
16 Ramus of ischium
17 Body of pubis
18 Intestinal gases

Fig. 434. Acetabulum, shown in top view. Position: patient prone, the healthy side lifted by about 50°. The central ray is aimed 12° cranial onto the film-near acetabulum. This radiograph allows a better view into the acetabulum; the posterior superior acetabular margin is shown especially well.

To Figs. 430 and 434.
The anterior margin and the posterior margin normally surround $^2/_3$ to $^4/_5$ of the femoral head. Its fixation in the acetabulum is achieved by the articular capsule and the strong ischiofemoral and pubofemoral ligaments and the iliofemoral ligament (Figs. 411 and 412). The capsule inserts at the acetabular rim and encloses the head down to the neck of the femur (Fig. 412). A shallow acetabulum (Fig. 430) predestinates for luxation; a deep acetabulum is often caused by protrusion of the acetabulum (see Fig. 490).

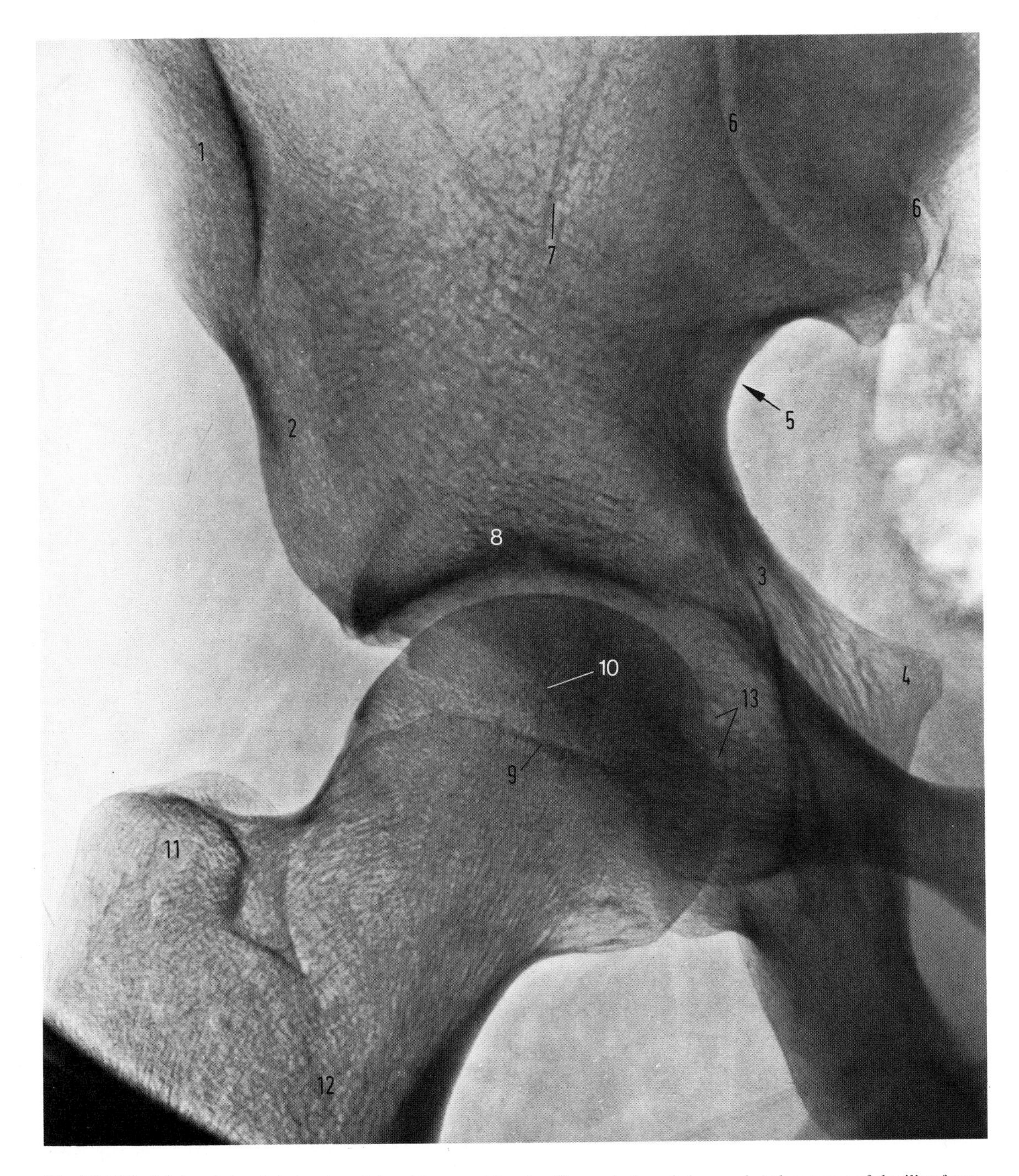

Fig. 435. Hip joint, pelvis rotated outward, in a 21-year-old male. The central ray is beamed at the center of the iliac fossa.

1 Anterior superior iliac spine
2 Anterior inferior iliac spine
3 Wall of the lesser pelvis
4 Ischial spine
5 Greater sciatic notch (↖)
6 Sacroiliac joint
7 Nutritive canal (sometimes Y-shaped); see Fig. 442 (n)
8 Roof of acetabulum
9 Anterior rim of acetabulum
10 Posterior rim of acetabulum
11 Greater trochanter
12 Intertrochanteric crest
13 Cyst-like artifacts

According to *Zseböck,* the intracapsular position of the femoral head and neck conditions the intracapsular fractures of the neck of the femur and also, in juveniles, the intracapsular epiphysiolyses; the blood supply is worsened by the intracapsular position. The blood vessels run partly from the diaphysis, partly through the ligamentum teres femoris into the interior of the head and neck. As the vessels of the ligamentum teres femoris, which reach into the acetabular fossa, often close with advancing age, one of the causes for the poor healing of fractures of the femoral neck in the aged can be seen here.

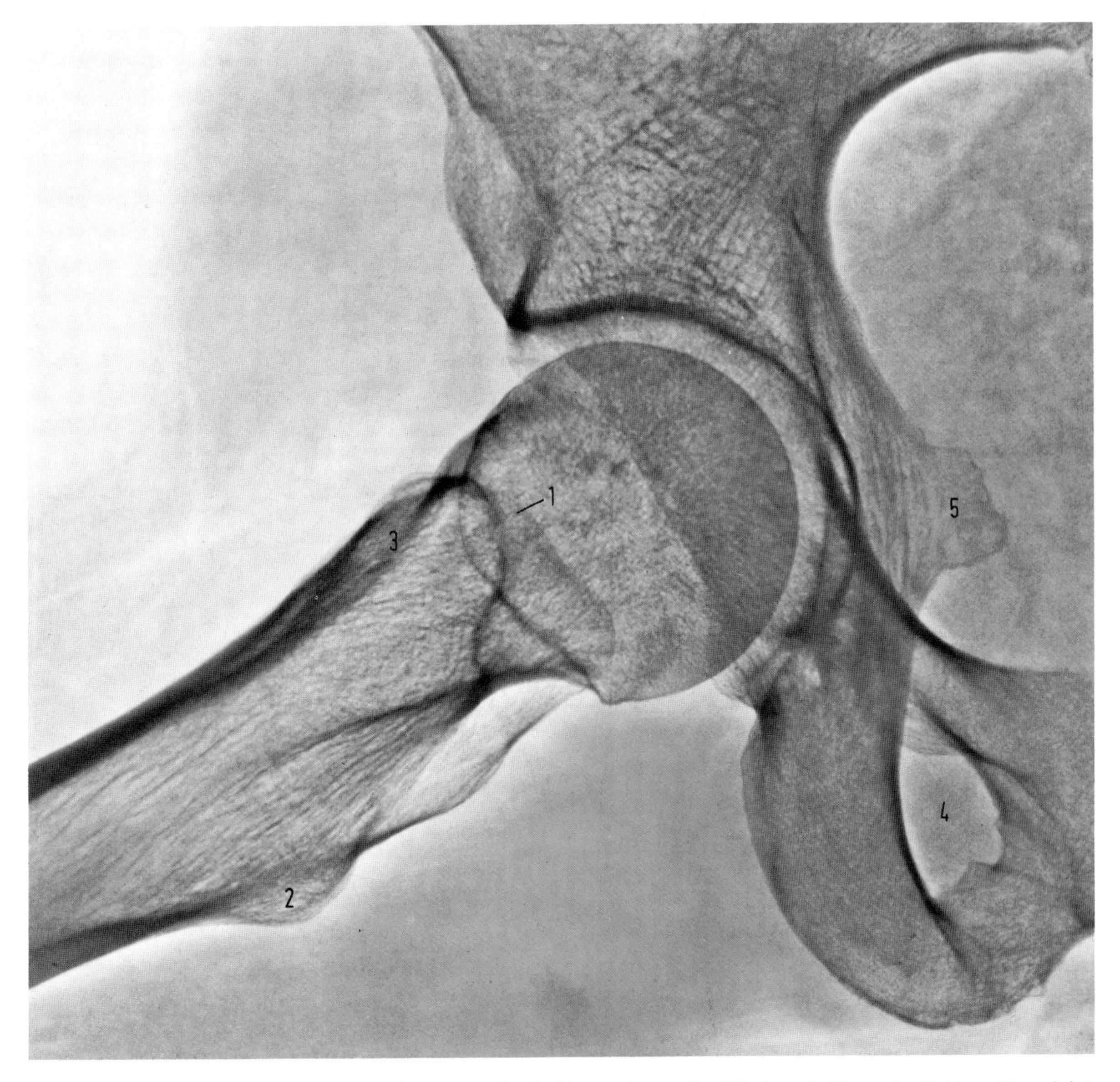

Fig. 436. Hip joint, in flexion and abduction, after *Lauenstein.* Position: patient supine. The leg to be X-rayed, with hip and knee joints bent, is rotated so far outward that it lies with its lateral surface on the film; the healthy pelvic half and the healthy leg are to be slightly lifted. The central ray is aimed vertically onto the middle of the groin (see Fig. 437). In this position, an incongruity of the articular surfaces may occur which will cause a vacuum phenomenon, rarely found in the hip *(Seyss).*

1 Tip of greater trochanter
2 Lesser trochanter
3 Dorsal surface of femoral neck
4 Obturator foramen
5 Ischial spine, much broadened by ossification of the insertion of the sacrospinous ligament. This occurs with tearing out of the ligament or by a partial tear, as well as in fluorosis. Ossification of the whole ligament has also been described as an anomaly *(Busch).* For the significance of this in obstetrics and gynecology, see also Fig. 411.

Fig. 437

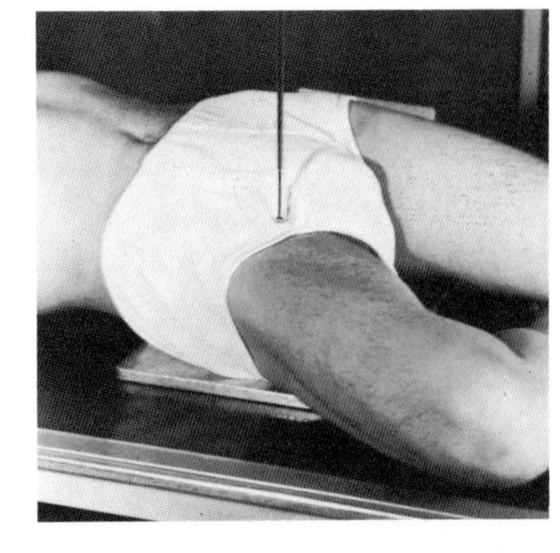

This radiograph is well suited for an early diagnosis of epiphysiolysis of the femoral head *(Esser)* for example. *Bernbeck* recommends a special exposure for radiologic diagnosis of torsion of the femur in luxated hips, with bending of the hip at right angles and with maximal internal rotation and abduction of the legs. Through this technique, anteroposterior curvings of the femoral neck and forward or backward shifts of the head of the femur can also be seen.

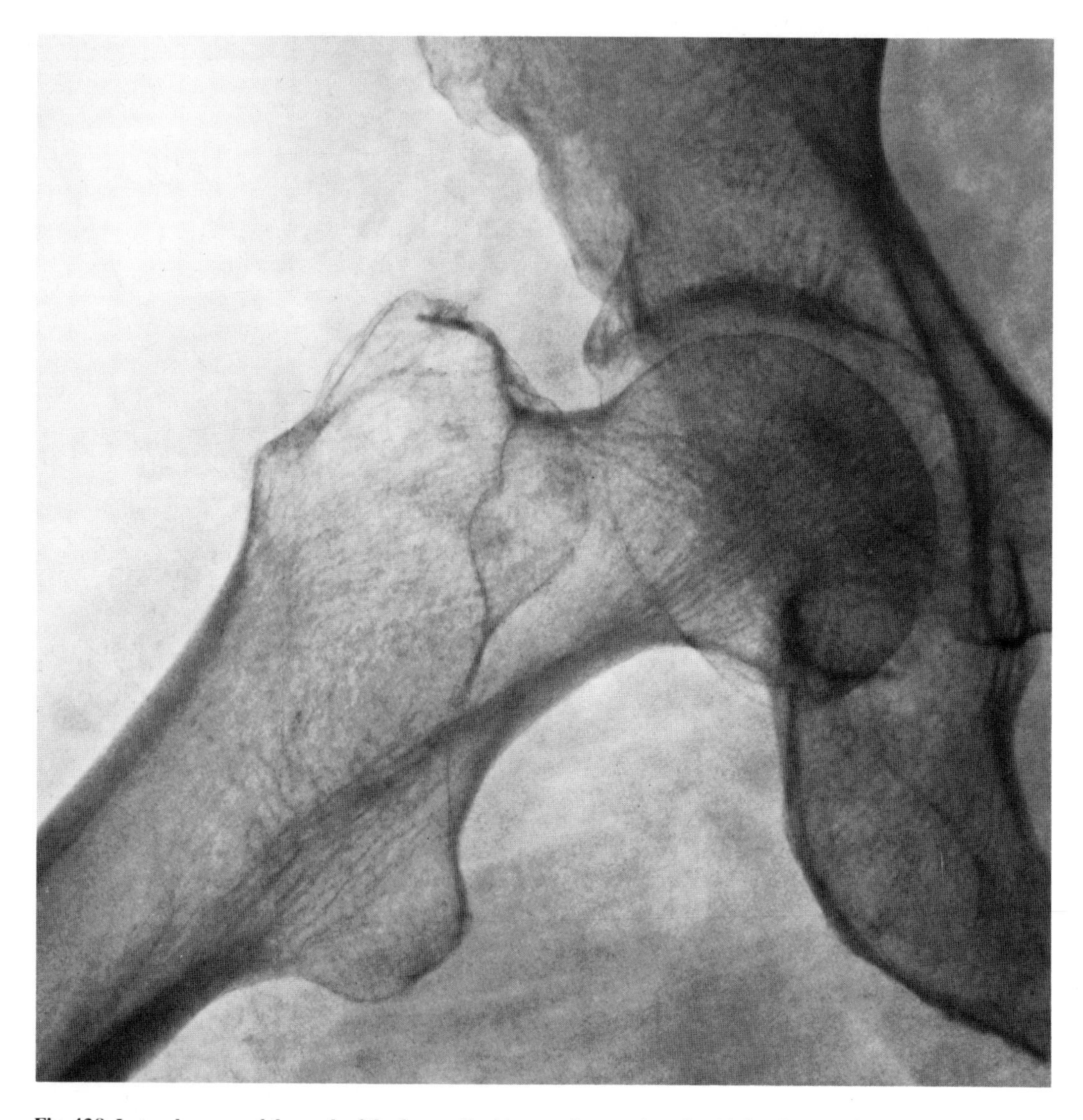

Fig. 438. Lateral survey of the neck of the femur. Position: patient supine; the thigh to be examined is abducted at 45° and lifted 60°. The central ray is directed 15° caudally onto the center of the femoral neck. In this position superimposition of the two trochanters is avoided. In this way even delicate fissures in the femoral neck become visible. Simulated holes in the femoral head may be mimicked by the lower border of the acetabulum, by a marked posterior rim of the ascending ramus of the ischim or, at the ramus of the ischium, by a coarseness for muscular insertion.

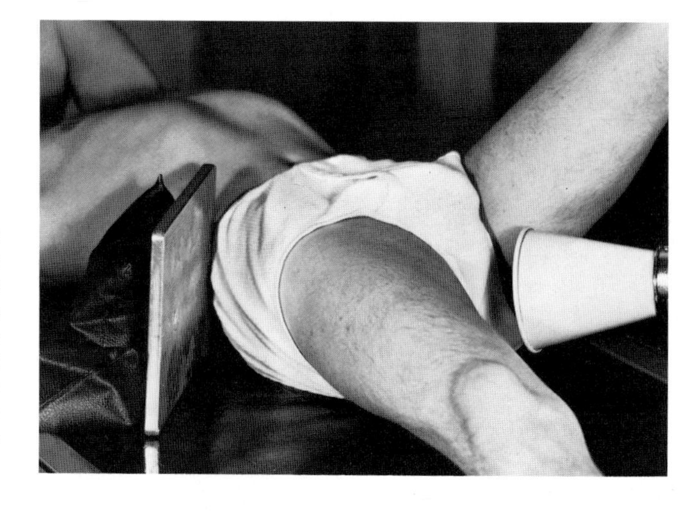

Fig. 439. Axial demonstration of the hip joint. Position: patient supine; the leg to be examined is laterally abducted, the healthy leg is lifted. The cassette is pressed between pelvic crest and costal arch, parallel to the axis of the femoral neck. The central ray is aimed at the inner side of the thigh to be examined, into the groin (gonads radioprotection). This radiograph will ascertain any displacement of fragments or kinking of the axis in fractures of the neck of the femur. In cases of impacted fractures, their age can be determined by means of this radiograph; furthermore, it is suitable for analysis of faulty positions (coxa vara or valga).

1 Profunda femoris artery
2 Femoral artery,
3 Lateral femoral circumflex artery; on this view it somewhat winds at first in a cranial direction and then laterally; it arises from the first part of the profunda femoris artery
4 Ischial tuberosity, with ossification of the insertion of the adductor magnus muscle

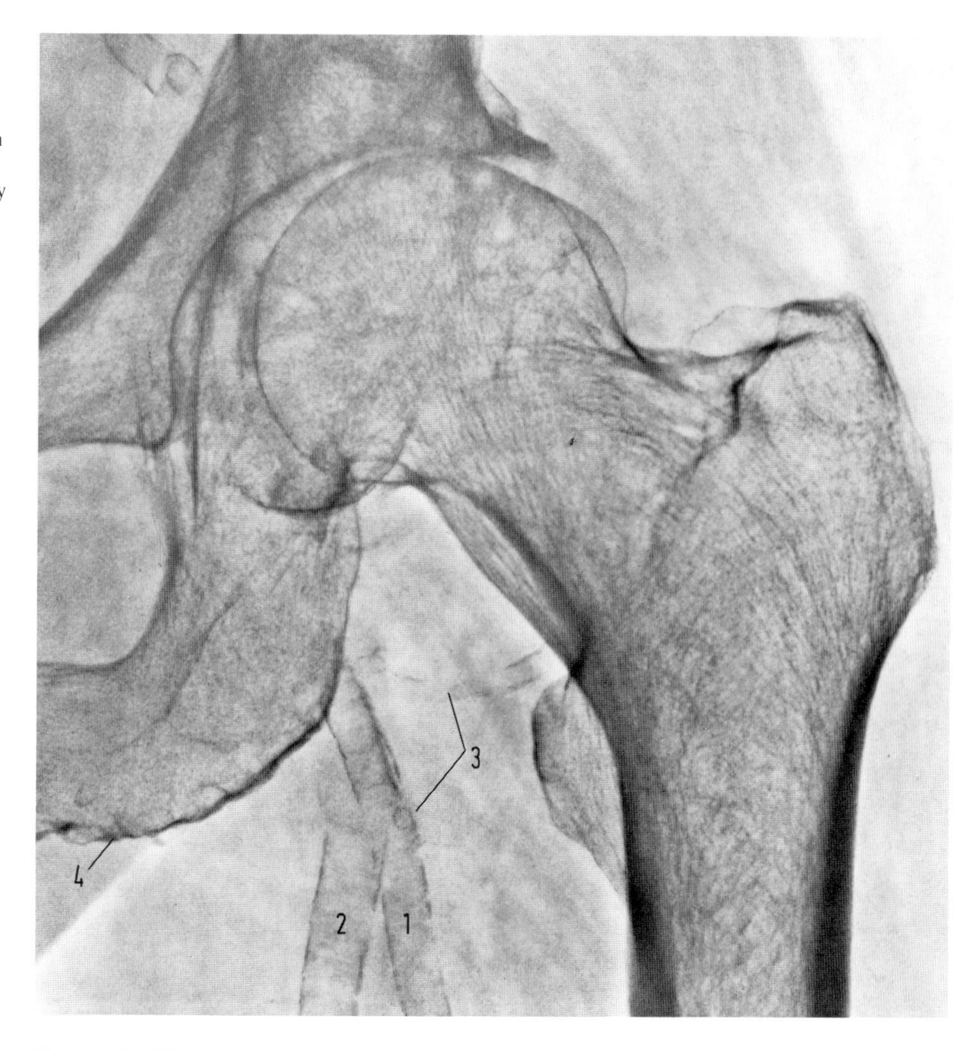

Fig. 440. Calcified arteries of pelvis and thigh in a 73-year-old female. Apart from atrophy of bones (osteoporosis of involution) due to advanced age, there is an arthrosis of the left hip joint with much narrowing of the articular space in its upper region. The femoral head is flattened and contains vacuolar zones of reconstruction (see Fig. 442, No. 132).

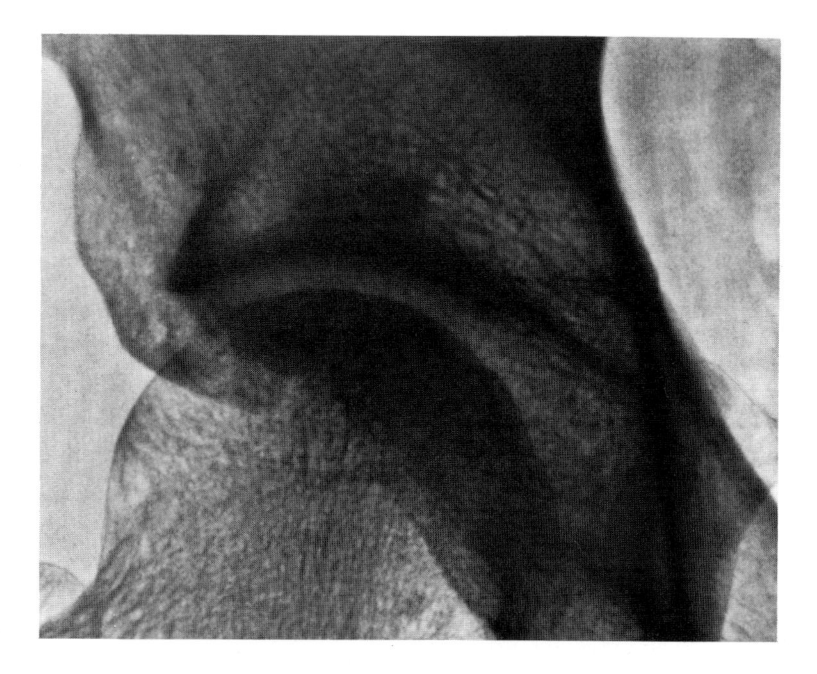

Fig. 441. Exostosis-shaped bony bulge at the upper rim of the right hip joint in the region of the anterior inferior iliac spine (from the collection of *W. Werner,* Berlin). Generally, the exostoses at the anterior inferior iliac spine are peg-like and conical. The spine has its own apophyseal nucleus and sometimes also has a few accessory nuclei. Therefore, difficulties of differential diagnosis, i. e., to distinguish them from aseptic bone necroses or tear-off fractures during adolescence (tear-off of the rectus femoris muscle), may arise. Because several nuclei may be present, a great variability of exostosis-like bony protrusions may be encountered. In this case, fusion of the exostotic bulge with the apophysis of the acetabular rim is still possible. Exostosis-like ossifications of the lower acetabular rim are more frequent, especially as a consequence of coxarthroses. From the anterior inferior iliac spine, the strongest ligament of the body, the iliofemoral ligament, arises directly from the bone (see Fig. 412). It supposedly ossifies, but the very sparse literature on the subject does not clarify this point.

Variants and Sources of Diagnostic Error of the Lumbar Spine, Pelvis and Hip Joint*

To Figs. 442 and 443:

51 Peg-shaped ossification of the tip of the 12th rib; embedded calcifications as a symptom of general degeneration; simulation of a pathological process in the 12th rib by superimposed, calcified anterior costal cartilage.

51* Independent nucleus of ossification (not to be mistaken for a kidney stone in cases of a short rib)

99 Separation of margin of vertebra (see Figs. 389–391). This rarely occurs on a traumatic basis; no disturbance of ossification of the epiphyses of the vertebral body; prolapse of disk into the cancellous tissue

100 Shrunken or underdeveloped presacral disk

101 Nodule of *Schmorl,* found mainly dorsally in the base of the vertebral body (prolapsed nucleus)

102 Deforming spondylosis (Figs. 380, 390); the most frequent degenerative indication of "wear and tear"

103 Ossification in the annulus fibrosus (Fig. 393); to be differentiated from separation of the vertebral margin (see No. 99)

104 Calcification within the nucleus pulposus (Figs. 392, 393)

105 Independent apophysis of spinous process; see Fig. 463 b. This appears between ages 11 and 14, and fuses around age 25; may be mistaken for a fracture or for calcification of soft tissues.

106 Joint-like approximation of spinous processes of the lower lumbar spine *(Baastrup, Schumann* and *Trautmann);* see Fig. 446

107 *Hahn's* vascular canal in juveniles; occurs only isolated in the adult, on a single or on several vertebrae (see Fig. 332 a)

108 Massive ledge of transverse process, sometimes with bridge or pseudoarticular space; see Fig. 456. To be differentiated from late traumatic and inflammatory-degenerative changes.

108* Isolated transverse process or rudimentary rib (see Figs. 396, 452); if unilateral, may simulate a fracture (excluded by its smooth border)

109 Cleft in the spinous process of L I. For details on cleft formations see Figs. 384, 459.

110 Styloid process (see Figs. 455, 460 and 462); elongated accessory process

111 Spaces of the intervertebral articulations, vertical and curved (see Figs. 396, 402); frequently very asymmetrical

111* Mamillary process (above) i.e. inconstant accessory nucleus during 11th to 14th years of life; if persistent, may simulate a fracture. Accessory process (below)

112 Cleft formation in the lower articular process of L II (see also Figs. 470 a, 461). It represents mostly a persistent apophysis; differential diagnosis for fracture or calcification of the capsula. *Ravelli,* among others, reported on malformations at arches and articular processes; *Pfeiffer* described persistent apophyses of the articular processes of the lumbar vertebrae.

112* Hole-like increased radiolucencies in the lower vertebral bodies, mainly bilateral and symmetrical *(Reinhardt);* see also Fig. 470 b

113 Cleft formation in vertebral arch (interarticular part). This disposes to spondolisthesis, most frequently in the 5th, more rarely in the 4th lumbar vertebrae (see *Schmorl-Junghanns, Brocher* and Fig. 471); oblique radiographs are required.

114 Asymmetrical closure of arch, easily mistaken for a fracture; should not be confused with spina bifida (see Figs. 470 a, 457, 458 and 466)

115 Complete transverse cleft in the sacrum, having the appearance of a branching-off of the sacroiliac joint, with assimilation of L V onto the sacrum (sacralized 5th lumbar vertebra); see Fig. 470; occurs especially in case of a transitional lumbosacral vertebra

115* Accessory sacroiliac joint (see Fig. 451); not infrequently arthrotic

116 Ossified iliolumbar ligament (see Fig. 446 and Fig. 411); quite asymmetrical; inflammatory processes and constitutional anomalies of development (e.g., ossification occurs even in youth) must be assumed as causes of ossification

116* Start of ossification of the iliolumbar ligament (see Figs. 446 and 411)

117 Edge of psoas muscle (see Figs. 396, 455); pseudofracture, pseudoapophyses

118 Outer edge of erector spinae muscle

118* Outer edge of quadratus lumborum muscle (see Fig. 448)

119 Lengthened sacral hiatus; cleft in sacrum (see Fig. 469)

120 Paraglenoid sulcus of ilium and sacrum (see Fig. 450 a, b); preformed spur, but no ossification of insertion; should not be mistaken for arthrotic spikes. *Cuveland,* as well as *Doesel* described an abnormal process at the same spot without paraglenoid sulcus.

121 Lateral sacral cleft, i.e., missing of the lateral wall of a sacral foramen (see Fig. 414); should not be confused with infraction

122 Ischial tuberosity (see Figs. 436, 440) where the musculus adductor magnus arises

122* Calcified sacrotuberous ligament (see *P. Fischer; Teichert,* 1957; *Thamm;* and Figs. 411, 412

122** Exostosis of musculus gracilis (see Fig. 500); if unilateral, may be mistaken for an osseus sarcoma. A gracilis syndrome may arise, either acute (by overexertion, e.g., extreme abduction in sportsmen or in women during labor, a painful condition at the insertion of the tendon) or chronic (erosion of the margin of the bone becoming visible on the radiograph at this localization). Also, a post-traumatic ischiopubic osteochondrosis may occur at this spot.

123 Symphysis (Figs. 410, 425, 427, 498 and 501). Irregular contours and variants of shape are normal; unequal height of the symphysis occurs mainly with loosening of the pelvic girdle. Next to it, the gluteal fold (W).

123* Bony bridge of symphysis (see Fig. 498); on calcification in the symphyseal cartilage, see *Hilliger* and *Schwenkenbecher.* As with changes in the intervertebral disks, degenerative and senile changes also arise in the symphysis and its surroundings, e.g., streaky, spotty calcifications, ossifications and bridge formations (Fig. 498), as well as vacuolar, sclerosing and ankylosing processes (Fig. 499 b).

123** Isolated bony nucleus at the lower end of the symphyseal cleft (see also *Kuehne*); differential diagnosis for post-traumatic osteochondrotic necrosis of the cartilage (e.g., in football players) or simple splintered fracture (Fig. 501)

124 Spikes at the obturator foramen; sometimes part of a "spiky pelvis." Ossification of the tendinous insertion of the obturator externus muscle. A spiky anterior and posterior obturator tubercle is also observed (see *Seyss* and p. 218 f).

* The letters in heavy type are to be found also (or only) on the lateral view (Fig. 443).

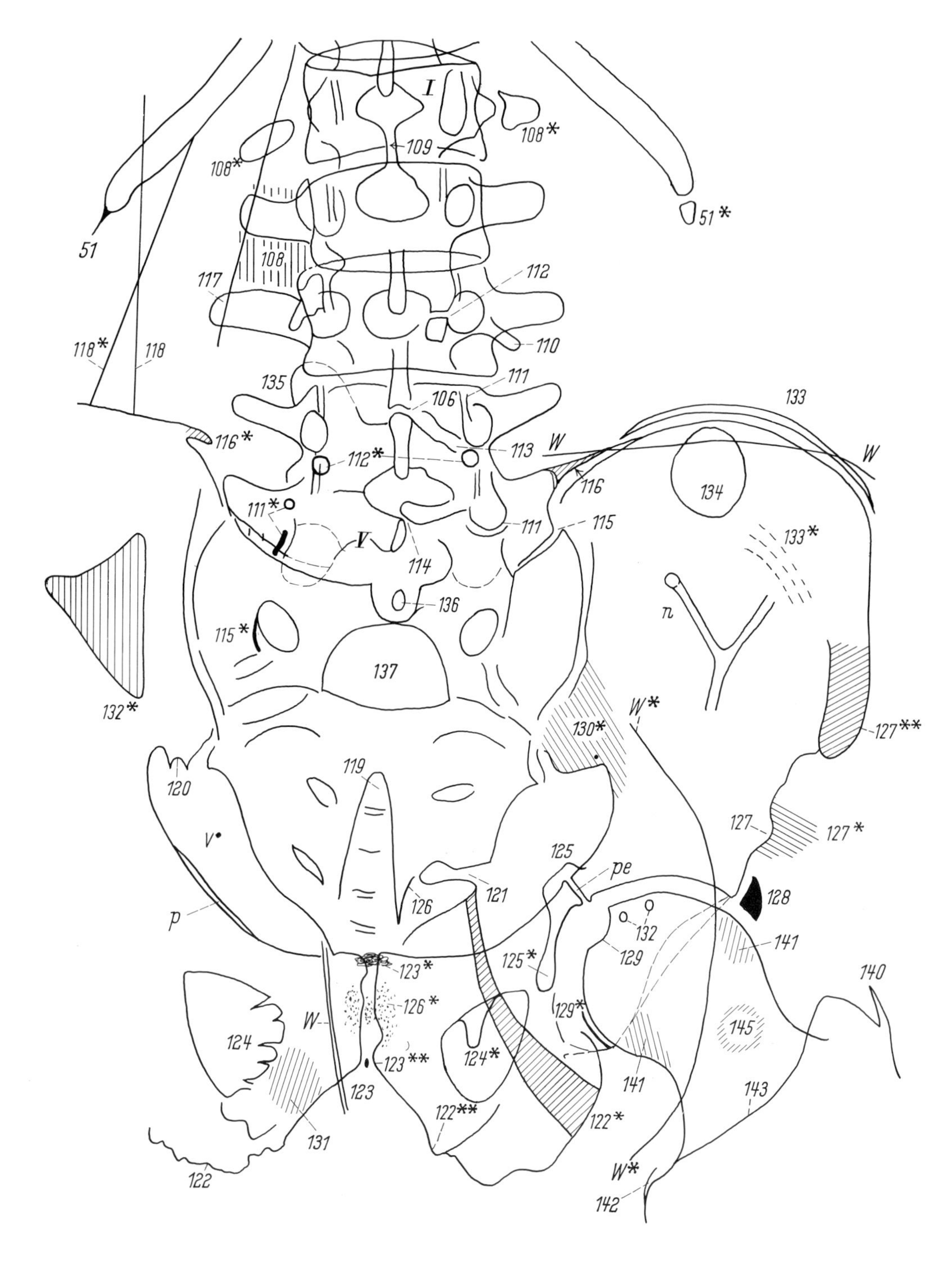

Fig. 442. Variants and sources of diagnostic error of lumbar spine, pelvis and hip joint.

W — Gluteal fold

WW — Soft tissue contour, upper edge of gluteal region

W*W* — Contour of the soft tissues lying on the support (see Fig. 429)

pe — Persistent Y-cleft (see *Schönreich);* closes normally during puberty; standard deviation up to age 17 (Fig. 1142)

p — Pseudoperiostitis (or pseudocallus) (Fig. 429)

V — Phlebolith (Fig. 429)

n — Nutritive canal in ilium (see Fig. 479)

124* — Unusual shape of an anterior obturator tubercle (see *Maurer* and p. 218 f, also *Rokay* and *Horváth)*

125 — Broadened ischial spine (see Fig. 410)

125* — *Köhler's* teardrop (see Fig. 430); drop-shaped elongated figure from structures of the acetabular floor (due to projection)

126 — Calcified seminal ducts (Figs. 444 and 445) occur as senile changes or because of chronic inflammation (e.g., gonorrhea, tuberculosis) or diabetes

126* — Calcium formation in the prostate (see Fig. 499)

(continued on p. 200)

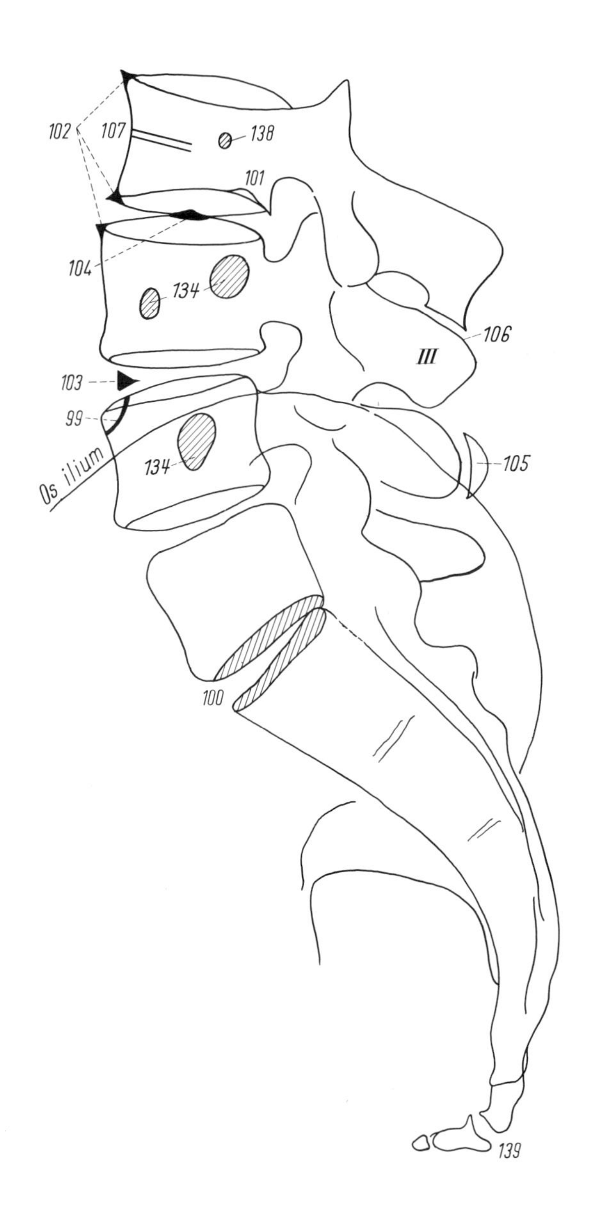

Fig. 443. Variants and sources of diagnostic error of lumbar spine and sacrum.

127 Anterior inferior iliac spine (Fig. 435, see also Fig. 441); medial from it, an atrophic zone

127* Ossification within the iliofemoral ligament (see Figs. 411, 412)

127** Calcified origin of ligament (inguinal ligament) on the anterior superior iliac spine; this is a preferential locus for bone metastases (see Fig. 411)

128 Bone next to acetabulum (see Fig. 485, also Fig. 487); may be a traumatic splintering-off, arthrotic osteophytes, zones of reconstruction or a post-traumatic metaplastic ossification with deforming arthrosis

129 Fovea capitis femoris; may simulate a focus of increased radiolucency in the femoral head *(Ueberschaer)* when taken with the *Lauenstein* technique (see also Fig. 434)

129* Acetabular notch (see Fig. 431)

130* Condensing iliitis, (Iliitis condensans), often presenting more extensively as sacroiliitis; arises mainly as bilateral sclerosis of the spongy bone tissue, with enriched calcium content, and occurs more often in females, perhaps as a consequence of pregnancy (Figs. 482, 483)

131 Normal increased radiolucency at the border between sacrum and ischium; here stress fractures may occur, as well as a harmless chondropathy (Fig. 500)

132 Vacuole-like "zone of reconstruction," especially in deforming arthrosis (see Fig. 440)

132* Iliac horn (see Figs. 482, 483 and 484); exostosis on the outer pelvic wall. In this drawing, unilateral *(Birkner),* but mostly symmetrical; dominantly hereditary, no prevalence by sex.

133 Apophysis at the iliac crest (Fig. 396); occurs in juveniles up to the age of 25. Until now, a persistent apophysis has been described only once, by *J. Petersen.* May be mistaken for an atraumatic ossification at the insertion of soft tissues.

133* Remnants of metal-containing injections

134 Spots of intestinal gases (see Figs. 429 and 434); should not be mistaken for osteolytic metastases or calcified shadows after subcutaneous injection

135 Simulated clamp formation, by sideways-projected articular processes; may occur on asymmetrical projection or in scoliosis

136 Isolated apophysis of the (absent) spinous process of the 1st sacral vertebra; arose from an accessory bony nucleus (see Fig. 457)

137 Projection in transverse section of the upper sacral vertebrae, seen especially on projection at a higher level or in hyperlordosis (see Fig. 469)

138 Kidney stone, simulating calcified osseus tumor

139 Normal shape of coccyx, very variable (see Fig. 421 and Figs. 410, 419)

140 Spur on trochanter; calcification of insertion of glutaeus medius muscle (Fig. 438)

141 Normal zones of lesser calcium content; in these, bony atrophy is recognizable early

142 Spur on the lesser trochanter, an ossified insertion of soft tissues; should not be mistaken for a persistent accessory nucleus (Fig. 778)

143 Intertrochanteric crest (see Figs. 429, 430)

145 "Ring shadow" (if a cyst is suspected, tomography should be used), without pathological significance (see also Fig. 438)

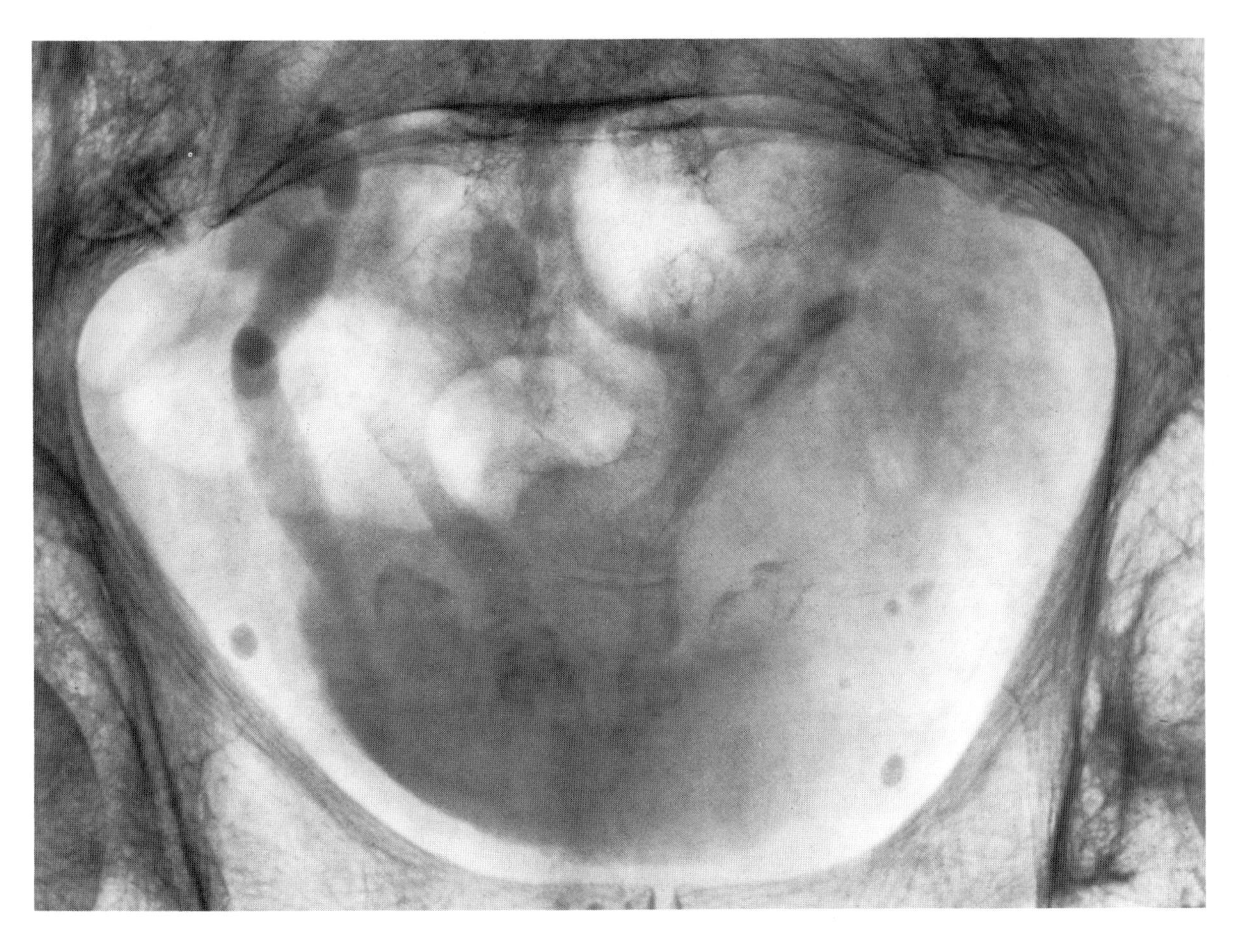

Fig. 444. Calcification of both ejaculatory ducts, with seminal vesiculae and concurrent contrast demonstration of a right hydroureter.

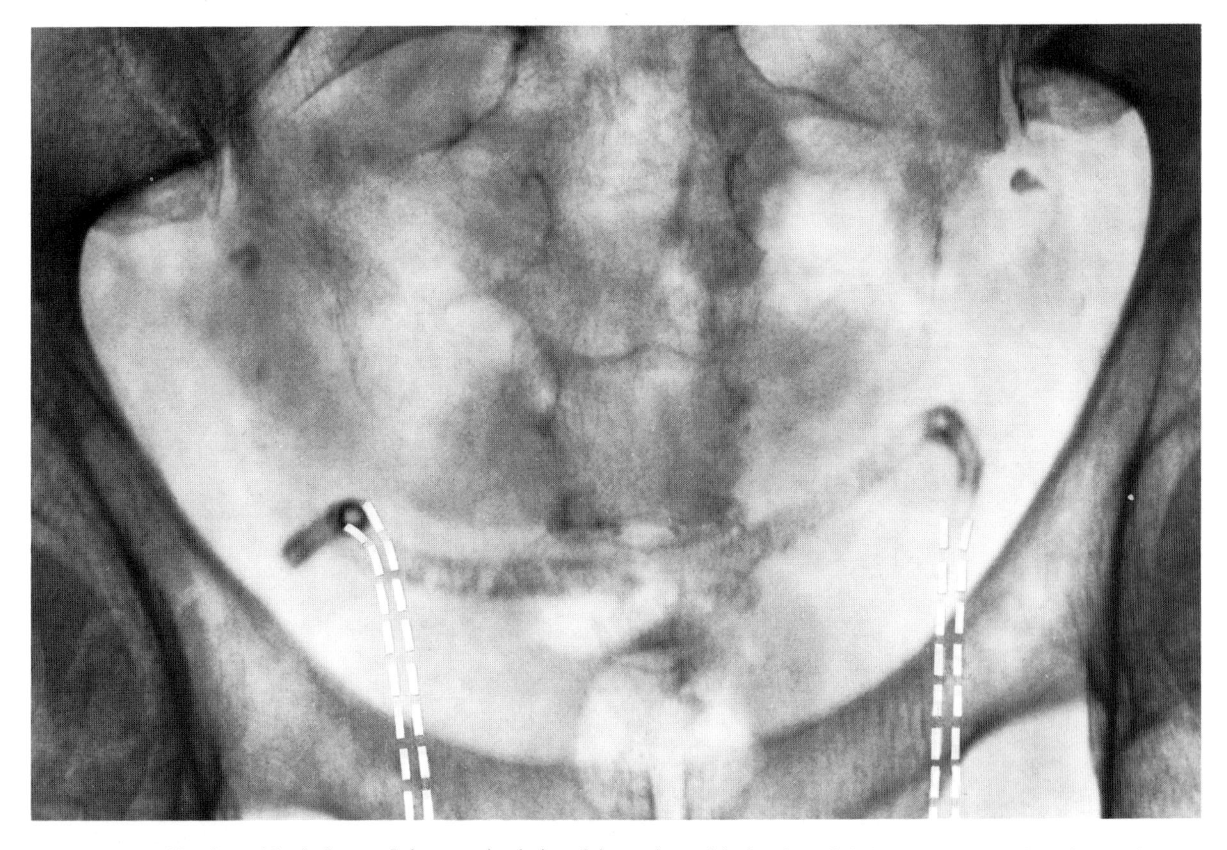

Fig. 445. Calcification of both ductus deferentes in their pelvic section, with drawing of their presumed continuation to the testes.

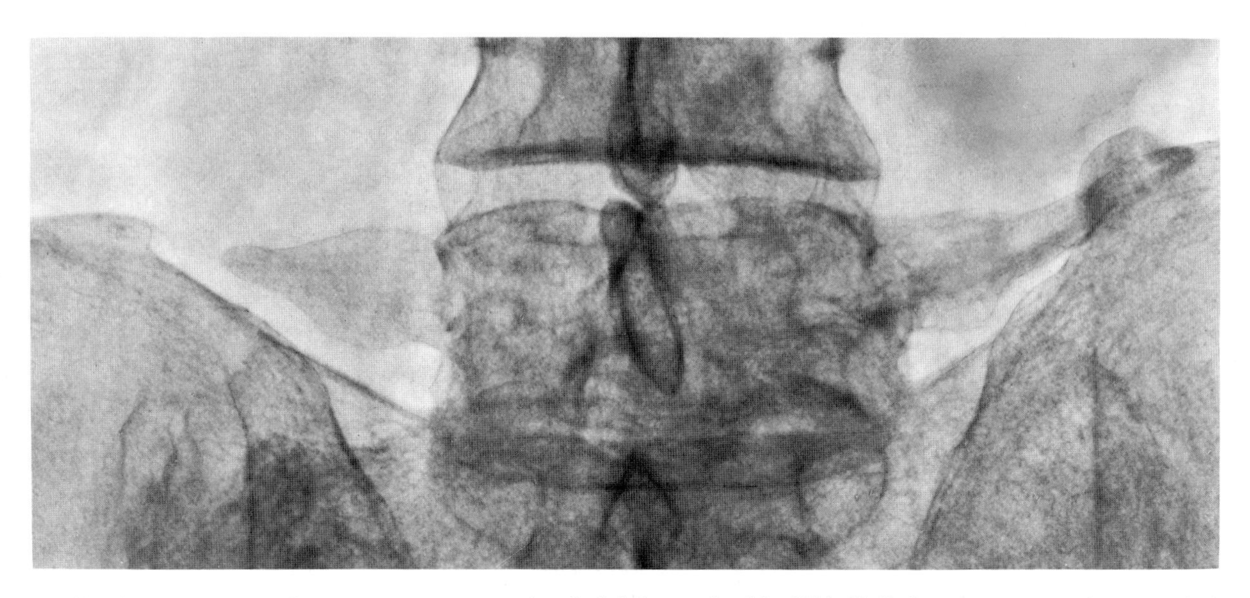

Fig. 446. Ossified iliolumbar ligament, more pronounced on the left than on the right. With this finding, there appears almost regularly a so-called long transverse process of L V, which may cause a nearthrosis. For ossifications of the ligaments of the pelvic floor (sacrotuberous, sacrospinous), see *P. Fischer.* Ground-off spinous process between 4th and 5th lumbar vertebral bodies (interspinal pseudarthrosis *Baastrup).*

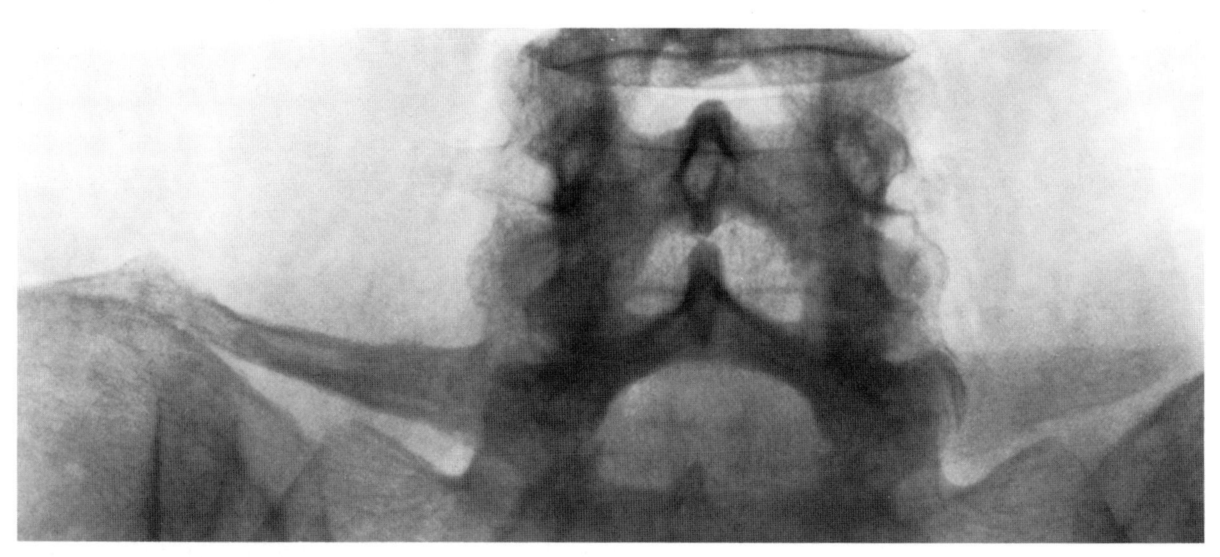

Fig. 447. Dorsally stretched, short transverse processes of L IV. Abnormally long transverse processes of L V; on the right, a bony ligamental iliolumbar connection (not to be confused with transition vertebra); on the left, persistent apophysis of the transverse process. Ossification of the iliolumbar ligament is often associated with condensing osteitis of the ilium and occurs also after traumata. The loosening of the pelvic girdle may point to damage through overloading. In cases of condensing osteitis, connections with hormone metabolism are also considered; estrogens enhance the activity of osteoblasts.

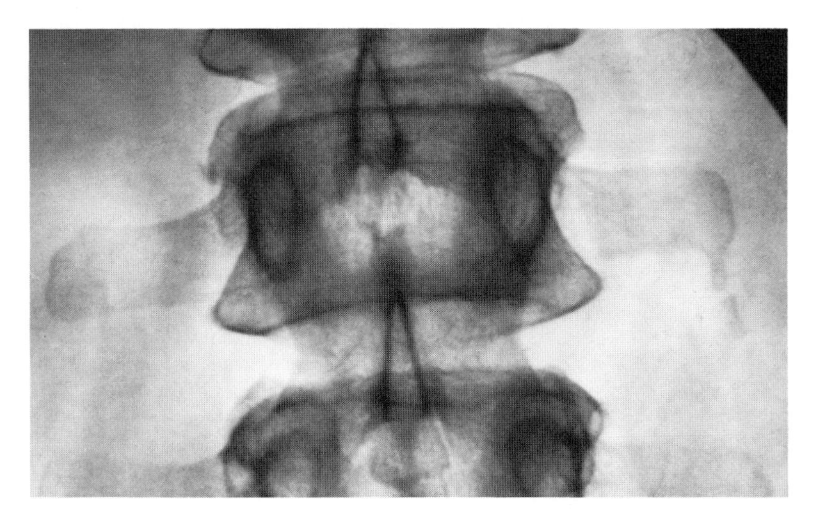

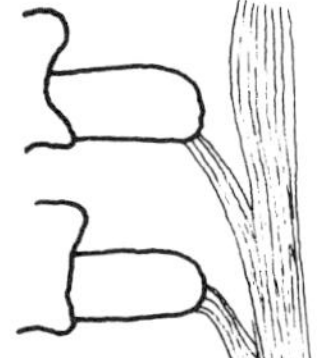

Fig. 449. Bundle-shaped musculotendinous insertion of the quadratus lumborum muscle at the lower tips of the costal processes.

Fig. 448. Rare spur formation at the lower rim of a tip of a lumbar transverse process (L II). Pseudoarticulation-like union with an adjoining bony spur, a possible ossification of the insertion of the quadratus lumborum muscle after trauma.

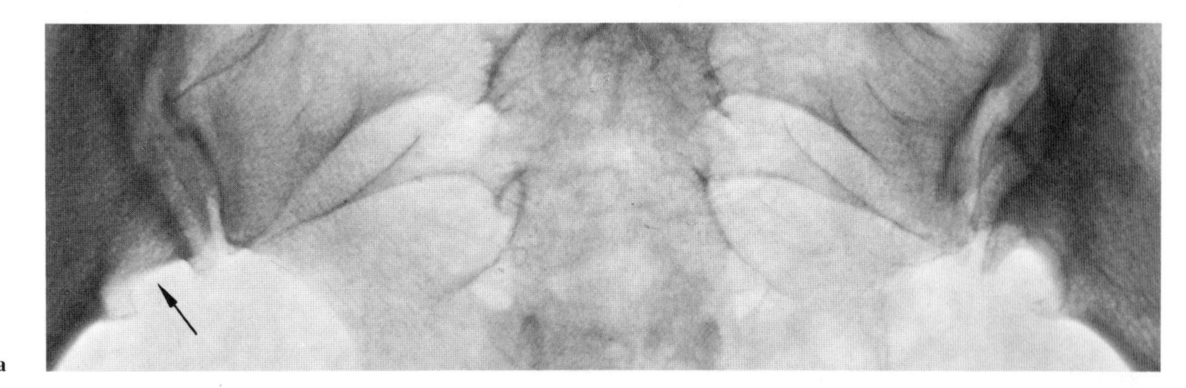

Fig. 450 a

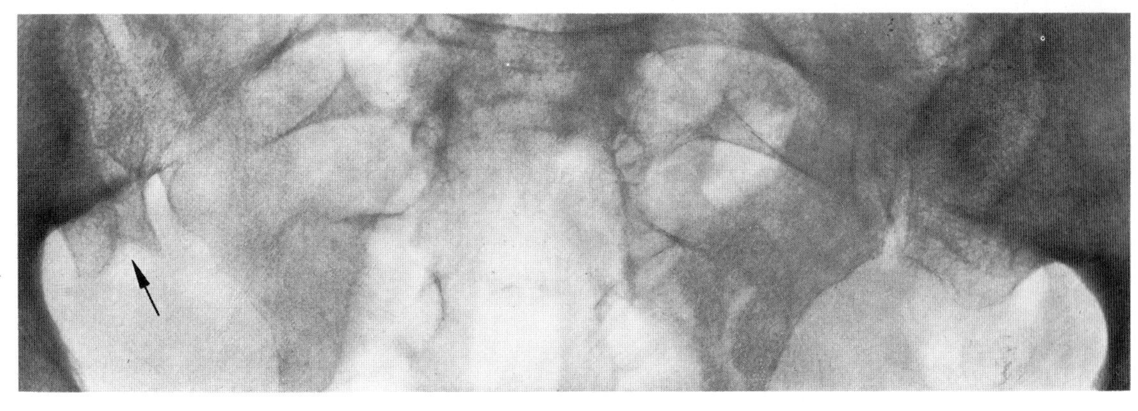

Fig. 450 b

Fig. 450. Bilateral paraglenoid sulcus, lateral to the right and left sacroiliac joint (↖); see also Fig. 442, No. 120. The spikes at its borders are often mistaken for osteoarthrotic spikes, for which there is no exact proof as yet. The paraglenoid sulcus (BNA), also called juxta-auricular sulcus (JNA), is no longer mentioned in the Paris nomenclature. This variant occurs in several forms; the sulcus (Fig. 450 a) which may close to a ring, the blunt plate (Fig. 450 b, left) and the two-cornered protuberance (Fig. 450 b, right). This may develop from wrenching of ligaments (micro-traumata of the ventral sacroiliac ligaments). The paraglenoid sulcus is not a vascular conduit (in any case, not always and not only) for the superior gluteal artery, which seems to run variably further medially (see also *de Cuveland, Hofer, Dihlmann, Maurer).*

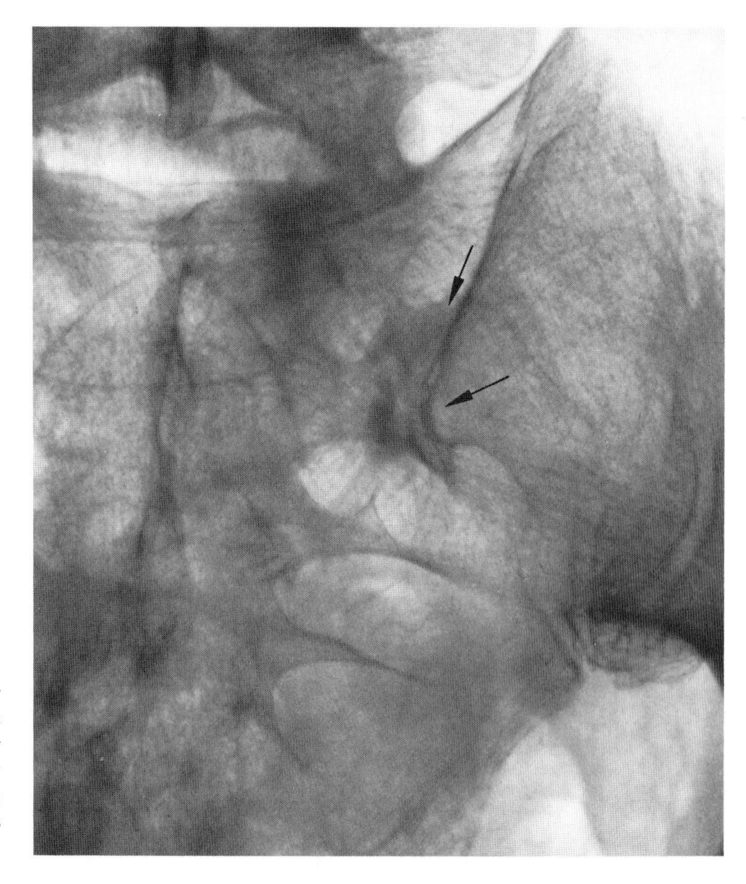

Fig. 451. Accessory sacroiliac joint (↙↙). These are articular connections between ilium and sacrum, lying dorsally to the proper sacroilial joint. The course of the joint is oblique or horizontal, medial from the sacroiliac joint; it is not infrequently arthrotic. *Schneider* found such an accessory sacroiliac joint in 14% of 1100 radiographs studied; this radiograph is a part of his work.

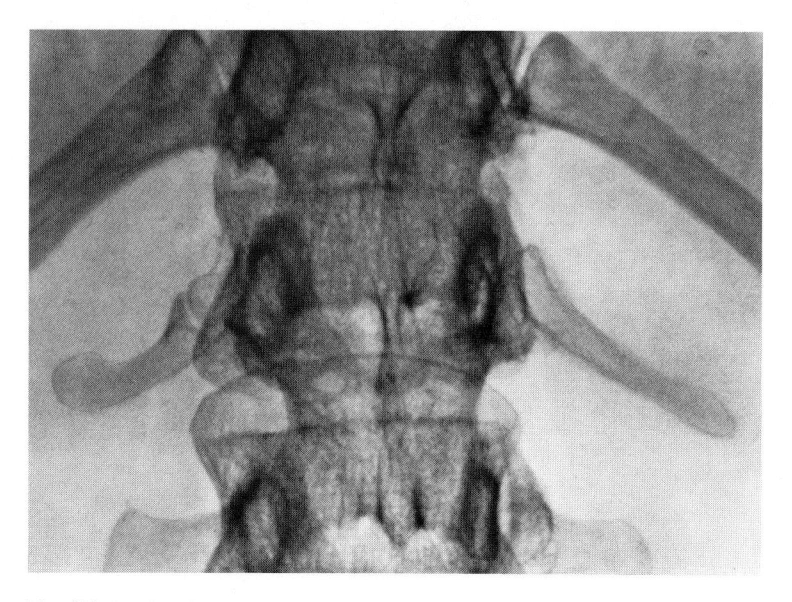

Fig. 452. Lumbar form of a caudal variant. Rib and transverse process of L I articulate on the right side and are fused into one unit on the left. The frequency of lumbar ribs amounts to 7–8% (see also p. 183).

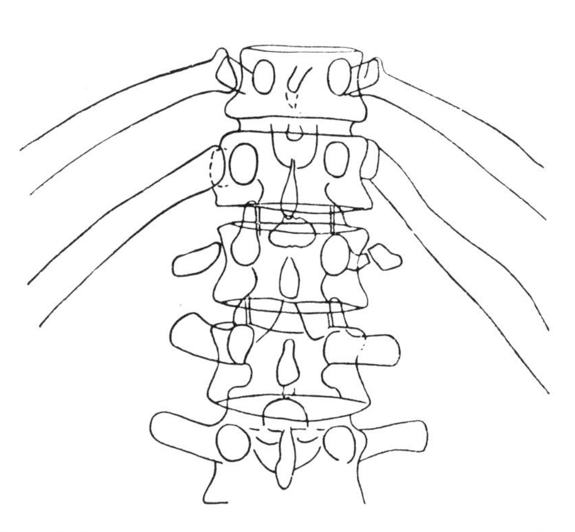

Fig. 453. Pseudoarticulating transverse process on the right of L I, rudimentary lumbar rib on the left.

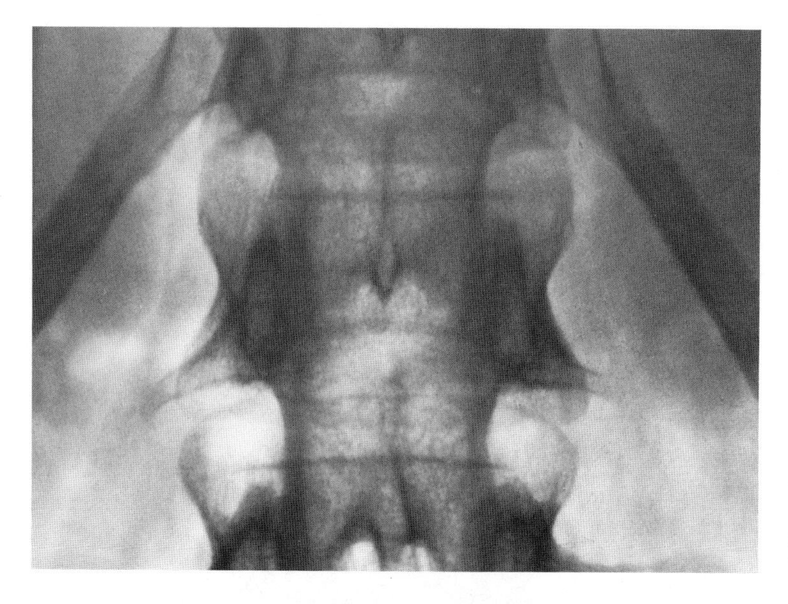

Fig. 454. Rudimentary, low-sitting transverse processes at L I, fused into a unit with a rudimentarily developed rib. This fusion takes place with the ventrolateral tubercle of the transverse process, while the head and neck of the rib have regressed or styloid processes on both sides at aplastic transverse processes.

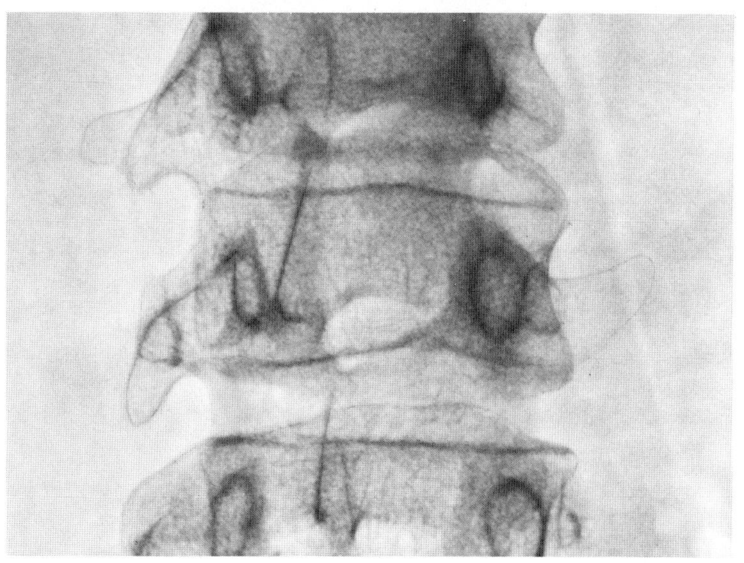

Fig. 455. Styloid process on the right side of several lumbar vertebrae. In this case, in addition to a formation of butterfly and wedging vertebrae, an occult spina bifida and costal malformations occurred. *Rubaschewa* found a styloid process in 7.9% of 1000 radiographs, most frequently on the lower lumbar vertebrae. The styloid process is simply an extra-long accessory process which arises at the base of the transverse process at the transition to the upper articular process (i.e., a spiky rudiment of an articular process). Phylogenetically and ontogenetically, it is a tubercle for (origin or insertion of) muscles; the musculi intertransversarii mediales lumborum extend from it to the mamillary process, a rudimentary articular process, of the neighboring vertebra *(Sobotta-Becher)*. The difference in size of the process may be explained by the inconstancy of these muscular structures (see also Fig. 463 a, b). On the left, the distinct shadow of the edge of the psoas muscle, simulating a fracture or an apophysis at the transverse process (from the collection of *W. Werner,* Berlin).

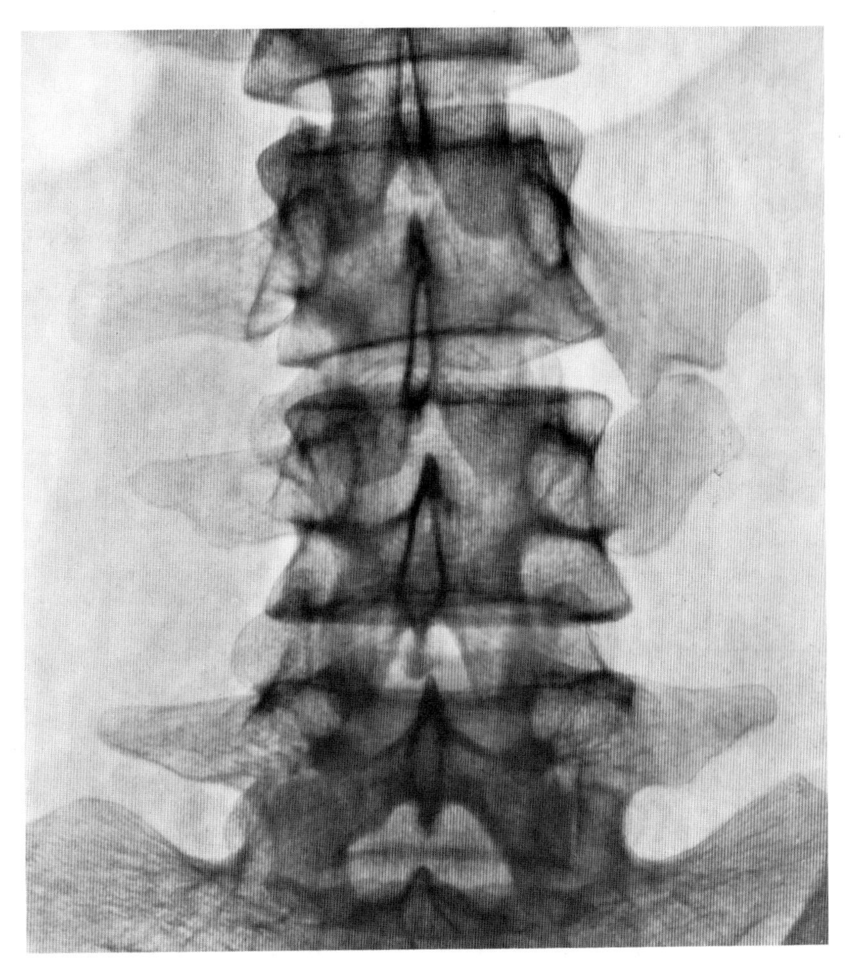

Fig. 456. Bridge formation on the left side between the transverse processes of the bodies of the 3rd and 4th lumbar vertebrae with a joint-like connection. *De Cuveland* reported on bridge formation between transverse processes of lumbar vertebrae; he pointed out the differentiation between congenital connections of transverse processes and of bony clasps, caused by trauma. In our case, the shovel-shaped transverse processes, facing one another, indicate a congenital origin. In 1974 *Haas* described the formation of bony clasps between the left transverse processes of L III and L IV many years after a trauma, and impressively demonstrated the bony fixation of those segments. He believes a post-traumatic ossifying myositis to be the essential cause.

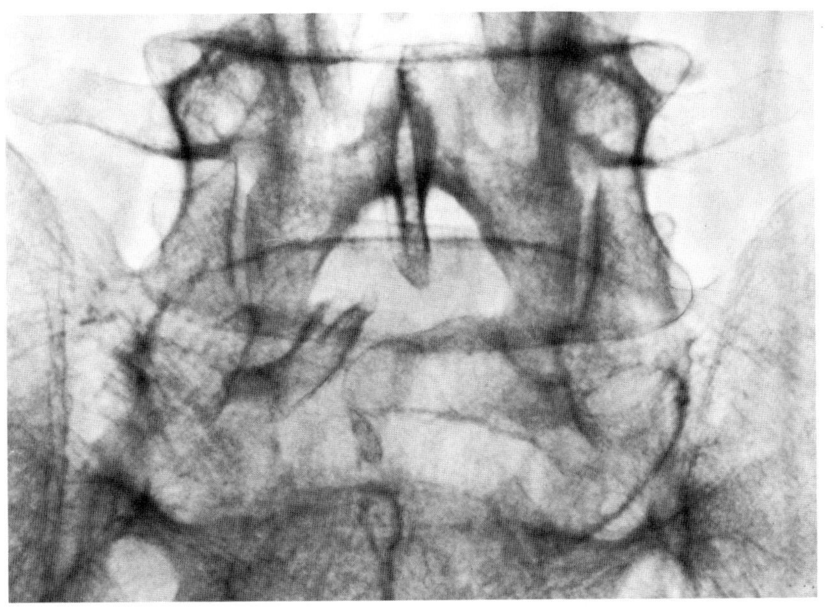

A contrasting condition to malformations in the region of the vertebral arches is aplasia of the vertebral body (asoma), being neither cartilaginous nor bony, while the vertebral arches exist *(Putti, Liechti, Diethelm, Reinhardt)*.

Fig. 457. Cleft formation in the first sacral vertebra. The cleft formation lies in the region of the vertebral arch, runs obliquely and arose because the two halves of the arch grew past one another. Below the cleft is the isolated apophysis of the spinous process of the 1st sacral vertebra. It lies either in the cartilaginous tip of the spinous process or, if the chondral closure of the arch is absent, in the gap between the halves of the arch. (For further cleft formation see Fig. 459.)

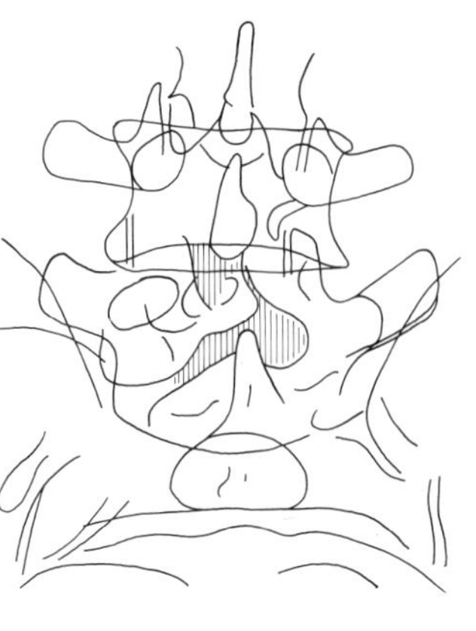

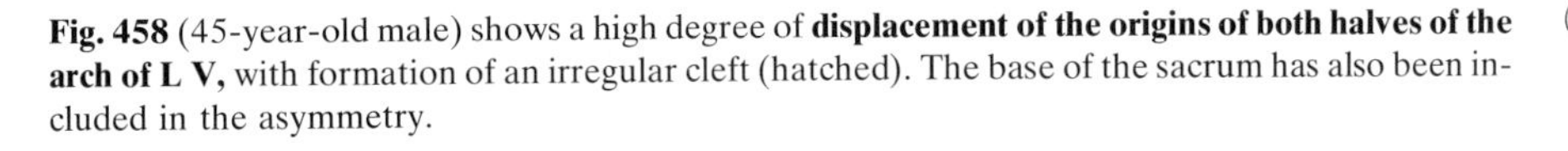

Fig. 458 (45-year-old male) shows a high degree of **displacement of the origins of both halves of the arch of L V,** with formation of an irregular cleft (hatched). The base of the sacrum has also been included in the asymmetry.

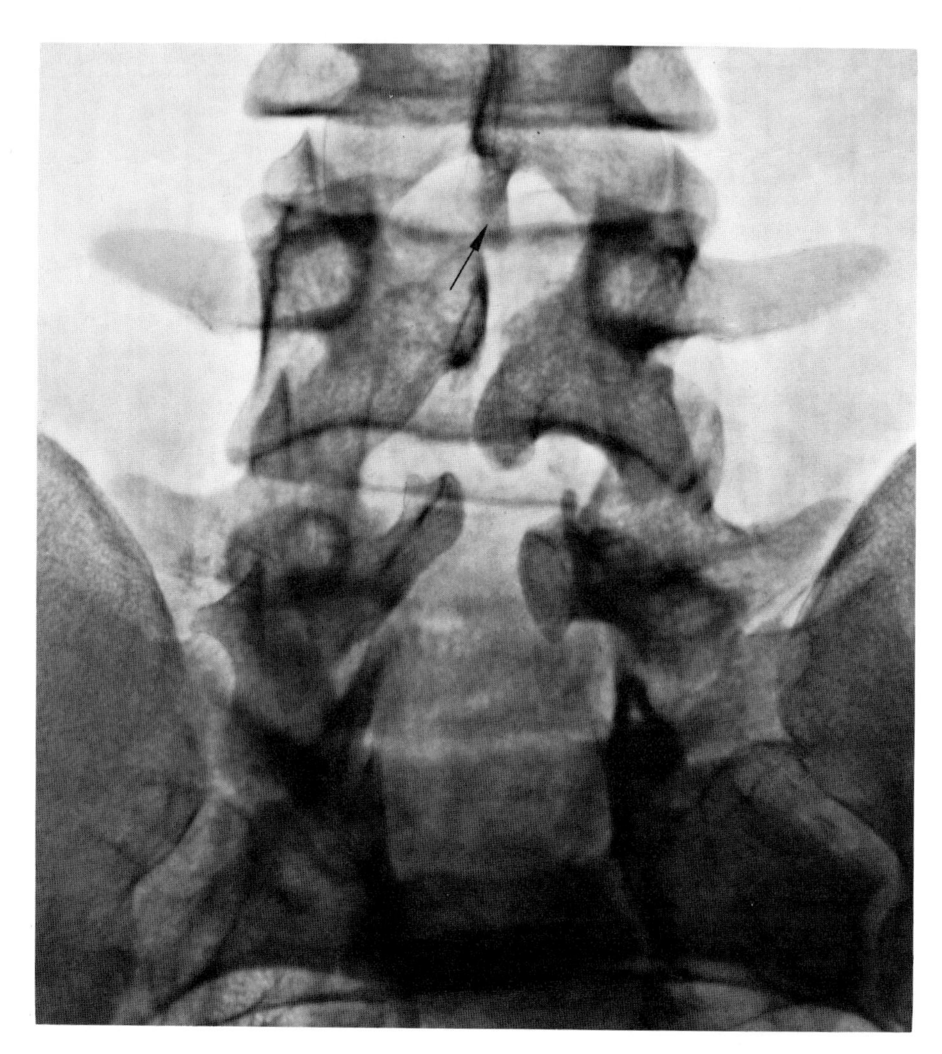

Fig. 459. Spina bifida at the arches of L IV and L V with extension into the sacrum. The spinous process of L III shows a small notch (↗) at its lower edge, but split formation did not occur (see Fig. 384 and Fig. 442, No. 109). *Giles* found a spina bifida in 23.9% of 1122 radiographs of the vertebral column. *Stein* and *Schmidt* found a frequency of only 14% in the female.

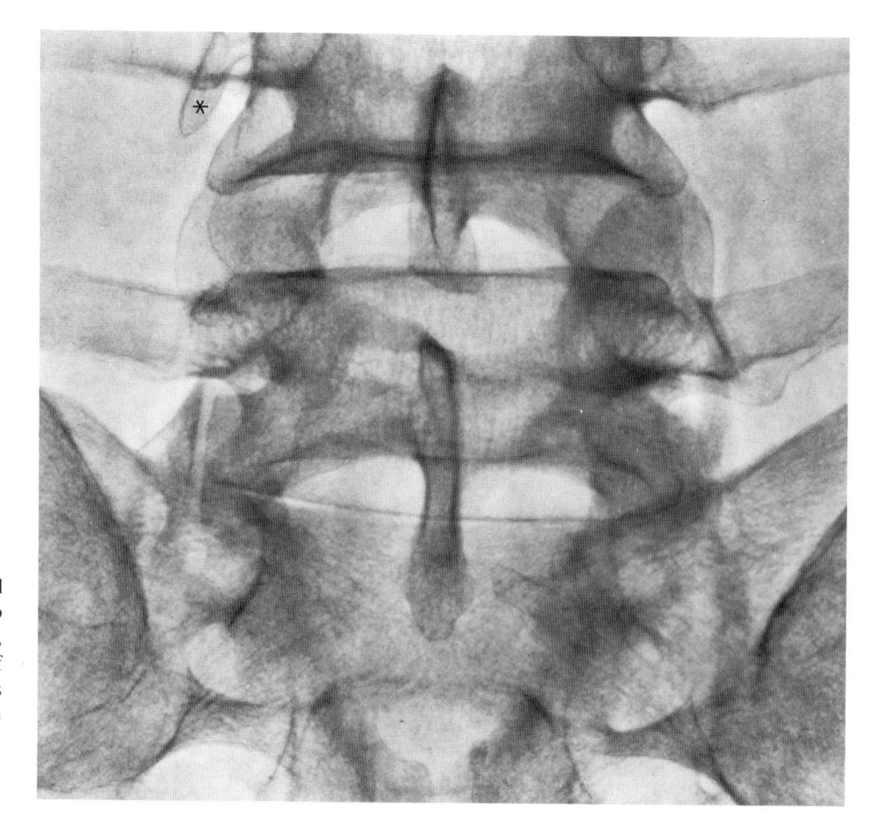

Fig. 460. Missing closure of the arch at the 1st and 2nd sacral vertebrae, in this case corresponding to an occult spina bifida. The spinous process of L V, apparently elongated by an adjoining apophysis of S I, protrudes into the broad gap of S I; it appears as a pseudofracture. A further variant is seen: a large styloid process at the right side of L IV (*); see Fig. 442, No. 110 and text to Fig. 455. Refer to *Rubaschewa.*

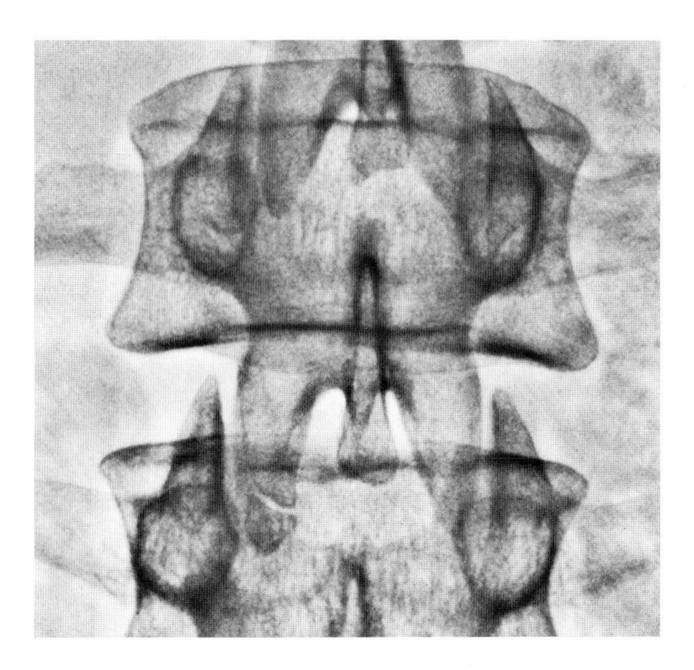

Fig. 461. Horizontal cleft formation in the right lower articular process of L III. This is not a fracture but a persistent apophysis *(Oppenheimer, Went, Pfeiffer).*

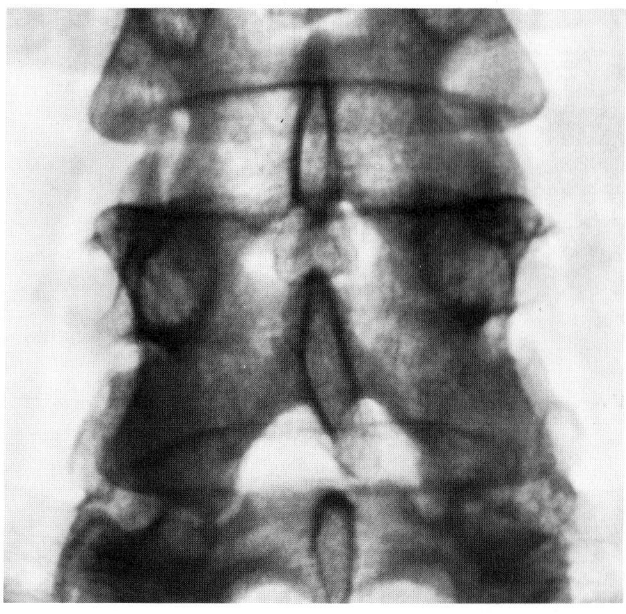

Fig. 462. Very short, hypoplastic transverse processes at L IV; this is a partial symptom of the cranial variant of the spine. In addition, on the right there is a styloid process (frequency about 8%; see Fig. 455).

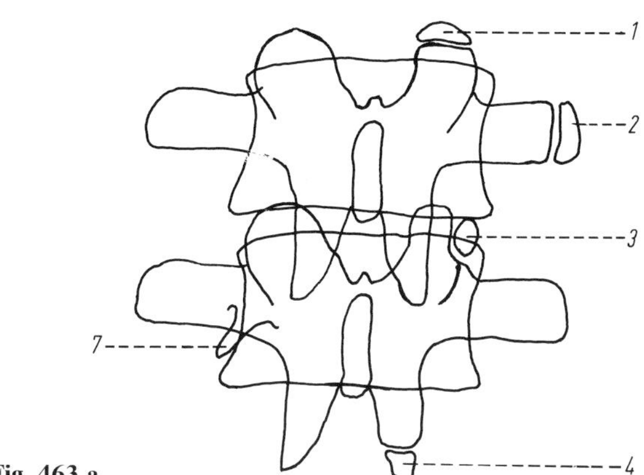

Fig. 463 a

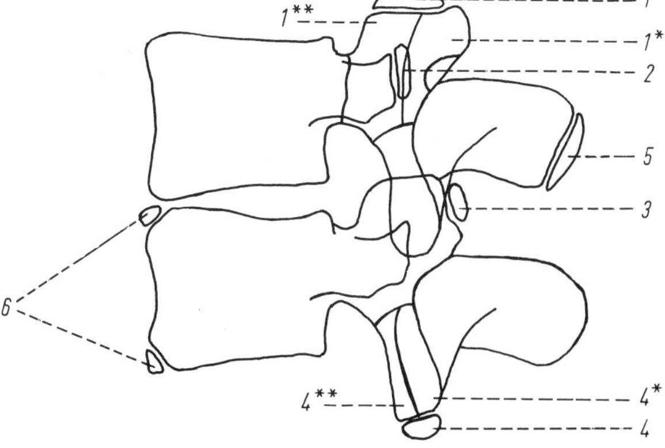

Fig. 463 b

1, 1* and 1** Persistent nuclei at the upper articular process, with lines of cleft
2 Persistent apophysis at the transverse process
3 Persistent apophysis at the mamillary process
4, 4* and 4** Persistent nuclei at the lower articular process, with lines of cleft
5 Persistent apophysis at the spinous process
6 Persistent marginal ledge at the anterior upper and lower margins of the vertebral body
7 Styloid process (enlarged accessory process)

Fig. 463. Vertebral anomalies (schema in Fig. 463 b supplemented according to *Oppenheimer);* see also cleft formation in the vertebral arch, Fig. 384.

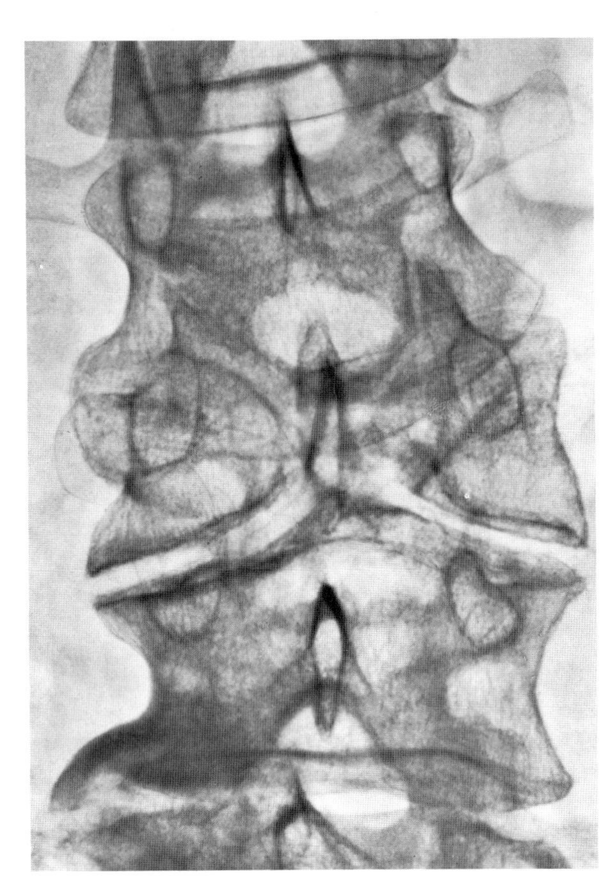

Fig. 464 a

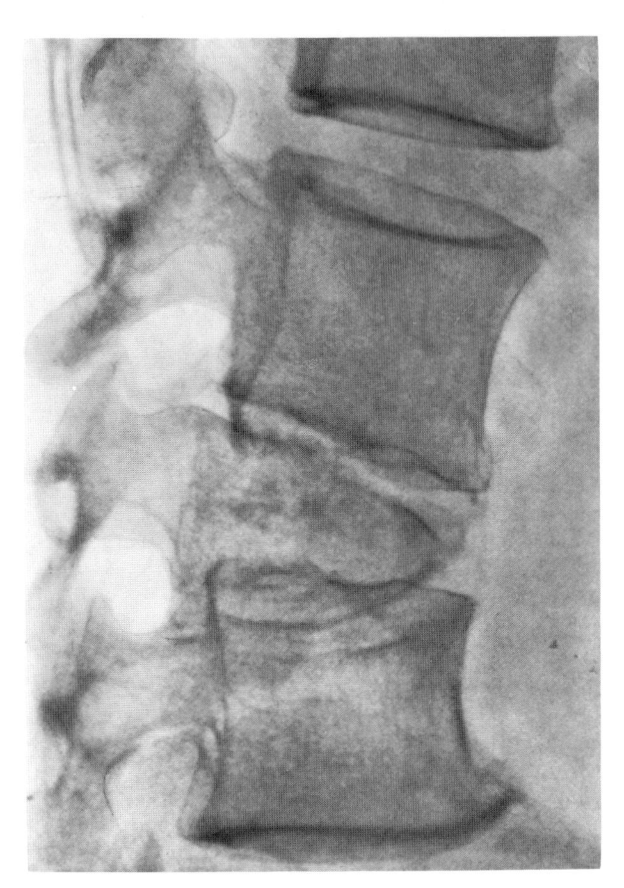

Fig. 464 b

Fig. 464. Dorsal hemisoma of L III. Congenital butterfly or wedging vertebra L III, caused by non-development of the anterior halves of the vertebral body, with widening of the vertebral bodies by an anterior sagittal cleft (see also *Diethelm*). Over the course of decades, the deformed wedging vertebra has been pushed backwards and the two neighboring vertebrae L II and L IV have approximated with sclerosing supports of the anterior margins (in a male, 30 years of age). (From the collection of *W. Werner*).

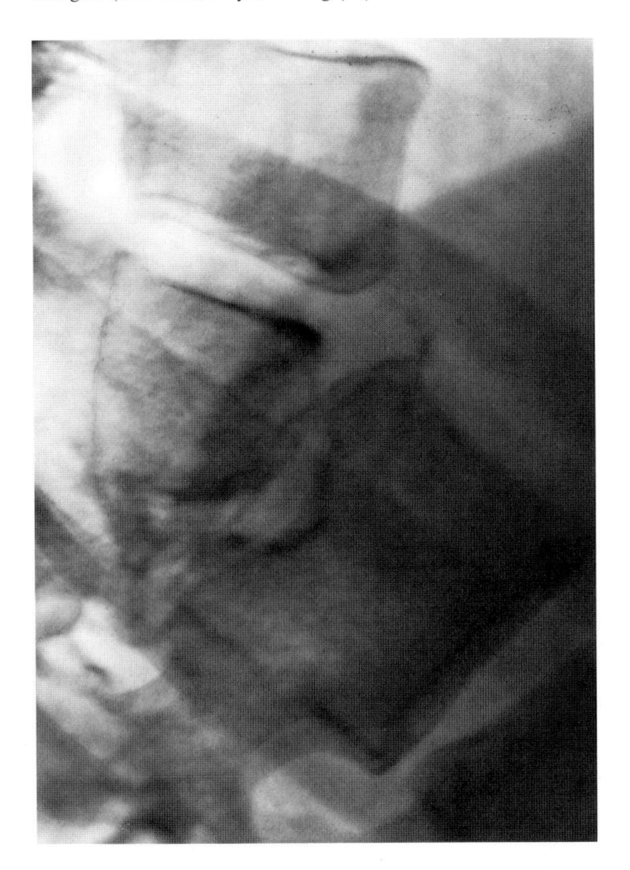

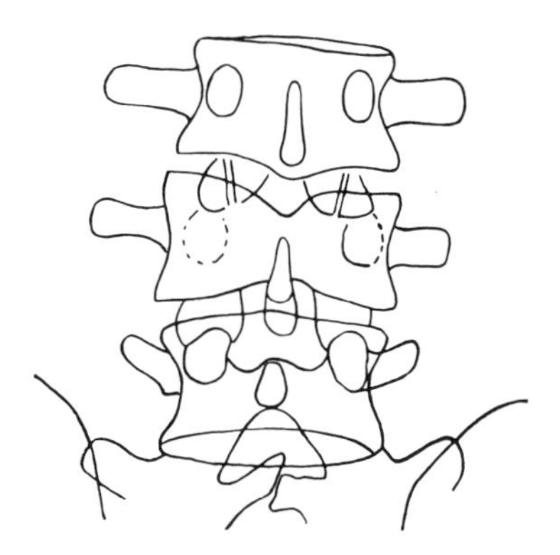

Fig. 466. Butterfly shape of L IV, with adapting shapes of the bodies of L III and L V (malformation). Cleft formation in the 1st sacral arch. By the term anterior spina bifida, the much rarer cleft formations in the vertebral body are meant, as opposed to the deficient dorsal closures of the arches. Butterfly vertebra with ventral or dorsal notch may be considered as a lesser degree of anterior spina bifida *(Reinhardt)*.

Fig. 465. Thoracic hemi- or wedging vertebra (TH XI). This causes a congenital gibbus *(Brocher, Schöneich)*. Intravertebral defects, in combination with the rare frontal cleft in the vertebral body, may signify a special form of chordal persistence *(Vielberg, 1970)*.

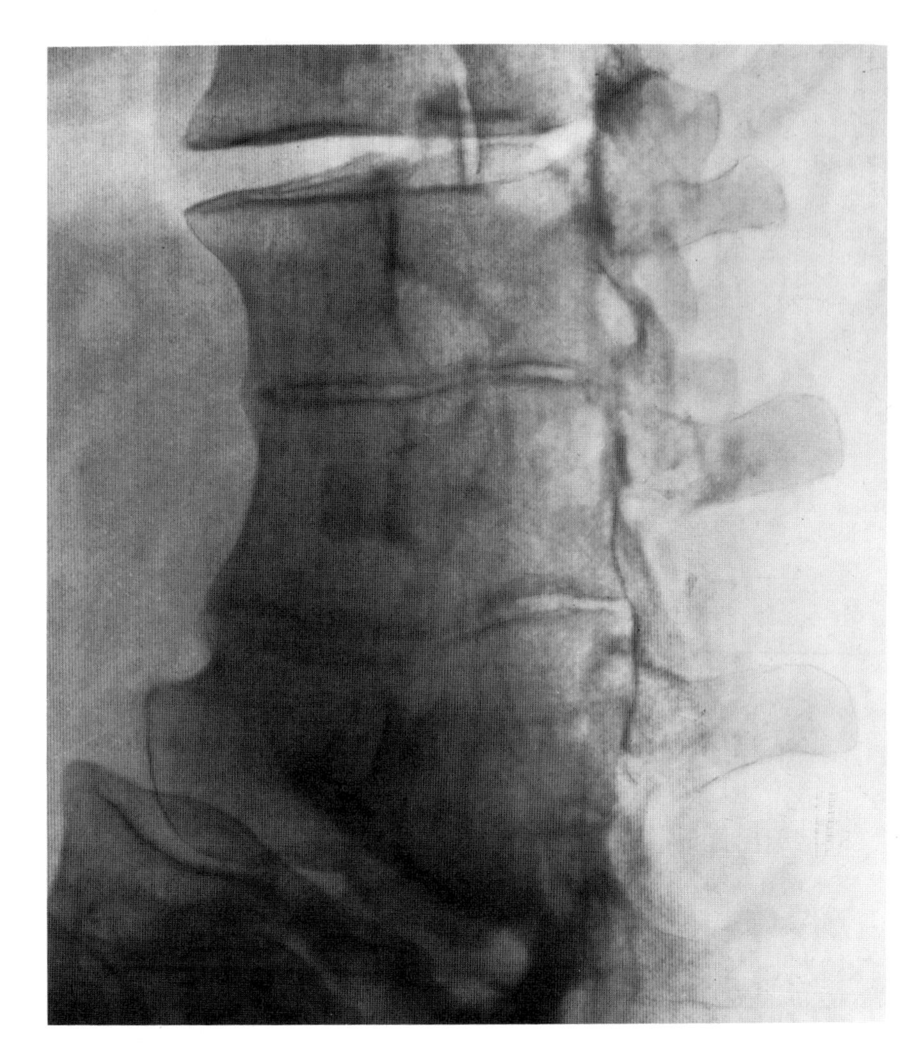

Fig. 467. Partial formation of block vertebrae L II to L IV through disturbance of development. This is a constantly recurring, quite definite type A (*Diethelm,* 1974), which shows fusion of the anterior 3rd, with wedge-shaped narrowing and indented concave anterior surface of the block vertebrae. Intervertebral spaces for the disks are still present but greatly narrowed. According to *Valentin* and *Putschar,* this finding is in conformity with the transformation of the sacral vertebrae into the sacrum. As these processes start only during post-fetal life, according to these authors, the concept of congenital block vertebrae should be replaced by that of dysontogenetic block vertebrae.

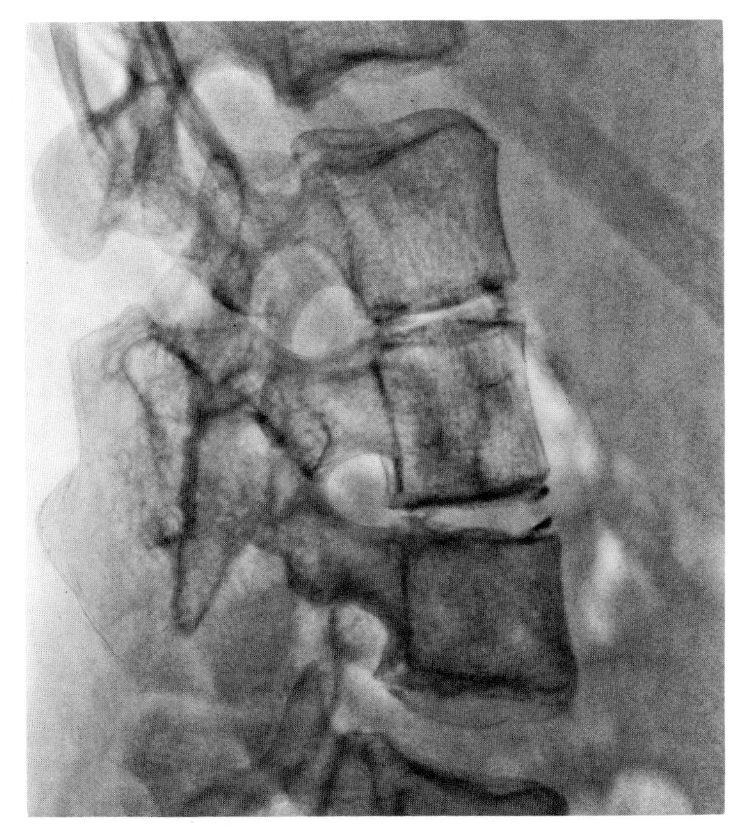

Fig. 468. Malformations of the vertebral arches cannot be systematized, neither with regard to their causal endogenous or exogenous geneses nor to their manifestations. In the present case, there were the following findings in a 10-year-old girl:

1. a rare, probably unilateral aplasia of the lower articular process,
2. a hypoplastic spinous process at L II and aplasia of the spinous processes L III and L IV,
3. fusion of remnants of the malformations into a bony plate, lateral to the arches, which passes over 2-½ segments.

Excessive width of the sacral hiatus points to the presence of a megacauda *(Pia),* which is accompanied by caudal symptoms and sciatic complaints. The megacauda represents a congenital dystic distension of the dural covering of the cauda equina. Concurrently, there is saccular distension of the respective sheaths of the nerve roots and an enlargement of the intervertebral foramina.

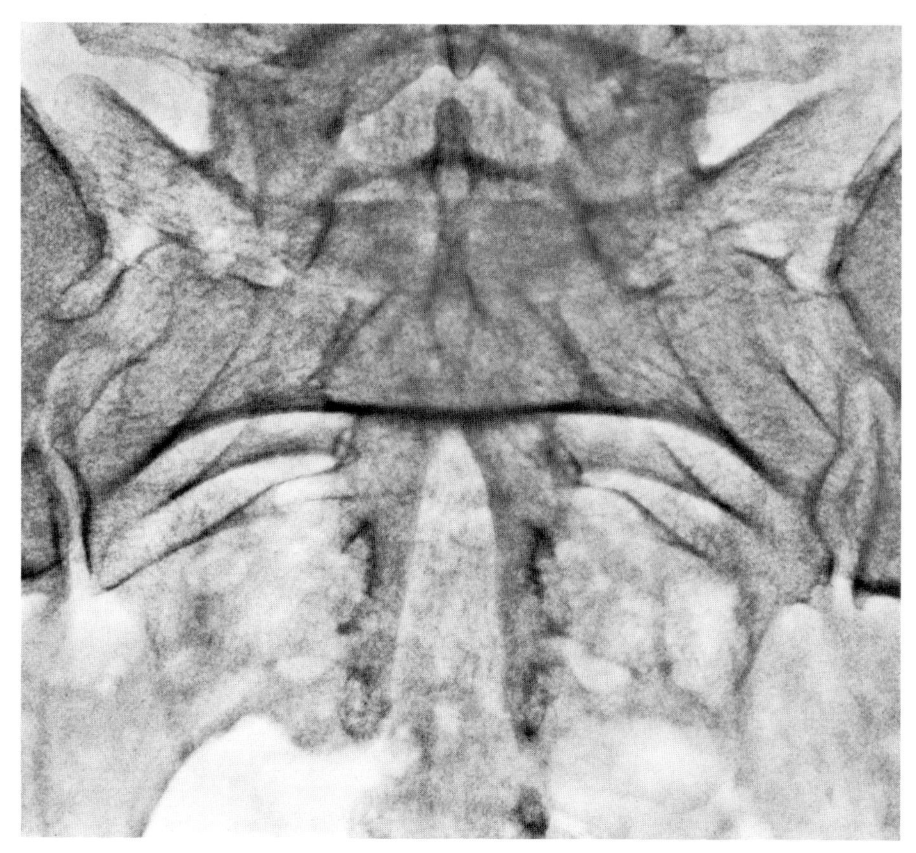

Fig. 469. Extended sacral hiatus (see Fig. 442, Nos. 119, 137). The upper sacral vertebrae are projected in cross section. The open sacral hiatus is one form of the congenital defects of sacrum and coccyx *(Kienböck* and *Zimmer).*

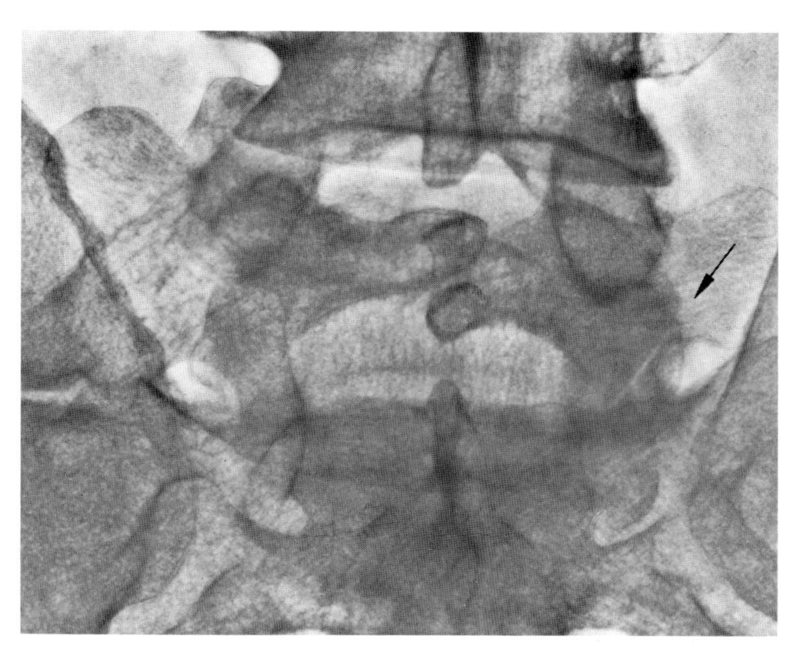

Fig. 470 a

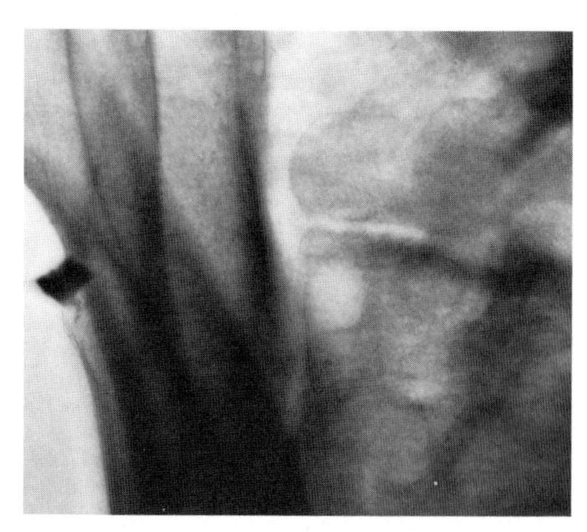

Fig. 470 b

Fig. 470. Lumbalization of the 1st sacral vertebra, which has been partially assimilated on the right and is only separated by an additional articular space. In addition, there is an incomplete closure of the arch of the 1st sacral vertebra, which should not be mistaken for a spina bifida. There is a persistent cleft of an apophysis at a lower articular process (↙), which is not a fracture line. **Fig. 470 b shows an articular space after outward rotation.** As an incidental finding, a shell splinter may be seen adjacent to the outer iliac wall. Finally, there appears in the cancellous tissue of the 1st sacral vertebra a round, amply pea-sized, not quite distinctly defined increased radiolucency which, after *Bortmann's* presentation, is to be considered as due to projection. This apparent "foraminal effect" can be clarified by tomography.

Fig. 471. Spondylolisthesis of the body of L IV (genuine sliding of a vertebral body). This is the result of interarticular spondylolysis. Its basis is a cleft (↘) which divides the arch into:

a) an anterior upper portion, consisting of the root of the arch, the upper articular process and the transverse process, and
b) a posterior lower portion, consisting of the lower articular process, the dorsal vertebral arch and the spinous process.

Spondylolysis may occur unilaterally or bilaterally. The defect in the interarticular portion is mostly congenital; its traumatic genesis is in dispute.

The transition from spondylolysis (defect of the arch) to spondylolisthesis (sliding of vertebral body, *Exner*) is favored by traumatic influences or heavy physical work *(Beeler; Collard* and *Brasseur)*. The forward shift of the vertebral body takes place towards the next caudal, healthy vertebra but sometimes also to the next higher one. In case of pseudospondylolisthesis, not only the vertebral body but the complete vertebra slides forward. Its premise is a bevelling and incline of the pertinent articular surfaces and a destruction of the pertinent disk, as in osteochondrotic degeneration of the disk *(Junghanns)*. Spondylolysis, followed by spondylolisthesis, also occurs in juveniles *(Francillon)*.

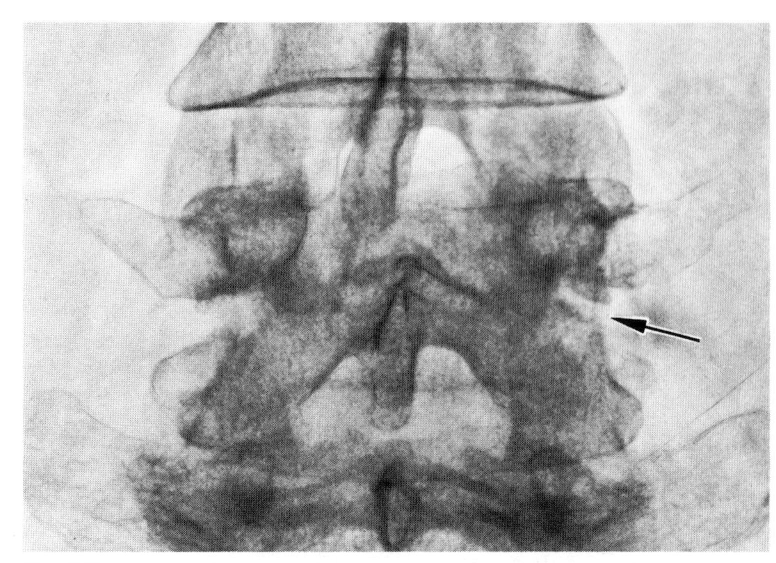

Fig. 471 a

In 1972 *Seegelken* and *Schulte* reported on a retrosomatic cleft at L II, in combination with spondylolysis of the opposite side of the same vertebra, both considered congenital anomalies.

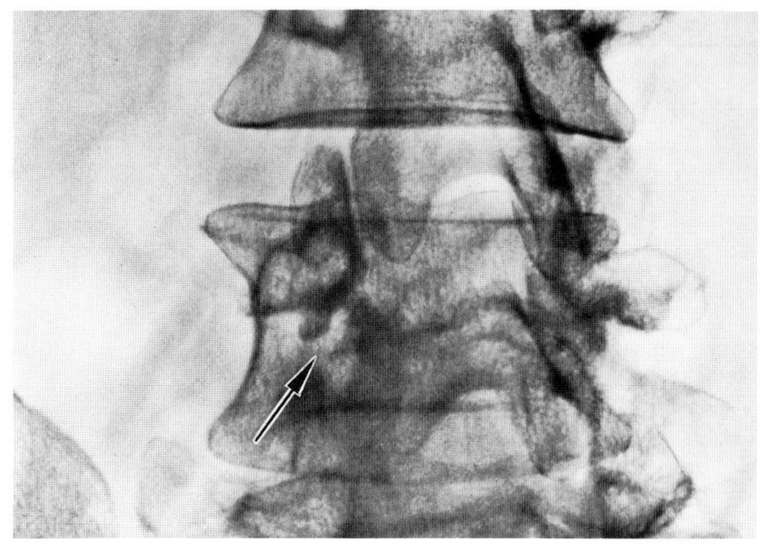

Fig. 471 b (Oblique projection)

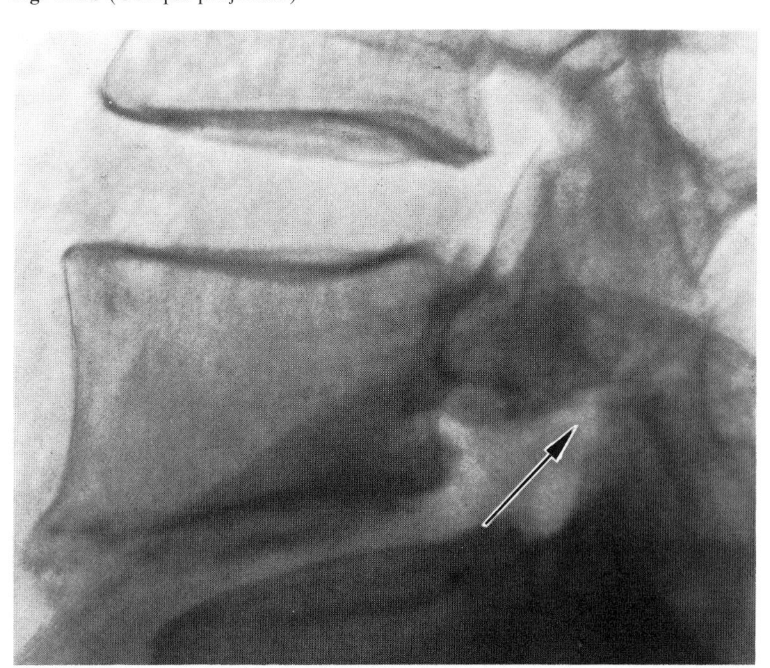

Fig. 471 c

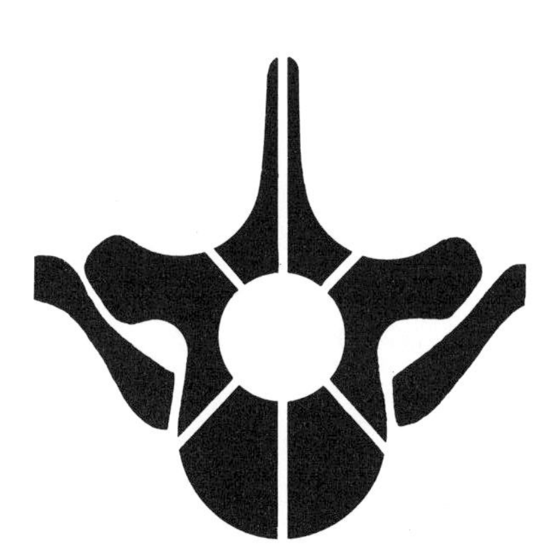

Fig. 472. Elementary vertebra, from *Putti*. Schematic view of a vertebra, from which the genesis of all vertebral malformations can be traced to impediments of fusion of those vertebral portions that originate in the precartilaginous period.

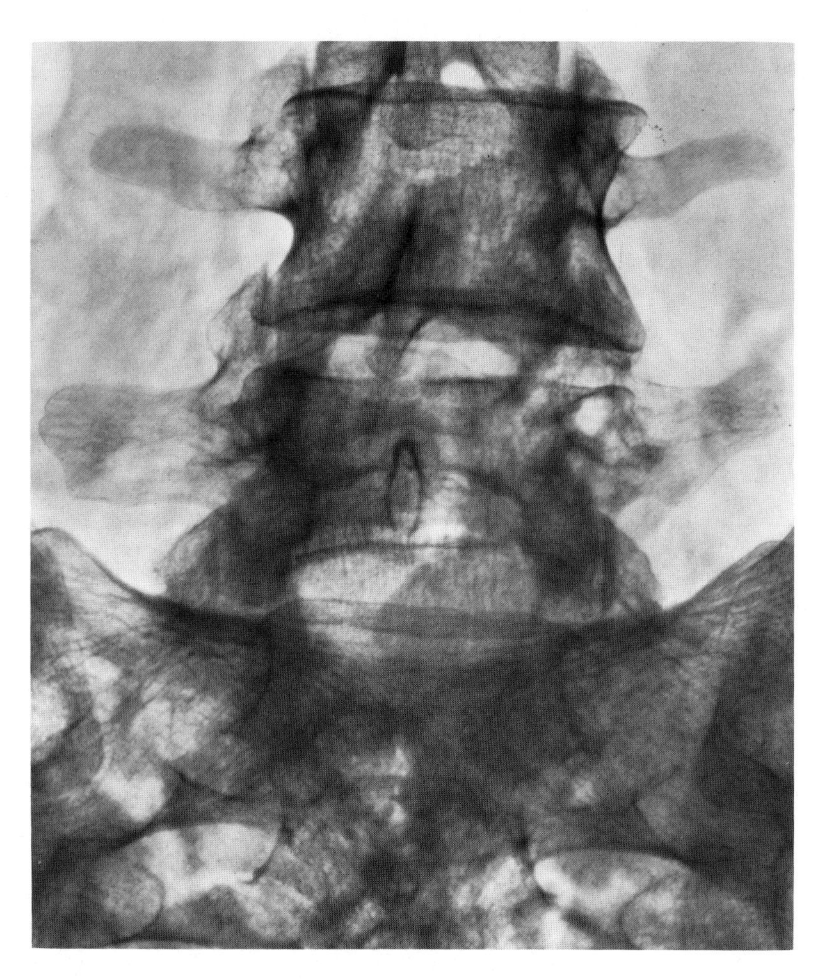

Fig. 473. General view of the lumbosacral transition.

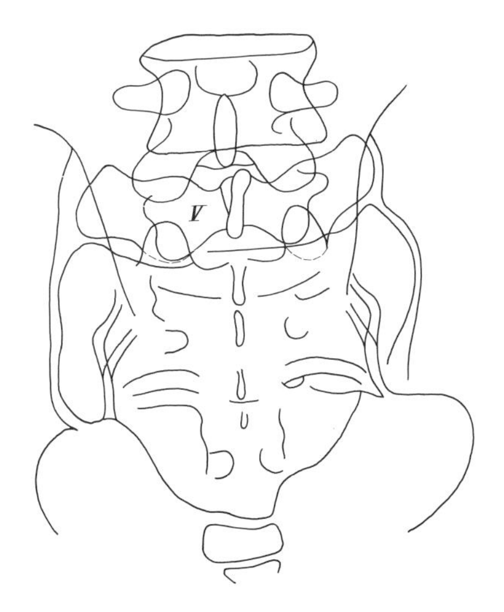

Fig. 474 shows a so-called transitional vertebra, a 5th lumbar vertebra assimilated onto the sacrum, i.e. **"sacralized."** Sacralization occurs at all stages; it appears at first as enlargement of the transverse processes, which lean on the ilia and the lateral masses of the sacrum and which lengthen the sacroiliac articulation more or less distinctly.

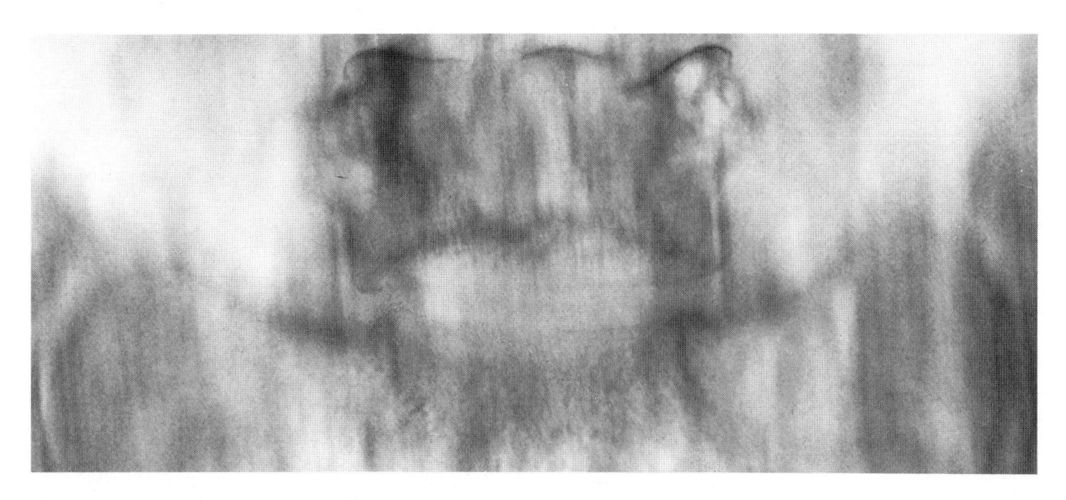

Fig. 475. Tomographic examination of the same case, under the same conditions of projection as in Fig. 473, taken ventrodorsally. The tomographic examination reveals a compression, caused by the infraction of the upper covering plate of L V, due to tumor metastasis. The bronchial primary tumor became manifest clinically and radiographically only some months later. Depth of layer 7.0 cm from dorsal.

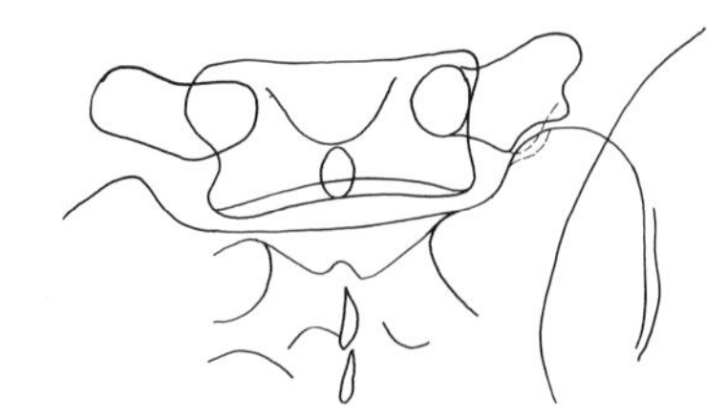

Fig. 477 shows a **hemilateral sacralized transverse process,** which articulates only downwards and not sideways.

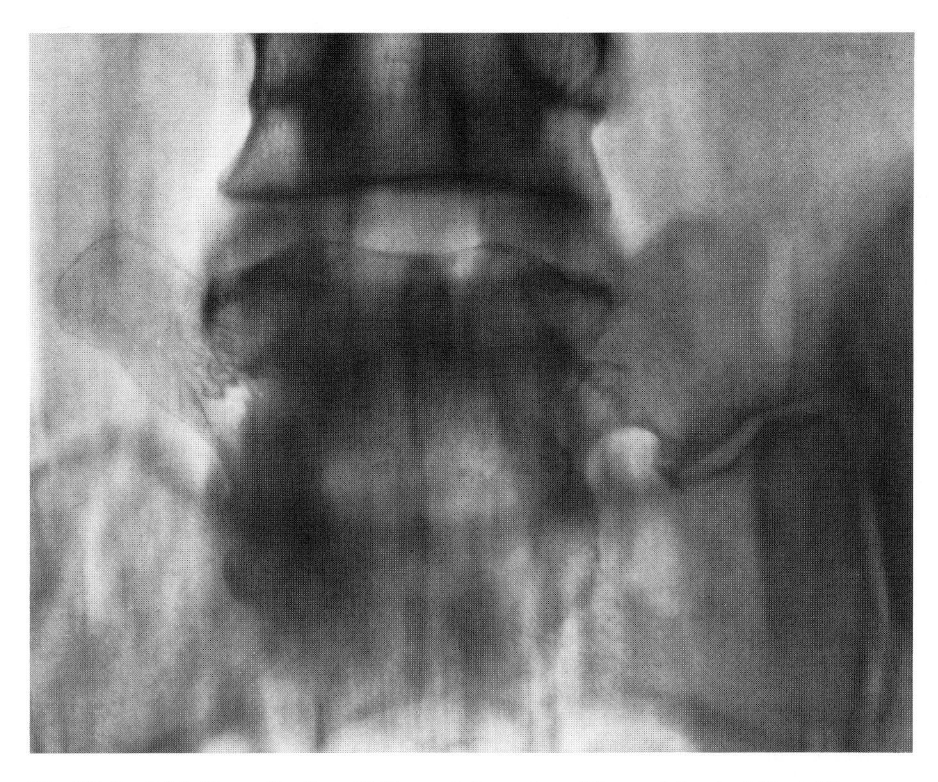

Fig. 476. Partial (left) sacralization of L V, a partial symptom of the cranial variant. The left transverse process of L V became attached to the sacrum by a joint-like connection, while at the right process the relations are normal. The term sacralization implies a complete, as well as a partial connection of the transverse processes with the sacrum, plus enlarged and broadened transverse processes of L V. Changes at the transverse processes of the upper lumbar spine with joint-like connections to one another, within the meaning of sacralization, are extremely rare.

Such a nearthrosis in cases of unilateral sacralization usually causes localized discomfort. Pains on the opposite side may be explained by faulty weight bearing. Therefore, surgical removal of hyperplastic transverse processes has given good results.

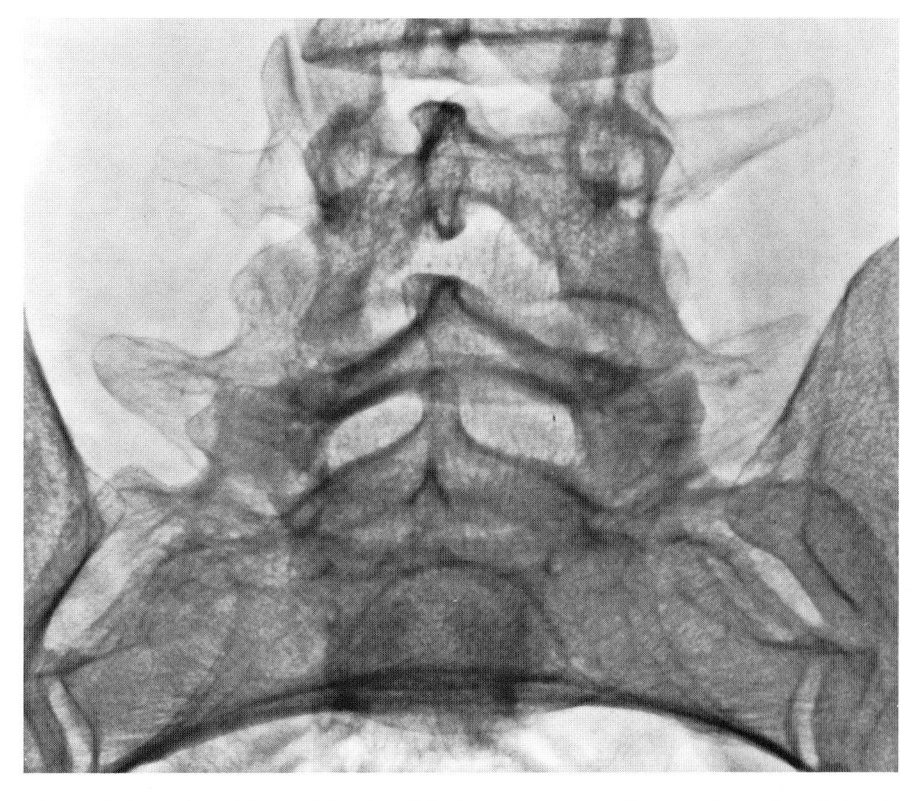

Fig. 478. Transition vertebra: lumbalization of S I, a partial symptom of the caudal variant. It is also necessary to evaluate as a formation of a transition vertebra the frequently observed underdevelopment of the disk between L V and S I, which is not infrequently thought to be a "damaged disk." It would be more correct to call it an "insufficiency of disk," as it can also be observed in other predisposed spinal segments as a preliminary step towards disk damage. The lumbalization of the 1st sacral vertebra (6th lumbar vertebrae) less frequently leads to complaints and is often a symptomless, accidental finding, e.g., on kidney examination. In the female, the lengthening of the lumbar spine may lead to increased lordosis, with correspondingly changed demands on muscles and ligaments, which may cause complaints.

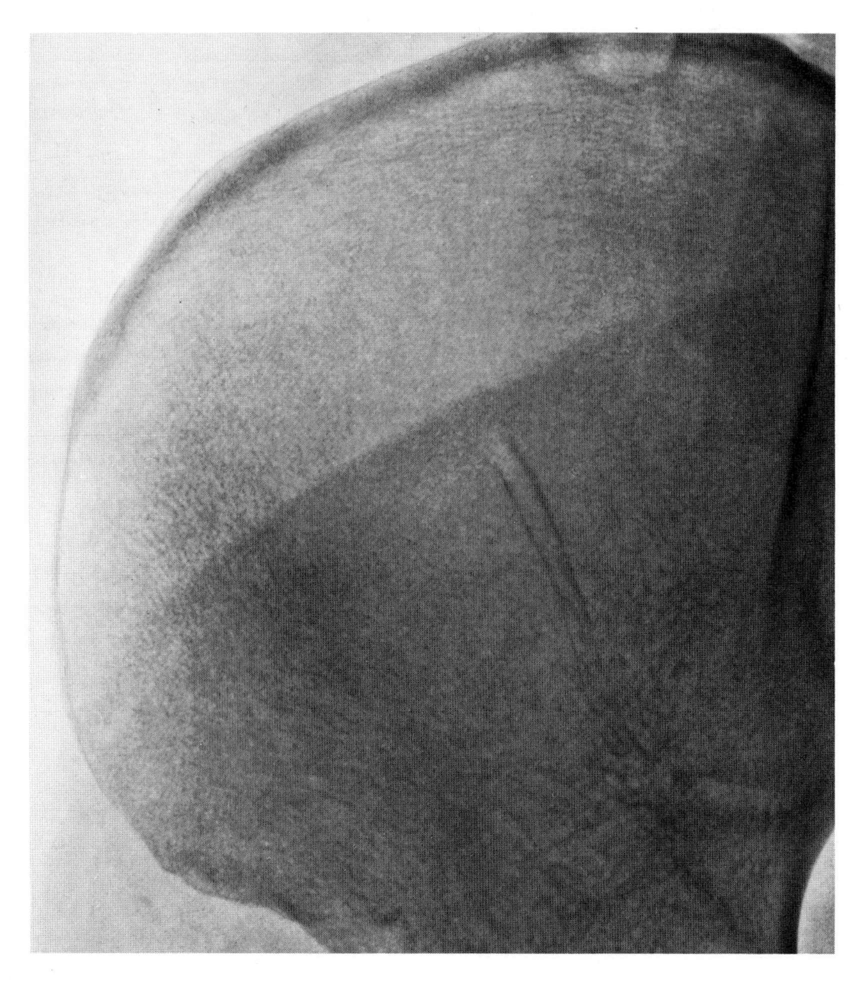

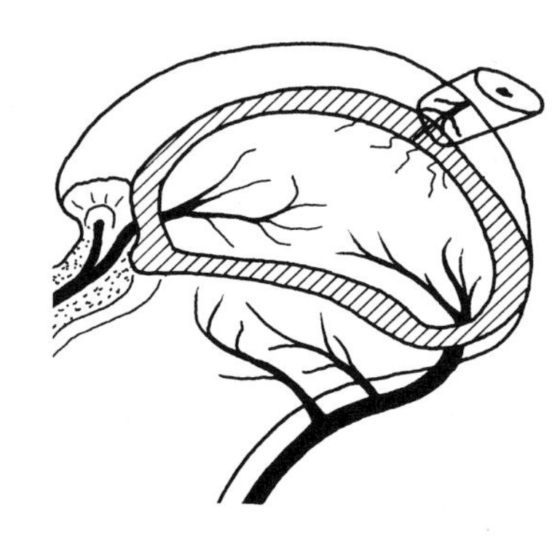

Fig. 480. Sketch showing the statically endangered vascular supply of the juvenile femoral head (from *Watermann*).

Fig. 479. Vascular canal in the center of the iliac fossa appears as a double-contoured band of increased radiolucency. This is often Y-shaped and sometimes "apparently" forked (see Fig. 442, n). In fact, it is only a crossing of two vascular canals which lie at different depths. Below the iliac crest a cyst-like semiglobular figure can be seen at the iliac fossa: it is a vesicle filled with intestinal gases, with an apparently sclerosed wall (see also Fig. 442, No. 134).

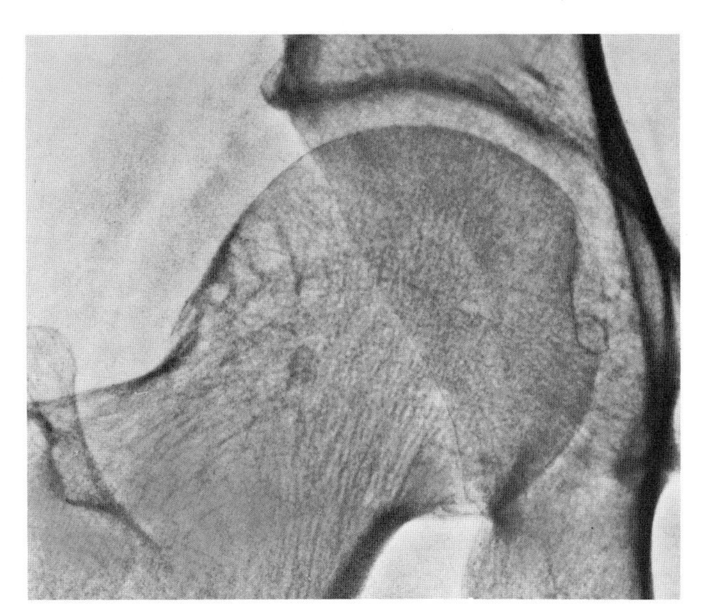

Fig. 481 a

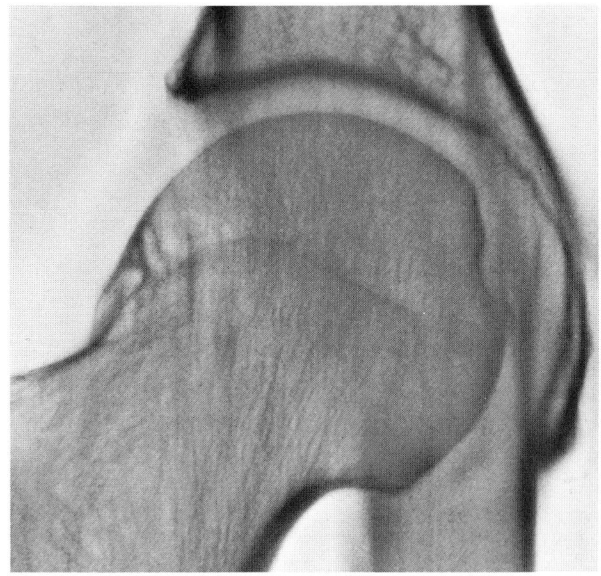

Fig. 481 b

Fig. 481. Thickening of the cortex of the upper contour of the femoral neck, caused by cystic-sclerotic reconstruction at the craniolateral and caudomedial angles of the region of neck and head of femur, seen here on general and tomographic views. At the epiphyseal spaces there are two statically endangered regions of blood supply, the craniolateral and the caudomedial angles of the epiphyseal space *(Bernbeck)*. The epiphyseal blood vessels of the head enter above these spaces; the metaphyseal blood vessels of the neck enter below. In this case, these marginal regions stand out as cystic-sclerotic zones of reconstruction. Disturbances of the vascular supply at this site may lead, in *Perthes'* disease, at the stage of reparation, to such regions of increased radiolucency and reconstruction. Also, in deforming arthrosis the early damage due to vascular disturbances begins at the cartilage at this point (see also Fig. 480).

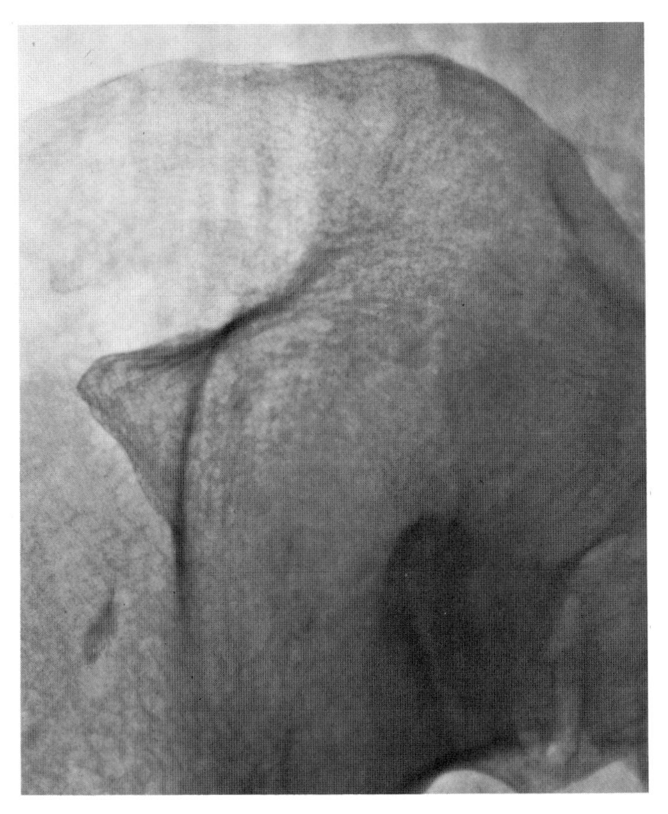

Fig. 482. Right side, anteroposterior. Here also, iliitis condensans.

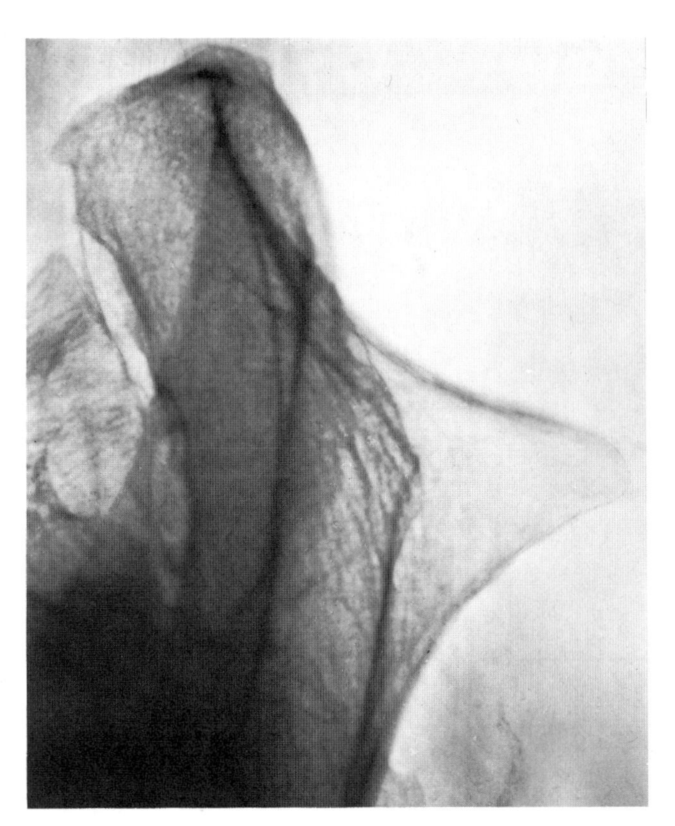

Fig. 483. Left side, lateral.

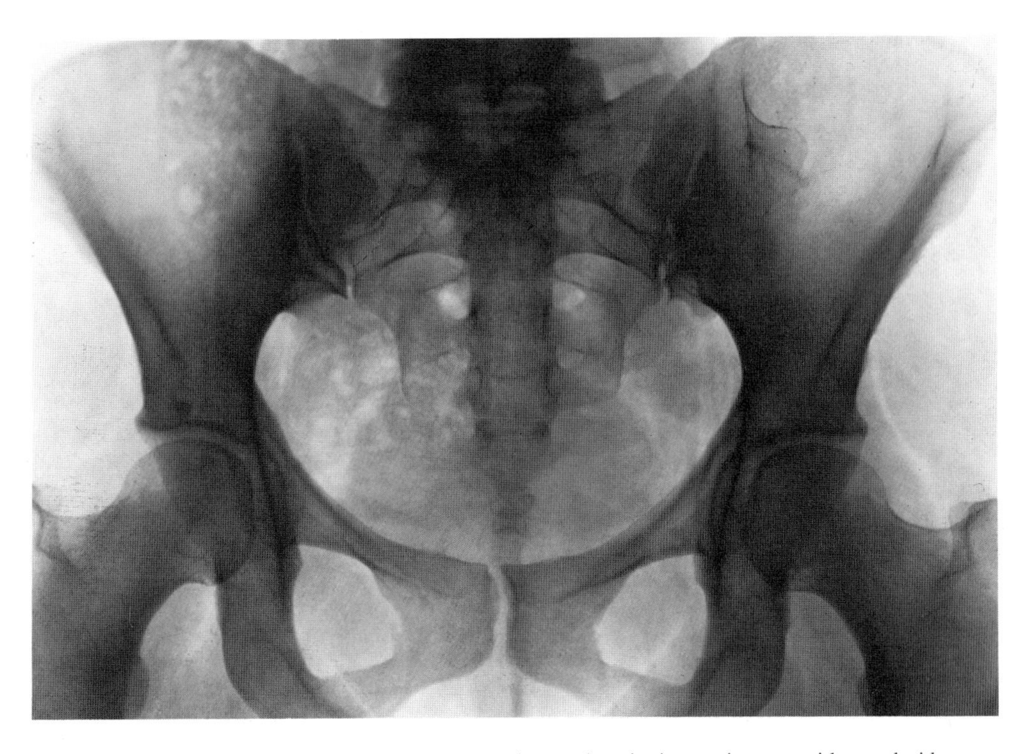

Fig. 484 shows the **rare case of a unilateral iliac horn** in an otherwise inconspicuous, neither android nor andropoid formation of the pelvis in a 44-year-old female *(Birkner)*.

Figs. 482–484. Iliac horns. They are mostly symmetrical, dominantly hereditary bony excrescences of the posterior surface of the ilium, lateral to the sacroiliac joints. These pelvic changes, first described in 1946 by the American *Fong,* are part of the general hereditary osteo-onychodysplasia *(Roeckerath),* which includes dysplasia of the pelvic girdle, dysplasia or aplasia of patellae, dysplasia of elbow with hypoplasia or aplasia of the head of the radius or the ulnar epicondyle, dysplasia of the hand as in *Madelung*'s deformity, dysplasia of nails, dysplasia of the shoulder girdle and dysplasia of the feet, with thickening of the ankles or clubfoot. The iliac horns are the connecting or main symptom of this hereditary osteo-onychodysplasia, which is not sex-linked. It is likely that they can also be observed isolated or unilaterally. Further work has been published by *Kaufmann* (1963), *Simay* and *Murányi* (1965), *Oláh* and *Fehérvári* (1968).

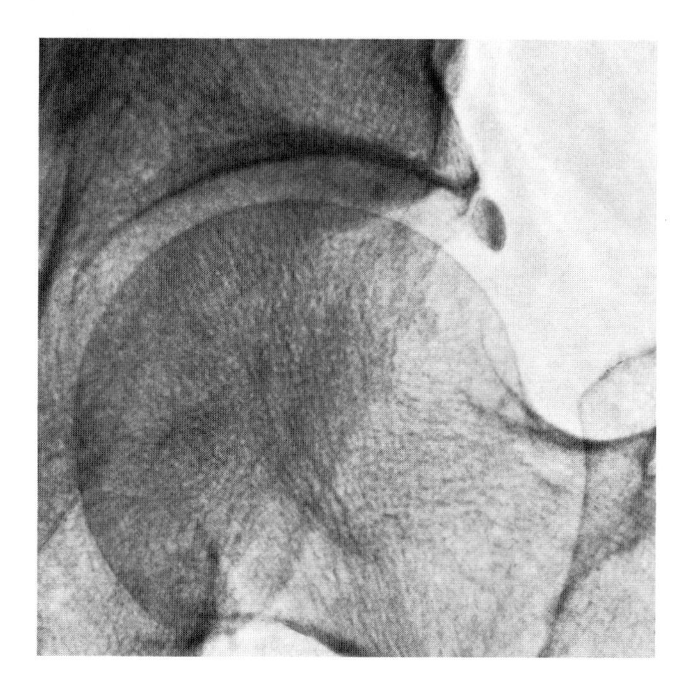

Fig. 485. Bone at the acetabulum or bone at the acetabular rim (= os acetabuli roentgenologicum) at the left hip joint. In the adult, this is a frequently demonstrable, rounded or pyramid-shaped, usually well-delimited shadow of bone next to the upper acetabular rim; it arises:
a) through separation of a bony part of the tip of the acetabular roof, caused by "zones of reconstruction"
b) through traumatic splintering-off of bone from the acetabulum
c) through splitting-off of arthrotic osteophytes
d) through metaplastic tissue ossification after trauma
e) occasionally through a persistent accessory nucleus.

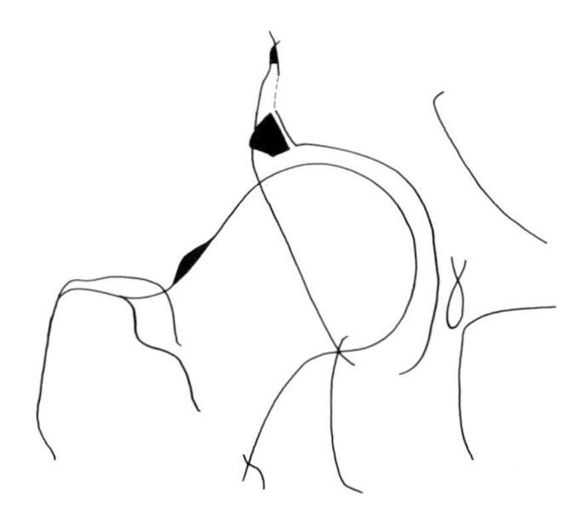

Fig. 487. Bone at acetabulum in a 37-year-old male who had never suffered from trauma or coxitis. It must be assumed that this formation stretches along the acetabular rim and is seen only at the upper end in cross section. The patient also carried such a bone at the other hip joint, and there he complained for ten years of occasional pains. The compression bulge at the upper contour of the femoral neck corresponds to an irregularity of the cortex which also occurs normally, usually as periostal thickening at the ventral surface, more rarely on the dorsal side of the femoral neck. (On the bone at acetabulum, see also the section on "Skeleton of the Infant," p. 489.)

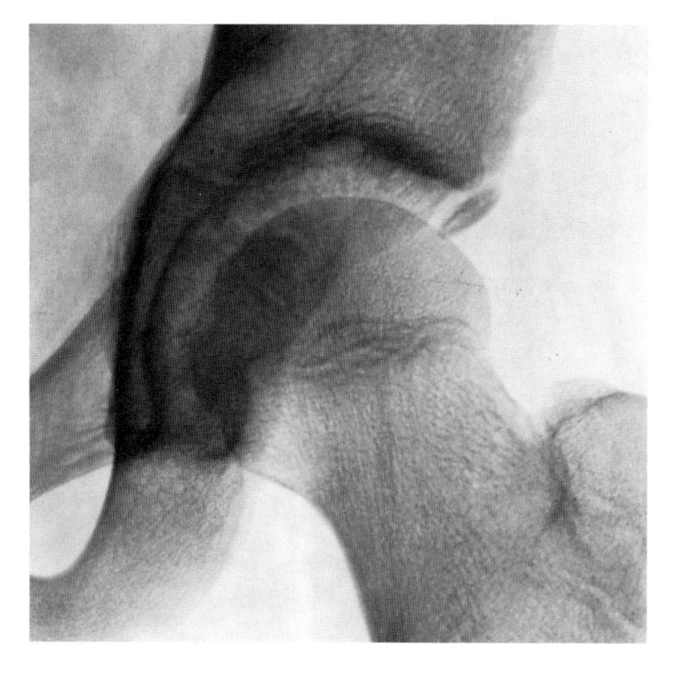

Fig. 486. Acetabular bone. Roentgenologically, an acetabular bone can only be demonstrated in the shape of a transitory, apparent formation of a supernumerary bone, as a so-called apophysis of the acetabular rim during late puberty. Very rarely, most likely due to hormonal disturbances of ossification, an acetabular bone persists in the adult (see *Schinz, Schmidt, Dyes*).

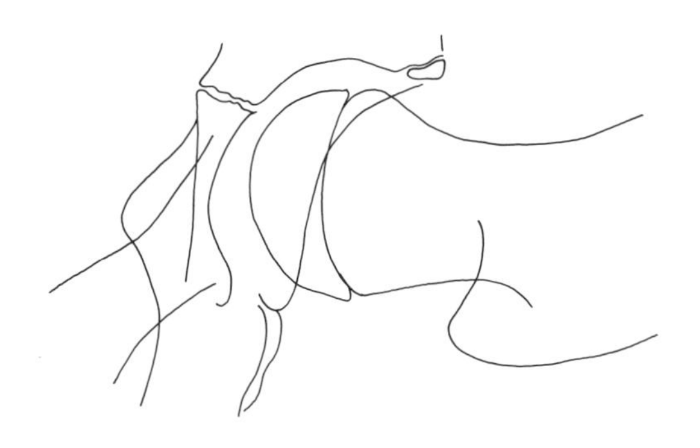

Fig. 488. Smallish apophysis of the **acetabular rim** (acetabular epiphysis), i.e., **acetabular bone** becomes distinctly visible as part of the acetabular rim. Here, too, a supernumerary bone is simulated, but in fact it represents a normal transitional stage in the ossification of the hip joint; very seldom, it may persist (persistent acetabular bone) or may be broken off by trauma or gradually separated by mechanically conditioned *Looser's* reconstruction (fatigue or permanent fracture).

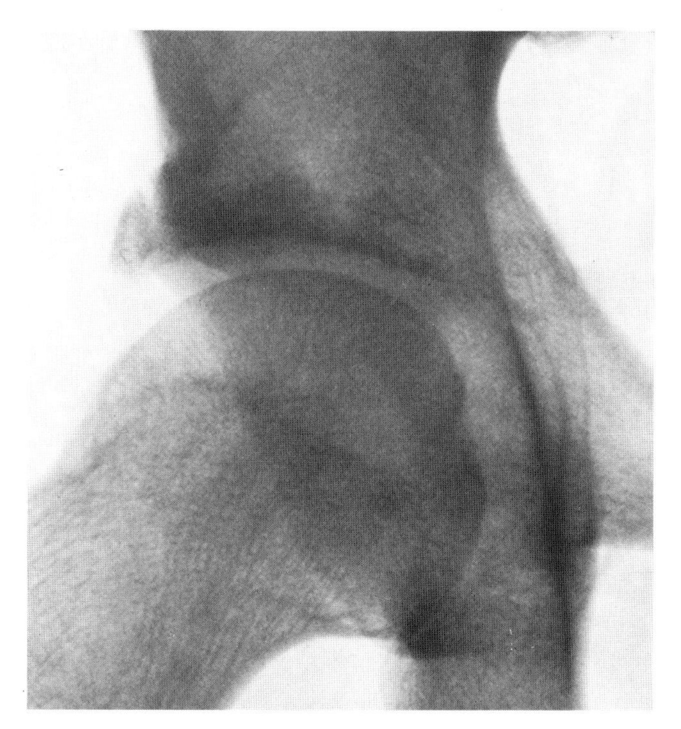

Fig. 489 a

Fig. 489 b

Fig. 489. Bilateral, still persistent acetabular bones, lying within the joint bones forming the acetabulum. Their bilateral occurrence is characteristic, although their size and shape may vary. Just as typical is the disappearance of the transitory acetabular bone at the end of the period of ossification coming, at the latest, during the 18th year of life.

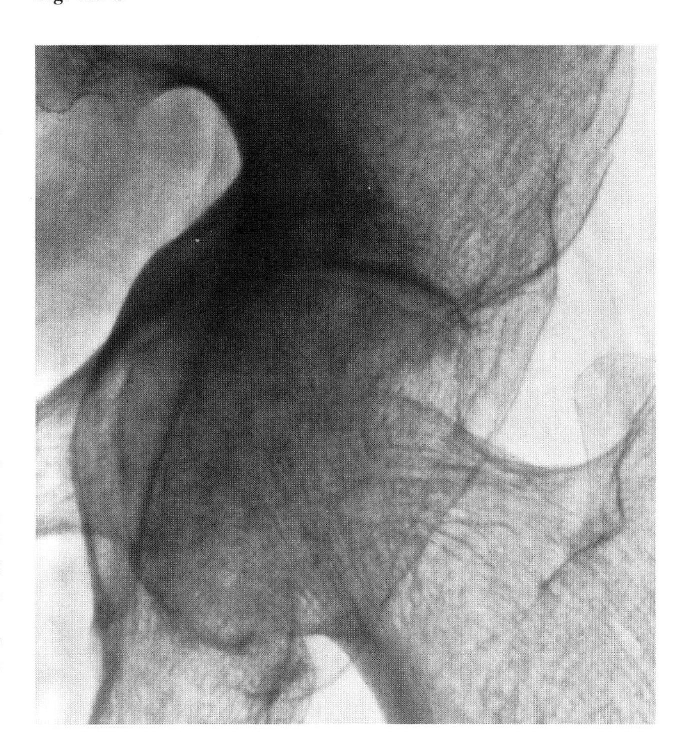

Fig. 490. Protrusion of the acetabulum in a 54-year-old female. This is a protrusion of the acetabular floor which occurs in both sexes in early infancy. Usually it disappears in adulthood. A more or less pronounced, persistent protrusion, whereby the shadow of the acetabular floor projects beyond the linea terminalis, may be a familiar condition occurring more often in the female. It may be acquired, unilaterally or bilaterally, through a disturbance of ossification, e.g., in rickets or in advanced age, in an osteoporotic or osteomalacic skeleton. Finally, the radiologically observed acetabular protrusion is today a not uncommon post-traumatic effect, i.e., a secondary protrusion of the acetabulum *(Klopfer, Schmidt)*.

The primary (idiopathic) protrusion of the acetabulum (after *Colin*):

A) In the child
Osteoarthritis
Asthenia
Osteochondritis
Abnormal ossification of the Y-cartilage
Congenitally deep acetabulum
Developmentally conditioned depth of the acetabulum

B) In the adult
Osteoarthritis
Late effects of a disease mentioned under A)
Generalized osteomalacia
Localized osteomalacia

Variants of the Bony Surroundings of the Obturator Foramen

The obturator foramen, whose bony rim is formed by ilium, ischium and pubis, shows the following inconstant and variable protuberances which are directed towards the obturator membrane:

1. The anterior obturator tubercle, a more or less raised hump at the anterior end of the obturator sulcus; therefore, it lies in the anterior upper part of the bony rim (Fig. 491).
2. The posterior obturator tubercle, which lies at the ventral margin of the body of the ischium, therefore, also in the upper part of the bony rim (see Fig. 491); it is not always well defined *(Rauber-Kopsch)* and rarely readily visible on radiographs.
3. Occasionally, spiky exostoses are found at the middle to lower rim of the obturator foramen, mainly bilaterally. *Seyss* considers such exostoses as variants, and proposes for them the collective designation of ischiopubic tubercle (see Figs. 496, 497).

After studying the pertinent standard anatomical references (*Waldeyer, Spalteholz-Spanner, Rauber-Kopsch),* one has to regard the multiple, spiky, bizarre exostoses of varying heights as ossifications of the muscular-tendinous insertion of the external obturator muscle, which is fixed at the medial lower and upper rim as well as at the outer surface of the obturator membrane (*Birkner* and *Consentius,* 1977). According to *H. Schneider,* spur-shaped bony additions are possible at any insertion of tendon or muscle and may even begin to develop at the beginning of adulthood.

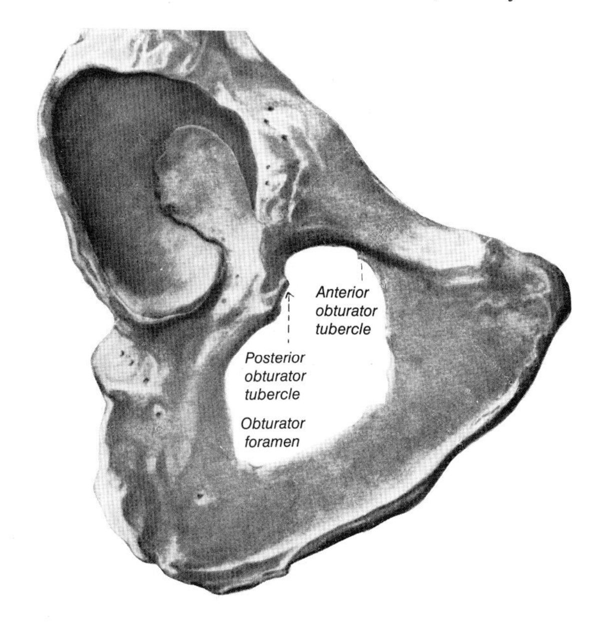

Fig. 491. Right hip bone, from front and below (from *Spalteholz-Spanner*).

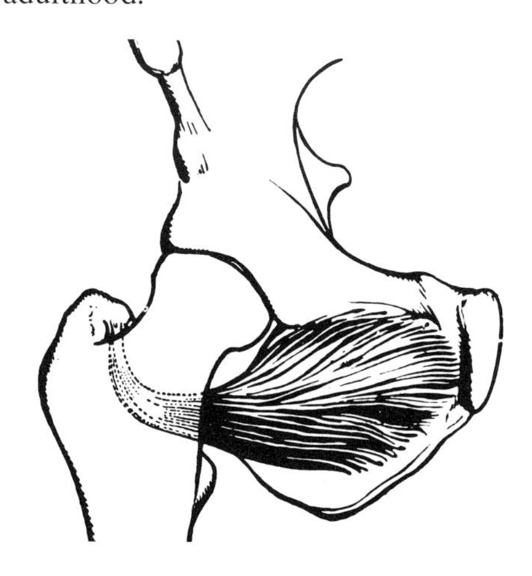

Fig. 492 demonstrates the course of the external obturator muscle. The insertions of its fibers at the medial rim of the obturator foramen correspond distinctly to the direction of the course of the multiple bony spurs. The field of origin of the external obturator muscle is situated on the outer side of the obturator membrane and on the medial part of the bony frame of the obturator foramen; see also Figs. 411 and 412 (from *Benninghoff-Goerttler,* 11th Edition).

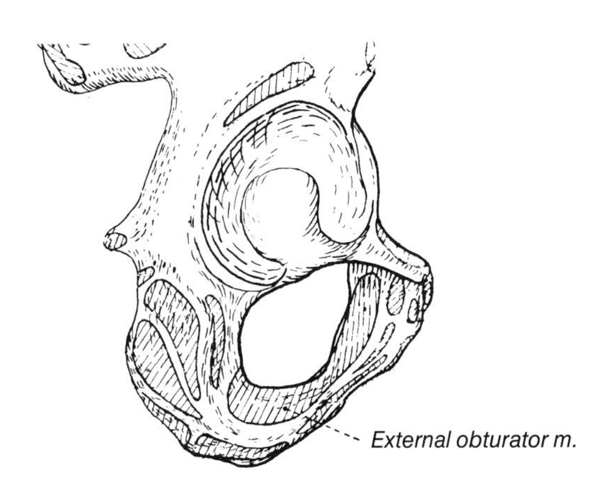

Fig. 493. Right hip bone. Origin of the external obturator muscle at the outer surface (from *Rauber-Kopsch*).

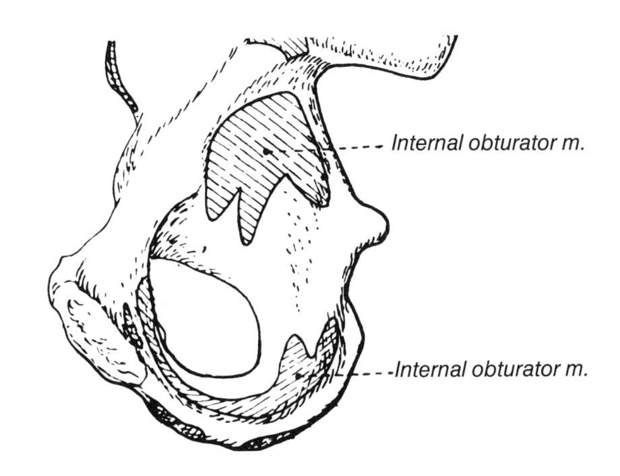

Fig. 494. Right hip bone, origin of the internal obturator muscle on the inner surface (from *Rauber-Kopsch*).

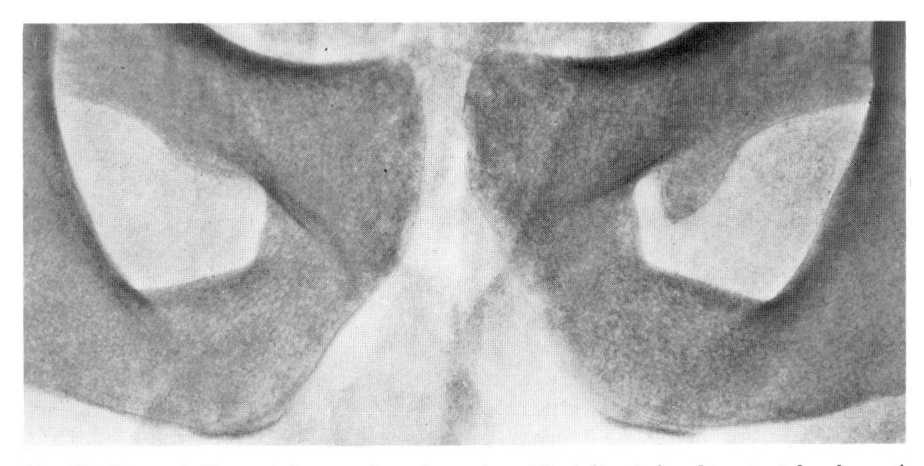

Fig. 495. Exostosis-like protuberance from the region of the left anterior obturator tubercle; on the right, a flatter tubercle. Male, 20 years of age. The apophyses at the ischial tuberosity have not yet fused; fusion occurs between the 20th and 25th years of life.

The fibers of the obturator membrane are fixed to special ligamental apophyses of the bone at the posterior obturator crest, at the anterior obturator tubercle, at the inner margin of the upper pubic ramus and at the posterior obturator tubercle, which is less constant *(Braus)*.

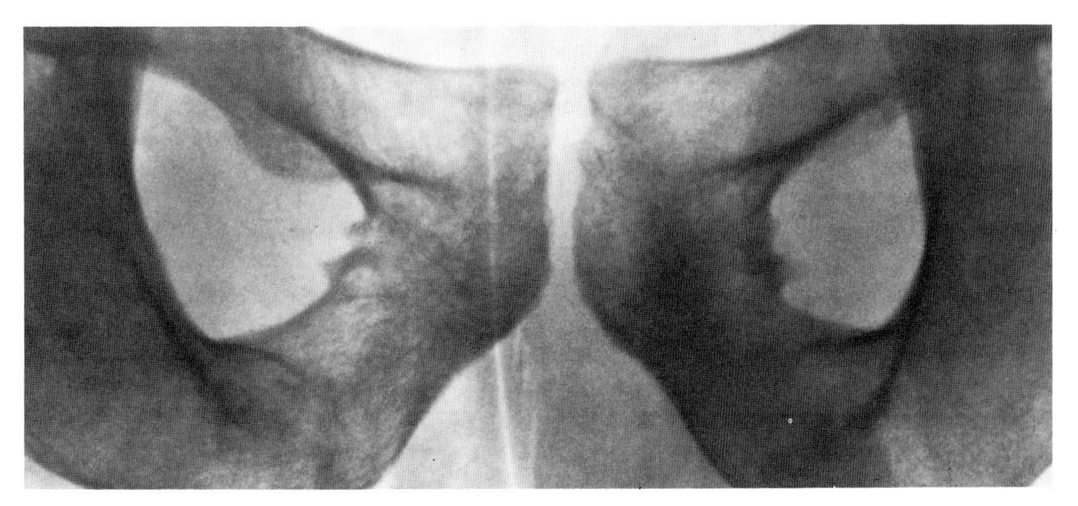

Fig. 496. Multiple exostoses at the medial rim of the obturator foramen (ossification of muscle or of insertion of the external obturator muscle).

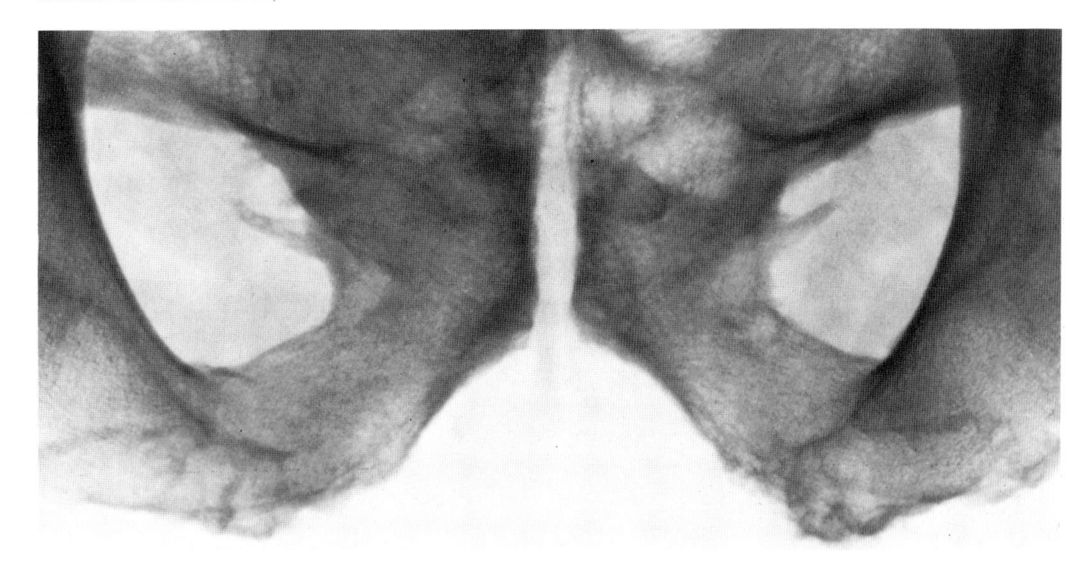

Fig. 497. 78-year-old male. **Multiple ossifications of tendon insertions at both ischial tuberositae (origin of the adductor magnus muscle) and at the medial bony rim of the obturator foramen (origin of the external obturator muscle).**

A roughening of the ischial tuberosity may develop from micro-traumata of the strong muscles which insert there (the semi-membranosus, semi-tendinosus, adductor magnus, biceps femoris muscles). They may also be caused in sportsmen by former necroses of apophyses after traumata and micro-traumata. Finally, chronic inflammations may be the cause.

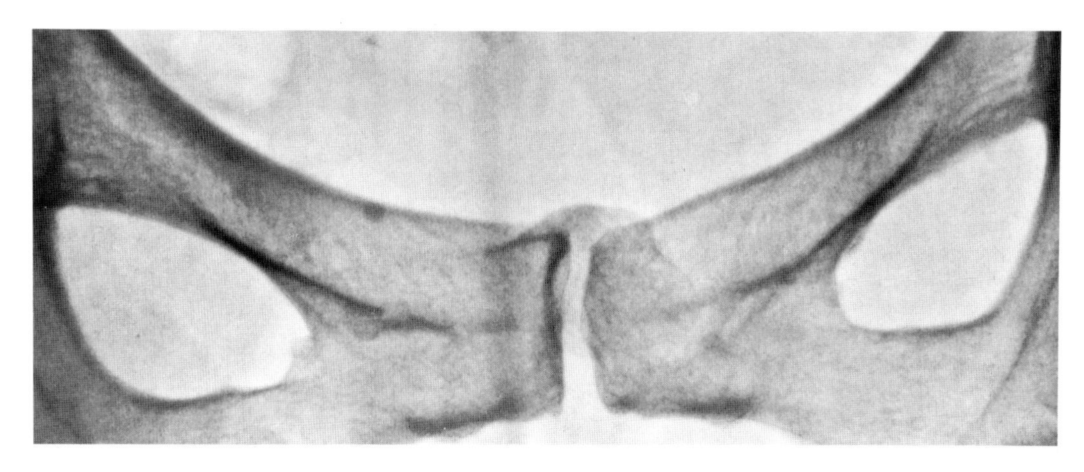

Fig. 498. Bony bridge across the symphysis, caused by an ossified superior pubic ligament; (see Fig. 442, No. 123*). In addition, ossifications of the tendinous insertions at the medial rim of the obturator foramen are observed (from the collection of *W. Werner).*

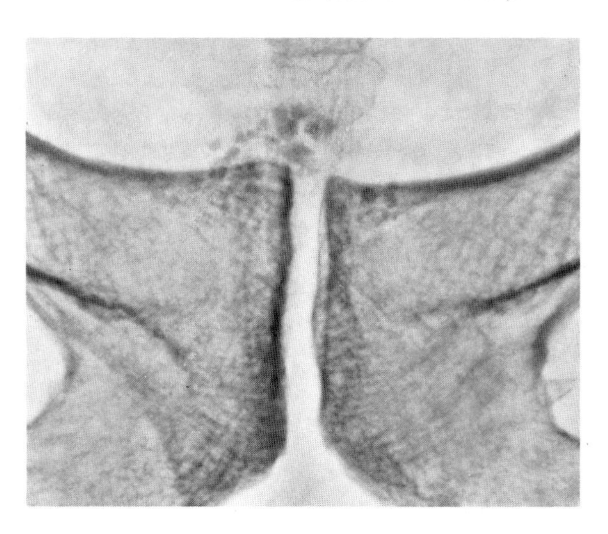

Fig. 499 a

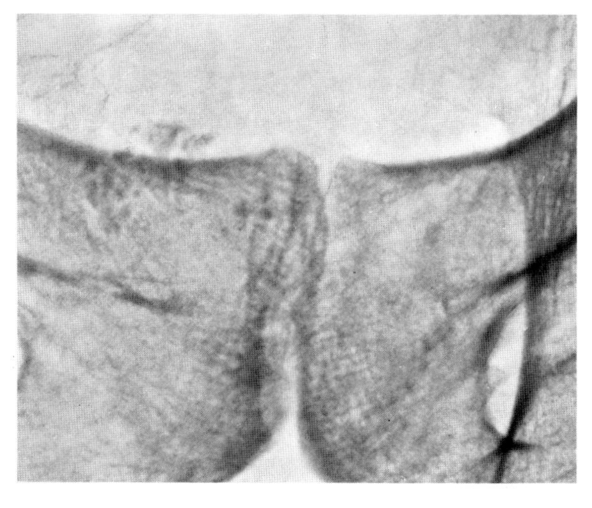

Fig. 499 b

Fig. 499. Calcified prostate in a 54-year-old male. On the anteroposterior view the typically speckled calcification is partly projected into the upper cleft of the symphysis. On Fig. 499b (picture in 1st oblique diameter) the calcification on the right, behind the symphyseal cleft, can be seen. The identity of the calcification is thereby clarified; see Fig. 442, No 126*, p. 199.

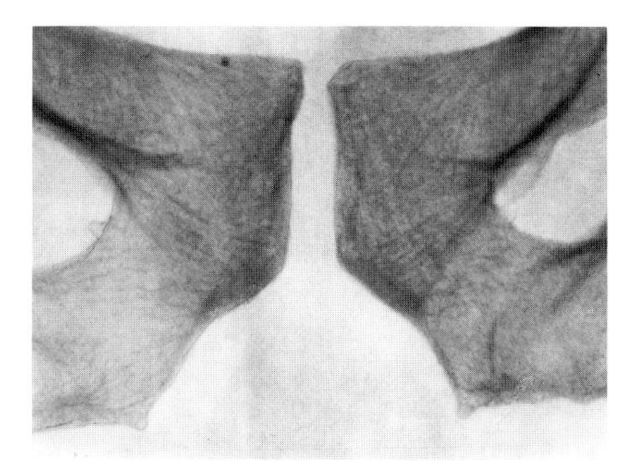

Fig. 500. Exostosis of gracilis, a frequent finding in the aged. This is an exostosis-shaped, bony elongation at the lower side of the ischial tuberosity, in the region of the tendinous origin of the gracilis muscle. If it is unilateral, it should not be mistaken for a pathological neoplastic bone formation (osteoma, sarcoma); see also Fig. 442, No. 122**, p. 199.

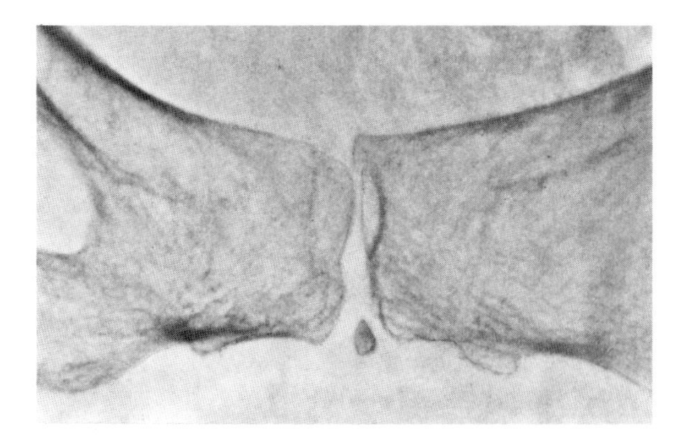

Fig. 501. Isolated bony nucleus at the lower symphyseal cleft; should not be mistaken for calcification of the prostate or for a prostatic stone (see Fig. 442, No. 123**, p. 199). For a differential diagnosis, an osteochondrotic, post-traumatic necrosis of the cartilage (e.g., in football players) or a simple splintered-off fracture should be considered.

III. Upper Extremities, Including the Shoulder Girdle

Radiographic Anatomy and Radiographs of the Clavicle and Shoulder Joint

Clavicle

For demonstration of the clavicle, the prone position is best. Care must be taken to ensure that the cassette lies on the clavicle, but due to the curvature of the clavicle this possibility is limited. If the medial part of the clavicle is to be shown, the patient is placed in the prone position; the cassette is raised on the outer side and projects vertically onto the clavicle. With this technique, the sternoclavicular joint shows well. With the patient prone, if the projection is median onto the spinal column, at about the height of the jugular notch, both sternoclavicular articulations are seen. The focus-film distance must not be too short or else the shadow of the spine becomes too broad. To survey exactly the acromial part of the clavicle with its particular space, it is useful to place the patient on his chest and to raise the cassette on the lateral side (Fig. 502). For injured patients the prone position is often uncomfortable. In that case, either ventrodorsal pictures with the patient supine or a dorsoventral picture with the patient sitting at the lung screen are taken. In this way, the desired view is usually achieved with sufficient distinctness (Fig. 503). If possible, all pictures of the clavicle should be taken with the patient holding his breath, or at least taking small breaths, and with the shoulder pulled upwards. A good illustration of the sternal manubrium with both clavicular joints often succeeds with a very oblique projection (in the second oblique thoracic diameter, i.e., in prone position with lifting of the right side). See also the views of the sternum in Figures 334 and 343.

Shoulder Joint

Radiographs of the shoulder joint are generally taken in supine position.

For radiographs of the shoulder joint and the scapula, the following projections are used:

1. sagittal
   a) ventrodorsal
   b) dorsoventral
2. sagittal oblique, with shifting of the X-ray tube in cranial or caudal direction
3. axial
   a) craniocaudal
   b) caudocranial
4. frontal, for demonstration of the scapula.

For all these projections the arm must be placed in internal or external rotation or in intermediate position, according to the needs of the case.

With maximal external rotation the lesser tubercle moves outwards and the greater tubercle backwards. For demonstration of the greater tubercle, the intermediate position is used (Fig. 517). With inward rotation of the arm, neither the greater nor the lesser tubercle is projected free. With exact sagittal projection of the head of the humerus, the acromion and the head partly cover each other. If the oblique sagittal projection with the tube shifted cranially is chosen, the head of the humerus is projected freely (Fig. 519). The lesser tubercle is projected into the margin of the axilla when the abducted arm is rotated inward. If the abducted arm is greatly supinated (axial projection), the lesser tubercle appears above and marginally (see Figs. 504 and 549).

To imitate the cranioventrodorsal pathway of the rays if the patient is prone, the central ray must be aimed nearer to the angle of the scapula and obliquely caudodorsoventral. On these oblique views the humeral head appears to be distorted (Fig. 518).

The coracoid process and the scapular spine are well projected with caudoventrodorsal direction of the rays (Fig. 522) and the lower angle of the scapula shares well with the arm in abduction.

When axial radiographs of the shoulder joint are taken, the cassette lies in the axilla (path of rays craniocaudal) or on the shoulder (path of rays caudocranial); see Fig. 520.

The frontal radiograph for demonstration of the scapula is taken with the patient supine or standing with the arm drawn right across the chest (see Fig. 514). As the articular space of the acromioclavicular joint stands obliquely, not sagittally, one best aims the central ray from a dorsal position, obliquely into the joint. In juveniles the articular space appears wider than in adults.

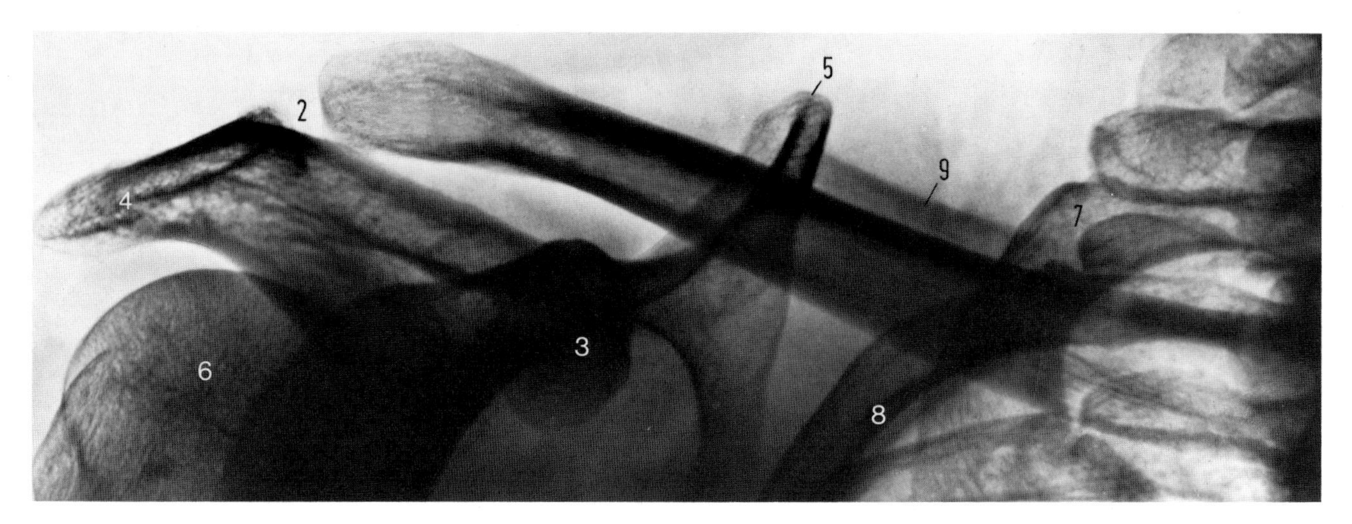

Fig. 502. Clavicle, dorsoventral. Projection: patient prone, the clavicle lies next to the cassette, the head is turned towards the healthy side, the upper arm of the side to be examined is rotated slightly inward. The central ray is aimed onto the center of the clavicle vertically to the film.

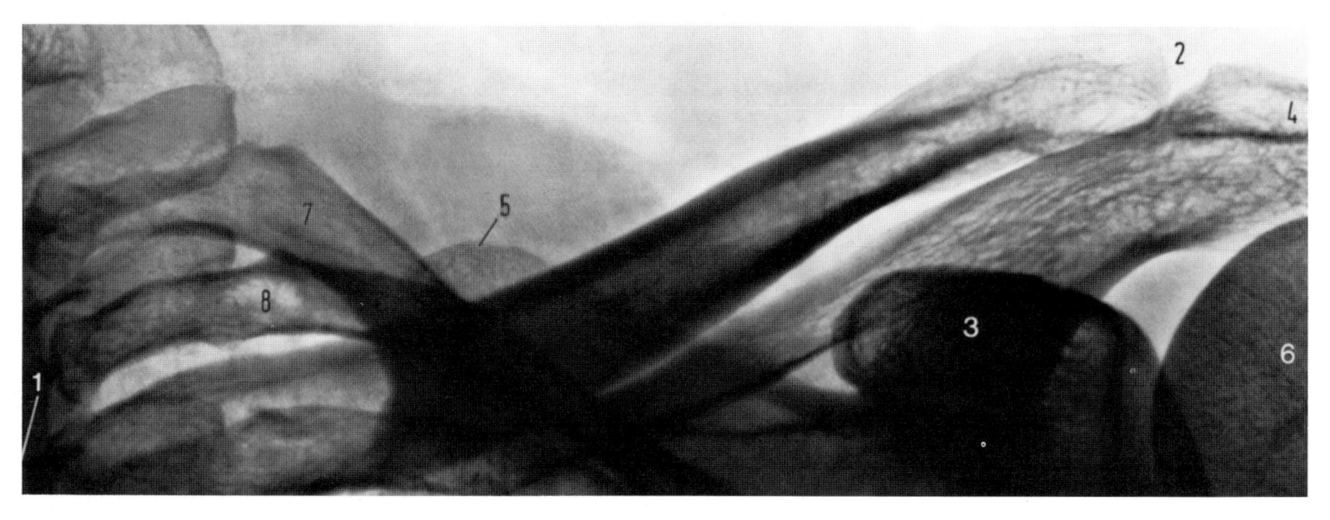

Fig. 503. Clavicle, ventrodorsal. Projection: patient supine, otherwise as in Fig. 502.

1 Sternoclavicular joint
2 Acromioclavicular joint
3 Coracoid process
4 Acromion
5 Superior scapular angle
6 Head of humerus
7 1st rib
8 2nd rib
9 Accompanying shadow against the subclavian triangle (greater supraclavicular fossa); may sometimes be concave (see also Fig. 509).

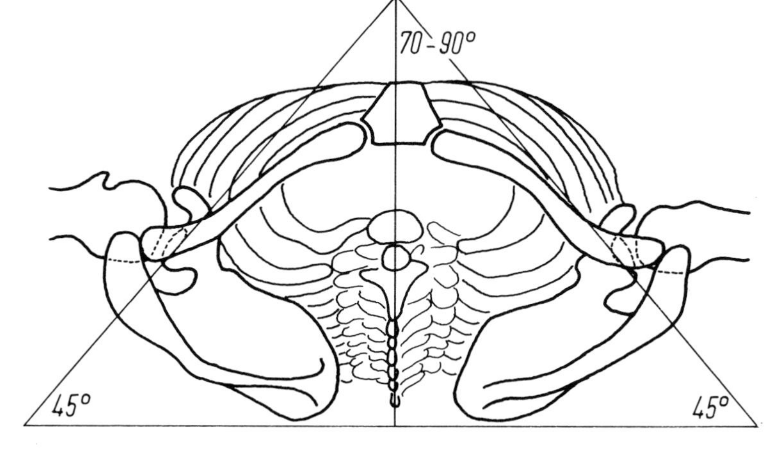

Fig. 504. Relation of the humeroscapular joints to the horizontal plane of the supine patient (after *Viehweger*), with the arm supinated and rotated outward, as in an axial radiograph of the shoulder joint. The lesser tubercle forms an edge ventrally.
On all views taken in the supine position, the articular surfaces of the glenoid cavities are turned ventrally by about 40–45°. Therefore, radiographs of both shoulders, taken for comparison, are often difficult to interpret roentgenotopographically; the various processes may take very different positions, e.g., on axial views.

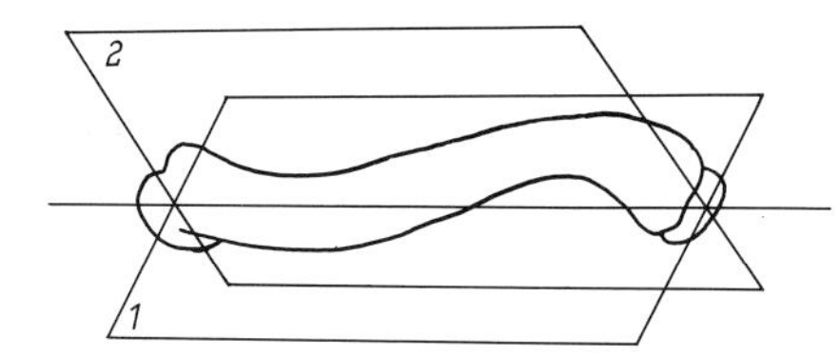

Fig. 505 shows the planes of projection in Figs. 506 and 507 (from *Schönbauer*).

1 First main plane: central ray ventrocaudocranial, vertical to film (Fig. 506)
2 Second main plane: central ray dorsocaudocranial, transthoracic, vertical to film (Fig. 507)

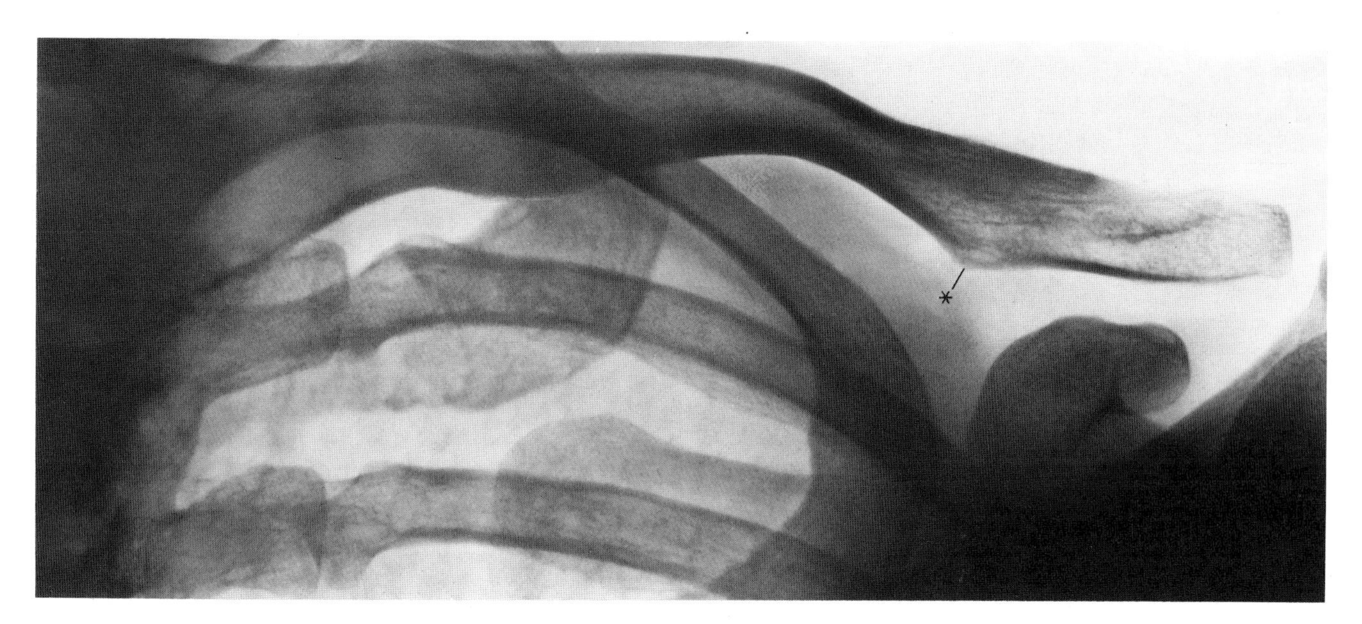

Fig. 506. Left clavicle, ventrocranial. * = conoid tubercle (see No. 67, Fig. 525)

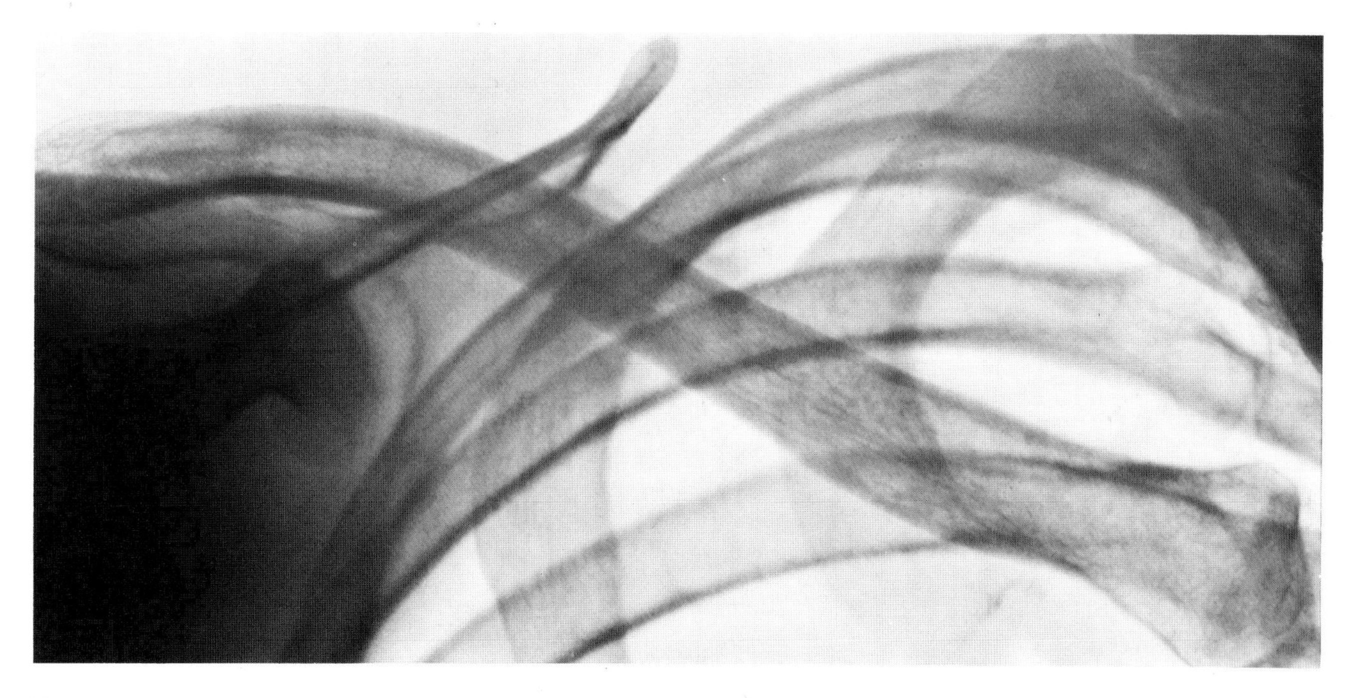

Fig. 507. Left clavicle, dorsocaudocranial.

Figs. 506 and 507. Left clavicle in two planes *(Schönbauer)*. This technique, though it cannot be applied in all cases, offers the possibility of determining the actual shift and kinking of the axis of the fractured parts.
Because of the curvature of the clavicle, two main planes can be defined: the first lies in the plane of the curvature, the second is vertical to it (see Fig. 505).
Seyffarth and *Heppe* have reported techniques for radiography of the clavicle in the second plane.

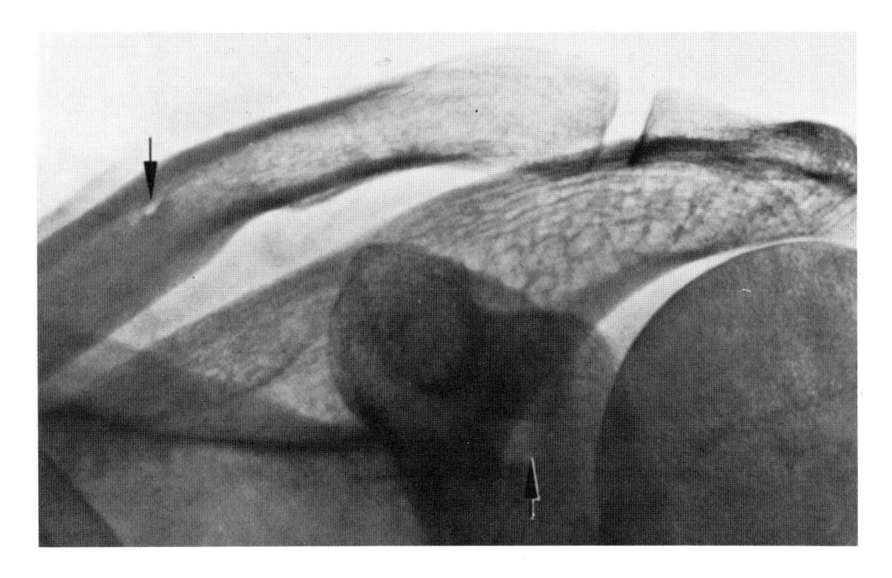

(↓) Nerve canal of the clavicle *(Pahl)*
(↑) Increased radiolucency in the upper angle of the glenoid cavity, simulated by adjacent superimpositions (see also No. 65, Fig. 525)

Fig. 508. Nerve canal of the clavicle (↓). Exit of the supraclavicular nerve from the 4th cervical segment; it provides the sensory supply for the thoracic skin above the two first intercostal spaces and for the sternoclavicular joint. The frequency of its occurrence is about 6%; it occurs twice as often on the left side as on the right and may also be present double in the clavicle. It may be mistaken for osteolyses, e.g., metastases. See also No. 62*, Fig. 525.

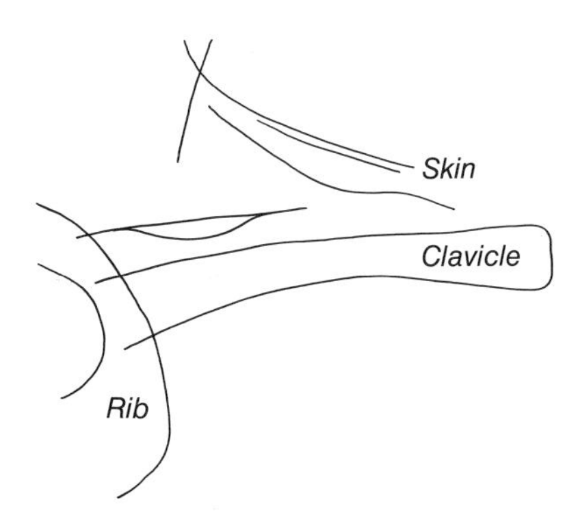

Fig. 509. Trigonum omoclaviculare (subclavian triangle).

A shadow that accompanies the clavicula in lean people corresponds to the border of the skin against the subclavian triangle (greater supraclavicular fossa); see Fig. 510, h. It may be projected concavely (see Fig. 509), as the floor of the fossa may also form a line. Crossing of shadows (Fig. 510) may simulate fibrous adhesions in a pneumothorax.

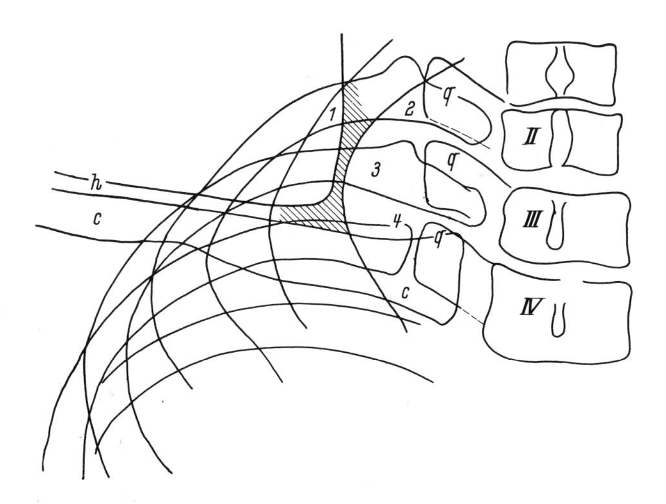

Fig. 510. Crossing of shadows in the supraclavicular fossa (hatched).

II–IV	Bodies of 2nd to 4th thoracic vertebrae
q	Transverse process
c	Clavicle
h	Skin covering the clavicle
1, 2, 3, 4,	1st to 4th ribs

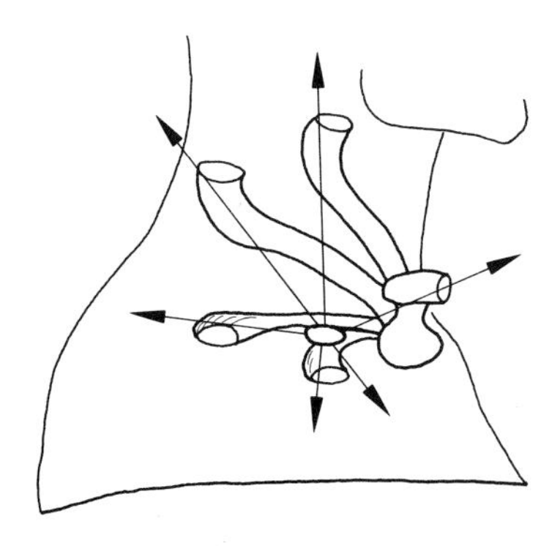

Fig. 511. Range of movements of the sternoclavicular joint (after *Lanz* and *Wachsmuth*). Any number of movements of the sternoclavicular joint are possible, around an infinite number of axes centering through the middle of the clavicle. It may be considered to be an inexact rotary joint; only its isolated voluntary rotation is excluded in the lining *(R. Fick)*.

Fig. 512. Scapula, ventrodorsal. For projection see Fig. 513. The arm is raised in order to rotate the scapula out of the bony thorax. The central ray is aimed onto the center of the scapula.

- 1 Head of humerus
- 1* Lesser tubercle
- 1** Greater tubercle
- 2 Acromion
- 3 Coracoid process
- 4 Center of clavicle with
- * Conoid tubercle
- 5 Neck of scapula
- 5* Infraglenoid tubercle
- 6 Glenoid cavity
- 7 Lateral angle (of scapula)
- 8 Scapular spine
- 9 Upper margin, near the superior angle (of scapula)
- 10 Axillary border of scapula
- 11 Vertebral border of scapula
- 12 Inferior angle of scapula
- I–VIII 1st to 8th ribs

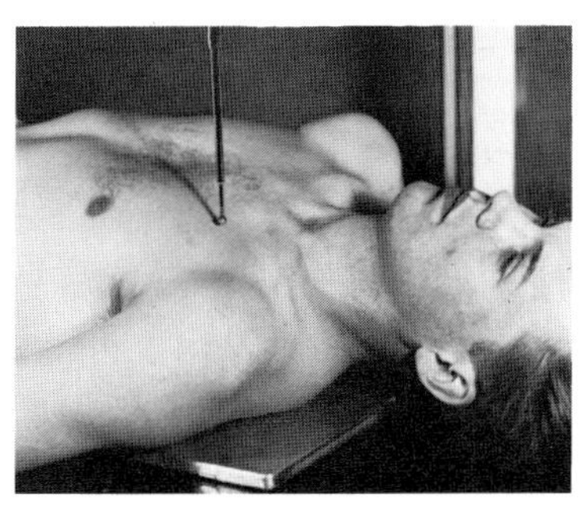

Fig. 513. The scapula moves somewhat away from the superimposition by the thorax; this results in a semi-oblique view of the scapula, similar to the lateroventrodorsal radiographs.

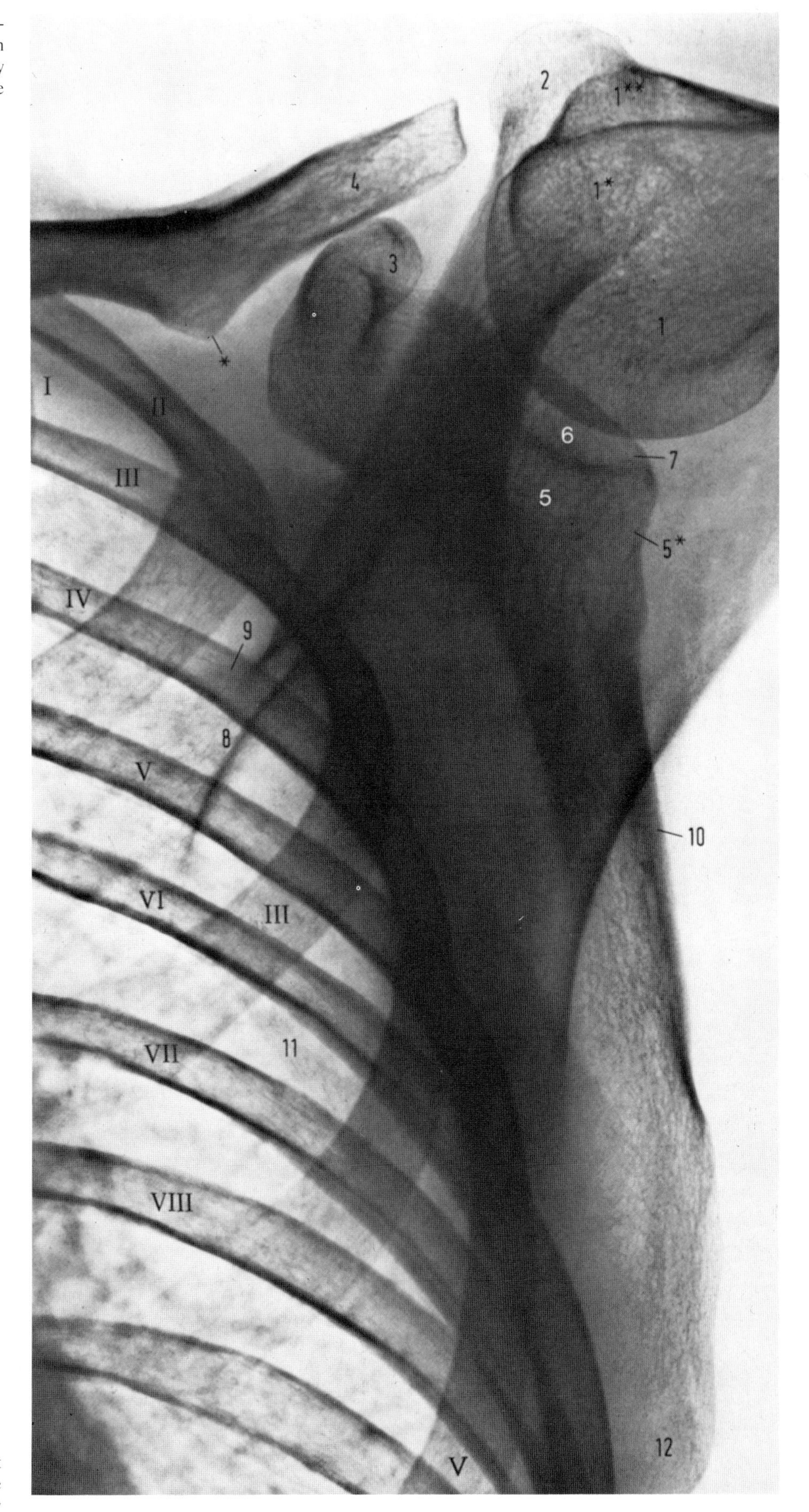

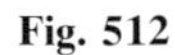
Fig. 512

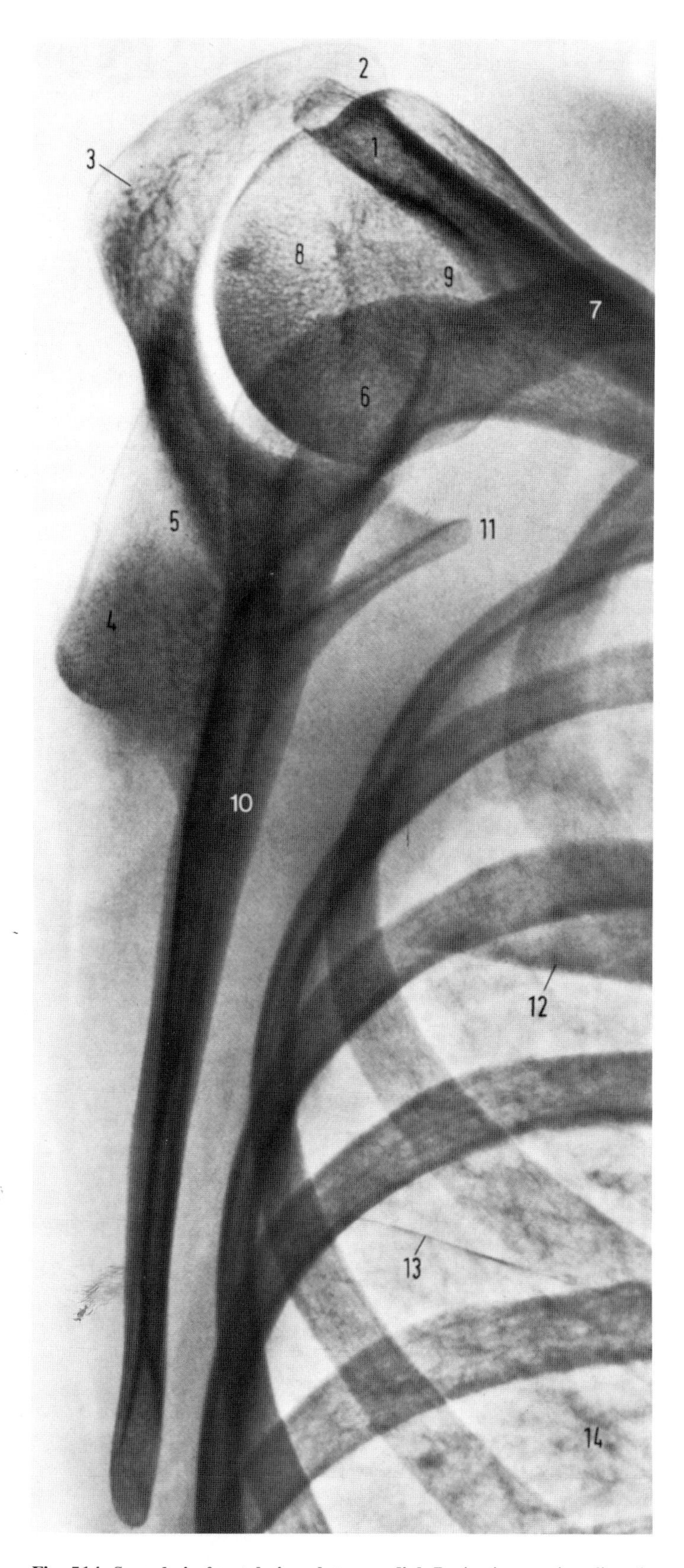

Fig. 514. Scapula in frontal view, lateromedial. Projection: patient lies obliquely, the arm of the diseased side is pulled forward until the lateral and medial margins of the scapula rest vertically above one another. The central ray is directed onto the center of the scapula.

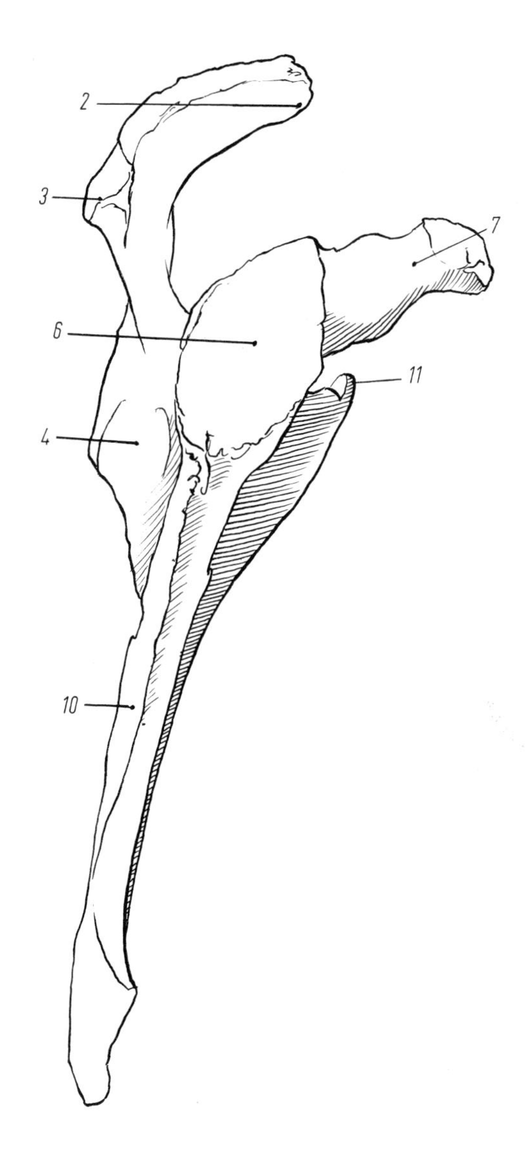

Fig. 515 shows the scapula in the same projection as Fig. 514.

1 Acromial end of clavicle
2 Articular end of acromion; the articular space is taken obliquely and is therefore not visible
3 Lateral edge of the acromion
4 Scapular spine
5 Base of scapular spine, superimposed on glenoidal labrum
6 Glenoid cavity, superimposed by head of humerus
7 Coracoid process
8 Head of humerus
9 Surgical neck of humerus
10 Body of scapula
11 Superior angle of scapula
12 Lower edge of soft tissue of upper arm
13 Interlobar cleft, seen orthograde
14 Normal vascular design of lung

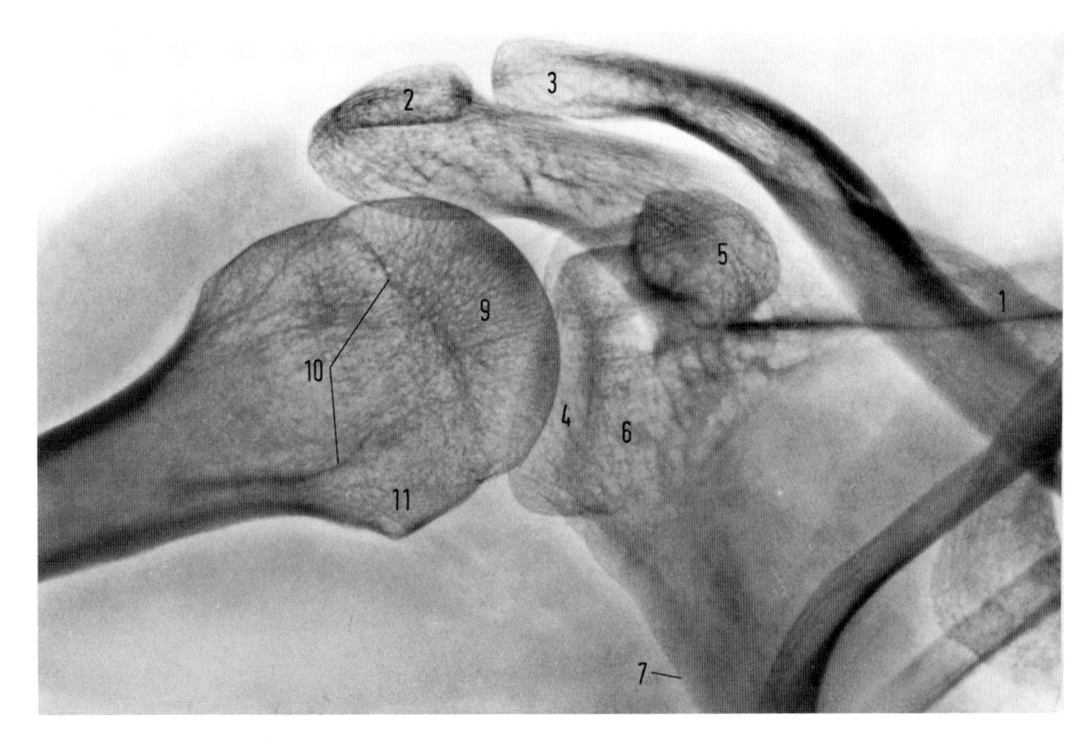

Fig. 516. Shoulder joint, ventrodorsal. Projection: patient supine, the upper arm is abducted and internally rotated. The central ray is aimed vertically onto the shoulder joint. In this position, the lesser tubercle (11) is projected freely into the axilla, and the greater tubercle (10) onto the anatomical neck, in reverse from Fig. 517. The tip of the coracoid process is projected into the upper part of the articular space of the shoulder.

1 Base (line for insertion) of the scapular spine
2 Acromion
3 Acromial end of clavicle
4 Glenoid cavity and lateral angle of scapula
5 Coracoid process
6 Neck of scapula
7 Lateral margin of scapula
8 Infraglenoid tubercle
9 Head of humerus
10 Greater tubercle
11 Lesser tubercle

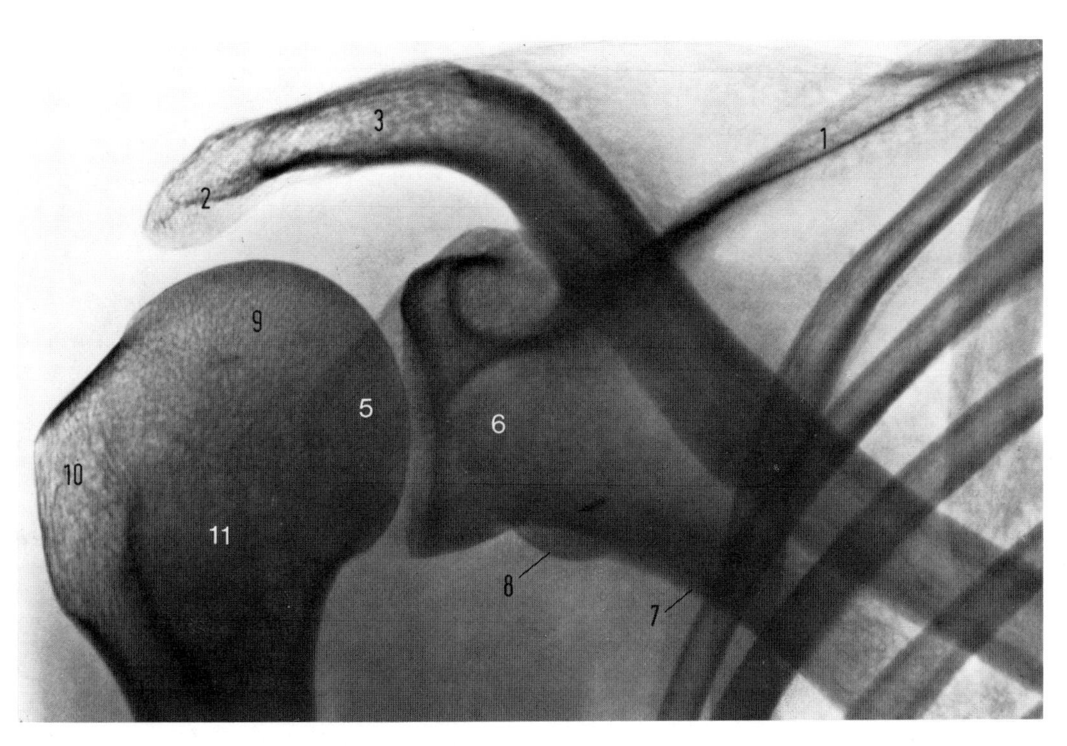

Fig. 517. Shoulder joint, cranioventrodorsal. Projection: patient supine, the healthy side is slightly lifted in order to place the diseased shoulder flat onto the cassette. The upper arm is in middle position of rotation. The central ray is aimed 25° craniocaudally and 15° laterally onto the shoulder joint. See also Figs. 504 and 519.

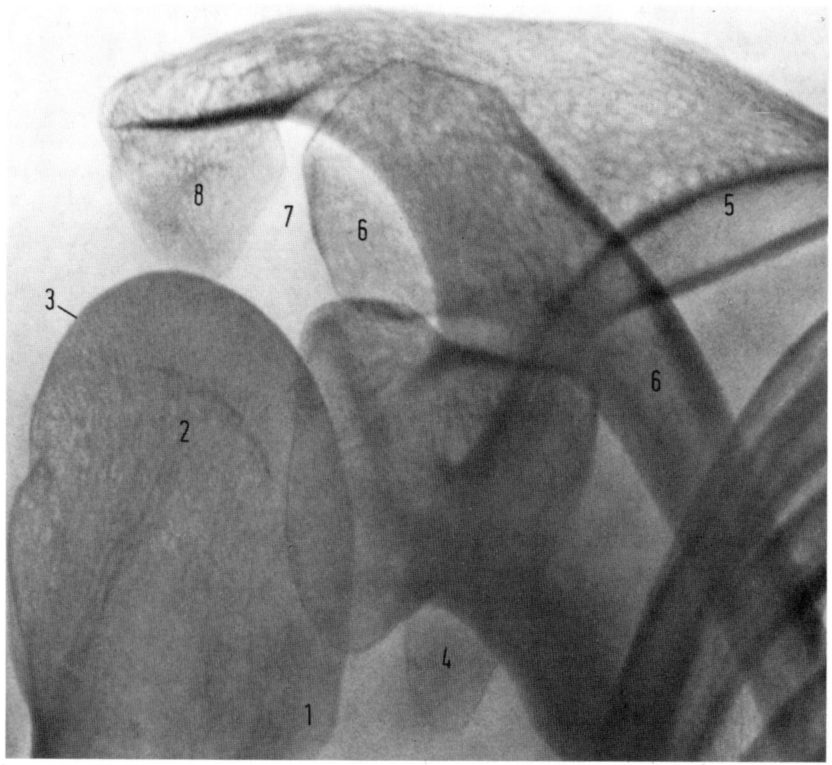

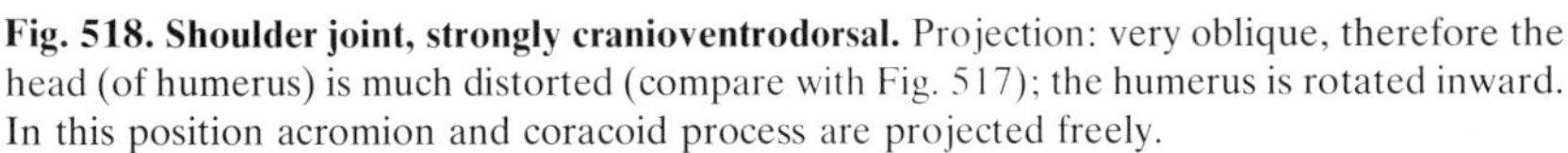

Fig. 518. Shoulder joint, strongly cranioventrodorsal. Projection: very oblique, therefore the head (of humerus) is much distorted (compare with Fig. 517); the humerus is rotated inward. In this position acromion and coracoid process are projected freely.

1 Lesser tubercle
2 Greater tubercle
3 Posterior periphery of head
4 Coracoid process
5 Base line in the groove between scapular spine and anterior margin
6 Clavicle
7 Acromioclavicular joint
8 Acromion

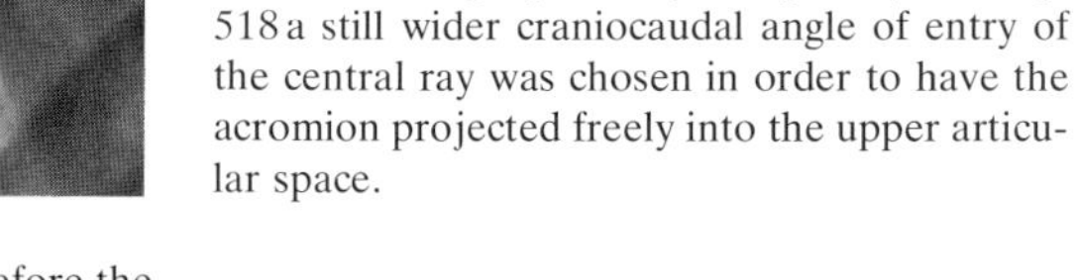

Fig. 519 shows how obliquely the central ray must be directed between acromion (1) and coracoid process (2) to bring the shadow of the head into free projection (see Fig. 517). For Fig. 518a still wider craniocaudal angle of entry of the central ray was chosen in order to have the acromion projected freely into the upper articular space.

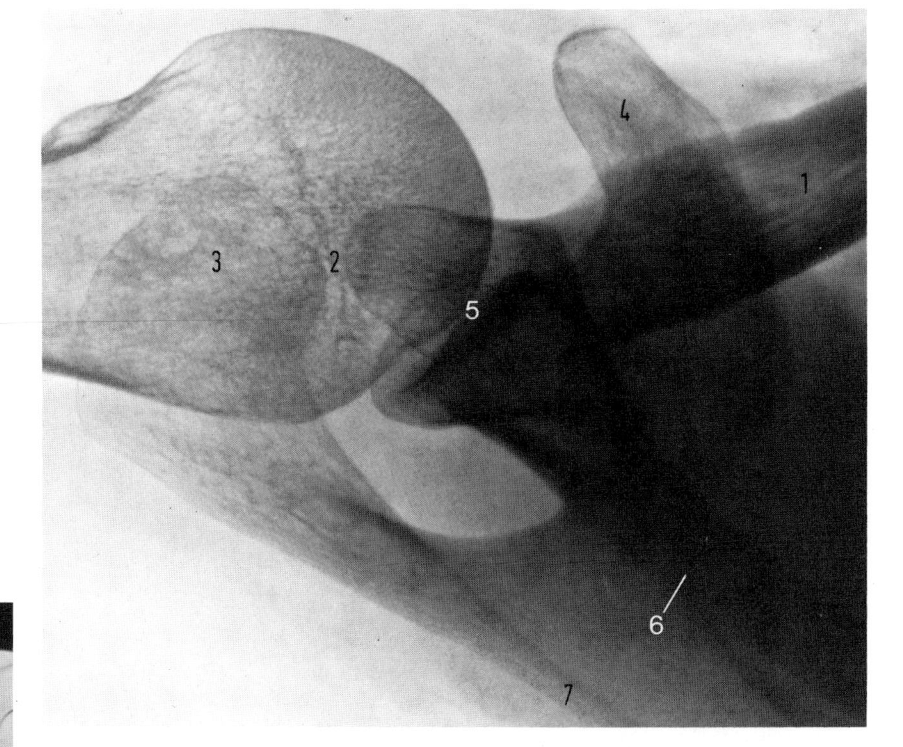

Fig. 520. Shoulder joint, axial. For projection see Fig. 521.

1 Clavicle
2 Acromioclavicular joint
3 Acromion
4 Coracoid process
5 Glenoid cavity
6 Axillary border (of scapula)
7 Scapular spine

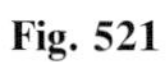

Fig. 521

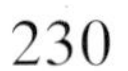

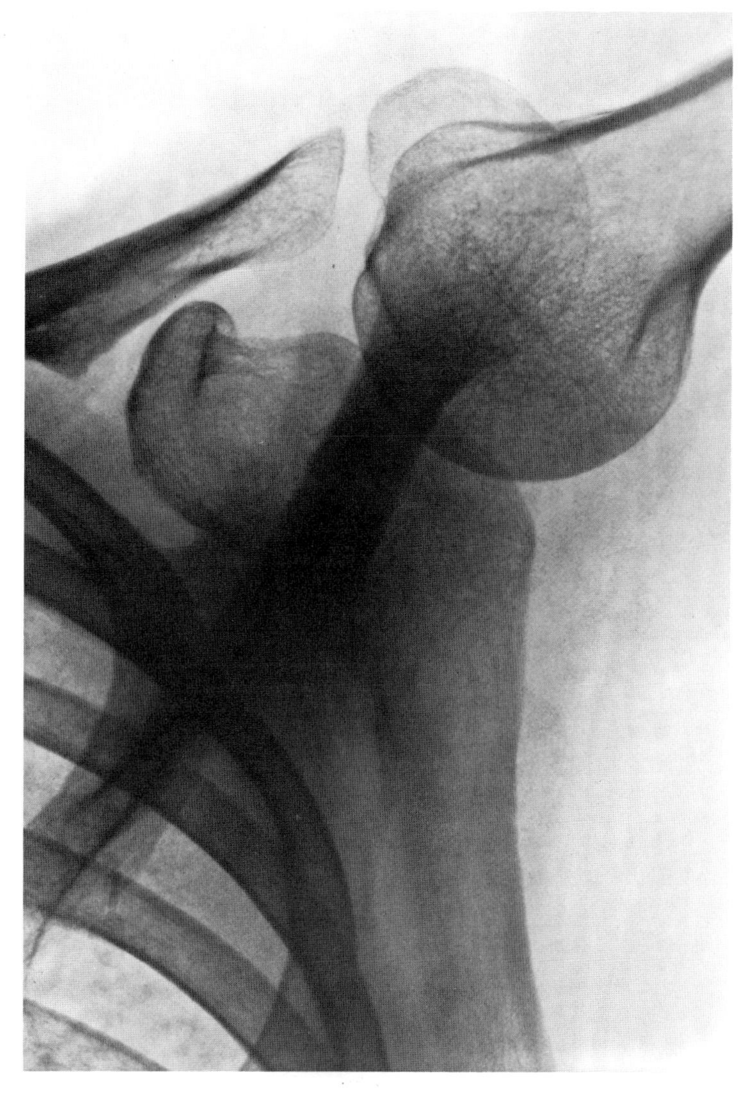

Fig. 522. Shoulder joint, caudoventrodorsal. The arm is raised and in external rotation. This radiograph shows the glenoid cavity and the neck of the scapula, as well as the coracoid process, especially distinct. When the arm is raised, the joint gapes widely and, therefore, fractures of the coracoid process are better shown. Fractures of this process are rare; they occur mainly near the base and are difficult to demonstrate with any other technique.

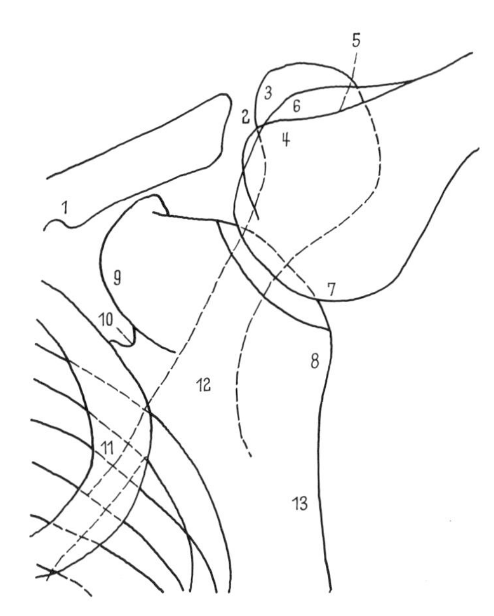

Fig. 523

1 Conoid tubercle (insertion of the conoid ligament from the coracoclavicular ligament)
2 Acromioclavicular joint
3 Acromion
4 Lesser tubercle
5 Intertubercular groove
6 Greater tubercle
7 Head of humerus
8 Neck of scapula, with infraglenoid tubercle
9 Coracoid process
10 Great scapula notch
11 2nd rib
12 Scapular spine
13 Axillary border of scapula

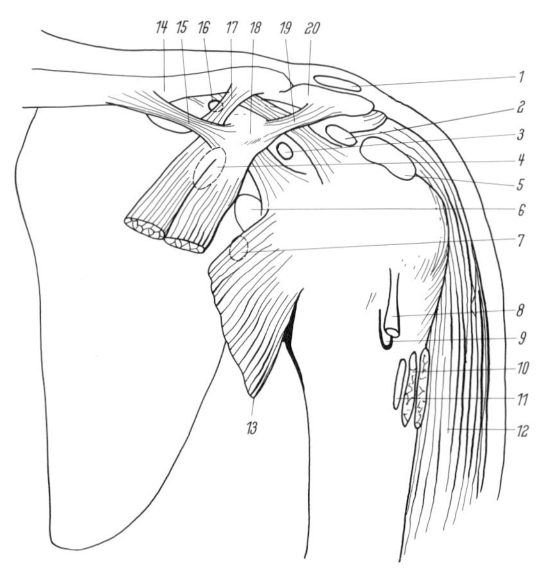

Fig. 524. Bursae of the shoulder joint (from *F. Merkel*).

1 Subcutaneous acromial bursa
2 Subacromial bursa
3 Subtendinous bursa of the supraspinatus muscle
4 Bursa of coracobrachial muscle
5 Subdeltoid bursa
6 Subcoracoid bursa
7 Subtendinous bursa of the subscapular muscle
8 Biceps tendon
9 Synovial intertubercular sheath
10 Tendon of major pectoral muscle
11 Subtendinous bursa of the major pectoral muscle
12 Deltoid muscle
13 Subscapular muscle
14 Clavicle
15 Conoid ligament
16 Bursa of coracoclavicular ligament
17 Trapezoid ligament
18 Coracoid process
19 Coracoacromial ligament
20 Acromion

Variants and Sources of Diagnostic Error of the Shoulder Girdle, Including the Upper Thoracic Region

50 Ossified cartilage of 1st rib, of mainly crumbly structure; see Fig. 334. Often there are one or two joint-like clefts; once the thorax becomes rigid, the clefts ankylose. Frequently, the pseudojoints undergo arthrotic degeneration.
50* Joint-like, calcium-free zone; see Figs. 337, 344
50** Parasternal bone (see Fig. 380); rudimentary costal remnant or nucleus of the sternal costal process
51 Ossifying costal cartilages (see Figs. 334, 337); sometimes ossification starts as early as the third decade of life, partly cloak-shaped, with upper and lower marginal shadow, partly as embedded spots and stripes *(E. Fischer)*. Here, too, there are pseudojoints or their precursors in the shape of marginal spikes in an ossified costal cartilage.
52 Cleft formation in the 1st rib, sometimes bilateral; the 2nd rib may also be split. In the literature it is considered a fatigue fracture, a constitutional hemiarthrosis *(Kipshoven)*; see also Fig. 362. On costosternal osteochondrosis C I–IV *(Tietze* syndrome), see Fig. 369.
53 Tubercle of the anterior scalenus muscle, usually well demonstrable at the upper edge of the rib
53* Tuberosity of the serratus anterior muscle, which can be shown radiographically only if of sufficient size and with tangential path of the rays, as it is seated anteriorly on the 2nd rib
54 Suprasternal bond (also episternal), often found double (see Fig. 381); may be connected to the articular disk via the interclavicular ligaments
54* Ligamental fossa (see Fig. 557); a normal depression of the costoclavicular ligament (not to be mistaken for *Friedrich*'s syndrome, a rare aseptic necrosis of the epiphysis of the sternal end of the clavicle)
56 Costal sulci (see Fig. 349), may simulate periostitis
56* Hole within a rib (see Fig. 375); frequently found in the osteochondral border zone; may simulate pulmonary cavity or bronchiectasis; if it occurs in the lower ribs, *Buelau*'s drainage might be considered
57 Bifurcated rib (Figs. 372, 363, 366, 369)
58 Bony bridge across ribs (between Th I and Th II, a form of Srb anomaly; see also *Wenz* and *Geipert*)
58* Bridge across ribs, with pseudojoint (see Fig. 361); differential diagnosis for bridging callus or inflammatory neoplastic bone formation
60 Acromial bone (see Figs. 549–551); occurs mostly bilaterally, may consist of several nuclei; in cases of a unilateral apophysis of the acromion it may therefore be mistaken for a broken-off fracture. The persistent fragment of the acromial end or an ossification of a bursa in the shape of an acromial tip is called an atypical acromial bone.
60* Coracoid process, taken orthograde. It develops from its own nucleus and fuses late, after puberty. If it does not fuse, it becomes a coracoid bone. A false coracoid bone may be a fractured and unhealed coracoid process; see Figs. 546–548.
61 Glenoid bone, corresponds to the bone next to acetabulum of the hip joint; see Fig. 532. The infracoracoid bone is also said to be part of the apophysis of the glenoidal labrum (see Fig. 543).
61* Ossicle in the acromioclavicular joint; may be a traumatic splitting-off, an arthrotic marginal spike, a congenital supernumerary bone or a calcified disk *(Schulte, Mörike)*
61** Persistent medial clavicular apophysis. Until the third decade of life, it should not be mistaken for effects of injury; see Fig. 1018 *(E. Fischer)*.
62 Humeroscapular periarthritis with calcified subdeltoid bursa. This is often the consequence of damage through overloading, which is accompanied by inflammation of soft tissues, capsulae or insertions of tendons (calcifying peritendinitis) or by degeneration; see Figs. 538 and 544–545 (painful shoulder).
62* Nerve canal (see Fig. 508), may occur double; not to be mistaken for an osteolytic metastasis (see also *Pahl*)
63 Persistent apophysis at the inferior angle (see Fig. 534); normally, this is only visible between the 16th and 18th years of life (see Fig. 1057).
The author has never seen a persistent apophysis at the vertebral border of the scapula *(Maassen)* and, with *Aumann* and *Neiss*, does not believe its occurrence has been proven.
63** Persistent apophysis at the superior angle, described in 1953 by *Ochs* as occurring very irregularly between the 16th and 18th years. *Viehweger* (1968, p. 414) shows a view (24) that is supposed to present a persistent bony nucleus at the superior scapular angle; however the present author has never seen any such persistence. Also, an independent apophysis at the superior angle is not mentioned in standard anatomical works *(Rauber-Kopsch, Braus, Benninghoff-Goerttler, Spalteholz, Pernkopf)*. See also text on p. 440.
63** Thickening of the inferior angle through forceful insertion of the anterior serratus muscle
64 Increased radiolucency in the head of humerus (see Fig. 530); this represents a normal pre-senile thinning of the compact tissue. Incorrect diagnoses may be made of osteomyelitis or sarcoma.
65 Increased radiolucency in the upper angle of the glenoid cavity (see Fig. 508), caused by bordering superimpositions
66/1 Hole-shaped defects in scapula; see Figs. 554, 555
66/2 According to *Viehweger,* they are acquired through atrophy of compact tissue, but *Fazekas* and *Ferjentsik* believe them to be congenital.
67 Conoid tubercle (see Figs. 506, 512, 540); if much developed, may simulate callus formation of periostitis; in rare cases a hole for the cephalic vein (Fig. 553) may be found
67* Coracoclavicular joint (see Figs. 540 and 542); shows post-traumatic ossification of the bipartite coracoclavicular ligament (severe arthrosis); If occurs bilaterally, might be an anomaly *(Schulte)*
68 Deltoid tuberosity (see Fig. 526); may simulate tumor
68* Radiolucent zone (see Fig. 530), caused by overlapping contours of soft tissues (W*)
a Sternoclavicular joint; its contours do not run parallel to each other (disk!). With the arm hanging down, the medial edge of the clavicle protrudes upwards; may simulate dislocation.
C Islet of compact tissue, not to be mistaken for bony infraction
p Pseudoperiostitic accompanying shadow at the surgical neck of humerus and at the neck of the glenoid cavity
S/1 Disk of fibrous cartilage between menubrium and body of the sternum (see Figs. 334 and 339)
S/2 Persistent segmentation
S/3 Compare with Figs. 336 and 376
n Nutritive canal within the scapula
III–VI 3rd to 6th ribs
W,W Soft tissue contour of the neck passing into the accompanying clavicle shadow, which is formed by the covering skin
W*, W* Intruding soft tissue contours of the cutaneous surface, e.g., of the mamma (Fig. 526)

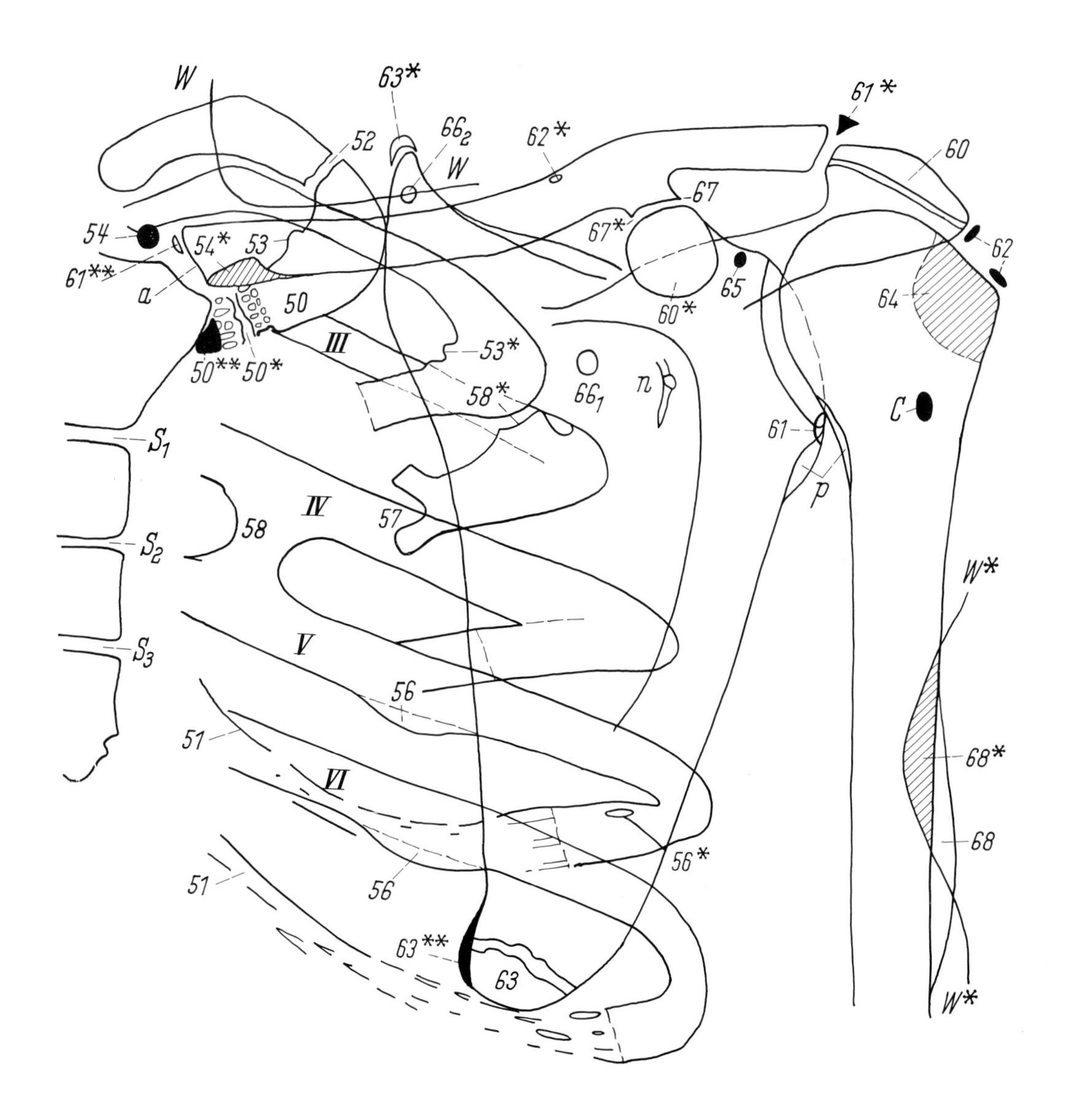

Fig. 525. Variants and sources of diagnostic error of the shoulder girdle and upper thoracic region.

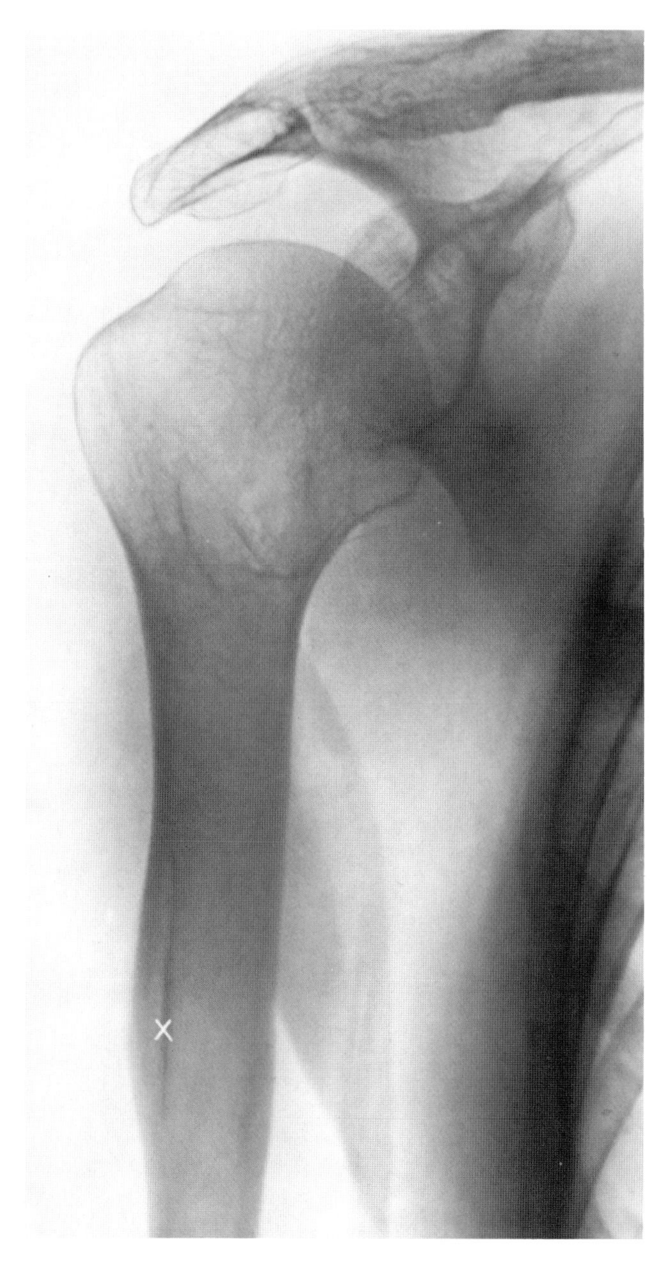

Fig. 526. **Tumor-like thickening of the deltoid tuberosity** (×) in a 69-year-old female. This thickening at the insertion of the deltoid muscle is almost always seen, more or less pronounced. Frequently a cystic translucency below the outer shell is found. Sometimes this thickened zone has a changed, osteoma-like structure, or the same view is obtained as in ossifying periostitis or with a callus after fracture. Striking, boomerang-shaped metaphyseal blood vessel in the neck of the humerus.

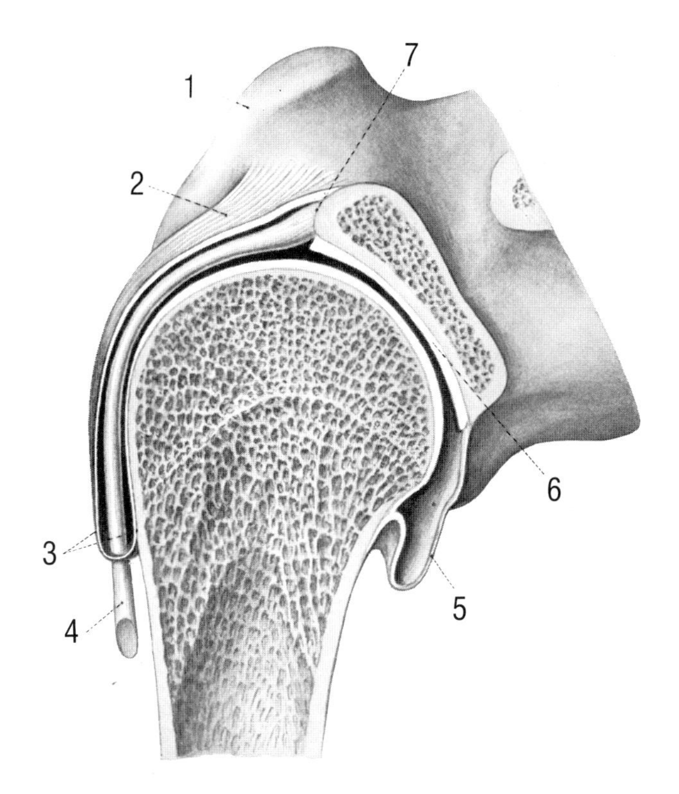

Fig. 527. Frontal section through the shoulder joint. Dorsal view (from *Sobotta-Becher,* 15th Edition).

1 Coracoid process
2 Coracohumeral ligament
3 Intertubercular synovial sheath
4 Biceps tendon (long head)
5 Articular capsule
6 Glenoid cavity
7 Insertion of the biceps tendon (long head)

Fig. 528. The semicircular limitation of the shadow arises when the upper arm is angled backwards so that the central ray is aimed into the marrow cavity of the shaft (of the humerus). The head rests correctly in the glenoid cavity when its medial contour runs parallel to one glenoidal labrum and leaves a normally wide articular space and, further, when the axis of the glenoidal ellipse in its continuation meets the center of the head.

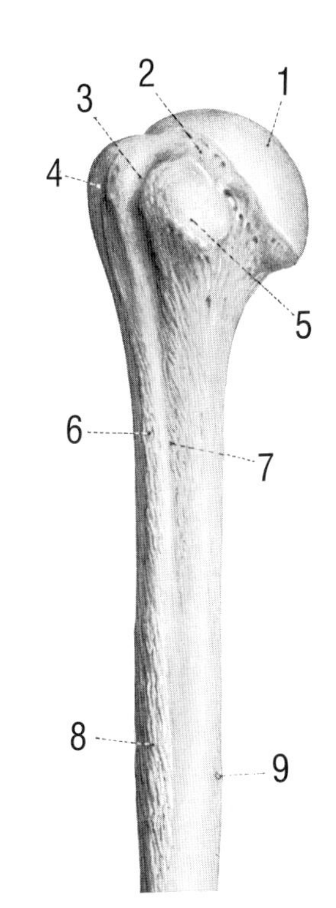

1 Head of humerus
2 Anatomical neck of humerus
3 Intertubercular groove
4 Greater tubercle
5 Lesser tubercle
6 Crest of greater tubercle
7 Crest of lesser tubercle
8 Deltoid tuberosity
9 Nutritive foramen

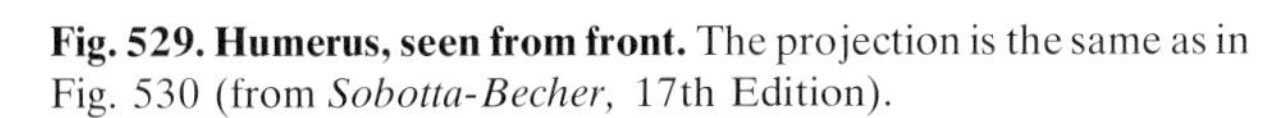

Fig. 529. Humerus, seen from front. The projection is the same as in Fig. 530 (from *Sobotta-Becher,* 17th Edition).

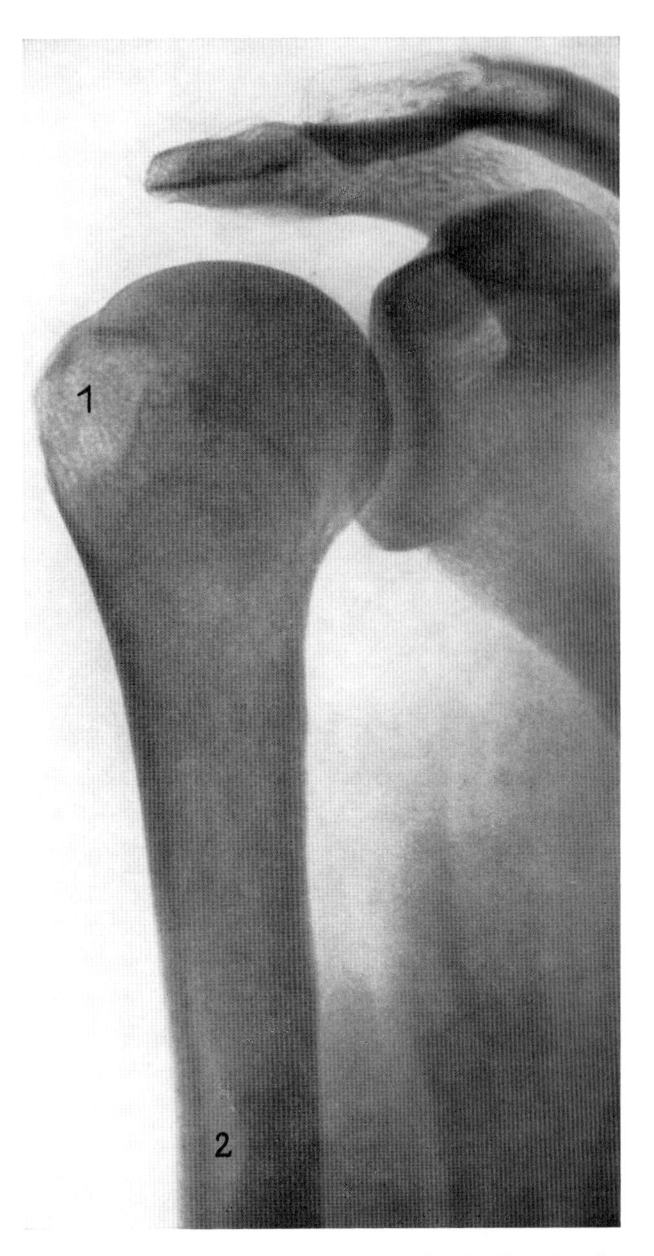

Fig. 530. Right shoulder joint, 42-year-old female. The soft radiograph shows two frequent peculiarities that easily cause errors (cf. Fig. 525, Nos. 64 and 68*).

1 Pre-senile increased radiolucency in the region of the greater tubercle. The lamellar and trabecular structures in the basal region of the greater tubercle become rarefied around age 35 to 40 *(Bruno).* Osteomyelits or sarcoma may be wrongly diagnosed.
2 Light zone at the lateral edge of the anterior axillary fold (pectoralis major muscle) which from that point curves into the outer contour of the mamma. Close above it, the "periostal thickening" caused by the deltoid tuberosity is frequently found (cf. Fig. 526). Here, too, suspicion of pathological calcium catabolism in the bone may be aroused. Absence of periostal added layers speaks against an abscess.

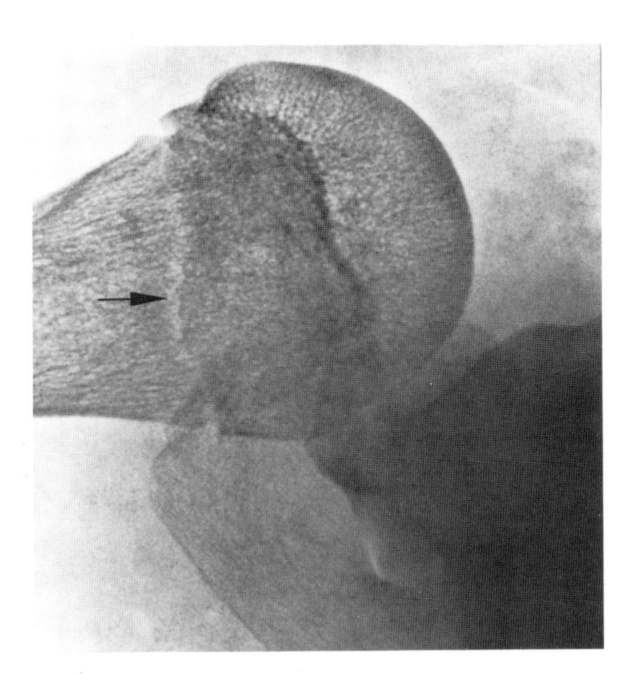

Fig. 531. Shoulder joint, axial, with "fracture" due to projection (→), in a 16 year old.
The epiphyseal plate appears here (as in Fig. 1049) in the shape of a step-like bent disk, whose anterior edge is projected separately from the posterior one.

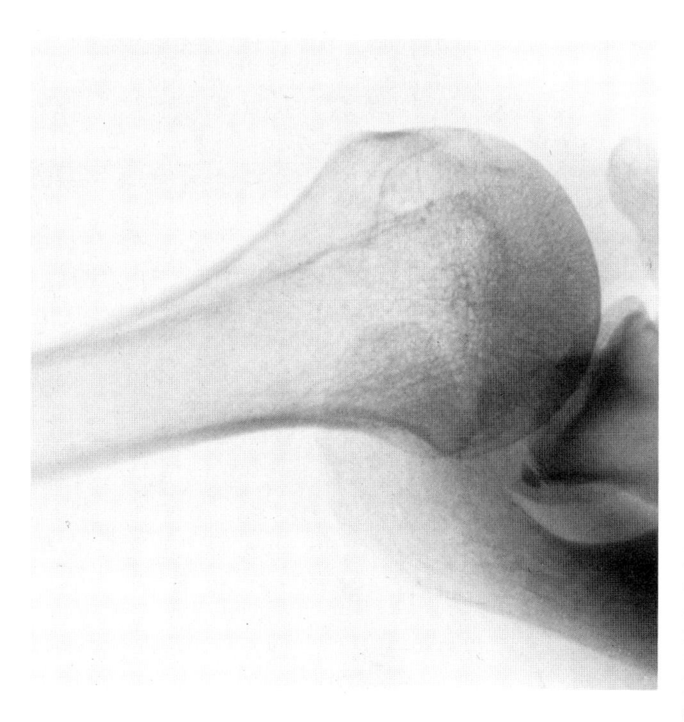

Fig. 532. **Glenoid bone, right shoulder joint,** axial (in maximal supination).

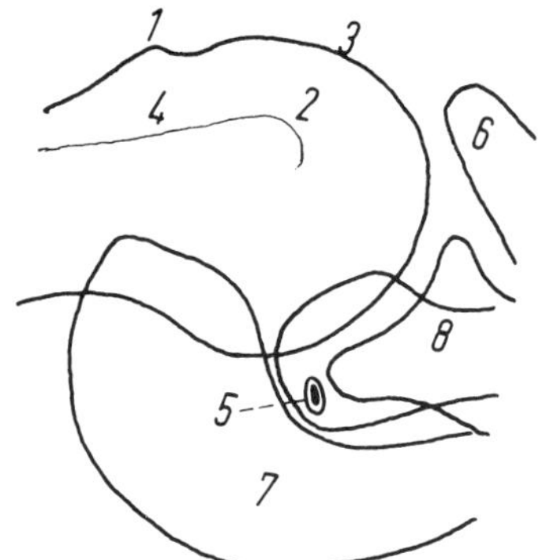

1 Lesser tubercle
2 Greater tubercle
3 Anatomical neck
4 Intertubercular groove
5 Glenoid bone
6 Coracoid process
7 Acromion
8 Clavicle

Fig. 533. Sketch to Fig. 532.

During development of the glenoid cavity of the shoulder, there is an apophyseal ring or an apophyseal marginal ledge, similar to the marginal ledge of the vertebral bodies. This ledge, or a piece of it, which remains isolated for a short time only, is very rarely visible and then mainly only at the lower rim. Occasionally, a part of the apophyseal ledge persists at this lower margin of the glenoid cavity as an isolated ossicle, which we call the glenoid bone. The sometimes visible infracoracoid bone at the upper rim of the glenoid cavity may represent an isolated ossified part of the apophysis of the glenoidal labrum.

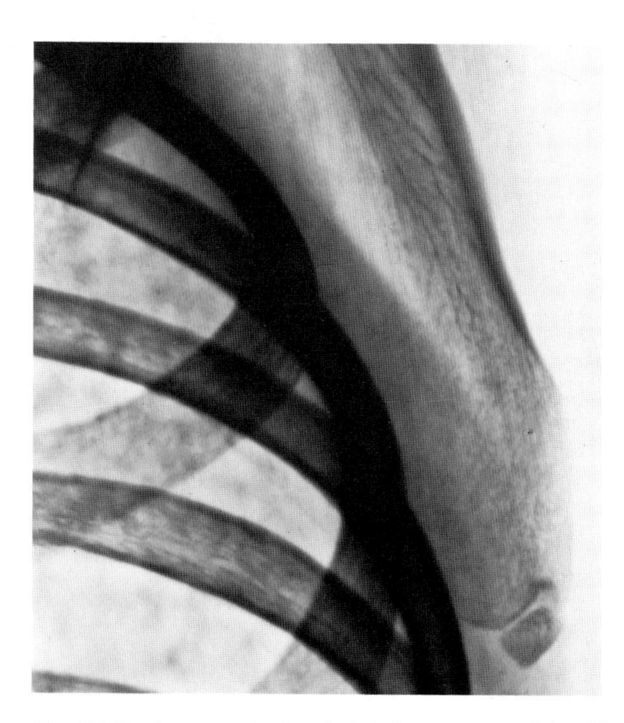

Fig. 534. Persistent apophysis at the inferior scapular angle in a 35-year-old male; after *Zimmer:* infrascapular bone. Usually, the apophysis is only visible between the 16th and 18th years of life. It may be mistaken for a fracture. See Fig. 525, No. 63 and Fig. 1057. The present author equates apophyses that appear this late with secondary centers of ossification, if they remain isolated.

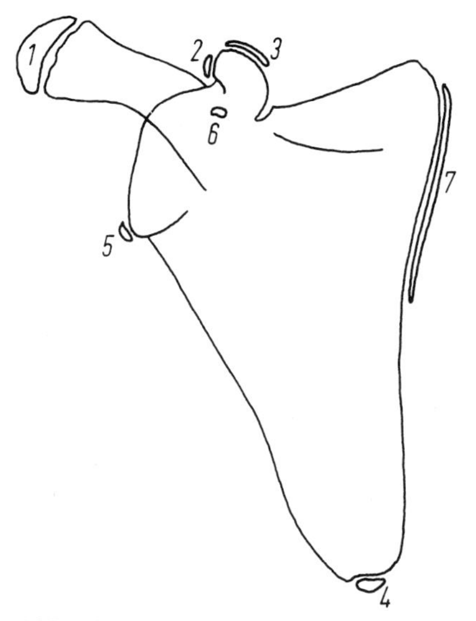

Fig. 535. Primary and secondary centers of ossification in the scapular region (schematic).

1 Acromial apophysis
2 Coracoid apophysis, at the tip
3 Coracoid apophysis, at the "knee"
4 Apophysis of the inferior scapular angle
5 Glenoid bone (a persistent piece of the apophyseal ledge)
6 Infracoracoid bone (perhaps also an isolated piece of the apophyseal ledge)
7 Apophysis at the vertebral border

Although the persistence of this apophysis, maintained by *Maassen,* is denied by *Neiss* and *Aumann* as well as by myself as not having been proven radiographically, the present author considers it important to mention this "apophysis" since this conception has not yet disappeared from the anatomical and radiographic literature.

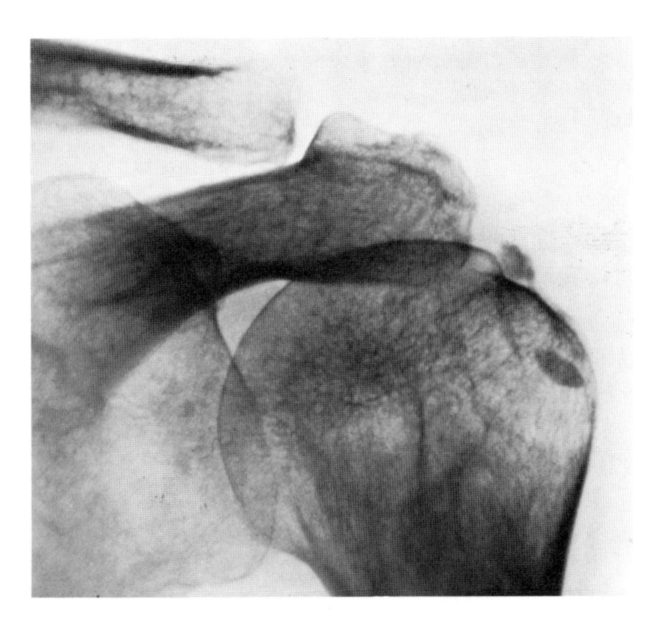

Fig. 536. "Painful shoulder" caused by calcified subacromial and subdeltoid bursitis (see Fig. 524). For a long time there has been objection to the existence and misuse of the concept of humeroscapular periarthritis *(Milner,* 1932). The present author considers the collective designation "painful shoulder" or "frozen shoulder" in the Anglo-American literature *(Ennevaara)* to be more correct.

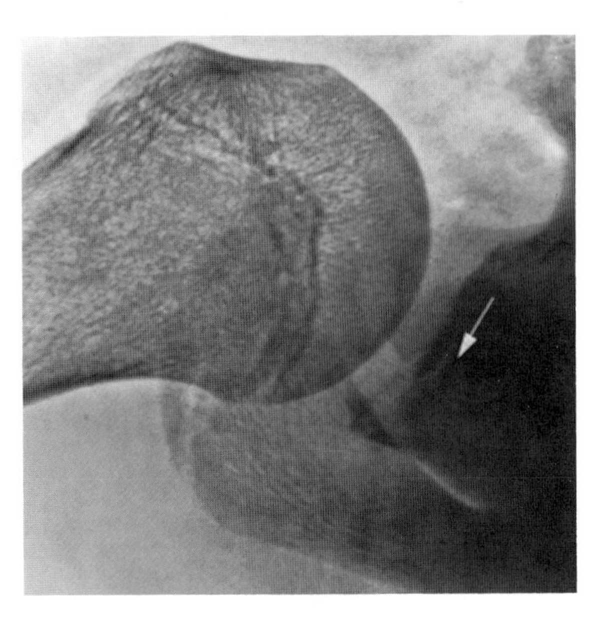

Fig. 537. Fracture, simulated by apophyseal cleft at the glenoidal labrum, in a 16 year old (↙).
This is a piece of apophysis of the glenoidal labrum that remains isolated for a short time only between the 16th and 18th years of life, and became visible on an incidental projection. In addition, a still-visible nucleus of the acromial apophysis can be seen.

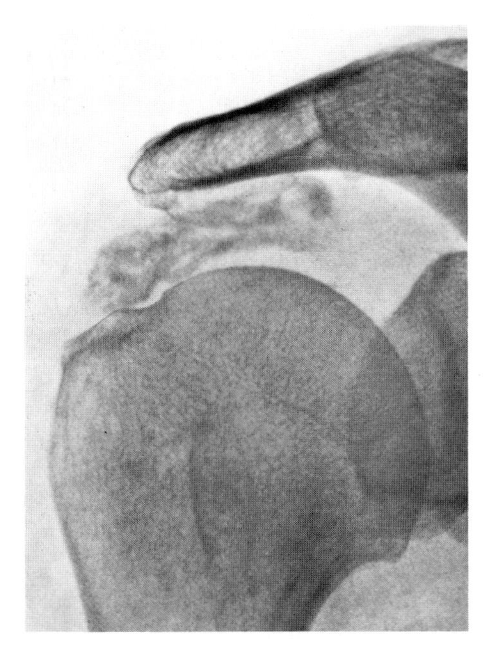

Fig. 538. Painful shoulder. Humeroscapular periarthritis *(Duplay),* **caused by calcifying peritendinitis of the supraspinatus muscle.** This condition is said to be initiated by acute or chronic traumata; psychogenic factors may be of importance. Frequent early symptoms are roughenings of the points of insertion of the capsula as well as of the contour of the greater tubercle, and roughenings of the contour of the acromioclavicular joint. Narrowings of the articular space as well as of the contour of the articular space of the humeroscapular joint, especially between humerus and acromion, are symptomatic. Late effects are calcifications in bursae or in degenerating necrotic tendinous insertions, as in this case; therefore, calcifying peritendinitis is also seen here.

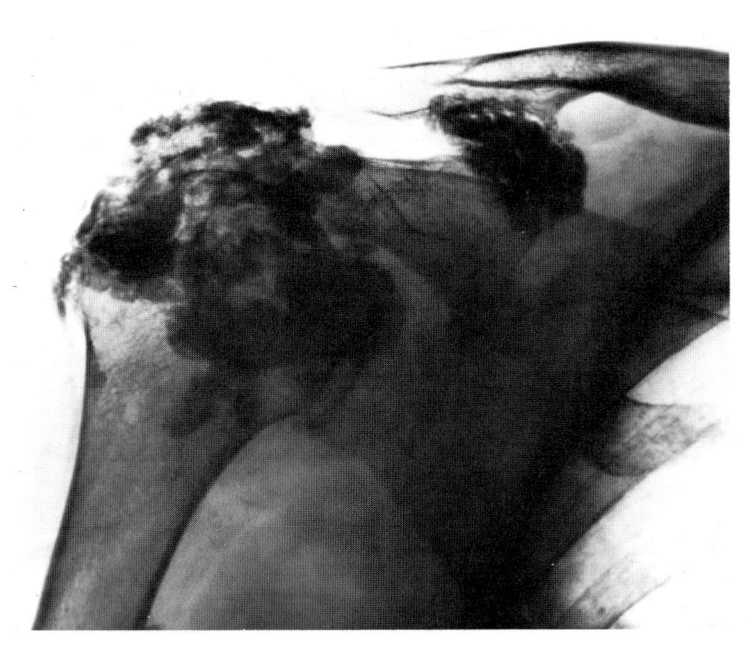

Fig. 539. Periarticular tissue calcifications. A calcific bridge exists between clavicle and coracoid process; *Villányi* described it as an isolated post-traumatic calcification. In this case, where trauma had not occurred, the enormous calciferous deposits in the periarticular tissue aroused suspicion *(Poppel* and *Zeitel)* of a *Burnett* syndrome (milk-drinkers' disease); in these cases, apart from these characteristic clod-like periarticular calcifications, early vascular calcifications occur. Further, in severe cases, calcifications develop in the eyes (cornea and conjunctive) and in the kidneys, with renal insufficiency *(Rühlmann et al.).*

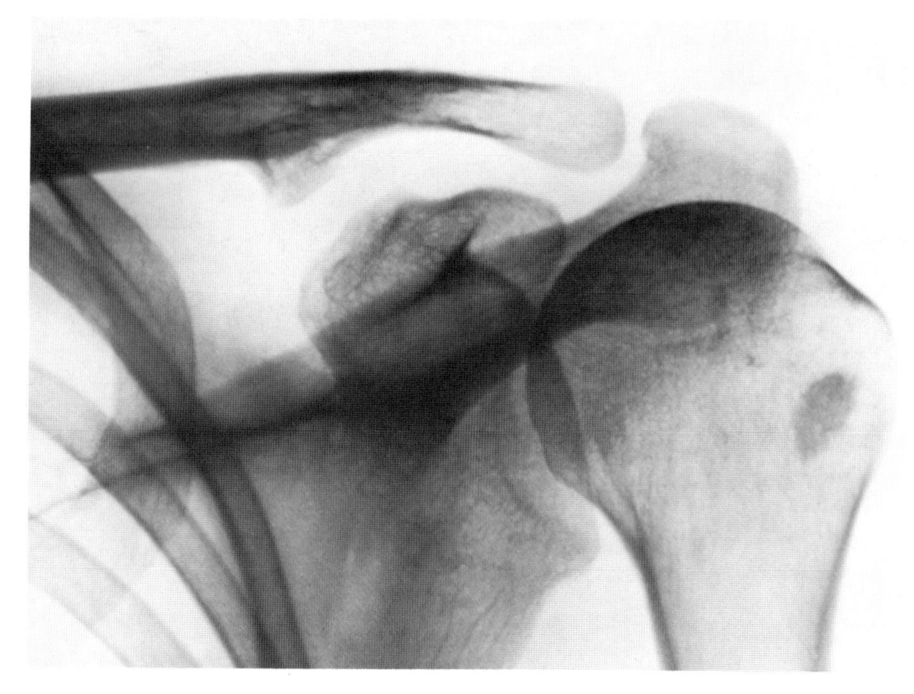

Fig. 540. "Coracoclavicular joint." In cases of a very prominent conoid tubercle, approximation to the coracoid process may take place and may even form a coracoclavicular joint (see No. 67* in Fig. 525). The system of ligaments between these two bony salients may partly ossify or calcify, especially after traumata, e.g., after dislocation of the acromioclavicular joint. If a so-called coracoclavicular joint is present, the then-existing coracoclavicular bursa may also calcify, following bursitis. A ring cyst at the insertion of the coracoid and an older bone infarction in the cancellous tissue of the greater tubercle can be seen. In addition, there is a shell-like ledge at the lower margin of the acromion (secondary accessory acromial bone?).

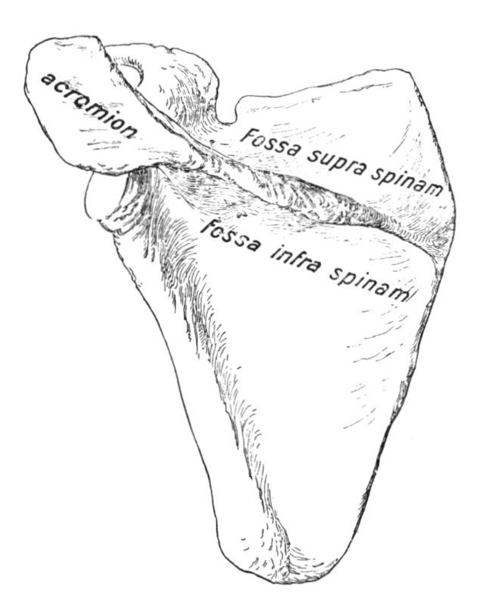

Fig. 541. Left scapula from dorsal; shows mainly the development of the labrum-shaped double contour of the upper edge of the scapular spine (from *Sobotta-Becher,* 15th Edition).

The humeroscapular periarthritis *(Duplay)* – **painful shoulder** – develops, according to *Zetkin* and *Schaldach,*
from inflammatory-degenerative processes,
adhesions of the capsula, through enforced resting position,
degenerative changes of the supraspinatus tendon,
inflammations of bursae,
inflammations of apophyses (inflammations of the coracoid process),
arthrosis in the acromioclavicular joint,
osteochondrosis of the cervical spine,
vegetative irritation of the articular capsule,
micro- and macro-traumata, and
from overexertion.

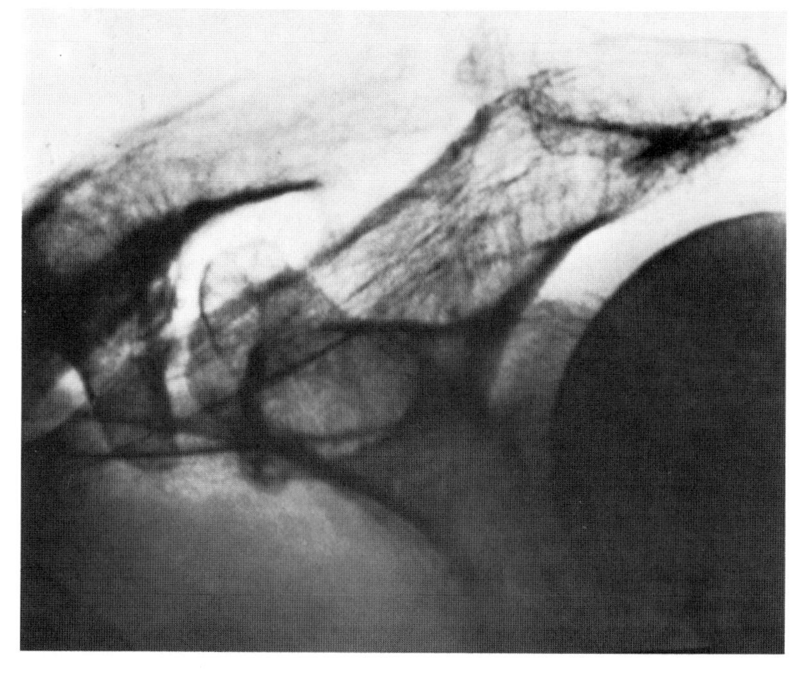

Fig. 542. Severe arthrosis of the so-called coracoclavicular joint. Together with a giant spur-like conoid tubercle and a very prominent coracoid process; the contours of the coracoclavicular joint are greatly arthrotically deformed and jagged.

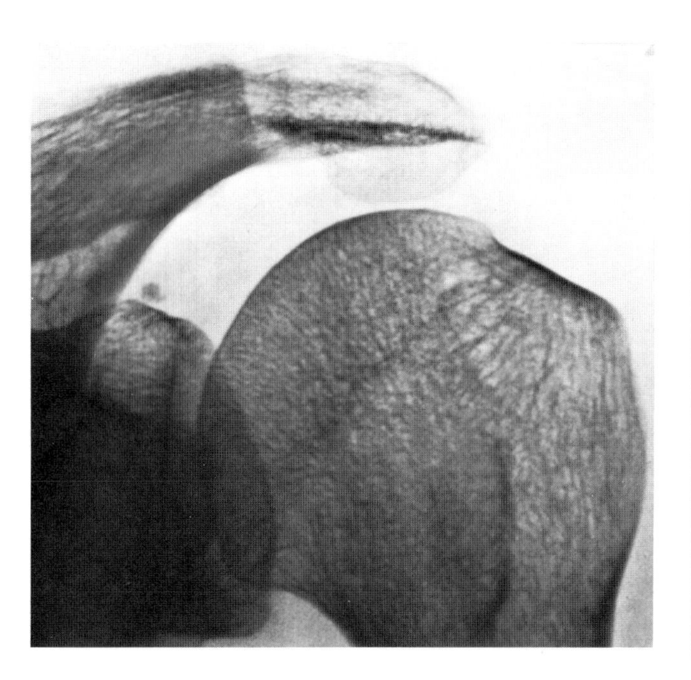

Fig. 543 a. Left shoulder, ventrodorsal.

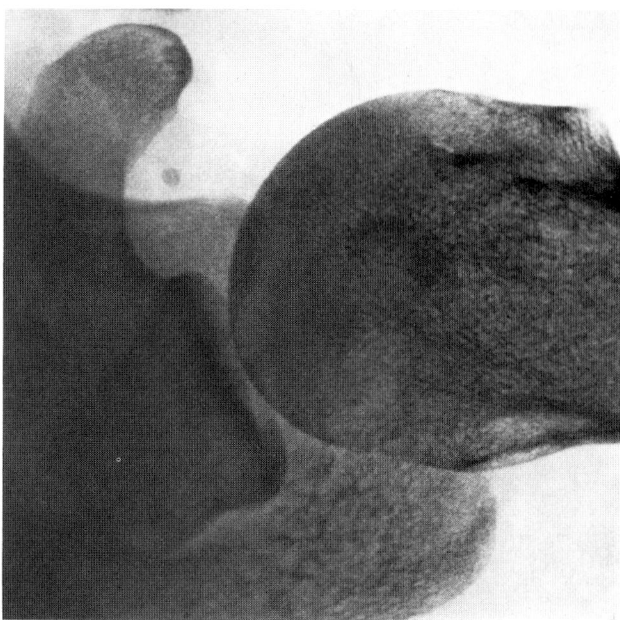

Fig. 543 b. Left shoulder, axial.

Fig. 543. Infracoracoid bone? The infracoracoid bone may be located between the coracoid process and the upper rim of the glenoid cavity of the shoulder. If an infracoracoid bone were really a persistent part of the apophysis of the glenoidal labrum, in this case a genuine infracoracoid bone could not be assumed as it is located much too far medially and above the glenoid margin. It remains an open question whether this roundish ossicle is a product of either a traumatic splintering-off or of an osteochondrosis dissecans.

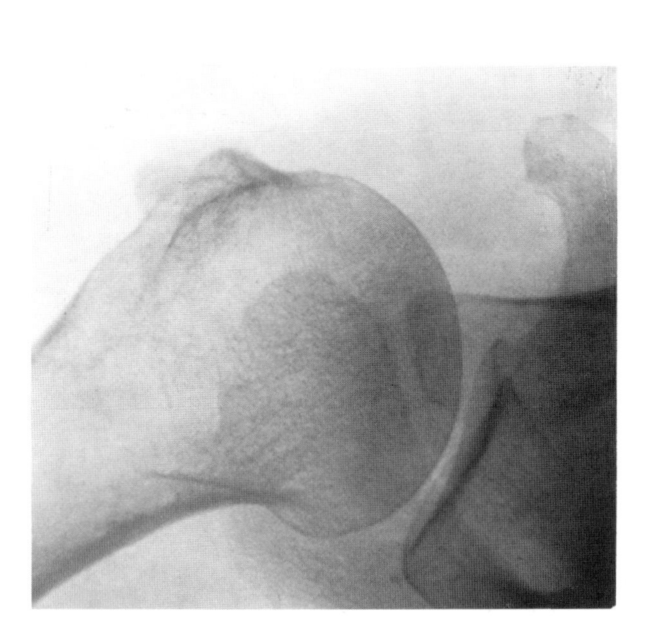

Fig. 544. Calcification of bursa above the greater tubercle of the head of the right humerus, or an isolated splintered-off greater tubercle after previous fracture-dislocation; see also Fig. 524. Such separations occur in 12–15% of all dislocations, with the axillary infraglenoidal as well as with the subcoracoidal type, whereby the humeral head is dislocated beneath the coracoid process. It might also be a genuine avulsion fracture, caused by the tendon of the head of the biceps muscle. The torn-off tubercle may be dislocated right below the glenoid cavity of the shoulder, remain there and become an impediment to repositioning.

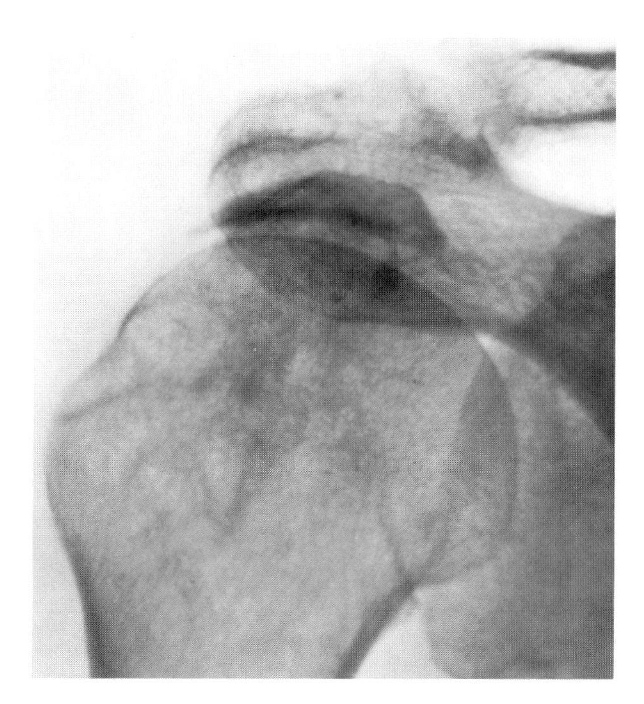

Fig. 545. Cap-like calcification between acromion and the upper dome-like portion of the humeral head, i.e., calcification of the supraspinatus tendon. One sees the typical narrowing of the subacromial space through shrinking tendinitis and peritendinitis of the supraspinatus muscle. In this case, the so-called periarthritis humeroscapularis led to cystic-sclerosing reconstruction of the bone.

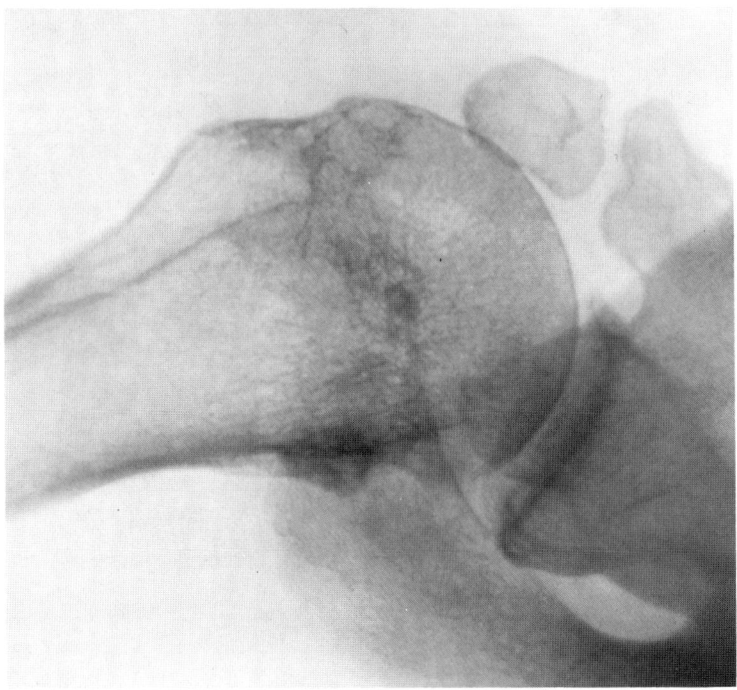

Fig. 546. **Coracoid bone.** Right shoulder, axial.

The coracoid process develops from its own bony nucleus; in reptiles and birds, it remains independent, as the coracoid bone. In man, fusion with the scapula occurs, though only late (after puberty), until the 20th year of life. If, in very rare cases, this fusion does not come about, a free coracoid bone results. A "false" coracoid bone develops when a coracoid process, broken off through trauma, does not reunite *(Schaefer)*. At the knee and tip of the coracoid process, apophyseal protrusions, developed from accessory nuclei, may persist if fusion of these additional spaces fails.

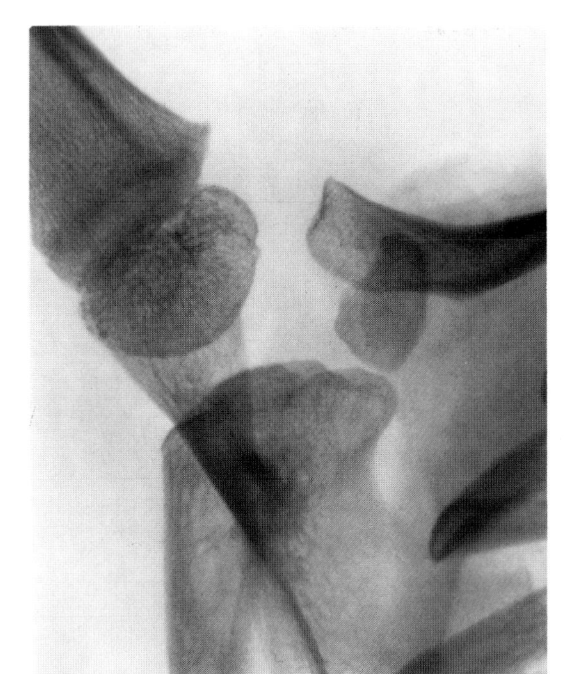

Fig. 547. Coracoid process, still free, in a 12 year old. Right shoulder, ventrodorsal, with the arm raised (see also *Günsel, Ravelli*).

1 Coracoid process; if persistent, then coracoid bone
2 Apophysis at the tip of the coracoid (may persist)
3 Apophysis at the knee of the coracoid (may persist)
4 Main cleft
5 Ancillary cleft at knee
6 Ancillary cleft at tip
7 Clavicle
8 Head of humerus
9 Rib
10 Superior border of scapula
11 Scapular spine
12 Glenoid cavity

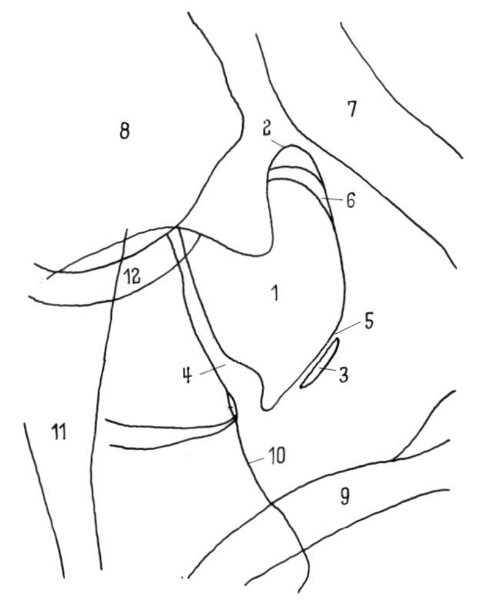

Fig. 548 (Sketch based on Fig. 1 from *Ravelli*). **Radiograph of right shoulder, ventrodorsal,** with the arm raised, in a 16 year old. Three nuclei for bone development and, respectively, three open clefts on the coracoid process are to be seen: the main cleft near the root and the supplementary clefts at knee and tip.

Acromial bone. The acromial bone occurs more often than the coracoid bone (7–15%), mainly bilaterally. As the acromial apophysis develops from two, three or more bony nuclei (see Fig. 552), there are different types of acromial bones, depending on which ancillary cleft fusion fails or whether the acromial bone is composed of all fused nuclei; therefore, the differential diagnosis between acromial bone and chip fracture may become very difficult. In cases of persistence of a broken-off, non-reunited acromial end or of osteoarthrotic layers on the acromion or sometimes even with calcified bursae, the designation is atypical acromial bone.

Fig. 549 requires further explanation:

1. It is an incidental radiographic finding; therefore, further exposures, especially of the other side, are lacking.
2. The irregularity of the bordering surfaces points to fractures through overloading or to pseudarthroses between fragments.
3. The unusual exostosis at the lesser tubercle may also indicate old, post-traumatic periarticular changes.

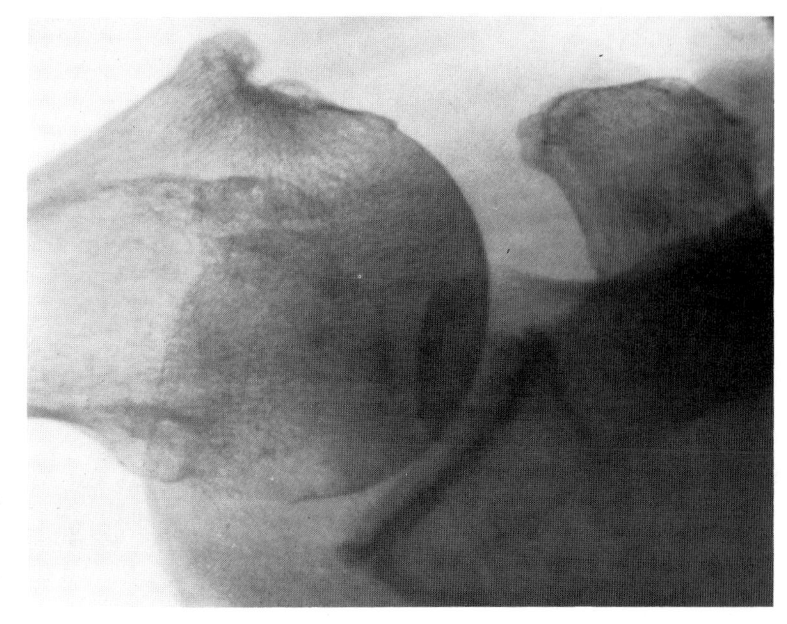

Fig. 549. Semi-coalesced, multipartite acromial bone. Exostoses at the lesser tubercle.

1 Multipartite acromial bone
2 Acromion
3 Scapular spine
4 Glenoid cavity of shoulder
5 Clavicle
6 Coracoid
7 Exostosis of lesser tubercle

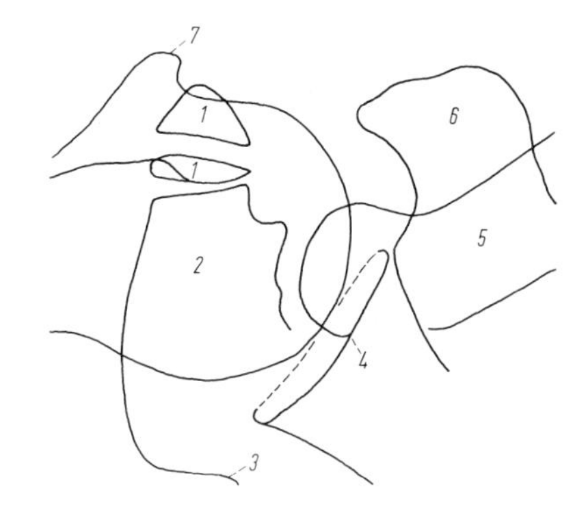

Fig. 550. Sketch to Fig. 549.

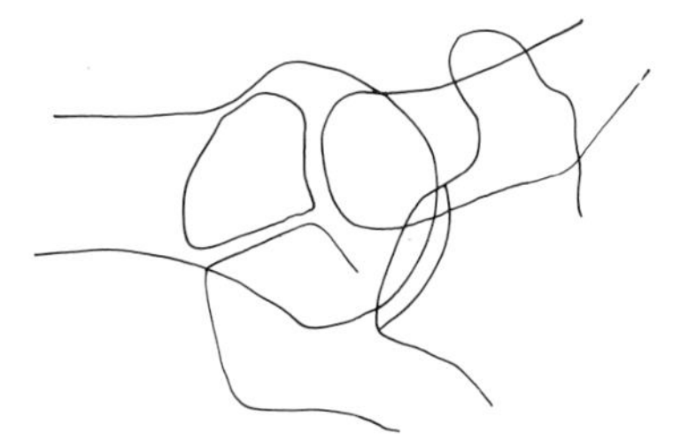

Fig. 551. Acromial bone in axial projection.

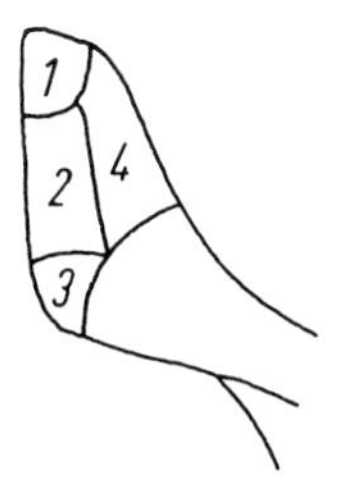

Fig. 552. Ossification centers of acromion (after *Bernardeau*).

1 Preacromion
2 Mesacromion
3 Metacromion
4 Cartilage

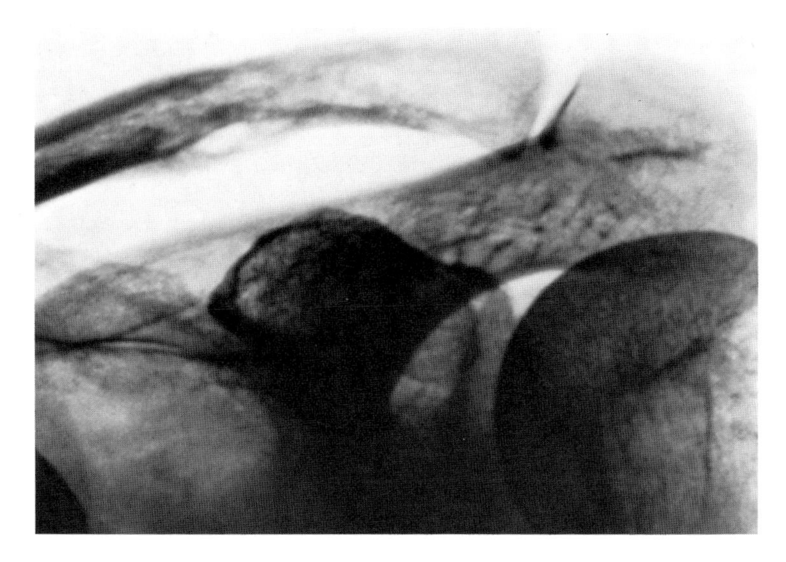

Fig. 553. Partial ossification of the conoid ligament, with hole formation. The medial share of the coracoclavicular ligament, the conoid ligament, together with the clavipectoral fascia form part of the deltoideopectoral triangle (*Mohrenheim*'s fossa). The cephalic vein and the thoracoacromial artery break through this ligamental-fascial plate which is partially ossified here, right below the clavicular margin. Ossification may be the consequence of macrotraumata, e.g., dislocations, or of micro-traumata, which develop from constant strain of pull and pressure on this functionally most important ligament.
Viehweger shows, in the Handbuch der Medizinischen Radiologie, bony appositions of the insertion of the coracoclavicular ligament at the clavicle. His Fig. 13 b shows a concave depression from below, without any explanation. *Viehweger*'s figure may be attributable, in this author's opinion, to an incomplete bony enclosure of the cephalic vein and the thoracoacromial artery, since in this figure it is apparently complete.

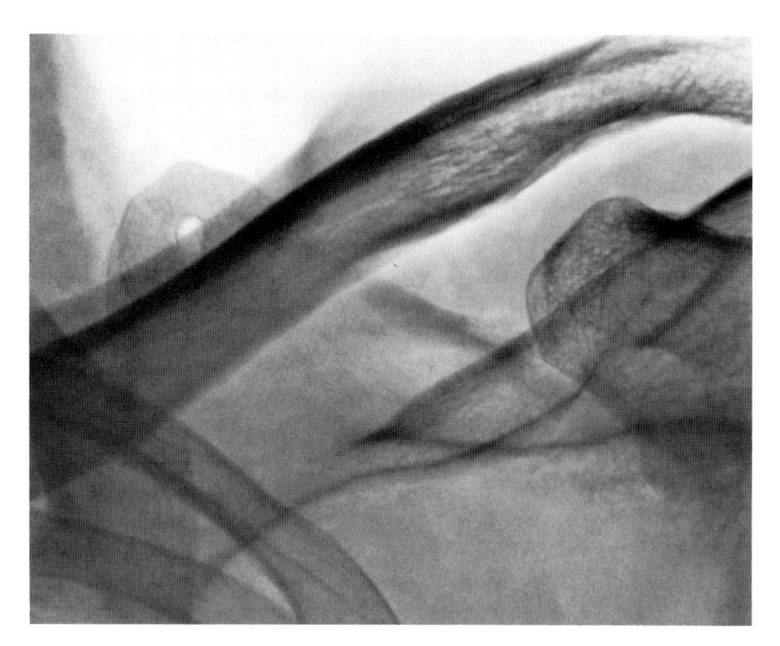

Fig. 554. Hole-like defect within the superior scapular angle. This is an incidental finding without a known cause. It should not be confused with the more common roundish defect at the scapular neck or at the beginning of the coracoid process, a vascular canal taken orthograde (see *E. Fischer*); cf. Fig. 525, No. 66/2. According to *Viehweger,* thinning of the middle parts of the supra- and infraspinatus fossae occurs constantly throughout life, therefore local bony atrophy will occur in circumscribed spots.

Fazekas and *Ferjentsik* showed a defect of about 10 mm (1dime) diameter in the infraspinatous fossa, with a swallow-tail-like deformity of the inferior scapular angle, concurrent with abnormal width of the scapula. They consider the simultaneous occurrence of both changes, which they described for the first time, as proof of a common congenital origin.

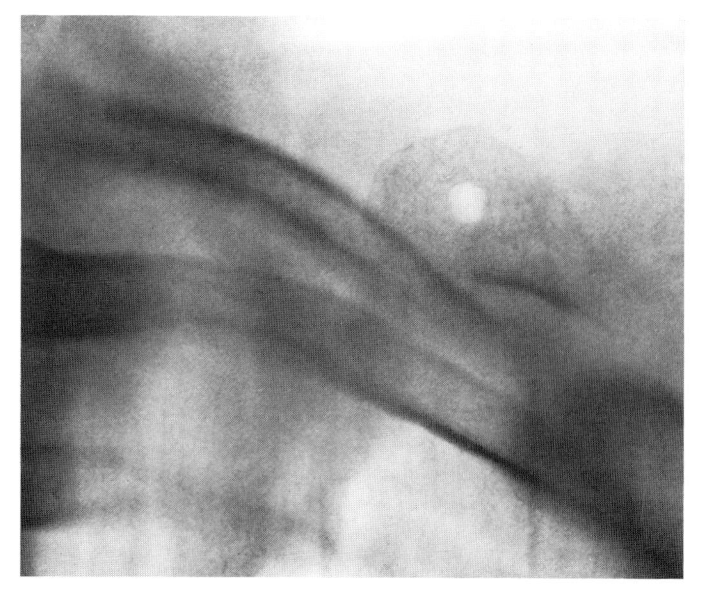

Fig. 555. Tomographic presentation of the above case.

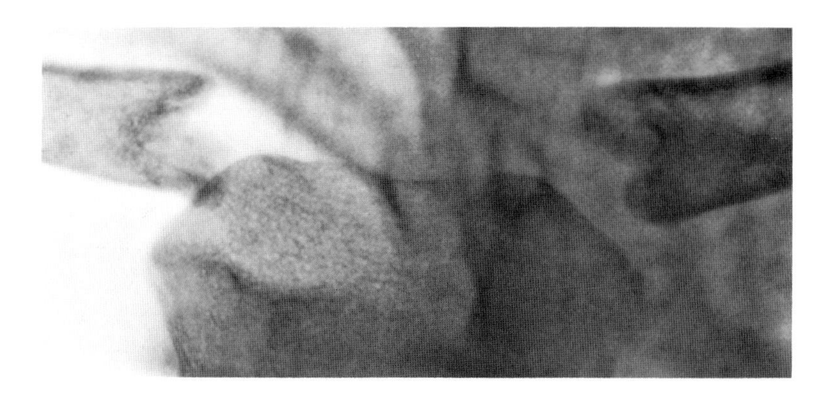

Fig. 556. Variants of the "fish-mouth shape" of the sternal ends of the clavicle. On the right, shape of a shark's mouth; on the left, a toothless fish mouth. The bilateral occurrence almost excludes a pathological process. The frequent, often unilateral, club-shaped and cup-shaped or mushroom-shaped intumescence of the sternal end of the clavicle with subjective complaints must be differentiated from tuberculous caries, osteomyelitis, deforming arthrosis, etc., all possible in this location. If the finding is unilateral, osteosarcoma should be considered.

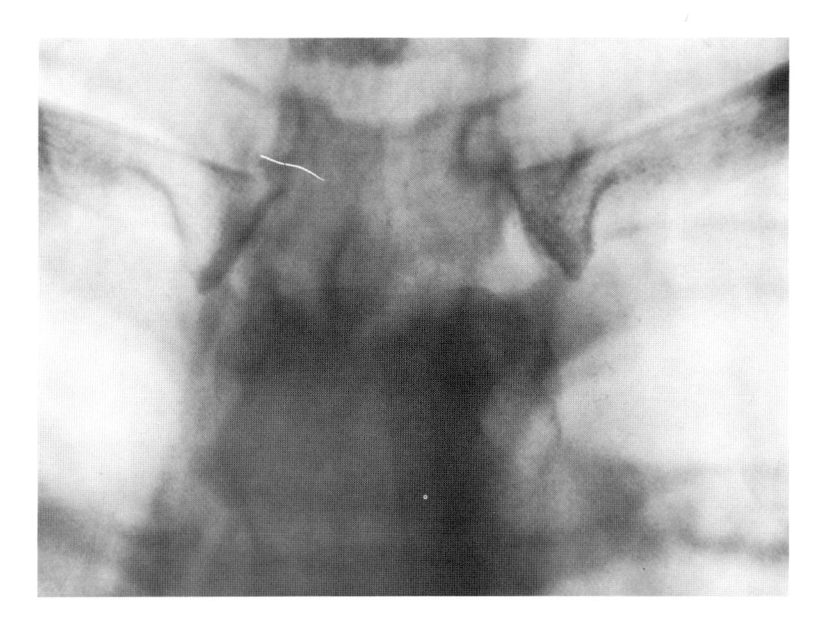

Fig. 557. Sternoclavicular joints with unusually pronounced bilateral ligamental fossae. These are irregular, notched ligamental fossae, impressions of the costoclavicular ligaments, which, in spite of their great variability, are neither a variant nor an anomaly. These thumbhead-shaped notches at the medial lower edge of the clavicle were thought to be tumor and aseptic bone defects (*Friedrich* syndrome), although their bilateral occurrence should have excluded a causative pathological process.
Horváth described such "usurations" as due to mechanical factors, microtraumata or atypical insertion of the costoclavicular ligament (rhomboid ligament). A destructive process of inflammatory or carious genesis is thus simulated.

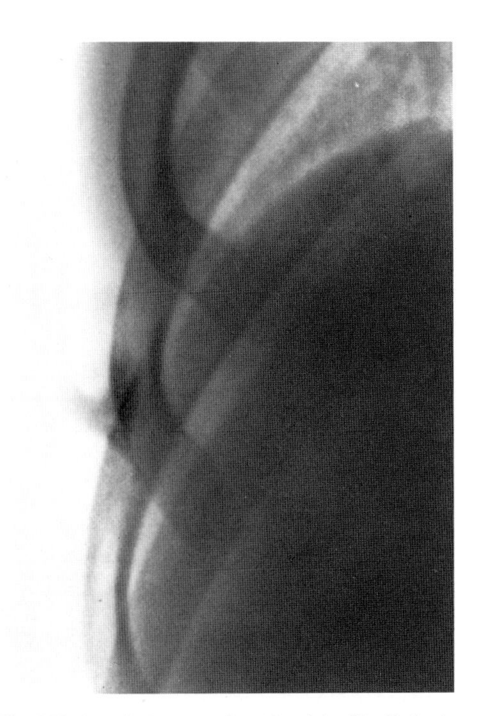

Fig. 558. Atypical exostosis at the right 6th rib, in the axilla.

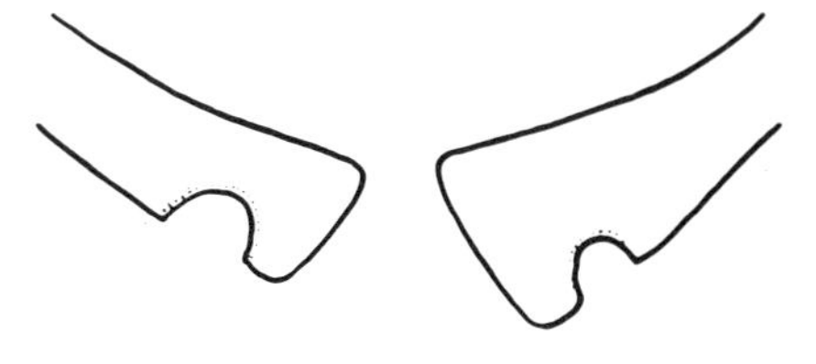

Fig. 559. Sketches of ligamental fossae, after *Simon (Ravelli)*.

Reinhardt described a bilateral anomaly at the distal third of the clavicle, which has so far not been published, consisting of a curved duplication of the clavicle in the direction towards the coracoid. Thus, he added to the rare anomalies of the clavicle a further unusual faulty development, which might be traced to the very complicated phylogenesis of this bone.

Figs. 560–565. Clasp-like cranial border of the scapula, caused by a hole in the supraspinatous fossa.

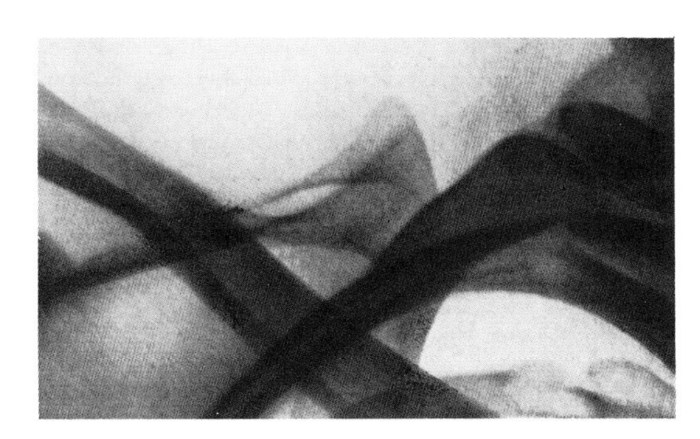

Fig. 560

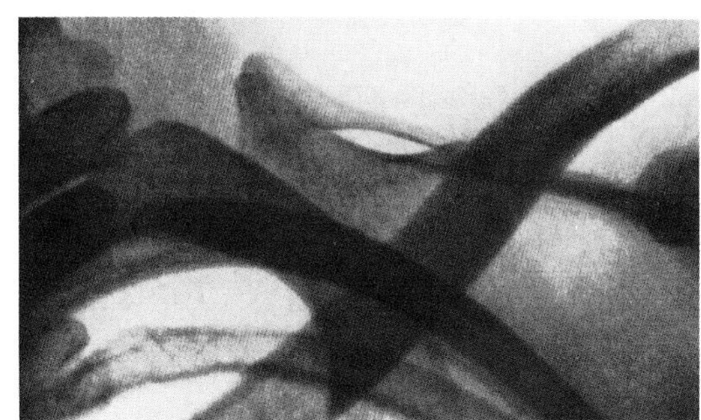

Fig. 561

Figs. 560 and 561. Hole formation in the supraspinatous fossa (developmental defect).

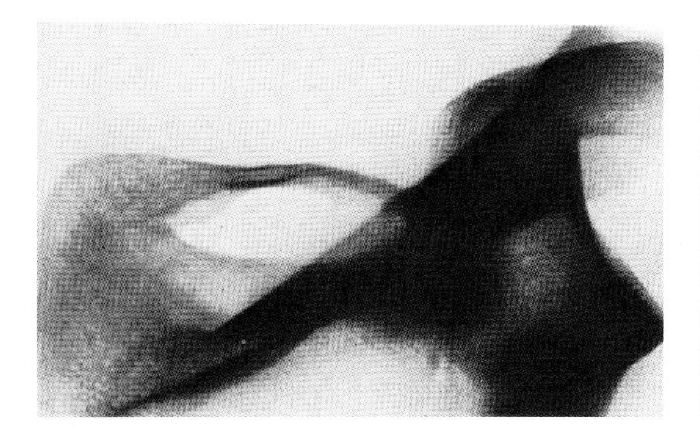

Fig. 562

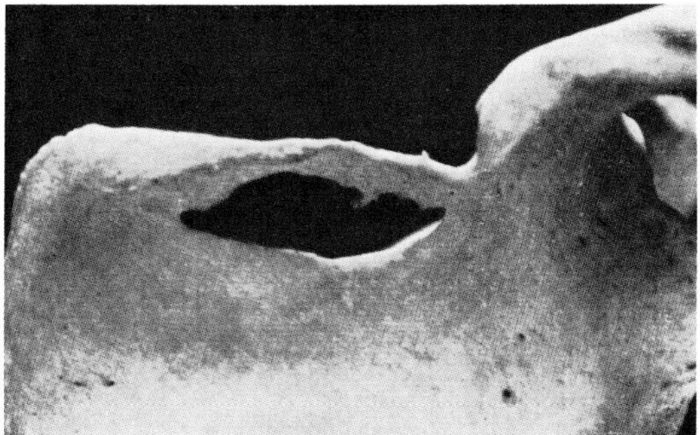

Fig. 563

Figs. 562 and 563. Skeletonized left scapula, shown radiographically and photographically. It becomes clear that this is not a case of an ossification of the transverse scapular ligament across the great scapular notch, which is found more laterally; rather, the bony plate of the supraspinatous fossa had not been preformed.

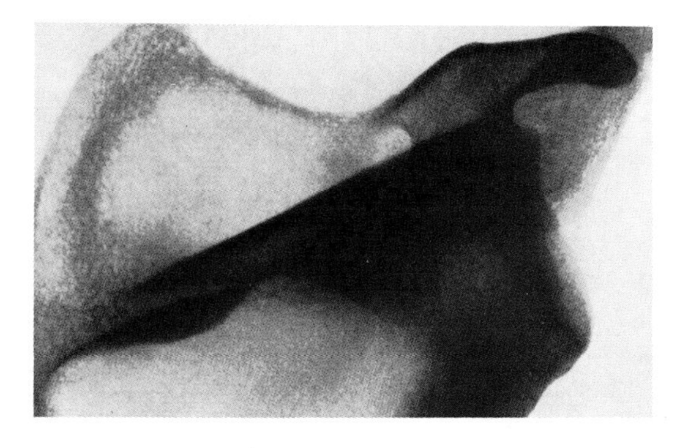

Fig. 564

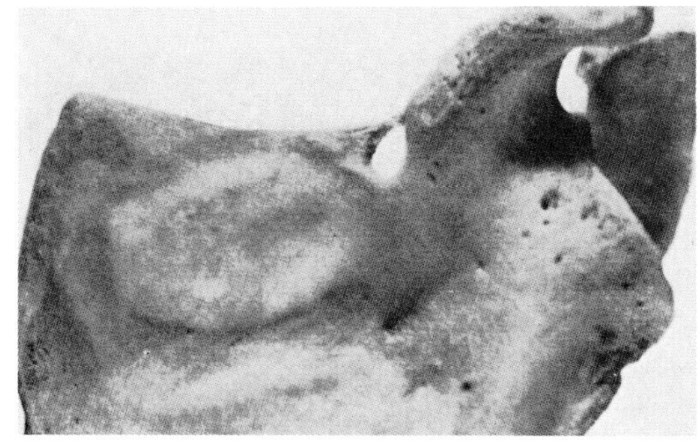

Fig. 565

Figs. 564 and 565. In contrast to the above views, this is a radiograph of a skeletonized clavicle with an ossified superior transverse scapular ligament (left). The photograph on the right simultaneously demonstrates the thin lamellar bony plate of the supraspinatous fossa in the light impinging upon it.

Radiographic Anatomy and Radiographs of the Elbow and Forearm, Including Exposure Techniques

Main directions of radiograph – elbow joint

1. *lateral*
   a) radioulnar
   b) ulnoradial; both pictures are taken with the elbow joint bent, in either pronation or supination
2. *sagittal*
   a) volodorsal
   b) dorsovolar; both exposures with the joint in extension, pronation or supination
3. *oblique radiograph,* oblique from outside, dorsoulnoradial
4. *sagittal radiograph* with the joint bent (e.g., in contracture)
5. *axial radiograph* of olecranon

Main directions of radiograph – forearm

1. *sagittal*
   a) volodorsal in supination
   b) dorsovolar in pronation
2. *lateral,* radioulnar

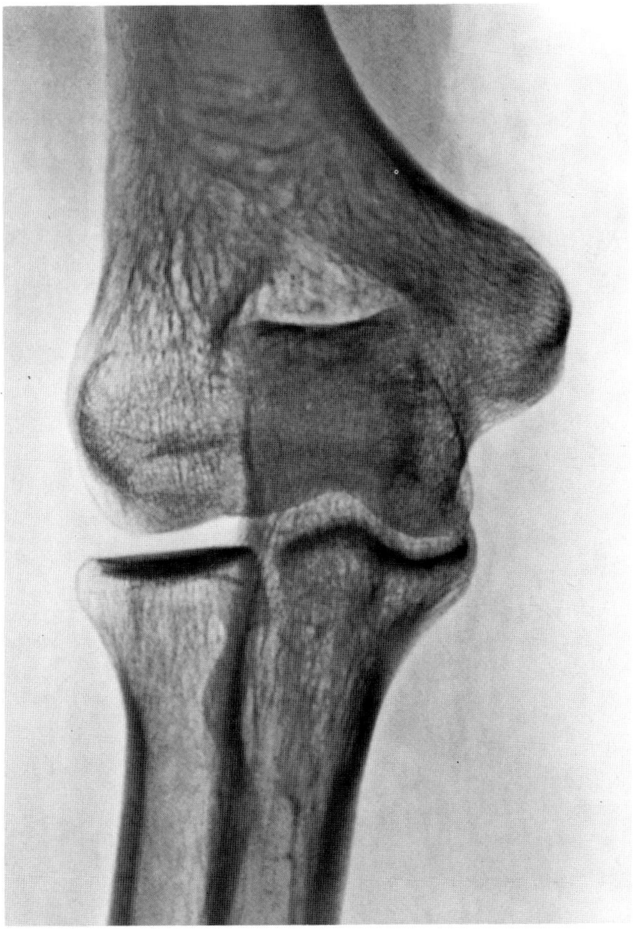

Fig. 566. Elbow joint, sagittal, volodorsal. Physiological cubitus valgus in a female, 22 years of age. Projection: forearm extended, supinated. The central ray is directed onto the center of the articular space.

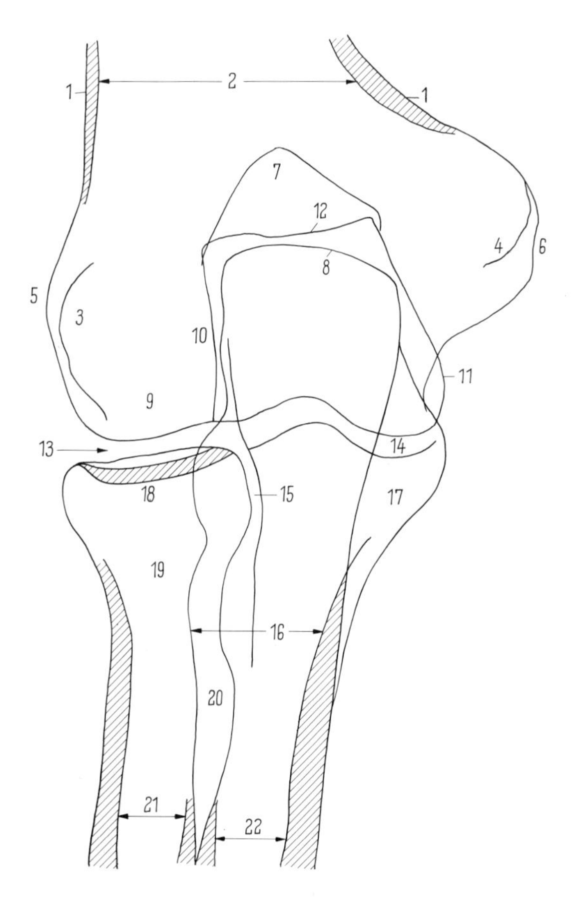

Fig. 567. Sketch to Fig. 566.

1 Medial and lateral edge of humerus
2 Medullary cavity
3 Lateral part of humeral condylus
4 Medial part of humeral condylus
5 Lateral epicondylus of humerus
6 Medial epicondylus of humerus
7 Olecranon fossa (line of upper border)
8 Olecranon (line of upper border)
9 Capitulum of humerus
10 Radial margin of trochlea
11 Ulnar margin of trochlea
12 Proximal margin of trochlea
13 Humeroradial articulation
14 Humeroulnar articulation
15 Proximal radioulnar articulation
16 Shaft of ulna, complete width
17 Coronoid process
18 Head of radius
19 Neck of radius
20 Radial tuberosity
21 Body of radius (medullary cavity)
22 Body of ulna (medullary cavity)

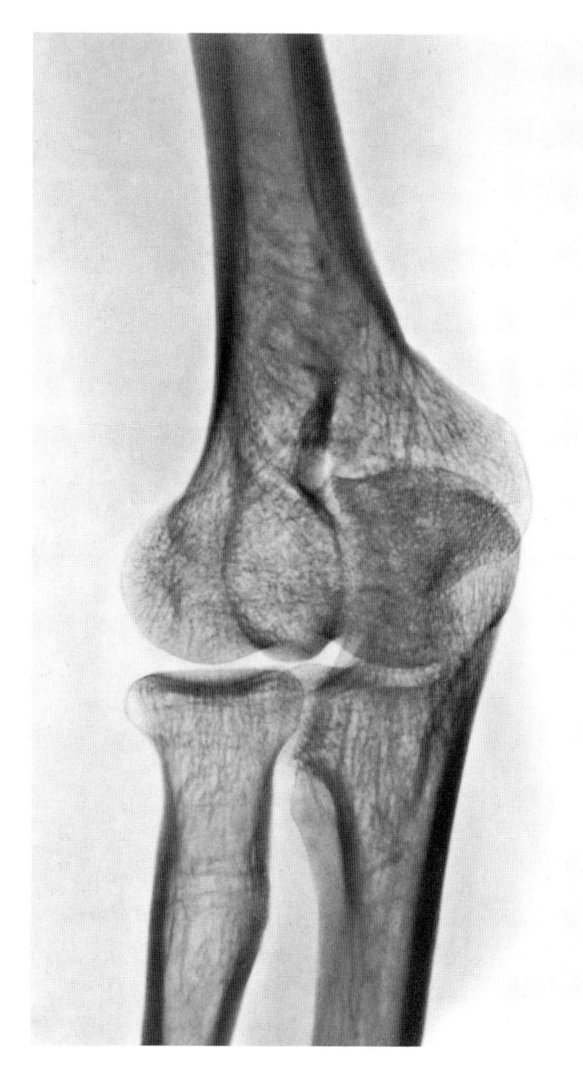

Fig. 568. **View of head of radius.** Projection: the arm is rotated outward until olecranon and lateral epicondylus of the humerus lie on the cassette. The central ray is aimed onto the center of the articular space.

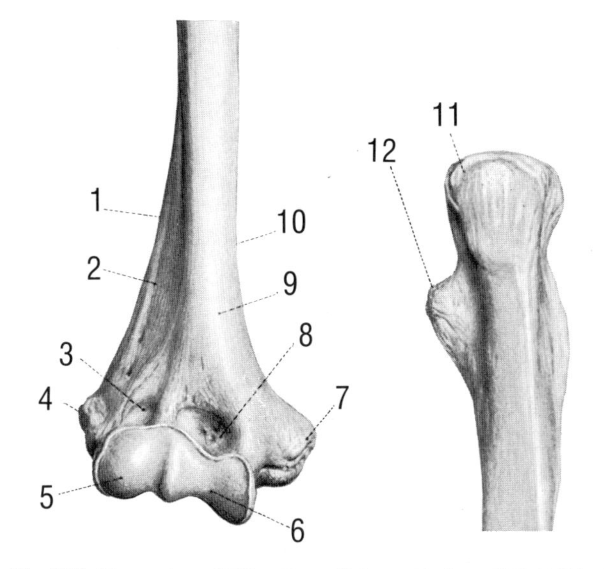

Fig. 569. Humenis and Ulna (from *Sobotta-Becher,* 17th Edition).

1 Lateral margin of humerus
2 Anterior lateral surface
3 Radial fossa
4 Lateral epicondylus of humerus
5 Capitulum of humerus
6 Trochlea
7 Medial epicondylus of humerus
8 Coronoid fossa
9 Anterior medial surface
10 Medial margin of humerus
11 Olecranon
12 Coronoid process of ulna

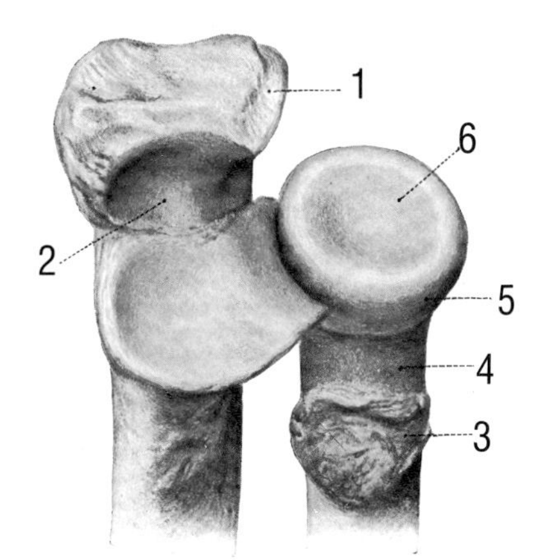

1 Olecranon
2 Semilunar notch
3 Radial tuberosity
4 Neck of radius
5 Articular circumference
6 Fovea of the radial head

Fig. 570. Proximal ends of radius and ulna; view into the joint obliquely from above (from *Sobotta-Becher,* 17th Edition).

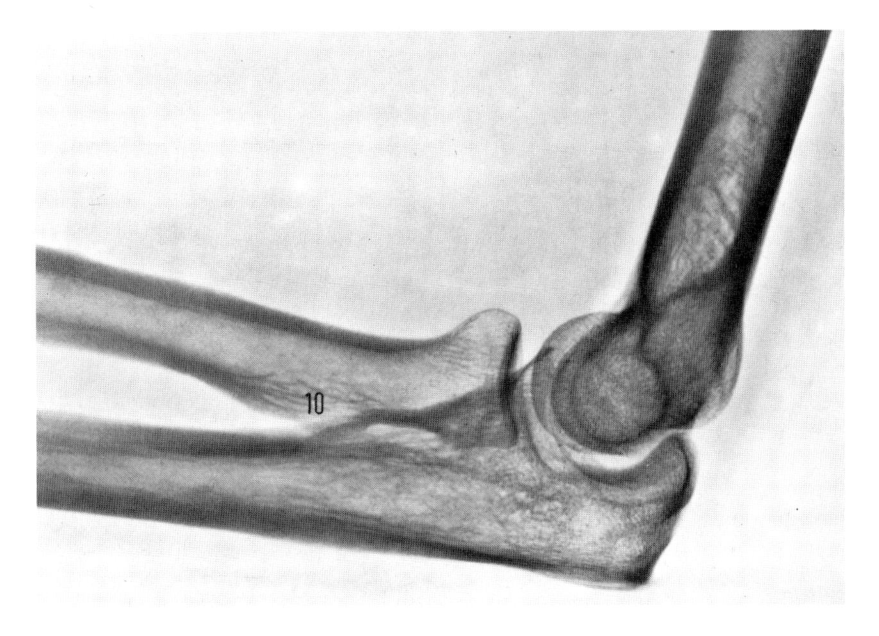

Fig. 571. Elbow joint, lateral, radioulnar. The forearm is supinated. For projection see Fig. 572. The central ray is aimed at the center of the elbow joint.

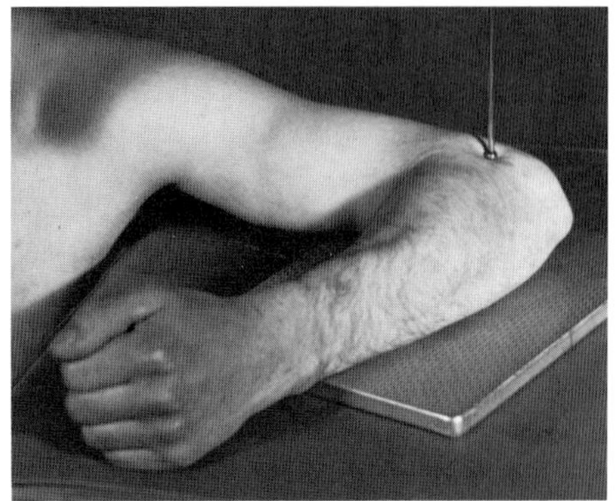

Fig. 572. Position for Fig. 571.

1 Coronoid fossa
2 Olecranon fossa
3 Medial epicondylus of humerus
4 Joint between humerus and radius
5 Joint between humerus and ulna
6 Coronoid process of ulna
7 Olecranon
8 Head of radius
9 Neck of radius
10 Radial tuberosity
x Radial tuberosity corresponds to the center of rotation of the joint. 4 and 5 are curved concentrically towards it; a line which vertically cuts the contours of the joints that belong together (arrow) must be directed at point X. In this way, dislocations can be recognized immediately and subluxations can be recognized with reasonable certainty. One must take into consideration that in supination (Fig. 571) the very flatly curved radial articular surface may normally deviate a little lateral-proximally, especially if a not infrequent incongruity of the articular surfaces should be conspicuous on sagittal inspection.

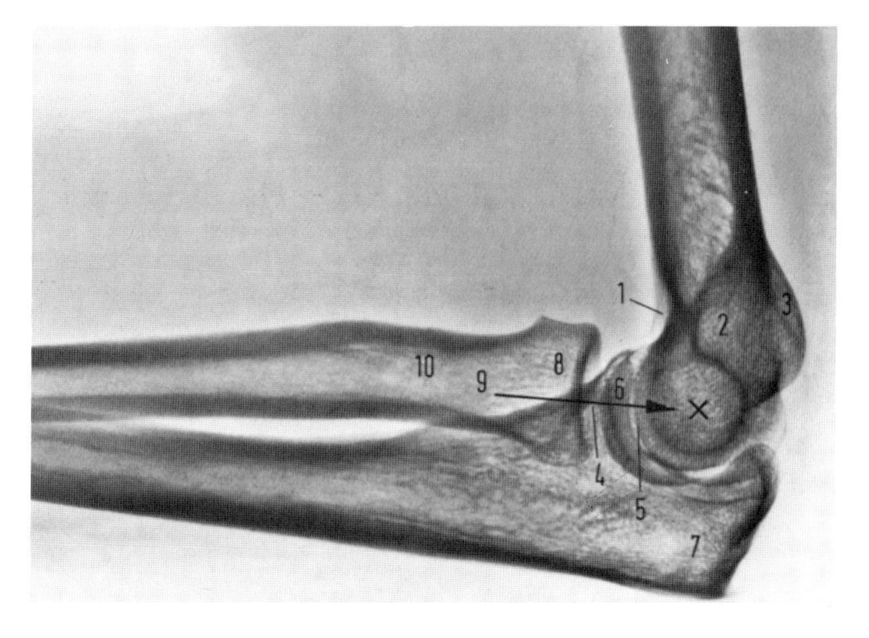

Fig. 573. Elbow joint, lateral, radioulnar. Forearm pronated, projection as in Fig. 572, only the volar side of the hand must lie on the cassette.

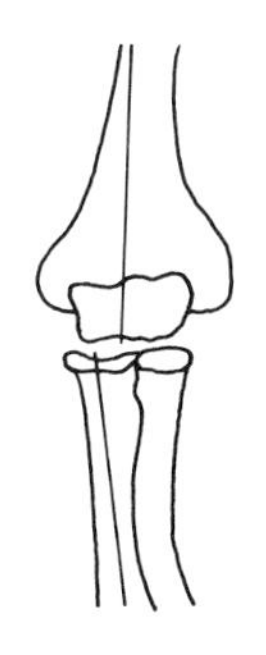
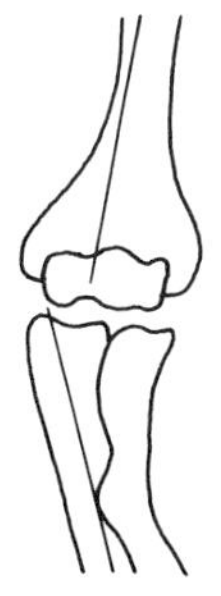
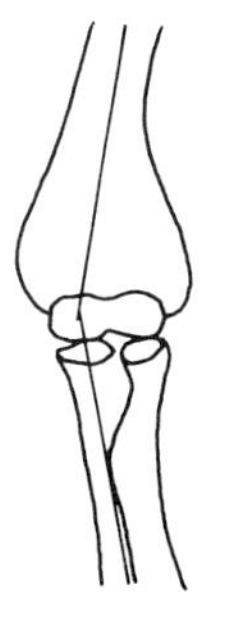
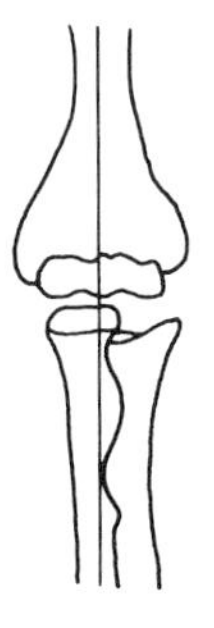
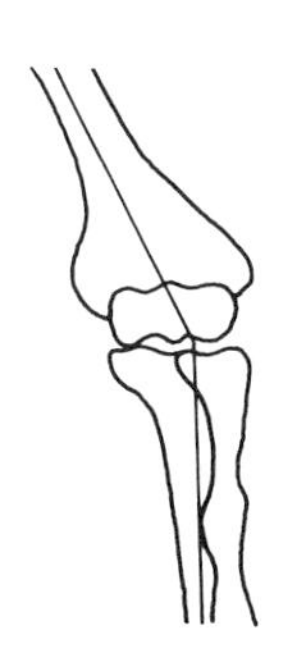

physiological cubitus valgus (male) | physiological cubitus valgus (female) | pathological cubitus valgus (male) | cubitus rectus | cubitus varus

Fig. 574. Varus – valgus positions, according to *von Keiser.*

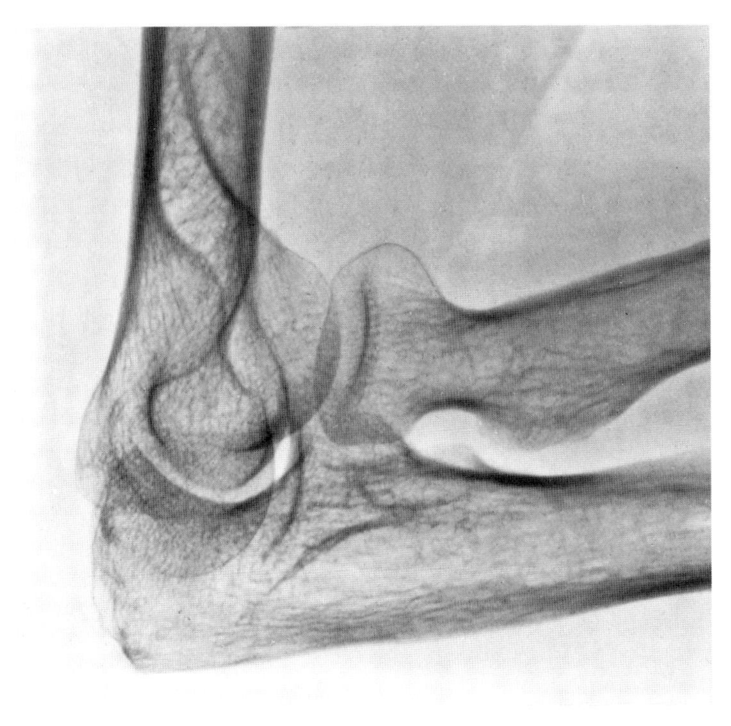

Fig. 575. **Elbow joint, dorsoulnoradial.** Position as in Fig. 572, with the forearm pronated. The central ray is aimed obliquely from the rear and laterally at an angle of 40–45°, onto the elbow joint. This radiograph is recommended for soft tissue diseases (soft rays should be applied), e.g., in the region of the ulnar nerve and the intratendinous bursa of the olecranon.

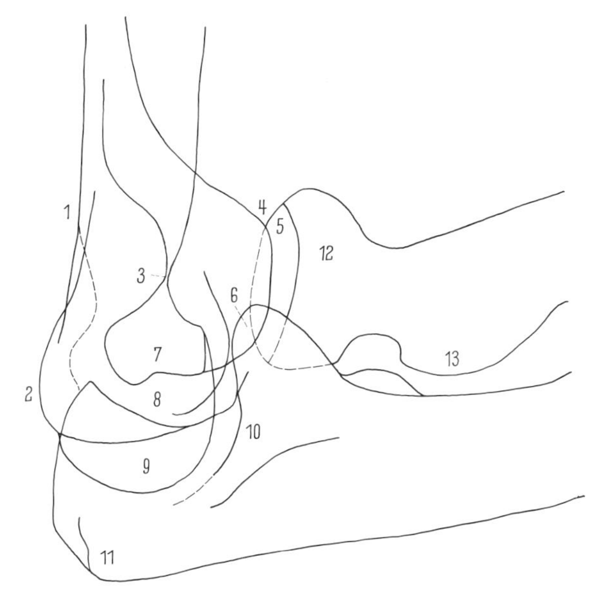

Fig. 576. Sketch to Fig. 575.

1 Contour of dorsal humeral surface
2 Medial part of humeral condylus
3 Bridge between olecranon fossa and coronoid fossa
4 Capitulum of the humerus
5 Humeroradial joint
6 Coronoid process
7 Contour of trochlea
8 Trochlear notch
9 Ulnar edge of trochlea
10 Medial contour of glenoid cavity
11 Roughness on olecranon (for insertion of triceps)
12 Head of radius
13 Radial tuberosity

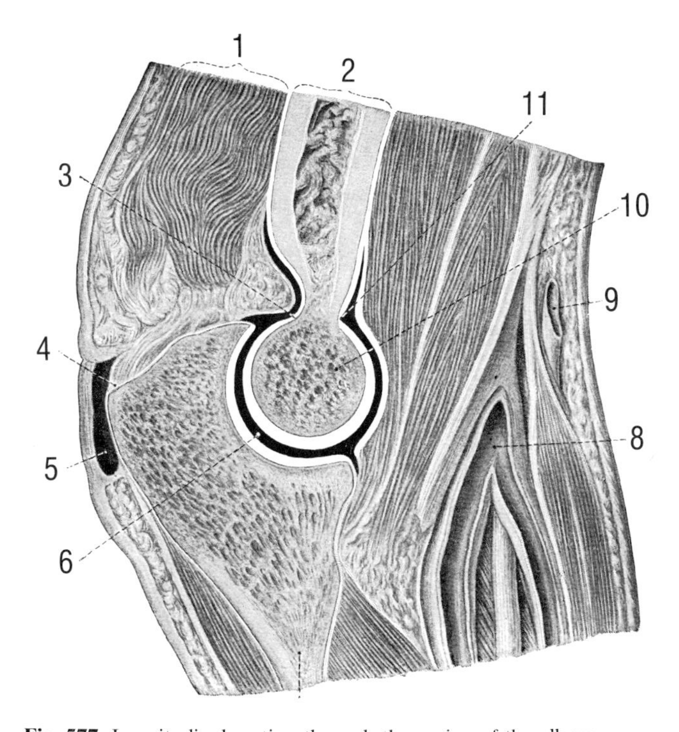

Fig. 577. Longitudinal section through the region of the elbow.

1 Humerus
2 Triceps brachii muscle
3 Olecranon fossa
4 Triceps tendon
5 Subcutaneous olecranon bursa
6 Articular space
7 Ulna
8 Brachial artery
9 Vena mediana cubiti
10 Trochlea of humerus
11 Coronoid fossa

Chronic bursitis is a symptom of inflammatory or post-traumatic illness of the elbow region; like changes at insertions or origins of muscles, tendons and ligaments, as well as in bones and joints; it is counted among occupational diseases which may lead to a reduction in earning capacity.

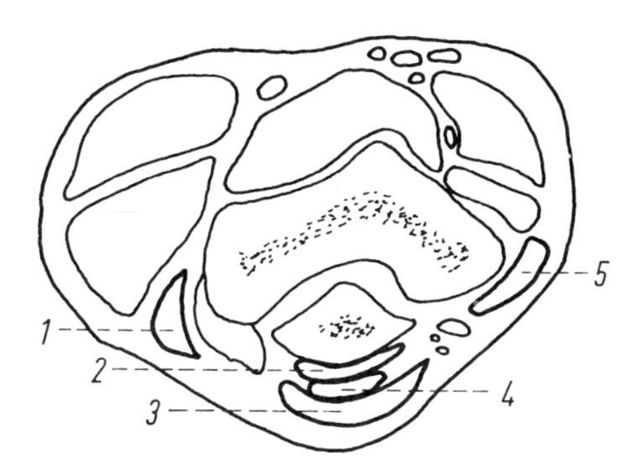

Fig. 578. The bursae of the elbow joint. Cross section through the left upper arm at the level of the epicondyles (from *Springorum,* 1957).

1 Subcutaneous bursa of the radial epicondyle
2 Subtendinous bursa of the olecranon
3 Subcutaneous bursa of the olecranon
4 Bursa of the triceps tendon
5 Subcutaneous bursa of the ulnar epicondylus

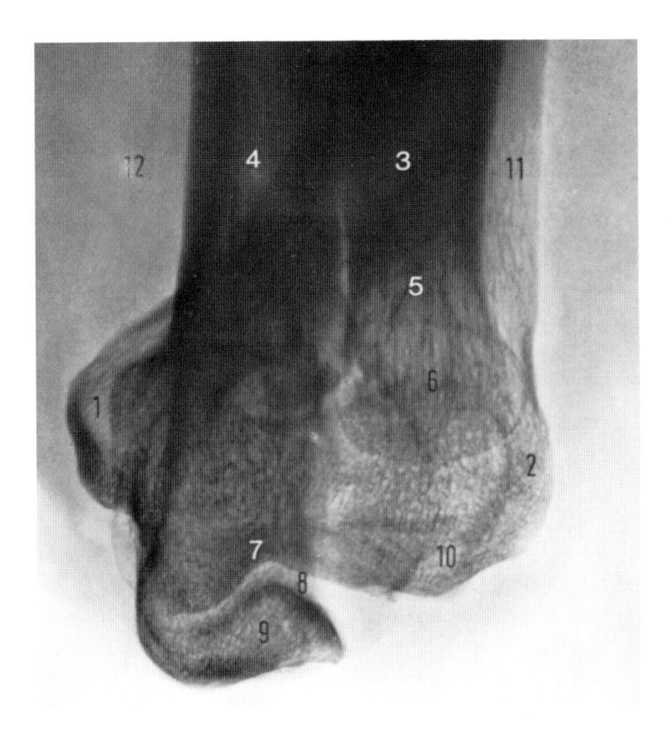

1 Medial epicondylus of humerus
2 Lateral epicondylus of humerus
3 Shaft of radius
4 Shaft of ulna
5 Radial neck
6 Radial head
7 Contour of trochanter
8 Articular space
9 Olecranon
10 Capitulum of humerus
11 Shaft of humerus
12 Musculature of upper arm and forearm, projected upon one another

Fig. 579. Axial radiograph of the olecranon, with bent elbow. The central ray is aimed between olecranon and posterior surface of the humeral condylus (see Fig. 580).

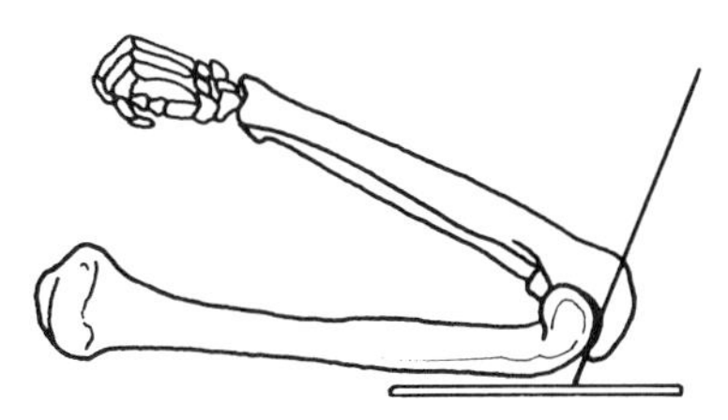

Fig. 580

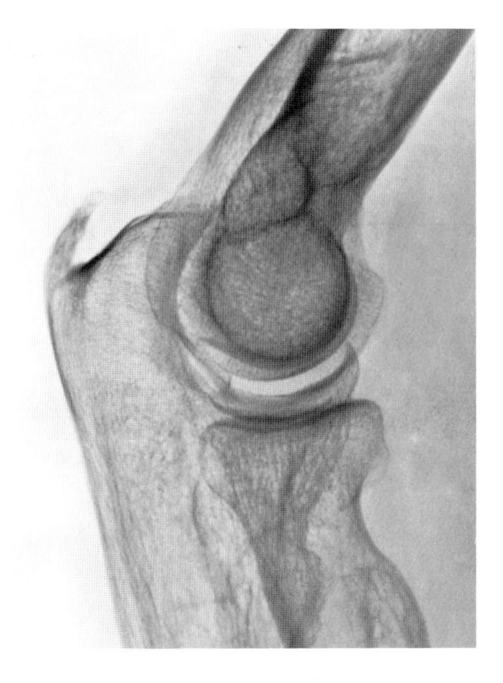

Fig. 581. Spur of olecranon. In the usual views this formation appears to be a spur, while in fact it is developed in lamellae and arises with a broad base from the olecranon, as can be shown with axial projection. Those who exert their triceps heavily and regularly seem prone to formation of an olecranon spur *(Rauber)*. At the base a cleft formation sometimes appears, which may make one think of a primary isolated skeletal element, with pseudoarticular connection to the olecranon. In rare cases the spur may break off, perhaps followed by formation of a pseudarthrosis. If the triceps is overworked, changes such as zones of reconstruction may occur, and long-term suffering is a frequent effect.

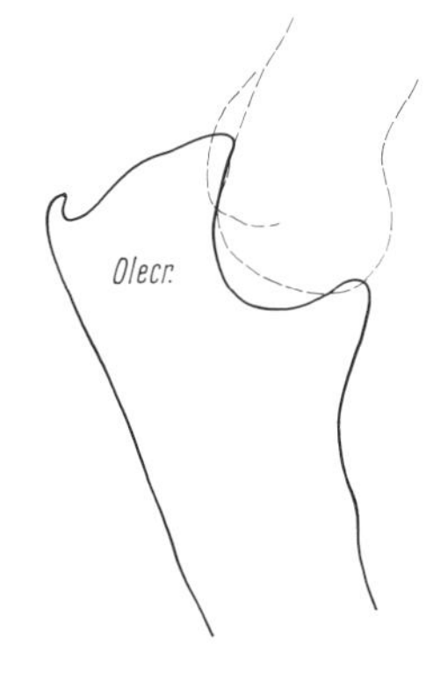

Fig. 582 shows an olecranon spur (male, 33 years old), which is not pathological in itself but, through pressure from outside or through friction, may favor the appearance of symptoms of irritation or of bursitis, similar to a calcaneus spur. In cases of deforming arthrosis it may become enlarged and deformed. Its length is 0.5–2.5 cm.

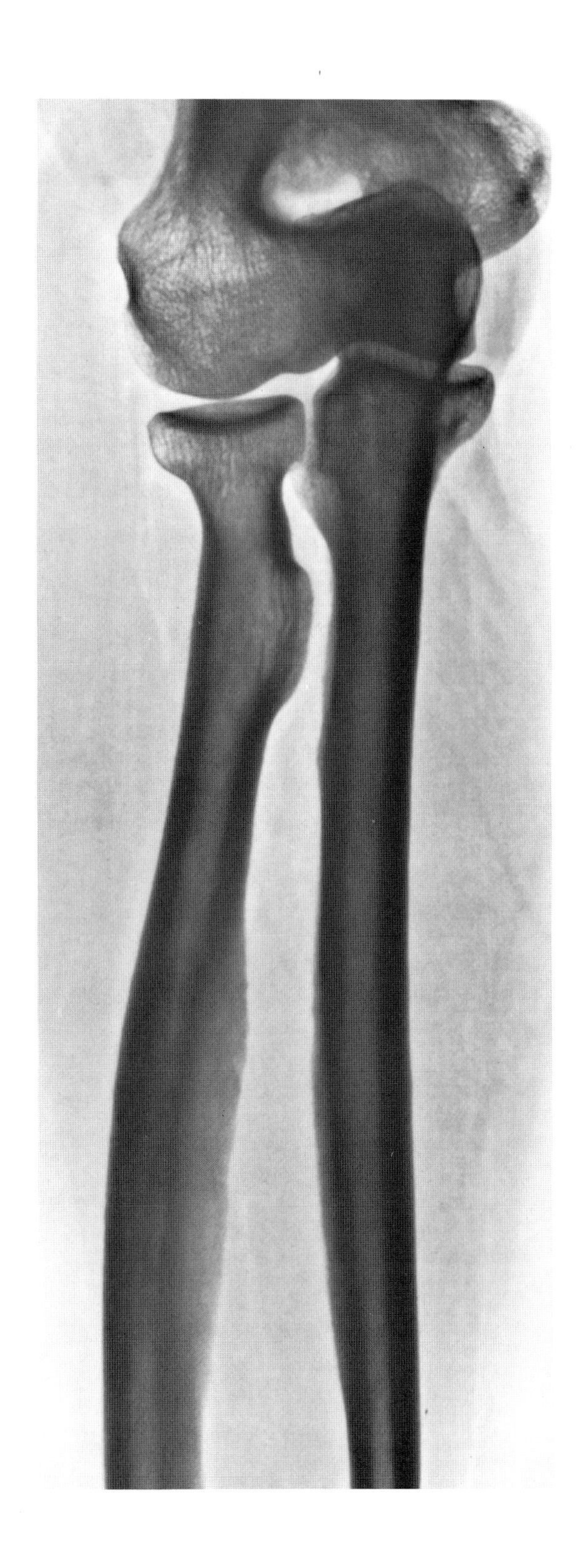

Fig. 583. **Forearm, volodorsal, in supination.** The central ray is aimed at the interosseus space.

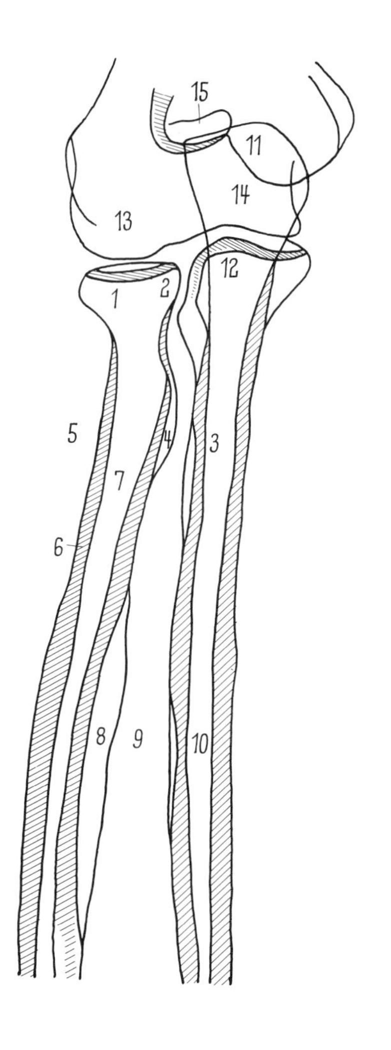

Fig. 584. Sketch to Fig. 583.

1 Head of radius
2 Annular circumference
3 Shaft of ulna
4 Radial tuberosity
5 Muscles
6 Radial cortex
7 Medullary cavity of radius
8 Interosseus margin, irregular, often looks like a pathological swelling. Radius as well as ulna of the adult show this kind of pseudoperiostitis. The interosseus membrane is fixed to this bony ledge.
9 Interosseus space
10 Medullary cavity of ulna
11 Olecranon
12 Coronoid process; at the radial side, below it an oval increased radiolucency, caused by the insertion of the annular radial ligament (see Fig. 585, g)
13 Capitulum of humerus
14 Trochlea of humerus
15 Olecranon fossa

Variants and Sources of Diagnostic Error of the Elbow and Forearm*

Especially in the region of the elbow, the possibilities of variants can so easily be confused with post-traumatic and post-inflammatory changes that, in the following, an effort will be made to indicate the most frequent opinions and to interpret them as far as possible. Because it is known that one-third of the cases of sportsmen with radiologically demonstrable changes with splintering-off, ossifications, calcifications, etc. can often be found only after a few years, interpretation of the findings must be adapted to individual cases.

69 Supracondylar process (frequency 2%), see Fig. 589. This is a phylogenetic remnant and may undergo avulsion fracture. In most cases, the median nerve and the brachial artery pass below the supracondyloid process.

70 Patella of elbow, i.e., sesamoid bone within the triceps tendon. This is a phylogenetic rudiment, usually bilateral and hereditary. Differential diagnosis for isolated apophysis of olecranon, traumatic splintering-off or osteochondrosis dissecans.

70* Anterior elbow bone (coronoid bone of ulna, fabella of elbow) is an accessory bone, present for a short time only, but may persist (see Fig. 594); a shearing-off fracture would have to be excluded

70** Sesamoid bone of elbow (see Fig. 602), i.e., osteochondrosis dissecans of the supratrochlear septum (aseptic necrosis), a spheric loose body in the olecranon fossa. Differential diagnosis for splintering-off in deforming arthrosis.

71 In cases of epicondylitis (tennis elbow), soft tissue calcifications next to the bone may occur due to advanced age or after chronic traumata (Figs. 590–592)

71* Vascular canal above a radiographic supratrochlear foramen (see Fig. 595)

71** Non-ossified area in the brachial medial intermuscular septum at the spot where the insertions of the pronator teres and the brachialis muscle meet *(Viehweger)*; see Fig. 605

72 Spur of olecranon (see Figs. 581, 582); this may be due to ossification of the insertion of the triceps tendon in chronic tendinitis after traumata or may be degenerative calcification. Perhaps this is a skeletal variant with its own bony nucleus.

72* Normal thinning of cortex (see Figs. 599, 601); should not be mistaken for osteomyelitis, sarcoma and other conditions

73 Accessory ossicle (see Fig. 590): split-off spophyseal nucleus? chondromatosis? or ossification of the insertion of the collateral ulnar ligament? See Fig. 592 (tennis elbow).

73* Persistent apophysis at the medial epicondylus *(Günsel, Sieckel)*; may be traumatic or a congenital anomaly

74 Thickened interosseous margin (see Fig. 583); a pseudoperiostitis; differential diagnosis against periostitis or callus

74* Normal spike, simulated by the middle bulge of the sharp contour of the radial edge of the trochlea (Figs. 586, 588)

n Nutritive canal

p Pseudoperiostitis (see also Fig. 583, where the finding is on the radius)

j Incongruity of the articular surfaces (apparent subluxation of the head of the radius; a very frequent occurrence, cf. Fig. 595)

g Ligamental fossa (insertion of the annular ligament of the radius); may cause a rounded or oval increased radiolucency of the cortex of the radial side of the ulna, below the ulnar coronoid process (see Figs. 583, 584)

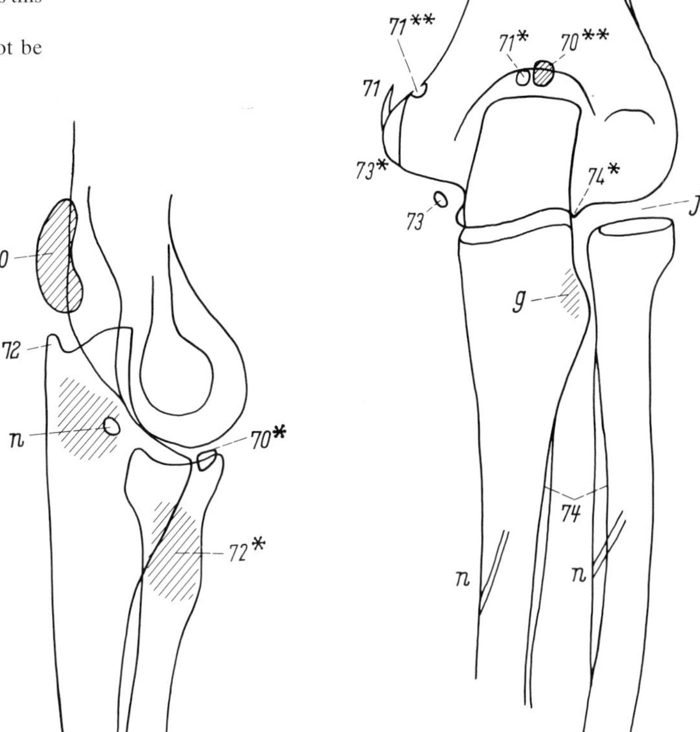

Fig. 585. Variants and sources of diagnostic error of elbow and forearm.

* The numbers in bold type relate only to the lateral view.

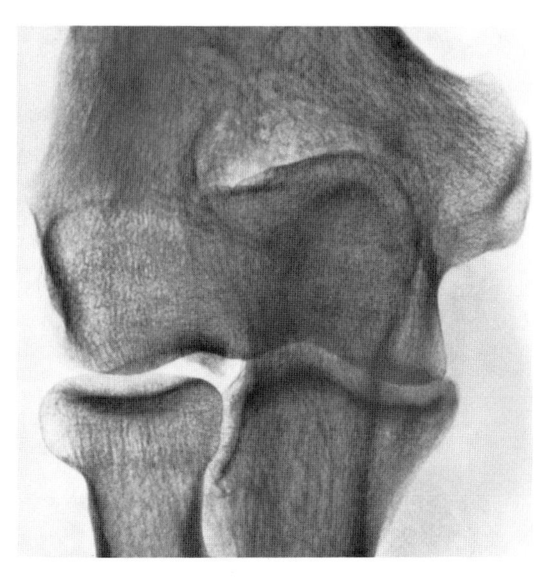

Fig. 586 a

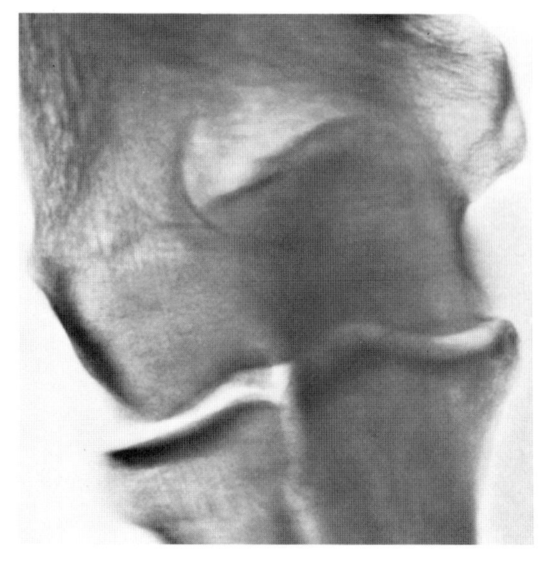

Fig. 586 b

Fig. 586. Spike at the border between trochlea and capitulum of humerus, cf. Figs. 588 (↙) and 585, No. 74*. No deforming arthrosis is present. Probably this is a variant emphasized by projection, a sharply set-off middle bulge of the radial edge of the trochlea *(Köhler-Zimmer)*. A similar spike in the same position, although somewhat flatter, can be seen in Fig. 591.

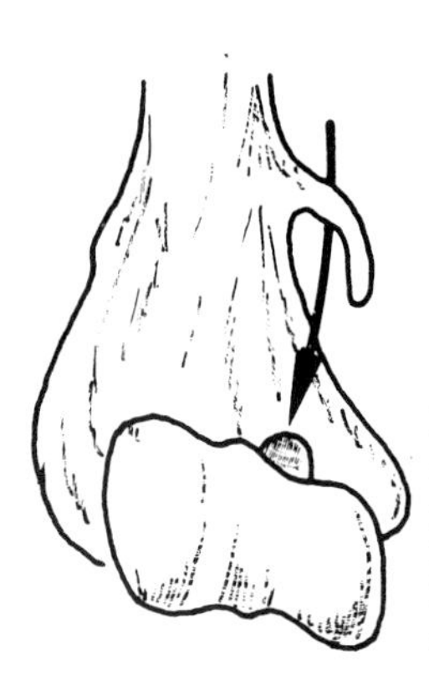

Fig. 587 (after *Braus*). **Course of the brachial artery and the median nerve** below the supracondylar process of the humerus (arrow). From its tip, a ligamental connection to the humeral epicondylus may be present and may possibly ossify.

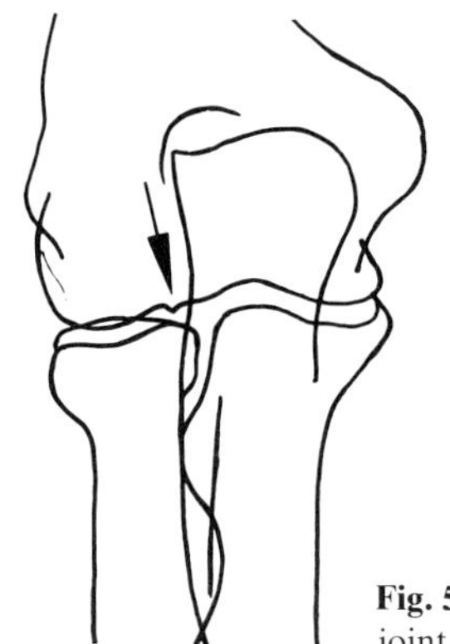

Fig. 588. Spike at the contour of an arthrotic joint of the humerus.

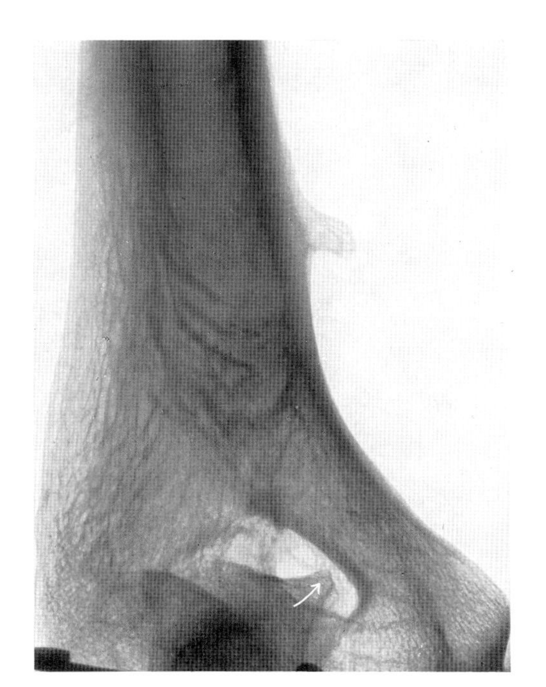

The supracondylar process protrudes best with slight inward rotation, as its position is medioventral. Sometimes a compact ligamental strand draws from it to the medial condyle; from this ligament part of the pronator teres muscle arises. Behind the process, the median nerve and the brachial artery run medially and distally through the space between the more or less narrowed process and the ligament. Depending on its anatomical relationships, the process may attain pathological significance, either spontaneously or after traumata, either neurogenous (due to compression of the nerve) or as an effect of disturbed vascular supply by the brachial artery. Familial occurrence has not yet been proven *(Köhler-Zimmer)* but manifestations among blood relatives have become known *(Reinhardt)*. Avulsion fractures of this process were described by *Ganz* and *Neiss*, i.a. The arrow (↗) shows the angular contours of the olecranon.

Fig. 589. Supracondylar process of humerus. Its frequency is about 1%; it denotes a phylogenetic remnant (Fig. 585, No. 69).

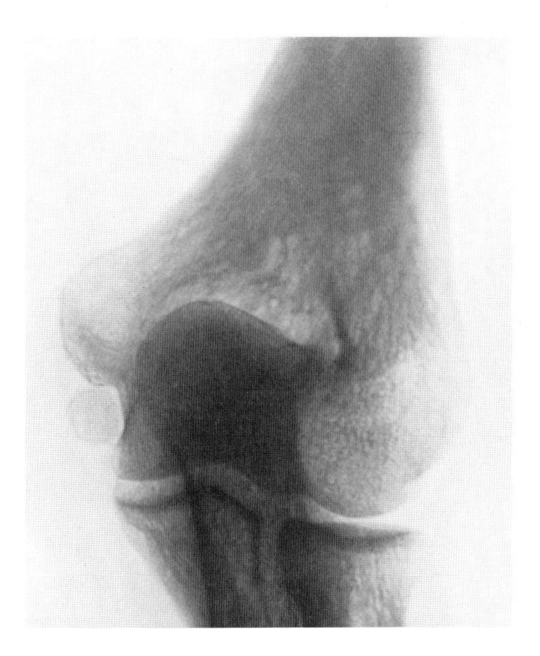

Fig. 590. Isolated supernumerary ossicle below the medial epicondylus *(Bánki)*. If it occurs bilaterally, a congenital anomaly (persistent bony nuclei) may be assumed (see *Viehweger)*; if unilateral, a juvenile trauma may be the cause *(Sieckel)*. The following interpretations are possible:

1 persistent apophysis from one of the two main nuclei of the olecranon (most likely)
2 accessory bone
3 chondromatosis
4 ossification of the insertion of the collateral ulnar ligament. Neoplastic bone formations within the medial and lateral collateral ligaments and in insertions of tendons are very frequent (up to 30%) among professional sportsmen.

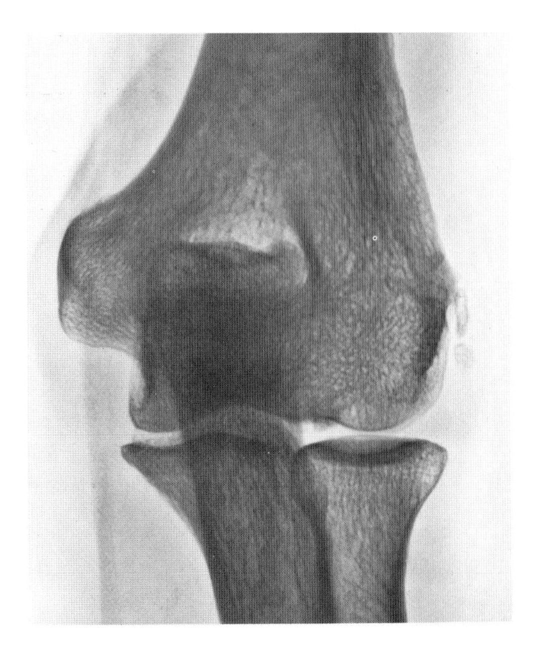

Fig. 591. Accessory bones at the lateral epicondylus (from the collection of *W. Werner,* Berlin); see also Fig. 585, No. 71. Accessory bones at the lateral and medial epicondylus may occur congenitally and are then mostly bilateral; when they are post-traumatic *(Brauer),* they are mainly unilateral. Finally, a unilateral ossification at the ligamental insertion may look like an isolated ossicle. It may also be the consequence of a chronic traumatic epicondylitis in ball-playing sportsmen (tennis elbow).

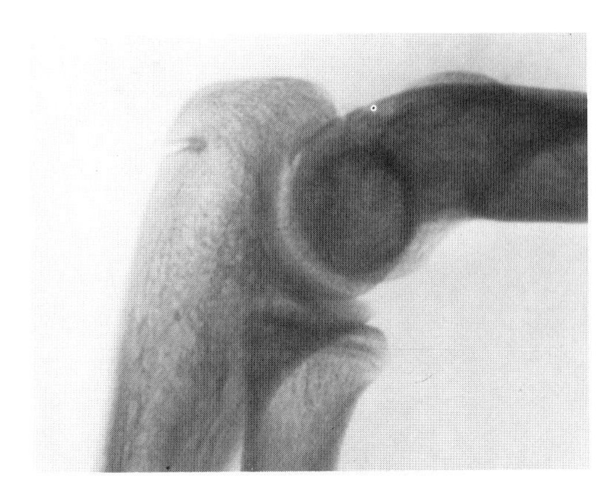

Fig. 593. The final fusion of the dorsal cleft, shown here in a 13-year-old boy. It may be postponed far beyond the 20th year of life (normally between the 16th and 20th years, see Fig. 1080 a, b). **Pseudo-loosening of the olecranon epiphysis!** *(Schmitt)*.

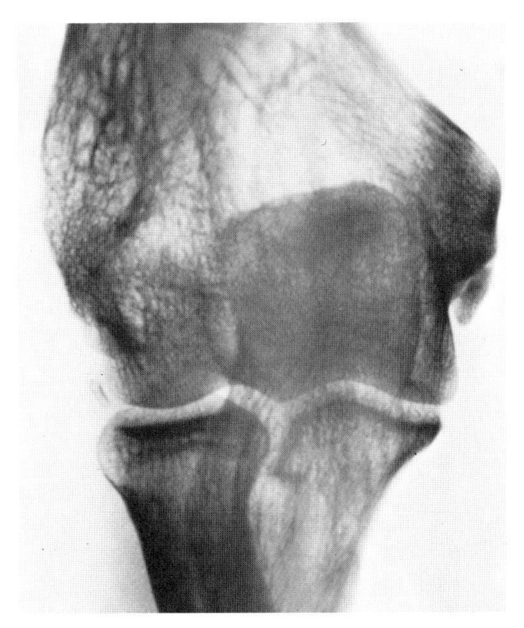

Fig. 592. Ossification of the insertion of the ulnar collateral ligament at the medial epicondylus (see also Fig. 585, No. 71).

Calcification in the radial collateral ligament *(Bánki)*. Calcification in the radial collateral ligament, in cases of epicondylitis, is typical not only for tennis elbow but generally for overwork of the extensor muscles, which arise at the radial epicondylus. Therefore, it also occurs in typists, dentists, etc. (from the collection of *H. Hiltemann,* Münster).

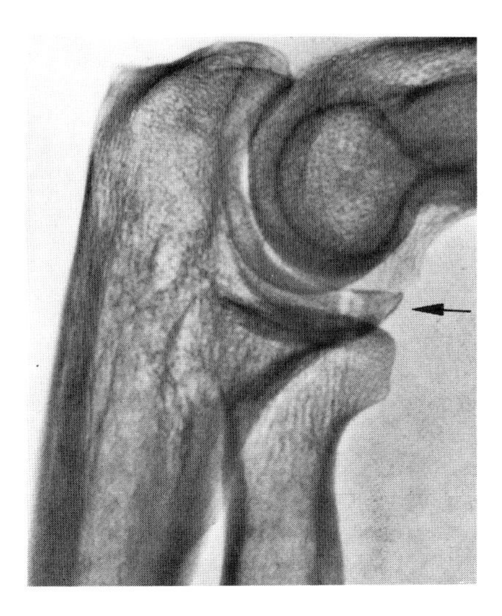

Fig. 594. An anterior elbow bone (←) (ulnar coronoid bone, fabella cubiti); see also Fig. 585, No. 70*. Should not be mistaken for a fracture occurring at the same spot (shearing-off fracture). In the literature some authors question the existence of an elbow bone as a persistent center of ossification, e. g., *Maurer, Neiss*. We have seen such isolated bodies quite frequently without a preceding trauma. In our opinion, the traumatic splintering-off of the coronoid process is very rare, as *Rumpold*, too, has ascertained.

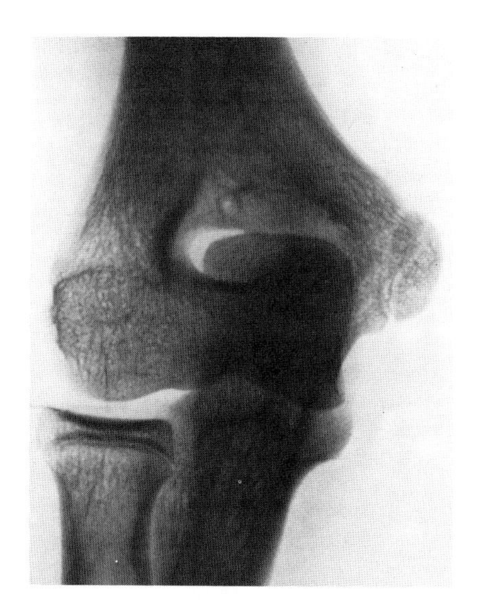

Fig. 595. Roentgenologic supratrochlear foramen (see also Figs. 1066, 1070 b, 1072 b, 1076 b). The supratrochlear foramen is a rare anatomical variant. Whether a roentgenologic supratrochlear foramen corresponds, in fact to an anatomical one, can only be decided when the radiologic diagnosis is followed by surgery, as a very thin supratrochlear septum may appear as a hole on a radiograph. A genuine supratrochlear foramen, according to *Schinz,* denotes a phylogenetic remnant which may be hereditary. If it is large enough, hyperextensibility always seems to be present. Within the supratrochlear foramen, osteochondrosis dissecans may take place. The sesamoid elbow bone (see Fig. 602 b) is today frequently considered to be a free body within the supratrochlear fossa after such an osteochondrosis of the septum (see also *Kohlmann* and *Neumann).* If the septum sequestrates too, a secondary supratrochlear foramen develops. A vascular canal can be seen here above the foramen.

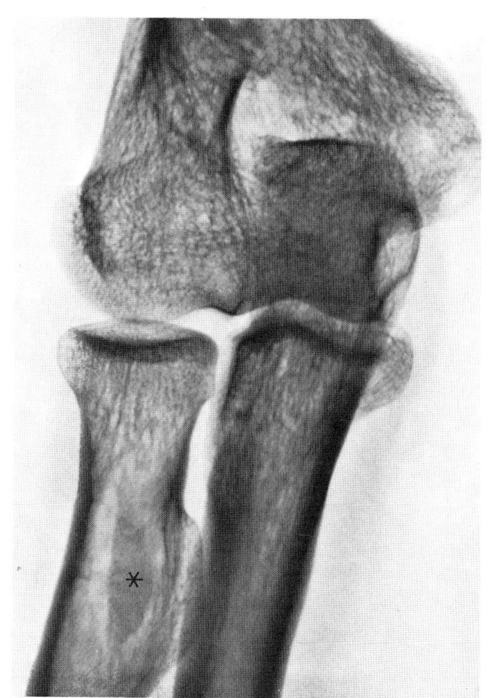

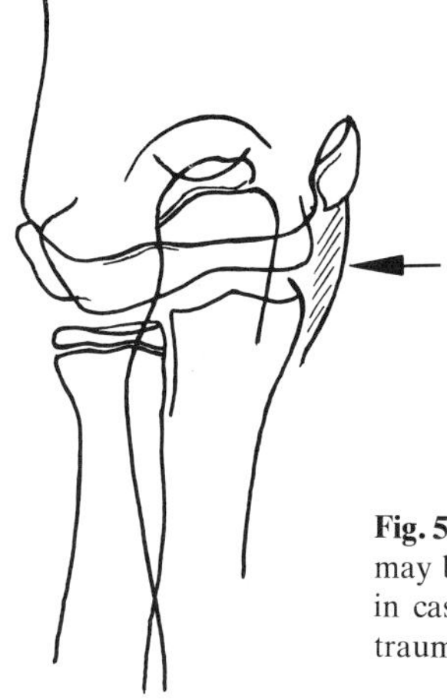

Fig. 597. The arrow indicates a soft tissue contour, which may become visible on soft-ray radiographs, especially in cases of soft tissue swellings (inflammatory edema, traumatic hematoma, effusion into a joint).

Fig. 596. Islet of compact tissue (*) in the proximal radial diaphysis; this must be differentiated from a bony infarction (extremely rare).

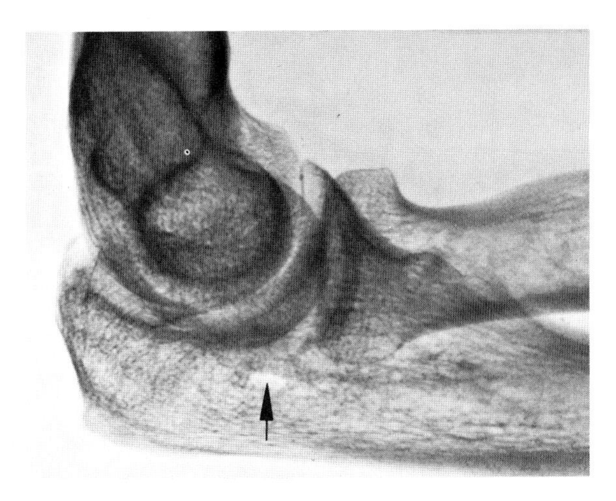

Fig. 598. Nutritive foramen, appearing as a cyst-like formation on a lateral view of the olecranon (↑). See letter n in Fig. 585. According to *Iannaccone* and *Barilla*, it occurs in about 12% of cases.

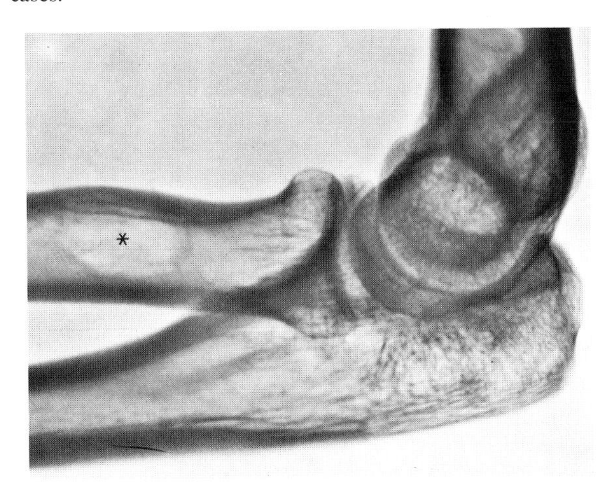

Fig. 599. Cyst-like increased radiolucency (*) in the proximal radial diaphysis. Confusion with osteomyelitis, fibrous osteitis or sarcoma is possible (see also Fig. 585, No. 72*).

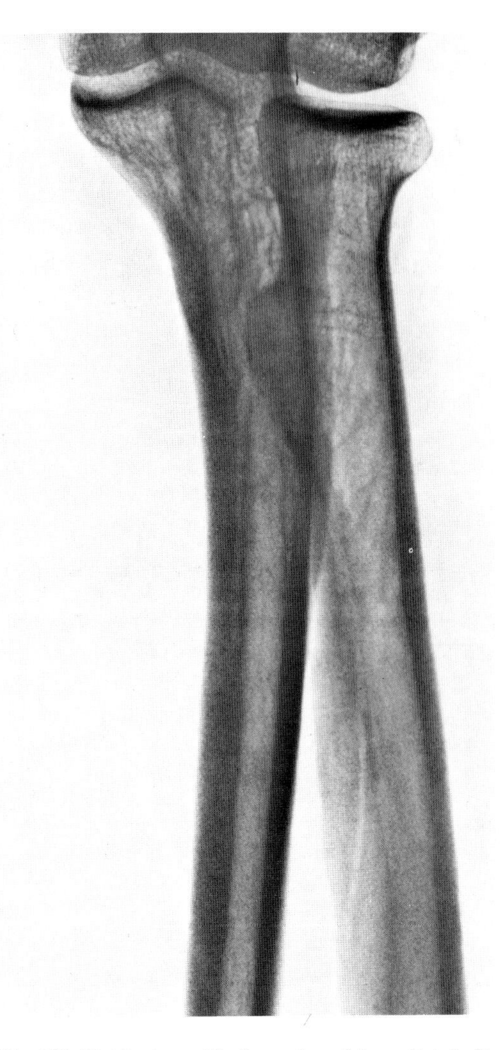

Fig. 600. Nutrient canal in the region of the radial shaft, simulating a fracture. Similar observations can be made in other long bones, especially frequent in the region of the ulnar and femoral shafts. See letter n in Fig. 585.

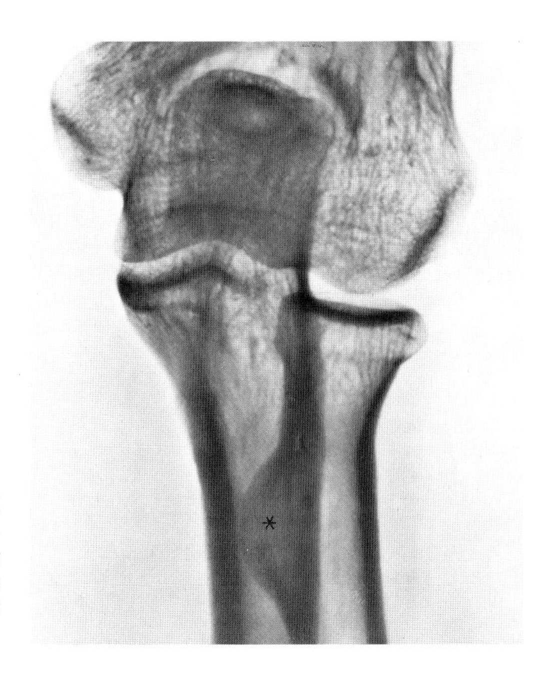

Fig. 601. Supplementary radiograph to Fig. 599. The volodorsal radiograph of the same elbow joint shows that the cyst-like increased translucency in the radius is a deceptive effect, caused by the orthograde presentation of the radial tuberosity (*). At this location the cortex is much thinned, resulting in an apparent "brightening of structures" on an overall view.

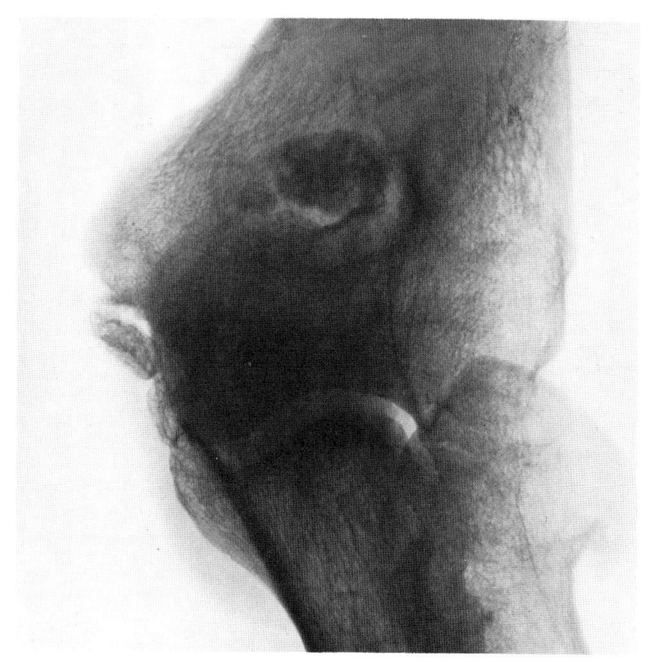

Fig. 602 a

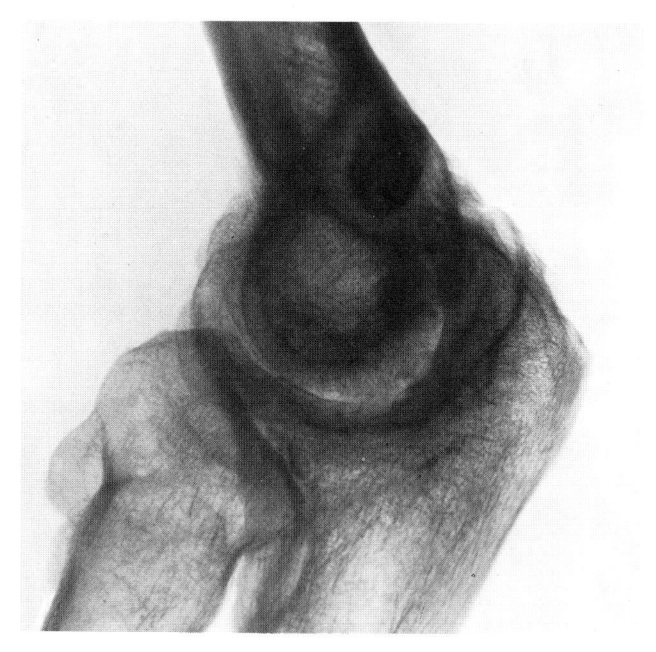

Fig. 602 b

Fig. 602. Sesamoid bone of elbow. Occasionally, one finds in the olecranon fossa a free body with smooth borders (No. 70**, Fig. 585). *Pfitzner* called it a sesamoid bone of the elbow. It may develop from an osteochodrosis dissecans *(Elingshausen, Hillger),* which is very frequent in the elbow region, or from other local processes (trauma). In our case, in addition there is a persistent apophysis at the medial epicondyle. In connection with previous traumata which also led to severe deformity of the head of the radius, a traumatic cause for both sesamoid bone and free medial apophysis cannot be excluded. However, *Canigiani et al.* do not consider the traumatic and osteochondritic cause as proven and speak definitely of a supratrochlear "bone." Such a bone may undergo secondary necrosis, which explains the incorrect designation of osteochondritis or osteochondrosis dissecans.

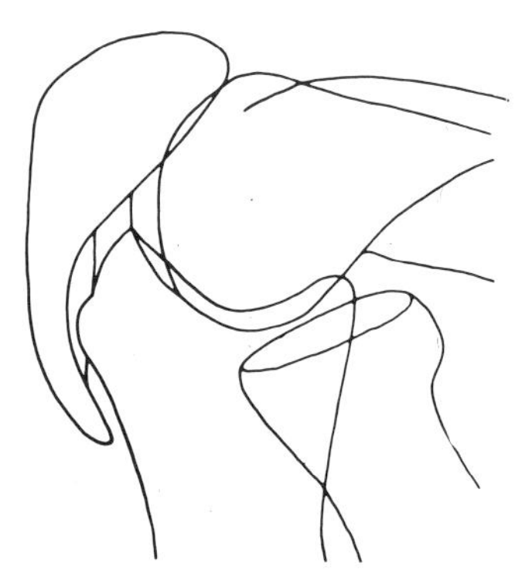

Fig. 603. Sesamoid bone of elbow, also called patella of elbow or elbow disk *(Pfitzner, Kienböck, Kremser).* Sketch based on a radiograph by *Odessky* and *Melnikowa.* This is probably a sesamoid bone in the triceps tendon (and therefore equated with the patella of the knee joint and a sesamoid bone in the quadriceps tendon). Similar signs may also develop in cases of a persistent and enlarged olecranon nucleus or a non-united fracture of the olecranon; then, it might be termed a pseudosesamoid. Further references are cited by *Buse.*

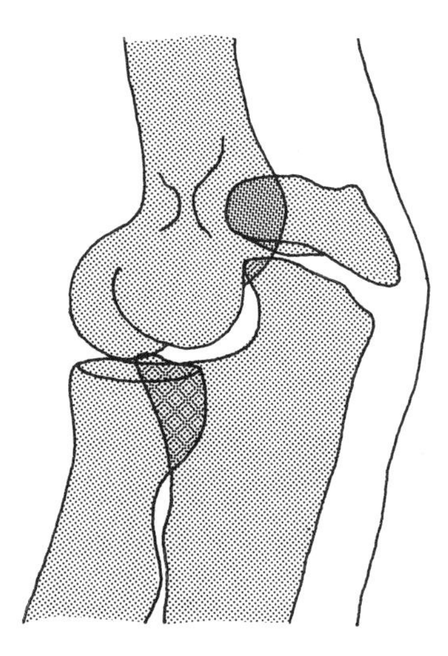

Fig. 604. Pseudosesamoid after avulsion fracture (sketch from *Kienböck).*

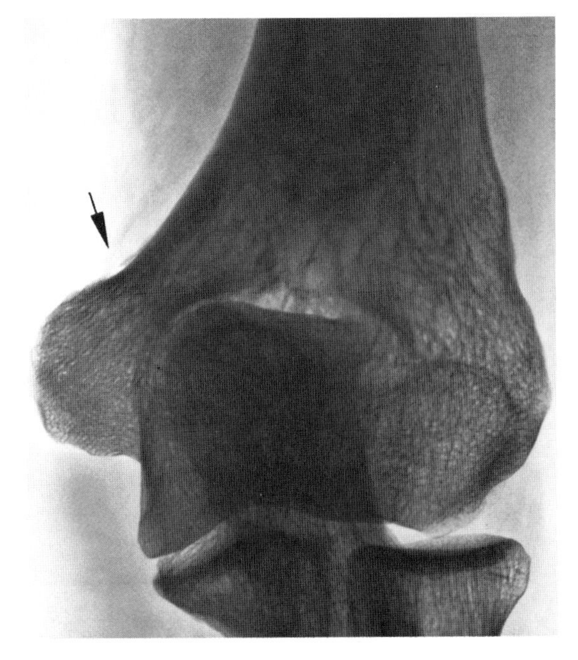

Fig. 605. Foveola at the medial epicondyle of the humerus (see Fig. 585, No. 71**). This smallish depression was still considered as etiologically unexplained in 1967 by *Köhler-Zimmer.* The same radiologic finding, as our own, is presented in Handbuch der Medizinischen Radiologie IV/2, p. 315 *(Viehweger).* There, a shallow depression is shown. Neither nerve nor blood vessels are found in this region. *Viehweger* hypothesizes, that for functional reasons, parts within the ossifications are left out, in this case at the border between the region of insertion of the brachial and the pronator teres muscles (from the collection of *H. Hiltemann,* Münster).

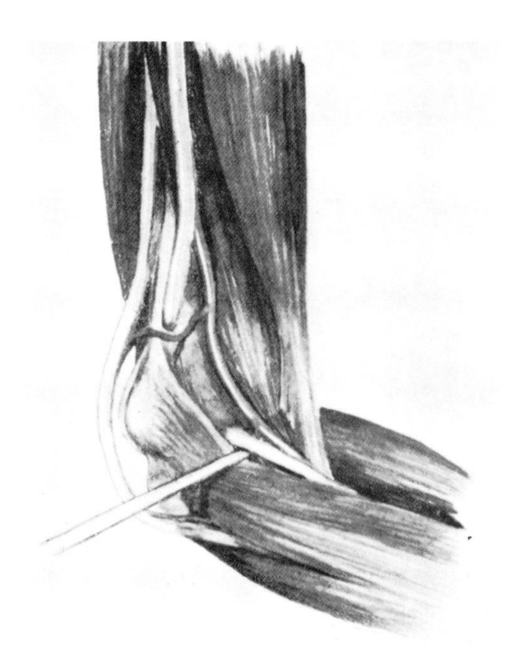

Fig. 606 (from *Roaf).*

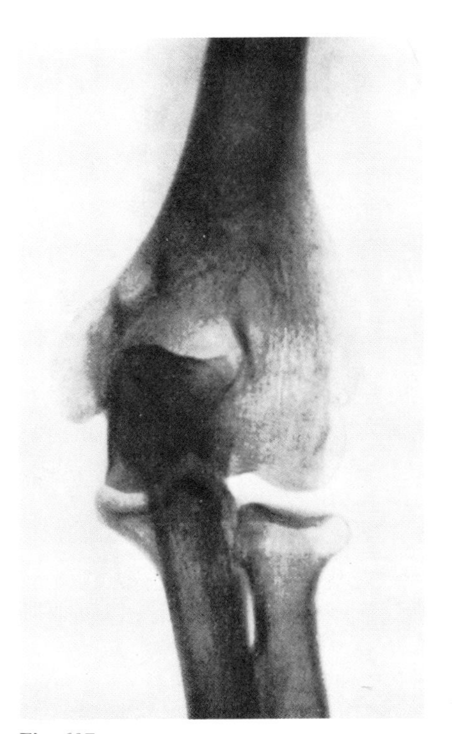

Fig. 607 a

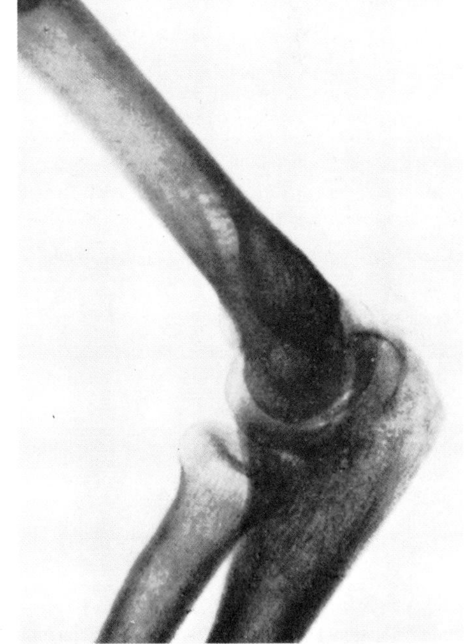

Fig. 607 b

Fig. 607. Post-traumatic hole formation at the medial margin of the distal end of the humerus; see Fig. 605. The strange and, in part, not yet clarified relationships at the margin of this bone are shown in a case presented by *Boaf* (from whose paper Figs. 606 and 607 have been taken). According to *Roaf's* report of the operation, a foramen developed at about the level of the above foveola, after an accident 8 years previously; this foramen enclosed parts of the median nerve. Below its exit between the trochlea and the olecranon a neurinoma had developed.

Radiographic Anatomy and Radiographs of the Wrist, Metacarpus and Fingers, Including Exposure Techniques

Radiographs of the **wrist** are taken:
1. in *sagittal* direction
   a) dorsovolar (the most frequent exposure)
   b) volodorsal (less frequent)
2. in *transverse* direction
   a) radioulnar (the most frequent exposure)
   b) ulnoradial (less frequent, and less comfortable for the patient)
3. *ulnodorsovolar,* in hyperpronation
4. *radiovolodorsal,* with the hand half-open

The positions mentioned do not always suffice to demonstrate the radius as needed. To examine it thoroughly, an additional view must be taken with the hand in hyperpronated position (ulnodorsovolar) (Fig. 623).

The lateral ulnoradial radiograph is suitable for isolated demonstration of the **pisiform bone,** which is covered by the neighboring bones when the hand is in normal position (Fig. 620).

In order to have a good view of the **hamate bone** and especially of the **hamulus** in the lateral position, the central ray must be aimed from distal onto the steeply placed wrist, passing between the well-abducted first and remaining metacarpal bones. Therefore, the hand is first placed for radioulnar projection, then it is raised into radial abduction with simultaneous lifting of the anterior edge of the cassette and the opposing thumb is put in abduction. The hamulus then moves out as required (Fig. 627).

The **trapezium (greater multangular bone)** and the trapezoid (lesser multangular bone) always cover each other on dorsovolar and volodorsal exposures. With radioulnar projection the greater multangular bone becomes free but, because of the greater distance from the film, it appears enlarged and blurred. To demonstrate it distinctly, the projection must be done exactly in reverse; therefore, the first metacarpal bone must be exposed from the ulnar edge, with the thumb opposing and in abduction (Fig. 625).

The **scaphoid bone (navicular bone)** must be taken in three different directions, in order not to miss transverse fractures. One then obtains Fig. 612, for which the technique of positioning has been described.

As radiographs of the wrist must be taken quite frequently, and as they have to furnish as much information as possible, considering the importance of the function of the hand, one must know the variants of its shape and structure (p. 270).

Radiographs of the **metacarpus** are taken:
1. in *sagittal* direction
   a) dorsovolar
   b) volodorsal
2. in *transverse* direction
   a) radioulnar
   b) ulnoradial, especially for the first metacarpal bone

It should be noted that, conforming to the curvature of the metacarpus, the 2nd and 5th metacarpal bones are shown better than the middle ones with projection 1. These appear more distinct when the back of the hand lies on the cassette. Further, it must be remembered that with dorsovolar exposure, the heads of the middle bones become distorted and show club-shaped enlargement if for some reason (contracture, bandage) they do not lie directly on the cassette. For the remaining exposures, the hand is placed as for radiographs of the wrist. One focuses onto the center of the metacarpus or onto the level of the proximal phalangeal joints if these are to appear as distinct clefts. The row of the proximal phalangeal joints is usually sought much too far distally; in fact, they are near to the distal transverse fold when the hand is bent.

In the usual radioulnar exposure (Fig. 617) the 1st metacarpal bone is seen sagittal but enlarged because of the great object-film distance. Therefore, the uncomfortable ulnoradial position of the hand must be used (Fig. 620), but with the thumb in abduction as described for the greater multangular bone (Fig. 625).

It must be briefly mentioned that the 4th metacarpal bone is generally conspicuously slim, that at the base of the 5th small apophyses are visible, that sesamoid bones in varying numbers as well as islets of compact bone tissue may occur, and that in contrast to the 2nd and 5th metacarpals, the epiphyseal cartilage of the 1st metacarpal bone is located proximally.

The usual exposures for **fingers** are:
1. *sagittal*
   a) dorsovolar
   b) volodorsal
2. *lateral,* radioulnar.

Occasionally, an oblique exposure may become necessary for tangential projection of a specific spot.

For demonstration of the proximal phalangeal joints, the same rules and aids as outlined for the metacarpus must be applied. If the hand is pressed hard against its support and at the same time is slightly pronated, the 4th proximal phalangeal joint is seen tangentially. This is similar to *Stauing*'s "zither player's position", in which the 2nd to 5th metacarpal bones and the proximal joints of the fingers are projected semi-obliquely (Fig. 633).

Demonstration of the **thumb** in sagittal direction is somewhat troublesome, especially for the proximal joint (see Fig. 645).

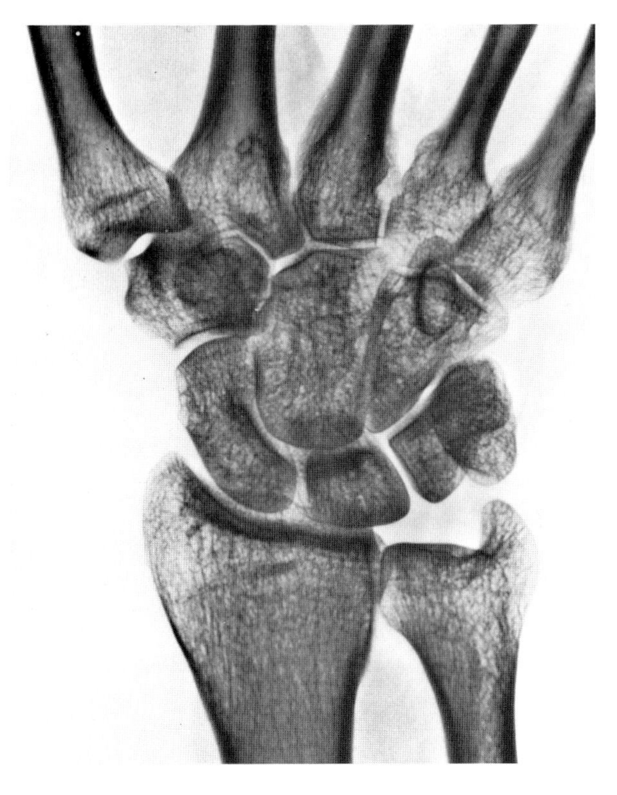

Fig. 608. **Right wrist, dorsovolar.** Projection: forearm extended, wrist and metacarpus lie with their volar side on the film. The central ray is aimed vertically onto the center of the wrist.

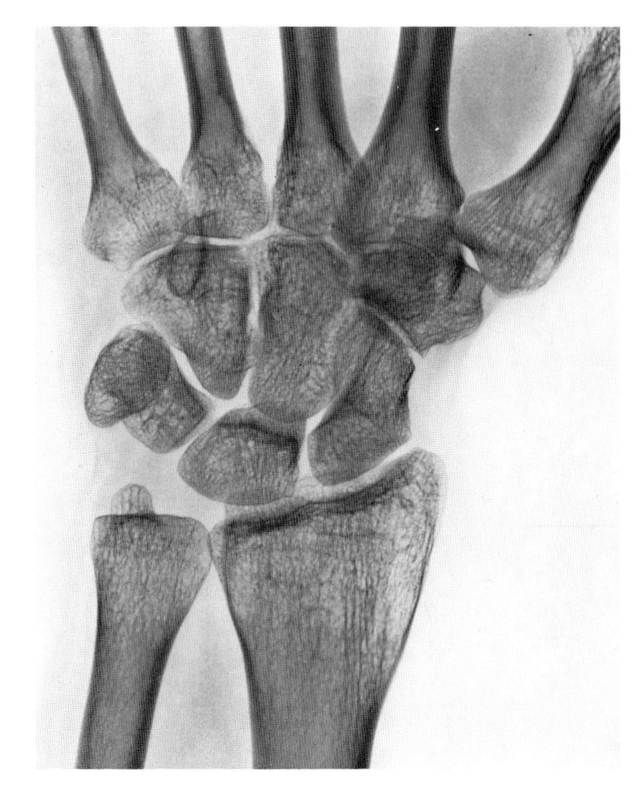

Fig. 609. Right wrist, volodorsal (rarer). Projection as in Fig. 608, only the forearm is in supination. The central ray is aimed vertically onto the center of the carpus.

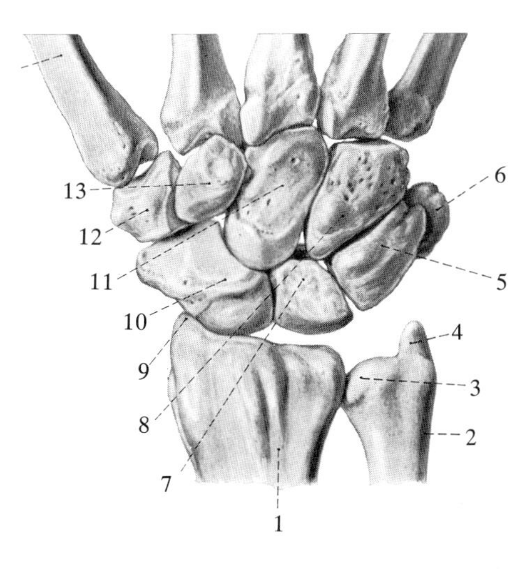

Fig. 610. Carpus, dorsal view (from *Sobotta-Becher,* 17th Edition).

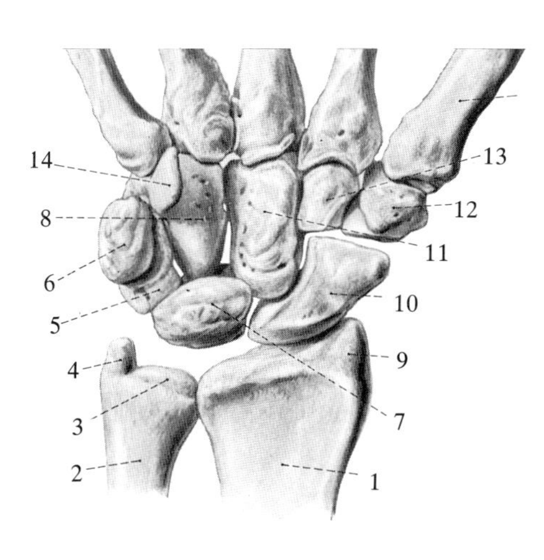

Fig. 611. Carpus, palmar view (from *Sobotta-Becher,* 17th Edition).

1 Radius
2 Ulna
3 Head of ulna
4 Styloid process of ulna
5 Triangular bone
6 Pisiform bone
7 Lunate bone
8 Hamate bone
9 Styloid process of radius
10 Scaphoid bone (navicular bone)
11 Capitate bone
12 Trapezium (greater multangular bone)
13 Trapezoid bone (lesser multangular bone)
14 Hamulus of hamate bone

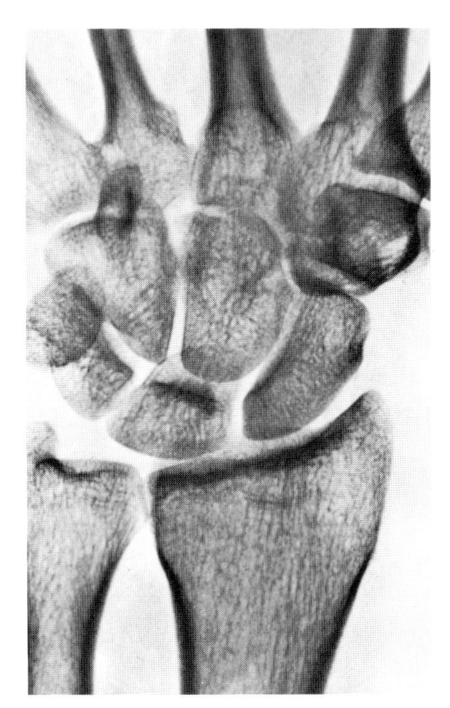

Fig. 612a. Projection: dorsovolar.

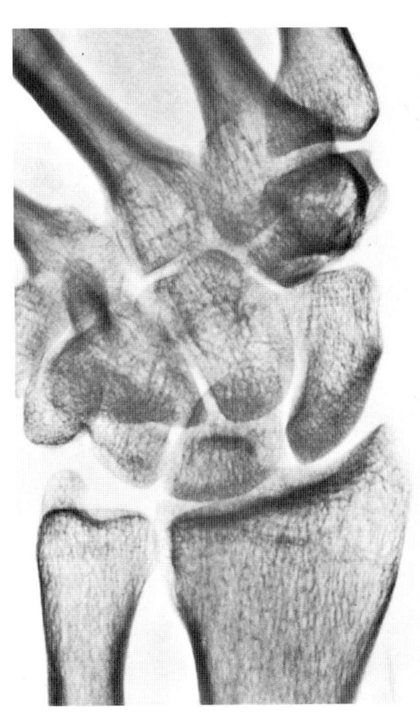

Fig. 612b. Projection: dorsovolar, but in semi-dorsiflexion (Figs. 613 and 616) and slight ulnar abduction.

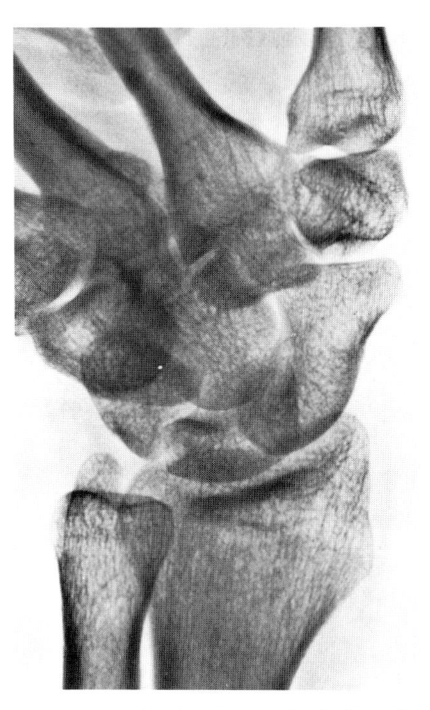

Fig. 612c. Projection: dorsovolar basic position, fingers bent, the hand supinated 45°, slight ulnar abduction (see Fig. 614).

Fig. 612. Special radiographs of the scaphoid bone (navicular bone) in three different projections. The central ray in all three exposures is aimed vertically onto the navicular bone.

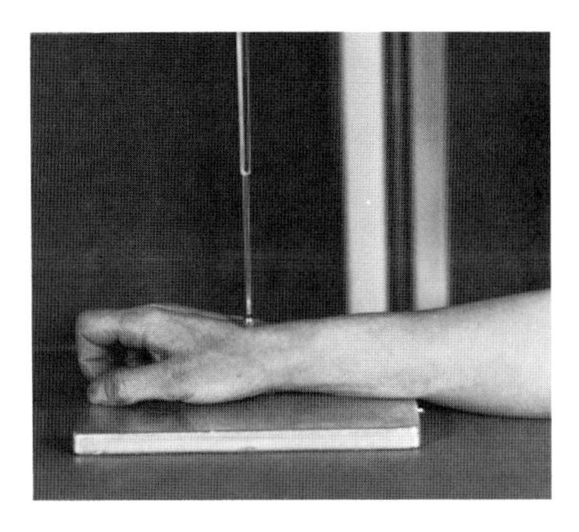

Fig. 613

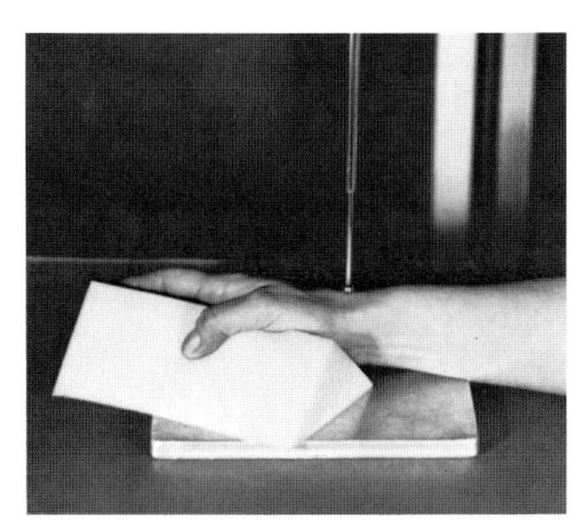

Fig. 614

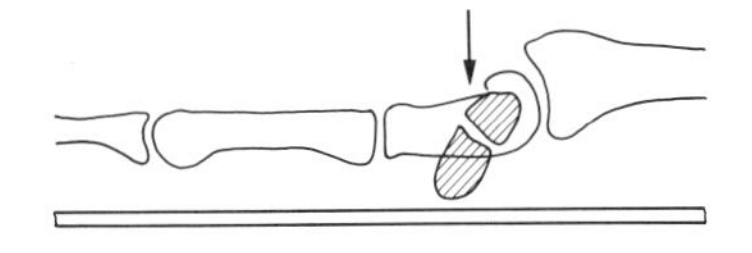

Fig. 615. Schema of projection of fracture of the scaphoid bone *(Agostini)*, with fingers outstretched.

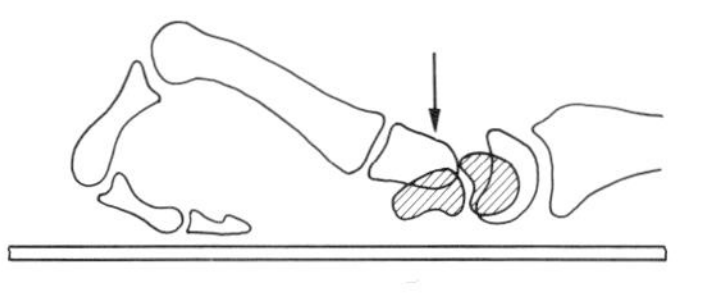

Fig. 616 shows that in this position the fracture of the scaphoid (navicular) bone (shown hatched) is projected more favorably than in the usual extended position (Fig. 615).

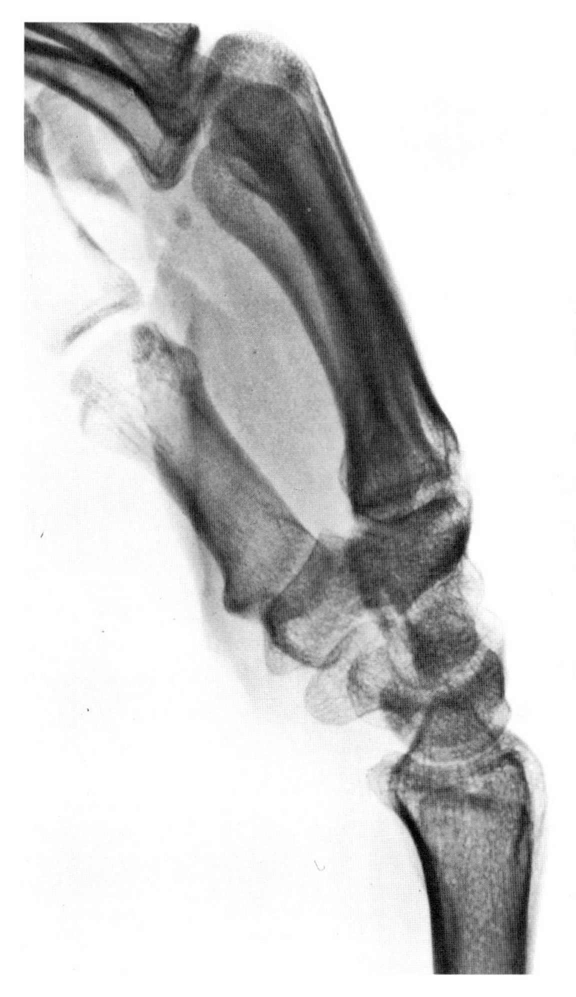

Fig. 617. **Right wrist, lateral, radioulnar.** For projection see Fig. 619. The central ray is aimed vertically onto the center of the wrist.

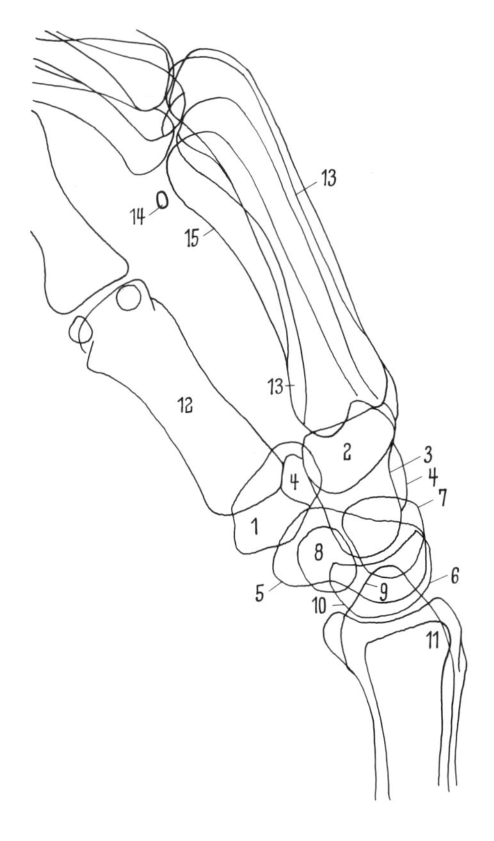

Fig. 618. Sketch to Fig. 617.

1 Trapezium (greater multangular bone), articulates with the 1st metacarpal bone (12)
2 Trapezoid bone (lesser multangular bone), articulates with the 2nd metacarpal bone (13)
3 Capitate bone, articulates with the 3rd metacarpal bone and with the lunate bone
4 Hamate bone, recognized by its hamulus
5 Scaphoid bone (navicular bone), recognizable by its shape and its articulations with the greater multangular bone
6 Lunate bone, recognizable by its shape and its articulation with the radius and head of the capitate bone
7 Triangular bone
8 Pisiform bone
9 Styloid process of radius
10 Articular space between radius and lunate bone
11 Styloid process of ulna
12 Metacarpal bone I
13 Metacarpal bone II
14 Sesamoid bone (inconstant)
15 Metacarpal bone V

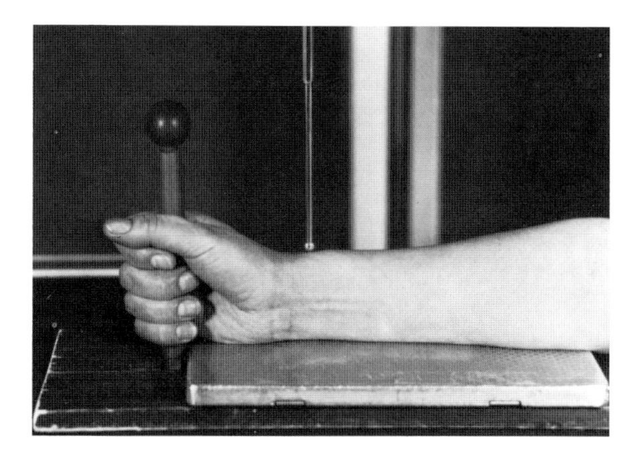

Fig. 619

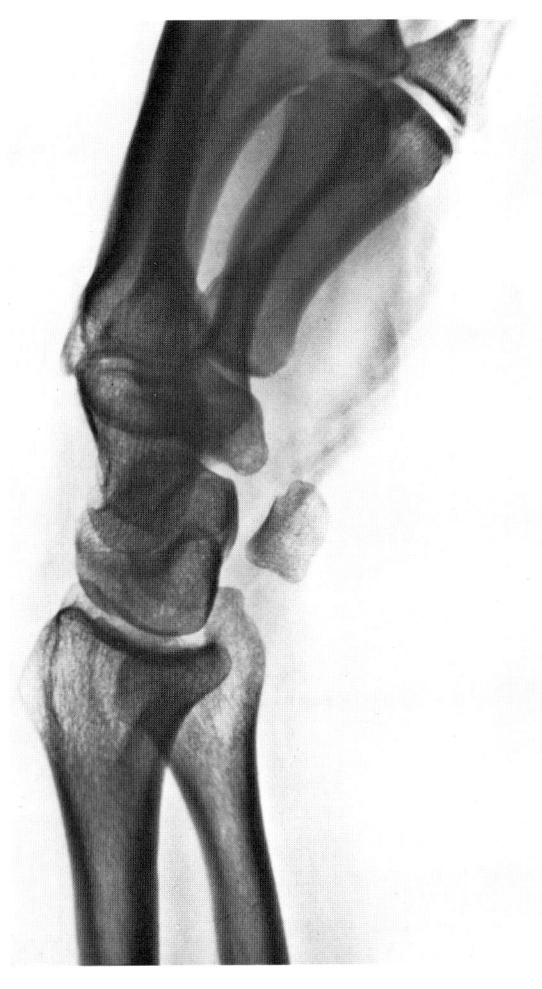

Fig. 620. Right wrist, lateral, ulnoradial. For projection see Fig. 622. The central ray is aimed vertically onto the center of the wrist.

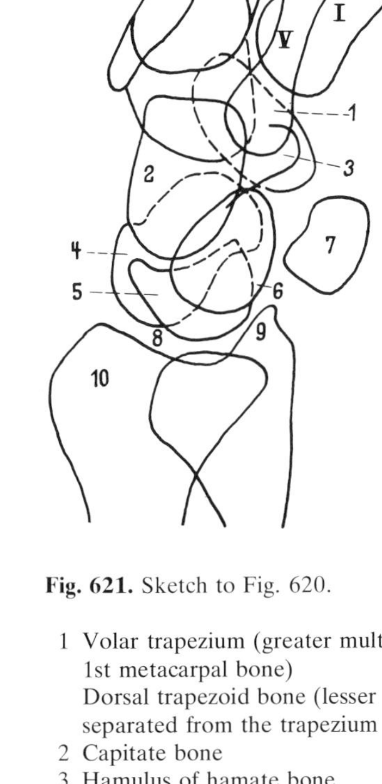

Fig. 621. Sketch to Fig. 620.

1 Volar trapezium (greater multangular bone, articulates with the 1st metacarpal bone)
Dorsal trapezoid bone (lesser multangular bone); cannot be separated from the trapezium
2 Capitate bone
3 Hamulus of hamate bone
4 Scaphoid bone (navicular bone)
5 Lunate bone
6 Triangular bone
7 Pisiform bone
8 Articular space between radius and lunate bone
9 Styloid process of ulna; appears enlarged, as it is film-distant
10 Distal epiphysis of radius
I Metacarpal bone I
V Metacarpal bone V

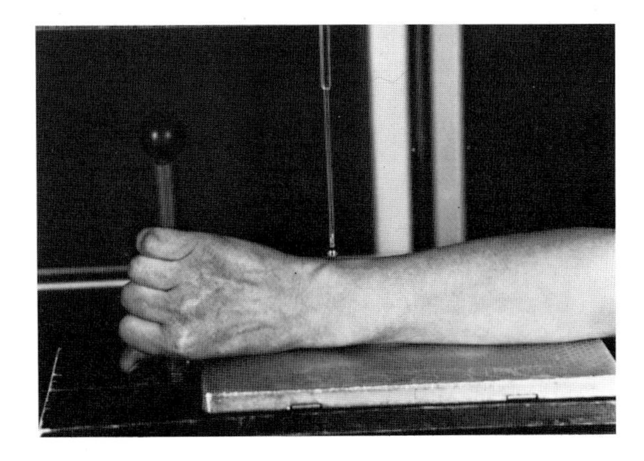

Fig. 622

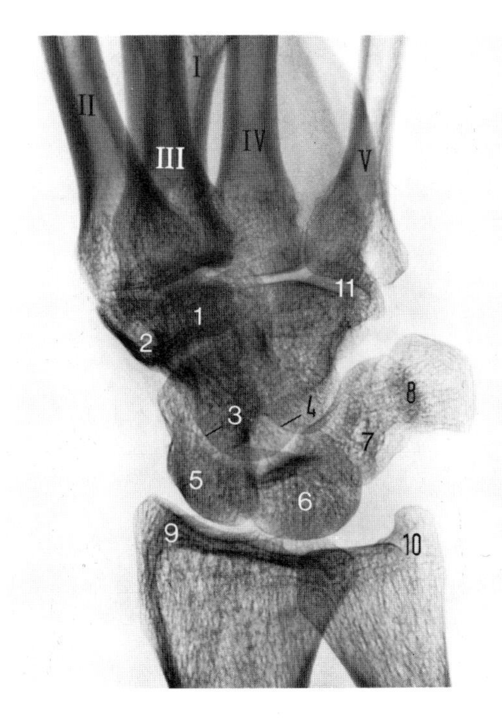

Fig. 623. Right wrist, oblique, ulnodorsal. Positioning as for an ulnoradial exposure of the wrist, except that the arm is not hyperpronated quite as much (see Fig. 624).

1 Trapezium (greater multangular bone)
2 Trapezoid bone (lesser multangular bone)
3 Capitate bone
4 Hamate bone
5 Scaphoid bone (navicular bone)
6 Lunate bone
7 Triangular bone
8 Pisiform bone
9 Styloid process of radius
10 Styloid process of ulna
11 Hamulus of hamate bone
I–V Metacarpal bones I–V

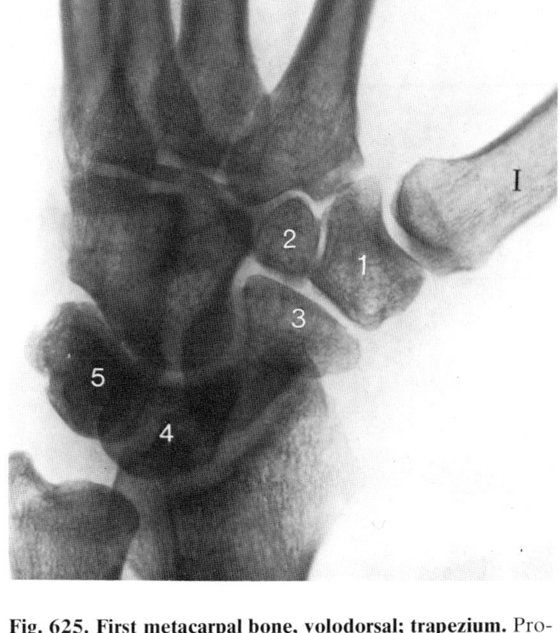

Fig. 625. First metacarpal bone, volodorsal; trapezium. Projection: forearm is hyperpronated so that the outstretched thumb lies with its dorsal side on the cassette. The central ray is aimed vertically onto the carpometacarpal joint I (see Fig. 626).

1 Trapezium (greater multangular bone)
2 Trapezoid bone (lesser multangular bone)
3 Scaphoid bone (navicular bone)
4 Lunate bone
5 Triangular bone

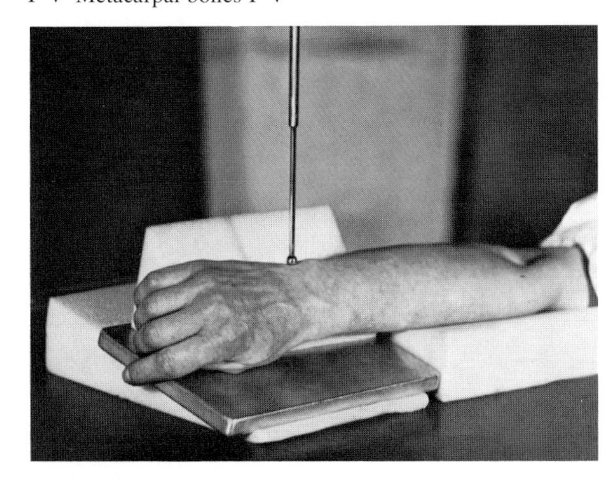

Fig. 624

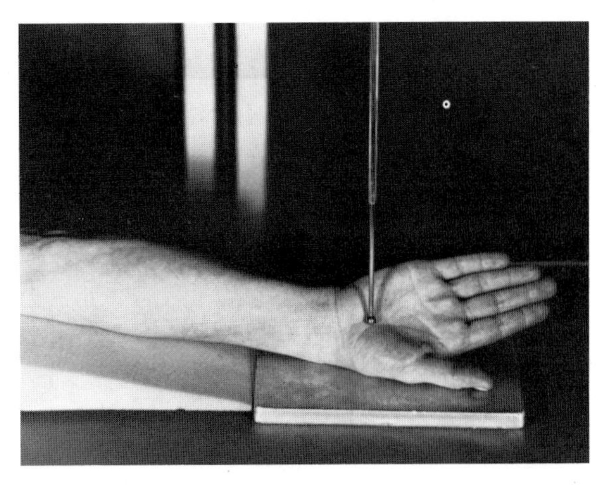

Fig. 626

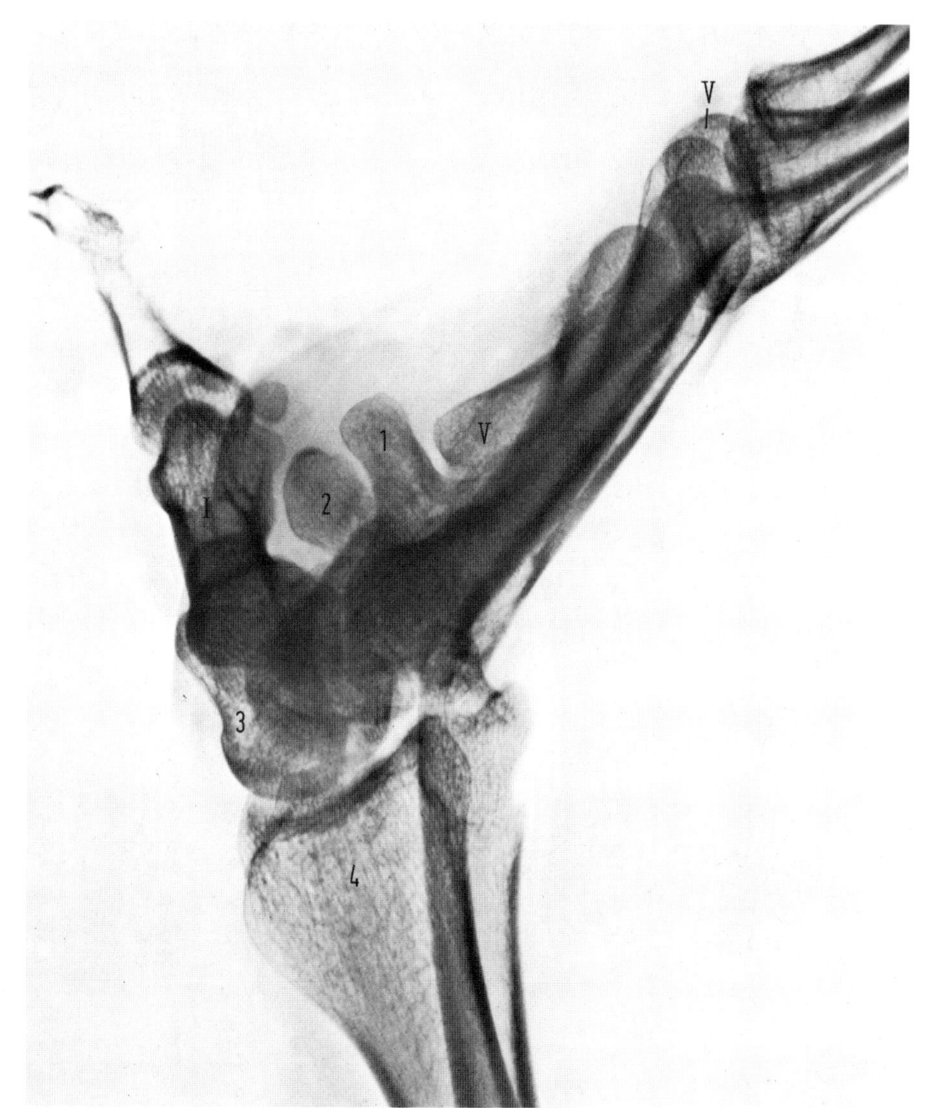

1 Hamulus of the hamate bone
2 Pisiform bone
3 Scaphoid bone (navicular bone)
4 Radius
I Metacarpal bone I
V Metacarpal bone V

Fig. 627. Right carpus, acroradioulnar. Demonstration of the hamulus of the hamate bone with the base of the 5th metacarpal bone. For projection see Fig. 628. The central ray is aimed from the fingertips obliquely onto the carpus.

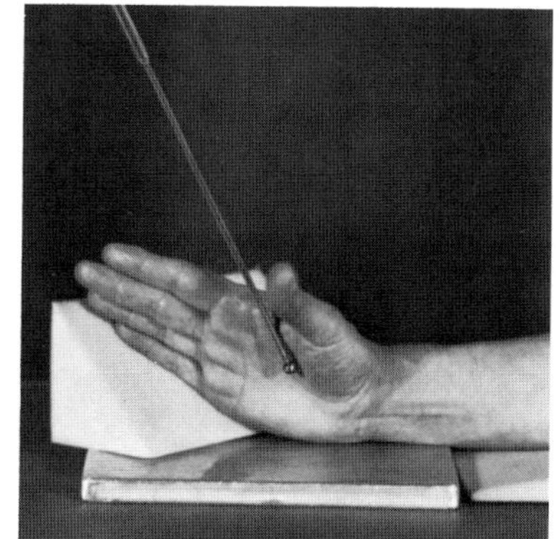

Fig. 628

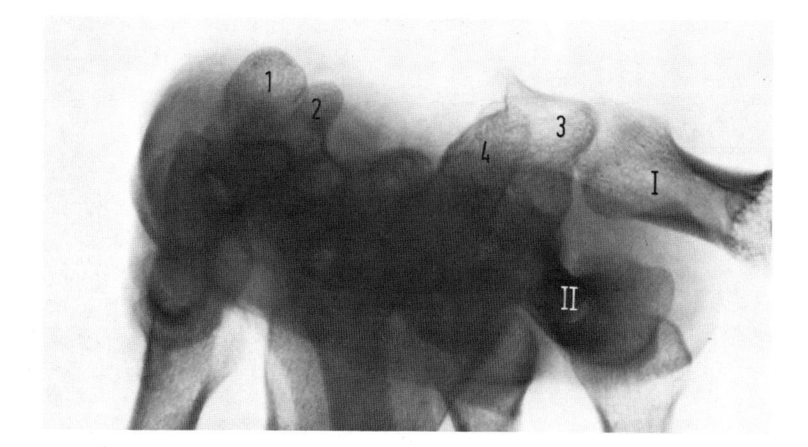

Fig. 629. Carpal canal, axial. For projection see Fig. 630.

1 Pisiform bone
2 Hamulus of hamate bone
3 Greater multangular bone
4 Navicular bone
I Metacarpal bone I
II Metacarpal bone II

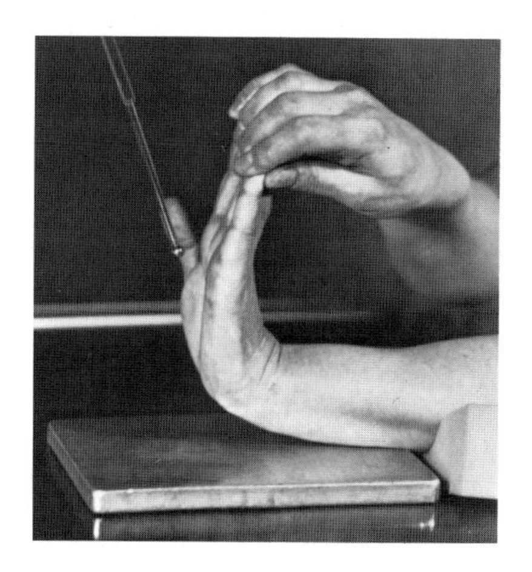

Fig. 630

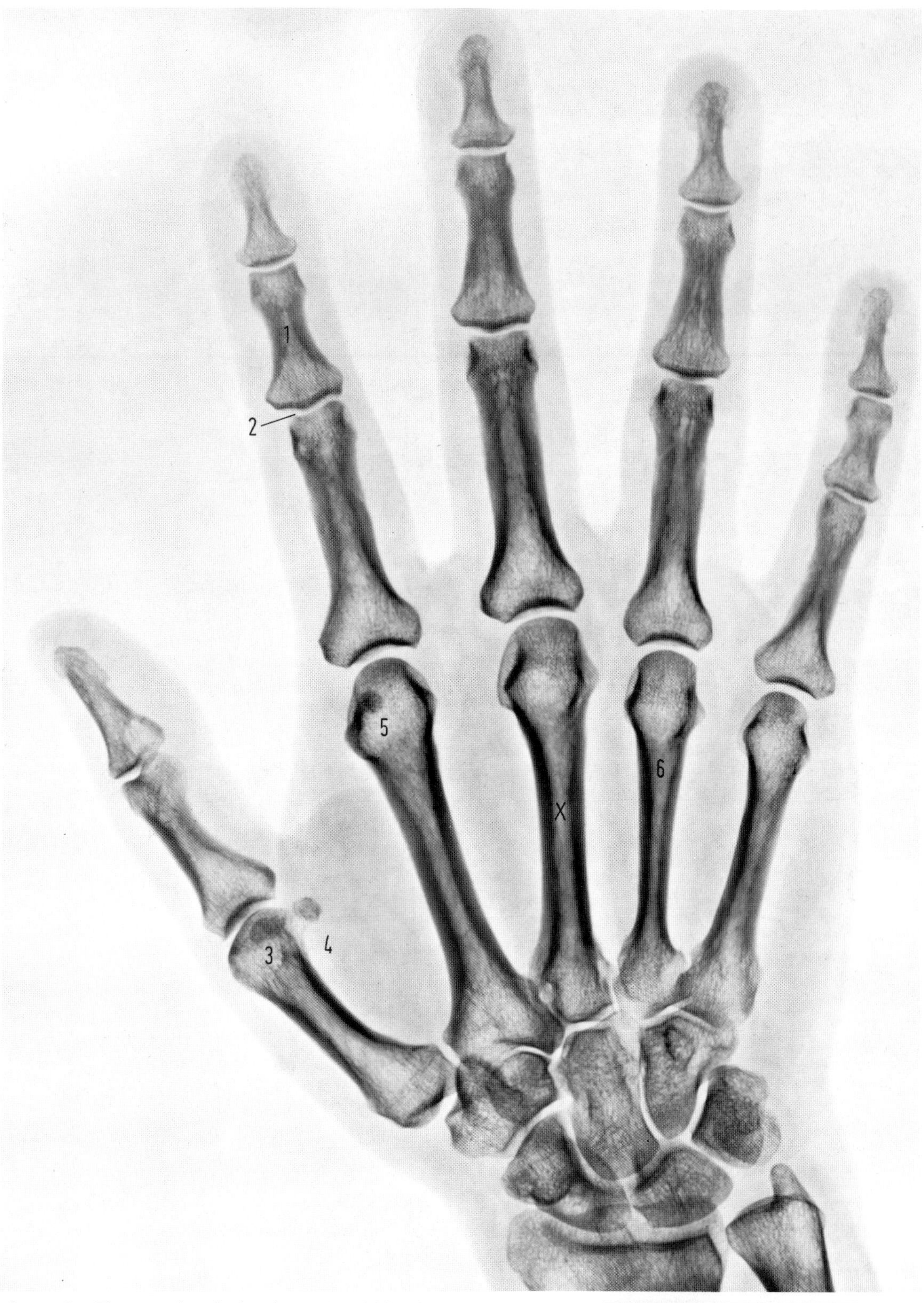

Fig. 631. Right hand, dorsovolar. The central ray is aimed onto the middle of the 3rd metacarpal bone (X). The 4th metacarpal bone is always slim; if the hand is held very hollowed or cannot be stretched completely, the 3rd metacarpal bone, because of its greater distance from the cassette, appears distorted, enlarged and, in its peripheral part, often club-shaped. On the outer side of the 5th metacarpal bone, at a point about the middle of its length, a bony tuberosity, which serves the insertion of the abductor digiti quinti muscle, is not infrequently found. This tubercle might be mistaken for a callus or for osteitis. For projection of the exposure, see Fig. 632.

1 Middle phalange
2 Proximal interphalangeal joint
3 and 4 Sesamoid bones at the basal joint of the thumb, lying within the flexor tendons
5 A rare sesamoid bone at the basal joint of the index finger
6 Metacarpal bone IV, remarkably slim.

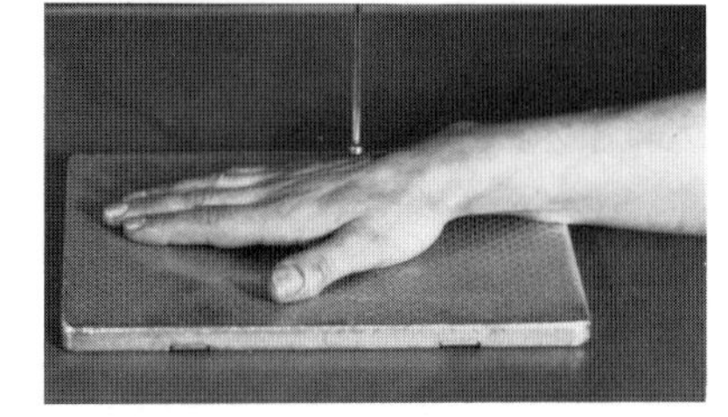

Fig. 632

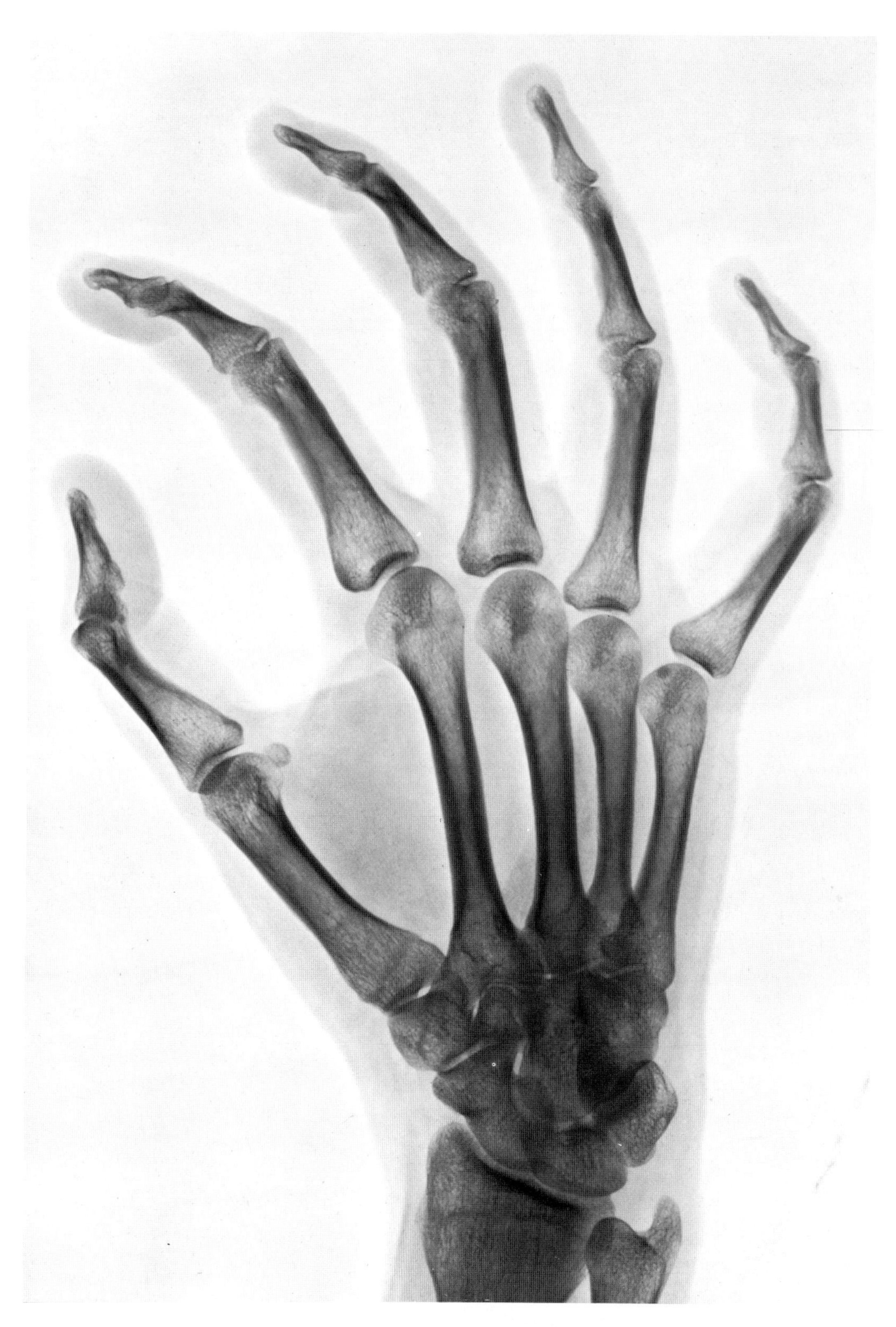

Fig. 633. Right wrist, semi-oblique ("zither player's position"). For projection see Figs. 634 and 635. The central ray is aimed vertically onto the basal joint of the 2nd finger.

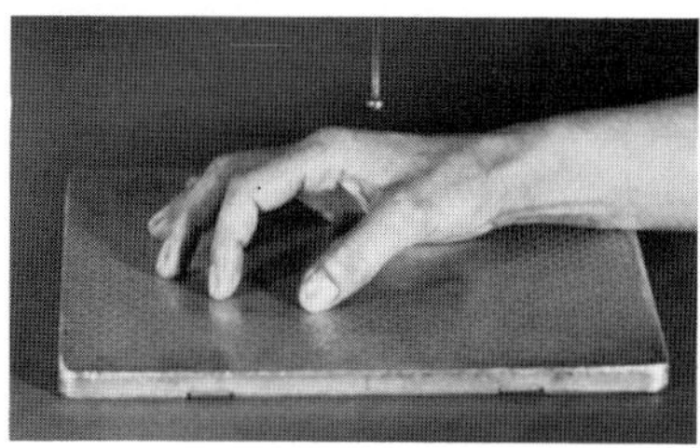

Fig. 634

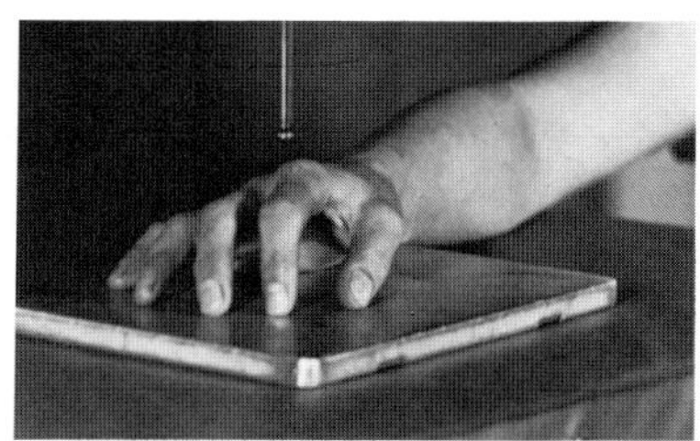

Fig. 635

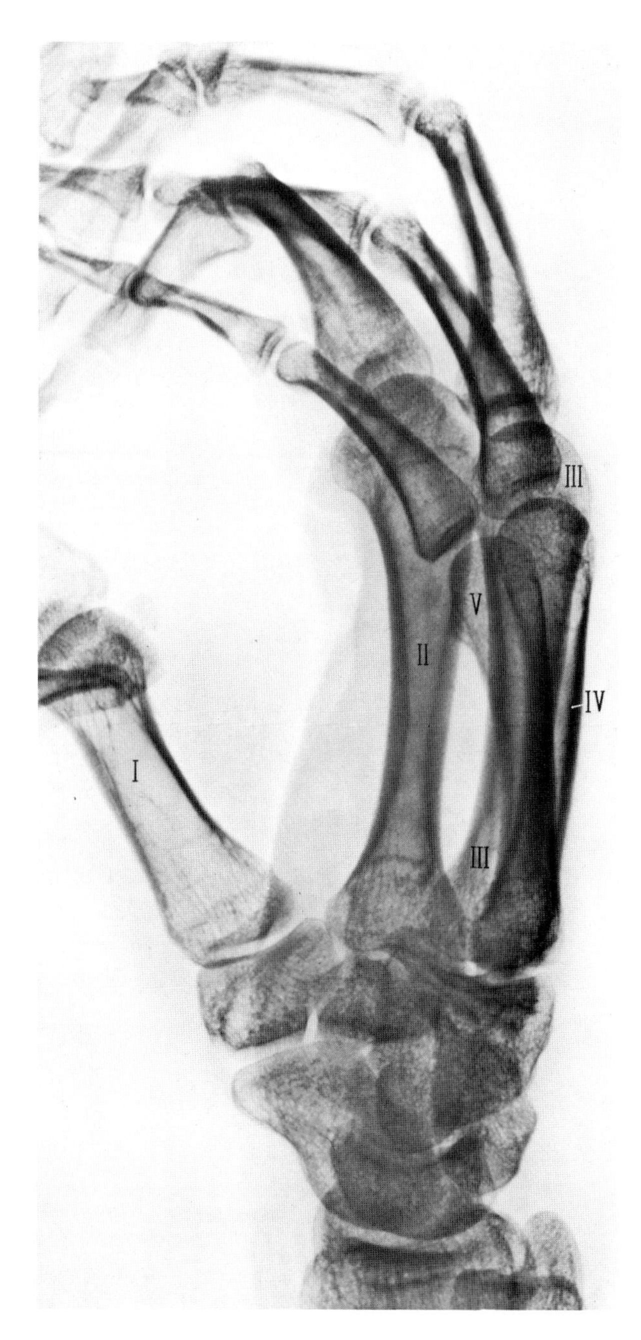

Fig. 636. **Metacarpus, lateral, radioulnar.** The hand to be examined is strongly compressed laterally by the other hand so that the metacarpal bones can move well away from each other (see Fig. 639). The central ray is aimed vertically onto the head of the 4th metacarpal bone.

I–V are the numbers of the metacarpal bones. V is the smallest; its finger shows the sharpest contours. The 4th finger, too, shows good contours and structure. The dorsal surface on the metacarpal bones is taken tangentially; its dorsal cortex stands out well. The 2rd metacarpal bone can be recognized from the trapezoid bone (lesser multangular bone); the remaining bone is then the 3rd metacarpal.

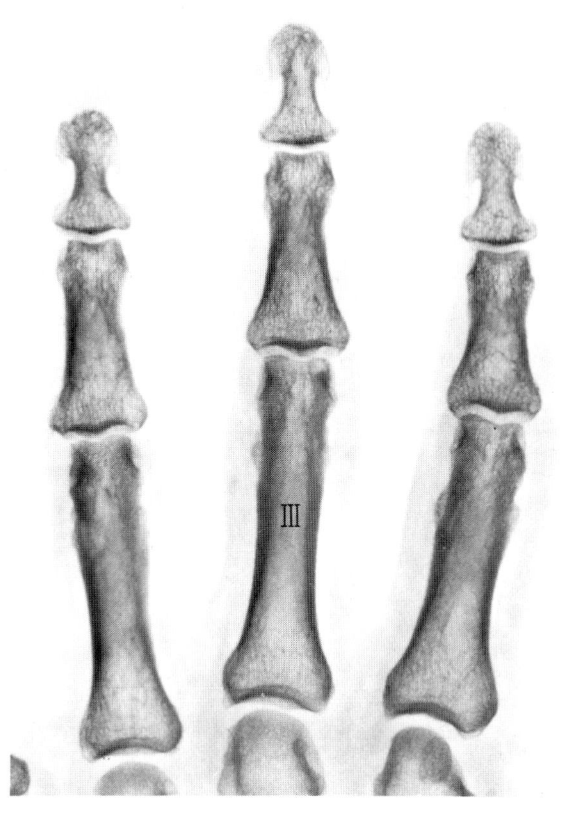

Fig. 637. 2nd to 4th fingers, right, dorsovolar. For projection see Fig. 638. The central ray is directed vertically onto the middle joint of the 2nd finger.

III designates the basal phalange of the 2nd finger. Attention must be given to the width of the articular space and to the even depth of the shadows of the phalangeal bones. The free end of the distal phalangeal tuberosity may be very rough.

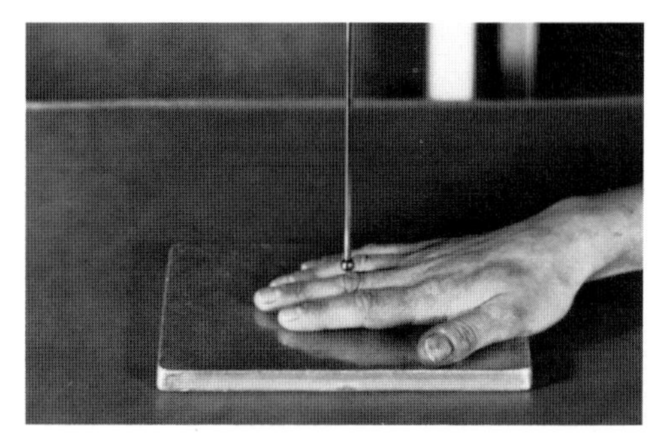

Fig. 638

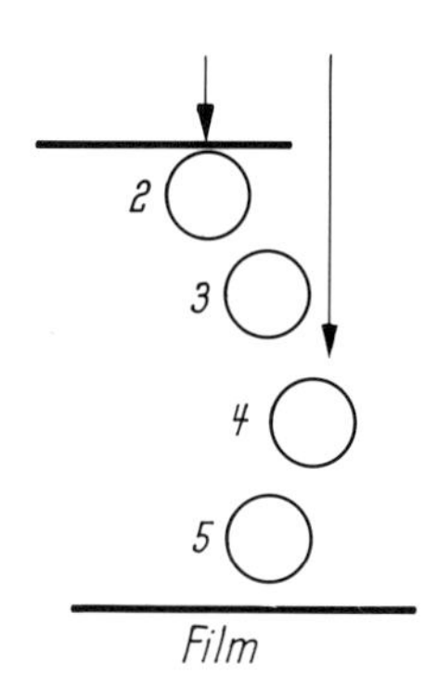

Fig. 639

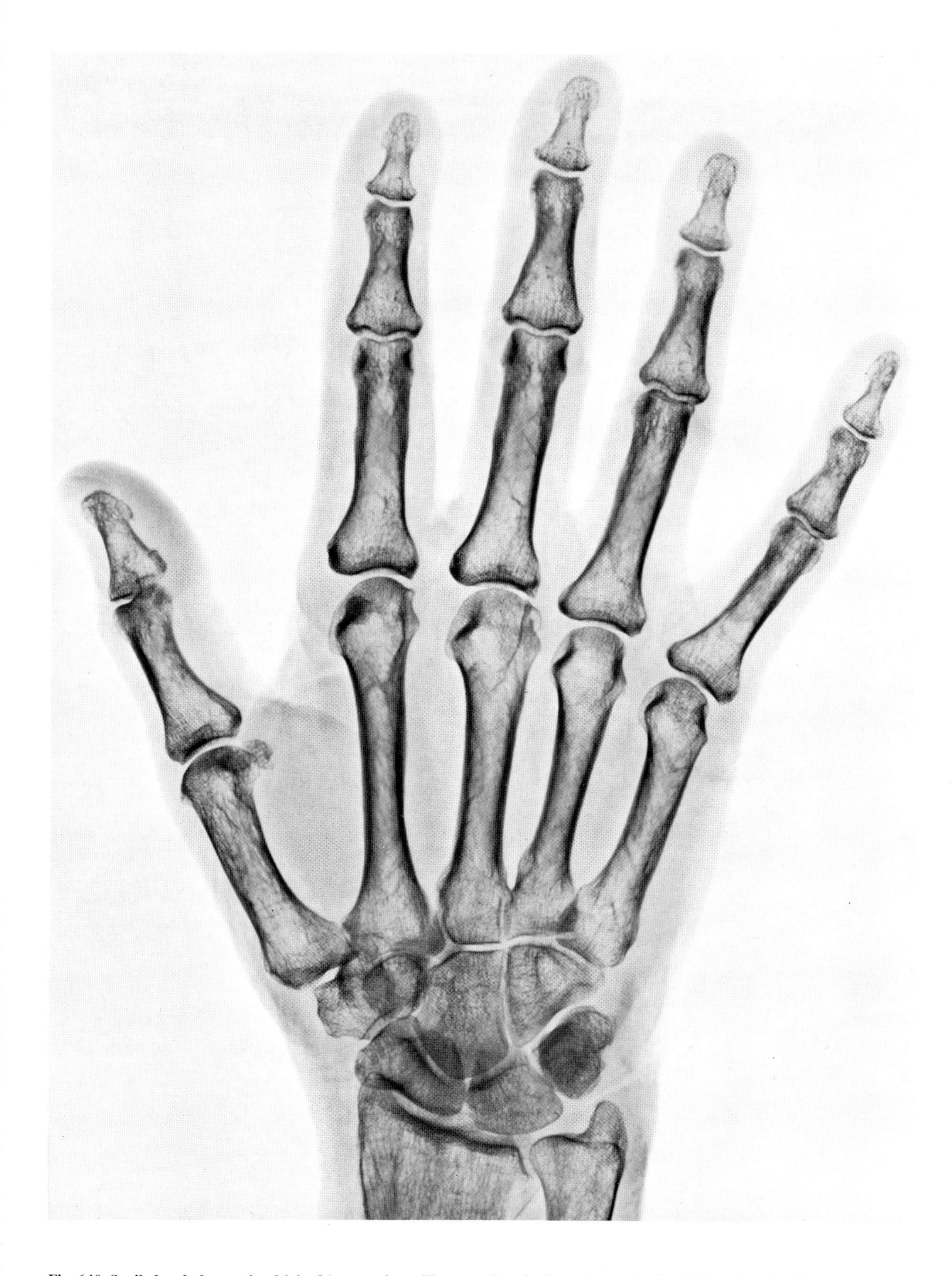

Fig. 640. Senile hand, dorsovolar. Male, 84 years of age. The central ray is directed onto the basal joint of the 2nd finger. The radiograph shows changes in the joints corresponding to advanced age (senile deforming arthrosis). Furthermore, one recognizes the very pronounced form of the so-called atrophy of old age, which is an expression of physiological involution of old age, non-pathological. One may assume true senile atrophy if no arthrotic or even arthritic changes can be found which cause pain or impediment of movement.

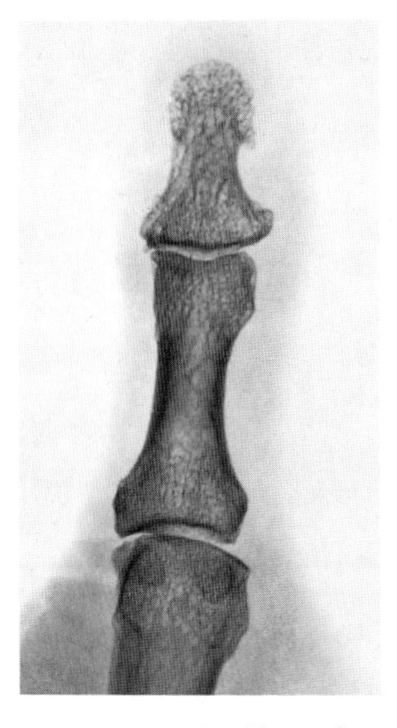

Fig. 641. **Thumb, dorsovolar.** For projection see Fig. 644. The central ray is aimed vertically onto the basal joint. At the head of the 1st metacarpal bone two sesamoid bones are seen.

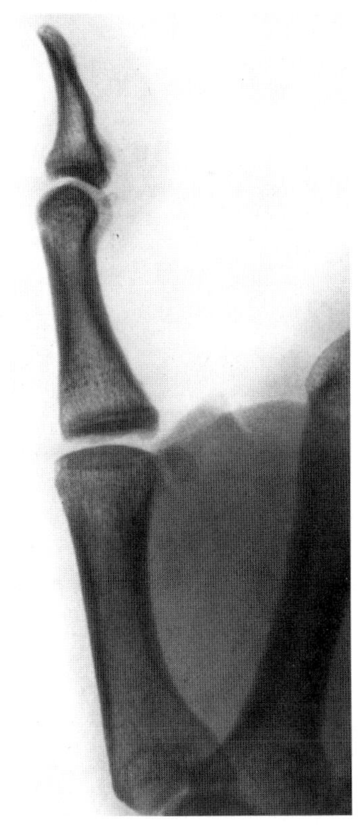

Fig. 642. Thumb, lateral. For projection see Fig. 645. The central ray is aimed vertically onto the basal joint. Next to the basal joint there is a sesamoid bone.

Fig. 642

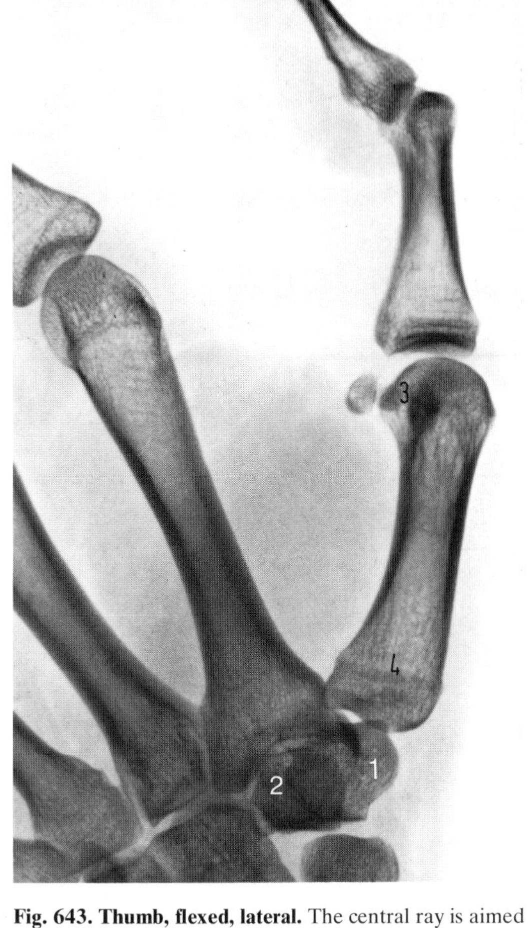

Fig. 643. Thumb, flexed, lateral. The central ray is aimed vertically onto the 1st metacarpophalangeal joint.

1 Greater multangular bone
2 Lesser multangular bone
3 Two sesamoid bones
4 Metacarpal bone I

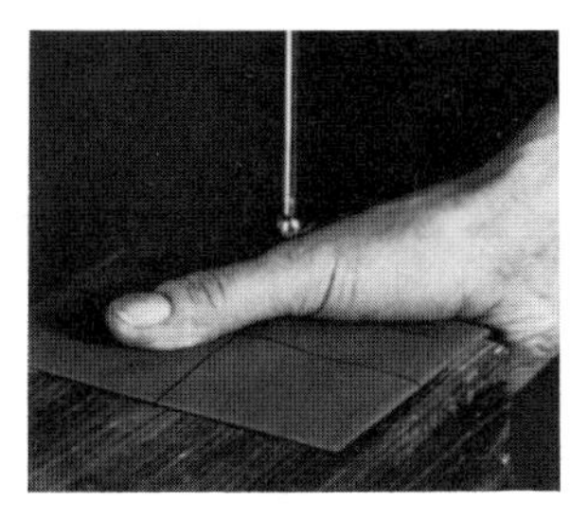

Fig. 644

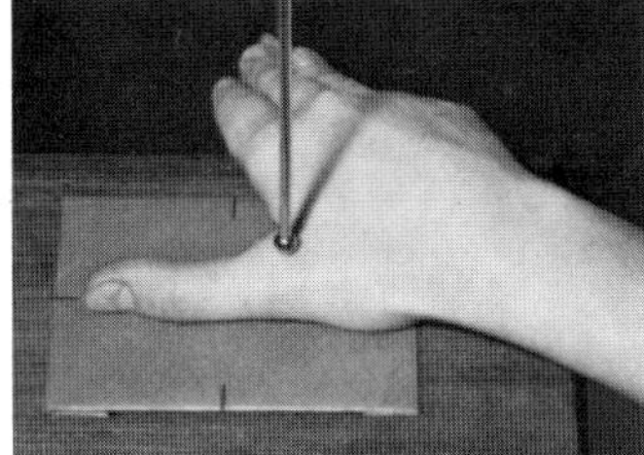

Fig. 645

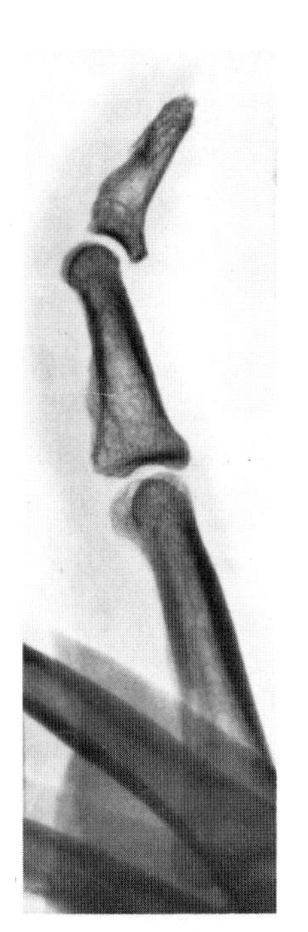

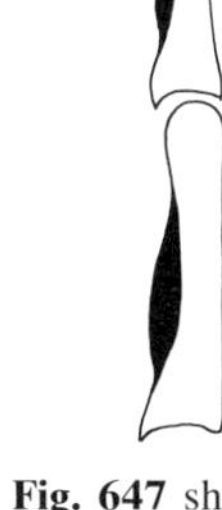

Fig. 647 shows volar bulges, occurring frequently at strong fingers during mature age, also at the basal joint. Wrong diagnoses may include periostitis, panaritium of the bone and callus.

Fig. 646. Index finger, lateral. It shows an abnormal hyperextensivity of the ungual phalange. The bony ledge on the flexor side of the middle phalange is normal.

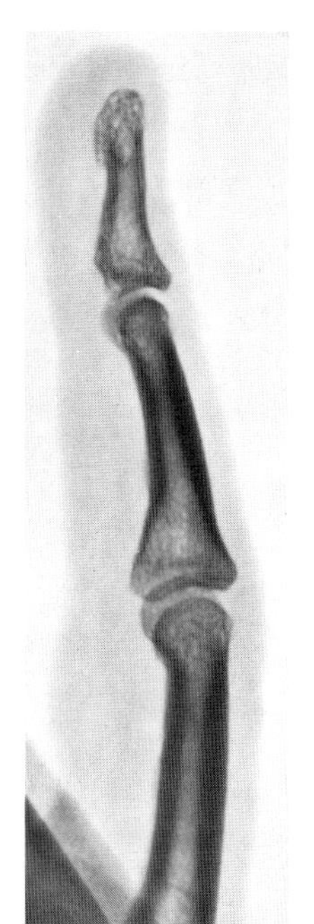

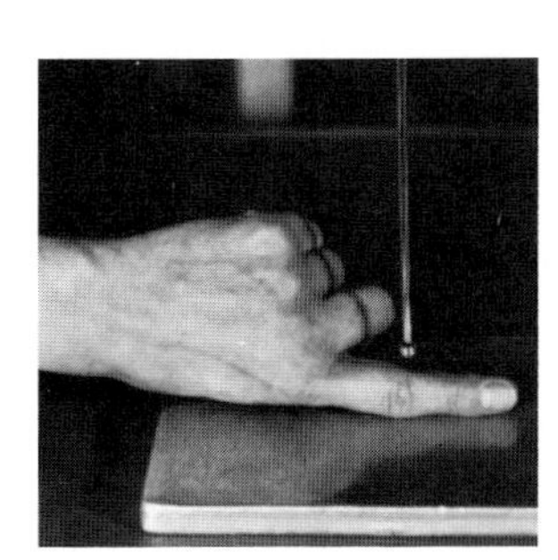

Fig. 649

◀ **Fig. 648. Index finger, lateral.** For projection see Fig. 649. The roughness at the tip of the unual phalange and the volar side of the base is normal.

Variants and Sources of Diagnostic Error of the Wrist, Metacarpus and Fingers*

A former collaborator *(A. Neiss)* of the present author proposed designating any bony particles which may occur in addition to the classical bones as "accessoria." He based this proposal upon research results from descriptive anatomy, ontogenesis and phylogenesis and traumatology. These results led to the decision to supplement the meritorious investigations by *W. Pfitzner* (1894–1902) on the morphologic elements of the skeleton of the hand with more recent roentgenologic knowledge. While *Pfitzner* described a total of at least 25 accessory ossicles, apart from the eight "canonical" bones, it has now been determined, in accordance with newer roentgenologic views, that there are only three "anatomically described, comparative-anatomically roentgenologically proven and generally recognized genuine accessory formations of bony structure" *(Rochlin* and *Zeitler):*

1. the os centrale as well as the os centrale bipartitum
2. the secondary trapezoid bone
3. the styloid bone

As *Neiss,* basing his work on developmental theories and anthropologic considerations, denies even these few bones the designation of primary, we intend to accept his non-commital conception of "accessorium" for all these frequently, occasionally or rarely appearing bones. The question of the genesis of these accessoria will not be dealt with in principle but only in individual cases.

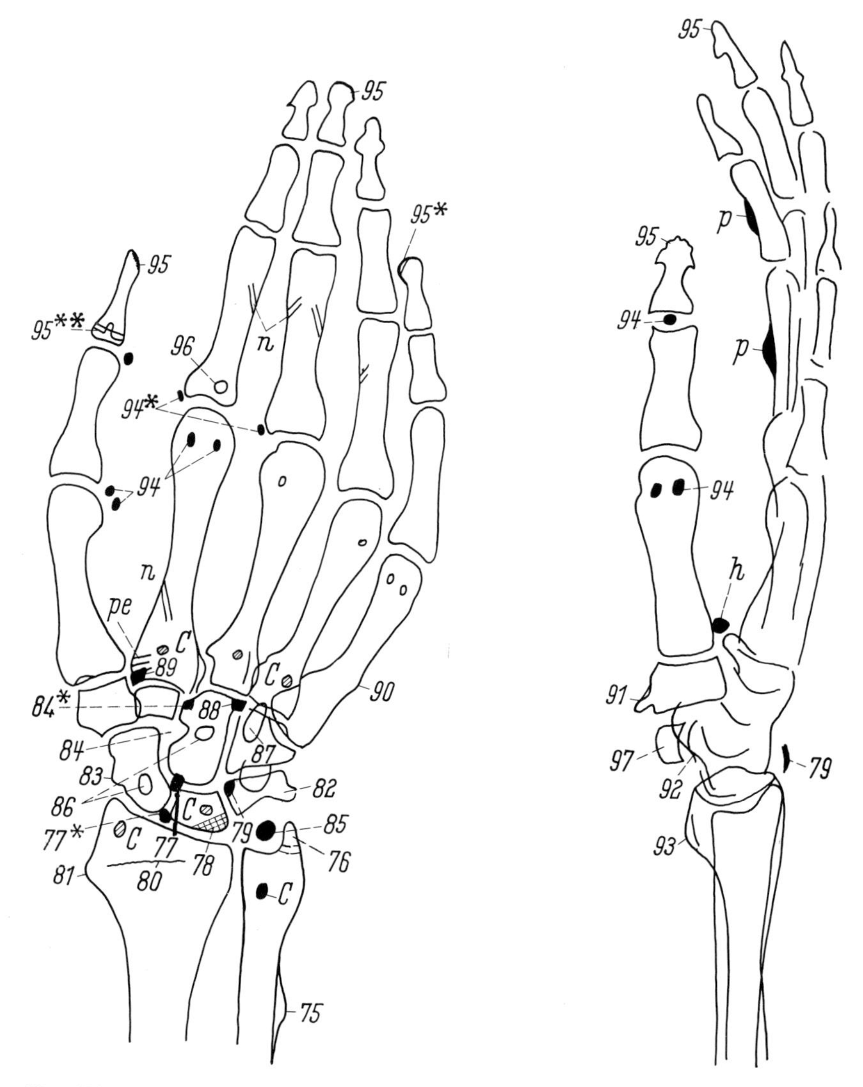

Figs. 650 and 651. Variants and sources of diagnostic error of the wrist, the metacarpus and the fingers, with special consideration of the so-called accessoria.

* The numbers in bold type are to be found also (or only) on the sketch of the lateral side.

pe Pseudoepiphysis, which is not pathognomonic for mongoloid idiocy, but also occurs in the healthy, and further multiple in cranioclidodyostosis
C Islets of compact tissue
h Special bone of hamulus
n Nutritive canal
p Pseudoperiostitis

75 Thickening at the distal part of the ulnar shaft, probably caused by local work hypertrophy due to excessive demand on the pronator teres muscle, whose plane of origin reaches up to the lateral margin of the ulna
76 Styloid bone of ulna (see Figs. 685–688); causes difficulties of differential diagnosis for avulsed fragment, triangular bone, aseptic necrosis, persistent apophysis of an ulnar apophysis originating from two nuclei
77 Hypolunate bone (see Fig. 657). This is a doubtful anatomical accessorium, and is probably only a post-traumatic formation. It may be confused with an islet of compact tissue.
77* "Os paralunatum," accessorium (?), radioproximal at the side of the lunate bone (Fig. 700)
78 Necrosis of lunate bone, after chronic traumatism *(Haslhofer)*
79 Epitriquetrum = epipyramis (see Fig. 697); seen only twice by the author, after previous accident
80 Rough ledge for insertion of the palmar radiocarpal ligament. The shadow band may be mistaken for an epiphyseal scar or an old fracture.
81 Normally thickened ledge of the radial tuberosity, for fixation (Anschmiegen) of the extensor carpi radialis longus muscle (Fig. 625)
82 Excrescence at the triangular bone; assimilated external ulnar bone (?) or ossification of insertion of ligament?
83 Tubercle of the navicular bone (see Figs. 609 and 678); Unilateral or bilateral aplasia of the navicular bone may occur
84 Lacuna for an os centrale, which is always preformed chondrogenically but ossifies only rarely *(Grashey),* Fig. 677; at its side a round increased radiolucency in the capitate bone, rarely pathological (see also Fig. 675)
84* Styloid bone of metacarpal bone III. The styloid process of the 3rd metacarpal bone remained independent. It cannot be distinguished from a meta- or parastyloid (Fig. 691).
85 Triangular bone (see Figs. 687, 670 and 689); may be the result of a fracture, a calcification of a disk or an accessorium
86 Cysts in the navicular and capitate bones; may be pathological (hemorrhagic cysts or necrotic foci), Fig. 655. They may occur in different small bones of the wrist, predominantly in the proximal sections of the capitate and hamate bones. Pathologically and anatomically, they are often circumscribed medullary fibroses, frequently without any significance (see Figs. 677, 673 a, 1114). According to *Ravelli,* it is a vascular canal taken axially.
87 Hamulus of hamate bone, sometimes extra large (see Fig. 627 and *Viehweger*). It may occur isolated as a special hamulate bone; then, the differential diagnosis is for pseudoarthrosis or fracture.
88 Secondary capitate bone; differential diagnosis for a *Gruber* ossicle, but it is probably an acquired accessorium
89 Secondary lesser multangular bone (see Fig. 693), a secondary accessorium after accident
90 Normal intumescence at the 5th metacarpal bone, an insertion of muscle (see Fig. 640)
91 Jutting-out tubercle of the greater multangular bone (see Fig. 617); this is a deception due to projection, making it appear as a split-off bony particle
92 Articular space at the pisiform bone (see Fig. 620); avoid confusing with dislocation
93 Normal thickening of the radial epiphysis (Fig. 617); after a previous trauma, it is suspect of callus formation
94 Sesamoid bones (see Figs. 631, 633, 659 and 1113–1117)
94* Rare localization of formation of subordinate nuclei in the hand *(Arenz);* differential diagnosis against avulsion fracture or aseptic necroses
95 Tuberosity of a distal phalange (see Figs. 637, 641)
95* Ungual endplate at the 4th finger, often stronger on the radial than on the ulnar side (Fig. 631)
95** Peg-like epiphyses are an expression of "peripheral dyostosis," often symmetrical, occurring on hands and feet (Fig. 706); a developmental disturbance of diverse genetic bases
96 Small, cyst-like increased radiolucency, caused by vascular canals (see also Fig. 655)
97 Pisiform bone (see Fig. 627); its hyperplasia is possible

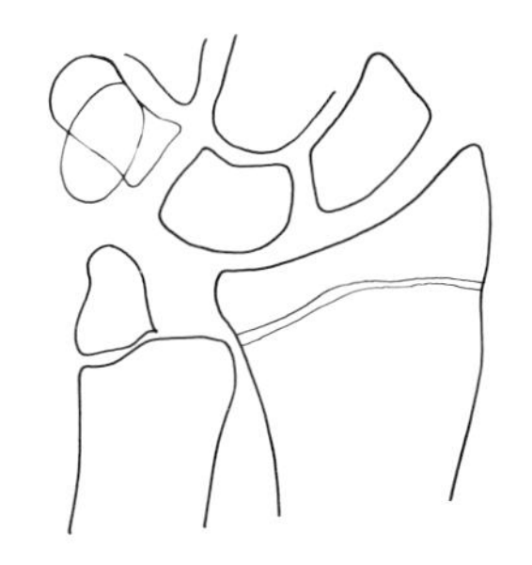

Fig. 652 (Juvenile bones). Usually, the shortening of the ulna is without significance, but it is said to favor necrosis of the lunate bone. With this shortening there is always an oblique position of the articular surface of the radius (so-called *Hultén*'s minus variant of the ulna; *Steinhäuser* and *Merhof).*

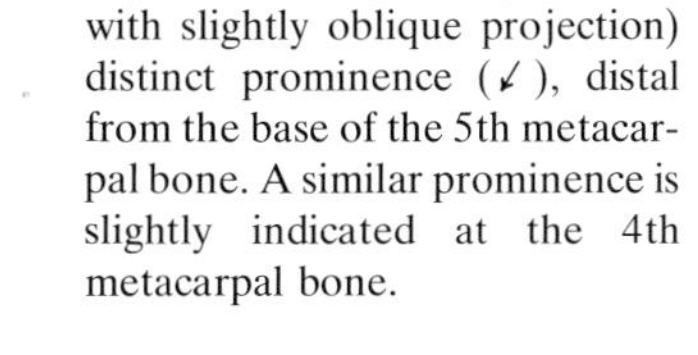

Fig. 654. Frequent (especially with slightly oblique projection) distinct prominence (↙), distal from the base of the 5th metacarpal bone. A similar prominence is slightly indicated at the 4th metacarpal bone.

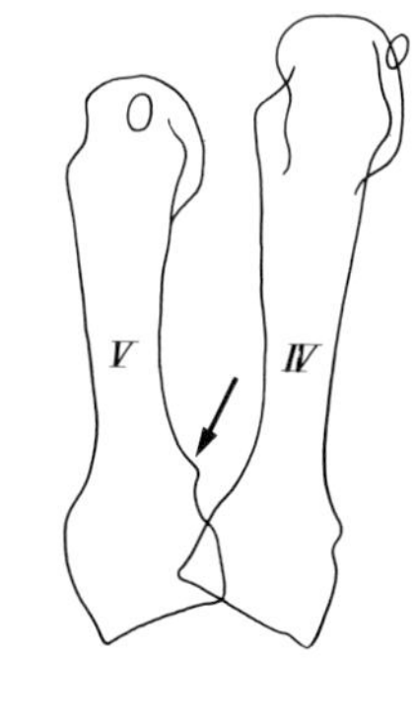

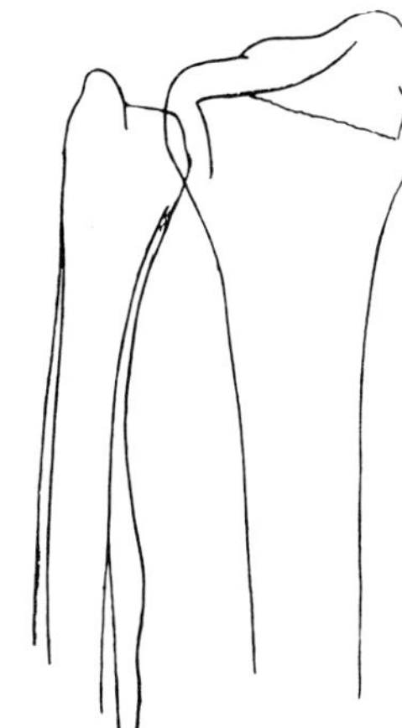

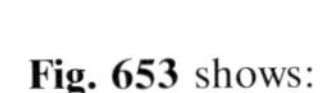

Fig. 653 shows:
1. at the lower end of the radius a sometimes conspicuously protruding tubercle (tuberosity),
2. an often visible oblique line of increased density (insertion of the palmar radiocarpal ligament), and
3. the interosseus margin of the ulna, which often protrudes like a callus.

Fig. 655. Localization of cystic increased radiolucencies in the skeleton of hand and forearm (after *Rochlin* and *Zeitler;* see also Figs. 677, 673 a, 1114). There are four possibilities for the development of such cysts:
1. cysts arising as herniae of the synovial membrane into the cancellous tissue,
2. necrobiotic pseudocysts (vascular disturbance),
3. post-traumatic hemorrhagic cysts, and
4. arthrotic marginal cysts caused by osteochondronecrosis.

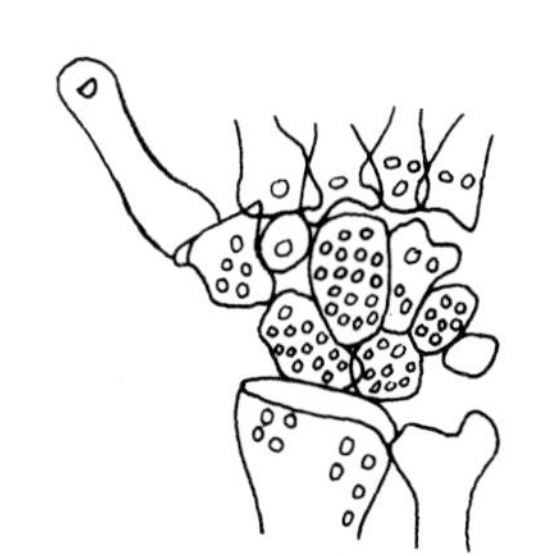

Figs. 656–658. Anomalies and variants of wrist and carpus (the most frequent accessoria are printed in italics) assembled according to *Pfitzner*.

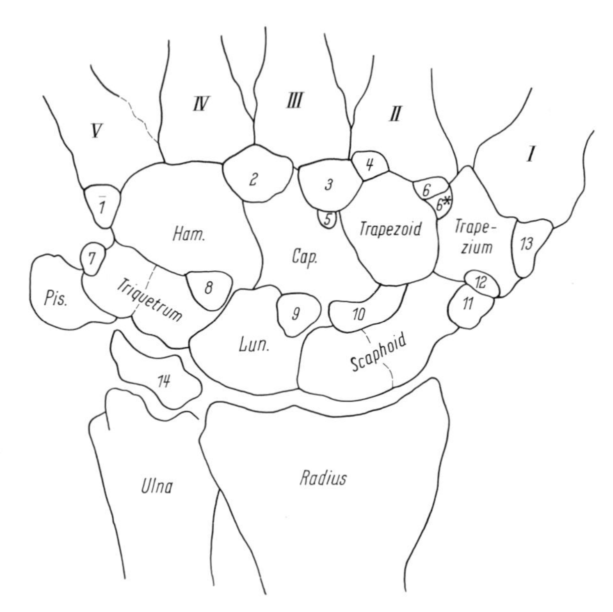

Fig. 656. Variants of the wrist, dorsal.

1 Vesalianum. According to *Neiss, de Cuveland* and others, this is an artificial construction as it has not been authenticated histoembryologically. It is either the product of an atypical ossification (persistent apophysis) or an avulsion of the tuberosity of the metacarpal bone V (Fig. 673).
2 Secondary capitate bone (Fig. 650, No. 88)
3 Styloid (see Fig. 650, No. 84*)
4 Parastyloid
5 Metastyloid
6 Secondary lesser multangular bone (see Figs. 693 and 650, No. 89)
6* Secondary greater multangular bone
7 External ulnar bone (see Fig. 668 and Fig. 650, No. 82)
8 Epipyramis (= epitriquetrum) (accessorium at triangular bone)
9 Epilunatum, appears mostly as tubercle at the radiodorsodistal corner
10 Central bone, may be bipartite. In its place one often finds a lacuna or notes that it has fused with the navicular bone as a prominence of this bone (see Fig. 677).
11 External radial bone, a non-united tubercle of the navicular bone (see Fig. 667). A bipartite navicular bone is shown in Fig. 694 a, b.
12 Epitrapezium (see Fig. 692)
13 Paratrapezium (see Fig. 674 a, b)
14 Triangular accessorium or intermediate antebrachial bone (see Figs. 687, 689 and 670)
15 Pretrapezium
16 Secondary capitate bone; effect of trauma? or anomaly?
17 Special bone of hamulus (see 650, No. 87)
18 Hypolunatum (see Fig. 650, No. 77)
19 Secondary pisiform bone (in synostosis); see Fig. 666
20 *Gruber*'s ossicle
21 Basal accessorium of hamulus

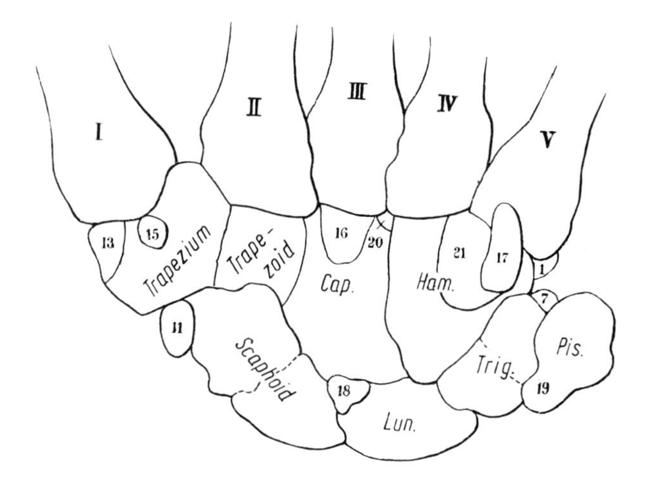

Fig. 657. Variants of the wrist, volar.

According to *Pfitzner,* divisions (ossa partita) occur at the scaphoid, triangular, greater and lesser multangular, pisiform and capitate bones.

Fusions have been described between lunate and triangular bone, greater multangular and scaphoid bone, lesser multangular and capitate bone, capitate and hamate bone, 3rd metacarpal and capitate bone, and lesser multangular and 2nd metacarpal bone. Through fusion of accessoria with the constant carpal bones, the latter obtain these small appendices, e.g., metacarpal bone I with paratrapezium (15), metacarpal III with styloid (3) (Figs. 656, 657, 664, 665).

Further fusions occur between the styloid process of the ulna and triangular plus pisiform bone, between lunate and hamate bone, between capitate bone and metacarpal IV, between greater multangular bone and metacarpal II, between metacarpal II and III, III and IV, between the styloid process of the 3rd metacarpal and the lesser multangular bone, and between lunate and triangular bone (Figs. 680, 681, 682). For fusions in the radiocarpal-metacarpal region, see also Fig. 1099.

With regard to the sequence of appearance of the bony nuclei for the carpal bones, see Fig. 1098.

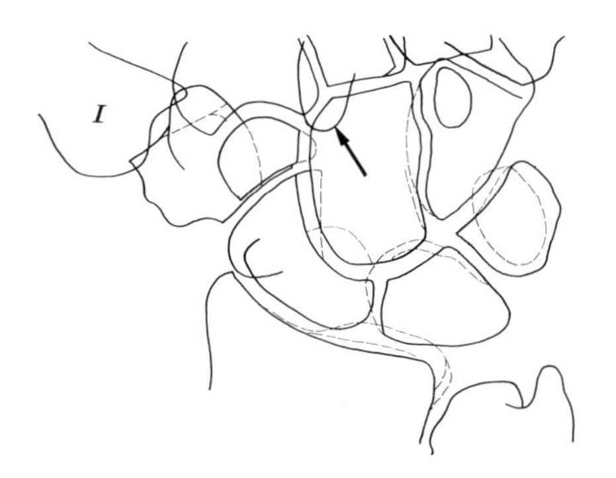

Fig. 658. If the central ray is directed somewhat peripherally onto the metacarpus, the shadow of the styloid process of the 3rd metacarpal bone (↖) falls onto the capitate bone, which may make one think there is an anomaly. I= metacarpal bone I.

Sesam bones of the human hand, after *Pfitzner* and *Stieda.* These sesam bones all lie on the volar side. In addition, there is an ulnar sesamum II, not marked here. In one case we saw radial sesamum II–IV, ulnar sesama II, V, and a distal interphalangeal sesamum I.

True sesam bones (sesama) are genuine, hyalin-cartilaginous preformed, enchondrally ossifying pieces of skeleton. In contrast, sesamoid bones are functionally conditioned thickenings, consisting of connective tissue and calciferous deposits within the tendons. The sesama are preformed before the beginning of joint formation, and their ossification starts in boys between the 8th and 10th years, and in girls after the 7th year of life. Only after the 13th to 16th years do they become visible on radiographs (see also *Kassatkin* and Figs. 1113–1117). The appearance of the first sesam bone on the ulnar side of the proximal joint of the thumb can be used as a sign of maturity and for evaluation of acceleration and retardation. One may find divisions, interpositions, fractures, inflammations (even gouty ones) and necroses of sesam bones with resulting arthrotic changes. The larger ones often show a texture of cancellous tissue; others, smaller ones, are frequently calcified.

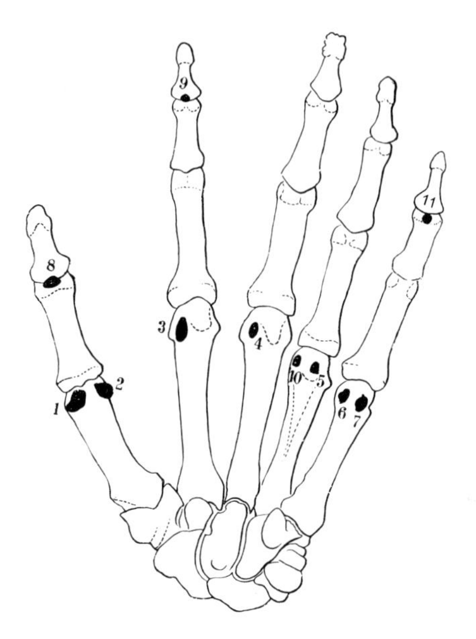

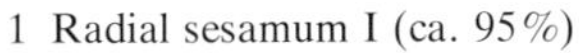

Fig. 659. Frequency of sesam bones of the hand (average values).

1 Radial sesamum I (ca. 95%)
2 Ulnar sesamum I (ca. 100%)
3 Radial sesamum II (ca. 50%)
4 Radial sesamum III (ca. 2%)
5 Ulnar sesamum IV (below 2%)
6 Radial sesamum V (ca. 3%)
7 Ulnar sesamum V (ca. 80%)
8 Interphalangeal distal sesamum I (ca. 70%)
9 Interphalangeal distal sesamum II (below 1%)
10 Radial sesamum IV (ca. 2%)
11 Interphalangeal distal sesamum V (below 1%)

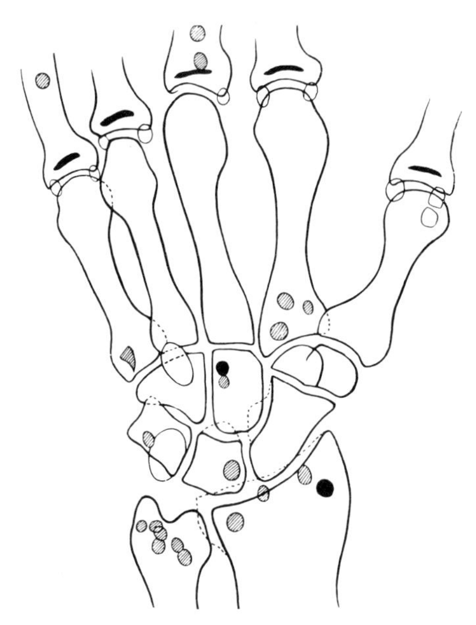

Fig. 660. Schematic survey of the most frequent islets of compact tissue and sesam bones of the hand. Hatched rings = findings from the work of *H. Fisher;* black rings = our own observations; hollow rings = sesam bones. For increase in size of the islets of compact tissue, see *Blank* and *Lieber.* Compact tissue islets are clinically harmless but important for radiographic differential diagnosis, monostotic osteoscleroses, closely related to osteopoikilosis, since the definition of *Albers-Schönberg.* They can occur in all parts of the skeleton and sometimes multiply, as in the skeleton of hand and foot but also in the bones of the forearm, calf, knee joint, femoral neck, head of humerus and acromion.

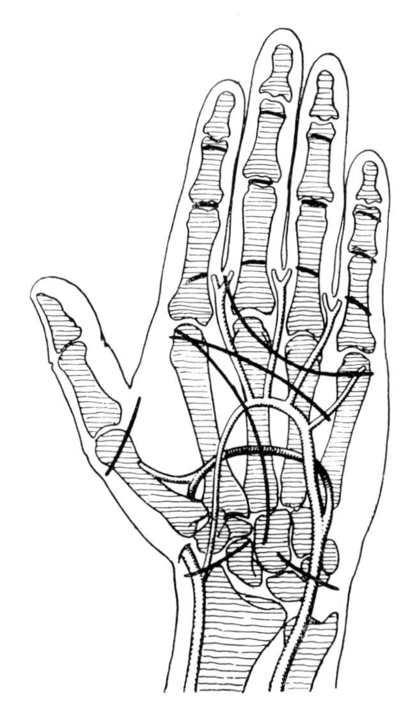

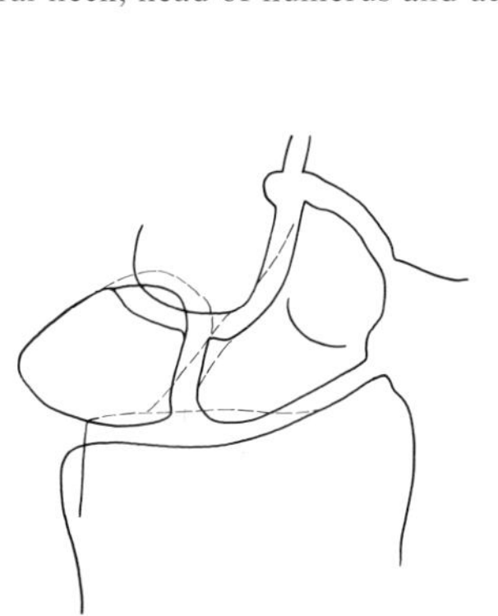

Fig. 661. With slightly oblique projection of the articular space between lunate and navicular bone (with little pronation), one obtains two double contours which cross one another. Especially if the views are not quite clearcut, one may think of traumatic displacement of deforming arthrosis. The articular space becomes visible only with suitable projection.

Fig. 662 shows the sagittal projection of the visible skin folds onto the bones and the palmar arches of the blood vessels, important for the evaluation of the position of foreign bodies (from *Corning*).

The folds of the joints of the hand and fingers may show easily on very soft radiographs. Different from lines of fissure, these lines pass beyond the margins of the bones. The middle fold of the bent fingers corresponds to the middle joint, while the distal joint lies distally and the basal joint proximally to the respective folds of the bent fingers.

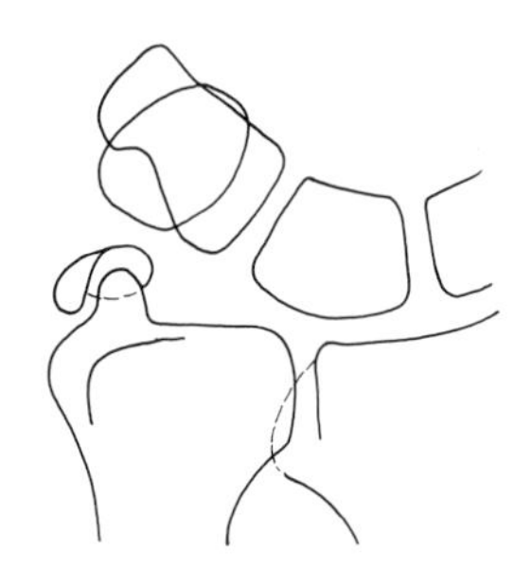

a) Male, 59 years

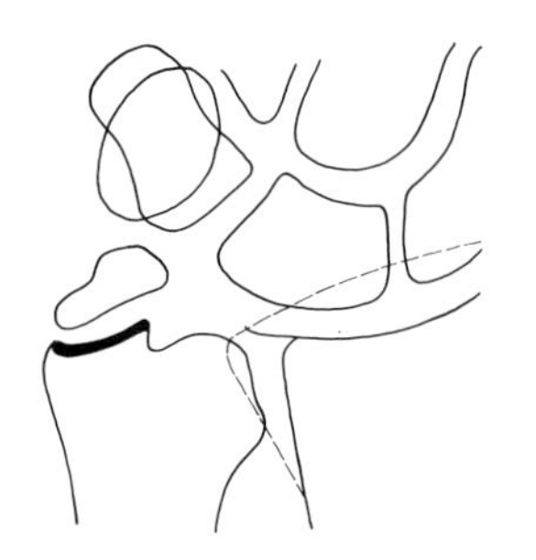

b) Male, 57 years

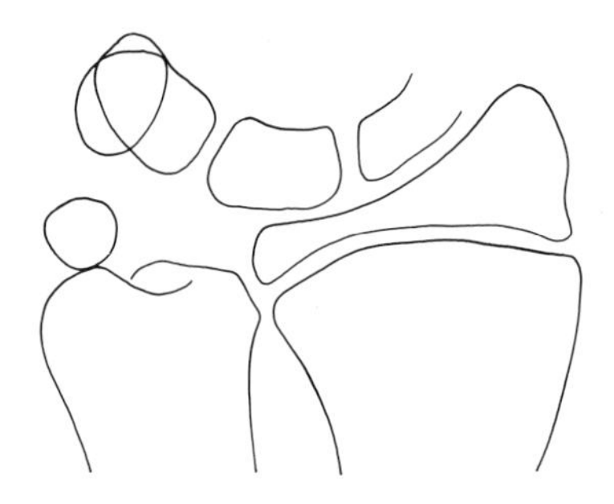

c) Male, 17 years

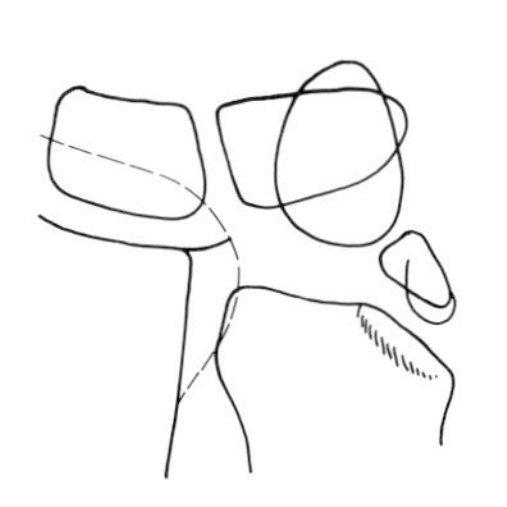

d) Male, 18 years

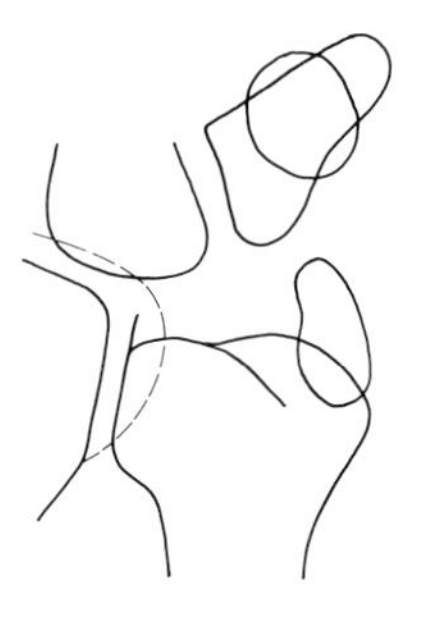

e) Male, 23 years

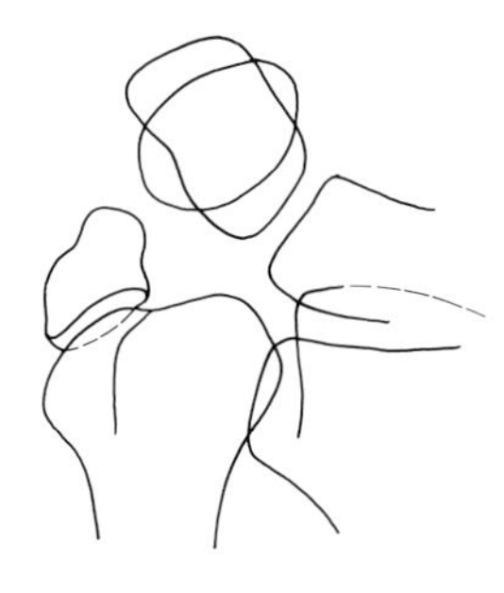

f) Sex and age unknown

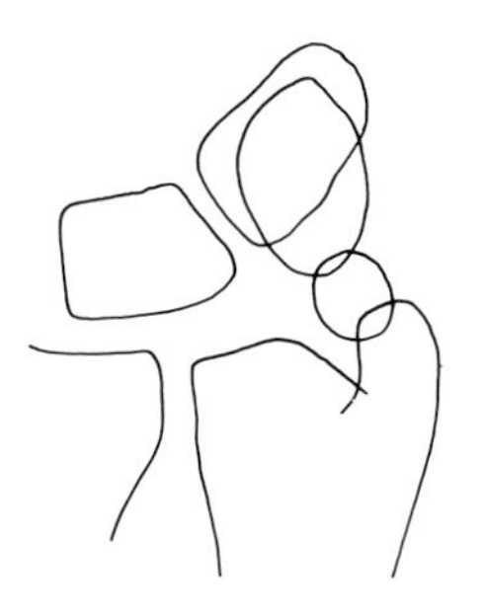

g) Male, 23 years

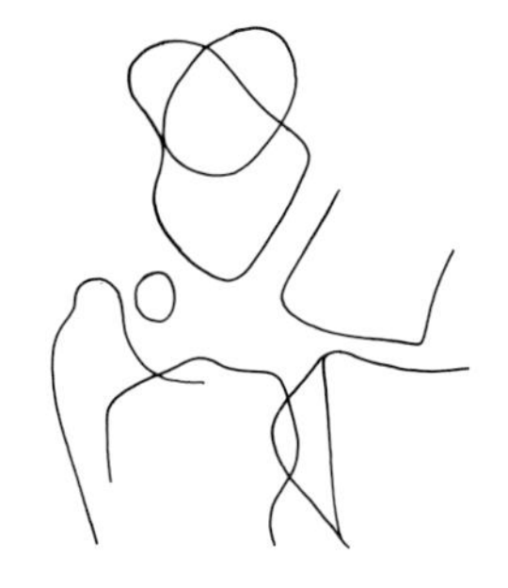

h) Male, 36 years

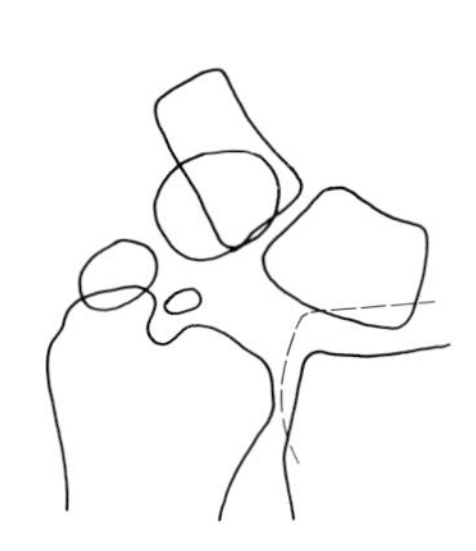

i) Female, age unknown

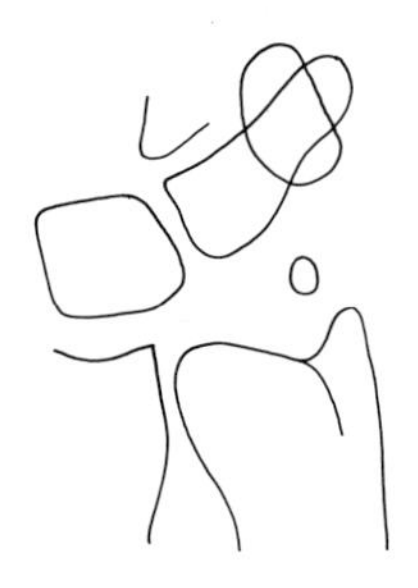

k) Female, 35 years

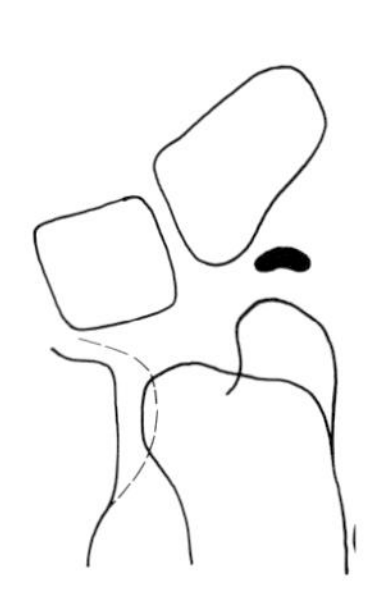

l) Female, 32 years

Fig. 663. Variants and accessoria in the radioulnar-carpal region. The drawings show the accessoria between ulna and the triangular and pisiform bones, which are quite variable in shape, size and position. While in cases of absence or hypoplasia of the styloid process, an independent, perhaps articulating, formation may certainly be considered to be a styloid bone (differential diagnosis for pseudoarthrosis after fracture), differentiation from a triangular bone with a well-developed styloid process may sometimes be difficult. Cf. Figs. 666, 670 and 685–688. If it occurs bilaterally, it always speaks for a triangular bone, according to *Riva,* while *Schinz* and *Grumbach* deny the independent existence of an os triangulare carpi, explaining it as a residual state after fractures of the ulnar styloid process. Obviously, both interpretations are correct. For differential diagnosis of variants in the region of the wrist, see also *Brauer* (cf. Fig. 666).

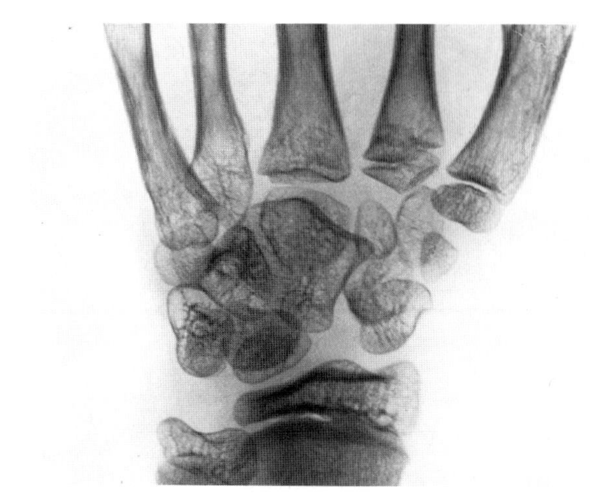

Fig. 664. Multiple carpal bones (from *Ruckensteiner*).

This wrist of a girl in her 8th year shows, in the carpal region, 14 nuclei of bones, which can be separated from each other. In addition, there is a normally developed epiphysis at the proximal end of the 2nd metacarpal bone. This multiplicity of origins of bony nuclei in the carpal region was found symmetrically in both hands.

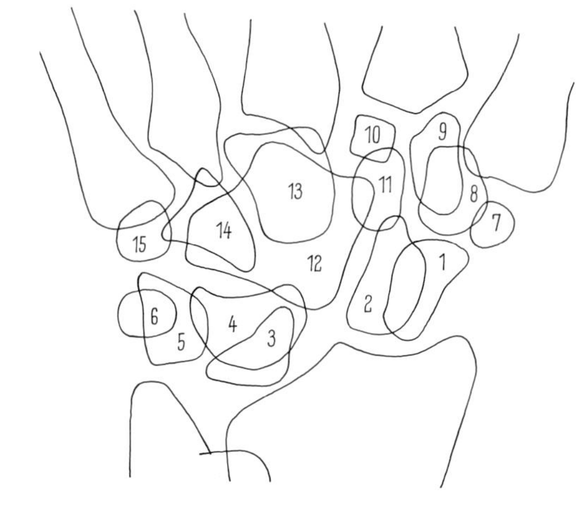

- 1 + 2 Bipartite navicular bone, where one bone (1) is placed radiovolar, the other (2) more dorsoulnar
- 3 + 4 Bipartite lunate bone; here, too, one bone (3) is lying more radiovolar, the other (4) more dorsoulnar
- 5 Triangular bone
- 6 Pisiform bone
- 7 + 8 Both correspond to the position of the greater multangular bone, probably a bipartition. But one may also consider the radially placed smaller bone (7) as paratrapezium, while the other larger one (8) may correspond to the greater multangular bone.
- 9 – 11 These three bones probably present a tripartite lesser multangular bone, a so-called tripartite trapezoid bone, but the proximal bone (11) may also have developed from an os centrale
- 12 + 13 Bipartite capitate bone, where the larger bone, the largest in the entire carpal region (12), lies more proximovolar, the other (13) more dorsodistal
- 14 Hamate bone
- 15 Os Vesalianum (a mistake; it is probably a basal hamate bone)

Fig. 665. The same patient as in Fig. 664, but in her 18th year of life. Now one can differentiate 15 carpal bones.

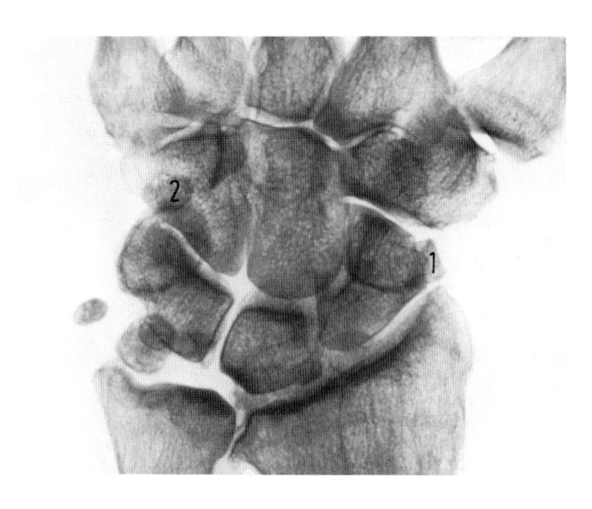

Fig. 666. Wrist with accessoria in the carpal region. At the radial side of the navicular bone there is, in a typical spot, an external radial bone (1), which may have developed from a splitting-off of the tubercle of the navicular bone (cf. Fig. 667, see also *Hennecke*). A not quite clarified finding, designated as external ulnar bone, is furnished by the calcification on the ulnar edge of the hamate bone (2); in this connection, *Köhler-Zimmer* mention the possibility of calcified tendons at the ulnar side. In addition, a pea-sized accessorium, the triangular bone, can be shown. Finally, a lentil-sized accessorium with smooth borders lies slightly lateroproximal from the pisiform bone, which might be a calcification of ulnar tendons or a secondary pisiform bone. *Brauer* was able to demonstrate unequivocally by a series of radiographs the post-traumatic origin of accessory ossicles of carpus and tarsus in two elderly patients. In one case, four months after a trauma a secondary triangular bone could be demonstrated; in another case, a subtibial bone, six years after injury. Radiographs taken immediately after the traumata excluded so-called avulsion fractures.

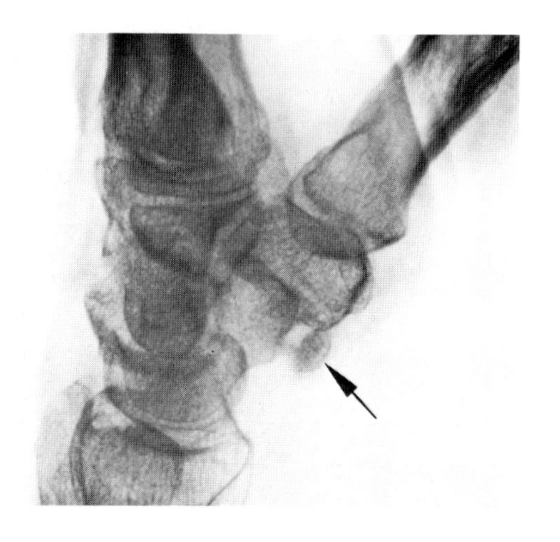

Fig. 667. External radial bone (↖), cf. Figs. 656, 657 and 666. While *Köhler-Zimmer* consider the external radial bone as a splitting-off of the tubercle of the navicular bone, *Terlep* was able to exclude previous trauma in a corresponding case. He described an extraordinarily large external radial bone. In our own case as well, no trauma had occurred in the patient's anamnesis. The cause for the development of such a small acessorium may be found in the failure of fusion of the nucleus of the navicular tubercle which is situated at this spot, as has also been stated by *Köhler-Zimmer*. The dorsal radial bone (at both carpi), described by *Rösli*, is found at the distal end of the radius, with which it forms a functional unit. Therefore, this accessorium must not be confused with the exernal radial bone shown in our radiograph. *Georgy* and *Hillger* endorse this author's opinion that this accessorium develops through failure of fusion of the tubercle of the navicular bone, though the cause has not been clarified.

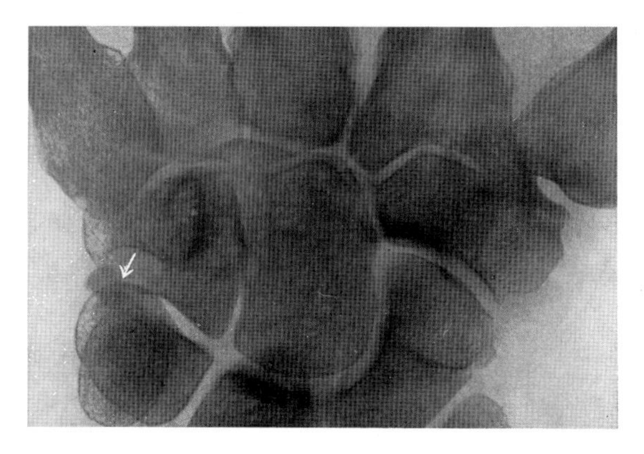

Fig. 668. External ulnar bone (↙), see Figs. 656, 657. Carpus of a 36-year-old male who fell on his hand. The clinical course was as in contusion. The independent character of this formation is demonstrated by the fact that the hamate bone exhibits a special hollowing for it. The size of the external ulnar bone is very variable, from pinhead to bean-size. The presence of a distinct, obviously very sturdy hamulus speaks against the conception of a "bone of the hamulus."

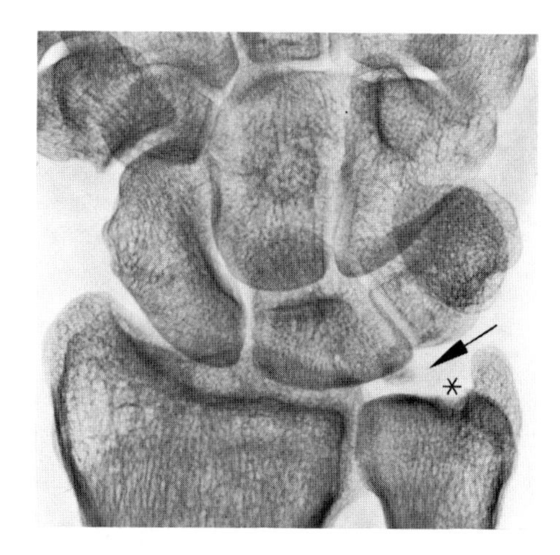

Fig. 669. Calcification of the articular disk in the ulnocarpal wrist (↙)? For differential diagnosis one has to consider a loose body in a hollowed osteochondritic groove (*) radial from the ulnar styloid process.

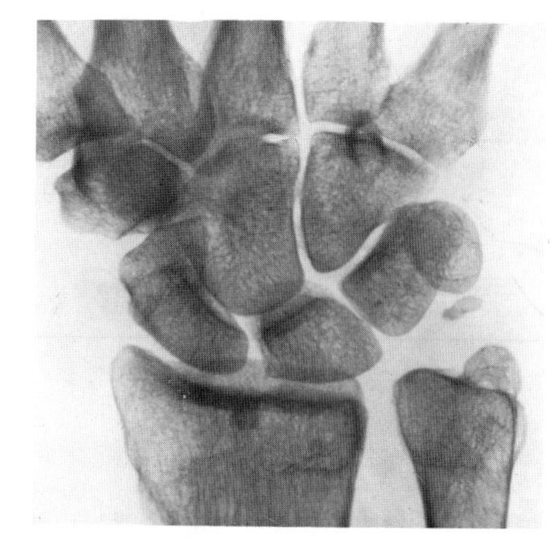

Fig. 670. Bipartite, very small triangular bone, cysts in the ulnar styloid process, two islets of compact tissue in the radial epiphysis (see also Fig. 650, No. 85). According to *Viehweger,* two bony nuclei may occasionally be found in the distal ulnar epiphysis, which may point to the fact that both nuclei share equally in the ossification of the distal ulnar epiphysis. *E. Fischer* described a bipartition of a so-called triangular bone caused by trauma.

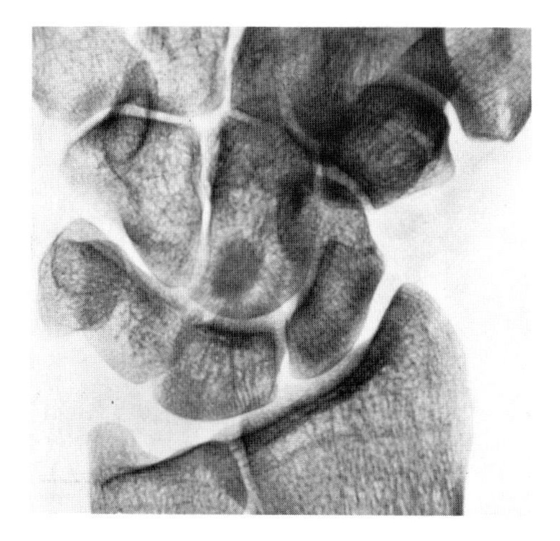

Fig. 671. Islet of compact tissue in the proximal part of the **capitate bone;** cf. Figs. 660 and 676.

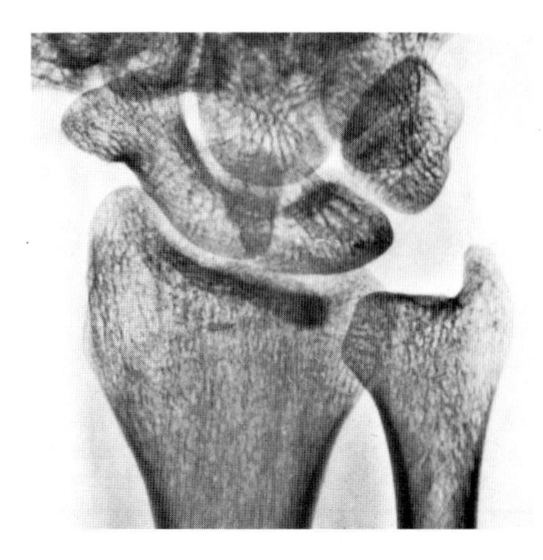

Fig. 672. Apparent sclerosis due to projection of the tissue near the joint in the distal radial epiphysis.

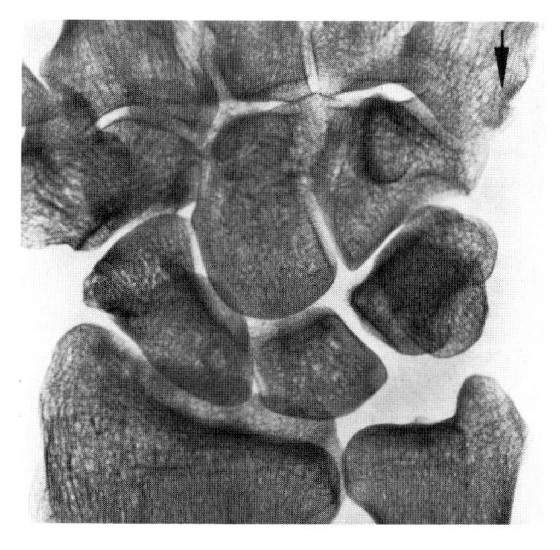

Fig. 673 a

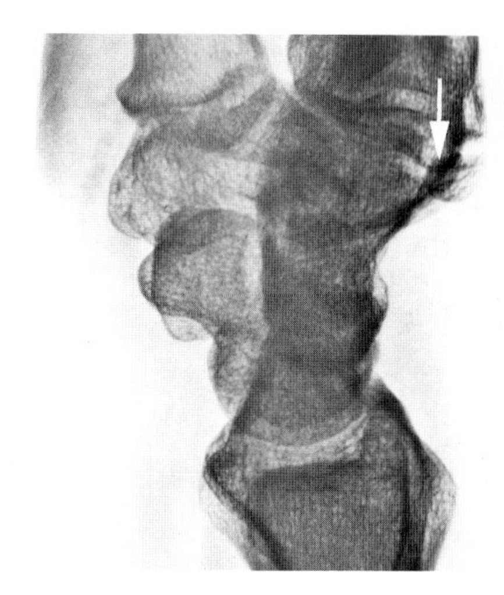

Fig. 673 b

Fig. 673. "Os Vesalium" (↓), see Figs. 656 and 657; so far not authenticated by any author. According to *Neiss, de Cuveland* and others, it is a persistent apophysis and/or avulsion of the tuberosity of the 5th metacarpal bone, after a known or long-forgotten trauma. Cyst in the navicular bone. Differential diagnosis for an axially taken vascular canal *(Ravelli)*. (From the collection of *W. Werner*, Berlin).

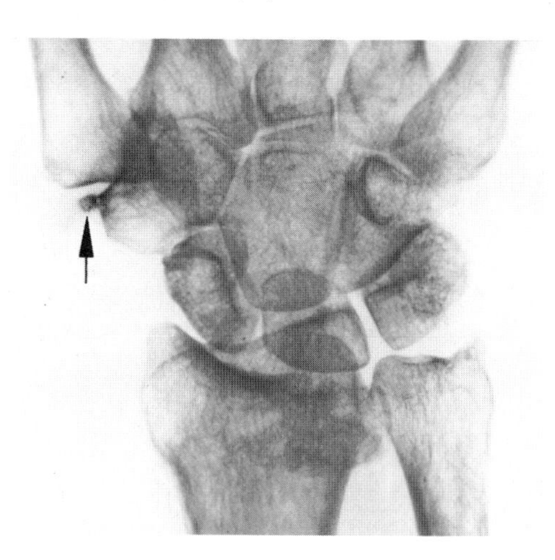

Fig. 674 a

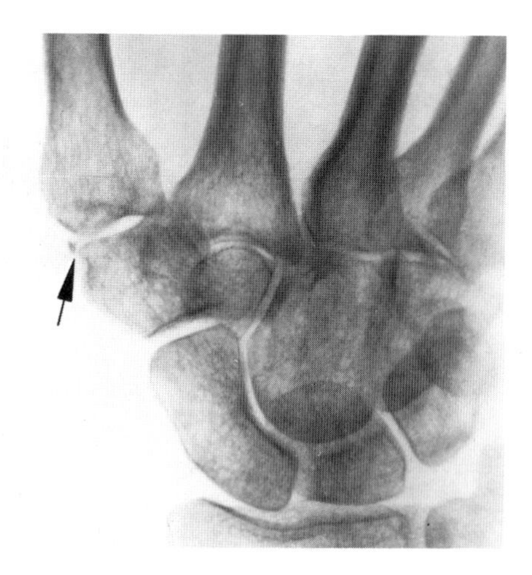

Fig. 674 b

Fig. 674. Paratrapezium (↑), see Figs. 656, 657. The views show wrists of two different patients. Both patients present the same finding: an accessorium at the distal radial edge of the greater multangular bone.

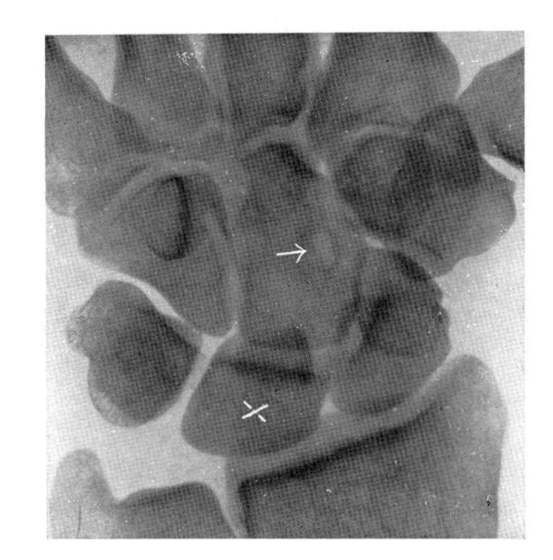

Fig. 675. Anomaly of structure in the capitate bone (→); see Fig. 650, No. 84. Wrist, dorsovolar, of a 33-year-old female. Central ray = x. At (→) there is a roundish tight spot, surrounded by increased density, which frequently can be found in absolutely normal bones, as well as in atrophic bones. Often it is placed more centrally within the bone. According to the position, this can only be a depression for a central carpal bone which has disappeared. A slightly abnormal edge of the navicular bone can also be seen.

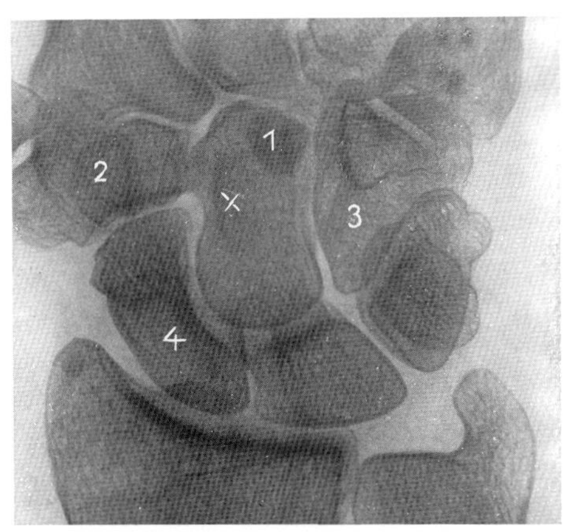

Fig. 676. Structural anomaly (?) of the capitate bone. Wrist, dorsovolar, of a 23-year-old male. There is suspicion of a ganglion. (Central ray = x)

1 Secondary capitate bone. According to recent opinion, this is a fragment developed through pathological causes (acquired accessorium). It may be mistaken for a large, very thick islet of compact tissue.
2 Greater and lesser multangular bones, covering one another
3 Hamate bone
4 Navicular bone

The ulnar styloid process is large and finger-shaped. Its shape and size are quite variable.

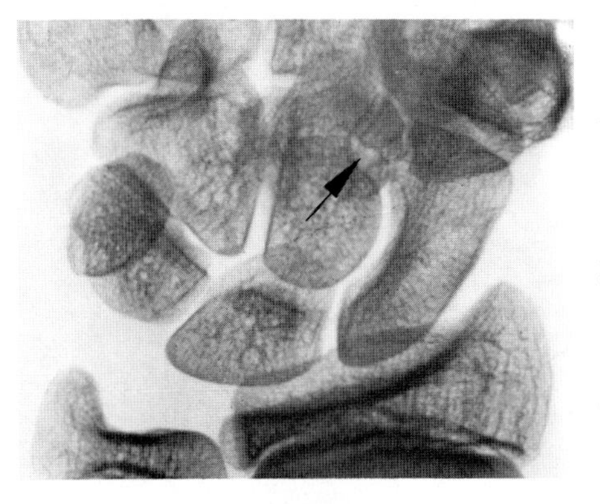

Fig. 677. Lacuna for the central carpal bone (↗); see Fig. 650, No. 84. A rare roundish or triangular formation the size of a small pea is visible in the space between the navicular, lesser multangular and capitate bones; sometimes there are two nuclei. Bilateral occurrence indicates an accessorium. Contrary to this opinion, according to the Wörterbuch der Medizin *(Zetkin-Schaldach),* it is an absolutely constant cartilaginous preformation; when it ossifies, fusion with the navicular bone occurs almost regularly. Numerous cysts in the carpal region can be seen, especially in the lunate, triangular, capitate and hamate bones (see Fig. 655).

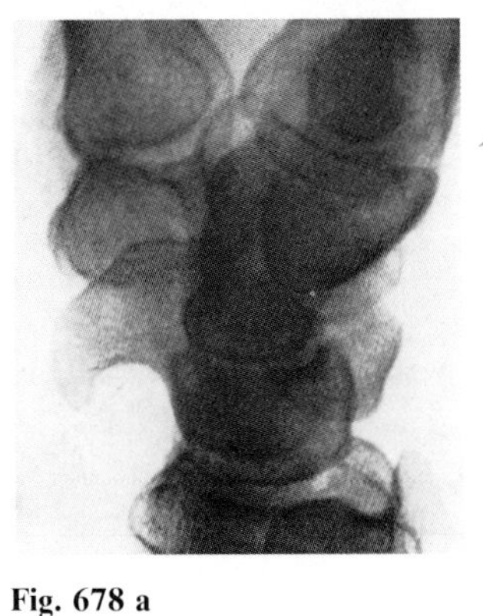

Fig. 678 a

Fig. 678 b

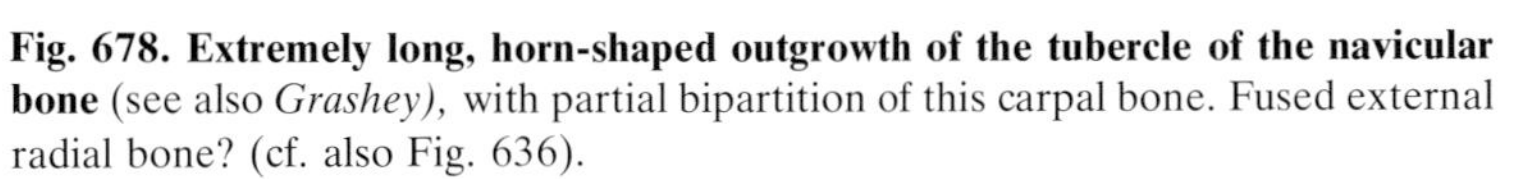

Fig. 678. Extremely long, horn-shaped outgrowth of the tubercle of the navicular bone (see also *Grashey),* with partial bipartition of this carpal bone. Fused external radial bone? (cf. also Fig. 636).

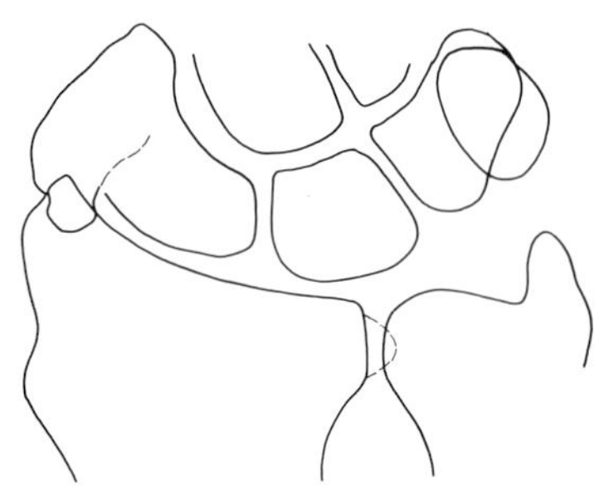

Fig. 679. Abnormally large tubercle of the navicular bone. Fused external radial bone? Roentgen sketch after *Grashey.*

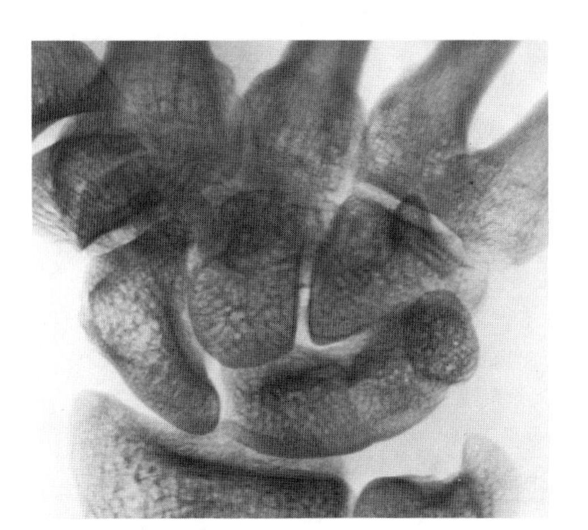

Fig. 680

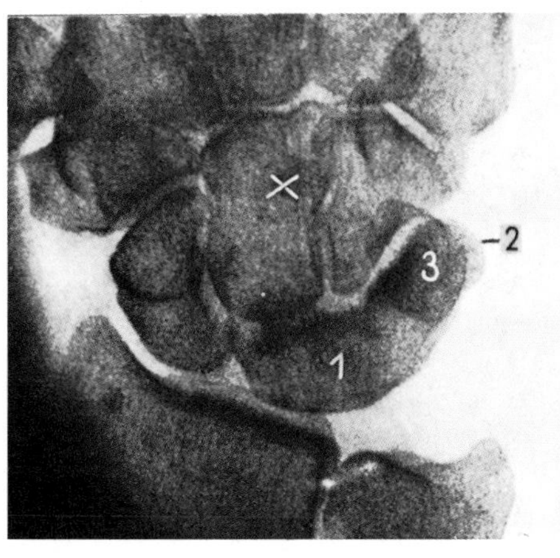

Fig. 681

1 Lunate bone
2 Triangular bone
3 Pisiform bone

Figs. 680 and 681. Synostosis between lunate and triangular bones. Central ray = x. The radiographs are those of two different patients but show the same anomaly: a synostosis between lunate and triangular bones. A notch of the distal contour, mainly visible between the two bones, is conspicuous. For the concrescences, see also Fig. 1099.

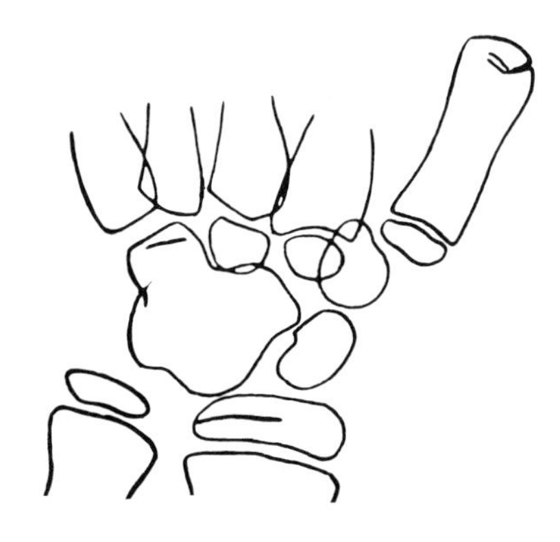

Fig. 682. Peculiar bilateral synostosis of lunate, triangular, hamate and part (?) of the capitate bone. In the same girl, bilateral synostoses of several tarsal bones were also found (see Fig. 838 a, b). According to *Arens,* synostosis between the lunate and triangular bones was established for the first time in 1903 by *Sömmering* and *Smith.* Concerning congenital synostoses of carpal and tarsal bones, see *Kewesch, Hoffmann* and *Dederich.* A rare pseudoepiphysis at the head of the first metacarpal bone: see Fig. 1110. *Marti* described a rare bony bridge between the greater multangular and the navicular bone, an anomaly which, according to the same author, can be ascertained more often in the corresponding tarsal region than in the carpus. *Neiss* was able to observe a bilateral synostosis between the lesser multangular and capitate bones. In 1971 *Buysch, Drewes,* and *Günther* published a further bilateral and unilateral case of the rare fusion of the lesser multangular and capitate bones.

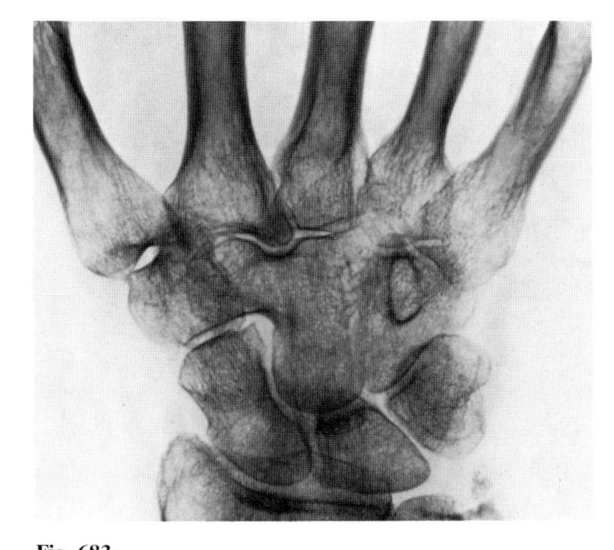

Fig. 683

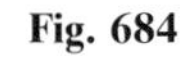

Fig. 684

Figs. 683 and 684. A concrescence of all distal carpal bones in both hands, with aplasia of joints, apart from a residual space between capitate and hamate bones, with completely free coalescing proximal carpal bones, never before been described. Partial fusion between the heads of the metacarpal bones II and III on one hand, and of the lesser multangular and capitate bones on the other. On the left, an ulnar styloid bone; on the right, a rudimentary styloid process. According to *Pfitzner,* coalescence is favored in the presence of accessoria. (See *Cockshott* on carpal fusions, taking into account racial differences, as well as *Fuhrmann, Steffens* and *Rompe,* who published a case of synostosing of the hand, combined with multiple additional malformations, under the aspect of genetic problems.)

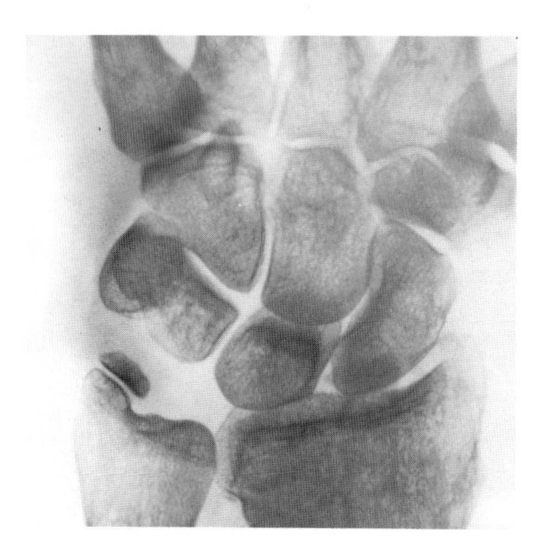

Fig. 685. Styloid bone. Carpus dorsovolar (see Fig. 650, No. 76). An accessorium rides on the sharply defined, smooth contours of the styloid process; it seems to form an articulation with the ulnar styloid process. As there is a concurrent fracture of the radius which is not quite new, one has to decide whether this represents a break-off at the styloid process or an isolated styloid bone. We believe that it must be concluded from the sharply defined contour that the isolation of this accessorium should not be connected with the fracture of the radius and that an isolated ulnar styloid bone must be assumed.

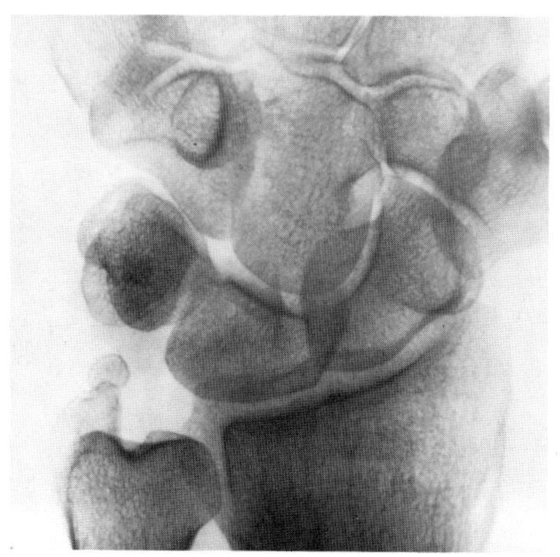

Fig. 686. Styloid bone? Triangular bone? In this view, too, an isolated accessorium is recognizable at the tip of the well-formed styloid process. It has a roundish shape, unusual for a triangular bone. On the other hand, a styloid bone is not to be expected at a styloid process that is so pronounced. Therefore, it cannot be definitely determined whether this is an independent styloid bone or a post-traumatic triangular bone (= an avulsion fracture of the ulnar styloid process). *Riva* pointed out a bilateral triangular bone with no known previous trauma.

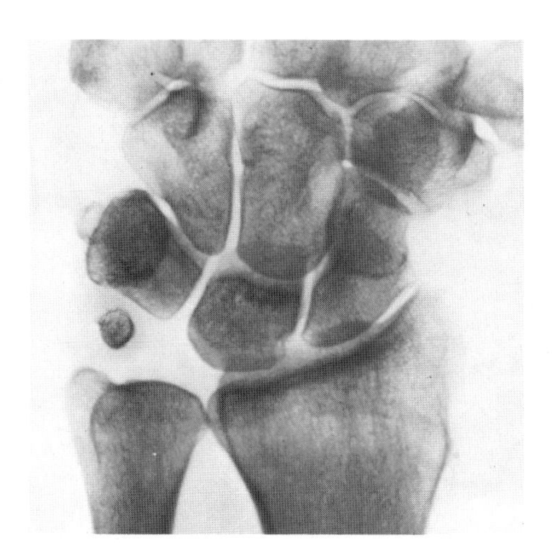

Fig. 687. Styloid bone? Triangular bone or intermediate antebrachial bone? Carpus, dorsovolar. In the present case, with a feebly developed styloid process, one finds an accessorium between ulna and triquetrum, which may conform by its position to a triangular bone. The shape, too, is somewhat unusual for a triangular bone. The hypoplasia of the styloid process speaks for a styloid bone.

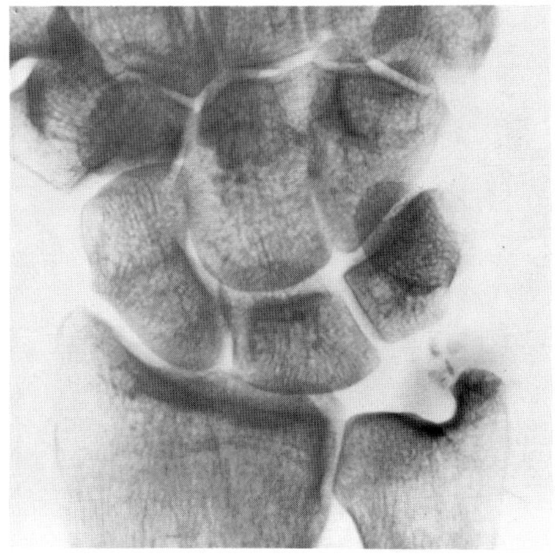

Fig. 688. Multiply divided styloid bone? Calcification of tendon or disk? Osteochondrosis dissecans? A previous trauma in the patient's history is not known. But, in this author's opinion, this case shows the fate of a very rare variant, a multiply divided preformation of a bony nucleus of an isolated ulnar styloid bone. This is certainly an interesting final state, reminiscent of the one which, in the case of a 14-year-old boy, *Jungblut* left open.

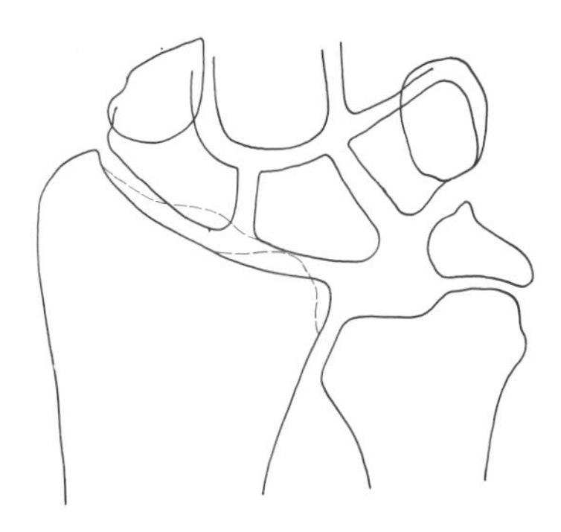

Fig. 689. Typical independent "os triquetrum" (triangular bone).

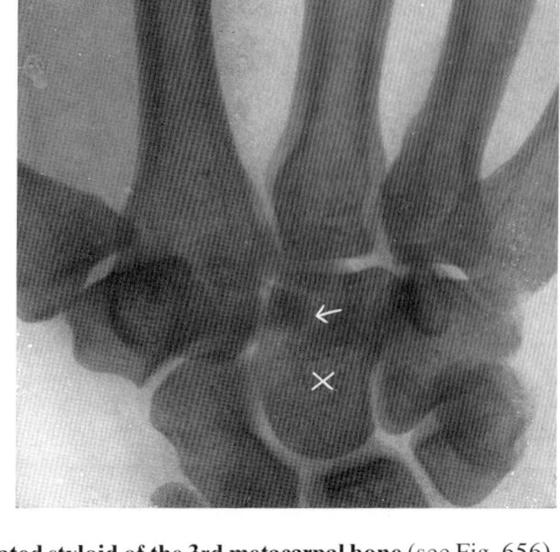

Fig. 691. Assimilated styloid of the 3rd metacarpal bone (see Fig. 656). Carpus, dorsovolar, of a 26-year-old female. The radiograph was taken because of inflammatory swelling of the soft tissues. Projection onto x. While usually the lesser multangular bone is well rounded, here, a process (←) that corresponds by its position to a styloid bone is seen. The increased radiolucency of the articular space makes this formation apparently independent. But thorough inspection shows an upper and lower connecting line that crosses the bright articular space. Therefore, the accessorium cannot be considered as assimilated. Radiographically, it cannot be differentiated from a metastyloid and parastyloid (post-traumatic accessoria).

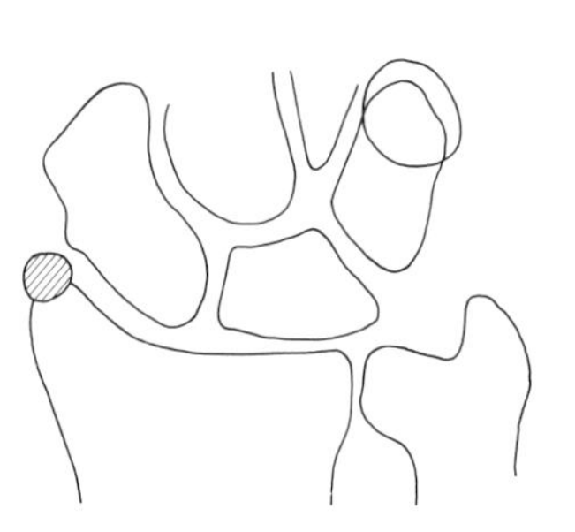

Fig. 690. Styloid bone of radius. An independent nucleus in the radial styloid process is said to occur; this may lead to persistence of an accessorium, possibly after damage to the cartilaginous joint, "but avulsions may lead to similar findings" *(Zimmer)*.

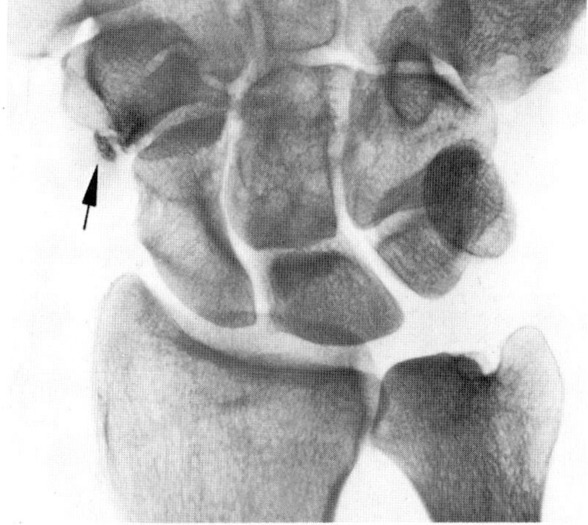

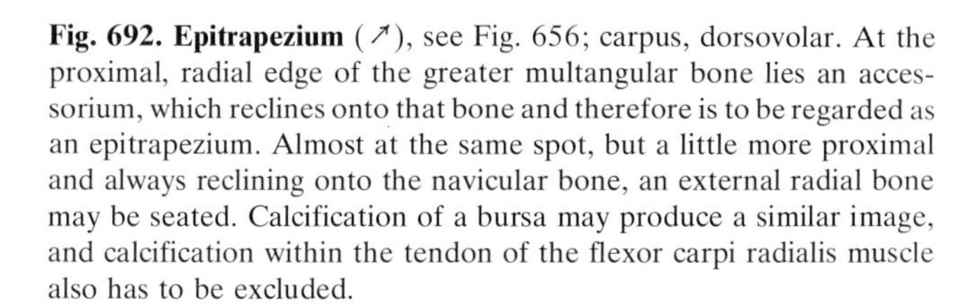

Fig. 692. Epitrapezium (↗), see Fig. 656; carpus, dorsovolar. At the proximal, radial edge of the greater multangular bone lies an accessorium, which reclines onto that bone and therefore is to be regarded as an epitrapezium. Almost at the same spot, but a little more proximal and always reclining onto the navicular bone, an external radial bone may be seated. Calcification of a bursa may produce a similar image, and calcification within the tendon of the flexor carpi radialis muscle also has to be excluded.

1 Greater multangular bone
2 Lesser multangular bone
3 Tubercle of navicular bone
4 Styloid process of radius
5 Triangular bone

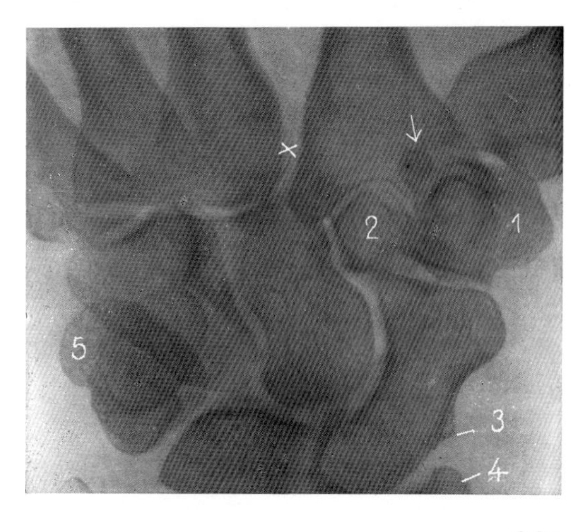

Fig. 693. Secondary trapezoid bone *(Pfitzner)*; see Fig. 656. Carpus, dorsovolar, of a 48-year-old male (fractures of radius and 3rd metacarpal bone through accident). Projection onto x, in this case a pathological diastasis of joint. At ↘ an accessorium, distinctly attached to the lesser multangular bone by an articular line, a secondary trapezoid, probably a "secondary accessorium."

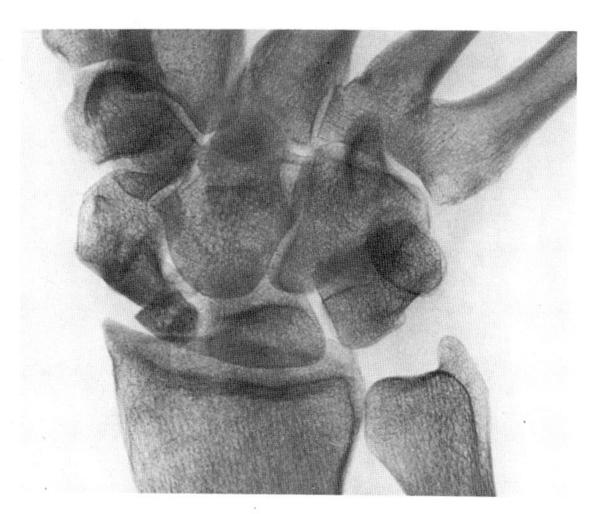

Abb. 694 a

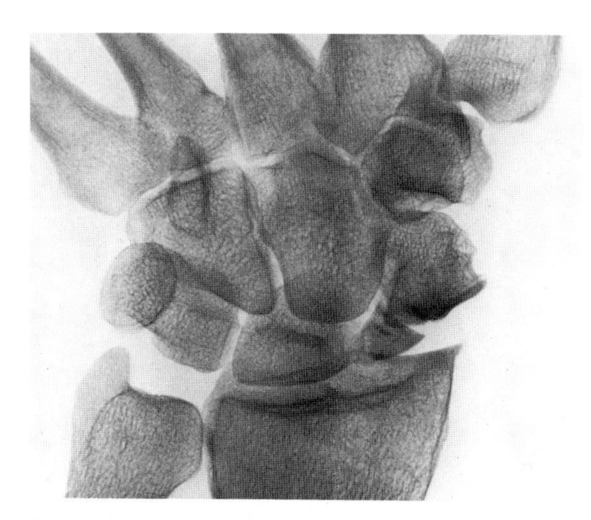

Fig. 694 b

Fig. 694. Bipartite navicular bone? Pseudarthrosis after fracture? Right wrist, dorsovolar and volodorsal. Generally, one ought to arrive at the clarification of the diagnosis by means of radiographs of both wrists, after exclusion of trauma. Findings in both wrists will then point to the very rare congenital bipartition *(Lange, Eggimann, Reckling, Gollasch).* In 1968 *Maes* reported on a unilateral aplasia of the navicular bone, which had been treated over the years with plaster casts as "necrosis of the navicular bone." This malformation of retardation develops, according to *Maes,* "e cause ignota." *Knákal* and *Chvojka* (1970) showed the very rare bilateral aplasia of the navicular bone.

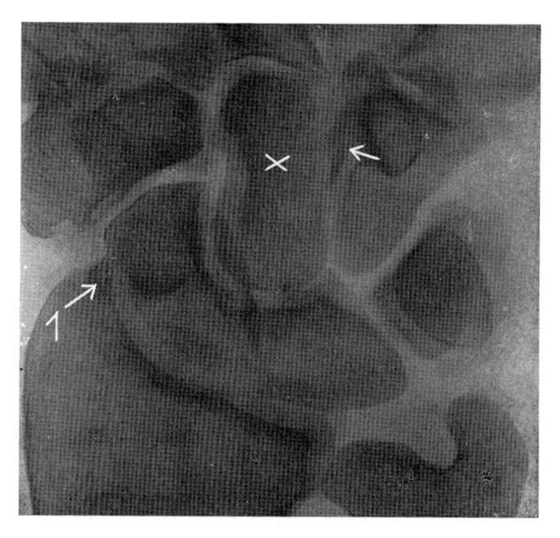

Fig. 695. Prominent tubercle of the navicular bone (1 ↗). Wrist, dorsovolar, of a 48-year-old male. Contusion of the wrist. Projection: onto x. With oblique projection the shadow of the tubercle of the navicular bone, which is quite prominent, covers the styloid process of the radius. The diamond-shaped bit (←) of increased density lies between two articular lines. As the articular space is projected obliquely, two spaces result. The doubtful shadow is caused by the two bones, which cover each other in this region. In 1974 *Lugger* described a pea-sized tubercle of the navicular bone.

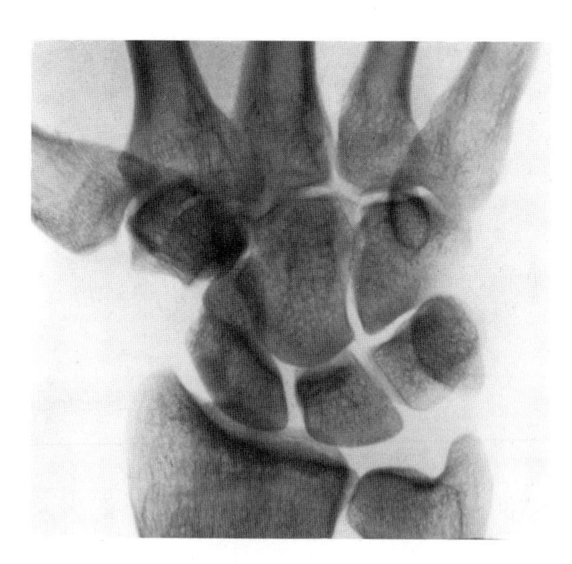

Fig. 696. Islet of compact tissue within the navicular bone; this is rare in children but more frequent in adults.

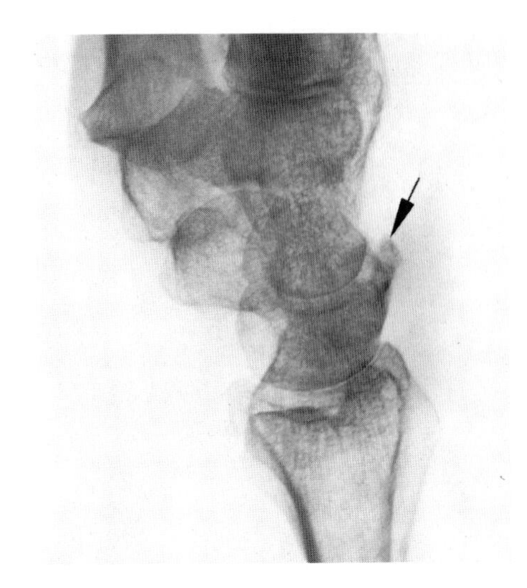

Fig. 697. Epitriquetrum (↙)? *Pfitzner* originally called it epipyramis. The hooklet, which often protrudes at the same spot on the dorsum of the triangular bone, may break off and then be mistaken for the anomaly of an epitriquetrum. Because in this case a free projection, as in *Thews'* sketch (Fig. 698), has not been achieved, the question of whether this is a small promontory of the triquetrum or an independent accessorium must remain open.

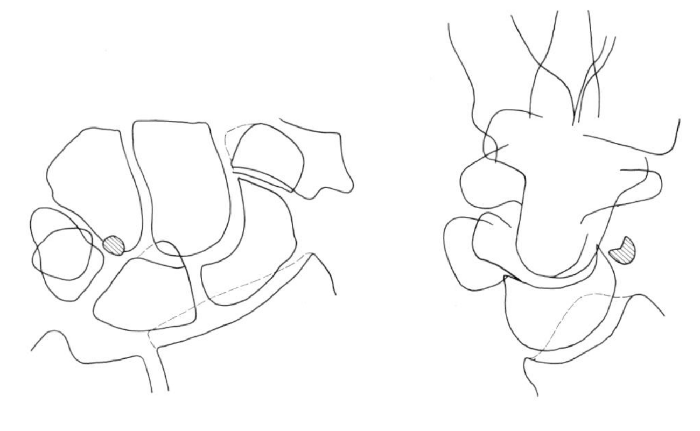

Fig. 698. Epitriquetrum = epipyramis (from *Thews,* Röntgenpraxis, 1939).

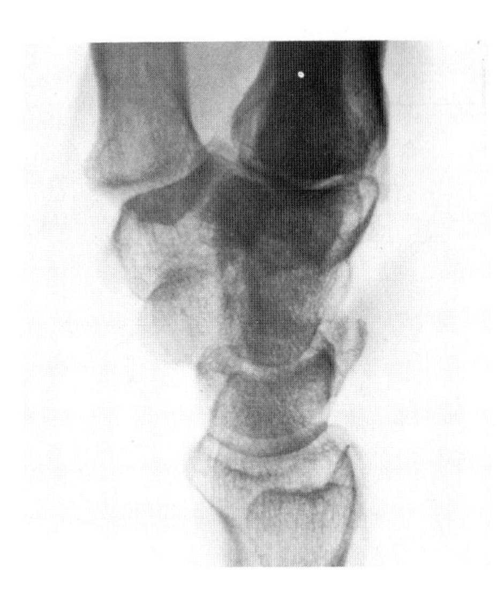

Fig. 699. Pronounced hook formation on the triangular bone. Wrist, radioulnar. The described hooklet on the dorsal surface of the triquetrum shows an especially bony formation of a promontory here.

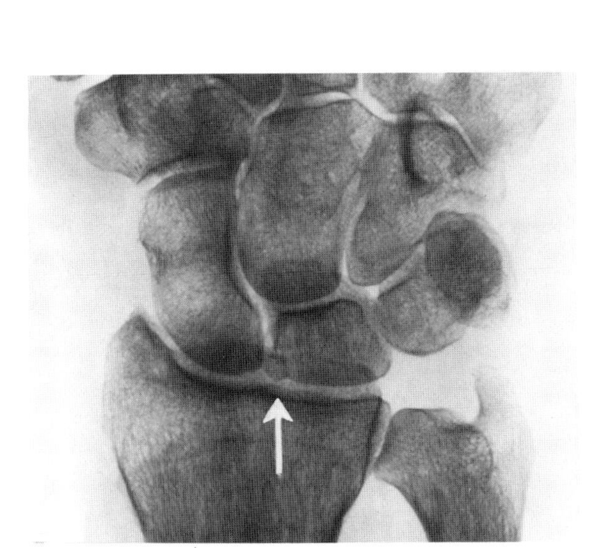

Fig. 700. Lentil-sized accessorium with smooth borders in the triangle of the articular space of the radiocarpal and navicular lunatum joint; it should not be mistaken for one of the known accessoria. Therefore, as an aid to diagnosis, it has been called "os paralunatum."

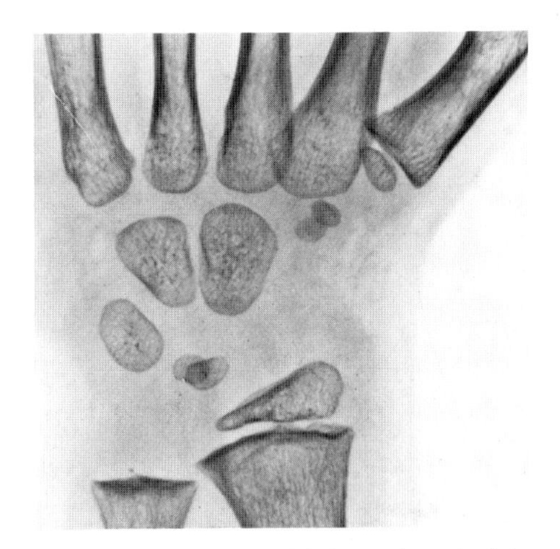

Fig. 701. Double preformation of the nucleus of the lunate bone (only in the right hand) in a 5 3/4-year-old boy *(Eggimann).* At this stage, it cannot yet be determined whether this is a passing or a final bipartition, possibly based on a hereditary disturbance. *Schaaf* and *Wagner* found the same duplications of the carpal bones in each of three siblings with polytope enchondral dyostosis, i.e., duplication of the lunate, triangular, lesser multangular, capitate and hamate bones.

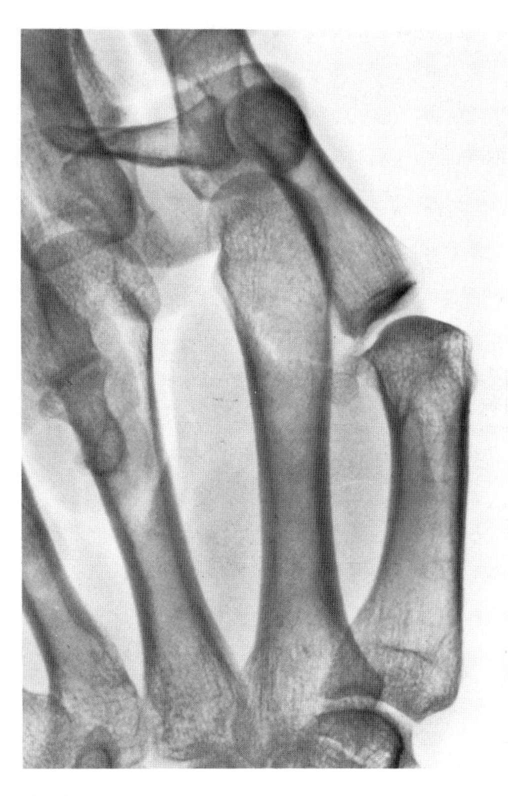

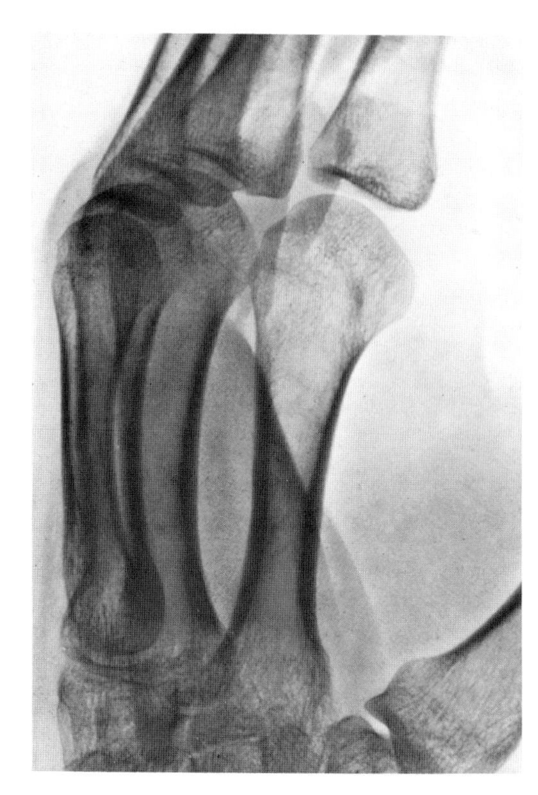

Fig. 702 a **Fig. 702 b**

Fig. 702. Fracture, simulated by *"Mach* **effect,"** in the 2nd metacarpal bone, caused by crossing of the soft tissues of the bent and opposing proximal joint of the thumb. The lateral view makes possible the exclusion of a fracture. This phenomenon may appear on radiographs as a dark or light band at the borders of crossing of differently blackened surfaces (quoted by *Köhler-Zimmer*).

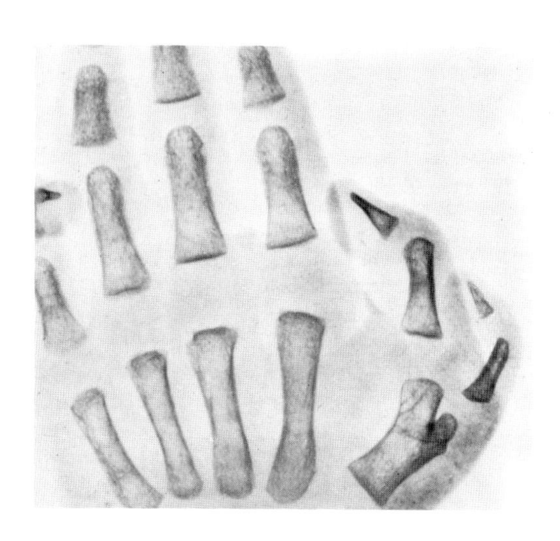

Fig. 703. Polydactylism of the thumb. This is counted among the multiple formations in the extremities and occurs particularly often in the region of thumb and 4th finger. Duplication of the formation of the 1st to 3rd fingers has also been observed (see *W. Müller* and *Werthemann*). *Witt, Cotta* and *Jäger* comprehensively described the congenital malformations of the hand and their operative treatment. In the present case we are dealing with a dominantly hereditary malformation, often accompanied by secondary syndactylism.

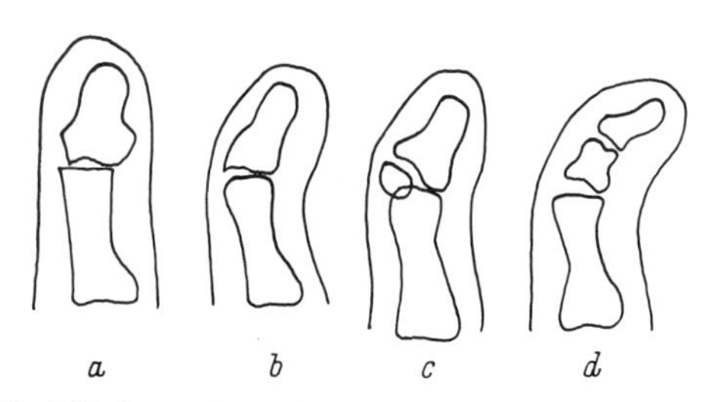

Fig. 704 shows the various malformations up to a thumb consisting of three phalanges *(from W. Müller).*

Brachydactylism of the fingers. The growth of the middle phalange of the 4th finger is not infrequently retarded; consequently, it is too short and mostly levelled at the head. Therefore, the obviously too-short finger appears slightly bent medial-convex. In such cases, the middle joint often shows a more or less pronounced (desmogene) flexion contracture. In cases of pronounced brachydactylism, one finds the shape of the middle phalange typically similar to the short middle phalanges of the toes. For measurements of the skeleton of the hand and their relations, see *Pfitzner.*

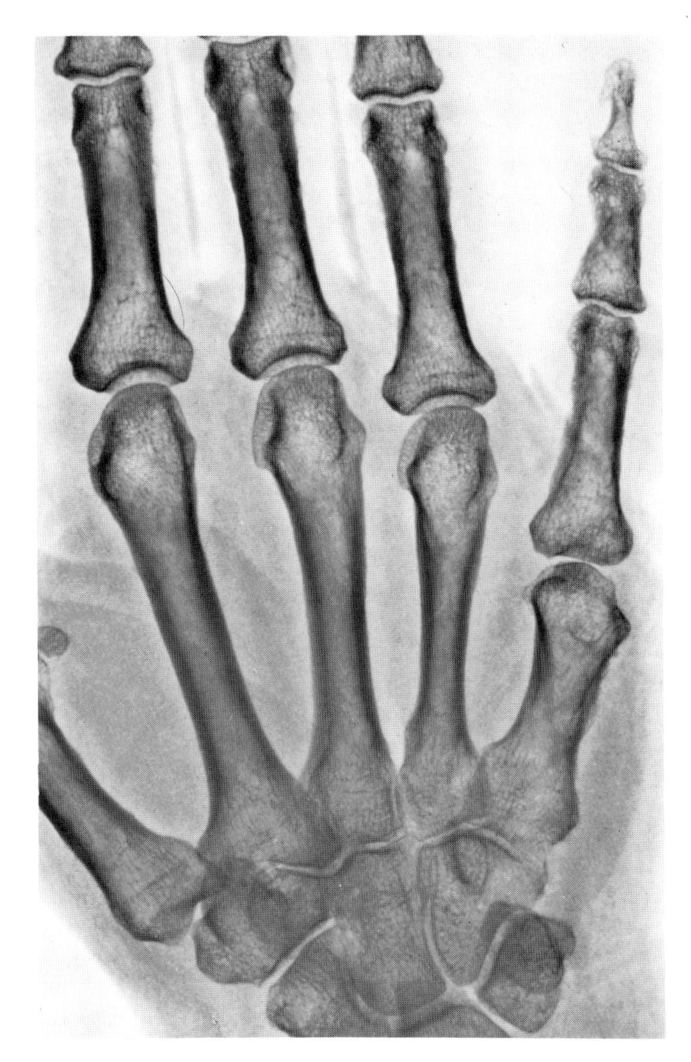

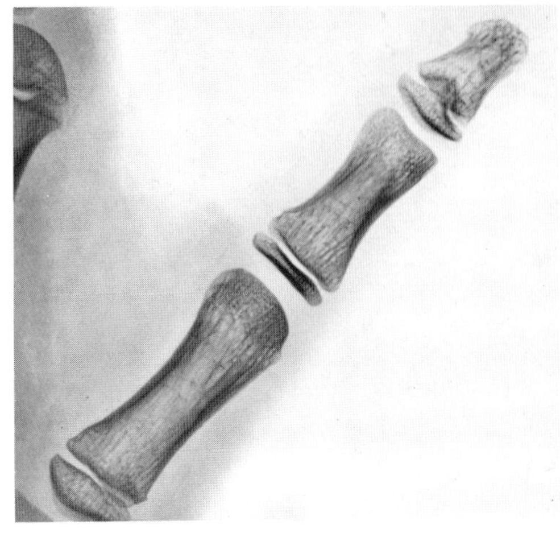

Fig. 706. Peg-like epiphysis of the distal phalange of the thumb. See also Fig. 650, No. 95**.
Disturbed development through inflammatory or traumatic damage to the growth zone; it may occur also in cases of hormonal dysfunction or, allegedly, in acute rickets.

Fig. 705. Brachydactylism, caused by brachyphalangia of metacarpal bone V. Cubic deformity of the distal epiphysis of the 5th metacarpal bone, as well as its shortening with plump deformity. Most frequently, one encounters the shortening of the 2nd finger. Brachydactylies are to be found at individual, or concurrently, at several metacarpals. *Arens* found bilateral brachydactylism of the 4th finger in two brothers. In our own case, the shortening of the 4th finger was observed only unilaterally in a 65-year-old female. Brachydactylism presents very different forms. We differentiate:

a) brachyphalangia (brachytele-, -meso-, -basophalangia),
b) brachymetapody, brachymetacarpy and brachymetatarsy, and
c) symbrachydactyly (see *Werthemann, Bucke, Fuhrmann et al.).*

All cases of brachydactylism are probably not independent local malformations but part of a general constitutional anomaly of the skeleton.

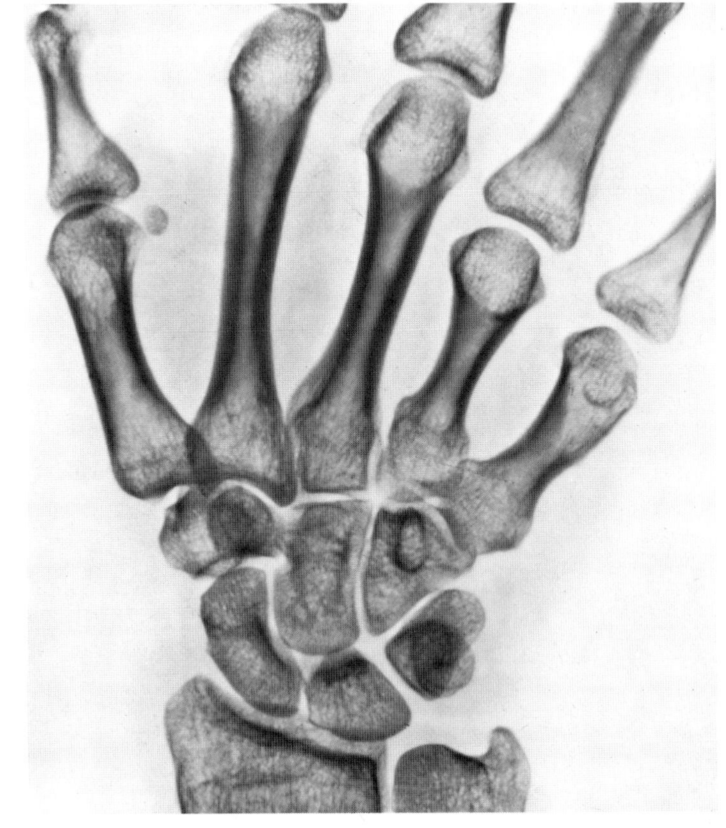

Fig. 707 shows **brachyphalangia of the metacarpal bones III to V,** with corresponding shortening of the fingers.

IV. Lower Extremities

Radiographic Anatomy and Radiographs of the Knee Joint and Calf, Including Exposure Techniques

Directions of exposure:

1. sagittal
   a) anteroposterior
   b) posteroanterior
2. transverse
   a) fibulotibial
   b) tibiofibular
3. oblique radiographs
4. special radiographs of the patella
   a) with lateral shift, path of rays fibuloanteroposterior
   b) with the joint bent, axial exposure
   c) short-distance radiographs
5. oblique, caudoanteroposterior radiograph of the intercondyloid space, after *Frik*.

Using the main directions, the projection is always directed onto the particular space, which one can usually feel distinctly laterally at the level of the apex of the patella, and which also corresponds to the skin fold of the bent knee. The sagittal radiographs are done with the leg stretched; the lateral ones are better taken with the knee slightly bent. Medium soft rays, and also soft ones, are used for views of soft tissues.

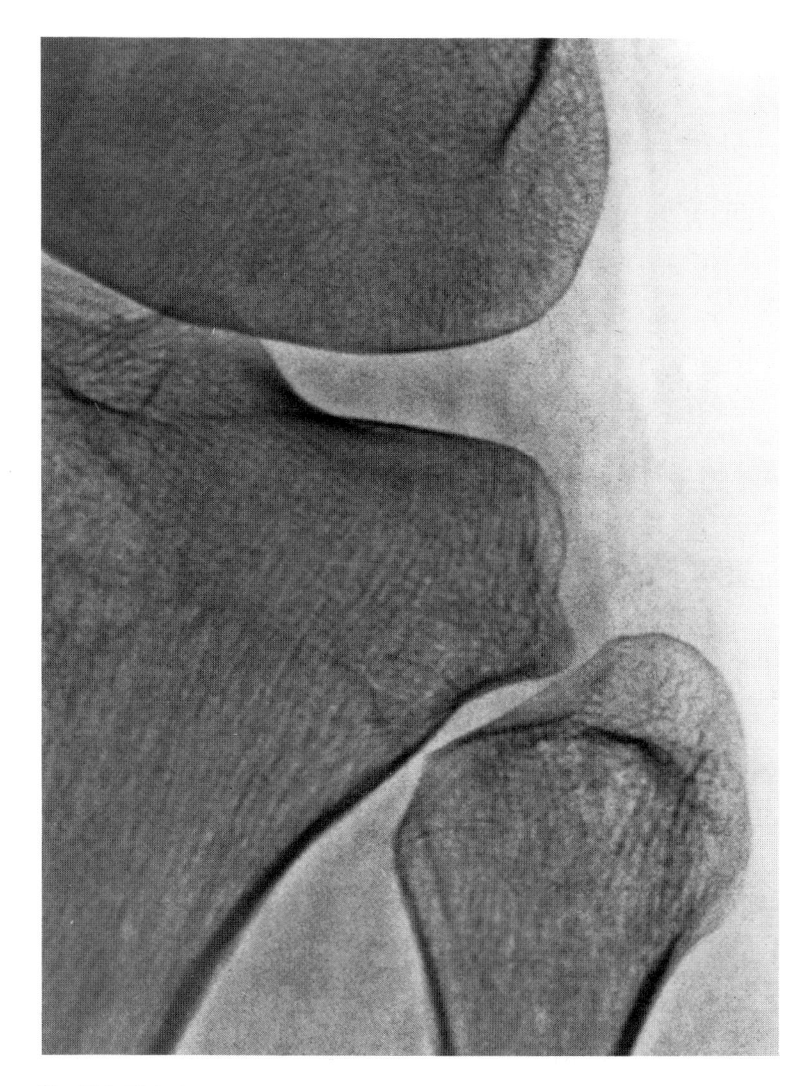

Fig. 708. Tibiofibular joint, taken with the most meticulous focus (see also Fig. 710). Patient supine, leg stretched; internal rotation of the calf by about 30°, which affords a free projection of the head of the fibula. The central ray is directed onto the head of the fibula, vertical to the cassette.

1 Tibiofibular articulation
2 Apex of the fibular head
3 Head of fibula
4 Lateral condyle of femur
5 Lateral intercondyloid tubercle of tibia
6 Lateral condylus of tibia

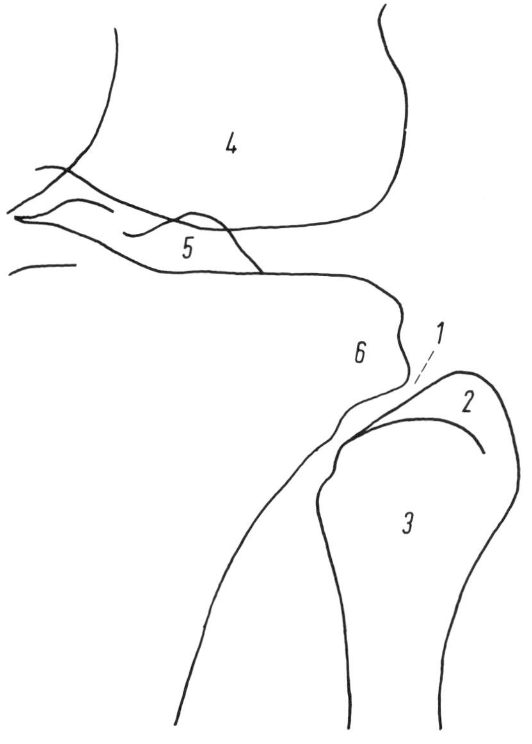

Fig. 709

The patella appears enlarged due to perspective. If the apex of the patella lies more distal or the tube stands more proximal, the apex of the patella, whose upper part is sometimes indistinct, may disturb by projecting into articular space. Within the articular space lies the radiolucent meniscus (fibro-cartilage).

Physiologically, the menisci and the cruciate ligaments are invisible without arthrography. However, their calcification, or deformities of the intercondyloid tubercles, point to pathological states. Similarly, the state of the insertions at the condyles of the collateral ligaments may provide a pointer for evaluation of these ligaments (small split-off particles), especially when a trauma had been sustained a considerable time ago. The tibiofibular joint may show steps in its space (see Fig. 708). The lateral tibial condyle often juts out laterally beyond the femoral condyle. This finding, sometimes wrongly diagnosed as "subluxation," is non-pathological. The tibial space of the knee joint can often be demonstrated as a bright line, without the use of contrast media (*Löhr* and *Hellpap*).

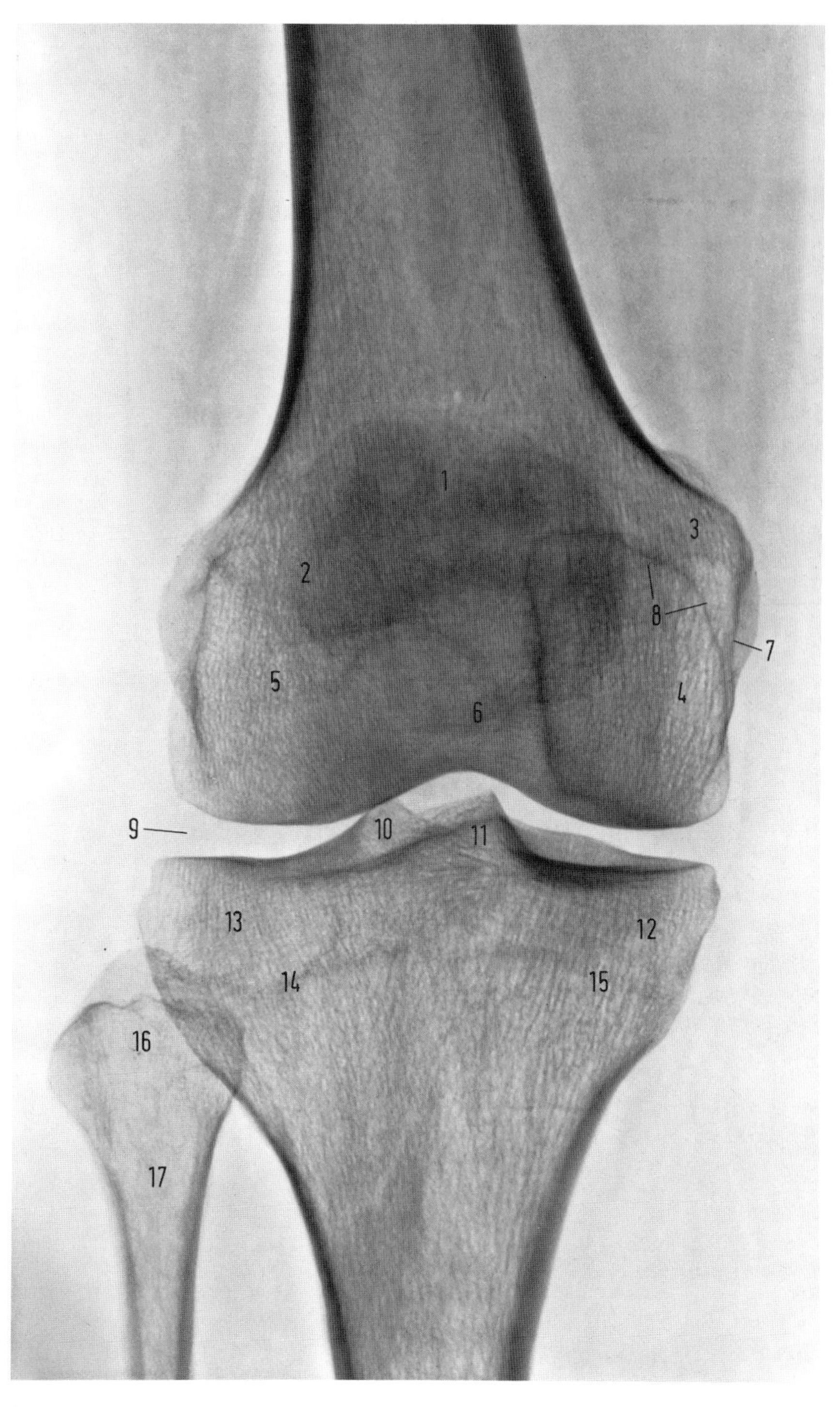

Fig. 710. Knee joint, anteroposterior (leg stretched). For projection see Fig. 711. The central ray is directed one finger's breadth below the apex of the patella, onto the center of the knee joint, vertical to the film.

1 Patella
2 to 3 Wavy epiphyseal line
4 Medial femoral condylus
5 Lateral femoral condylus
6 Intercondyloid fossa of femur
7 Anterior rim of the articular surface of the medial condyle
8 Posterior rim of the articular surface of the medial condyle
9 Apparent lateral articular space
10 Lateral intercondyloid tubercle of tibia
11 Medial intercondyloid tubercle of tibia
12 Medial tibial condylus
13 Lateral tibial condylus
14 to 15 Epiphyseal scar of tibia
16 Head of fibula
17 Neck of fibula

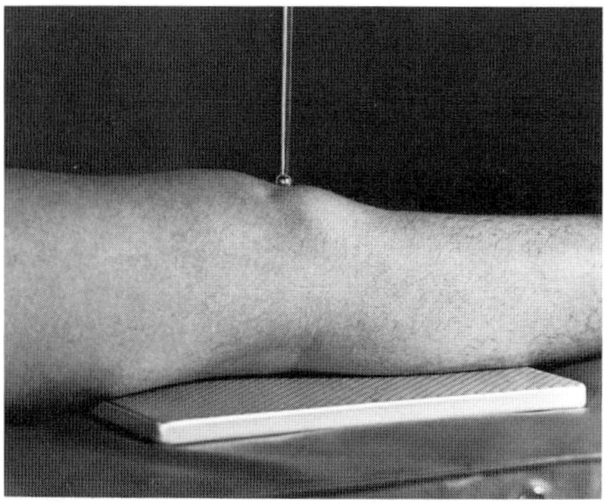

Fig. 711

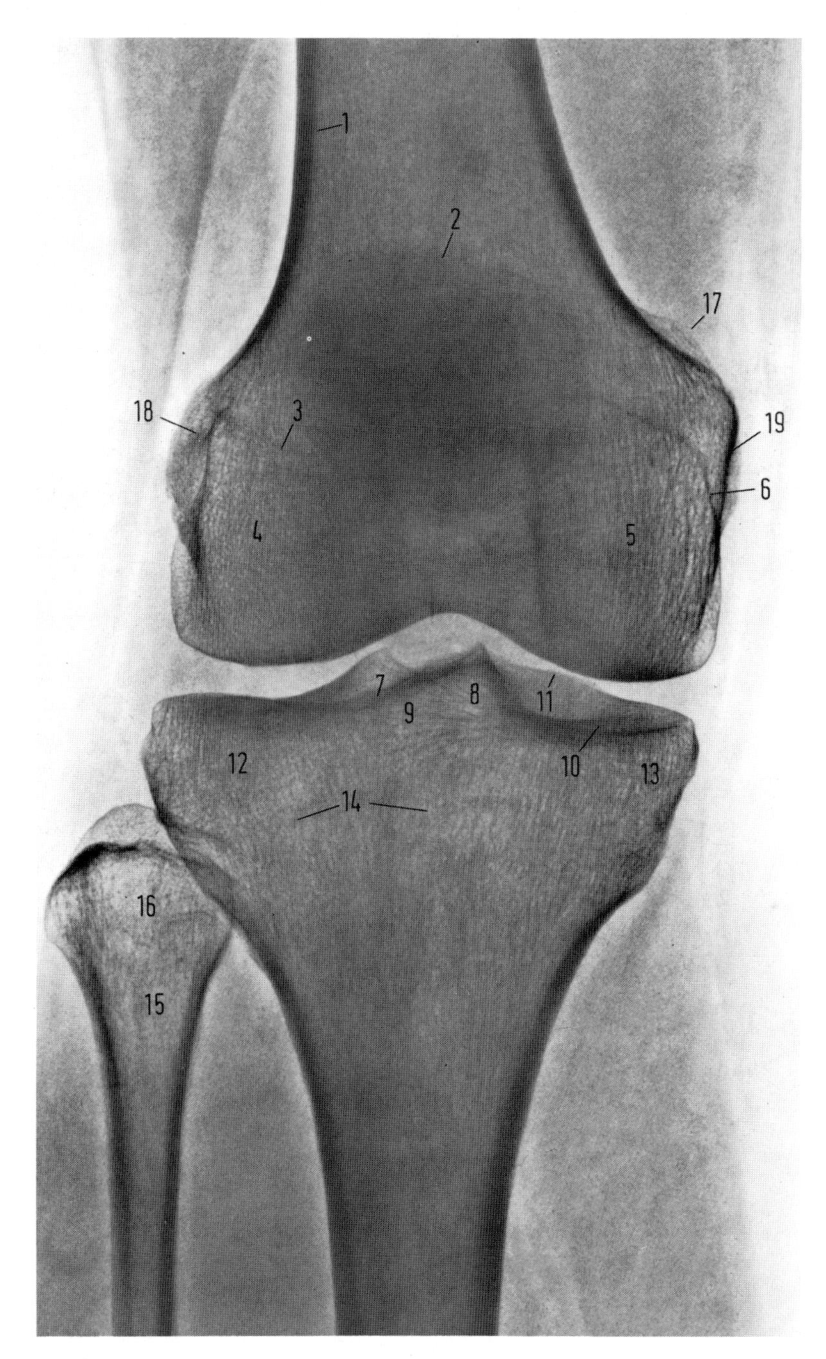

1 Cortex
2 Edge of the base of the patella (may have a double contour)
3 "Epiphyseal (cartilaginous) scar"
4 Lateral femoral condyle
5 Medial femoral condyle
6 Margin of medial condyle
7 Lateral intercondyloid tubercle of tibia
8 Medial intercondyloid tubercle of tibia
9 Intercondyloid eminence of tibia
10 Posterior edge of the articular surface
11 Anterior edge of the articular surface
12 Lateral tibial condylus
13 Medial tibial condylus
14 "Epiphyseal scar" (fused epiphyseal cartilaginous disk)
15 Neck of fibula
16 Head of fibula
17 Apparent periostal thickening
18 Lateral femoral epicondylus, rough outer contour for insertion of tendons (see Fig. 739, No. 153)
19 Medial epicondylus of femur

One recognizes from the distinct contour and structure of the patella that it was lying on the cassette. The lateral side is recognized by the fibula. If the fibula is not visible on the radiograph, one recognizes the medial femoral condylus because it is larger and juts out more. Usually, the lateral articular surface of the tibia protrudes slightly laterally; the medial epicondylus is the place for insertion of the tibial collateral ligament, which is normally not visible. Below the lateral epicondylus one can observe a groove closely above the articular space (a furrow for the tendon at the popliteal muscle). The sharp protrusion of the lateral margin of the medial condylus of the femur into the articular space is a frequent, conspicuous, normal finding. From this little spike one can follow an upward-running line which limits the medial condylus against the intercondyloid fossa.

Fig. 712. Knee joint, posteroanterior. Projection: patient prone, knee stretched, leg in middle position of rotation. The central ray is aimed vertically onto the apex of the patella.

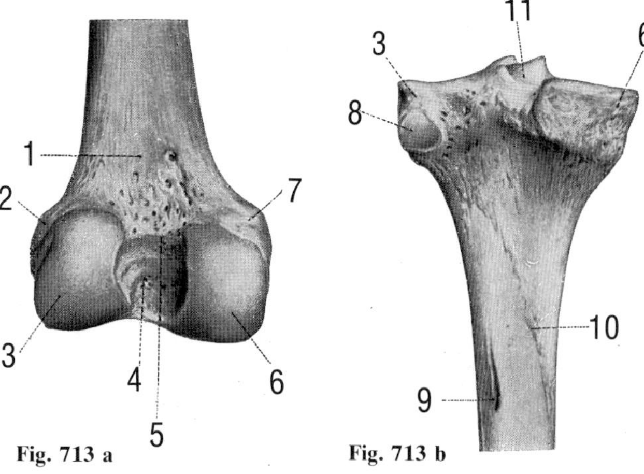

Fig. 713 a

Fig. 713 b

1 Popliteal surface
2 Lateral femoral epicondylus, rough
3 Lateral femoral condylus
4 Intercondyloid fossa of femur
5 Intercondyloid line of femur
6 Medial femoral condylus
7 Medial femoral epicondylus
8 Articular surface for fibula
9 Nutritive foramen
10 Line for soleus muscle
11 Intercondyloid eminence of tibia

Fig. 713 (from *Sobotta-Becher,* 17th Edition).

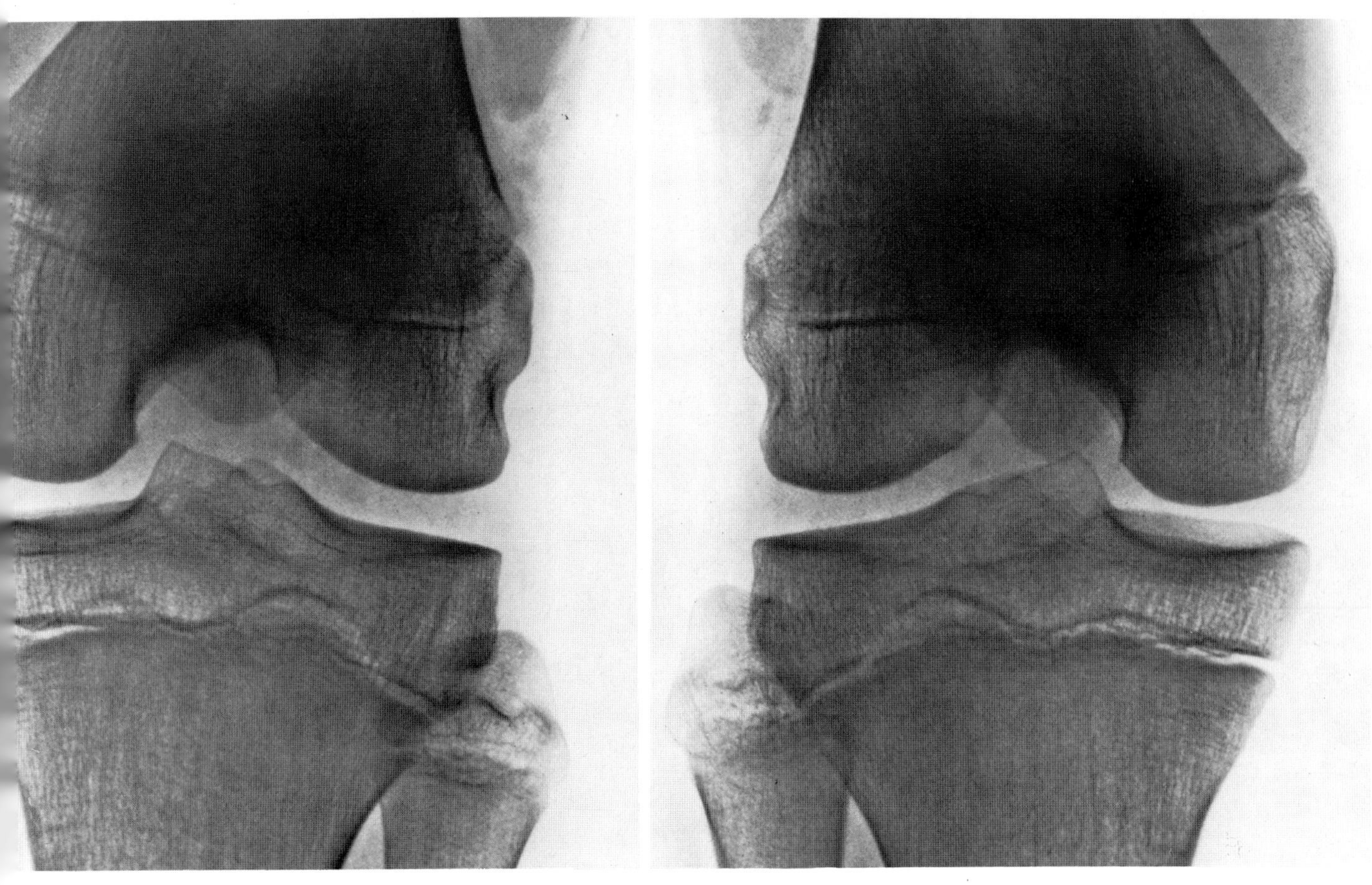

Fig. 714 a

Fig. 714 b

Fig. 714. Posteroanterior radiograph of both bent knee joints, for comparison. For projection see Fig. 715. With this projection one achieves under comparable conditions the isolated demonstration of the femoral condyles, as well as an unequivocal evaluation of the whole tibial articular surface, including the intercondyloid eminence.

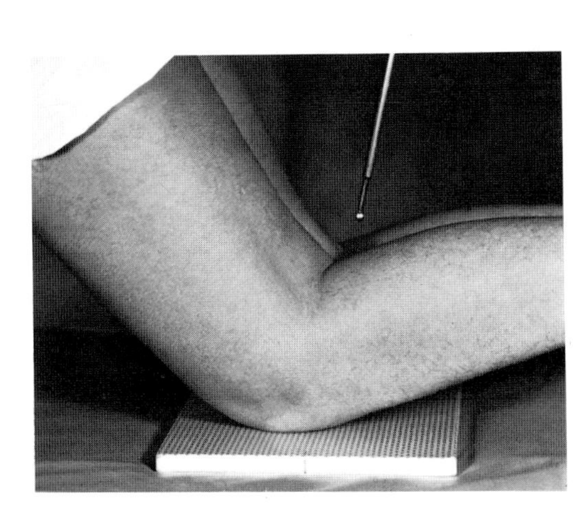

Fig. 715. The anterior surface of the knee joints lies on the cassette, and both legs are bent in the joint by about 70°. The central ray is aimed between the femoral condyles.

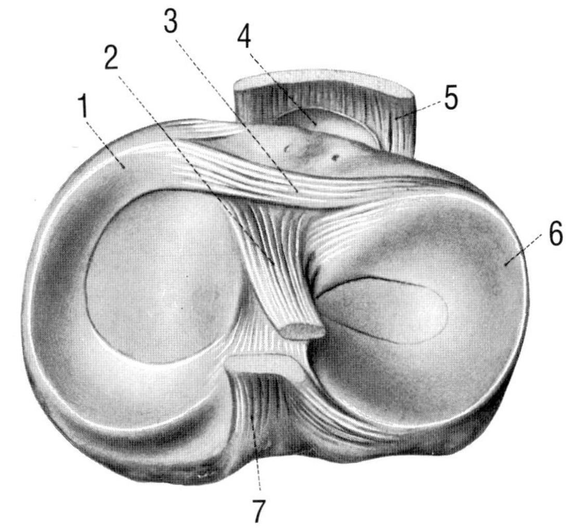

Fig. 716. Tibial condyles with both menisci and the cruciate ligaments of the knee (from *Sobotta-Becher,* 17th Edition).

1 Medial meniscus
2 Anterior cruciate ligament
3 Transverse ligament
4 Bursa infrapatellaris profunda
5 Ligamentum patellae
6 Lateral meniscus
7 Posterior cruciate ligament

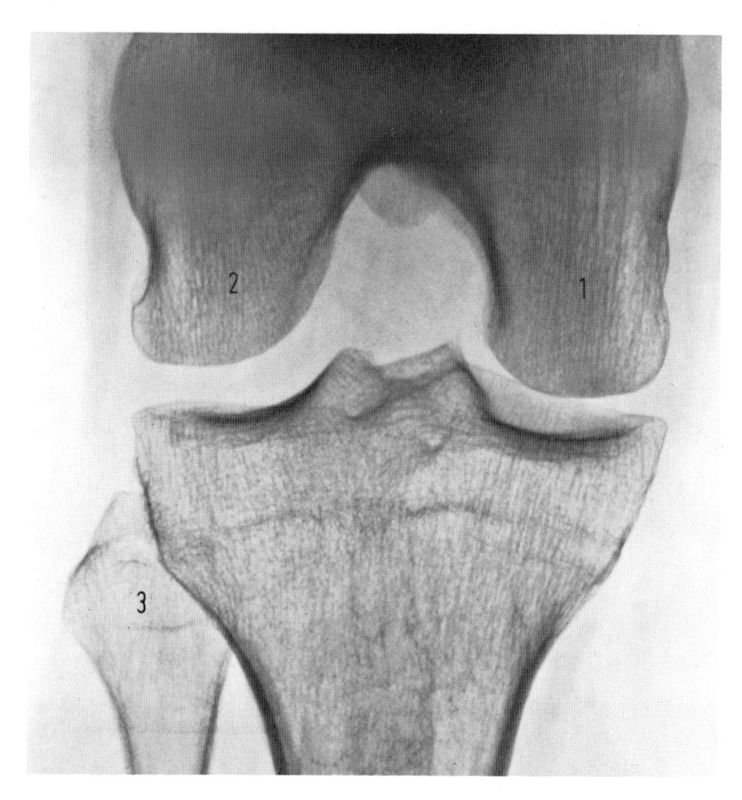

1 Medial femoral condyle
2 Lateral femoral condyle
3 Head of fibula

Fig. 717. Knee joint, caudoanteroposterior, for demonstration of the intercondyloid fossa of the femur, after *Frik* (see also *Kliemann*). For projection see Fig. 718. A flexible cassette is placed into the popliteal fossa. The arrow shows the direction of the central ray. This radiograph promotes the demonstration of injuries, loose bodies in the joint, foreign bodies and ossifications of soft tissues.

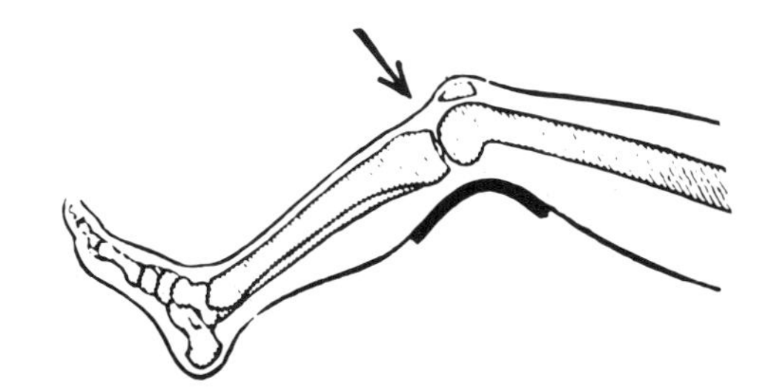

Fig. 718. One can obtain a similar possibility for demonstration with *Schoen's* bridge, the casette lying on the table (*H. Schoen,* 1960).

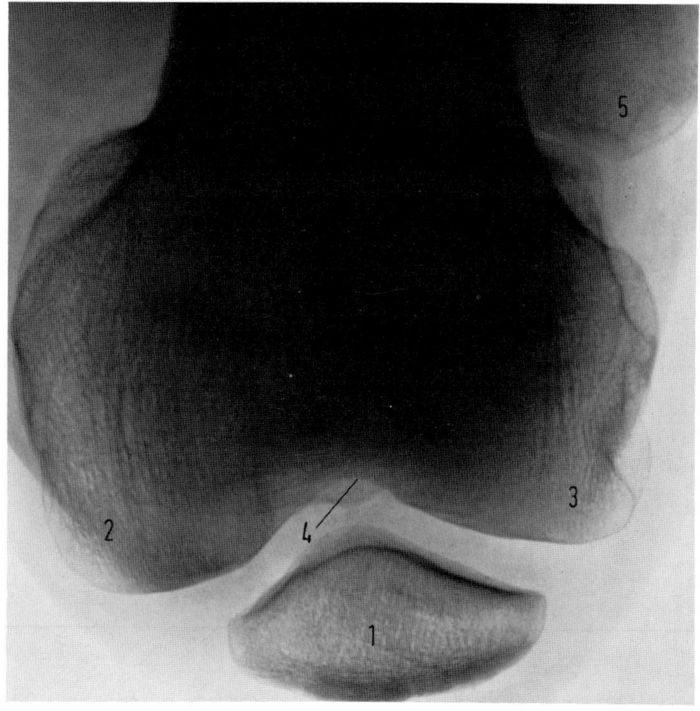

1 Patella
2 Medial femoral condylus
3 Lateral femoral condylus
4 Tibia
5 Head of fibula

Fig. 719. Patella, axial. Patient prone. For projection see Fig. 720. The central ray is aimed vertically onto the patella (↘). This projection gives good information on structure and articular surfaces of the patella.

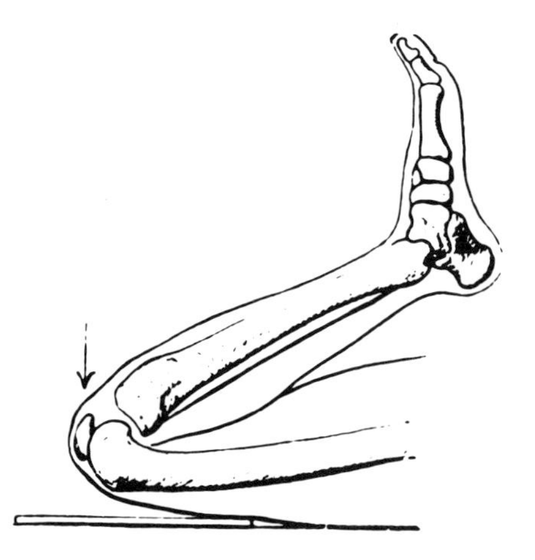

Fig. 720

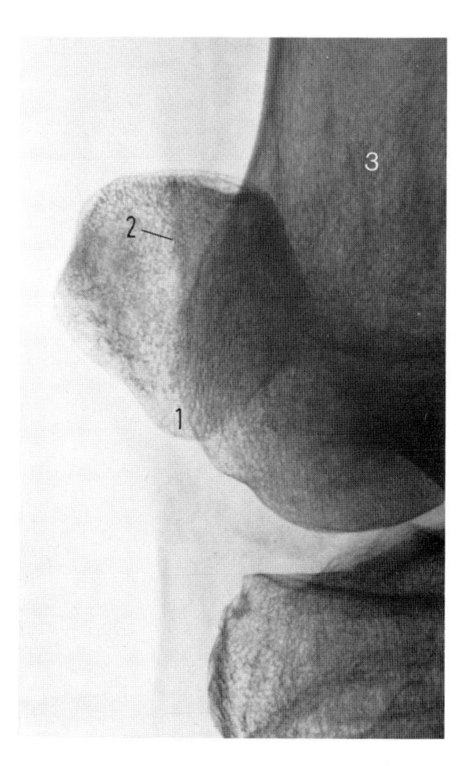

Fig. 721. Patella, fibuloposteroanterior (see Fig. 722). Very often the patella is so mobile that it can be dislocated far lateral and kept fixed in this position by compression from the popliteal fossa.

1 Apex of patella
2 Contours of the main mass of soft tissues, from where the patella had been pressed outward, covered only by a skin fold.
3 Femur

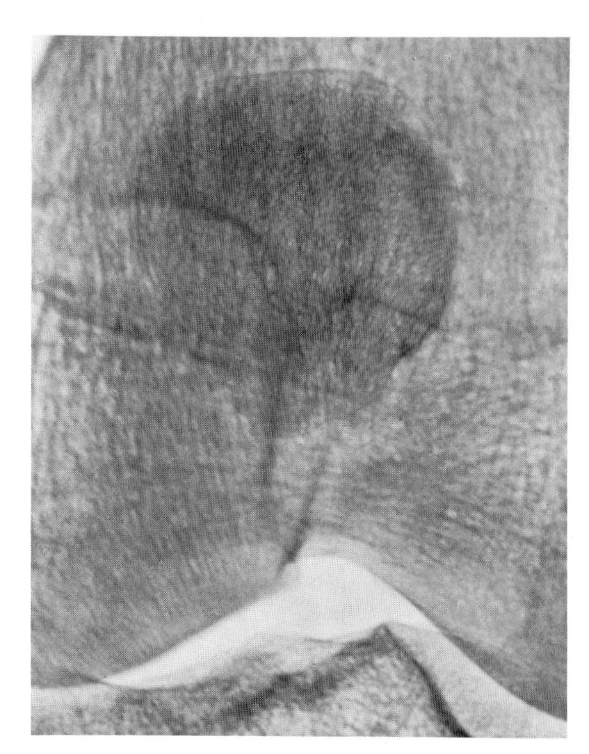

Fig. 723. Patella, posteroanterior contact radiograph. By means of the contact radiograph, the film-distant structures become blurred and the film-near patella is traced more distinctly (apparent hyperplasia).

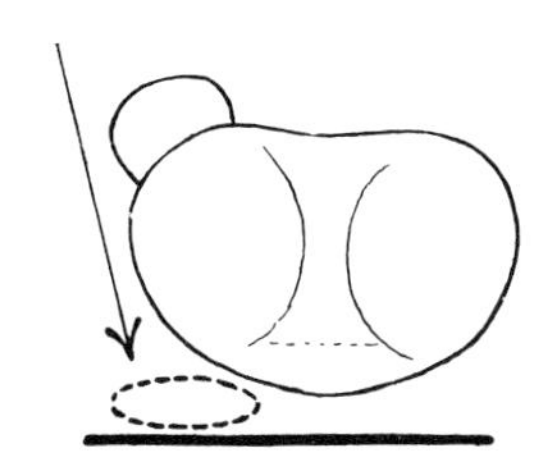

Fig. 722

While hyperplasias of the patella are always the consequence of pathological processes (*Paget*'s disease or inflammatory processes exclusively in the patella), bilateral aplasia is invariably combined with other malformations of the skeleton, sometimes in hereditary diseases. In bilateral hypoplasia, too, hereditary diseases play a special role, known as osteoonychodysplasia (see p. 215) (dysplasias of pelvis, elbow, fingernails and anomalies of pigmentation of the iris).

1 Articular surface of fibula
2 Intercondyloid eminence
3 Nutritive foramen
4 Posterior surface
5 Lateral surface

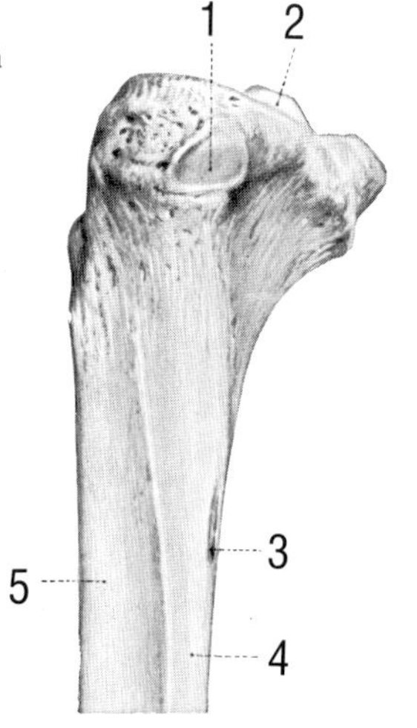

Fig. 724. Proximal end of tibia (from *Sobotta-Becher,* 17th Edition).

1 Popliteal surface
2 Medial epicondylus
3 Intercondyloid fossa
4 Lateral condylus
5 Medial condylus

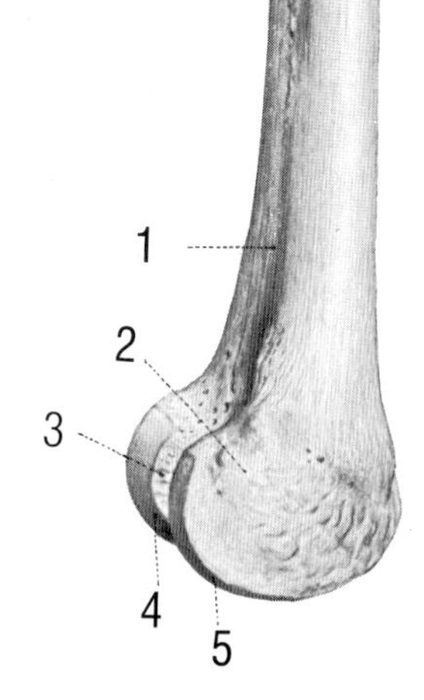

Fig. 725. Distal end of femur (from *Sobotta-Becher,* 17th Edition).

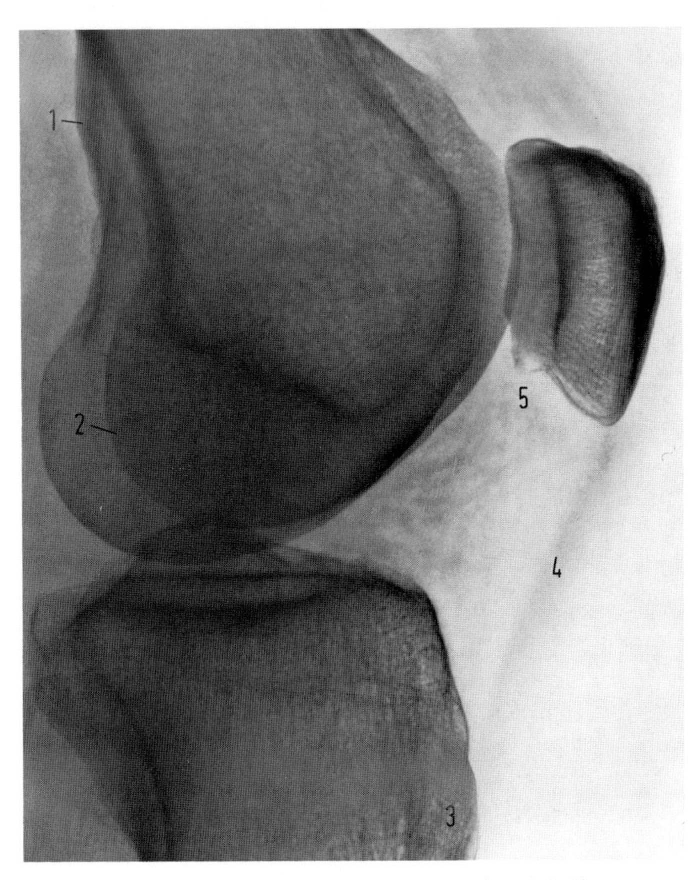

Fig. 726. Knee joint, dorsofibulotibial. Demonstration of the ligamentum patellae. For projection see Fig. 728.

1 Tubercle for origin of the medial head of the gastrocnemius muscle *(Grashey)*
2 Lateral femoral condylus
3 Tuberosity of tibia (see Fig. 727, 24-year-old male); may protrude still more and have a radial structure, like the greater tubercle of the humerus
4 Ligamentum patellae
5 Osteocartilaginous exostosis of the patella

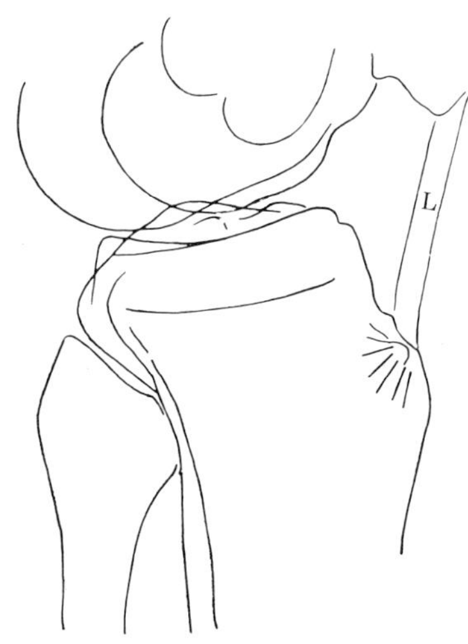

Fig. 727. L = ligamentum patellae.

Fig. 728

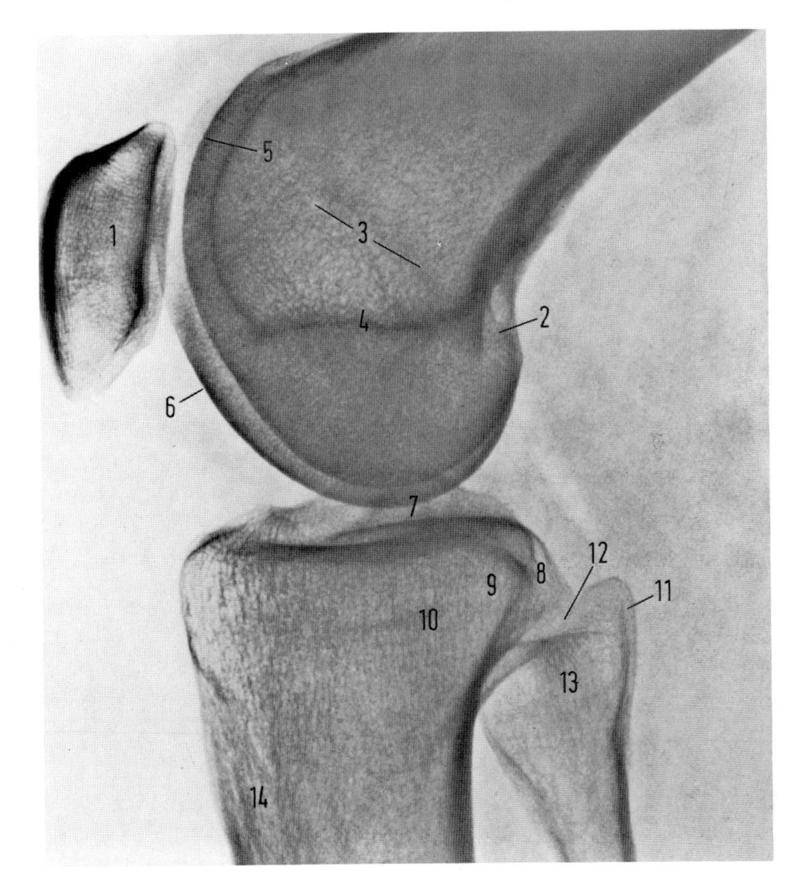

Fig. 729. Knee joint, tibiofibular. For projection, see Fig. 730.

1 Patella
2 Intercondyloid fossa of femur
3 Epiphyseal line
4 Inner contour of condyle, against the intercondyloid fossa (the adjacent epicondylus may also be included in this characteristic line)
5 Lateral femoral condyle
6 Medial femoral condyle
7 Intercondyloid eminence of tibia
8 Lateral tibial condylus, recognizable by its articulation with the fibula
9 Medial tibial condylus
10 Epiphyseal scar
11 Apex of head of fibulus
12 Tibiofibular articulation
13 Head of fibula
14 Tuberosity of tibia

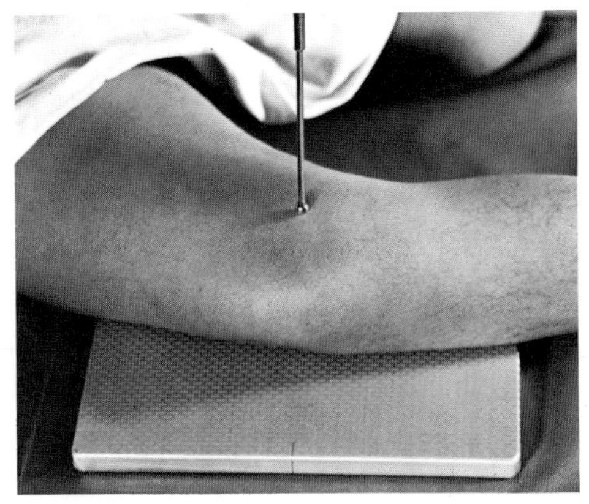

Fig. 730

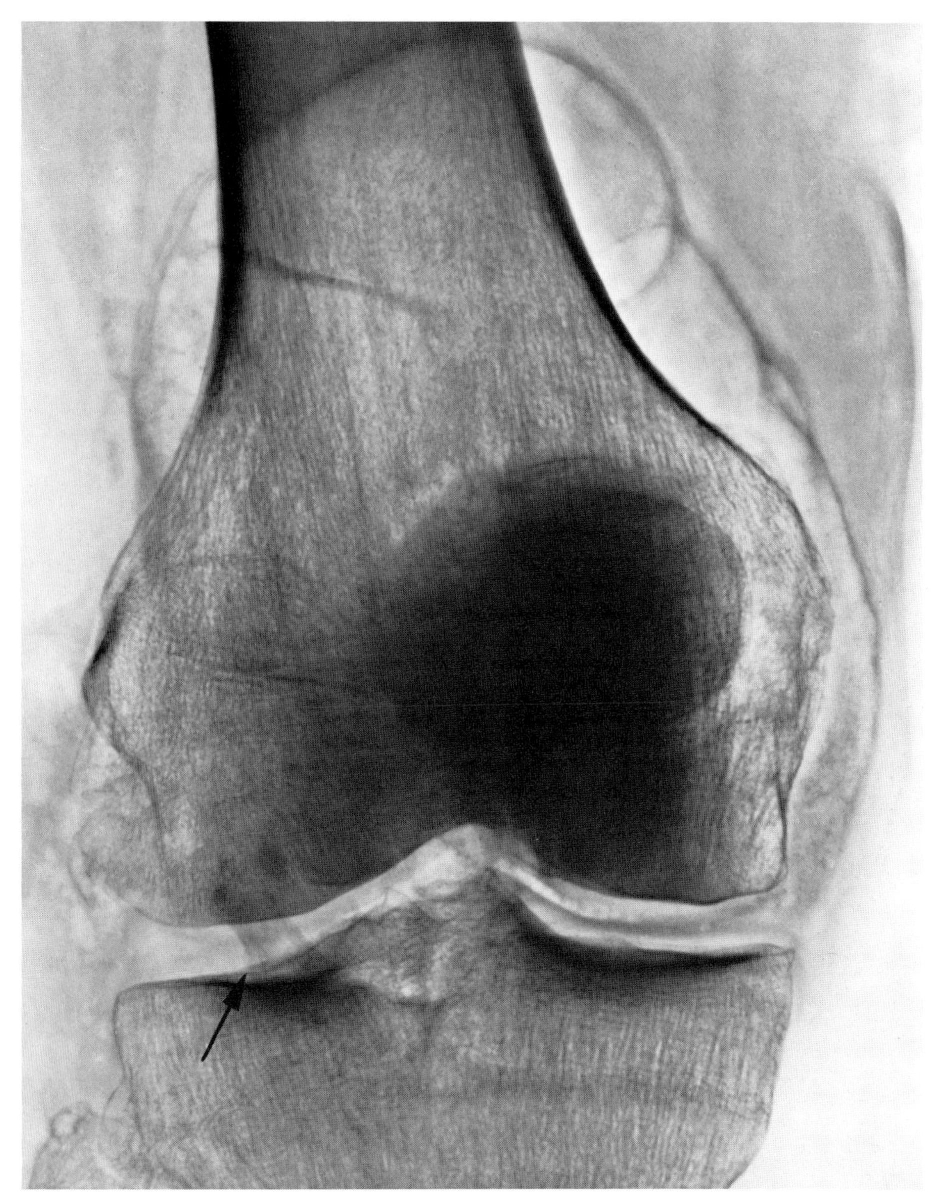

Fig. 731. **Right knee joint, anteroposterior. Double-contrast presentation,** effected by injection of 30 ccm air and 5 ml of a highly concentrated, triiodized water-soluble contrast medium, according to *Oberholzer,* after anesthesia of the point of injection with 1% procaine hydrochloride. A periarticular ossification (↗) is present.

Because of invisibility of the sensitive and vulnerable menisci and cruciate ligaments, **arthrography of the knee** is the most frequently indicated method of demonstration of joints *(Thiemann, Fischer* and *Mollowitz).*

For the puncture, one ought to use canulae as fine as possible after having withdrawn any exudate with a suitably wide canula. Most stringent asepsis is required. This method is excellently suitable for showing the menisci. It is recommended, according to the experience of the injector, to use either injection with air only or with a positive contrast medium, or to apply the double-contrast method.

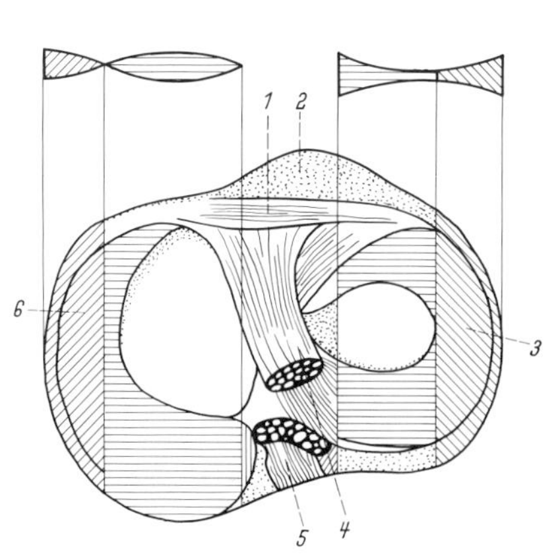

1 Transverse ligament
2 Tuberosity of tibia
3 Lateral meniscus
4 Anterior cruciate ligament
5 Posterior cruciate ligament
6 Medial meniscus

Fig. 732. Projection of the menisci (after *Laarmann*).

In 1970 *Kamprad* and *Hasert* showed how, through combination of arthrography and tomography with blurring in several dimensions, the method can be extended and enlarged, thus providing improved diagnostic possibilities, especially for smaller lesions of the cruciate ligaments.

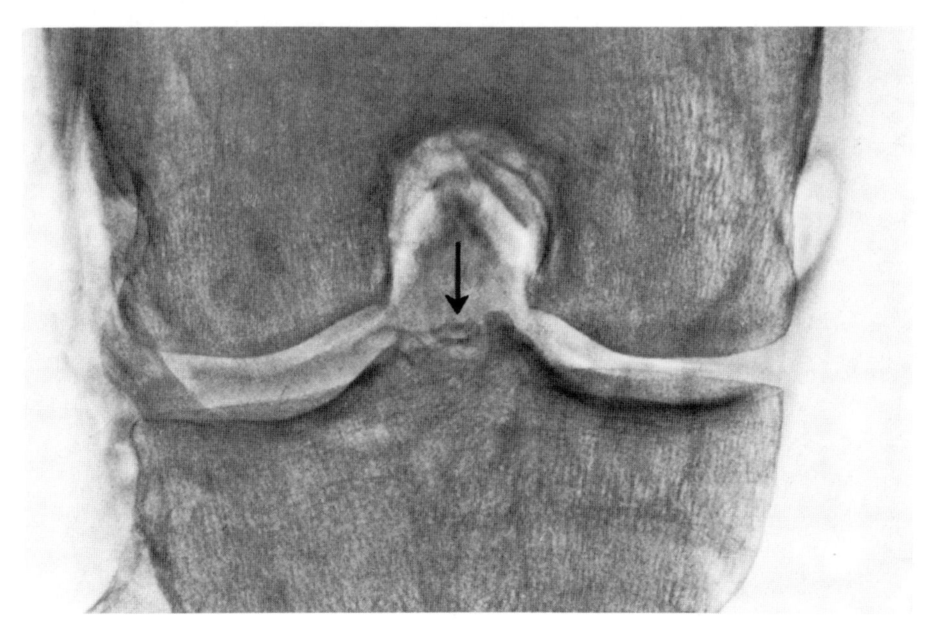

Fig. 733. Right knee joint, after *Frik* (for projection, see description of Fig. 717). Double-contrast demonstration of the cruciate ligaments of the knee, in the same patient as in Fig. 731. The intercondyloid eminence (↓) has been split off due to an old accident (the patient had been a ballet dancer). Additional damage to the collateral ligaments caused hypermobility.

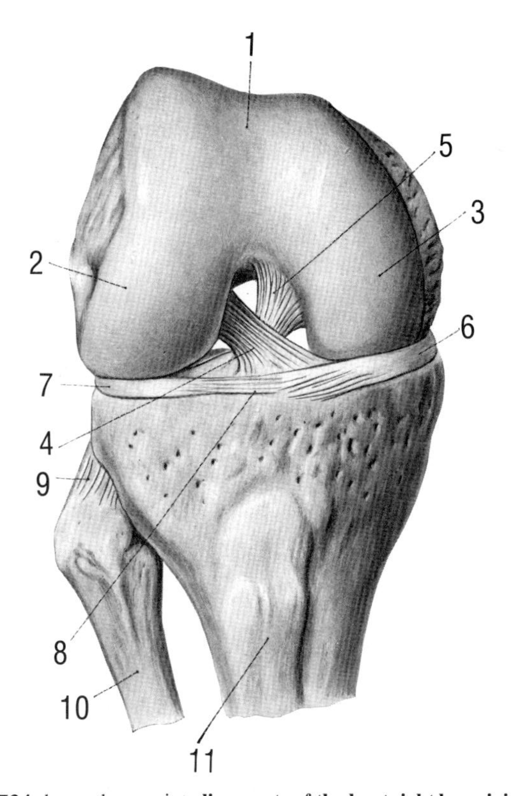

Fig. 734 shows the cruciate **ligaments of the bent right knee joint** (from *Sobotta-Becher,* 17th Edition).

1 Patellar surface of femur
2 Lateral femoral condyle
3 Medial femoral condyle
4 Anterior cruciate ligament
5 Posterior cruciate ligament
6 Medial meniscus
7 Lateral meniscus
8 Transverse ligament
9 Fibular collateral ligament
10 Fibula
11 Tuberosity of tibia

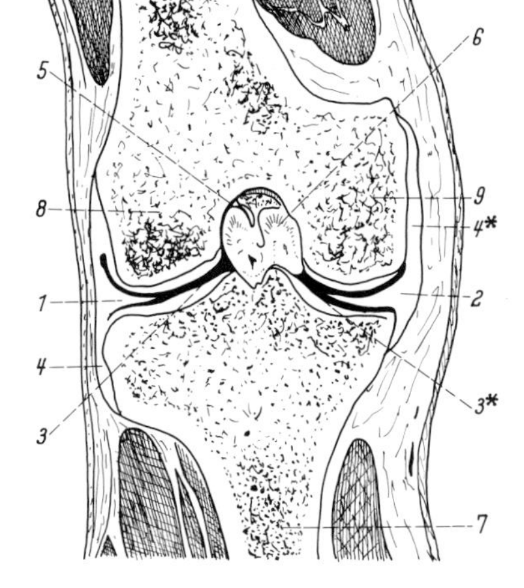

Fig. 735 shows the **fixation of the menisci to the capsule of the knee joint.** Frontal section to the stretched right knee joint (after *Corning*).

1 Lateral meniscus
2 Medial meniscus
3, 3* Articular space
4, 4* Capsule of the joint
5 Anterior cruciate ligament
6 Posterior cruciate ligament
7 Tibia
8 Lateral femoral condyle
9 Medial femoral condyle

Figs. 736 and 737. Serial meniscography according to the double-contrast method, after *van de Berg* and *Crèvecoeur,* (see also Figs. 731, 757 a, b). *Bessler* explains in detail the diagnostic possibilities of double-contrast arthrography.

The patient lies prone on the table; the calf is held free in the air by means of a padded roll placed under the thigh above the knee. Controlled by a fluoroscopy, the menisci are photographed slightly tangentially in series with the corresponding rotation of the leg into the positions shown in Fig. 738. ↓ = tear in the lateral meniscus, Fig. 737).

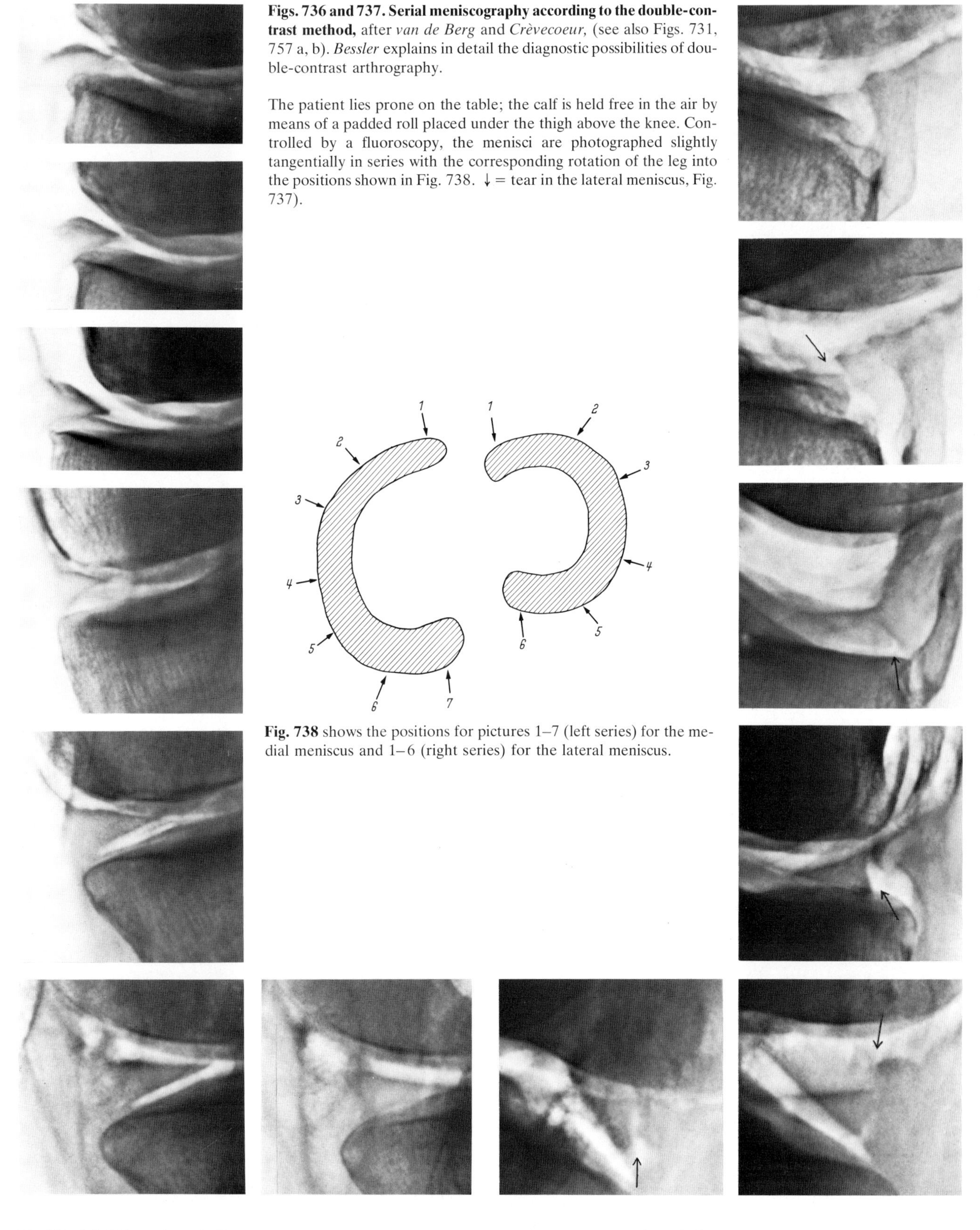

Fig. 738 shows the positions for pictures 1–7 (left series) for the medial meniscus and 1–6 (right series) for the lateral meniscus.

Fig. 736. Medial meniscus 1–7.

Fig. 737. Lateral meniscus 1–6.

Variants and Sources of Diagnostic Error of the Knee Joint and Calf*

To Figs. 739 a and b:

150 Fabella, most frequent sesamoid bone found in the lateral head of the gastrocnemious muscle; becomes visible only during puberty. In deforming arthrosis it occasionally becomes deformed; on an anteroposterior view it may appear like an islet of compact tissue (Fig. 774). Fractures and chondromalacia of the fabella may occur.

151 Lines of cleft in case of patella biparta (Figs. 758-761 and 1176). The smaller fragment is often shifted slightly dorsally. Care should be taken not to mistake it for a fracture or a patella duplex (see Fig. 762). The borders of the patella biparta are more regular; those of a fracture are irregular, with sharp edges. In cases of patella biparta with local osteochondronecrosis, one sees crateriform clefts.

152 Marginal bulge at the patella (see Figs. 712, 731). The double contour is caused by the visibility of its anterior and posterior edge. Confusion with healed chondromalacia should be avoided.

153 Roughness at the lateral femoral (popliteal sulcus) and tibial (insertion of the iliotibial tract) condyles (Fig. 712). During extension the tendon of the popliteal muscle clings to the popliteal sulcus. If the roughness is unilateral and without arthrotic changes, it points to *Rauber*'s sign for torn menisci (see Fig. 740).

153* Tertiary intercondyloid tubercle (Fig. 776); it is a tubercle in front of the intercondyloid eminence. Part of the anterior cruciate ligament may insert there *(Politzer* and *Pick).* It is not an arthrotic spike!

154 Ossification within a meniscus (Fig. 763), primarily due to advanced age and is not post-traumatic. Secondary post-traumatic calcifications may occur, especially in juveniles after injury to a meniscus. They occur throughout the meniscus or as foci, where the differential diagnosis against a loose body may become difficult. Already 3–4 months after an accident, secondary calcification may become visible. In cases of a wobbly joint, one can obtain a spontaneous demonstration of the vacuum phenomenon at this spot (= *Fick*'s sign, described for the first time at a carpal joint of a finger).

154* Quarternary intercondyloid tubercle. There is a small spur for insertion of the posterior cruciate ligament. See also *Teichert.* Not to be mistaken for osteoarthrosis.

155 Osteochondrosis dissecans; occurs mainly medially, less frequently laterally. Its most frequent localization is the knee joint. In about 20% of cases it occurs bilaterally, especially at the femoral condyles. Therefore, constitutional and endocrine causes are also likely (Fig. 765).

155* Spur-like exostosis at a typical spot (Fig. 768); therefore, it is not post-traumatic but may sometimes cause ostitic pains

155** Apophysis of the anterior lateral articular surface of the tibia *(Teichert),* but this is questionable. Could it be an enostoma or an islet of compact tissue?

156 Lines of growth, a consequence of growth disturbances (decrease in height, increased density, wavy cartilaginous joint) of the epiphysis, as they can also be observed in the distal epiphysis *(Hohmann et al.).* They are also called "intermediary bands" (Fig. 769), e.g., in sprue, *Möller-Barlow* disease, rickets, lead poisoning.

157 Spur at the upper margin of patella (ossified insertion of the quadriceps tendon). In cases of overwork it becomes visible as early as the 30th year of life, but normally only after the 60th year. Apex (and base) of the patella are often the seat of *Larsen-Johansson*'s osteopathy of the juvenile patella (see Fig. 761). A combination with *Osgood-Schlatter* disease is possible.

157* Osteocartilaginous exostosis of the patella (osteochondroma) (see also Fig. 726 and *Maurer*); this localization is rare. If the exostosis occurs bilaterally, it is a variant. Malignant degeneration might be possible.

158 Ossified insertion of the ligamentum patellae *(Feistmann-Lutterbeck, Lossen;*see also Fig. 741). It should not be mistaken for a persistent nucleus of the patellar apex (see Fig. 761). Ossification of the ligamentum patellae is always pathological (local nutritional disturbance, inflammation in periosteum and bones).

159 Calcified bursa (Fig. 774). Calcifications in prepatellar, infrapatellar and more distal smaller bursae of knee are post-traumatic (so-called housemaid's knee).

159* Normal zone of increased radiolucency (see Figs. 729 and 745), apparently atrophic but often due to overexposure

160 *Ludloff*'s spot, a calcium-rare zone *(Ludloff, Ravelli),* seen on lateral view in children and juveniles, non-pathological (see Fig. 1165 and 1168 a)

161 Dorsal supracondylar exostosis of femur *(Grashey),* after avulsion of the origin of the medial head of the gastrocnemius muscle (see also Fig. 726)

161* Not quite constant bordering groove on the medial condyle, as a distinguishing mark between the two condyles *(Ravelli);* see also *Teichert*

162 Normal roughness on the posterior surface of the medial tibial condyle; insertion of the semimembranosus muscle (Fig. 770 b)

163 Bone infarct *(Teichert);* see Figs. 777 and 778. Infarct of medulla; necrosis of infarct with later calcification, caused by embolism on the basis of capillary formation of thrombi, endocarditis or arteritis

164 *Stieda-Pellegrini* shadow, a post-traumatically ossified insertion of soft tissues; may also be a parosteotic neoplastic bone formation (see Figs. 756 and 757). An important fact for expert opinion is that secondary ossifications may often be visible as early as 2–6 weeks after a trauma; in that case the calciferous density will increase with time.

164* "Clothes-hanger" exostosis (Aufhängerexostose) (Fig. 767). These are solitary cartilaginous exostoses, as in 155*. They arise near the epiphyseal lines, but never after trauma.

165 Periarthritis calcarea of the knee (Fig. 731). This is an analogue to scapulohumeral periarthritis. Its genesis may be inflammatory, degenerative, traumatic or microtraumatic.

166 Interosseus margin (interosseus membrane of the calf); see Fig. 712 and Fig. 752. Manifestations of pseudoperiostitis occur mainly at the concave margins of bones *(Grashey).*

166* Pronounced hump of the tibial tuberosity (Figs. 764 a and 772 b). With slight external rotation it may be projected into the interosseus space and cause the accompanying shadow *(Ravelli, Birkner).*

166** Nutritive canal, widened in cases of varicosis *(Saupe)* (Fig. 1192 b)

167* Hollow depression in fibula, caused by thinning of the cortex, simulating defect

p Pseudoperiostitis (see Fig. 712)

n Above the center of the joint: nutritive canals which have been thought to be smallish osteomyelitic foci

o Secondary osteoma of capsule (Fig. 766)

---

* The numbers in bold type are also found (or only found) on the lateral view.

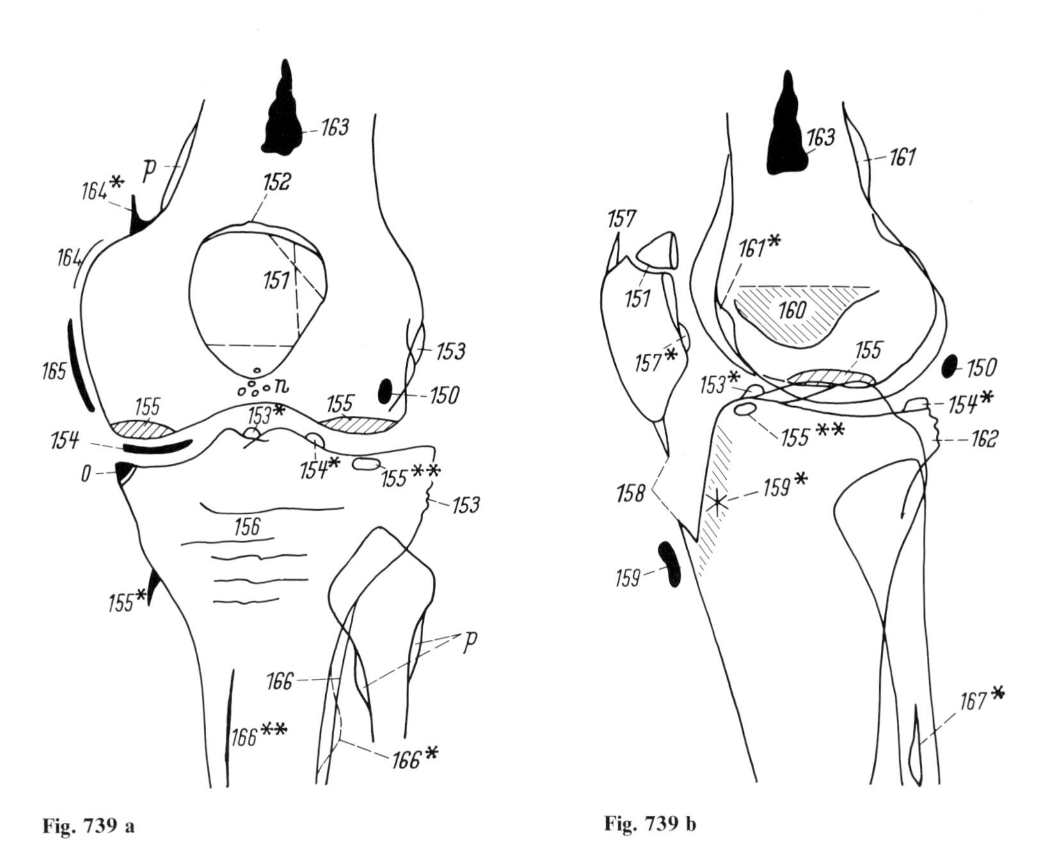

Fig. 739 a

Fig. 739 b

Fig. 739. Variants and sources of diagnostic error of knee joint and calf.

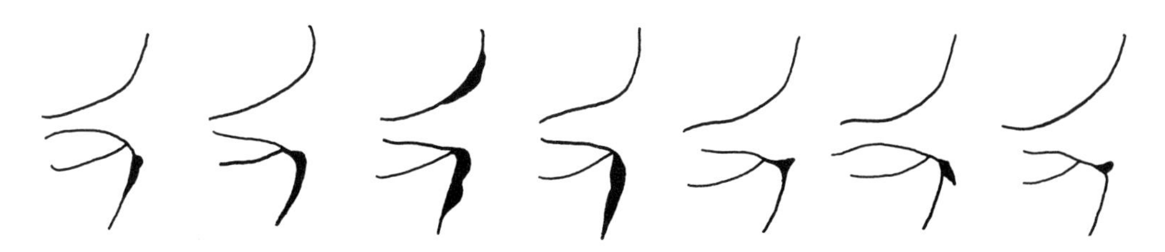

Fig. 740. Shapes of Rauber's sign *(Rauber's* console), after *Barucha. Barucha* found periostal thickenings and scleroses at the inner and outer sides of the tibia, respectively, in about 90% of medial and about 80% of lateral meniscus lesions, which were confirmed by surgery.

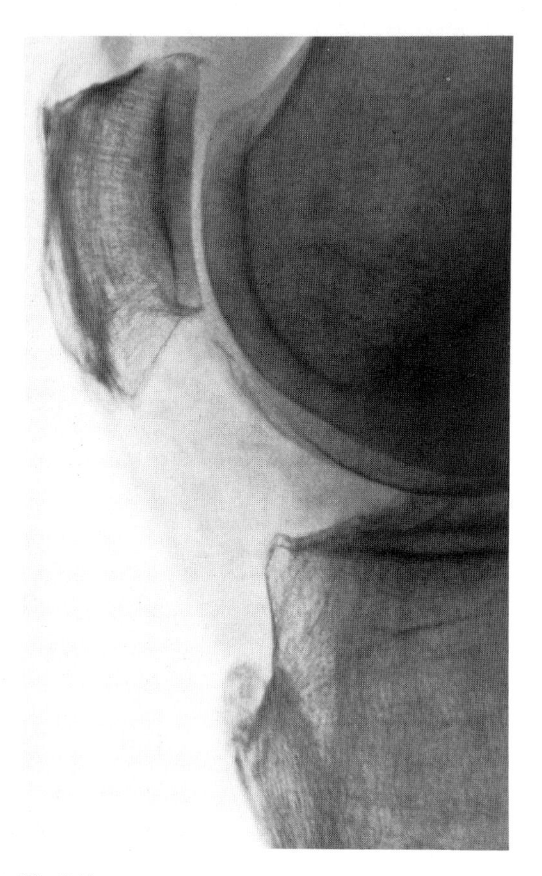

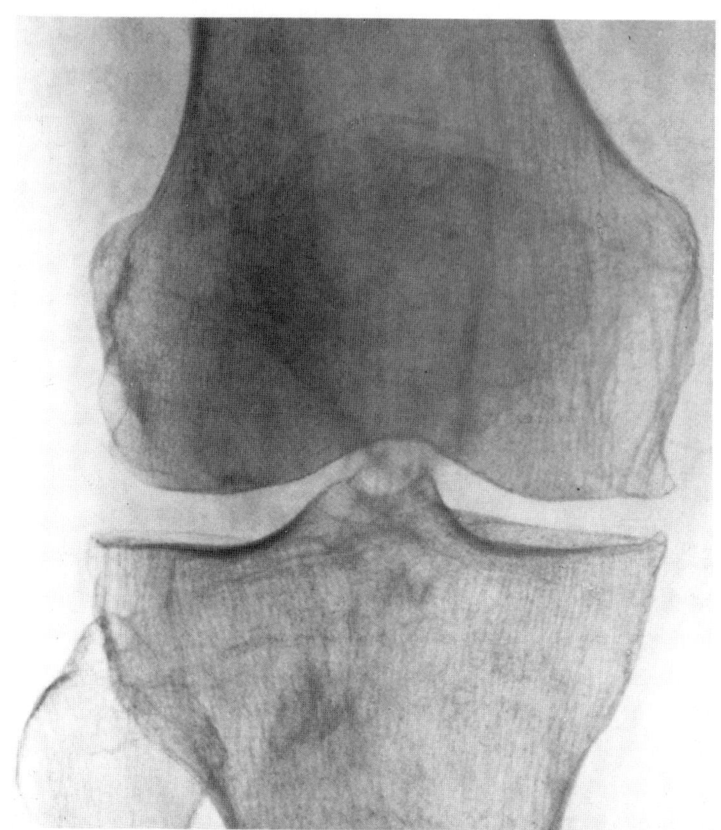

Fig. 741 a **Fig. 741 b**

Fig. 741. Ossified insertion of the ligamentum patellae. Calcifications of insertions of tendons or ligaments are often preceded by traumata (cf. Figs. 745, 746, 757 and their text). However, no previous trauma was noted in this case of a 68-year-old female. From such ossifications of tendon insertions one must differentiate the so-called "pophyseal nuclei," such as the one which can be seen in Fig. 742. In the present case, this calcification of the insertion of the tendon simulates on the anteroposterior view (Fig. 741 b) an islet of compact tissue in the head of the tibia. Regarding ossifications at this site see also *Feistmann-Lutterbeck* and *Lossen*. Furthermore, one must differentiate the state after *Osgood-Schlatter* disease in adults. *Laczay* and *Csapó* trace calcification of the ligamentum patellae exclusively to previous traumatic damages, e.g., *Osgood-Schlatter* necrosis of the tibial apophysis.

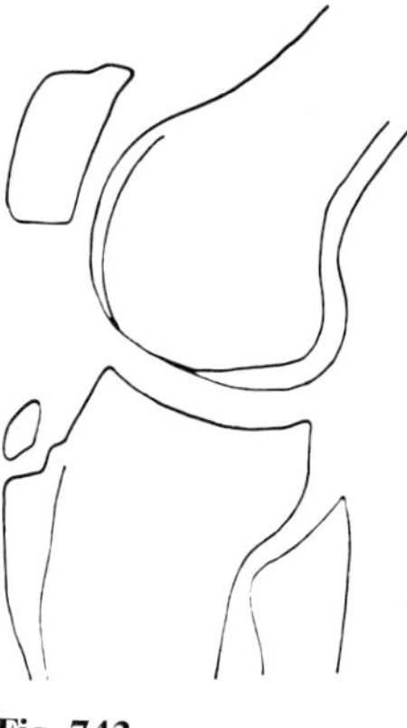

Fig. 742

Fig. 742 shows a not-infrequent **isolated bone shadow in the insertion of the ligamentum patellae** which may be found in the case of a much protruding tuberosity of the tibia. This is neither pathological nor a certain effect of *Schlatter*'s disease, but may be traced to an atypical or disturbed ossification during adolescence, as with other "persistent apophyseal nuclei." Regarding disturbances of ossification at the tibia and patella, see *Petersen, Heuck* and *Schumann*.

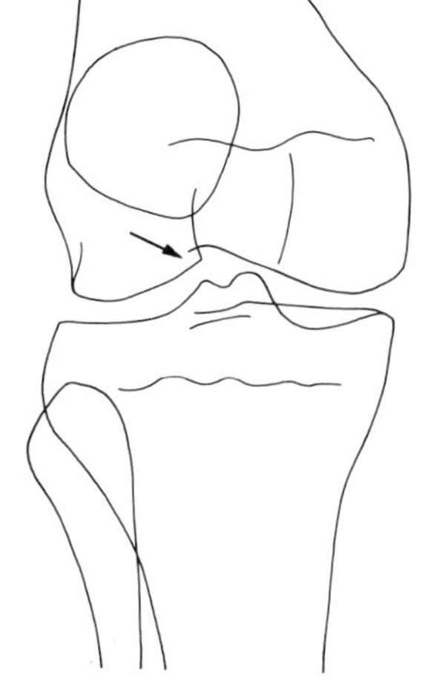

Fig. 743 shows an apparent **step formation in the joint** (↘). This is nothing but the result of an oblique projection, which can be recognized from the unequal breadth of the femoral condyles and also from the shift of the patellar shadow.

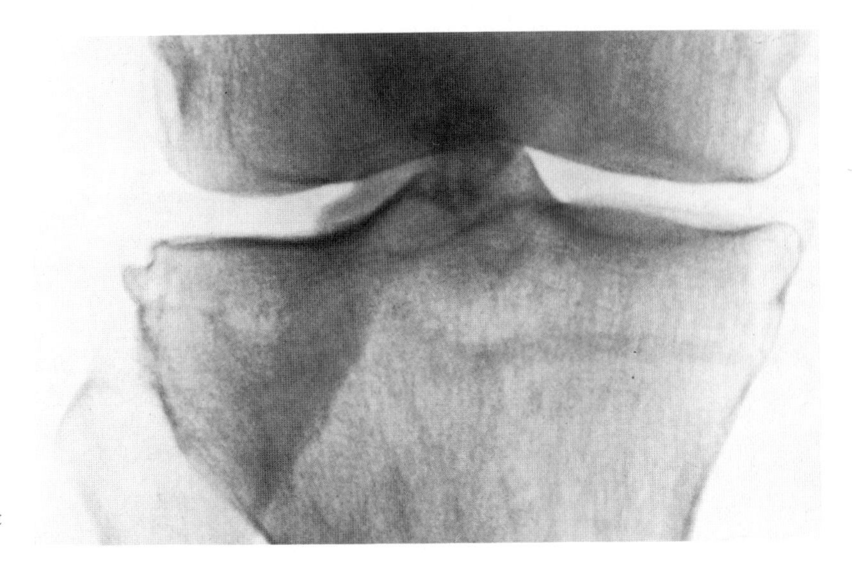

Fig. 744. Calcification of the cruciate ligament (from *Seyss*).

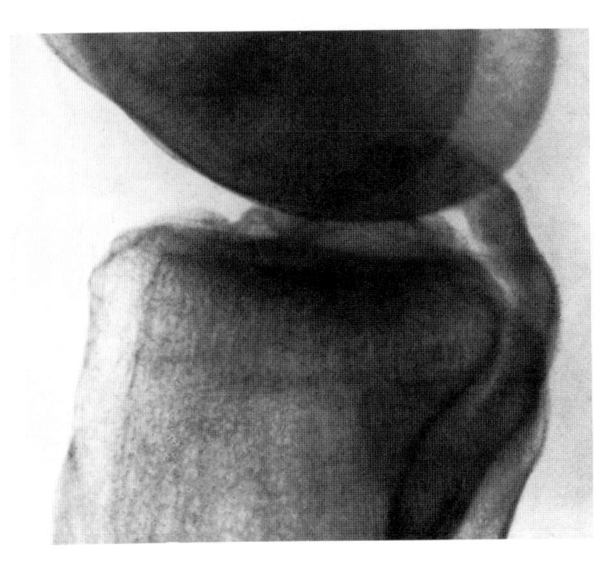

Fig. 745. Calcification of the ligamentum patellae (from *Seyss*). This lateral view shows, in addition, a sharply defined band of increased radiolucency at the anterior surface of the tibia, similar to the one in Fig. 746. It occurs in lean persons because this part is thin and does not lie on the cassette.

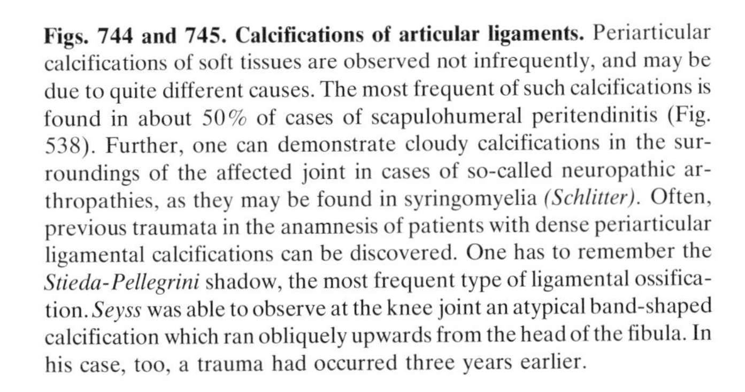

Figs. 744 and 745. Calcifications of articular ligaments. Periarticular calcifications of soft tissues are observed not infrequently, and may be due to quite different causes. The most frequent of such calcifications is found in about 50% of cases of scapulohumeral peritendinitis (Fig. 538). Further, one can demonstrate cloudy calcifications in the surroundings of the affected joint in cases of so-called neuropathic arthropathies, as they may be found in syringomyelia *(Schlitter)*. Often, previous traumata in the anamnesis of patients with dense periarticular ligamental calcifications can be discovered. One has to remember the *Stieda-Pellegrini* shadow, the most frequent type of ligamental ossification. *Seyss* was able to observe at the knee joint an atypical band-shaped calcification which ran obliquely upwards from the head of the fibula. In his case, too, a trauma had occurred three years earlier.

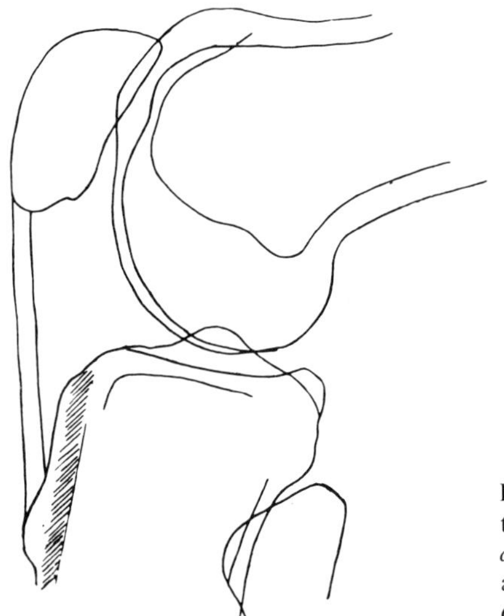

Fig. 746. *Tennef* and *Teichert*, i.a., reported on appearances of ossifications in the posterior cruciate ligament, and *Reisner* found them in the ligamentum patellae. The *Stieda-Pellegrini* shadow becomes visible between the 2nd and 4th weeks after trauma, and after the 3rd month trabecular structures are sometimes recognizable *(Guintoli* and *Chiappa)*.

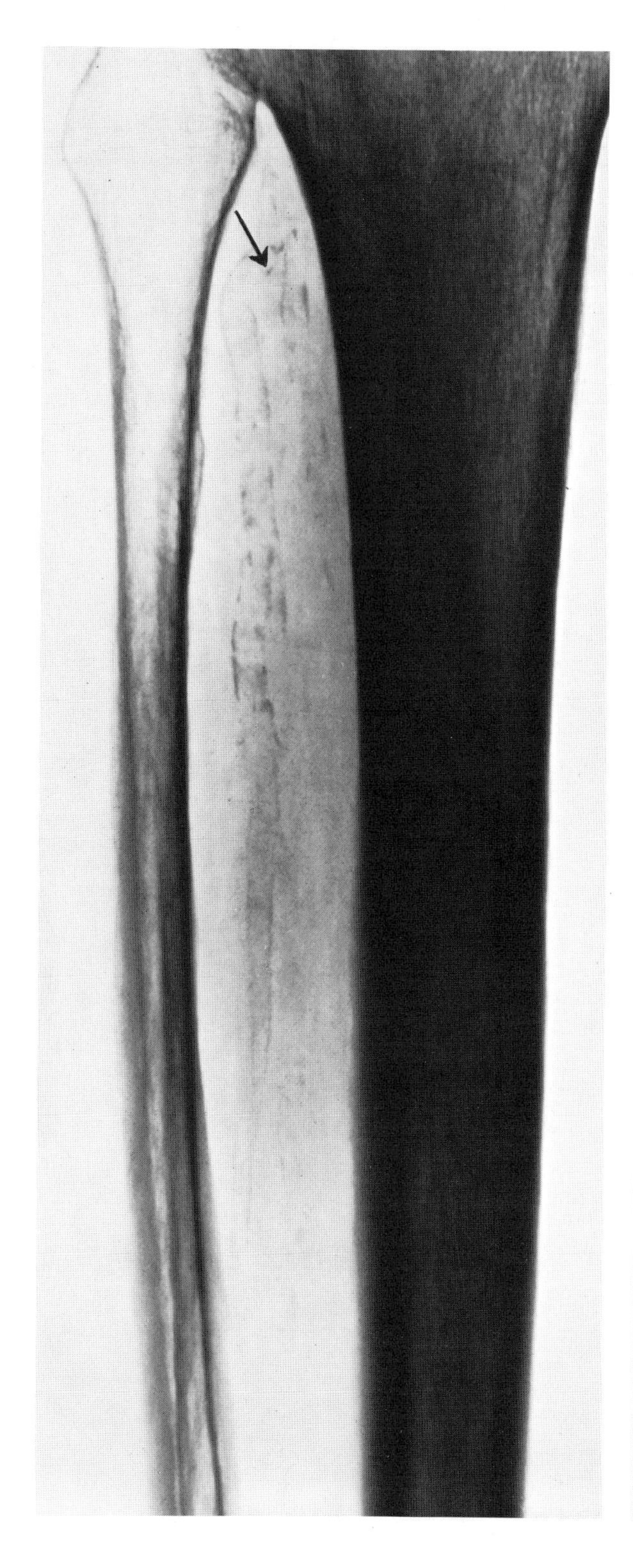

Fig. 747. Posteroanterior radiograph.

Fig. 748. Anteroposterior radiograph.

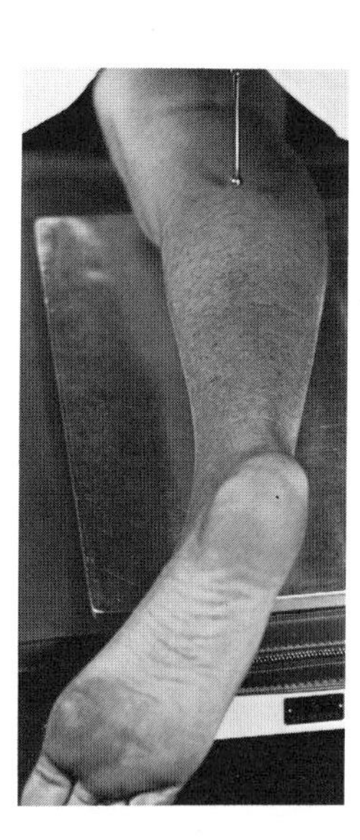

Fig. 749

Figs. 747 and 748. Right calf, interosseus space, posteroanterior (Fig. 747) of a 66-year-old female. (For comparison, the usual anteroposterior technique is shown in Fig. 748.) With this method of focusing (see Fig. 749), the fibula, which, when seen from front, lies slightly behind the tibia, is projected free, and a possibly present periostitis will become well recognizable. This radiograph, for which medium soft rays are recommended, is suitable for demonstration of vascular calcifications of the calf (↘).

Periosteal thickenings in cases of circulatory disturbances are demonstrable mainly in the lower extremities (see *A. Jakob, Seyss).* Such periosteal reactions can be shown not only in disturbances of circulation, on the basis of a complex of varicose symptoms, but also in tuberculosis or tuberculoid disease. *A. Jakab* points out that these periosteal thickenings can be explained exclusively by trophic disturbances due to blood influx (slowed-down circulation). See also *Graumann* and *Braband.*

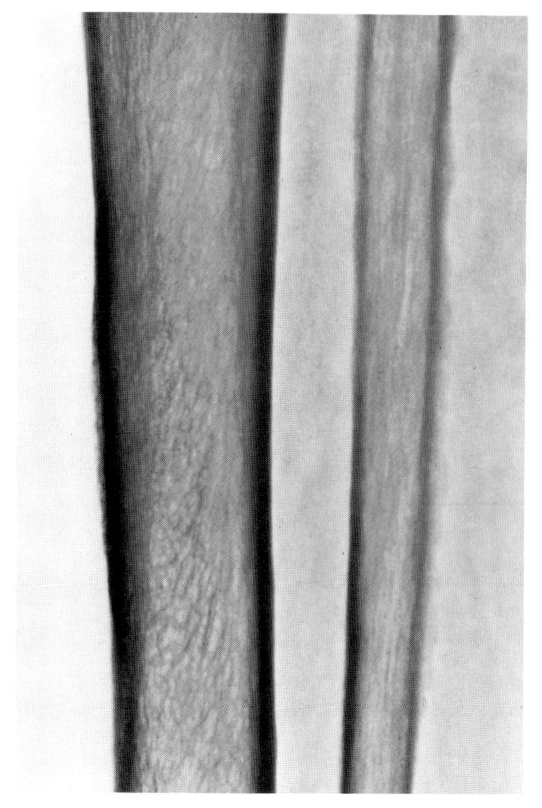

Fig. 750

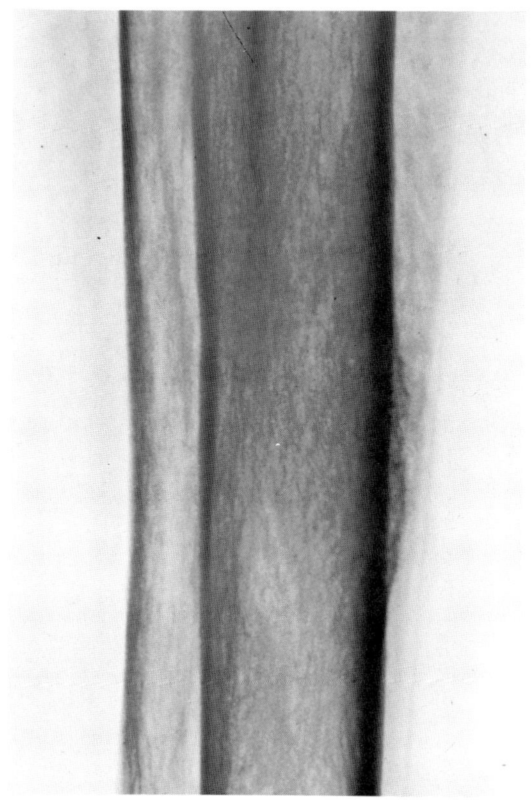

Fig. 751

Figs. 750 and 751. Periosteal reaction to circulatory disturbances. Periosteal proliferations at the middle third of the calf, at the medial and anterior surfaces of the tibia, as well as at the lateral surface of the fibula in a 71-year-old female suffering from circulatory disturbances in this leg.

1 Medial margin
2 Anterior margin
3 Interosseus margins
4 Anterior margin
5 Lateral margin
6 Medial crest

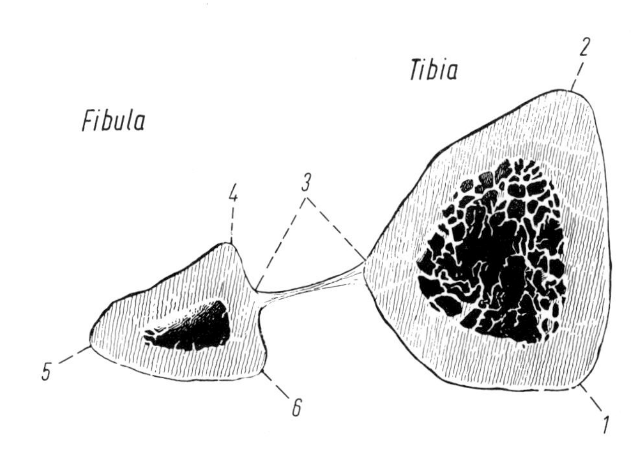

Fig. 752. Fibula and tibia (from *Sobotta-Becher,* 16th Edition). Position of the bones on transverse section (left calf seen from above). Therefore, the radiograph must be taken vertically to the interosseous membrane if a good survey of the interosseus space is required.

Figs. 753–755. Tomographic examination, for exact evaluation of the stability of the fracture. Figs. 753 and 754 show in the two standard planes a 5-month-old fracture of the left calf of a 44-year-old male. *Epstein* and *Sloven,* as well as *Wentzlik,* recommend the tomographic examination of fractures of the extremities even through a plaster case. Thereby, the interfering superimpositions of the plaster can be excluded (if the plaster is not too thick), and an unequivocal evaluation of the position of the fracture and of possible callus formation can be achieved. *Lob,* too, endorses the application of tomography in cases of fracture. *Seyss* further points out the value of tomographic examination with most meticulous focus radiographs of the extremities in inflammatory bone disease.

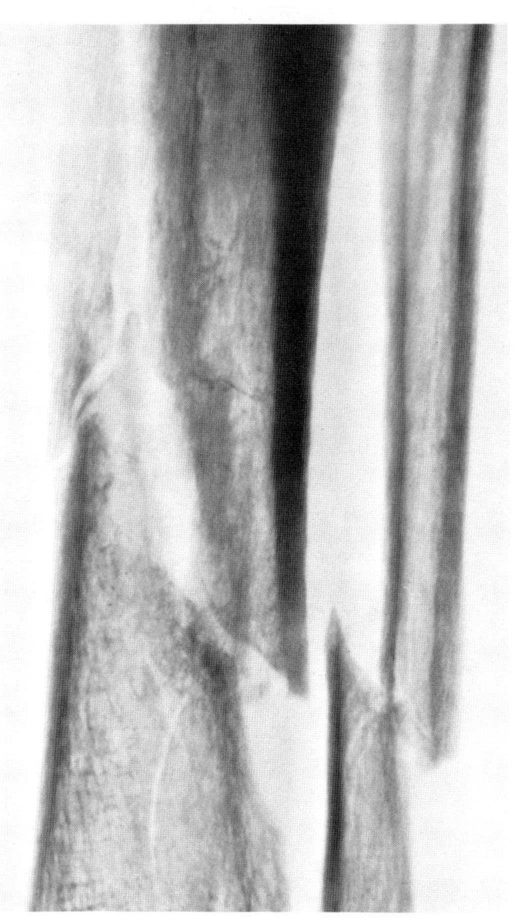

Fig. 753. Anteroposterior view.

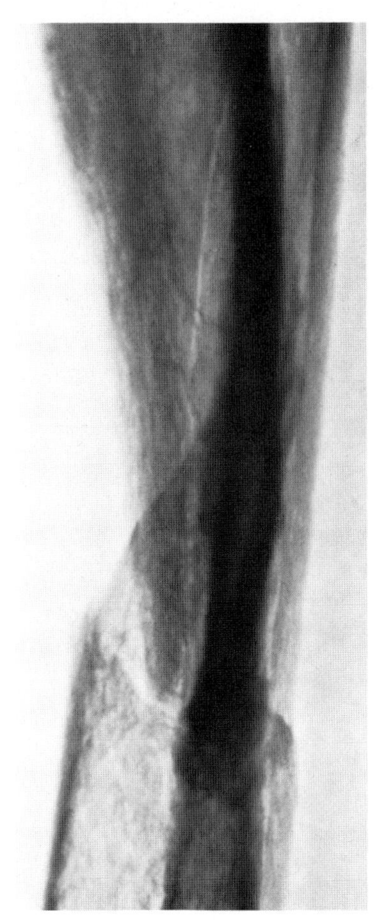

Fig. 754. Lateral view.

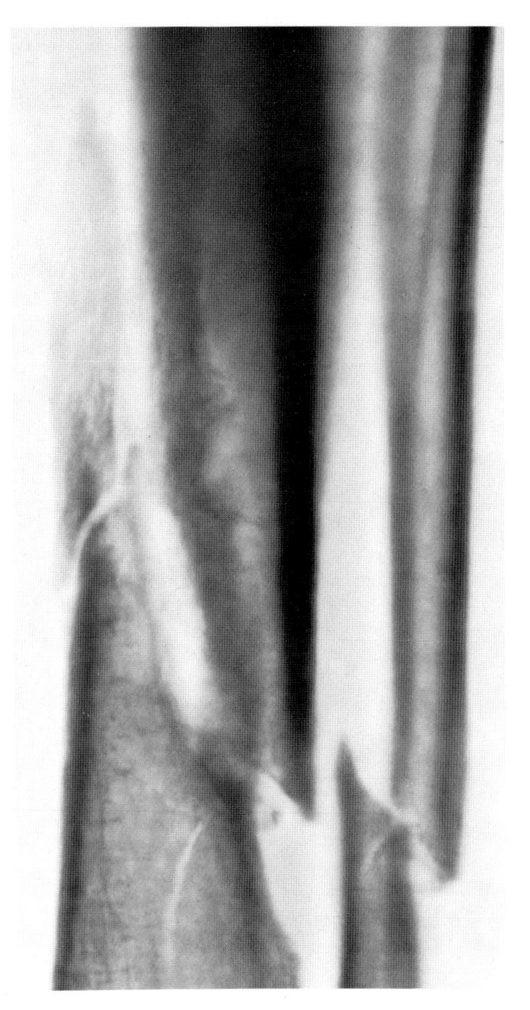

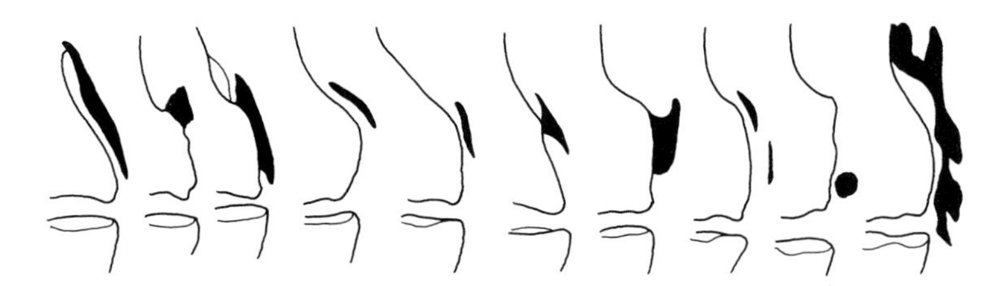

Fig. 756. Sketches of radiographs (after *Jonasch)* of the radiographically visible **calciferous shadows at the inner femoral condyle** *(Stieda-Pellegrini*-shadows).

Fig. 755. Tomography, anteroposterior, 6.26 cm.

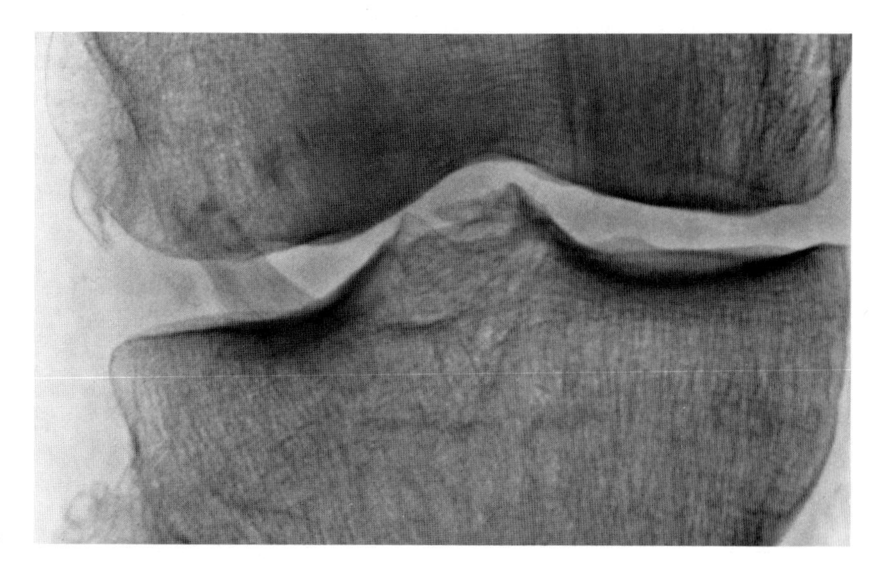

Fig. 757 a

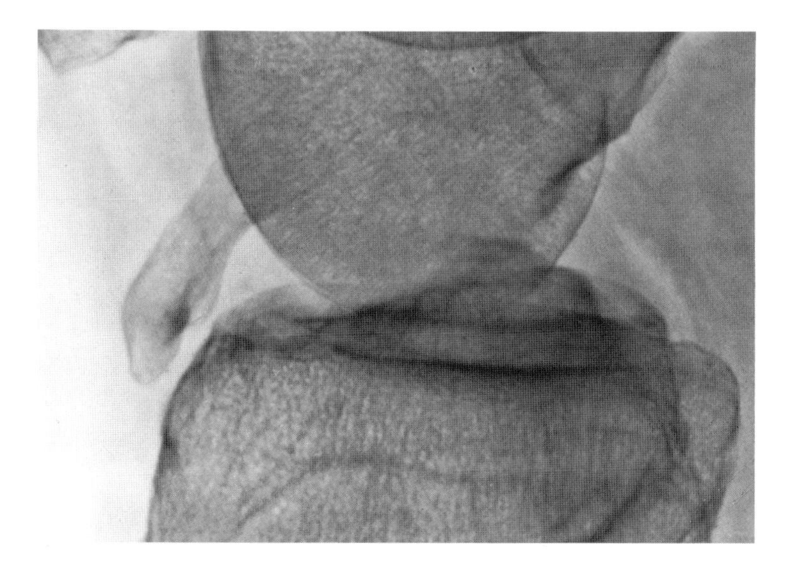

Fig. 757 b

Fig. 757. Particular ossification at the side and in front of the lateral condyle (very rare). In this connection, see Figs. 736 and 737. This is the right knee joint of a former ballet dancer who several years ago suffered, in addition to a tear in the outer collateral ligament with corresponding wobbly knee, a longitudinal tear in his outer meniscus along the insertion of the capsule (Fig. 737). This seems to be a similar ossification as in Figs. 744 and 746, particularly as a thorough examination under fluoroscopy did not provide any clue to a split-off. As a further defect, caused by trauma, a lentil-sized split-off from the intercondyloid eminence of the tibia can be seen.

Lüdeke reported on the multiple occurrence of parosteal neoplastic bone formations in paraplegics, which are mainly to be found on the medial surface of the distal end of the femur but are also seen in the surroundings of the hip joint. The parosteal ossifications in the region of the knee are always extracapsular, on the ventromedial surface of the medial femoral condyle. Anatomically and histologically, the *Stieda-Pellegrini* accompanying shadows and the parosteal neoplastic bone formations at the medial side of the knees of paraplegics are identical. The tearing of tissues by forced valgus kinking of the knee joint is also the cause in paraplegics of parosteal ossification at the inner side of the knee joint (see No. 164, Fig. 739 a).

Kolar and *Vrabec* observed para-articular calcifications and ossifications after injuries caused by electric current.

Jonash described a similar band-like ossification of the oblique popliteal ligament behind the lateral condyle as distinct from ossification of the posterior cruciate ligament.

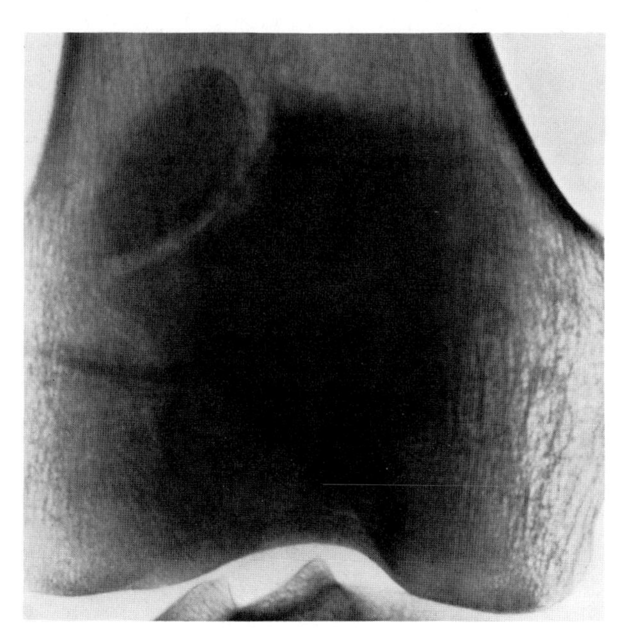

Fig. 758 a

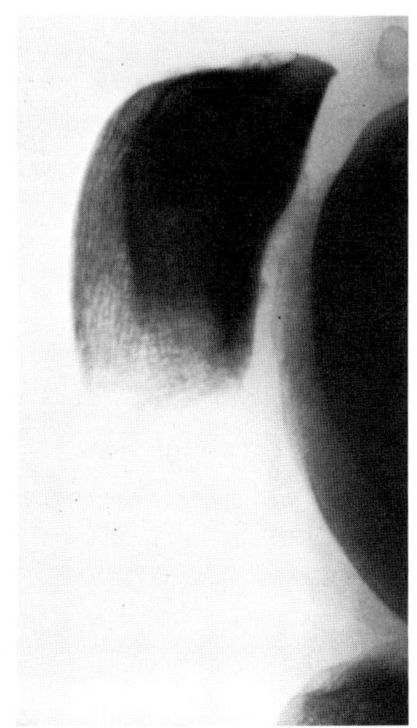

Fig. 758 b

Fig. 758. Patella biparta, sagittal and lateral. A bone segment has been separated by a sinuous cartilaginous cleft from the somewhat small patella at its upper lateral edge. The joints were not quite normal, showing signs of an early-acquired deforming arthrosis. The finding in the patella is not pathological but abnormal, and may instigate a search for further deviations from normal ossification. The usually bilateral abnormal state of the patella will prevent its being mistaken for a cleft of fracture; besides, the lines of separation are too even to be due to fracture. Wavy, rounded parallel contours are also otherwise characteristic for cartilaginous disks enclosed in bone (epiphyses).

Osteochondrosis dissecans may also occur *(Bauer)* but, according to *Marique,* it is rare and localized at the tibial facet of the patella. Numerous publications have appeared on the patella biparta (see *Köhler-Zimmer; Rinonapoli, Wütschke, Riess* and *Blankenburg).* Of importance is the differentiation from fractures for which a past trauma is the premise. Additional radiographs (contact radiographs, perhaps tomography) will aid the diagnosis; if it is still doubtful, a serial examination will show the later bony bridging of the cleft in cases of fracture.

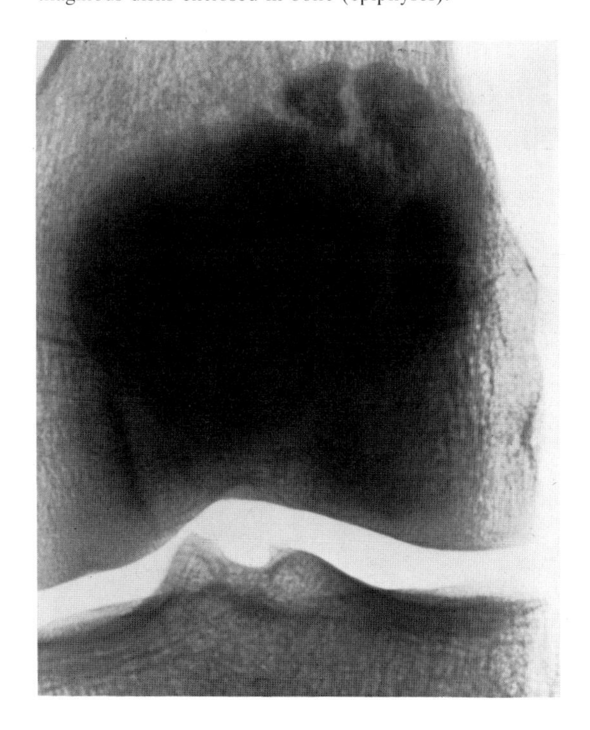

Fig. 759. Patella multiparta. The patella shows at its lateral cranial margin several isolated segments of varying size. The patient had not suffered any discomfort, nor had a trauma been sustained in the past. Malformations such as a patella biparta occur most often in the region of the upper outer quadrant. Severance of the lower tip is less frequent.

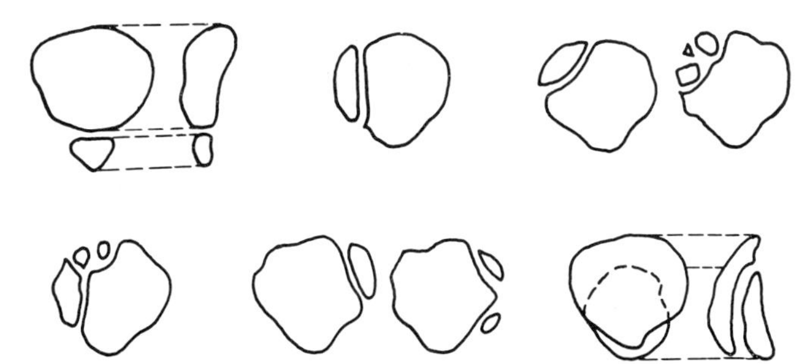

Fig. 760 shows the various **forms of a patella partita** (from *Schaer).*

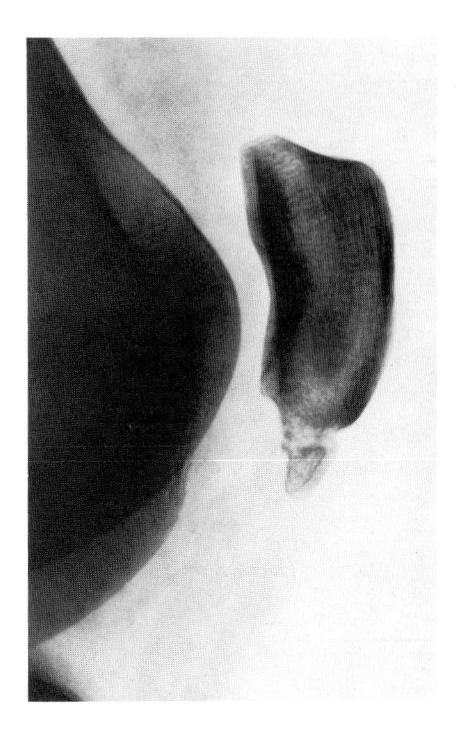

Fig. 761. Persistent nucleus of the patellar apex, female, 23 years of age. This was an incidental finding at the left knee joint, the right patella being normal. On the left, one sees atrophy of the cortical substance and secondary ossifying periostitis. These are not consequences of trauma; therefore, such a finding must not be considered as an effect of injury, when an expert opinion is given.

Such an isolated nucleus at the lower apex of the patella appears regularly during a short period (cf. Fig. 1165). It may persist now and then. If clinical symptoms are absent, this finding must not be mistaken for *Larsen-Johansson*'s disease, which connotes disturbances of ossification at the apex or base of the patella (counted amongst the epiphyseal necroses). *Larson-Johansson*'s disease generally heals at the beginning of puberty; it is often combined with *Osgood-Schlatter*'s disease.

Wütschke has demanded strict separation of the frequent patella biparta (whose divisions are always situated in the patellar region of normal size) from the very rare patella duplex (with the parts of the double patella always lying one below the other), and has based this demand on thorough studies of different ontogenetic theories.

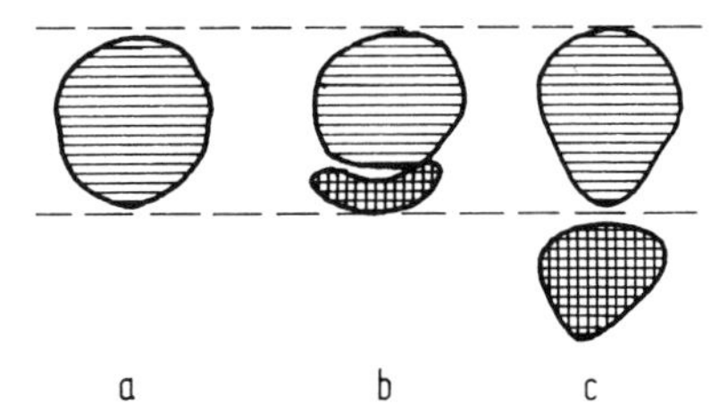

Fig. 762. Preformations of patella (after *Wütschke):* a) Normal patella, b) Patella biparta, c) Patella duplex.

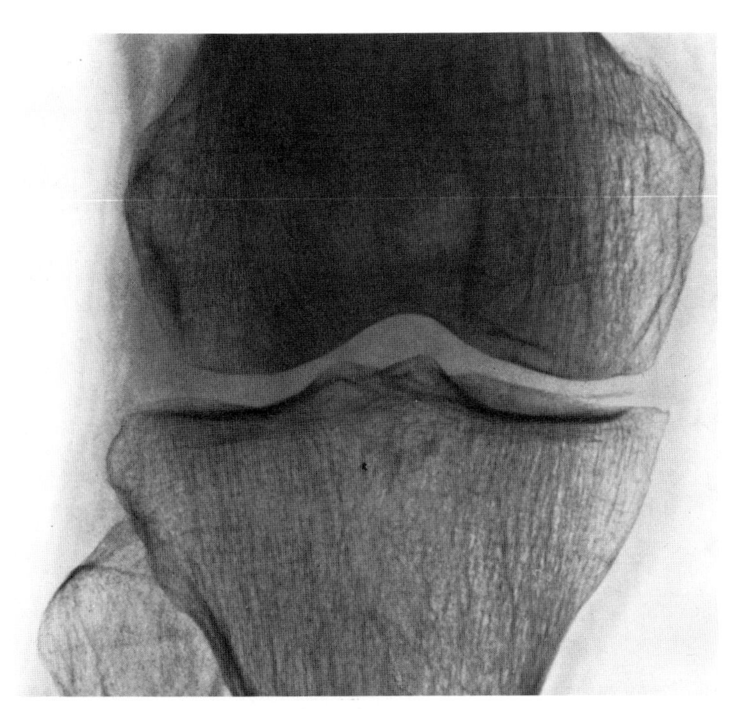

Fig. 763. Primary calcification in the medial meniscus, in a female, 73 years of age (chondrocalcinosis). See No. 154 in Fig. 739 a.

One finds calcifications of the menisci almost exclusively in people beyond the age of 50 *(Schulte).* Sometimes, there are concurrent calcifications of the intervertebral disks. According to *Schulte,* corresponding to statements in the literature, one finds calcification of menisci in 0.31% of examined knee joints. *Meyer-Borstel* was able to observe bilateral calcification of menisci. *Schrop* pointed to the significance of constitutional factors for the genesis of primary calcification of menisci by presenting the radiographs of two sisters. For further literature see *Jonasch. Tobler* found calciferous enclosures in 30% of 1400 histologically examined menisci. For changes in the knee joint in the shape of localized pressure atrophies, due to expansively growing meniscus ganglia, see *Albert.* They appear as a circumscribed, punched-out area at the border between bone and cartilage at the lateral margin of the tibial head, with smooth border of increased density, and as a more shallow recess at the lateral femoral condyle. *Fairbank* and *Lloyd* demonstrated pressure atrophies at the tibial head in cases of unusually large cystic changes at the lateral meniscus. Secondary calcifications of menisci, e.g., after sporting accidents, may often become visible in juveniles 3–4 months after the injury. *Jonasch* and *Rode* wrote about recognition and evaluation of meniscus injuries on the ordinary radiograph.

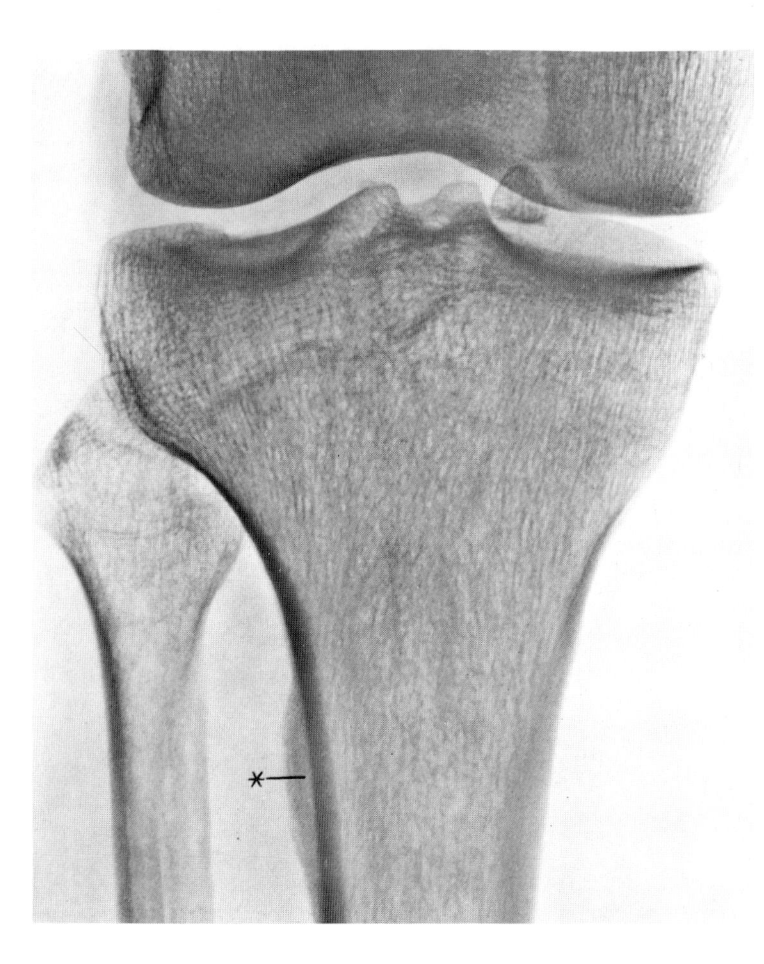

Fig. 764 a (from the collection of *W. Werner,* Berlin).

Fig. 764. Loose body of bony structure above the posterior part of the medial tibial condyle. A so-called "mouse-bed," a corresponding depression as the result of osteochondrosis dissecans, cannot be demonstrated, nor can an indication be found for a split-off (* = Tuberosity of tibia; cf. Fig. 739 a, No. 166*).

The following explanation is given for this concept: as bradythrophic tissue cannot produce an inflammatory reaction, one designates, according to *Pschyrembel* (1972), all types of osteochondrolysis as osteochondrosis and no longer as osteochondritis.

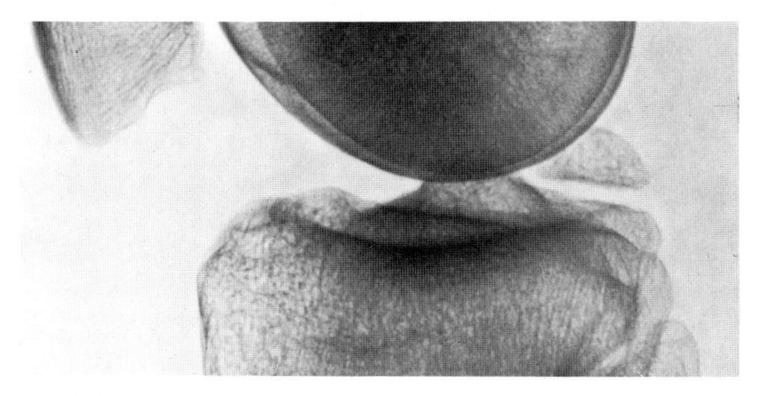

Fig. 764 b

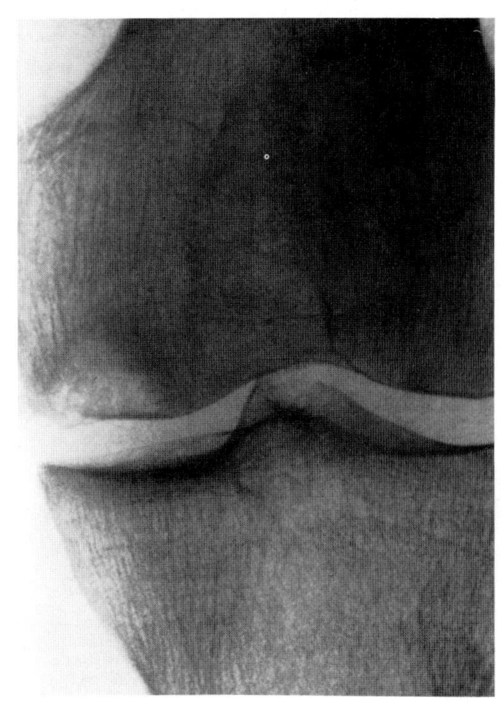

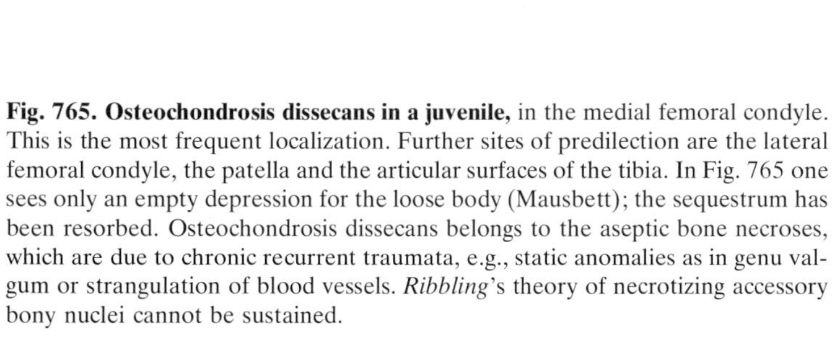

Fig. 765. Osteochondrosis dissecans in a juvenile, in the medial femoral condyle. This is the most frequent localization. Further sites of predilection are the lateral femoral condyle, the patella and the articular surfaces of the tibia. In Fig. 765 one sees only an empty depression for the loose body (Mausbett); the sequestrum has been resorbed. Osteochondrosis dissecans belongs to the aseptic bone necroses, which are due to chronic recurrent traumata, e.g., static anomalies as in genu valgum or strangulation of blood vessels. *Ribbling*'s theory of necrotizing accessory bony nuclei cannot be sustained.

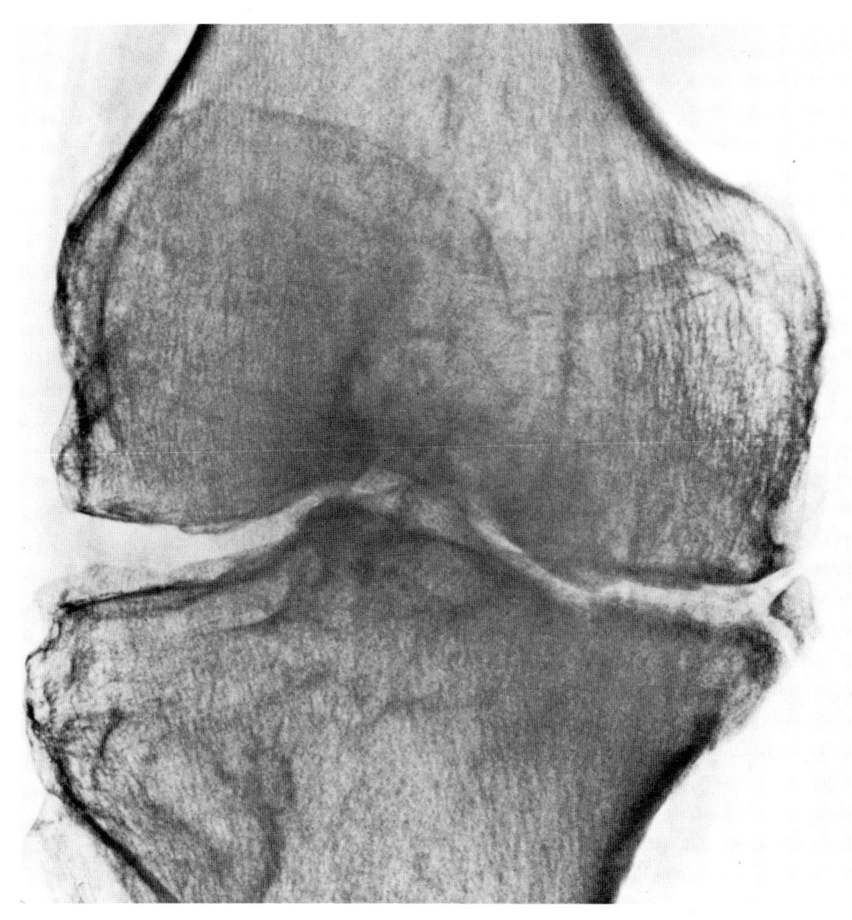

Fig. 766. Relatively rare secondary osteoma of capsule in deforming arthrosis of the knee joint, in a 69-year-old male. One had to consider the breaking-off of a bone excrescence of the margin at the late stage of a chondro-osteoarthrosis.

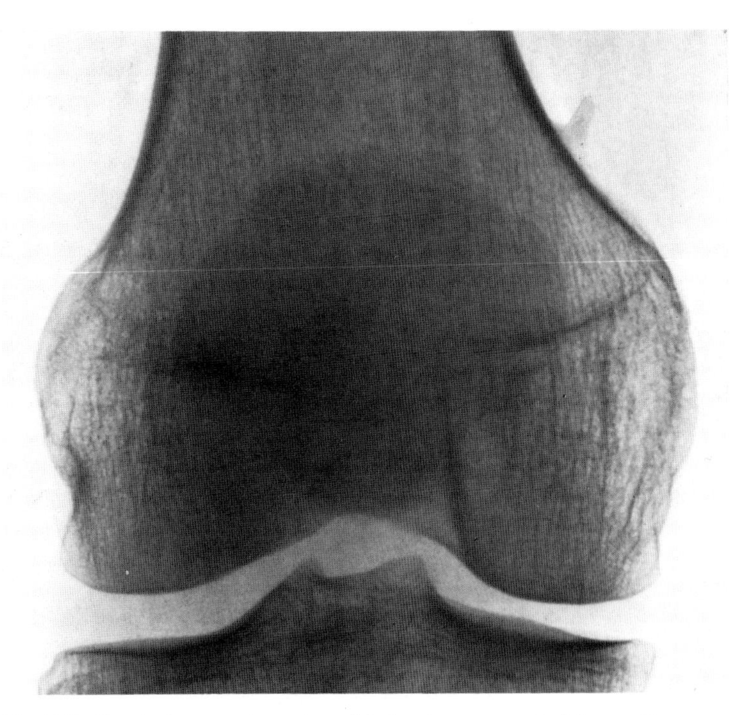

Fig. 767. Exostosis en portemanteau (clothes-hanger exostosis), a solitary cartilaginous exostosis at a typical site at the metaphyseal-diaphyseal transition. The multiple cartilaginous exostoses at similar sites of the bone shafts represent a dominant hereditary androtrope systemic disease (from the collection of *W. Werner*, Berlin).

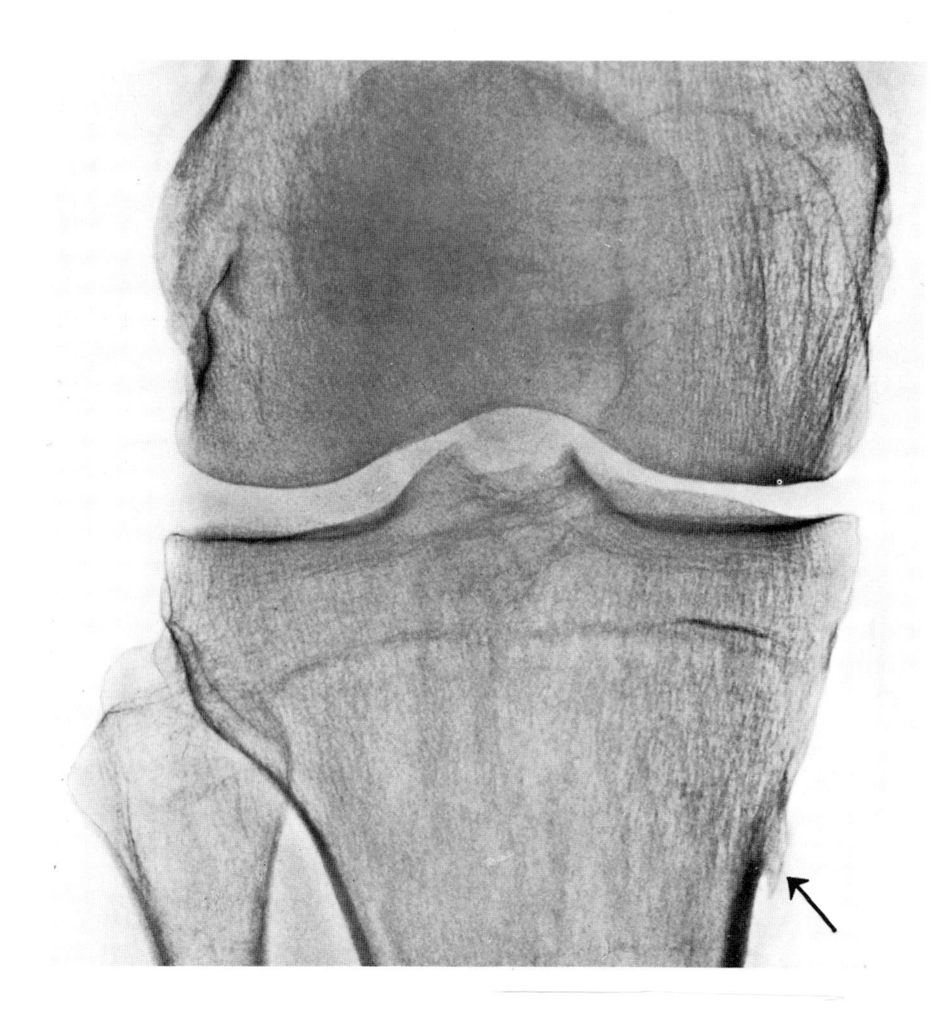

Fig. 768. "Epiphyseal scar" in the proximal tibial metaphysis in a male, 56 years of age. This is without any significance. An additional finding is a small, spur-like exostosis at a typical site (↖).

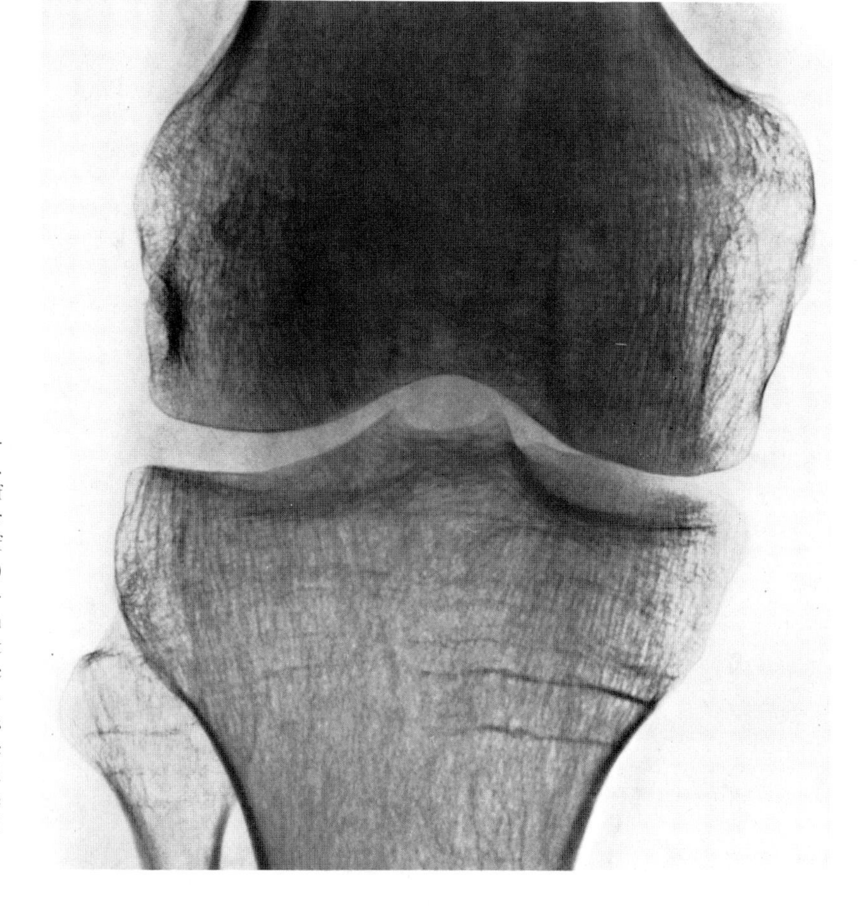

Fig. 769. "Intermediate band," the result of irregularly progressing ossification (in batches) (see Fig. 739 a, No. 156). These lines are also called lines of growth. Their causes can be manifold. The former assumption that they are a symptom exclusively of syphilitic bone disease (osteochondritis syphilitica) has been dropped on the basis of relevant examinations. Causes for the development of the changes in the bone are, e.g., illness of the mother (which might have passed unnoticed), dietetic and prophylactic measures taken during pregnancy, or even antirachitic or other therapy of the infant. Therefore, it is impossible to make the certain diagnosis of syphilitic bone disease from the radiograph alone *(Wolf* and *Psenner)*. These bands also occur after sprue, late rickets, *Möller-Barlow*'s disease, lead poisoning and juvenile chronic rheumatic fever.

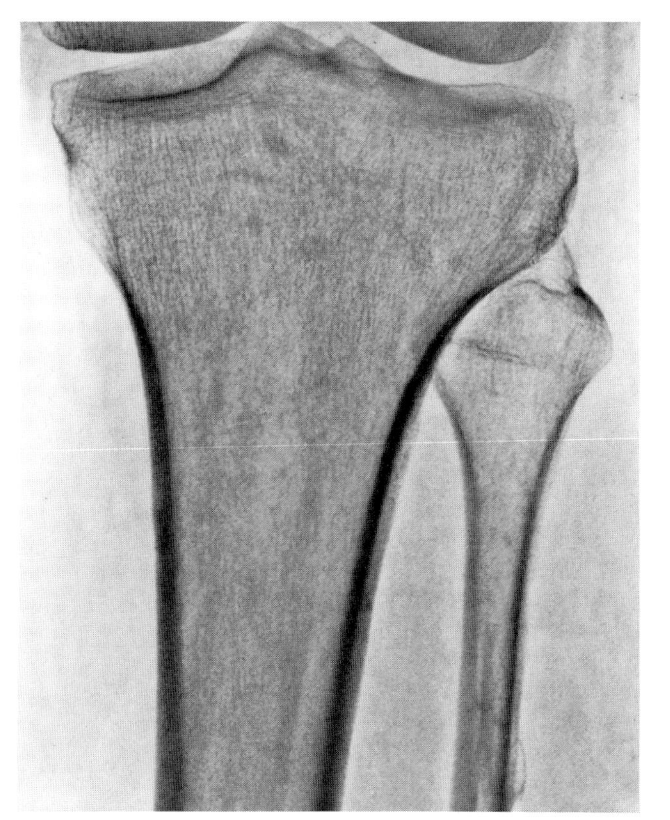

Fig. 770 a

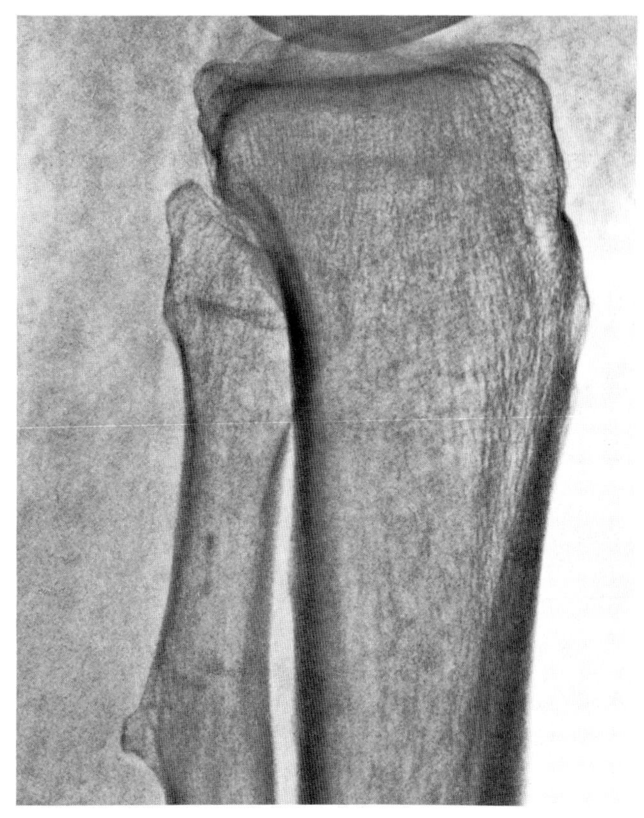

Fig. 770 b

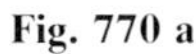

Fig. 770. Rare ostoid of the cortex at the proximal diaphysis of the fibula in advanced age (61-year-old female). Subchondral bone cyst in the medial tibial condyle, with thinning of the cortex. This arises from a juvenile development, from osteoid trabeculae and osteogenic connective tissue in the cancellous and compact bone, usually at the lower extremity. This formation, resembling a tumor, must be differentiated from sclerosing osteitis and traumatic periostitis, syphilis and sarcoma.

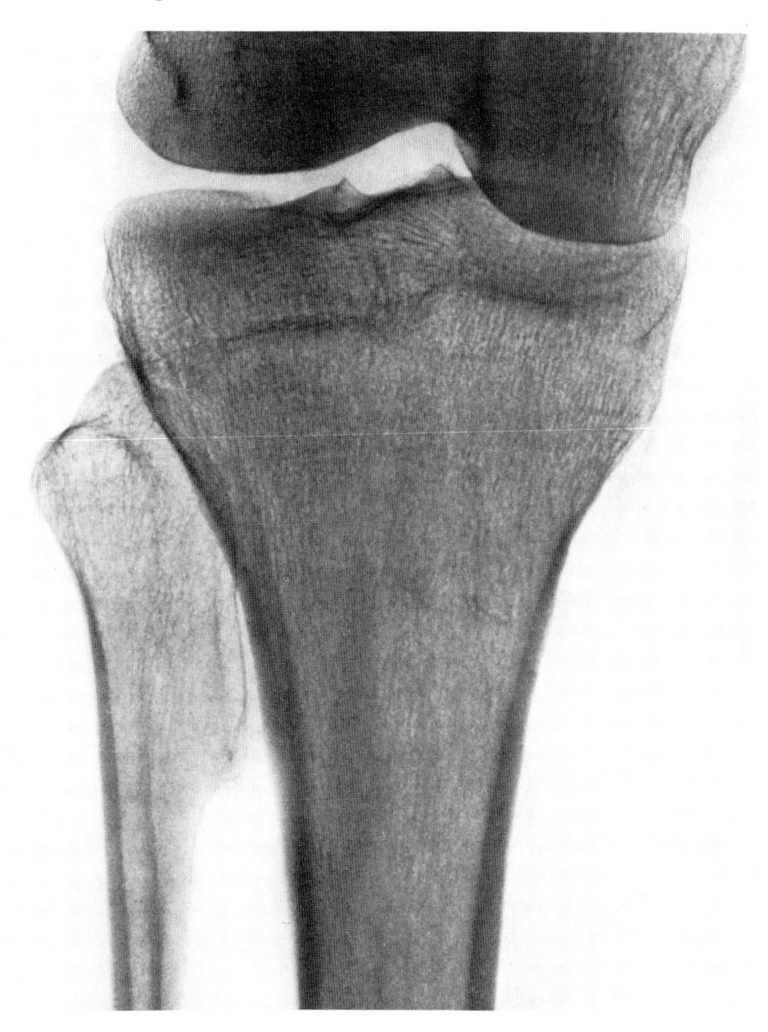

Fig. 771. Pronounced thickening of the periost below the head of the fibula in the region of the interosseus space (cf. Fig. 739 a, letter p). This is probably a transitional variant to the rare tibiofibular synostosis, described for the first time by *Rahm*. *Hippe* observed a further case of tibiofibular synostosis in the proximal part. Cases of synostoses between individual carpal and tarsal bones have been published a considerable number of times (see Figs. 683 and 684). More rarely, a congenital tibiofibular synostosis at the distal end or synostosis between radius and ulna can be found.

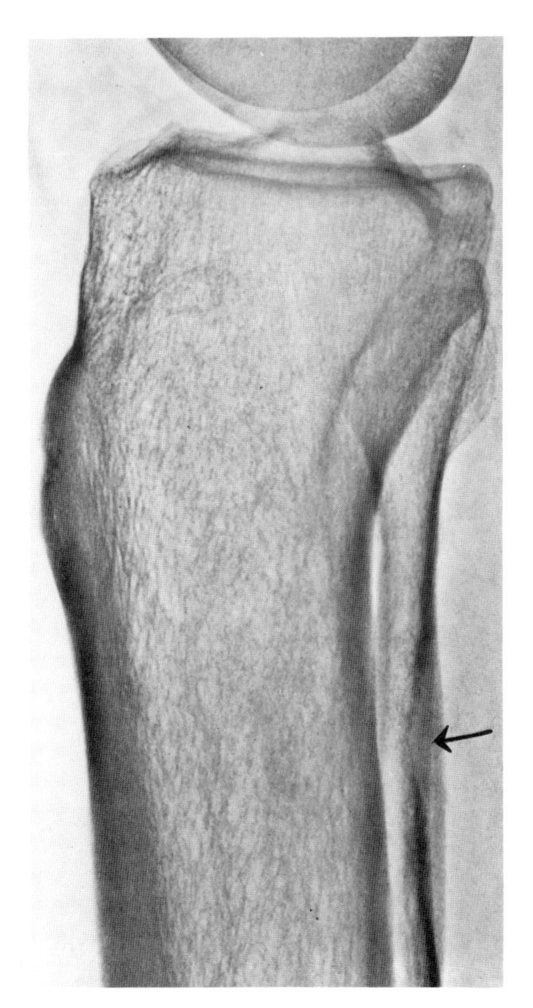

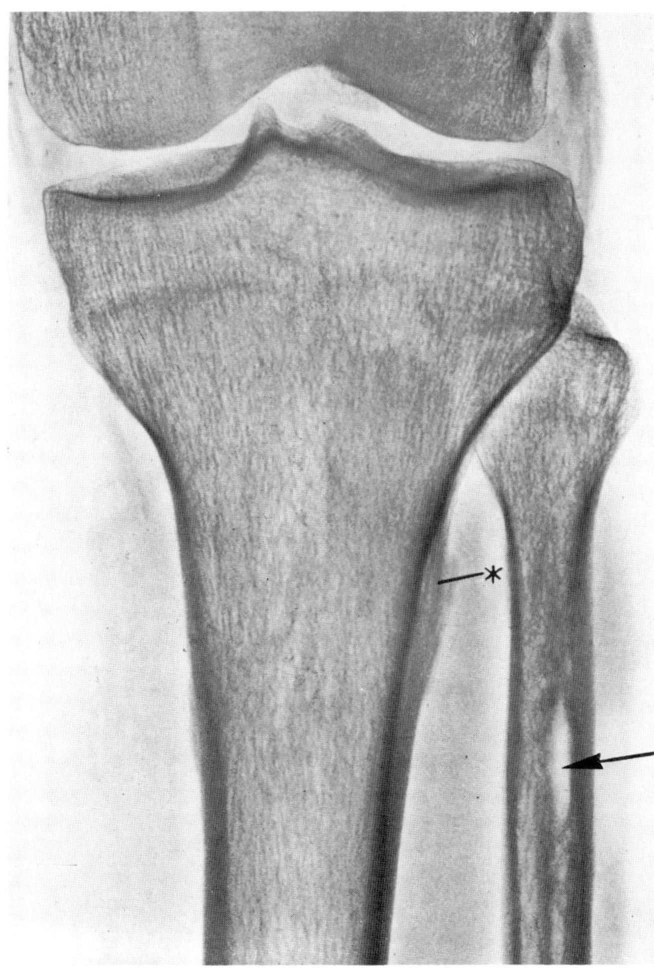

Fig. 772 a

Fig. 772 b. *=Tuberosity of tibia (see No. 166* in Fig. 739 a).

Fig. 772. Groovy notch in the proximal part of the fibular diaphysis, a non-ossifying bone fibroma (lateral view of Fig. 772 a). On the posteroanterior radiograph (Fig. 772 b) a defect, caused by thinning of the cortex at this site, is shown (←). Such defects are characteristic in the region of the knee joint, mainly in the metaphyses of femur and tibia, and more rarely, also in the fibula. They occur more frequently in men than in women, with diminishing frequency beyond the 30th year of life. It may be either a non-ossifying bone fibroma or a cortical sesmoid (hard fibroma). The characteristic radiographs do not leave much likelihood of confusion with condroma, giant cell tumors, bone cysts, sarcoma or osteolytic processes.

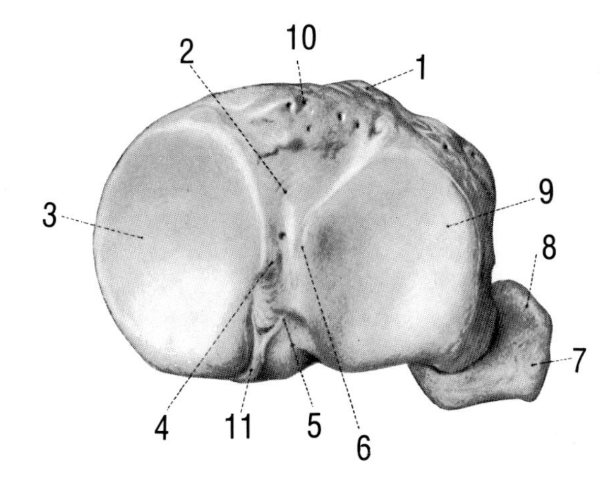

1 Tuberosity of tibia
2 Anterior intercondyloid region
3 Medial tibial condyle
4 Medial intercondyloid tubercle
5 Posterior intercondyloid area
6 Lateral intercondyloid tubercle
7 Apex of head of fibula
8 Head of fibula
9 Lateral tibial condyle
10 Region of the tertiary intercondyloid tubercle
11 Region of the quarternary intercondyloid tubercle

Fig. 773. The proximal ends of the right tibia and fibula (from *Sobotta-Becher,* 17th Edition).

To Figs. 774, 775. Calcified bursa. The subcutaneous infrapatellary bursa (see Fig. 739 b, No. 159) lies on the patellar ligament. The patient, a 48-year-old female, does not know of any previous bursitis; this is an incidental finding. In general, calcifications occur in the prepatellar bursa, in the infrapatellar bursa between tibia and ligamentum patellae, and in the superficial pretibial bursa above the insertion of the ligamentum patellae *(Norley* and *Bickel)*. The chronic prepatellar bursitis is also called "housemaid's knee." On chronic-purulent bursitis, see *Springorum*. The exact diagnosis of diseases of bursae is of special importance as chronic diseases of bursae caused by constant pressure during the patient's work lead to reduction of capability for gainful employment, or after accidents, such persons may in certain circumstances be eligible for compensation. An ancillary finding is a pea-sized **fabella** which appears in the anteroposterior view like an islet of compact tissue in the lateral femoral condyle (see also Fig. 739 b, No. 150). This is the most frequent inconstant sesamoid bone in the human body, and is almost always located in the lateral head of the gastrocnemius muscle. Its ossification takes place during puberty; it can be demonstrated unilaterally in 10–15% of cases but is not recognizable on radiographs before the 12th to 15th years of life. In contrast to free loose bodies, the fabella moves further distally when bending the knee by its flexor muscle.

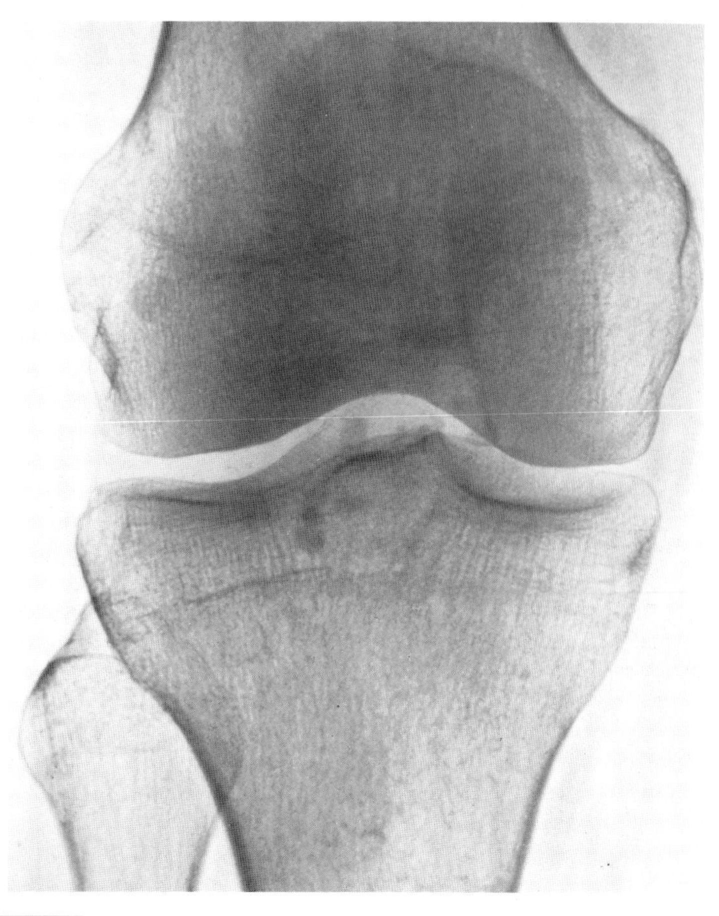

Fig. 774 a

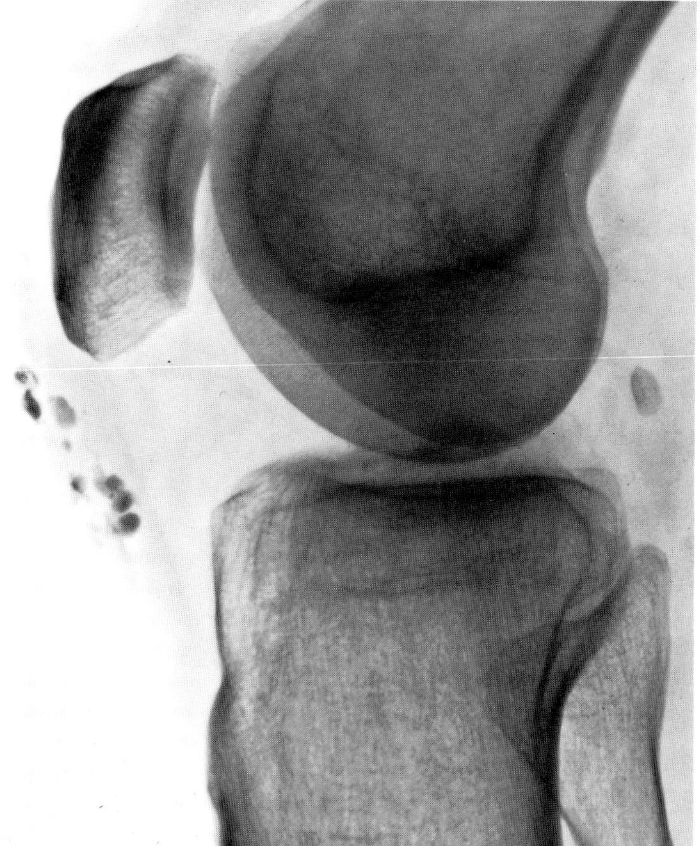

Fig. 774 b

1 Suprapatellar bursa
2 Subcutaneous prepatellar bursa
3 Subfascial prepatellar bursa
4 Subaponeurotic prepatellar bursa
5 Deep infrapatellar bursa
6 Subcutaneous infraprepatellar bursa
7 Bursa of the tuberosity of tibia
8 Bursa of the tibial gastrocnemius muscle
9 Bursa of the fibular gastrocnemius muscle
10 Bursa semimembranosa
11 Bursa anserina
12 Bursa propria of sartorius muscle

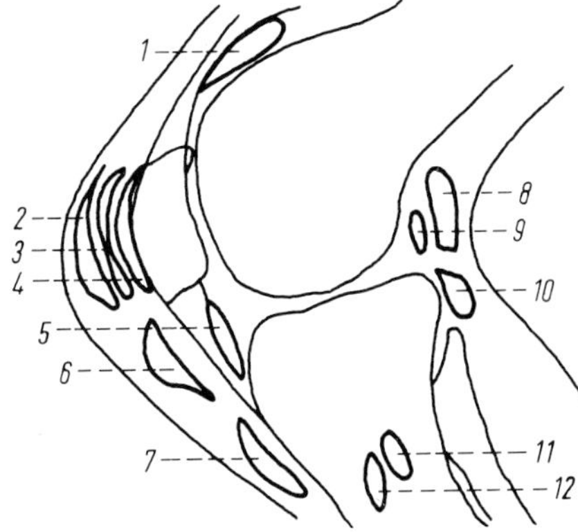

Fig. 775. The bursae of the knee joint, seen from inside the knee (after *Springorum* [1959]).

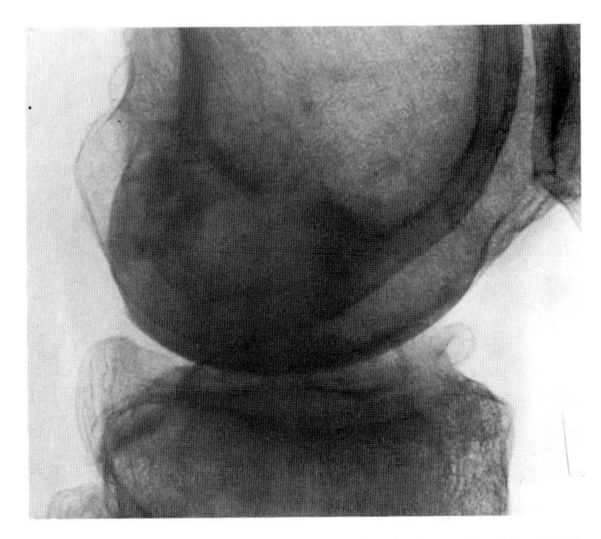

Fig. 776. Tertiary intercondyloid tubercle (see also No. 153*, Fig. 739). The tubercle is situated at the infraglenoid margin and serves as point of insertion of the anterior part of the anterior cruciate ligament. This insertion may be drawn out into a bony spur. According to *Oeser,* this represents a physiological sign of aging which must not be mistaken for a traumatic change. *Ravelli* found this tubercle in 3% of 1000 radiographs of the knee joint. On the anteroposterior view one recognizes it lying, in most cases, medial to the medial intercondyloid tibial tubercle.

Jonasch undertook research on the shape on radiographs of the tibial intercondyloid eminence and pointed out a difference in height of the tubercles which can often be observed. The largest difference between a higher medial intercondyloid tubercle and the lateral intercondyloid tubercle amounted to 5 mm. In the opposite case, the largest difference was 4 mm. *De Cuveland* was able to observe a complete congenital defect of the lateral spike of the eminence of the knee joint. *Haas* reported a case of impeded movement of the knee joint by an "exostosis" on the medial surface of the head of the tibia, where the tendon bundles of inserting muscles became chiselled off. The function of the joint was restored after this rare exostosis had been chiselled off.

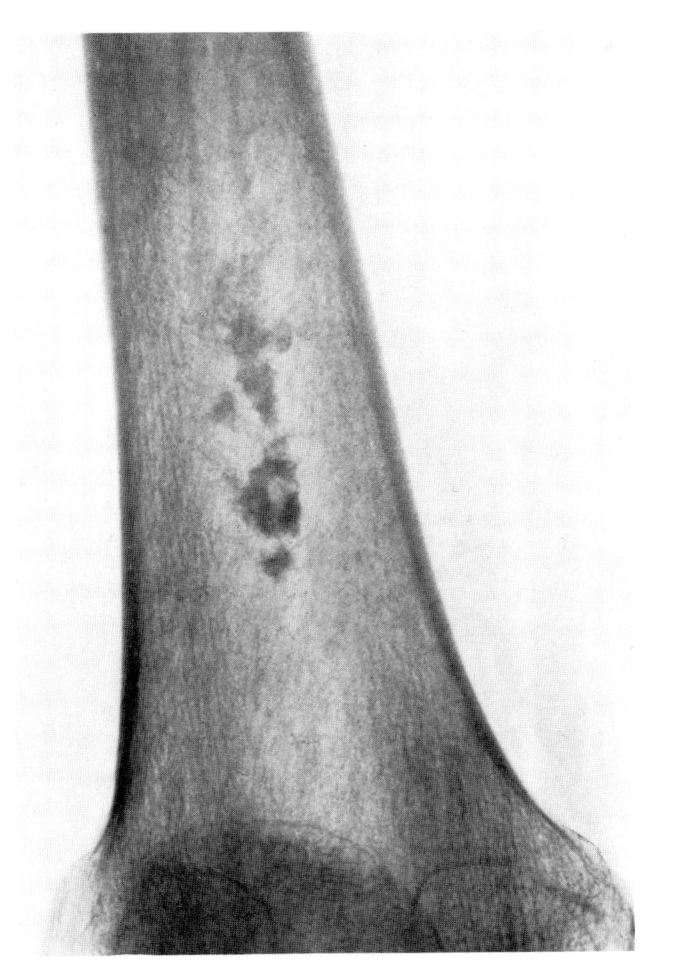

Fig. 777 a

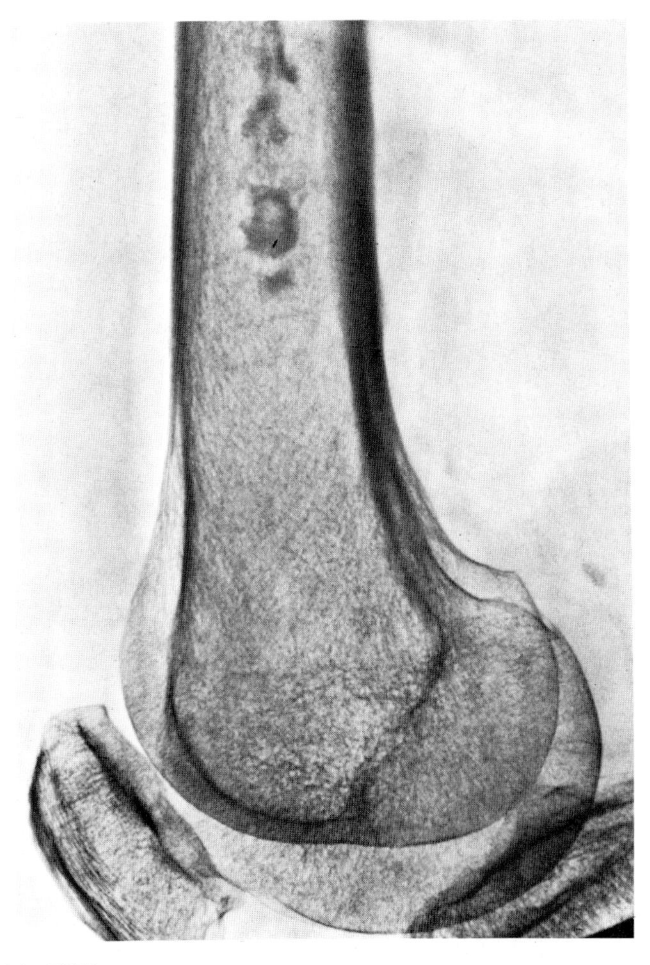

Fig. 777 b

Fig. 777. Bone infarct in the distal metaphysis of the femur, at the transition into the diaphysis, its most frequent localization (see No. 163, Fig. 739). For differential diagnosis, apart from calcified enchondroma or gumma, one should think of melorheostosis *(Spiegel* and *Koiransky, Brauer* and *Coutelle),* which often appears in the distal sections of the femur as a band-shaped or wax-drop-like formation, as an effect of enosteal or periosteal osteoscleroses (synonym: *Leri* syndrome).

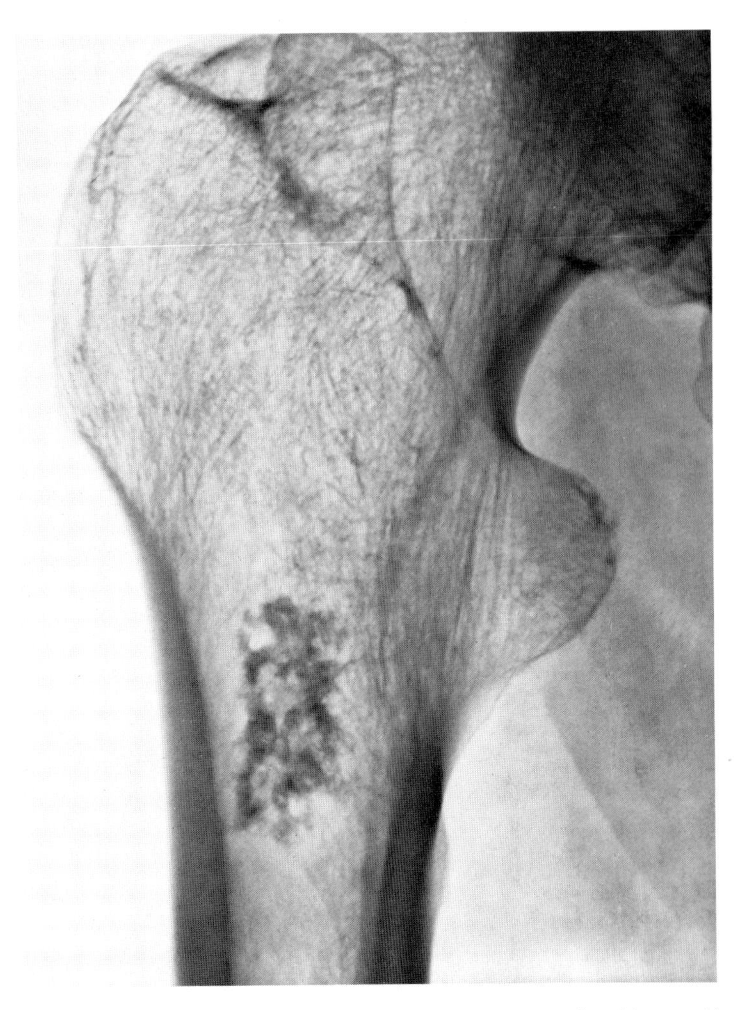

Fig. 778. Bone infarct in the proximal metaphysis of the femur in a 56-year-old male; this is the most frequent localization. One must differentiate it from calcified enchondroma *(Jakob)* and should also consider a gumma.

Primary bone infarcts are the result of the occlusion of a blood vessel, which may be due to quite different causes. The infarcts consist of a limited necrosis of the bone marrow and of regeneration of the osteocytes. Within the necrotic parts, deposits of calcium salts are formed which are, according to the research of *Schinz* and *Uehlinger,* a hydroxyapatite. These deposits can be demonstrated on radiographs in very different shapes: as central metadiaphyseal strands, porous ring shadows or calciferous rings in clusters or chain formation. Within the epiphyses, they are often wedge- or tongue-shaped. In these cases the base is formed by chondral calcified cartilage. The structure is irregularly spotty or striped.
Bone infarcts may manifest themselves clinically as undefined pain in bony regions near the joint. It is possible that some cases of osteochondrosis dissecans are based on a primary bone necrosis. Lately, necroses of the head of the femur have been observed after large doses of cortisone. The pathogenesis of the cortisone infarct has not been clarified *(Klümper et al.).*
Spur at the lesser trochanter, the insertion of the iliopsoas muscle: between bone and inserting tendon, the bursa subtendinea is placed. Occasionally, a persistent apophysis at the lesser trochanter may be observed which must not be confused with persistent accessory nuclei.

Radiographic Anatomy and Radiographs of the Talocrural Articulation, Malleoli, Tarsus and Toes, Including Exposure Techniques

The talocrural joint and malleoli are taken:

1. sagittal
   anteroposterior, for demonstration of talocrural joint, malleoli and talus
2. transverse
   a) fibulotibial, for demonstration of the internal malleolus, the talocrural joint and the tarsus
   b) tibiofibular, for demonstration of the talocrural joint, the tarsus and especially the lateral malleolus
   c) tibioposteroanterior projection.

The position of the talocrural joint should usually be at right angles. The projection is onto the center of the articular space, whereby it should be remembered that the most prominent point of the medial malleolus roughly corresponds to the articular space, while the outer malleolus reaches further distally. As a rule, one needs two radiographs: one anteroposterior (1) and one tibiofibular (2b) or fibulotibial, according to the site under review. In order to see the fibula well, one has to project the foot, apart from anteroposteriorly, obliquely from posterior and medial or reversed (Fig. 783). The fibula lies, in any case, somewhat behind the tibia. One has only to rotate the foot a little further to obtain a free projection of the posterior margin of the fibular shadow, which is of importance for the diagnosis of the frequent isolated fractures of the lateral malleolus.

When examining children, one can take both talocrural joints together and project onto the middle of a line connecting both joints. At a greater distance (100 cm), the distortion does not matter. With adults it is better to expose each joint separately; one can put them on one film, covering with lead the foot not to be exposed.

When a fibulotibial radiograph is taken, the patient lies on the side of the medial malleolus, with the knee slightly bent. A suitable support is placed below the knee and the whole calf, as for the analogous radiograph of the knee joint. Calf and foot must be well fixed.

On the lateral radiographs one sees distinctly the sinus tarsi and the individual tarsal bones. If the view of a particular small spot of the tarsus is required, the projection must be directed specially onto it. In this case further auxiliary radiographs are needed, dorsoplantar or plantodorsal radiographs of the metatarsus and additional special projections for the calcaneus.

The calcaneus is taken:

1. tibiofibularly, when it is best that the body of the calcaneus lies on the cassette (Fig. 788). This radiograph is also suitable for the neighboring bones,
2. fibulotibially, with the sustentaculum tali lying on the cassette (Fig. 791),
3. obliquely, from dorsal and above (Figs. 795 and 797),
4. obliquely, from ventral and below (Figs. 796 and 798).

The lateral radiographs show very well the contours of the sagittal sections of the calcaneus and the structure of the bone. But in spite of this, some changes of its shape (fractures) are not always clearly recognizable. Therefore, in order to exclude these with greater certainty, one must take an additional radiograph, vertical to the plane of the previous view.

For the navicular bone one lateromedial and one plantodorsal radiograph are usually needed; the same applies to the first cuneiform bone. For the cuboid bone a mediolateral and a plantodorsal radiograph are needed, rotating the foot as in Figure 785. When taking the dorsoplantar radiograph of the metatarsus, the tube must not be directed too much medially; otherwise, the cuneiform bones project too much one onto the other. Likewise with plantodorsal radiographs, one must move the tube more laterally and place the foot onto the cassette as flat as possible so on projection the individual tarsal bones move well away from one another.

The metatarsus and the small tarsal bones are taken:

1. dorsoplantarly (Fig. 805). With this method it is disturbing that the bones of the medial half are far away from the film and the row of the metatarsal bones slides down from the first to the fifth (see the transverse section on Fig. 779).

It follows, that with dorsoplantar projection the medial and proximal parts will appear less distinct, the interspaces will look narrowed and the bases of the metatarsal bones will appear pushed together. If one shifts the tube correspondingly laterally, the first three lateral intermetatarsal spaces will become more distinct but the first one remains superimposed. Therefore, this arrangement is chosen mainly when the demonstration of toes and metatarsal heads is essential. More frequently, the foot is placed

2. plantodorsally (Fig. 809). Then, the row of metatarsal bones lies fairly evenly on the film and the small tarsal bones stand out sharply.

To achieve a good radiograph of the basal interspace between the 1st and 2nd metatarsal bones, one also chooses the plantodorsal direction but turns the foot more straight so that the lateral margin of the foot rests away from the cassette: The central ray is aimed onto the 1st metatarsal bone or lateral from it. The arrows in Figure 779 show the most favorable projections for the various intermetatarsal spaces. It is obvious, that with a plantodorsal path of the rays these diverge in the same way as the interspaces between the bones; therefore, the spaces are better presented than with dorsoplantar projection.

Sometimes it is desirable to project the heads of the metatarsals laterally. If one places the foot onto its lateral margin, this succeeds fairly well, and if one simultaneously compresses the foot from the sides, the heads move sufficiently away from one another (see also Fig. 819).

The toes are well demonstrated with dorsoplantar projection, but as they are frequently found in positions of contracture, must be pressed down with ties or strips of gauze. Otherwise, considerable distortions may occur (Fig. 842). Lateral radiographs can be taken by wedging the film into the interdigital space (Fig. 820).

In order to demonstrate the sesamoid bones, or at least the lateral one at the base of the big toe, the first two toes are spread apart by the top of a bandage and one projects in fibulodorsoplantar direction. One can also fix the hallux in maximal dorsiflexion with stripes of bandage of adhesive plaster and then take radiographs of the sesamoid bones from above (Fig. 846).

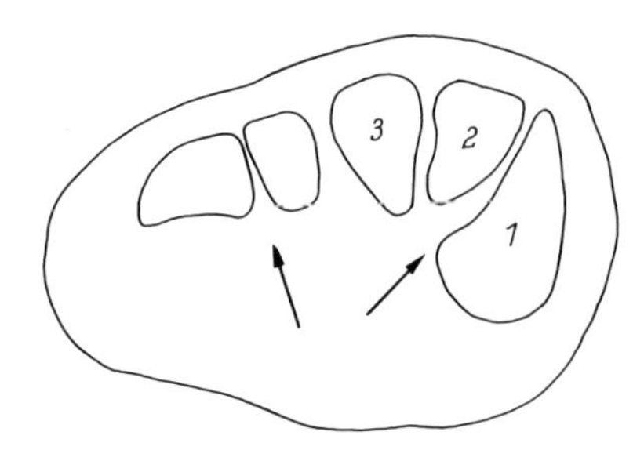

Fig. 779. Metatarsus, cross-section (after *Corning*).

The popliteal fossa should always be supported by a foam rubber pillow in order to avoid error through complete extension of the knee joint. An extended knee allows little torsion which goes beyond the physiological one, without displacement of the whole body. With much internal rotation, pronounced plantar flexion of the foot should be avoided. Otherwise, the calcaneal tuberosity and the tip of the lateral malleolus are superimposed upon each other, especially in cases of pes valgus.

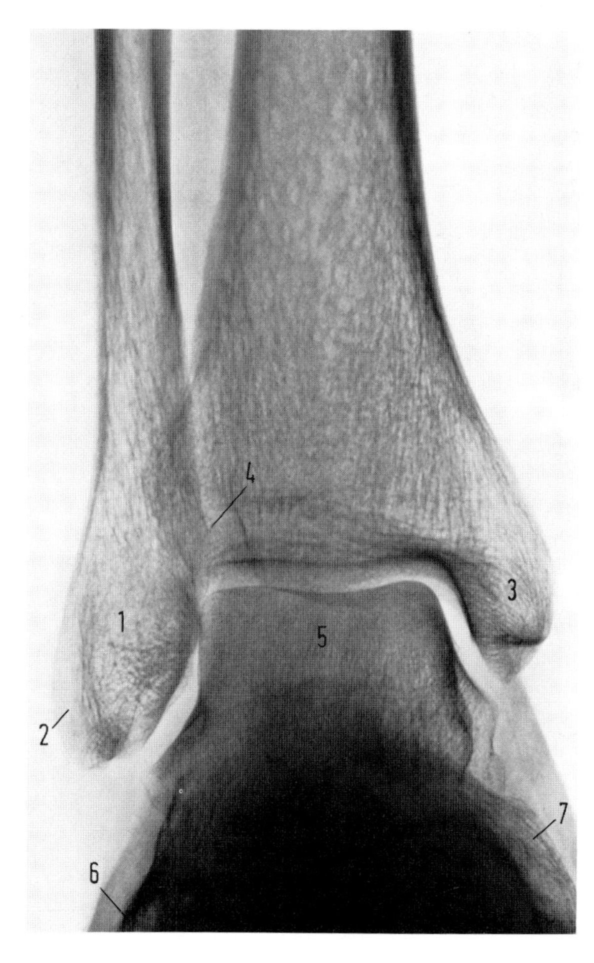

1 Lateral malleolus
2 Malleolar sulcus
3 Medial malleolus
4 Incisura fibularis
5 Trochlea of talus
6 Cuboid bone
7 Tuberosity of the navicular bone

Fig. 780. Talocrural joint, anteroposterior. For projection see Figs. 781, 782. The patient is supine, leg stretched, foot slightly drawn up.
After marking the tips of the malleoli, one draws a line from one to the other across the sole of the foot. This must run parallel to the cassette. The central ray is aimed vertically onto the center of the articular space of the talocrural joint *(Wentzlik)*. For anteroposterior radiographs of the talocrural joint, *Fürmaier* recommends an internal rotation of about 5°, with the central ray aimed vertically into the joint.

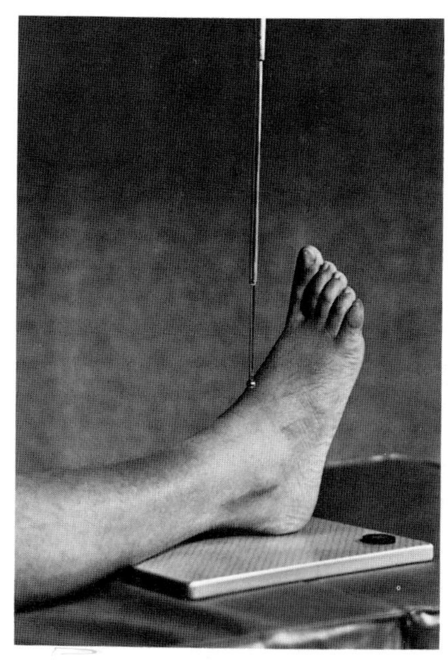

Fig. 781

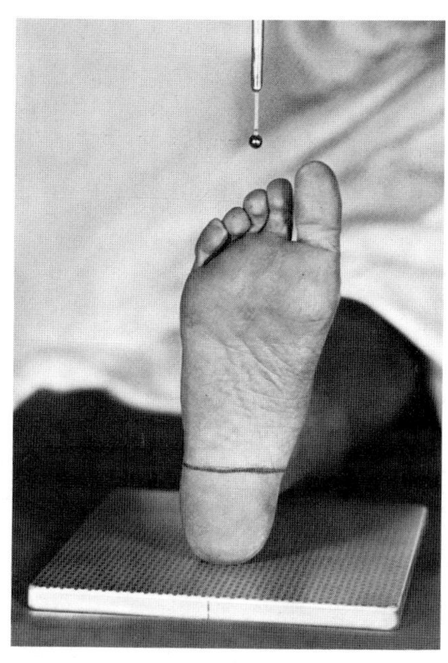

Fig. 782

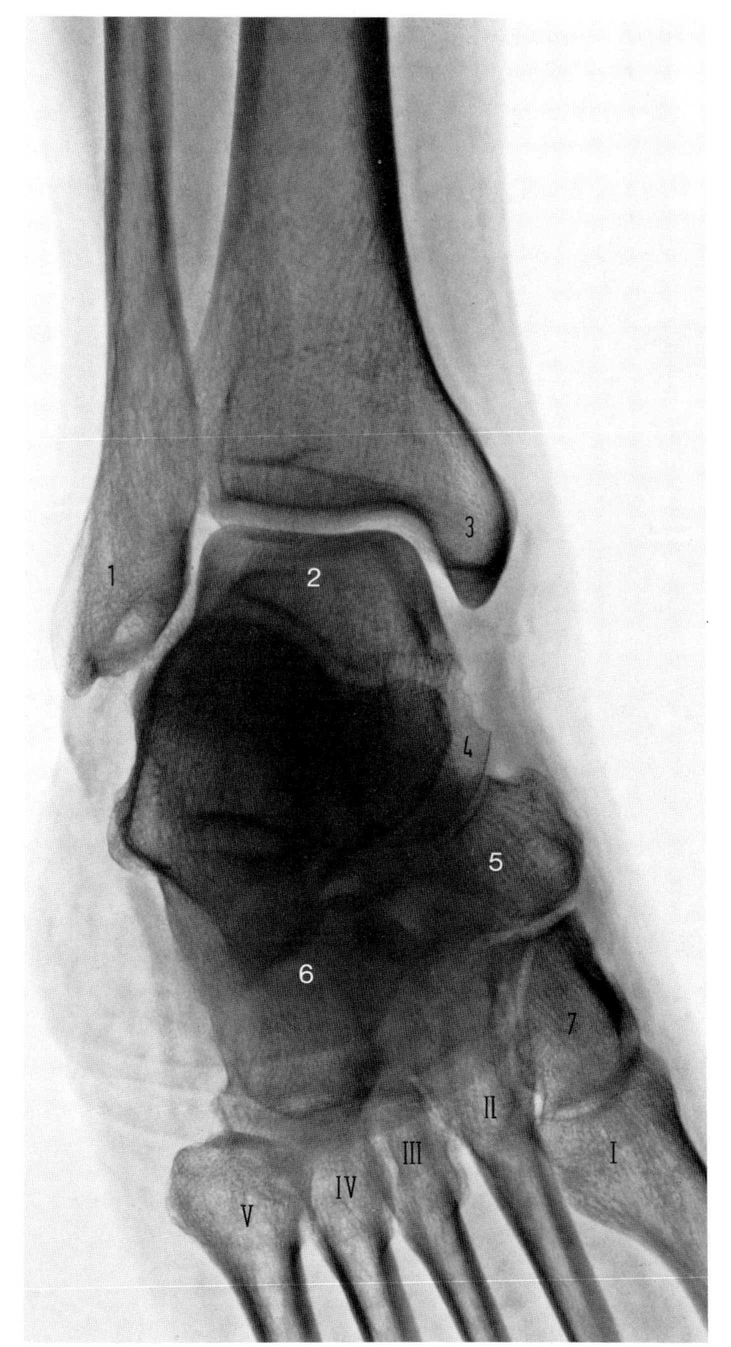

1 Lateral malleolus
2 Trochlea of talus
3 Medial malleolus
4 Head of talus
5 Navicular bone
6 Cuboid bone
7 Medial cuneiform bone (I)
I–V Bases of metatarsal bones

Fig. 783. Articular space between fibula and talus. For projection see Fig. 784. The extended leg is rotated inward by about 25–30°. The central ray is aimed vertically onto the articular space between fibula and talus.

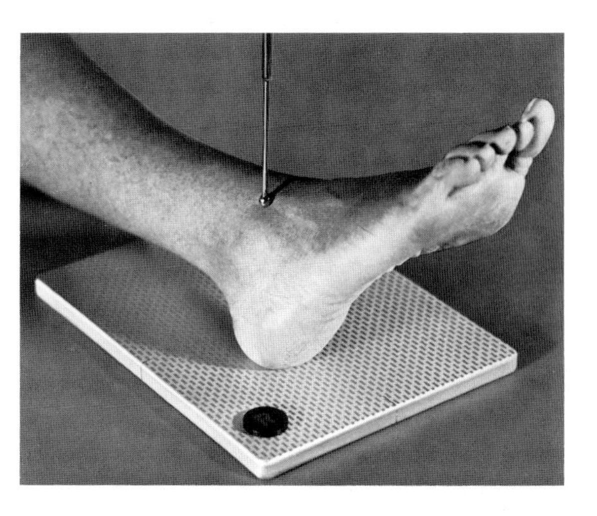

Fig. 784

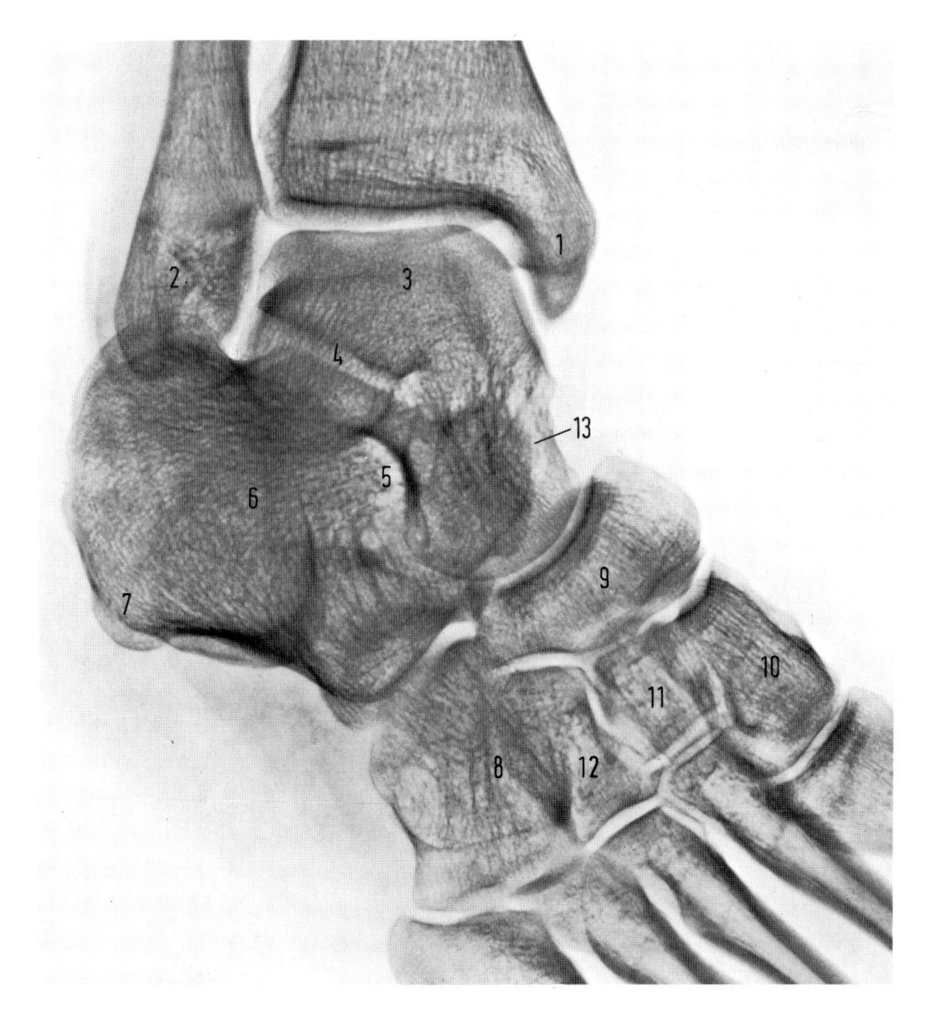

Fig. 785. Talocrural joint, tibioposteroanterior. It almost corresponds to Fig. 783, however the pathway of the rays has been reversed. Projection: patient prone, foot rotated much inward. The central ray passes through the talocrural articulation vertically onto the cassette. One can see well between tibia and fibula, i.e., into the joint and, respectively, into the syndesmosis in the upper part of the tibiofibular connection (cf. *Albers-Schönberg*).

1 Medial malleolus
2 Lateral malleolus
3 Trochlea of talus
4 Posterior articular space between talus and calcaneus
5 Sinus tarsi
6 Calcaneus
7 Lateral process of the calcaneal tuberosity
8 Cuboid bone
9 Navicular bone
10 Medial cuneiform bone (I)
11 Intermediate cuneiform bone (II)
12 Lateral cuneiform bone (III)
13 Neck of talus

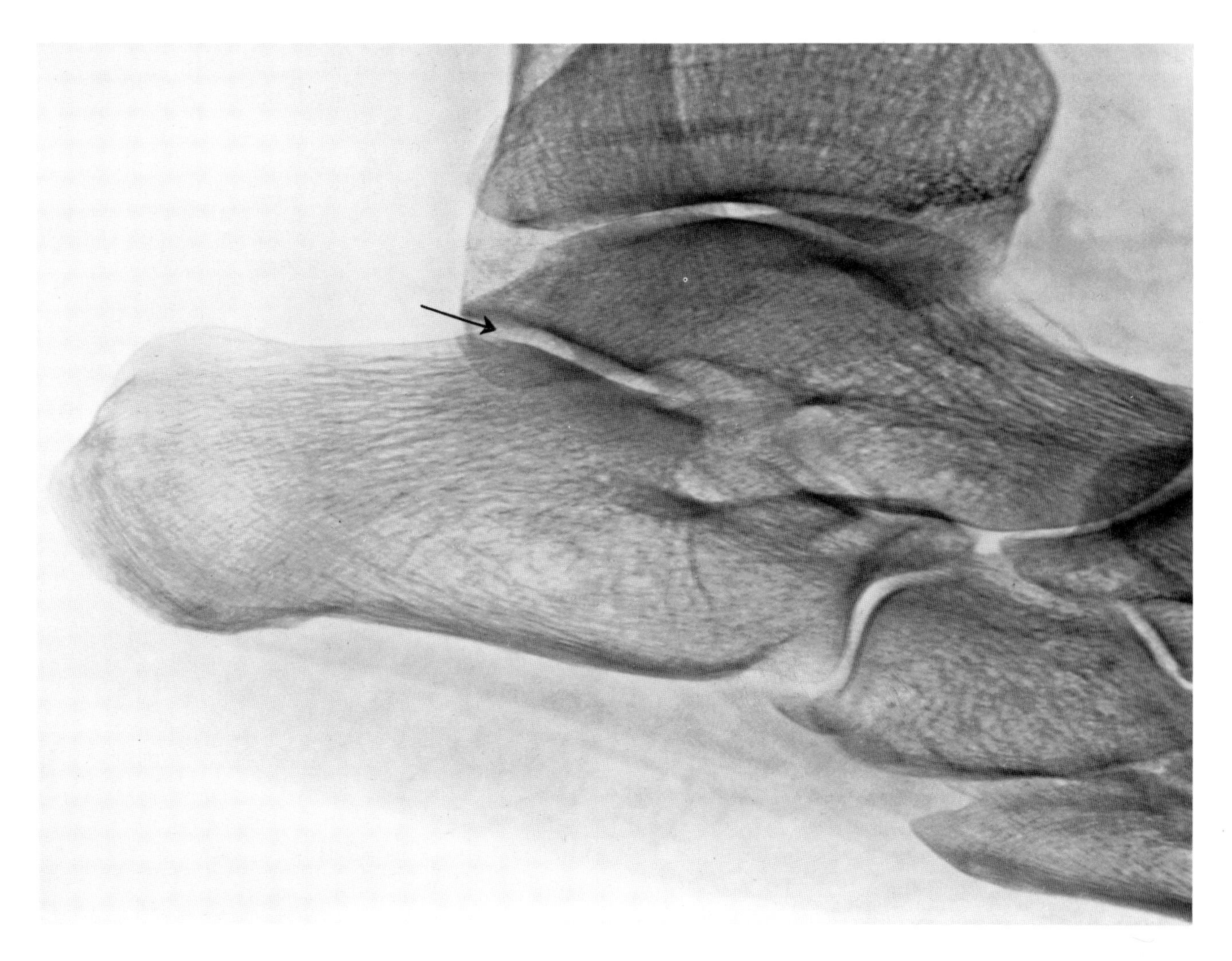

Fig. 786. Posterior part of the talocalcaneal articulation. For this view the central ray passes transversely through the posterior region of the joint (↘). The patient lies supine, the leg is rotated outward by 45°. The X-ray tube is inclined caudocranially by 30° against vertical, corresponding to 60° against the cassette (mean values), towards a point 2 cm caudoventral from the medial malleolus. This method originates from the Swede *Halgrimsson. Elsner* emphasizes its significance in clinical and accident medicine.

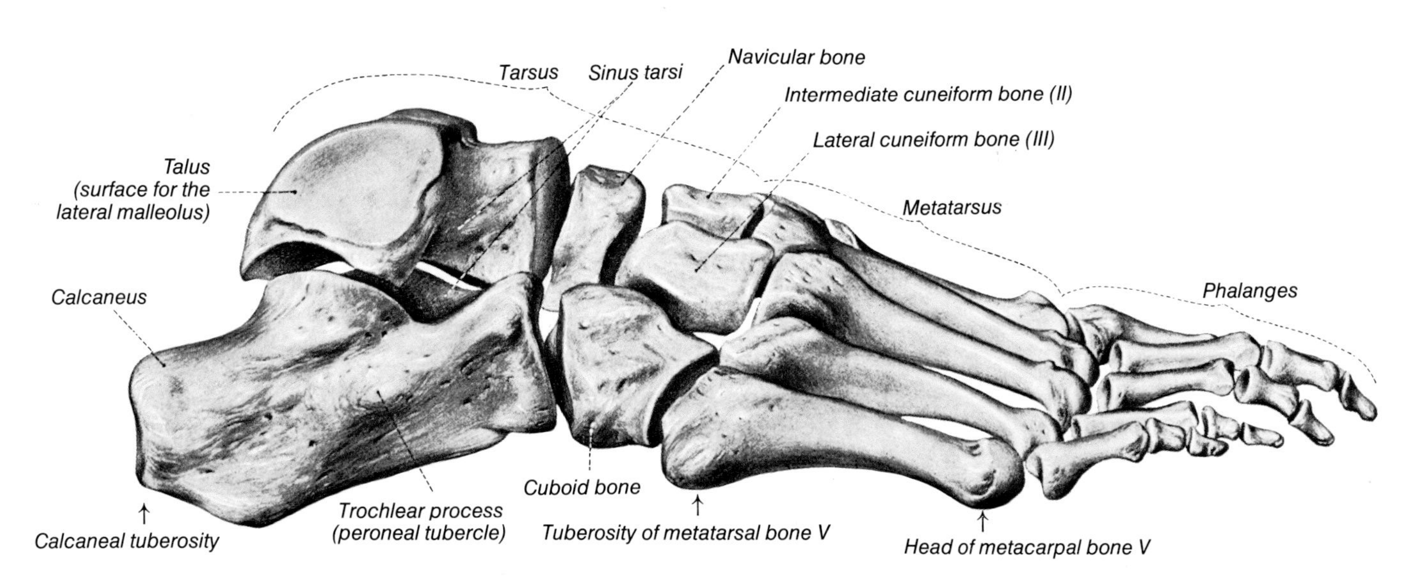

Fig. 787. Skeleton of the foot (from *Sobotta-Becher,* 17th Edition).

1 Tip of the medial malleolus
2 Tip of the lateral malleolus
3 Head of talus
4 Neck of talus
5 Trochlea of talus
6 Navicular bone
7 Base of metatarsal bone I
8 Cuboid bone
9 Anterior process of calcaneus
10 Body of calcaneus
11 Calcaneal tuberosity
12 Medial (and lateral) processes of the calcaneal tuberosity
13 Sinus tarsi; above it: posterior process of the talus
14 Sustentaculum tali
15 Pseudocystic triangle
16 *Haglund* exostosis.

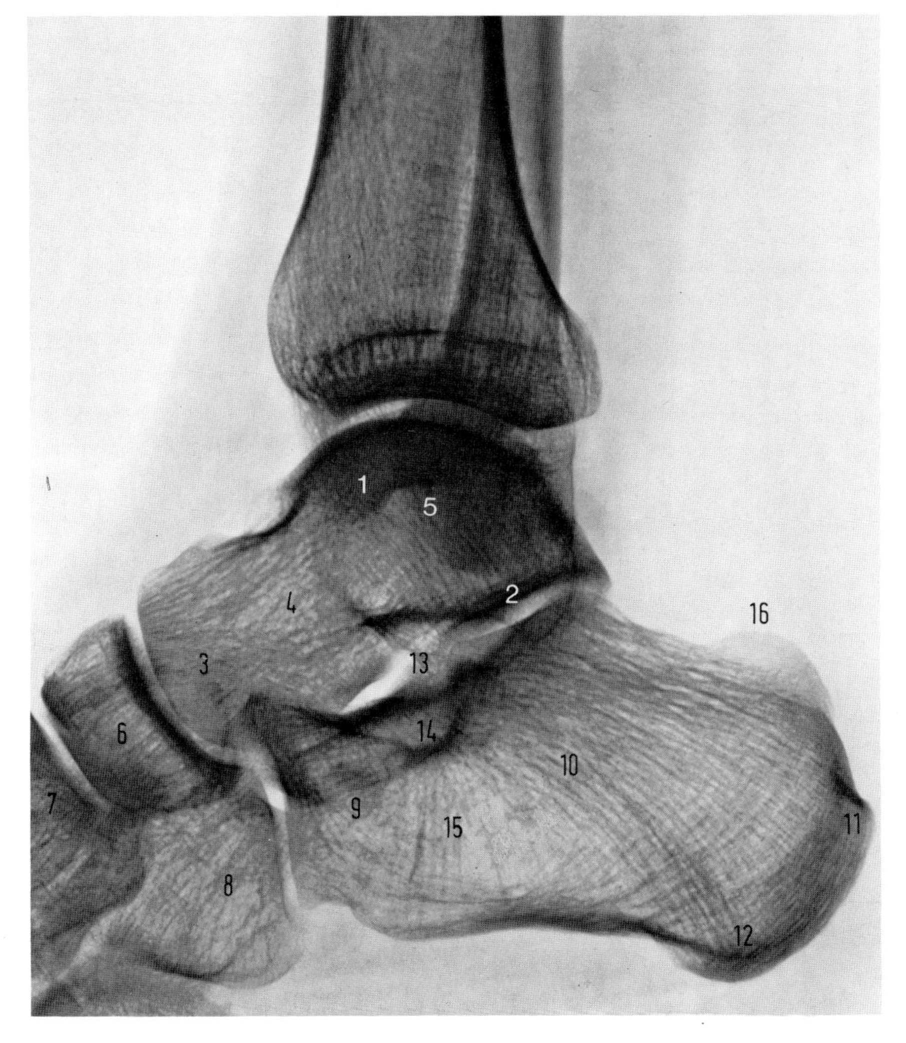

Fig. 788. Right talocrural joint (talocrural articulation, ankle joint), tibiofibular. For projection see Fig. 789. For the tibiofibular radiograph, *Fürmaier* recommends internal rotation of the foot by 5–10°, through slight raising of the tip of the foot. The central ray then enters slightly cranially from the tip of the medial malleolus. To examine whether ligaments of the ankle are intact, one needs radiographs in the maximal positions of pronation and supination. A *Haglund* exostosis can be seen on the upper surface of the calcaneal tuberosity (see also radiograph with meticulous focus, Fig. 792). One sees above the talocrural joint the epiphyseal scar, running parallel to the contour of the joint. The subtalar articulation (= posterior section) is separated from the talocalcaneonavicular articulation (= anterior section) by the sinus tarsi. Together, both form functionally the lower ankle joint. The posterior process of the talus is not developed. The prominence at the posterior contour of the calcaneus corresponds to the insertion of the Achilles tendons.

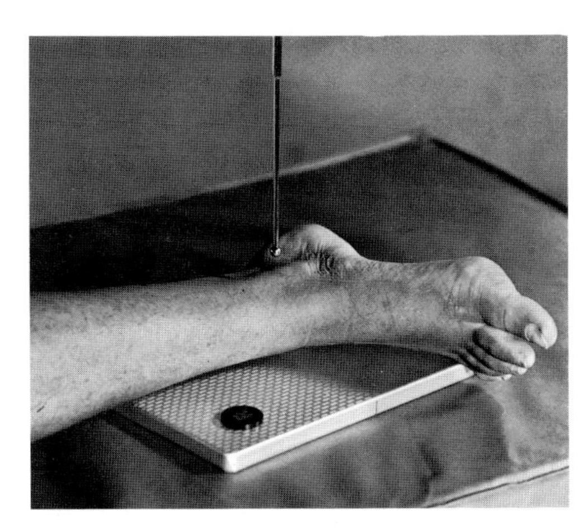

Fig. 789

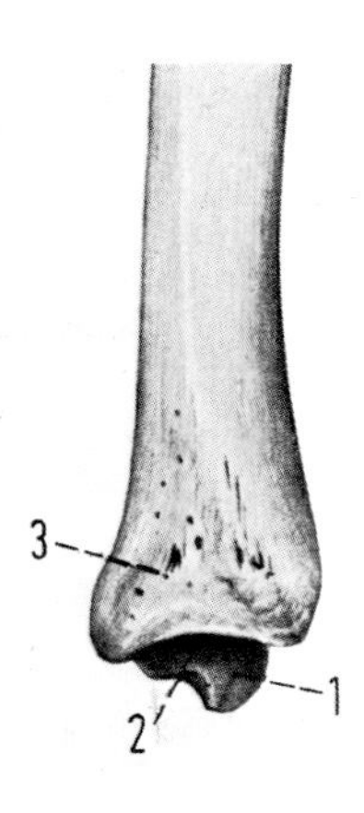

1 Lateral malleolar articular surface of tibia
2 Inferior articular surface of tibia
3 Incisura fibularis of tibia

Fig. 790. Right tibia, lateral view (from *Sobotta-Becher*, 17th Edition).

1 Tip of the medial malleolus
2 Tip of the lateral malleolus
3 Head of talus
4 Neck of talus
5 Trochlea of talus
6 Navicular bone
7 Base of metatarsal bone I
8 Cuboid bone
11 Calcaneal tuberosity
12 Medial (and lateral) processes of the calcaneal tuberosity
13 Sinus tarsi; above it: posterior process of talus
14 Sustentaculum tali
15 Pseudocystic triangle (see Fig. 823, No. 187)

(↙) Band of increased radiolucency, caused by superimposition: a pseudofissure, due to *Mach* effect

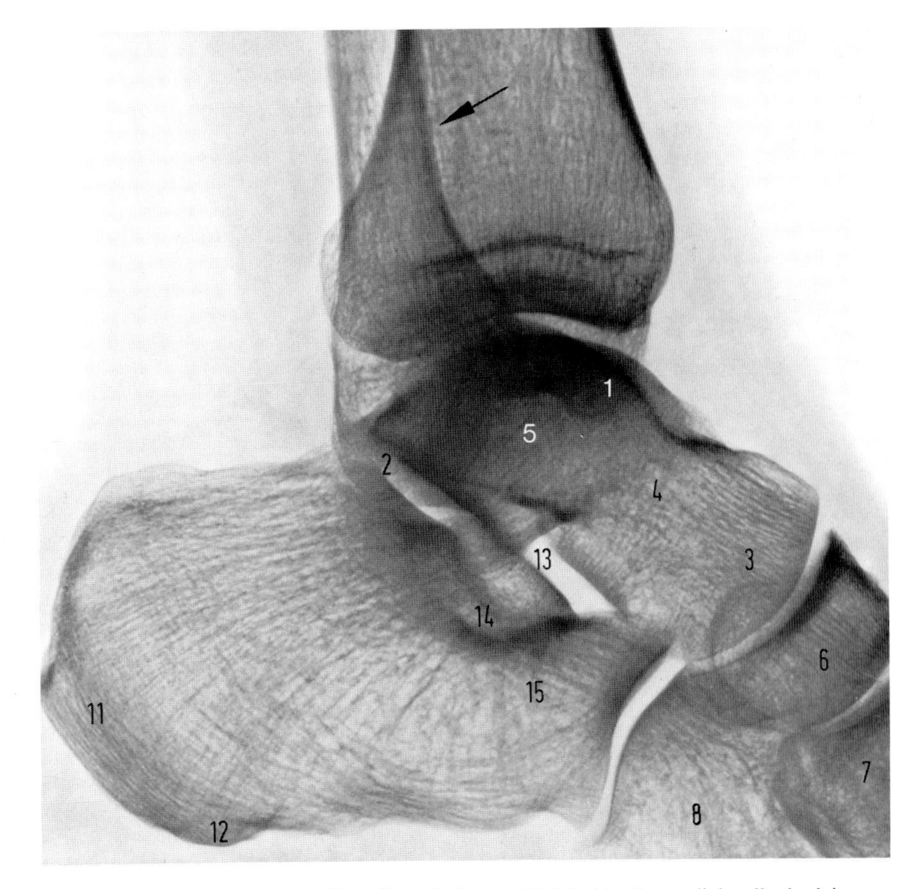

Fig. 791. Right talocrural joint, fibulotibial. Patient on his left side, the medial malleolus lying on the cassette. The central ray is aimed slightly in front of the base of the lateral malleolus (talocrural articulation). This view is quite similar to Fig. 788, however the parts of the foot which lie on the cassette appear sharper, as do the internal malleolus and the navicular bone.

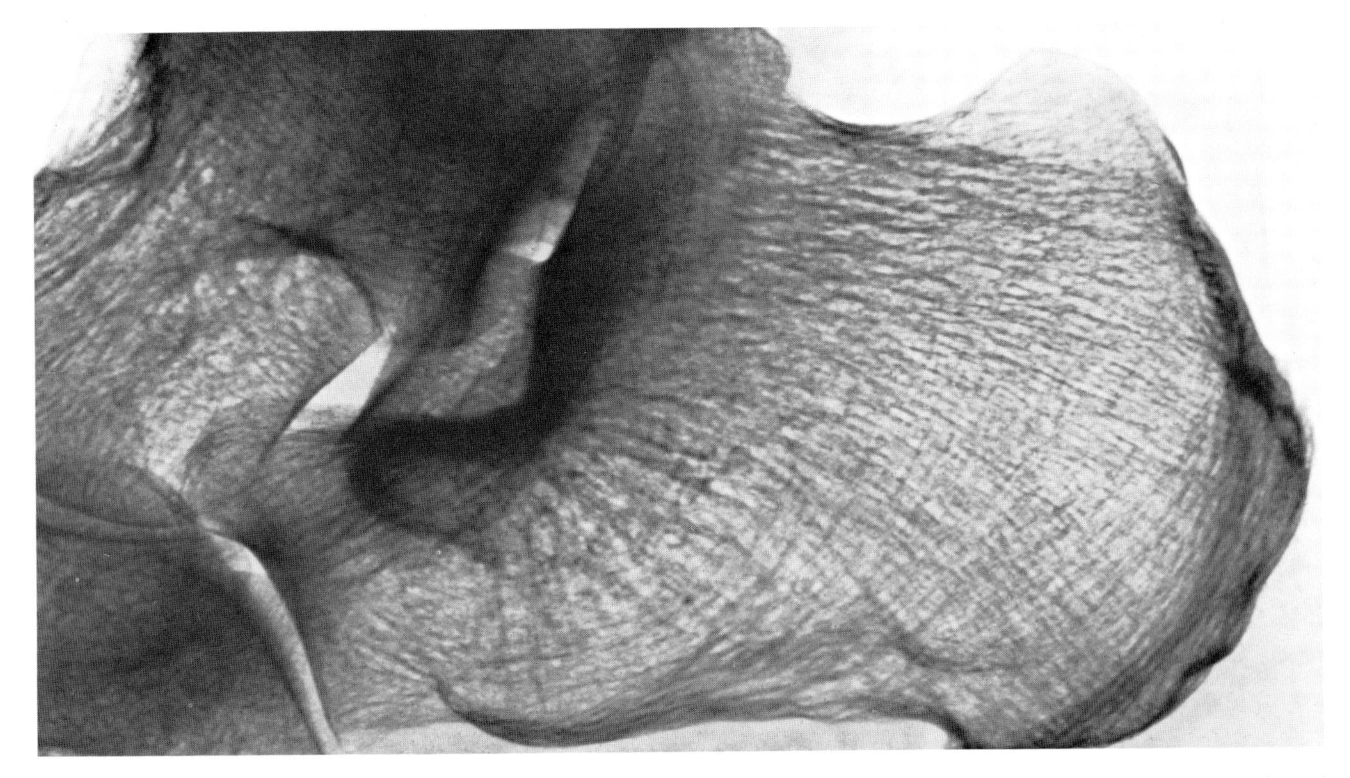

Fig. 792. Variant of shape of the posterior superior boundary of the calcaneus, showing as a hump-like exostosis at the upper pole of the calcaneal tuberosity *(Raspe)*. This is called a *Haglund* exostosis. The spur (due to advanced age) at the posterior surface (posterior calcaneal spur) is an ossification of ligamental and tendinous insertion; it is not a *Haglund* exostosis.

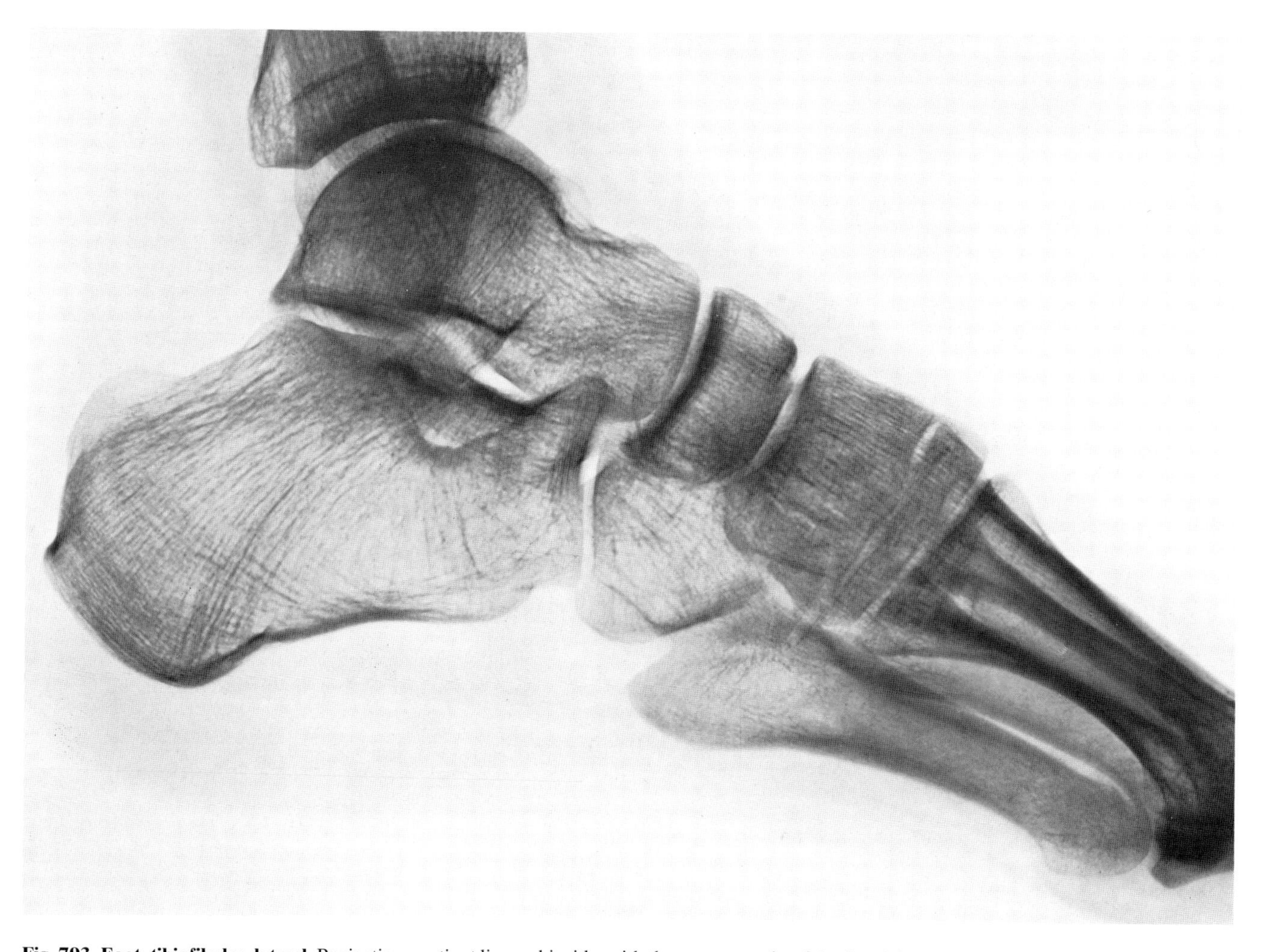

Fig. 793. Foot, tibiofibular, lateral. Projection : patient lies on his side, with the outer margin of the foot lying on the cassette. The central ray is directed onto the center of the tarsus.

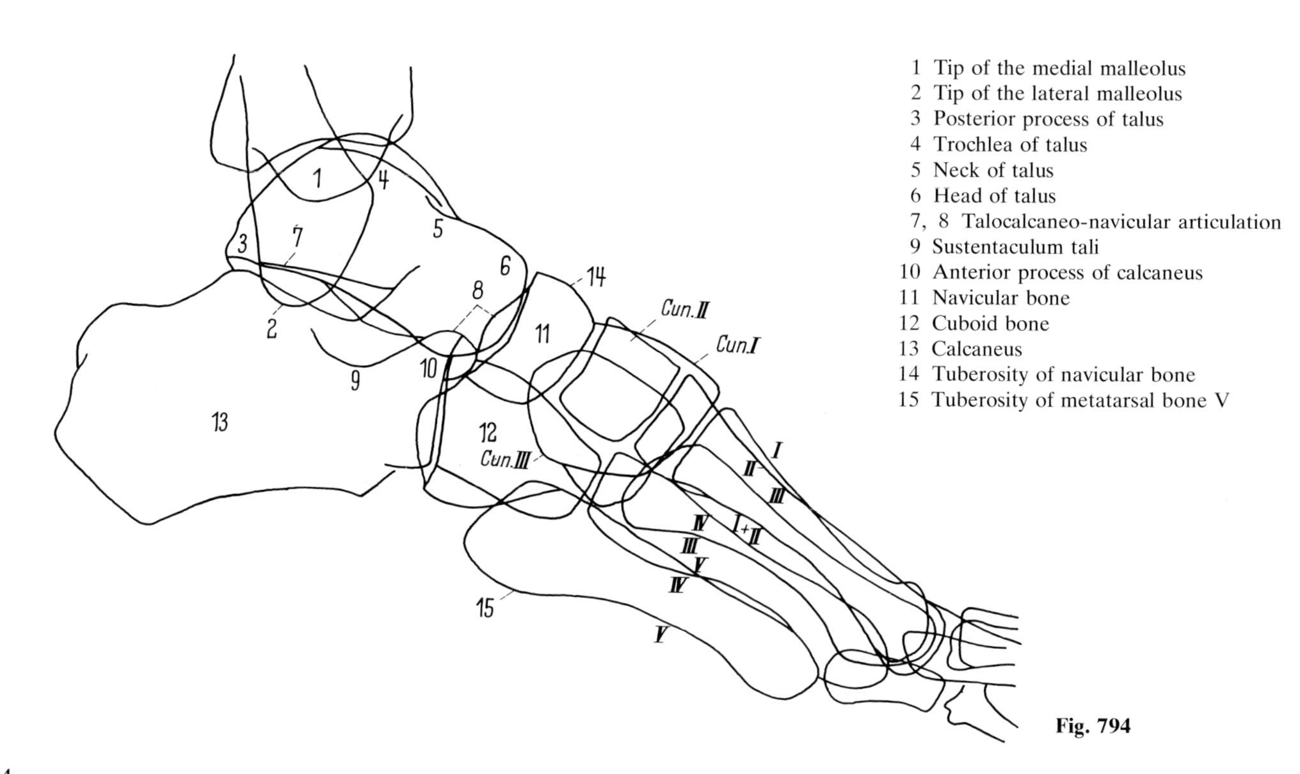

1 Tip of the medial malleolus
2 Tip of the lateral malleolus
3 Posterior process of talus
4 Trochlea of talus
5 Neck of talus
6 Head of talus
7, 8 Talocalcaneo-navicular articulation
9 Sustentaculum tali
10 Anterior process of calcaneus
11 Navicular bone
12 Cuboid bone
13 Calcaneus
14 Tuberosity of navicular bone
15 Tuberosity of metatarsal bone V

Fig. 794

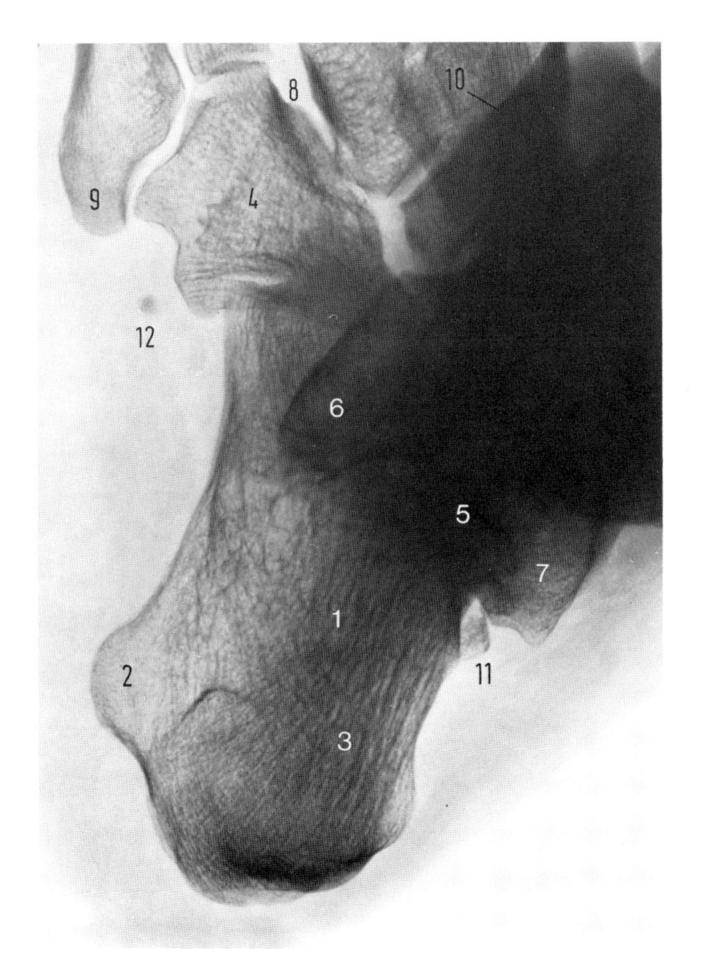

Fig. 795. Calcaneus, dorsocraniocaudal. For projection see Fig. 797.

1 Calcaneus
2 Lateral process of calcaneal tuberosity
3 Medial process of calcaneal tuberosity
4 Cuboid bone
5 Articulation between calcaneus and talus
6 Lateral malleolus
7 Posterior process of talus
8 Articulation between cuboid bone and lateral cuneiform bone (III)
9 Tuberosity of metatarsal bone V
10 Anterior margin of the soft tissues of the calf
11 Below the posterior process of the talus, a formation of bony density; query accessorium (os trigonum) or avulsion fragment of the posterior process of the talus
12 Accessorium under the cuboid bone; query os peroneum or calcification of a ligament

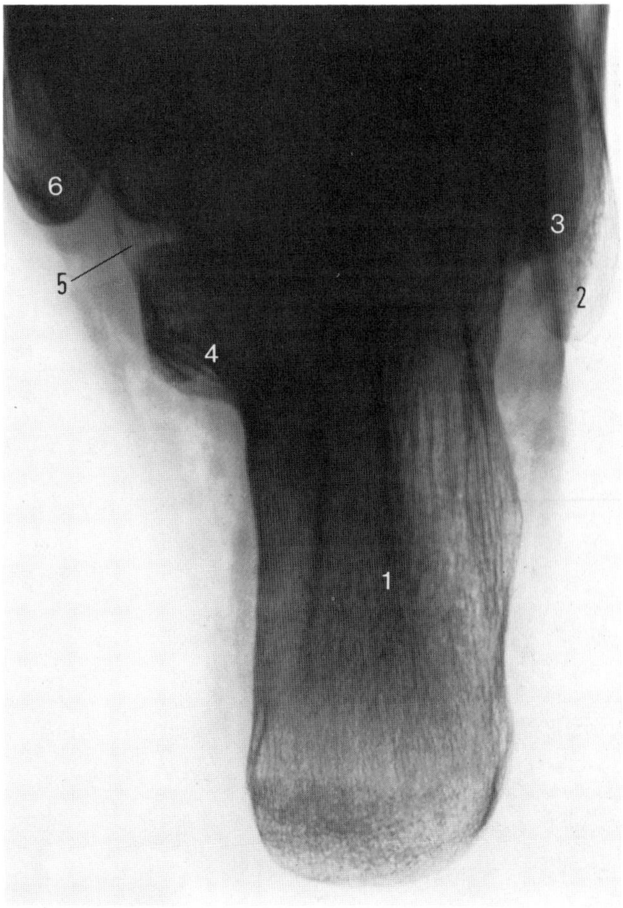

Fig. 796. Calcaneus, digitoplantodorsal. For projection see Fig. 798.

1 Calcaneus
2 Lateral malleolus
3 Tuberosity of metatarsal bone V
4 Sustentaculum tali and medial tubercle of the posterior process of talus
5 Head of talus
6 Tuberosity of navicular bone

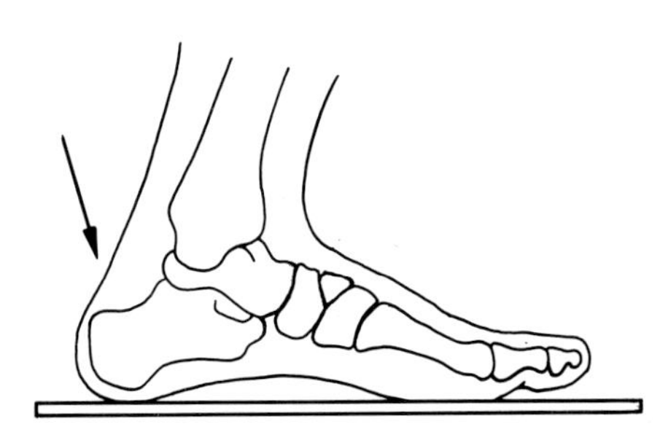

Fig. 797

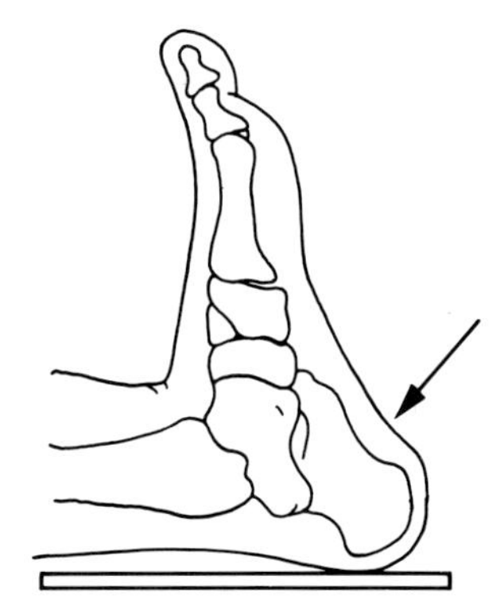

Fig. 798

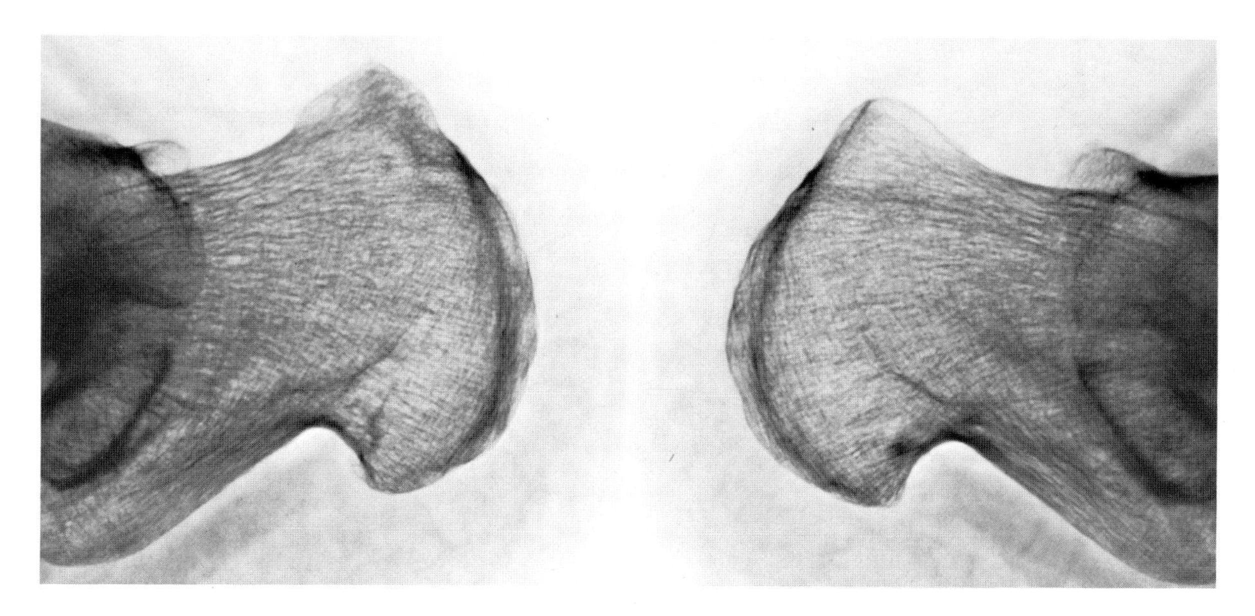

Fig. 799. Both calcanei, mediolateral (frog position). For projection see Fig. 800.

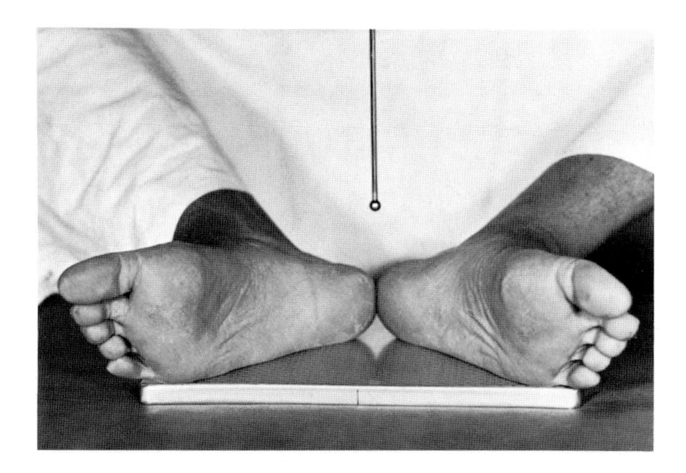

Fig. 800. This is an indispensable position for the diagnosis of an apophysitis of the calcaneus in juveniles *(Haglund* syndrome I) because of the comparability of both sides. Apophysitis is an aseptic necrotizing disease, especially in the flat-footed, which will later heal, leaving irregularly sclerosing, honeycomb or lamellar structures.

1 Posterior articular surface with talus
2 Medial articular surface with talus
3 Anterior articular surface with talus
4 Articular surface with cuboid bone
5 Sulcus for the tendon of the flexor hallucis longus muscle
6 Medial process of the calcaneal tuberosity
7 Calcaneal tuberosity
8 Sustentaculum tali

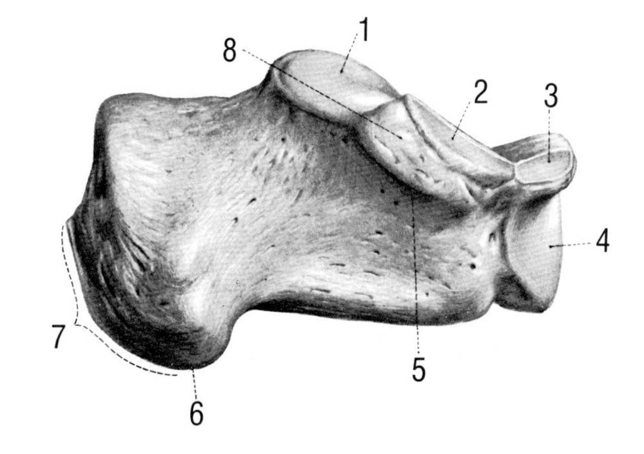

Fig. 801. Calcaneus, seen from medial, with sustentaculum tali (from *Sobotta-Becher,* 17th Edition, 1972).

Fig. 802. Metatarsus, semi-oblique, dorsoplantar. For projection see Fig. 804. This radiograph is important as a supplement to the usual dorsoplantar and lateral radiographs of the foot; it has the advantage that the metatarsotarsal joints are well visible and the anterior part of the foot is shown obliquely for detection of fractures. In addition, this view is useful to demonstrate the bony union between calcaneus and navicular bone. The sesamoid I of the fibula is divided into two (an exception); division of the sesamoid I of the tibia is more frequent. The cause of the divisions may be primary multiplicity of nuclei, osteochondrosis dissecans (osteochondropathy of juveniles) or an affect of traumatic fracture. If the division occurs after a fracture or after osteochondrosis dissecans, the sesamoids often contain necroses and are rather sensitive against pressure. Later on, these formations often take part in general osteoarthrotic processes (see also pp. 340–341).

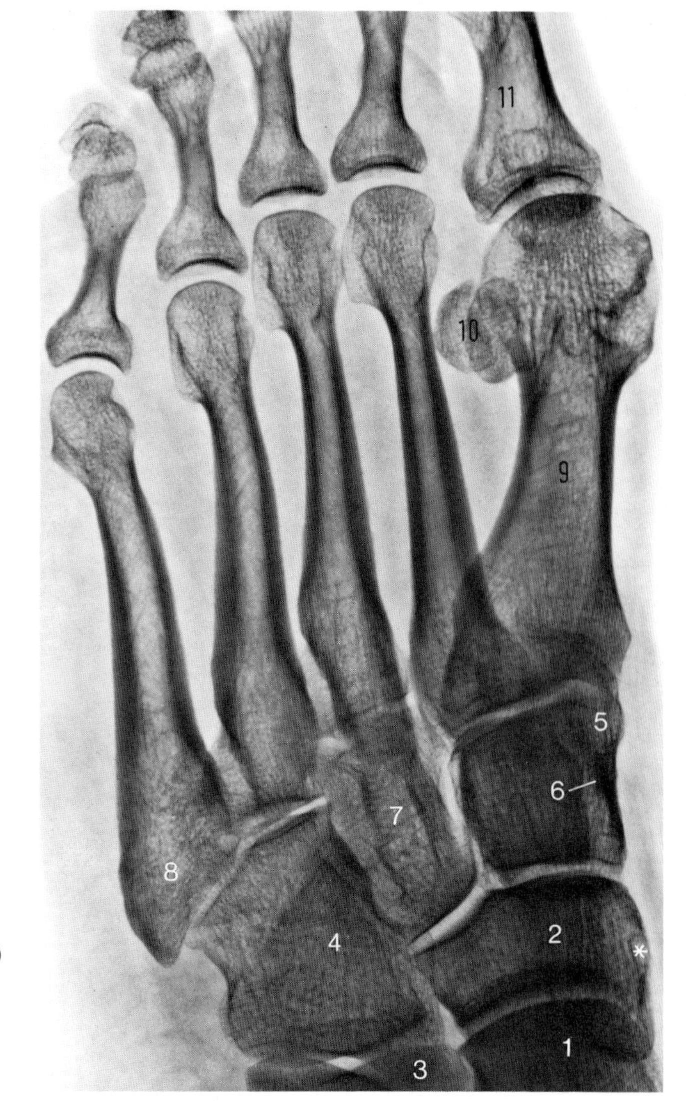

1 Head of talus
2 Navicular bone
* Tuberosity
3 Calcaneus
4 Cuboid bone
5 Medial cuneiform bone (I)
6 Intermediate cuneiform bone (II)
7 Lateral cuneiform bone (III)
8 Tuberosity of metatarsal bone V
9 Metatarsal bone I, with 10
10 Sesamoid bones
11 Proximal phalanx

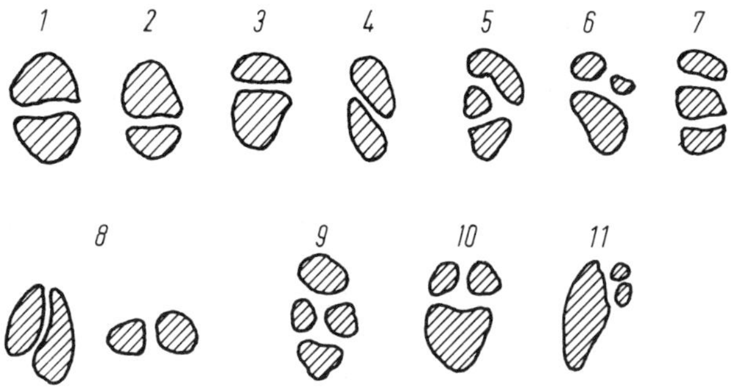

Fig. 803. Divisions of the sesamoid bones of the big toe, in order of frequency of their appearance (after *Kewenter).*

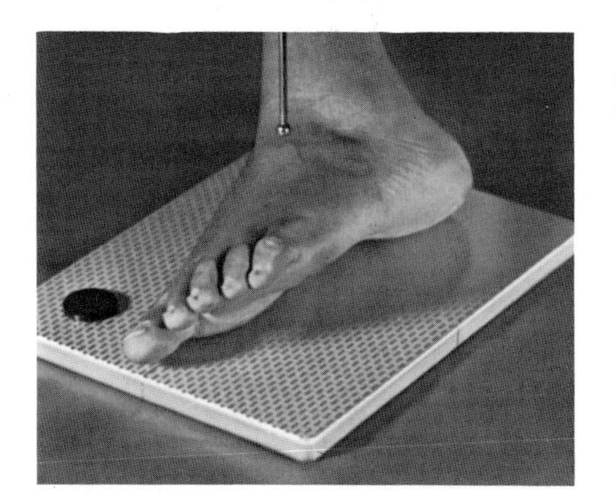

Fig. 804

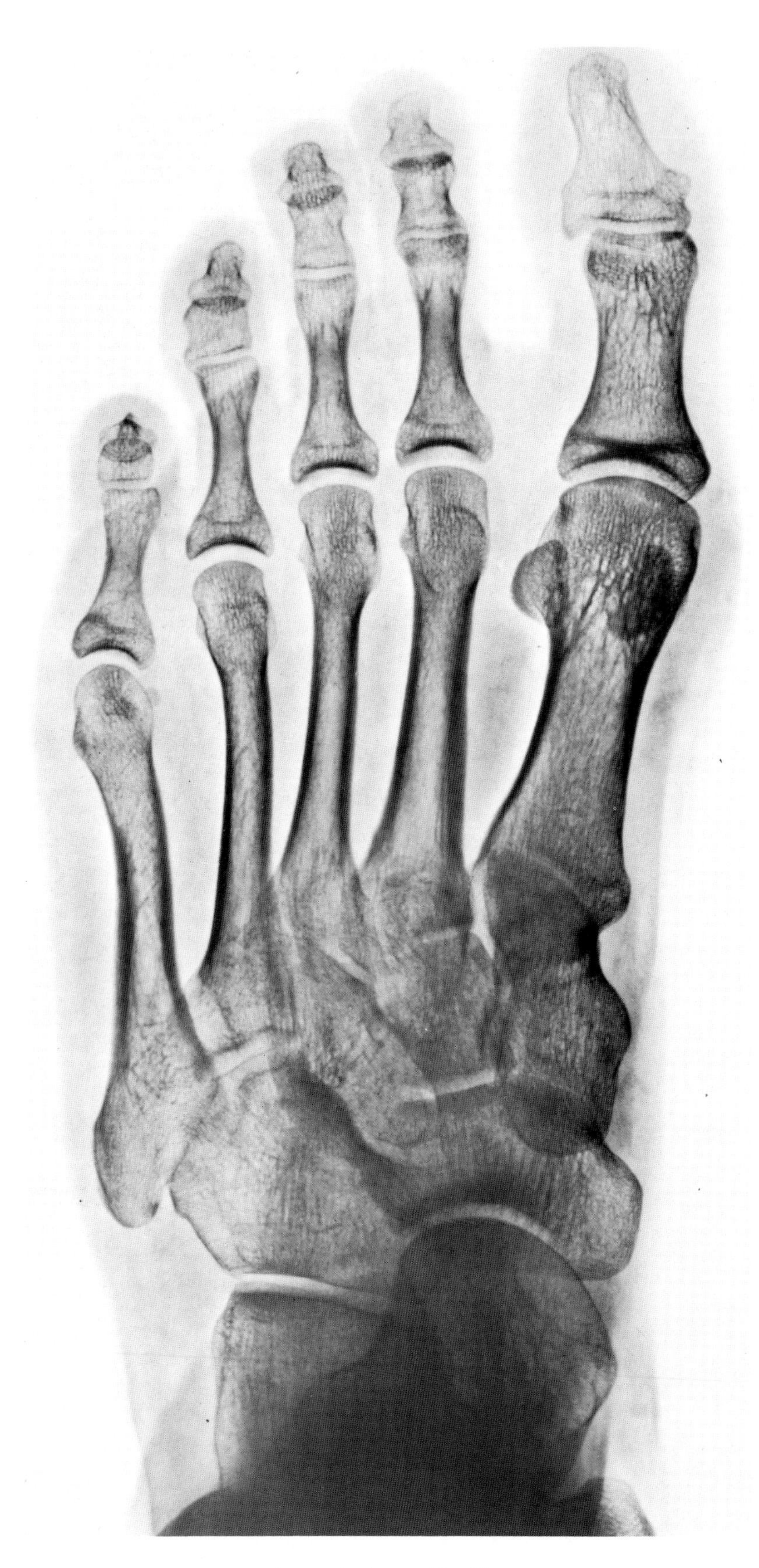

Fig. 805. Foot, dorsoplantar. For projection see Fig. 806.

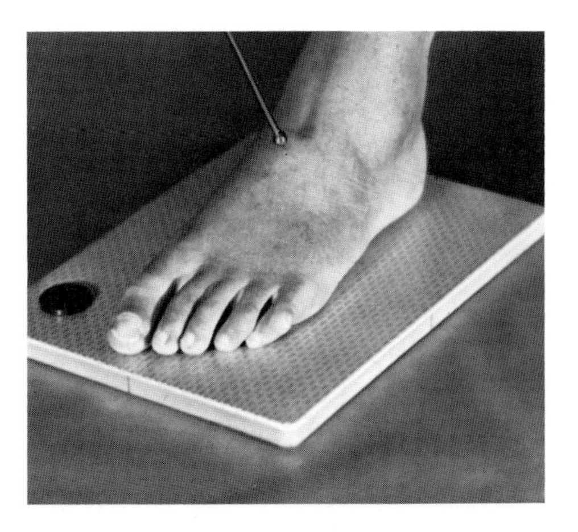

Fig. 806. The central ray is aimed onto the base of the 3rd metatarsal bone, at an angle of about 25°, inclined proximally (towards the heel); to achieve this, the articular spaces of the *Lisfranc* joints (i.e., the joints between tarsus and metatarsus) are taken as far tangentially as possible.

1 Medial cuneiform bone (I)
2 Intermediate cuneiform bone (II)
3 Lateral cuneiform bone (III)
4 Tuberosity of the navicular bone
5 Calcaneus
6 Lateral tubercle of talus
7 Trochlea
8 Head of talus
9 Cuboid bone
10 Tuberosity of metatarsal bone V

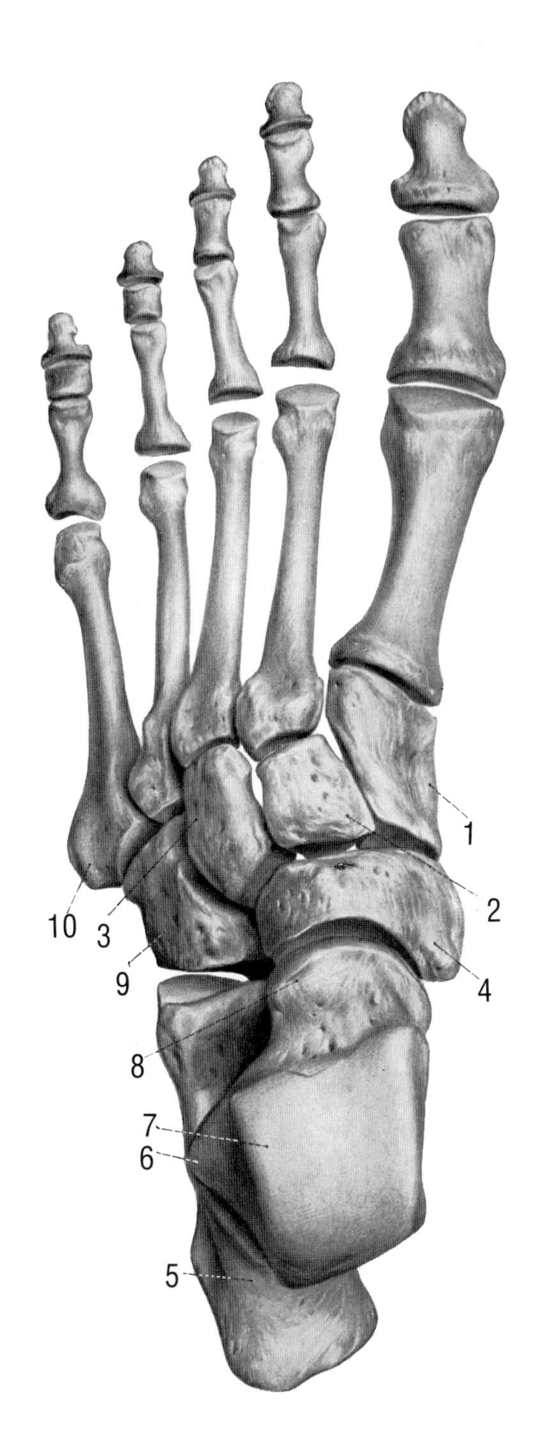

Fig. 807. Skeleton of the foot (from *Sobotta-Becher,* 17th Edition). This figure shows the foot as it is seen with the projection of Fig. 806 (i.e., from the direction of the central ray). With greater focus-film distance the projection is also fairly correct.

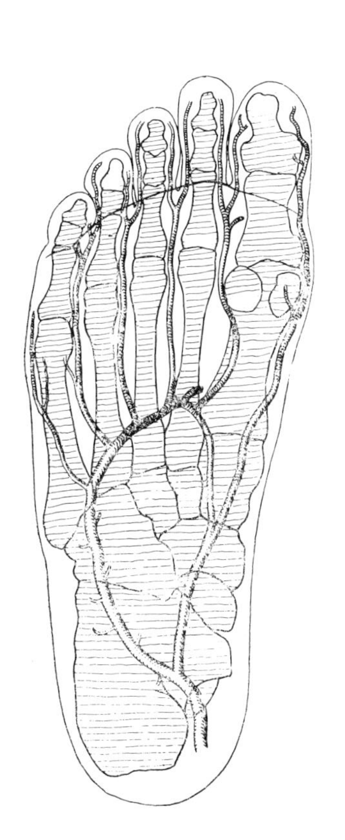

Fig. 808. Projection of the blood vessels onto a drawing of the bones (from *Corning).*

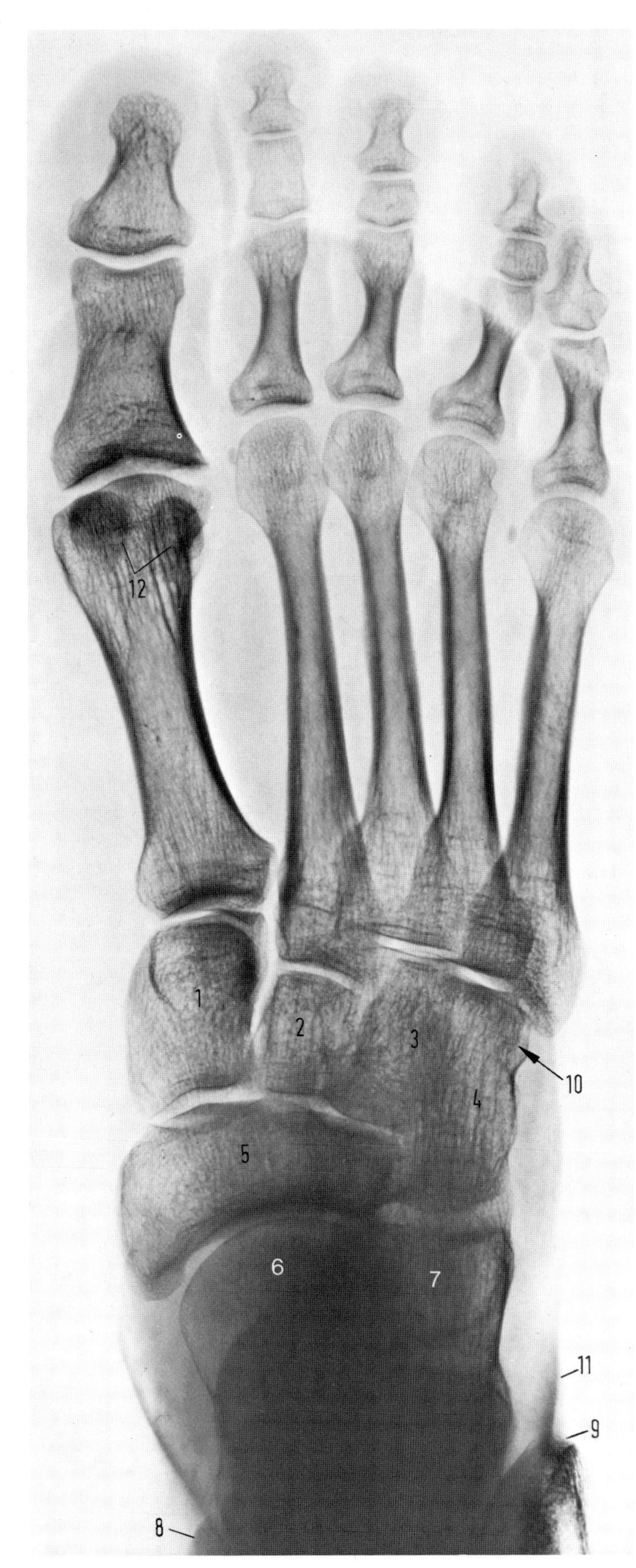

1, 2, 3 Cuneiform bones (I–III)
4 Cuboid bone
5 Navicular bone
6 Head of talus
7 Anterior calcaneal process
8 Tip of medial malleolus
9 Tip of lateral malleolus
10 Sulcus to the tendon of the peroneus longus muscle
11 Contour of soft tissues
12 Sesamoid bones; some additional small ones can be seen below the heads of the metatarsal bones II and V

Fig. 809. Foot, plantodorsal. For projection see Fig. 810. The central ray is aimed vertically onto the base of the metatarsal bones. *Lisfranc*'s articular line is well recognizable.

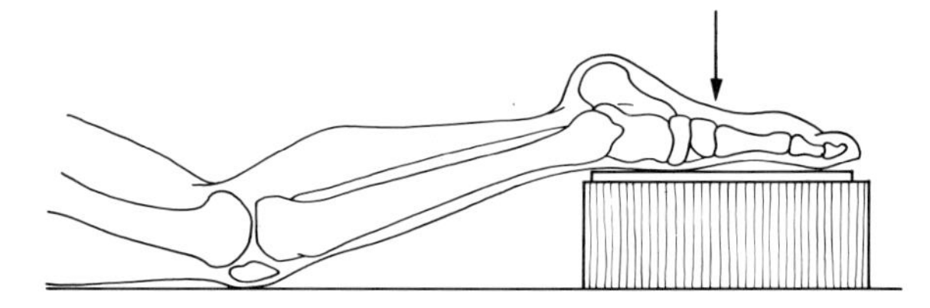

Fig. 810

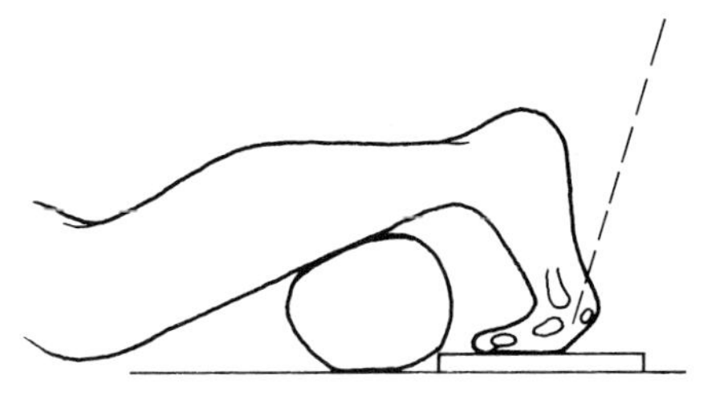

Fig. 811

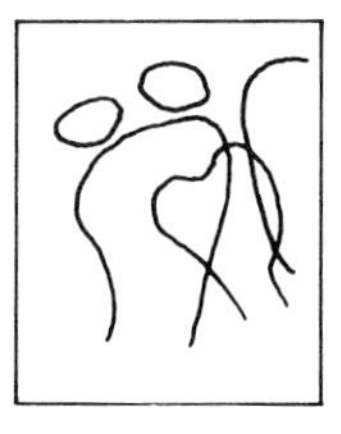

Fig. 812

Figs. 811 and 812. Sesamoid bones of the big toe. Technique of exposure according to *W. Müller* (see also Fig. 846, with technique of exposure).

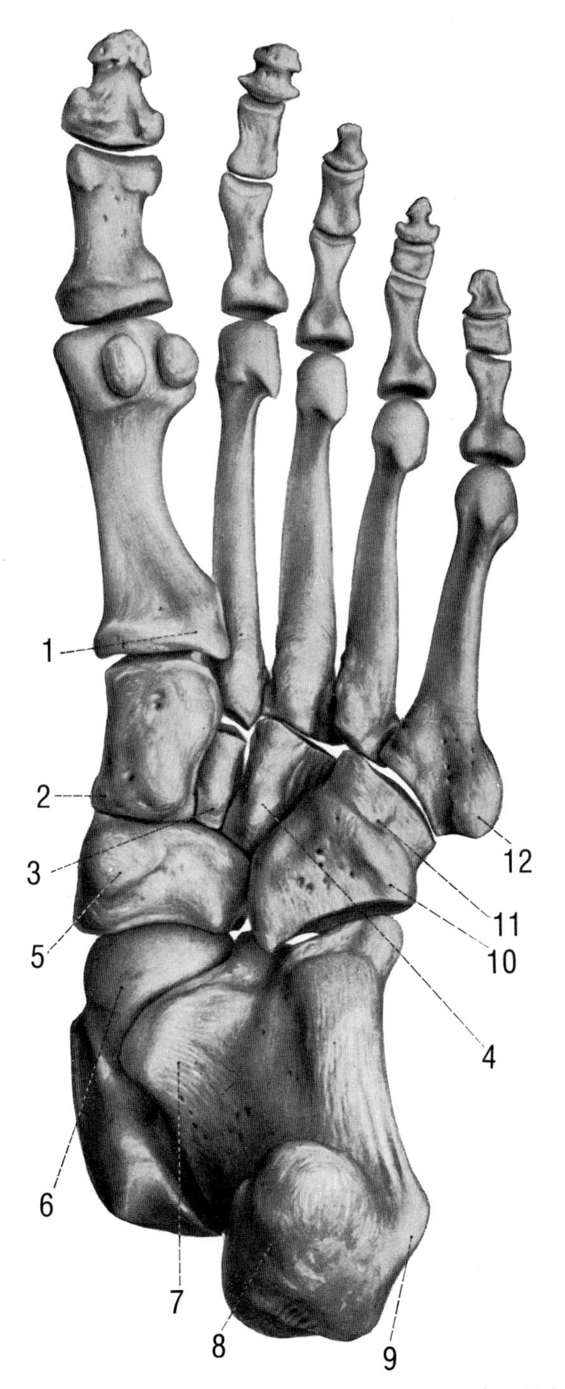

Fig. 813. Plantar view of the left foot (from *Sobotta-Becher,* 17th Edition).

1 Tuberosity of metatarsal bone I
2, 3, 4 Cuneiform bones (I–III)
5 Tuberosity of the navicular bone
6 Head of talus
7 Sustentaculum tali
8 Medial process of calcaneal tuberosity
9 Lateral process of calcaneal tuberosity
10 Tuberosity of cuboid bone
11 Sulcus of cuboid bone for tendon of peroneus longus muscle
12 Tuberosity of metatarsal bone V

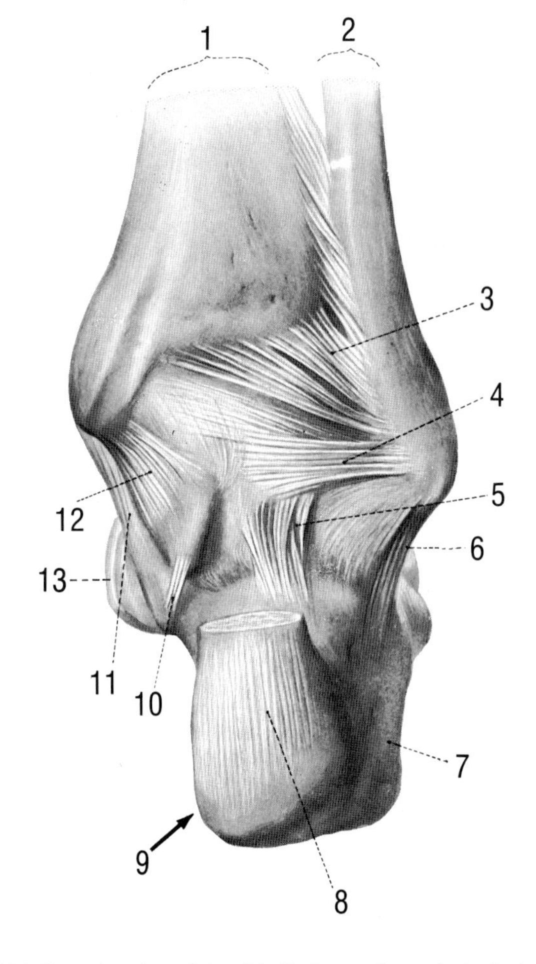

Fig. 814. Posterior view of the tibiofibular syndesmosis (articulation) **and of the talocrural articulation.** The tendo calcaneus has been cut (from *Sobotta-Becher,* 17th Edition).

1 Tibia
2 Fibula
3 Posterior tibiofibular ligament
4 Posterior talofibular ligament
5 Posterior talocalcaneal ligament
6 Calcaneofibular ligament
7 Calcaneus
8 Tendo calcaneus (Achilles tendon)
9 Calcaneal tuberosity
10 Medial talocalcaneal ligament
11 Calcaneotibial of part of deltoid ligament
12 Posterior talotibial part of deltoid ligament
13 Talus

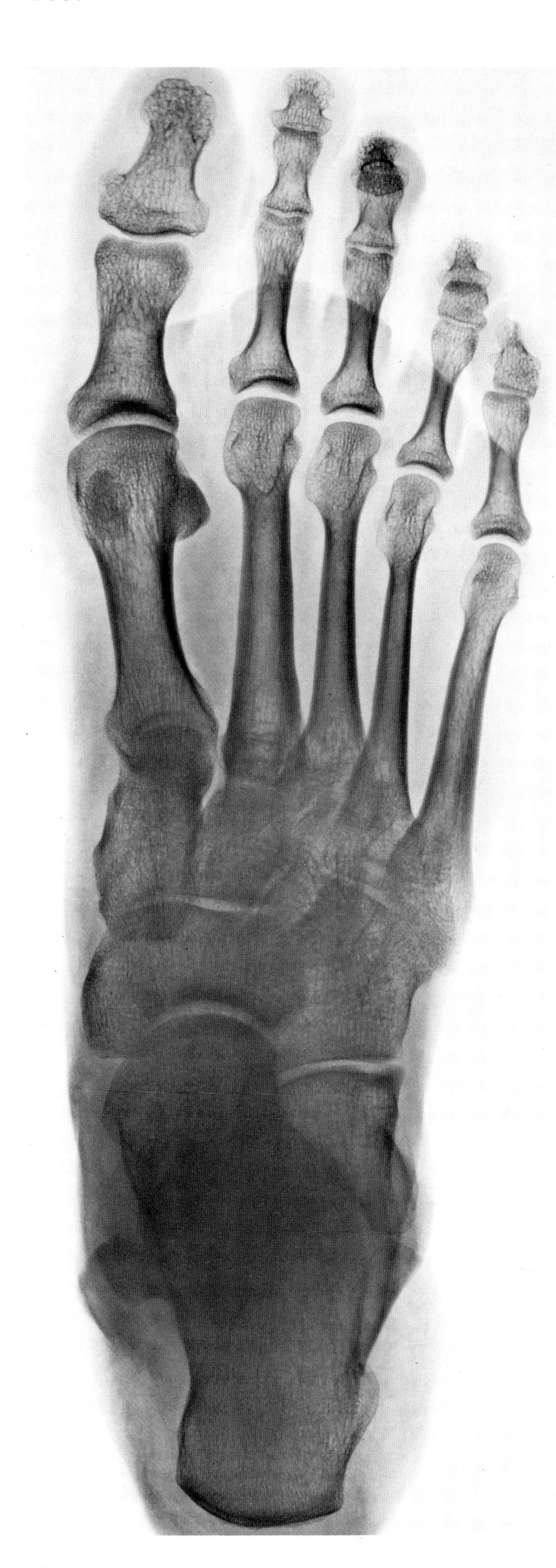

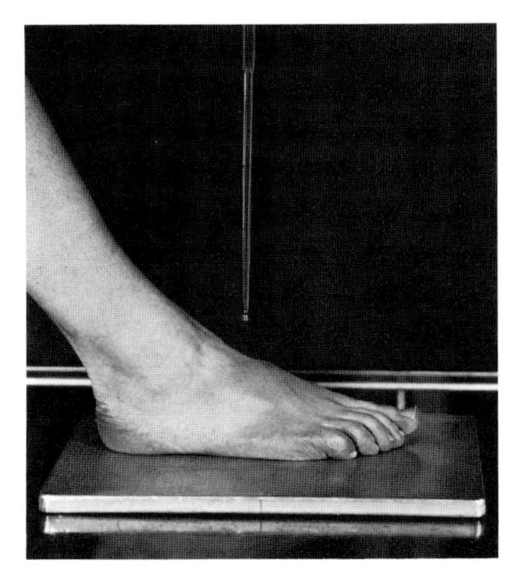

Fig. 816. First radiograph in pes equinus position, maximal plantar flexion. Focus–film distance 1 m.

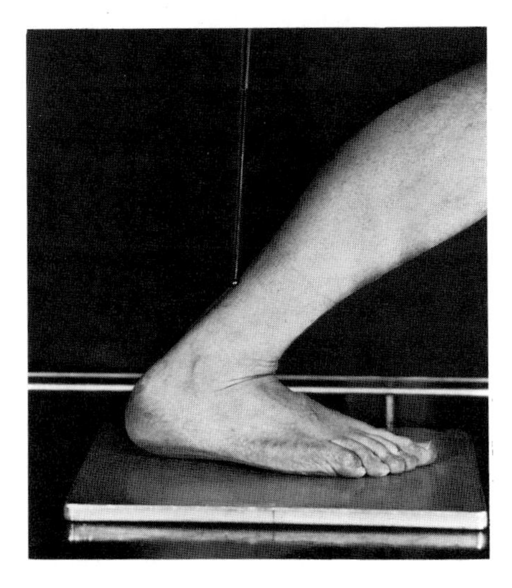

Fig. 817. Second radiograph in pes calcaneus position, maximal dorsiflexion of the foot, knee bent. The central ray is directed unchanged vertically to the film onto the region of the head of the talus. Focus–film distance 1 m. The foot is placed on the maximal fixed cassette, the central ray directed exactly vertically. At first the calf projects beyond the posterior margin of the cassette. The first radiograph (Fig. 816) is taken with a small dose. Then the patient must bend forward maximally, while the sole of the foot remains unchanged on the cassette (Fig. 817). Now the radiograph is taken with a greater dose.

Fig. 815. View of whole foot, dorsoplantar *(Fischer-Wasels).* For projection see Figs. 816 and 817.

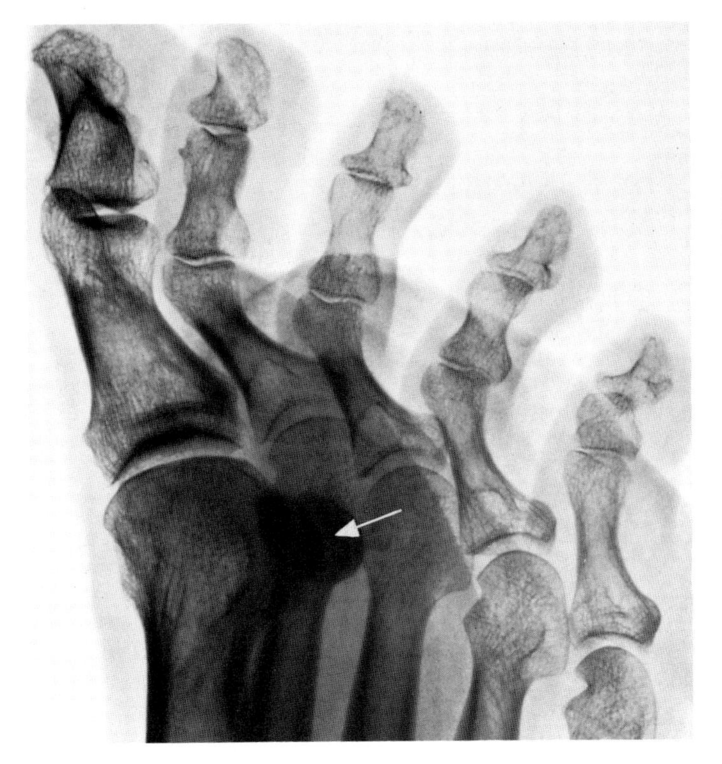

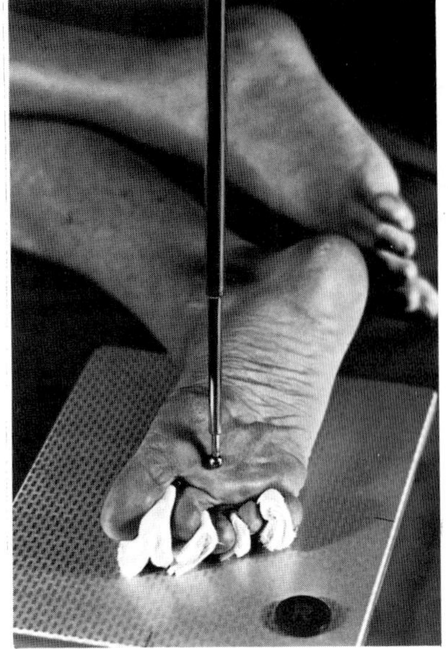

Fig. 818. Toes, semi-oblique; foot medilateral. For projection see Fig. 819. The central ray is aimed approximately onto the head of the metatarsal bone III. One sees the foot from the direction of the margin of the 5th toe. The peculiar pinioning of the metatarsal heads on the lateral view, especially that of the 5th, is remarkable. (↙) Two sesamoids at the 1st metatarsal head.

Fig. 819

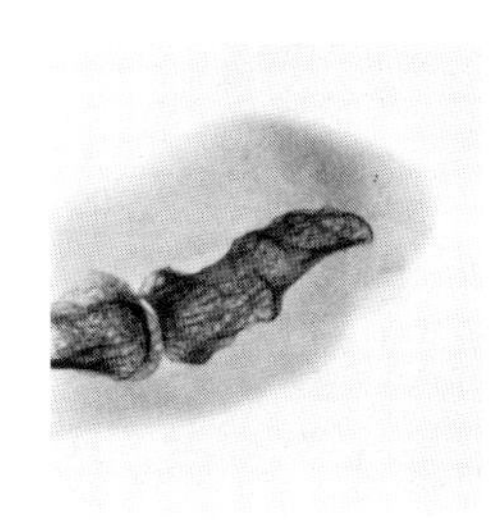

Fig. 820. Fifth toe, lateromedial. Dental film in the interdigital space. Articular space between the basal phalanx and the fused middle and ungual phalanges.

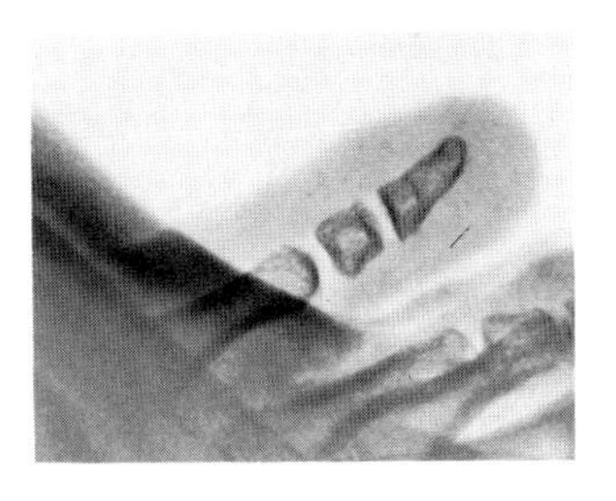

Fig. 821 a

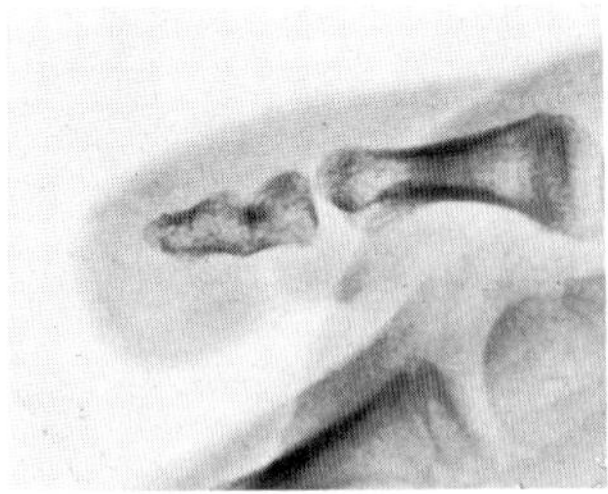

Fig. 821 b

Fig. 821. Fusion of ungual and middle phalanges of the right 5th toe (821 b), while the phalanges of the left 5th toe have developed normally. This fusion can be observed in about 1/3 or 1/4 of cases *(Köhler-Zimmer)*.

Variants and Sources of Diagnostic Error of the Talocrural Joint, the Ankle, Tarsus and Toes*

To Figs. 822 and 823:

168 Band of superimposition *(Mach* effect), see Figs. 788, 791; a pseudofissure *(Dihlmann)*

170 Os tibiale externum = an accessorium of the navicular bone. It lies in the tendon of the tibialis posterior muscle and, according to *Francillon,* may develop on the basis of connective, chondroid or cancellous tissue, as well as on a hyaline-cartilaginous basis. One finds a fully developed and a rudimentary form, a conglomeration of single shapeless particles, and a cartilaginous form. The os tibiale externum may be divided and may fracture *(Kienböck* and *Müller).* Its frequency is about 10% (Figs. 854, 855). See also *Schlevogt, Hensel.*

170* Os cuboideum secundarium? Not proven by radiography; has been mentioned by *Pfitzner* as an anatomical hypothesis only.

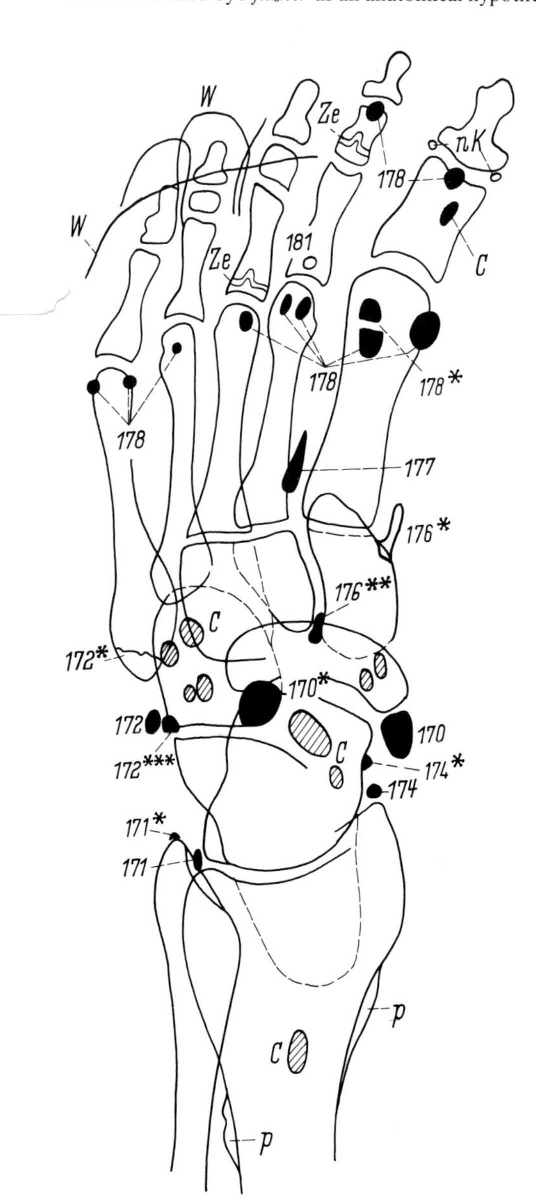

Fig. 822. Variants and sources of diagnostic error of the foot and malleoli (dorsoplantar view).

171 Intercalary bone between lateral malleolus and talus (Fig. 859)

171* Os subfibulare (see *de Cuveland, Brauer);* has its own center of ossification in the tip of the malleolus

172 Os peroneum = os cuboideum accessorium (see Figs. 865, 866). It may be divided several times. One sees a sesamoid in the tendon of the peroneus longus muscle (Fiebelkorn). *Gnilka* described the development of a similar ossicle from a fragment torn off the base of the metatarsal bone V. *Dittert* mentioned a peritendinitis calcarea of possibly similar appearance which vanished after radiation therapy. See also *Carey* and *Drexler; Sieckel.*

172* Persistent apophysis at the base of metatarsal bone V (Fig. 861); cf. also no. 185*

172** Accessory epiphysis, simulating a fracture (Fig. 1199)

172*** Os calcaneocuboideum laterale *(Teichert).* It has not been clarified whether it belongs to the calcaneus (persistent apophysis of the lateral upper margin) or to the cuboid bone.

174 Os subtibiale = accessory talus (Fig. 858). It may be divided; it represents a persistent inconstant nucleus in the tip of the medial malleolus. It may occur unilaterally or bilaterally, and has been found in about 14% of examined cases *(de Cuveland* and *Heuck, de Cuveland, Hoed, Volkmann, Waschulewski).* If it occurs unilaterally, one must decide whether this is an avulsion of bone, another effect of injury or an accessorium *(Brauer).*

174* Os sustentaculi (Fig. 881), a persistent apophysis

174** Os supratalare, here on a spur of the talus, though it may also occur in the absence of a spur. Differential diagnosis against ossification in the talocalcaneal ligament (Fig. 849).

175 Os supranaviculare (Fig. 877, differential diagnosis against Fig. 878). Might it be an effect of shearing-off or a persistent accessory nucleus of the navicular bone which had been preformed by several nuclei? Multiple accessory nuclei are liable to aseptic necrosis and to osteochondrosis *(Ueberschär)*

175* Stress fracture of calcaneous (Fig. 850); see *Rumpold*

176 Os cuneometatarsale II dorsale *(Schoen).* Persistent distal apophysis of the cuneiform bone II *(de Cuveland)* or result of trauma?

176* Supernumerary preformation of hallux *(Werthemann)*

176** Os intercuneiforme dorsale (Fig. 852). Regarding an os cuneometatarsale I dorsalefibulare, see *Marti.*

177 Os intermetatarsale I (Fig. 841). It may sometimes fracture; may show calcification of muscle or tendon, and can be simulated by calcification of blood vessels *(Faber, Haid).* Its frequency is 1–8%.

178 Sesamoids (Figs. 842, 843 and 846). Multiple divisions, diseases (aseptic necrosis) and injuries are possible: *Hubay, Kewenter*

178* Divided sesamoid (Figs. 839, 845 and 847); may be preformed primarily or develop secondarily after juvenile osteochondropathy or injury

179 Os trigonum = intermedium (Fig. 867); above it, query avulsion fragment out of the posterior process of talus or partition of the trigonum. It may occur divided (Fig. 870) or can fuse with the calcaneus (Fig. 871).

* The numbers in bold type are also (or only) to be found on the lateral (dorsoplantar) view.

Fig. 823. Variants and sources of diagnostic error of the foot (lateral view).

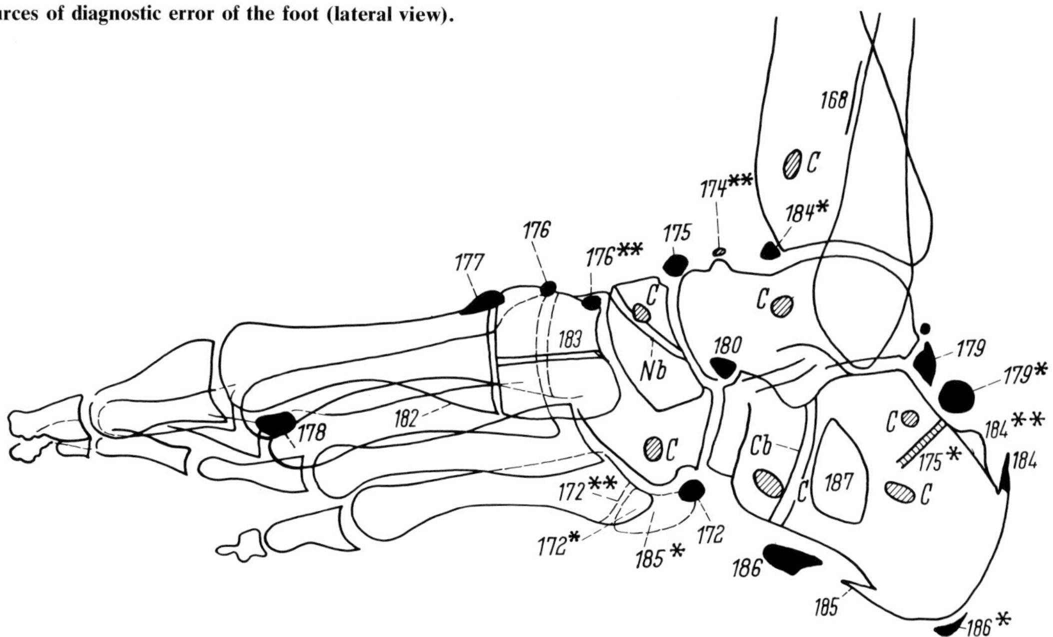

179* So-called os accessorium supracalcaneum (Fig. 872). It might be the posterior of two persistent nuclei of the posterior process of the talus, a dislodged os trigonum or an ossification of the bursa tendinis calcanei *(de Cuveland, Ravelli, Kremser, Schmitt).*

180 Calcaneus secundarius (Figs. 873, 874); must be differentiated from a fracture of the anterior calcaneal process or from an os tibiale externum *(Schoen, Porstmann* and *Arenz, Marti, Naumann)*

181 Small bone cyst (see Fig. 842); is without pathological significance and may occur multiply in primary chronic polyarthritis, syringomyelia and other diseases *(zur Verth)*

182 Band caused by superimposition of metatarsal bones, a pseudofissure (see Fig. 793)

183 Bipartite cuneiform bone (Fig. 1216); it occurs only with the medial cuneiform bone. According to *Pfitzner,* a persistent division into a plantar and a dorsal cuneiform bone can be observed in 0.3% of cases, and in twins and also bilaterally. See *Heidsieck, Barclay, Neumann.*

184 Spur on posterior calcaneus (Fig. 792), the ossified insertion of the Achilles tendon *(Haglund, Sack, Fröhlich).* Spurs developing with advanced age occur bilaterally, mostly without discomfort. In contrast, the inflammatory spur (bursitis achillea) is mainly unilateral and painful. *Volkmann* reported on a bilateral ossification within the Achilles tendon.

184* Os talotibiale; its existence is very questionable. Is it a piece of avulsed bone or a loose body in the joint? It must be differentiated from the os supratalare, which rests more distally on the dorsum of the talus.

184** *Haglund*'s exostosis is an atypical form of the dorsal section of the posterior process of the calcaneus, in the shape of a hump-like bulge (see Figs. 788, 792 and 880), caused by chronic pressure

185 Spur below calcaneus (Figs. 866, 867). It is usually a calcification of the insertion at the medial process of the calcaneal tuberosity, but may also be the result of an inflammation of the subcutaneous calcaneal bursa. It arises only rarely in the young, mainly between the 40th and 50th years of life. This ossification of the exostotic spur may also come about as the effect of degenerative damages of the insertion of the tendon at the tuberosity (especially with tendency to pes pronatus, pes planus or pes excavatus). See *Sack, Stucke, Seyss.*

185* "Os Vesalianum." According to *Schoen,* this is presumably a rare accessory bone. *Vesalius* described it "ad insertionem tendinis octavi pedem moventium musculi" (quoted by *de Cuveland),* which means a sesamoid at the place of insertion of the peroneus brevis muscle. In the present author's opinion, it represents an enlarged persistent apophysis of the metatarsal bone V, after trauma (see also Fig. 861).

186 Calcification within the plantar aponeurosis which may occur extensively and in multiplicity (Fig. 879); see *Jaroschy.*

186* "Os subcalcis or os tuberis calcanei" (accessorium); see *Millikan, Niemann, Heimerzheim.* It has no connection with the plantar aponeurosis.

187 Pseudocystic triangle (see Fig 788), in a normal calcaneus. It is well recognizable in 7% and moderately distinct in 22% *(Sirry),* but it may also occur in pathological states (deforming osteitis, enchondromata, arthritic cysts and other conditions).

C Islet of compact tissue; cf. Fig. 848 *(Fischer, H.)*

p Pseudoperiostitis, often at the points of insertion of tendons (Fig. 712)

NB Acquired bipartite navicular bone, after trauma. The division of this bone as a variant has not been proven (see *Zimmer, Schulte, Henssge).*

nk Accessory nuclei *(Ravelli)*

Ze Peg-shaped epiphyses *(Ravelli, Rossmann, Morscher,* see also Fig. 706)

Cb "Calcaneus bifidus" *(Smola, Schlüter, Bazant),* a temporary cleft formation in the anterior third of the calcaneus, vertical to its longitudinal axis *(Sever).* Fusion until the 5th year of life.

W Contour of soft tissues of toes and their overlying muscles

Bibliographies on variants, anomalies and accessoria may be found in *Pfitzner* (1896), *Schönkess* (1935), *Trolle* (1948), and *de Cuveland* (1957).

Figs. 824–826. Schema of variants for the skeleton of the human foot (after *Pfitzner)*.

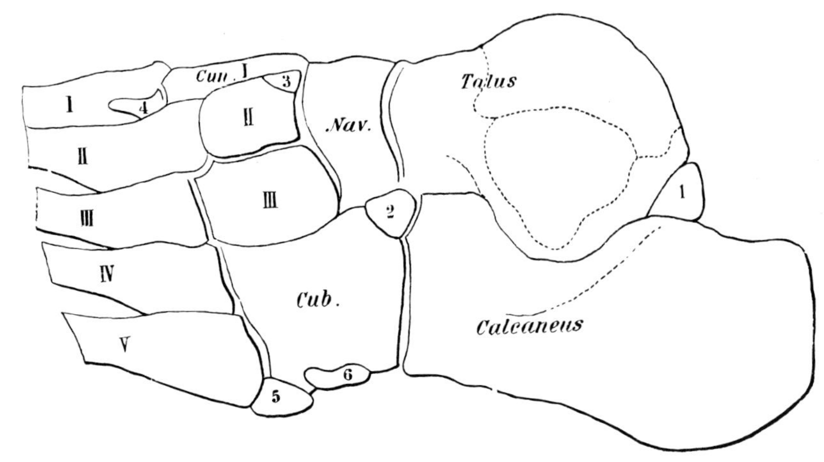

Fig. 824. Lateral view.

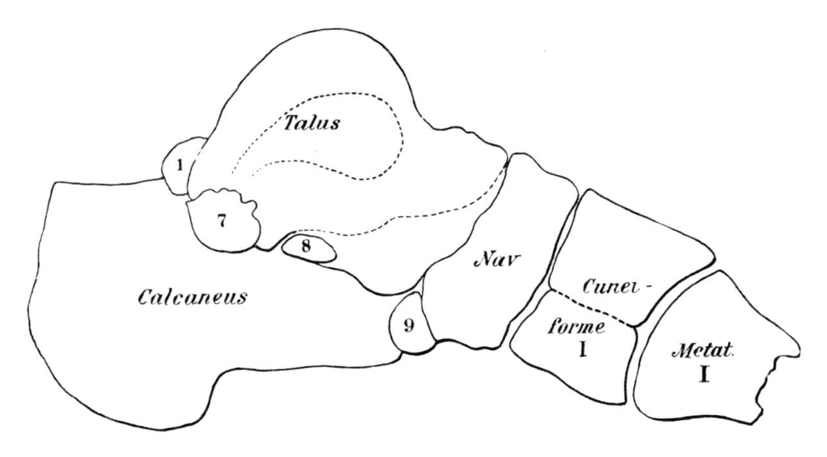

Fig. 825. Medial view.

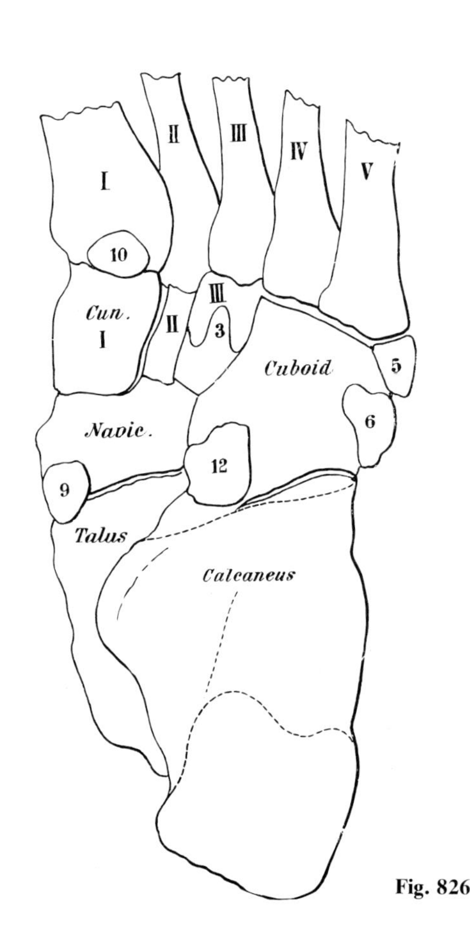

Fig. 826

1 Trigonum (intermedium cruris); see Figs. 867, 870 and 871 (synostosed), Fig. 823, No. 179
2 Calcaneus secundarius (a joint between calcaneus and navicular bone may occur); Fig. 823, No. 180, Figs. 873, 874
3 Intercuneiforme dorsale (Fig. 823, No. 176**, Fig. 852)
4 Intermetatarseum dorsale = os intermetatarsale I, Fig. 841; it may articulate, fuse with or move away from the cuneiform bone I or the metatarsal bone I
5 "Vesalianum"; see Fig. 823, No. 185*
6 Os peroneum (see Fig. 822, No. 172, Fig. 865) of the terminal tendon of the peroneus longus muscle; appears divided in Fig. 863
7 Talus accessorius = os subtibiale (Figs. 860, 858, 822, No. 174)
8 Os sustentaculi *(Grashey)*, Fig. 881. Occasionally, it is also visible on anteroposterior views of the talocrural joint. It is of clinical importance as it always causes discomfort.
9 Os tibiale externum (Fig. 854 a, b, Fig. 855), is found in the terminal tendon of the tibialis posterior muscle; it may be divided (Fig. 856, Fig. 822, No. 170)
10 Peroneal part of metatarsal bone I. *Maurer* also described the peroneal part of metatarsal bone II as an oval, button-like shadow above the base of metatarsal bone II
12 Cuboideum secundarium? Fig. 822, No. 170*

Abortive bipartition occurs with 1 and 6. If the inconstant bones become assimilated to the constant bones, these will show corresponding excrescences. On the other hand, apophyseal nuclei appear during adolescence. The apophysis at the base of the metatarsal bone V is found regularly (Fig. 861). Furthermore, we once saw a persistent supernumerary apophysis which separated the base of the metatarsal bone V in the shape of a transversely placed wedge (it may develop from a pseudoepiphysis; see Fig. 823, No. 172** and Fig. 1199).

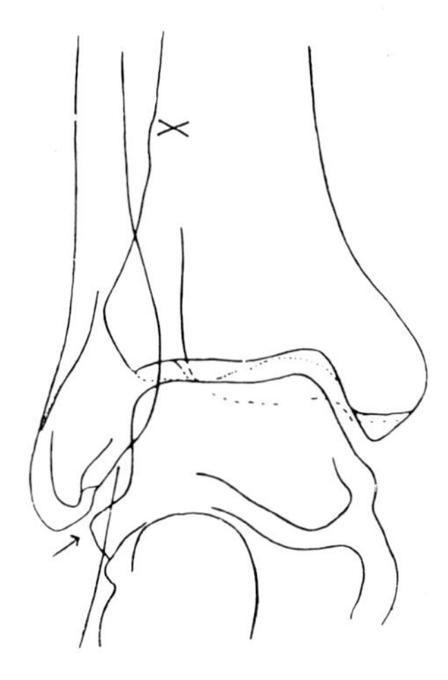

Fig. 827 (male, 39 years of age) shows at × a sometimes visible normal prominence. Occasionally, a longer stretch of the contour may be roughened. The arrow points to an occasionally pronounced, sharply jutting-out prominence of the talus.

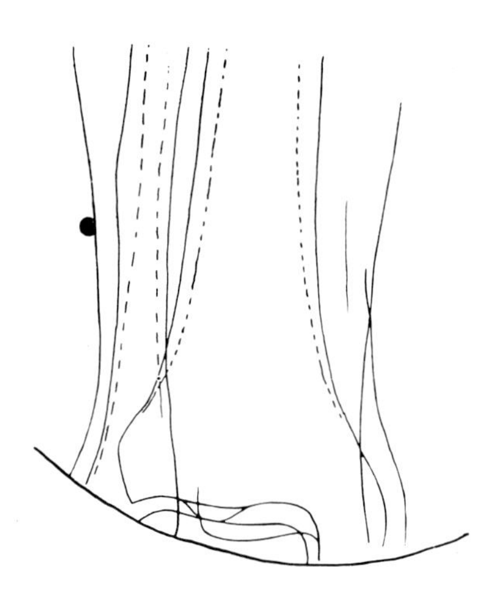

Fig. 828 shows at the lateral side of the fibula an often palpable spot, suspect of callus but in fact normal. Here, it is shown on the skin by a black dot.

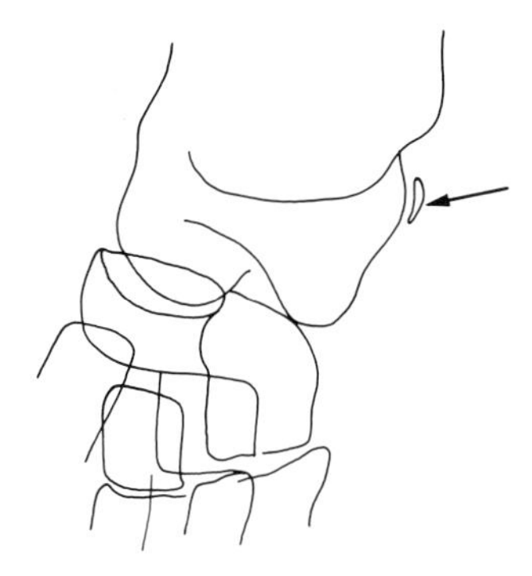

Fig. 829. Inconstant apophysis at the peroneal (fibular) trochlea, also called os trochleare calcanei or accessory calcaneus.

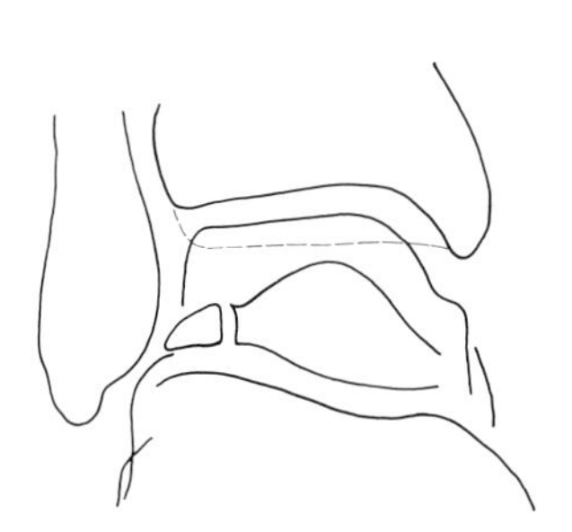

Fig. 830. Once we observed in the talus, above the articular space of the talocalcaneal joint, a cleft which we could not localize exactly. Apparently it had not been pathological.

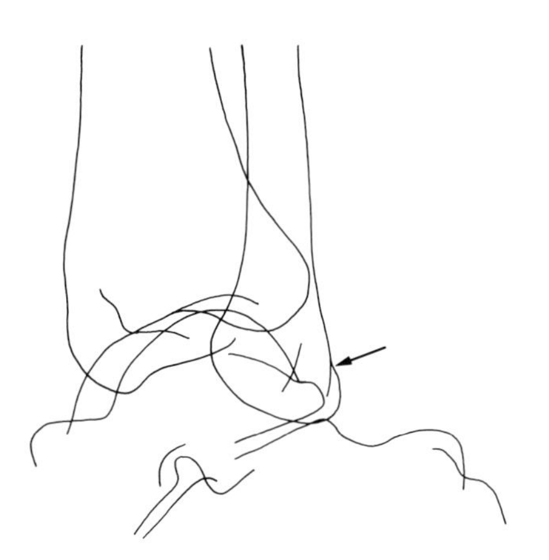

Fig. 831

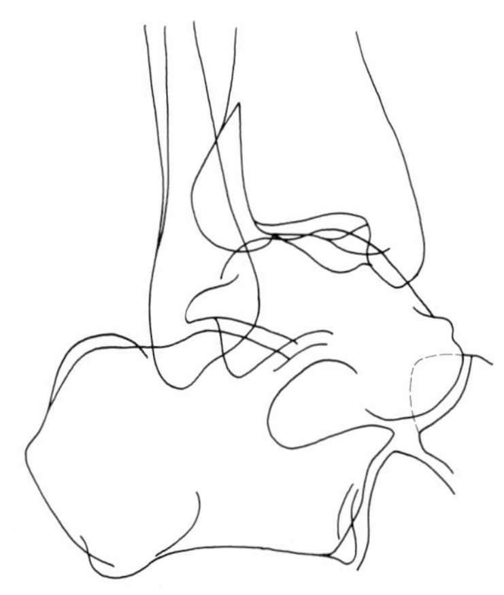

Fig. 832

Figs. 831 and 832. With this projection one sees quite often (Fig. 832) that surface of the tibia which turns towards the fibula distinctly set off, tapering off in cranial direction. Furthermore (Fig. 831, arrow), the lateral malleolus, taken obliquely, often shows a conspicuous prominence which may be taken for an avulsion fracture or a callus. For anomalies of the distal fibula, see *Petersen, F.*

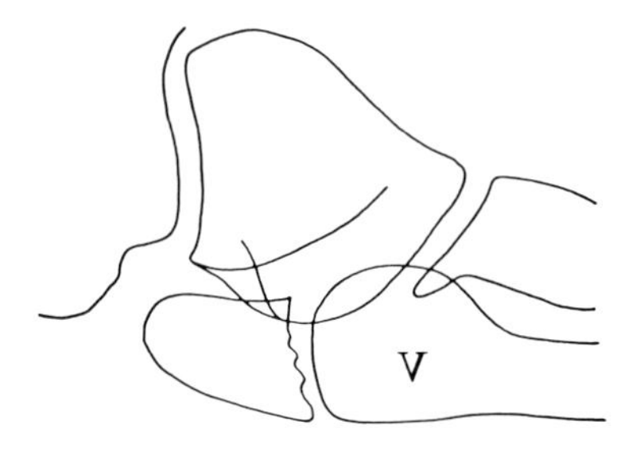

Fig. 833 a

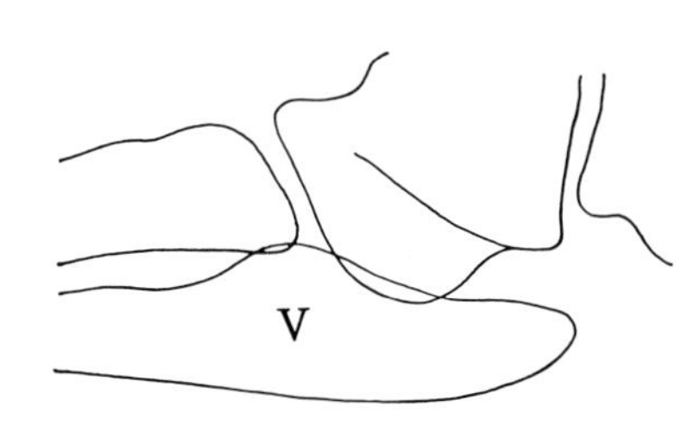

Fig. 833 b

Fig. 833. (Male, 28 years of age); a) right side avulsion or persistent apophysis at the base of metatarsal bone V; b) left side, apophysis, joined to the metatarsal bone V, much elongated either through anomaly or through trauma.

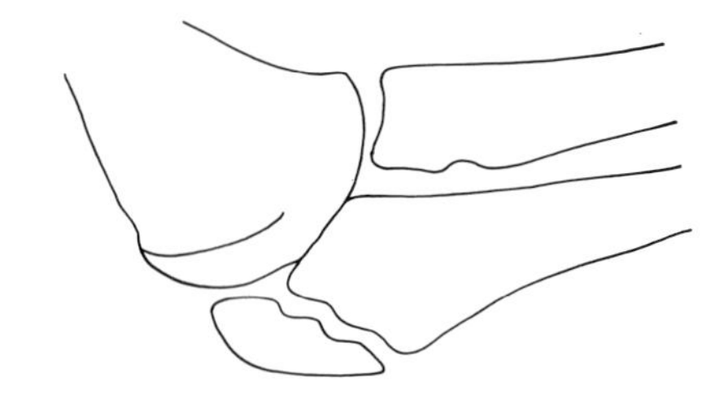

Fig. 834. (Male, 41 years of age); a classic example of a persistent apophysis of the metatarsal bone V, with oblique plane of coalescence (cf. Fig. 861).

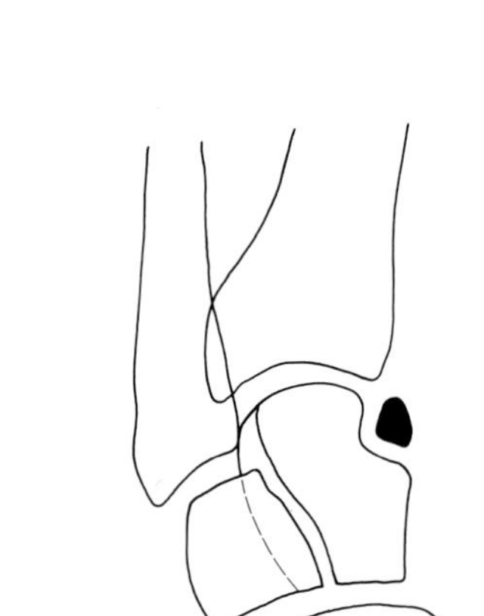

Fig. 835. (Male, 30 years of age); shows an indentation at the distal medial margin of the cuneiform bone I, to be considered a variant. This has been a bilateral finding.

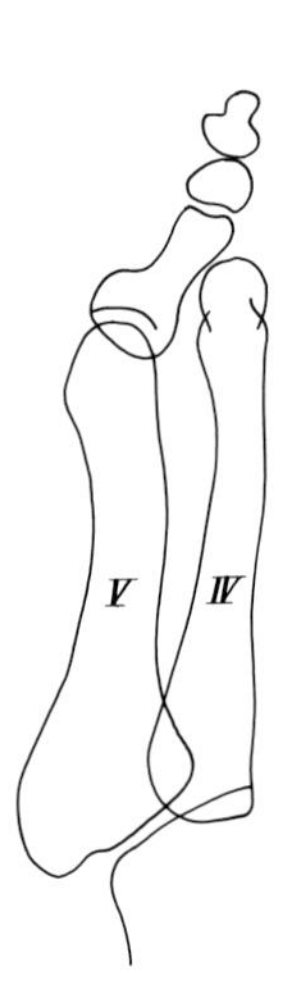

Fig. 836. (Male, 25 years of age). This is an example of the sometimes very peculiar, coarsely twisted shape of the metatarsal bone V, which often juts out at the base so far laterally that a subluxation is simulated.

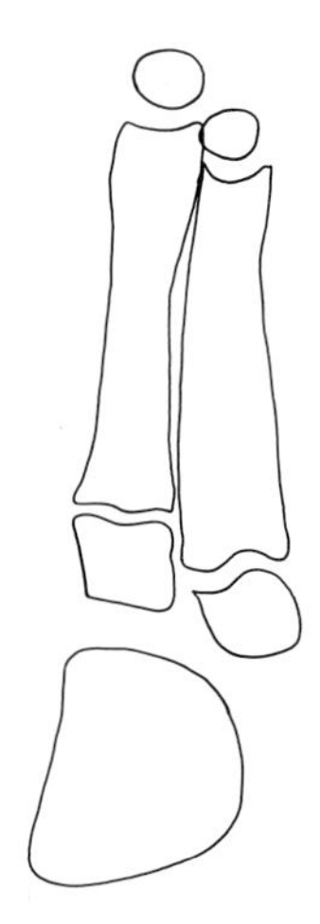

Fig. 837. (Boy, 7 years of age); showed proximal and distal epiphyses at all his metatarsal bones.

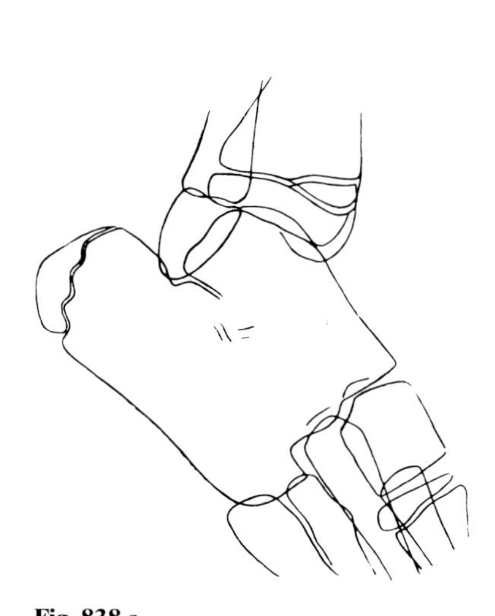

Fig. 838 a

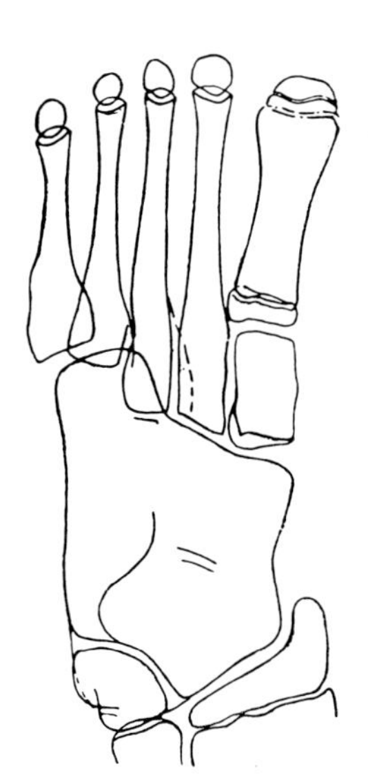

Fig. 838 b

Fig. 838. In this 11-year-old girl, who showed the conspicuous synostoses of carpus (Fig. 682), both tarsus also presented peculiar unions between talus, calcaneus, navicular bone, cuboid bone, further between cuneiform bone II and metatarsal bone II, as well as between cuneiform bone III and metatarsal bone III.

Further variants, according to Pfitzner, are:
Bipartition of the medial cuneiform bone (plantar and dorsal), navicular bone and calcaneus.
Union (concrescentia): talocalcaneal, partial and total; talonavicular, total; calcaneonavicular, calcaneocuboid, total; cubonavicular, intercuneiform II/III, cuneometatarsal II, total; cuneometatarsal III, partial and total; intermetatarsal I/II, the whole tarsus with metatarsal bone II/III; between middle and ungual phalanges, occurring in all four toes, very frequently in the 5th toe.

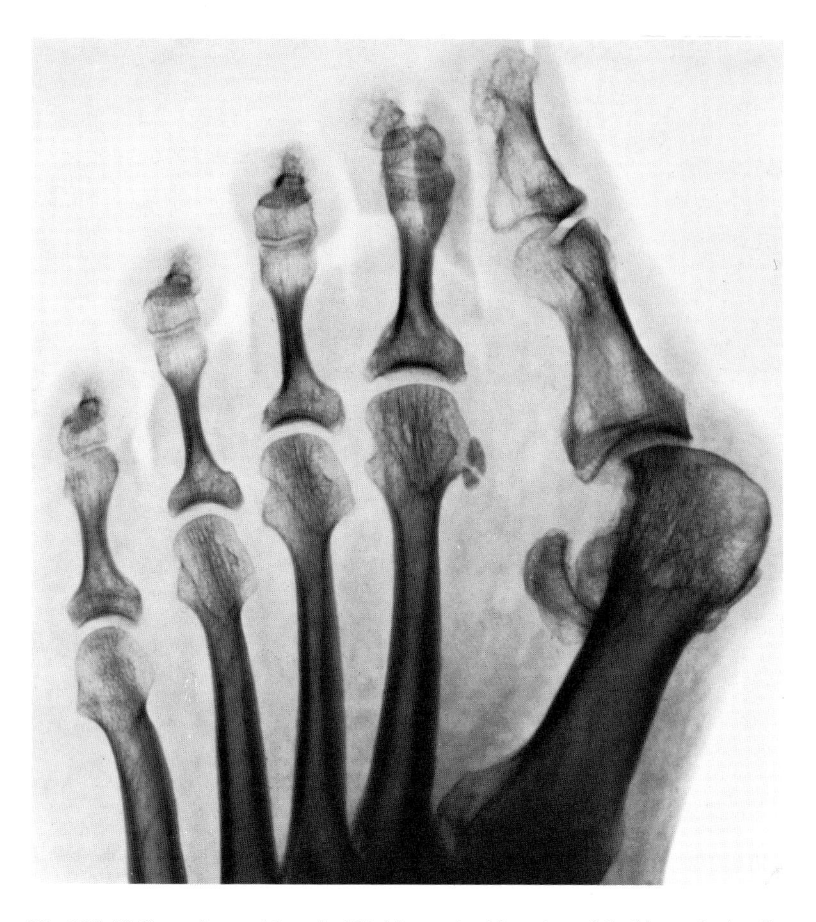

Fig. 839. Hallux valgus, with typical kinking and subluxation of the big toe in the direction towards the 5th toe. Arthrosis in the basal joint of the hallux, with correspondingly deformed sesamoids. Divided sesamoid below the head of the metatarsal bone II, missing anterior transverse arch of the foot. Hallux valgus occurs in about 6% of adults. Some lateral deviation of the basal phalanx of the hallux is always physiological and occurs even in the infant. On pathological hallux valgus, see *Haines* and *McDougall.*

Goodfellow investigated the hallux rigidus, which represents a partial stiffening of the basal joint of the big toe, on the basis of arthrosis deformans.

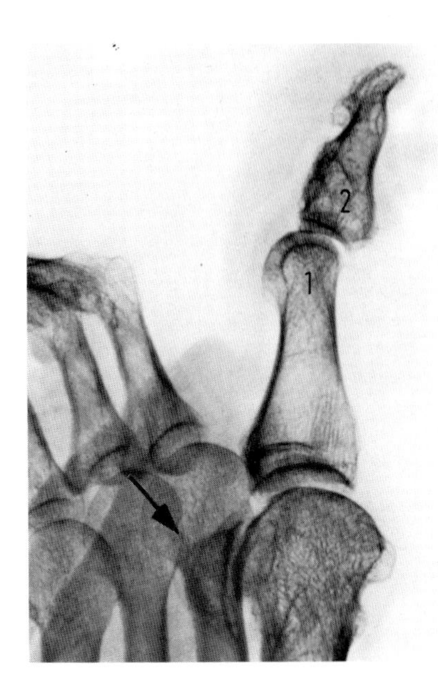

Fig. 840. Hallux, lateromedial. Hallux in dorsiflexion in an elderly patient suffering from hallux valgus and arthrosis in the basal joint. The big toe is tied to the cassette with bandages.

1 Basal Joint
2 Ungual joint
3 Sesamoid

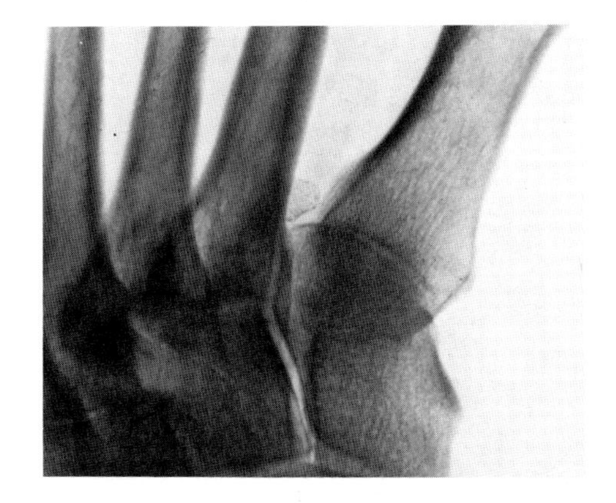

Fig 841 a

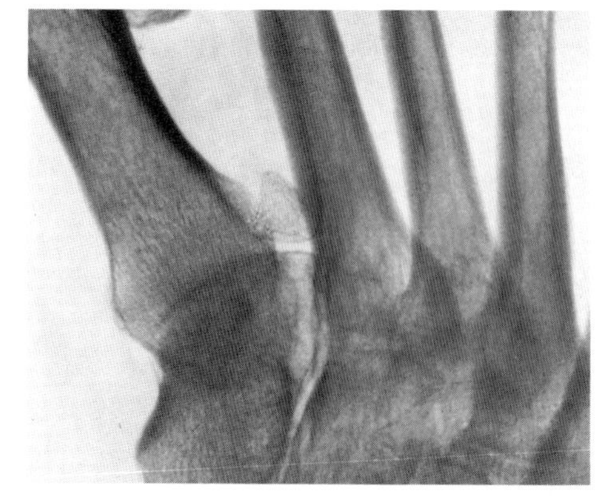

Fig. 841 b

Fig. 841. Bilateral os intermetatarsum. Cf. No. 177, Figs. 822 and 823.

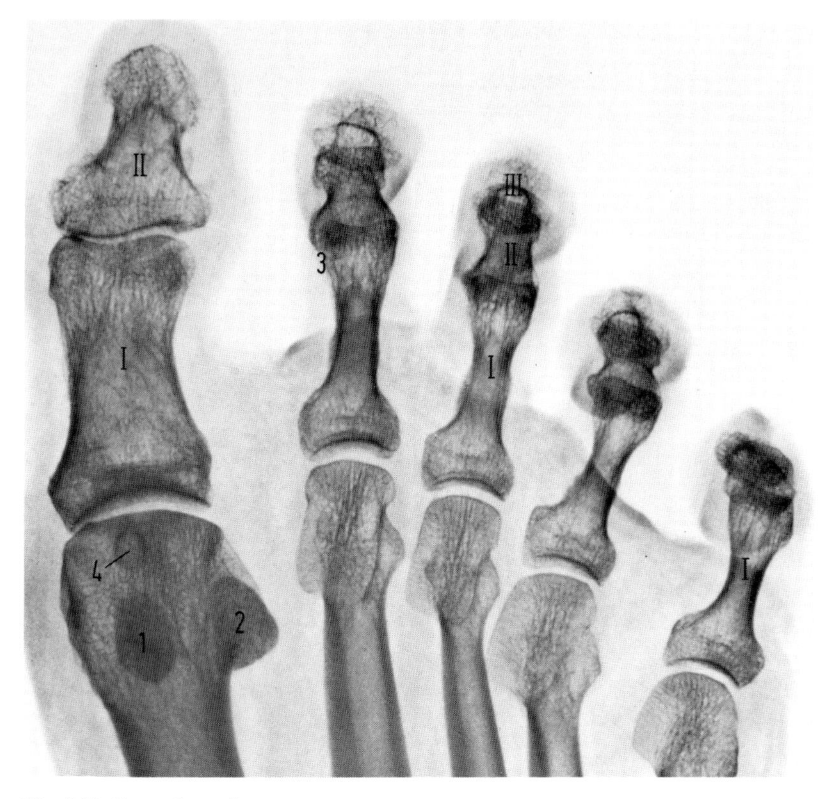

Fig. 842. Toes, dorsoplantar.
Variant: **fusion of the middle and ungual phalanges of the 5th toe** (see Fig. 820).

Fusions usually occur bilaterally. Interpretation of radiographs of the foot is not always easy. We observed a fracture of the fused two distal phalanges of the 5th toe (in the position of the normal articular space). Fusions may be simulated on insufficiently distinct radiographs. Usually, the middle phalanges become more rudimentary from medial towards lateral, and become shorter and plumper and also often somewhat bevelled. The irregular shape of the tuberosity of the distal phalanx is normal. The contour may appear moth-eaten.

Divided sesamoids occur; instead of the distal sesamoid I, *Stieda* once found two small ossicles which had moved apart laterally. Fractures of sesamoids may occur *(Stumme)*. Clefts of fracture appear on clear radiographs with jagged, irregular border lines, while bipartite sesamoids fit onto each other with smooth edges. In most cases divided sesamoids are together larger than one undivided. Islets of compact tissue may be mistaken for sesamoids (see Fig. 848). In juveniles osteochondropathy of sesamoids is frequent. Histologically, confluent necroses lead to osteochondrosis dissecans.

I, II, III Phalanges
1 Tibial sesamoid I
2 Fibular sesamoid I
3 Distal sesamoid II or islet of compact tissue
4 Solitary bone cyst in a case of hallux valgus with arthrotic narrowing of the articular space on the medial side

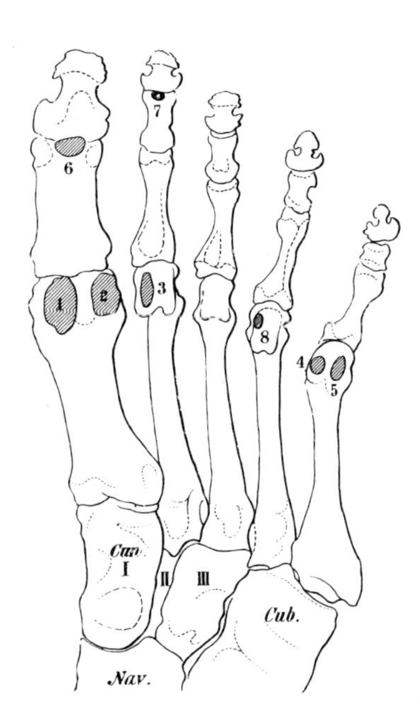

Fig. 843. The sesamoids of the human foot (after *Pfitzner* and *Stieda*).

1 Tibial sesamoid I
2 Fibular sesamoid I
3 Tibial sesamoid II
4 Tibial sesamoid V
5 Fibular sesamoid
6 Distal sesamoid I
7 Distal sesamoid II
8 Tibial sesamoid IV

There are, in addition, the fibular sesamoid II and the tibial sesamoid III.

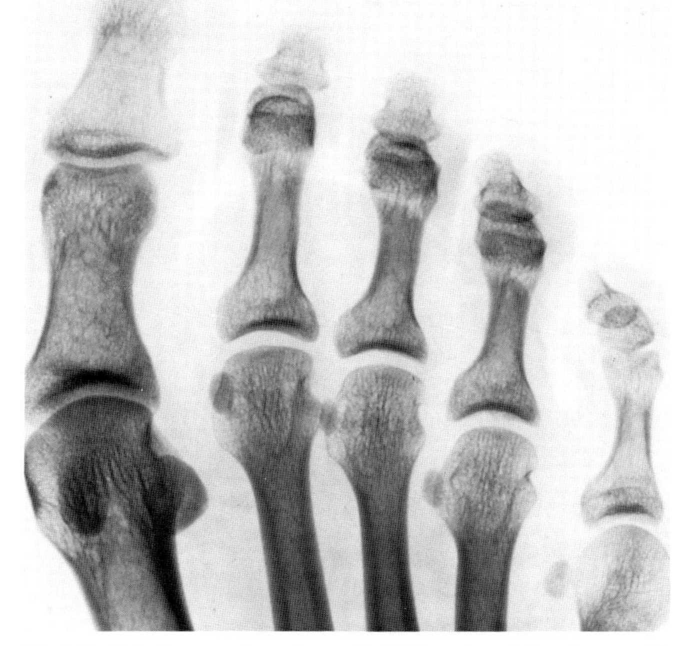

Fig. 844. Girl, 16 years of age, shows all of **Pfitzner's metatarsal sesamoids** bilaterally, with the clinical signs of sesamoidal chondropathy.

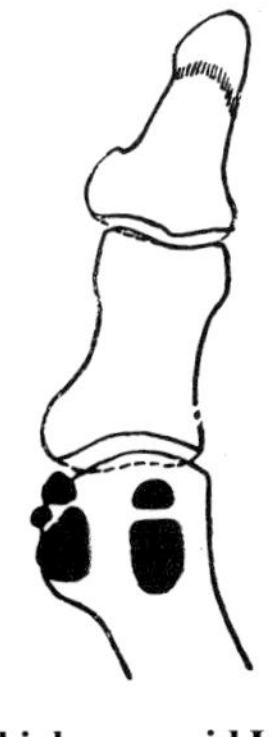

Fig. 845 shows a tripartite tibial sesamoid I and a bipartite fibular sesamoid I.

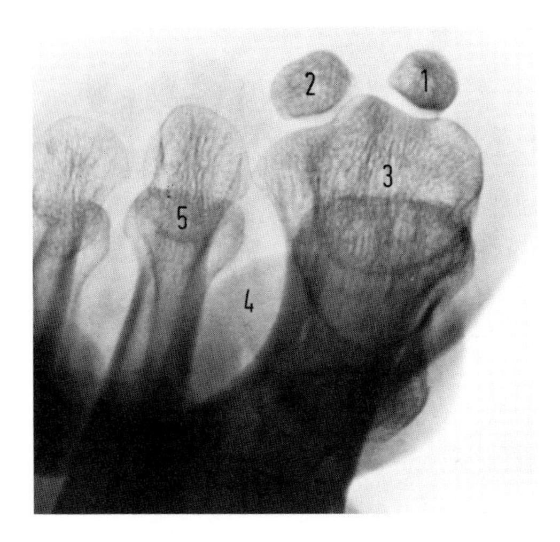

Fig. 846. Axial view of the sesamoids at the hallux. This radiograph is important for the diagnosis of several pathological changes at these sesamoids *(Müller, W.)*. The hallux is pulled by adhesive tape into such a position of overextension that the central ray is aimed between the metatarsal bone I and the sesamoids, showing the articular surfaces (see also Fig. 812).

1 Tibial sesamoid I
2 Fibular sesamoid I
3 Head of metatarsal bone I
4 Contour of the overextended hallux
5 Head of metatarsal bone II; basal phalanx of the second toe is dorsiflexed

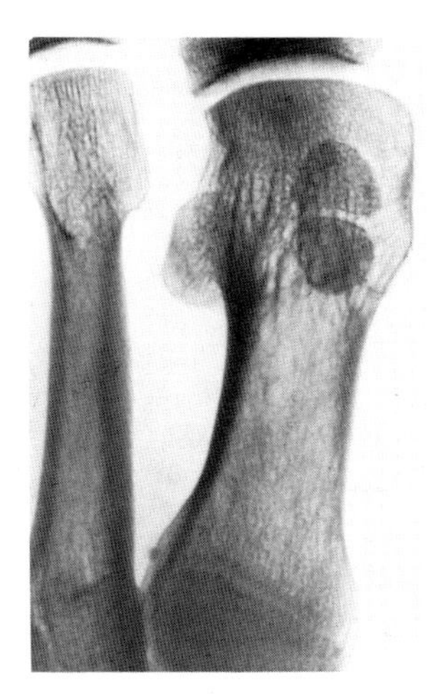

Fig. 847 a

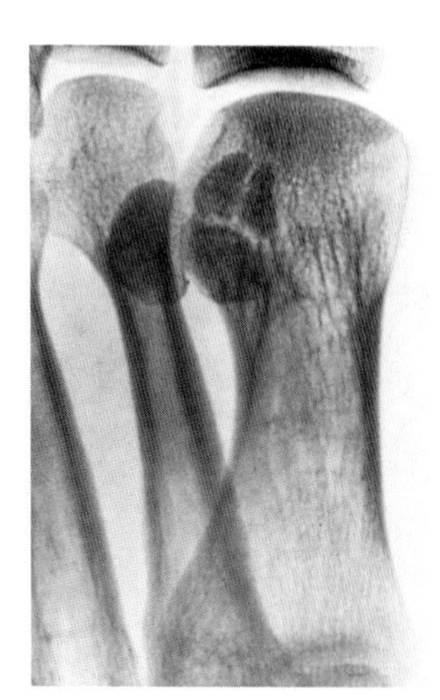

Fig. 847 b

Fig. 847. Bipartite and tripartite sesamoids of the foot; there had not been a trauma in the anamnesis. See Fig. 822, No. 178*, Figs. 843 and 845.

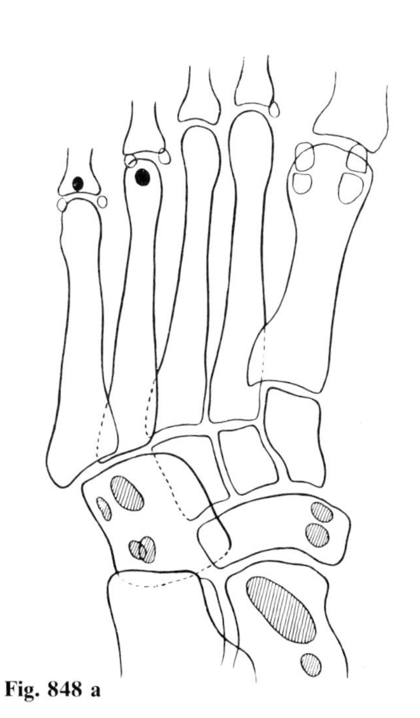

Fig. 848 a

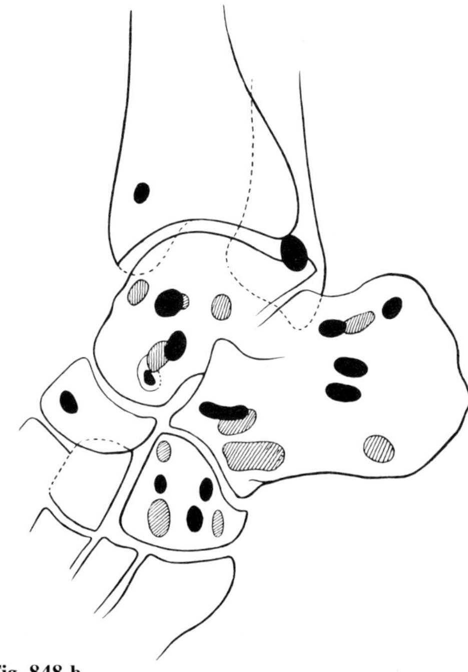

Fig. 848 b

Fig. 848. Islets of compact tissue in the foot. The figures show the localizations where islets of compact tissue may occur *(H. Fischer);* the more frequent spots are drawn in black (see also Fig. 853).

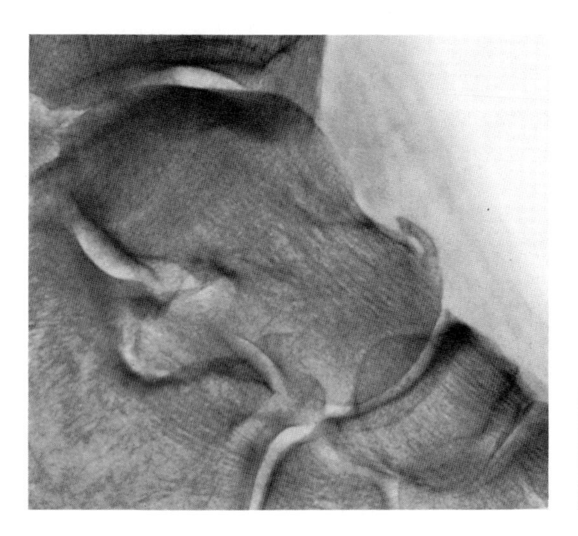

Fig. 849. Ossification in the talocalcaneal ligament, not to be confused with an os supratalare (see Fig. 823, No. 174**).

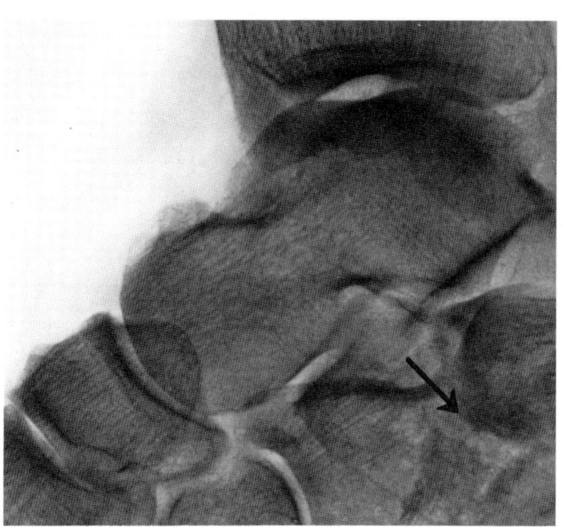

Fig. 850. Avulsion from the head of the talus, not a talar spur. The evaluation of this exostosis-like beak formation at the passage from the head to the neck of the talus has been quite variable. It has no connection with the joint *(Knoll)*. Avulsions have been described which may simulate an os supratalare (cf. Fig. 823, No. 174**). In our case both radiographs (Figs. 849 and 850) originate from the same patient. On the right, one sees in addition a fracture of the calcaneus (↘).

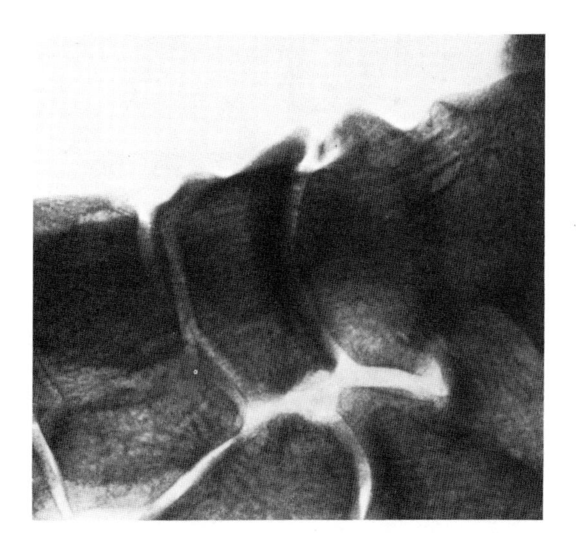

Fig. 851. Talar spur, with ossification of the talonavicular ligament. Opposite the spur one sees a rather large elongation at the articular margin of the navicular bone. It is an os supranaviculare, coalescing with the navicular bone (see Fig. 823, No. 175).

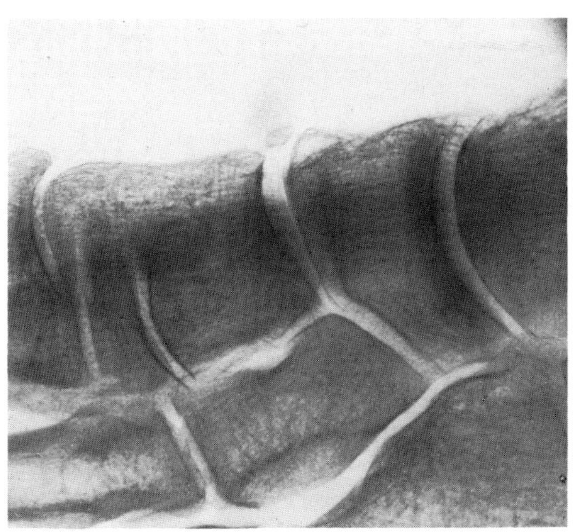

Fig. 852. Os intercuneiforme dorsale. An accessorium is lying on the dorsum of the foot between the cuneiform bones I and II *(Marti)*. There may also be an **os infranaviculare** above the naviculocuneiform I joint.

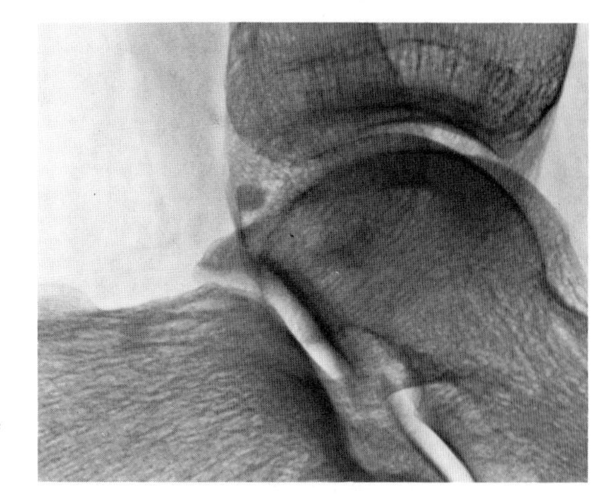

Fig. 853. Islet of compact tissue within the distal end of the fibula, towards the tip of the lateral malleolus (see Fig. 848b).

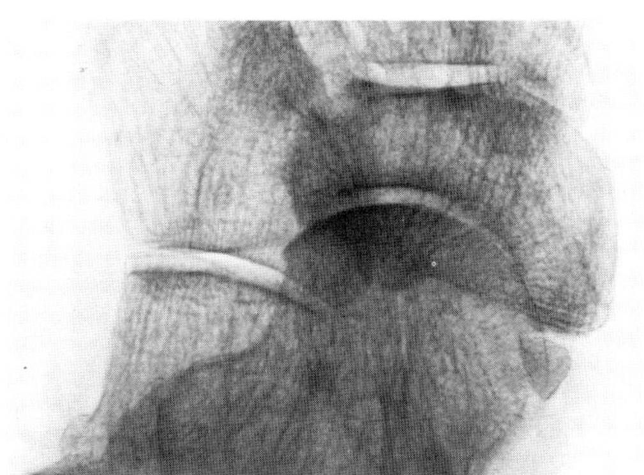

Fig. 854 a **Fig. 854 b**

Fig. 854. Bilateral os tibiale externum, most frequent, the right one is divided. Bilateral occurrence points to phylogenetic rudiments.
In juveniles the os tibiale externum remains cartilaginous for a long time and, therefore, becomes visible on the radiograph often only much later, after its ossification.

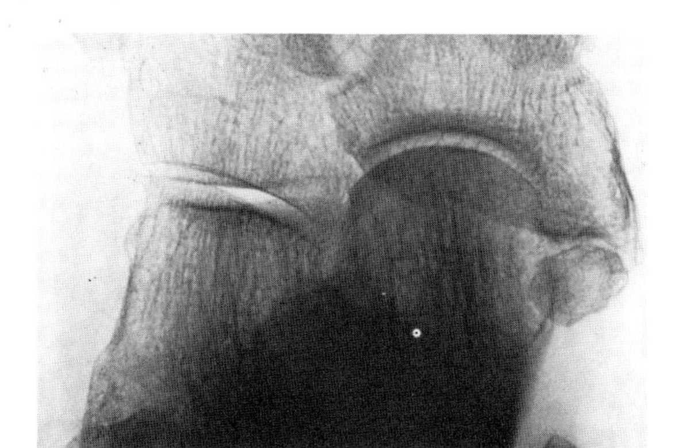

Fig. 855. Fairly large os tibiale externum (see Fig. 822, No. 170). This accessorium lies behind the tuberosity of the navicular bone and occurs in about 10% of all cases. Because of its size, it may be in this case an independent tuberosity of the navicular bone or an avulsion fragment.

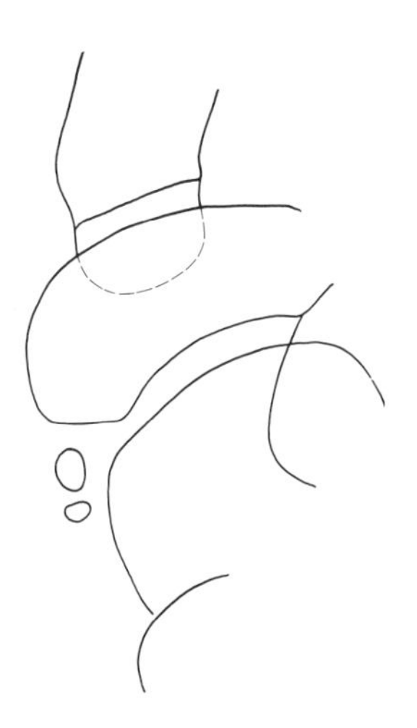

Fig. 856 shows **a bipartite os tibiale externum.**

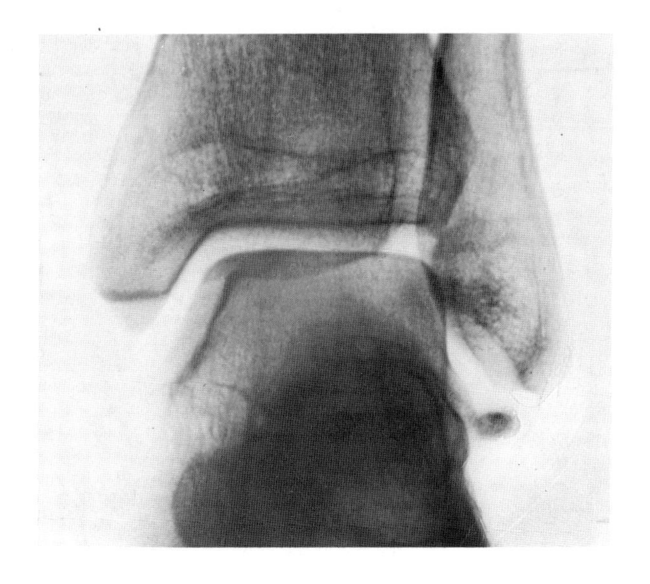

Fig. 857. Talus secundarius? An inconstant element of the skeleton? Or the result of a fracture, or a sesamoid within a ligament or a tendon?

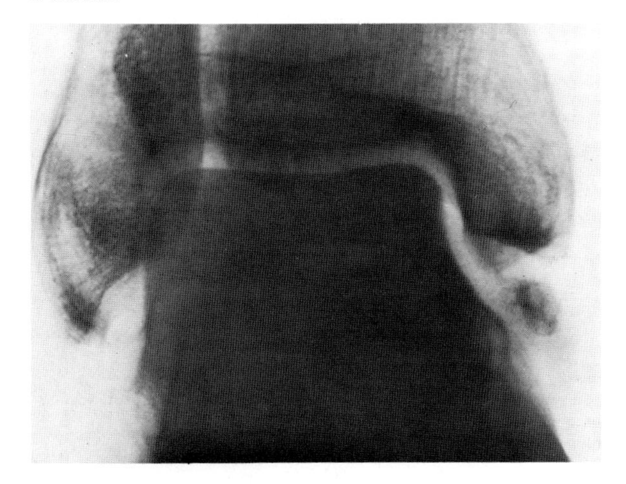

Fig. 858. Os subtibiale = talus accessorius. Differential diagnosis against split-off particles at the medial malleolus, ossifications within the deltoid ligament *(Bircher)* or bursitis calcarea. A special bony nucleus at the tip of the medial malleolus occurs frequently during the 8th to 9th years of life *(den Hoed, Helmes)*. See also Fig. 822, No. 174.

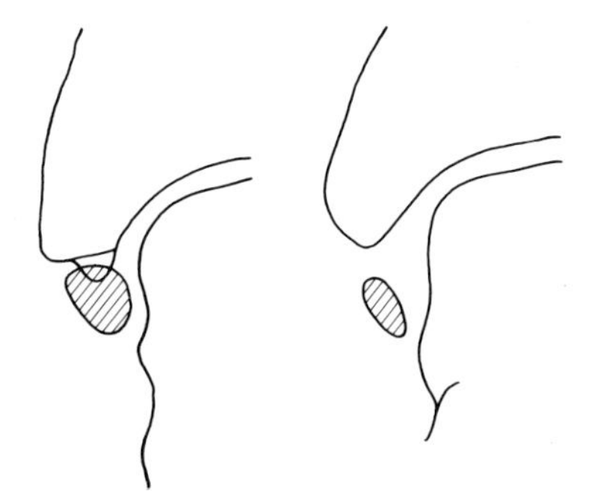

Fig. 860. Os subtibiale.

169 Soft tissue shadow = Achilles tendon and skin
169* Pseudoatrophic zones, overexposed because the malleoli had been placed in a hollow position
171 Intercalary bone between lateral malleolus and talus, a persistent anterior apophysis of the lateral malleolus
171* Os subfibulare, a persistent posterior apophysis of the lateral malleolus
174 Os subtibiale; in this connection, see *Brauer,* who observed the "development" of these ossicles after a trauma. According to *Henssge,* it is hypothetic to assume persistence of a juvenile bony nucleus into old age.

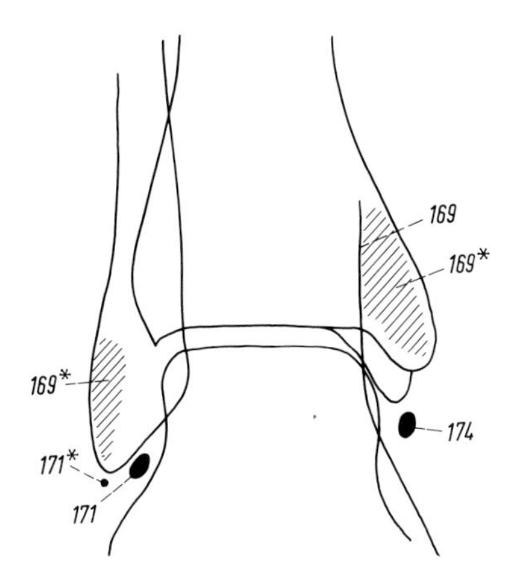

Fig. 859. Talocrural joint, anteroposterior.

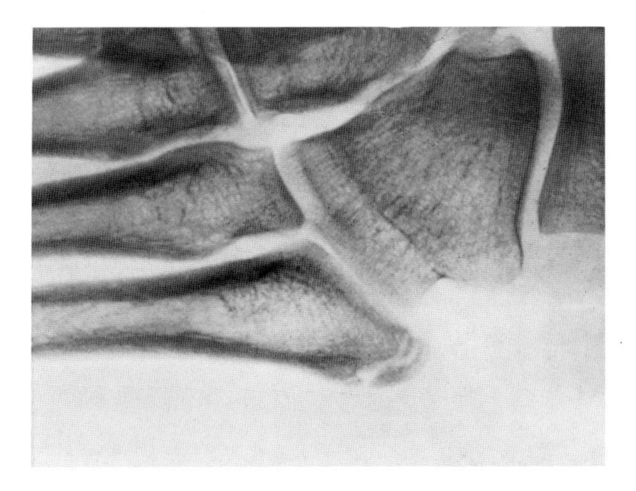

Fig. 861. Persistent apophysis. The tuberosity of the metatarsal bone V can persist as an isolated bone. It is often difficult to decide whether this is the result of a trauma. In doubtful cases comparative views of both feet may be of assistance (see also Fig. 822, No. 172* and Fig. 823, No. 185*).

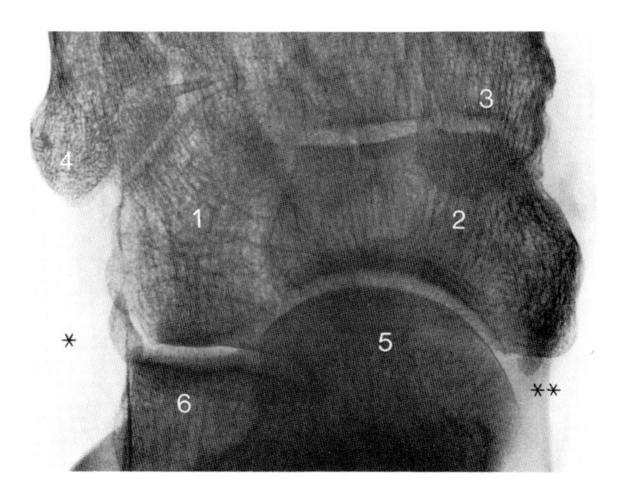

Fig. 862. Probably not an **os peroneum** (*), but an avulsion from the cuboid bone, because of the depression. Similar views are obtained in cases of peritendinitis calcarea.

1 Cuboid bone
2 Navicular bone
3 Medial cuneiform bone (I)
4 Tuberositas of metatarsal bone V
5 Head of talus
6 Calcaneus
** Os tibiale externum

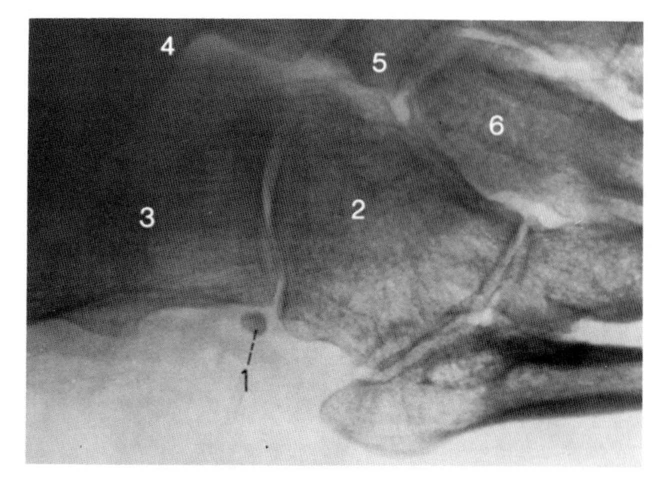

Fig. 865. Os peroneum. See Figs. 822 and 823, No. 172. It was described for the first time by *Vesalius* in 1555; according to *Weidenreich,* it is an ossified fibrocartilage within the tendon of the peroneus longus muscle.

1 Os peroneum
2 Cuboid bone
3 Calcaneus
4 Talus
5 Navicular bone
6 Lateral cuneiform bone III

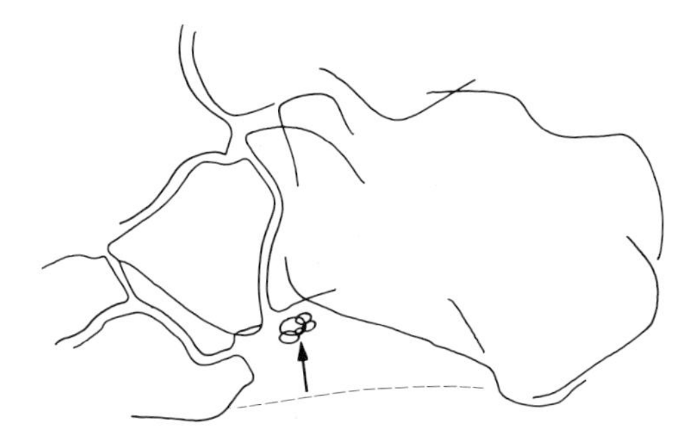

Fig. 863. (Male, 32 years of age). **Os peroneum,** consisting of several small pieces.

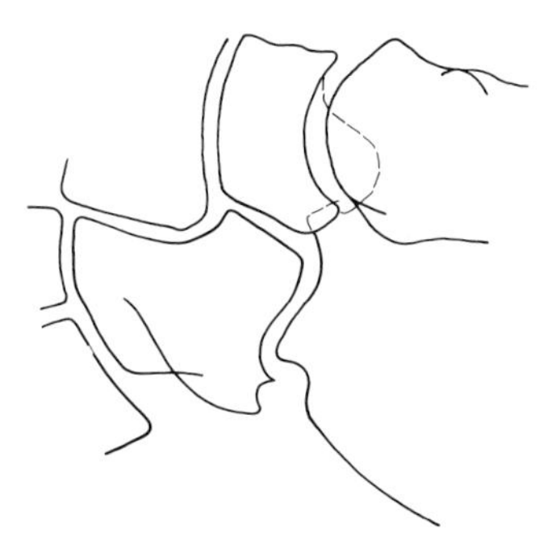

Fig. 864. The **cuboid bone** shows a groove which corresponds to a normal sulcus for a ligament (see also Fig. 866).

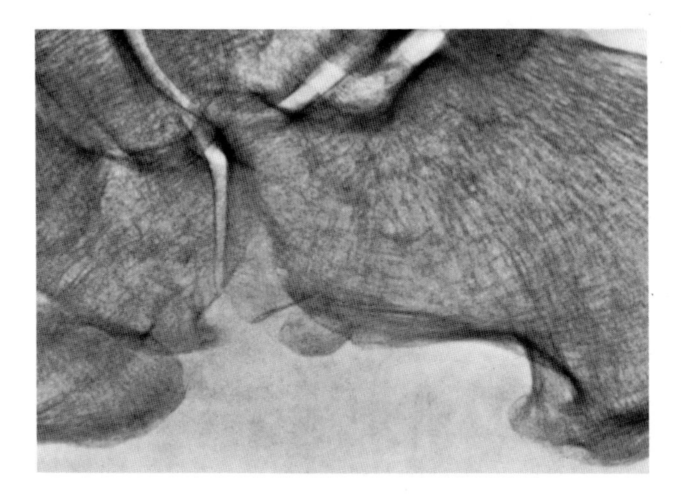

Fig. 866. Os peroneum. This diagnosis is supported by its sharply defined oval shape and its bony density. However, calcifying peritendinitis within the peroneus tendon cannot be excluded because there is likewise a ligamental ossification on the cuboid tuberosity which points to the accessorium. In addition, a spur below the calcaneus is seen.

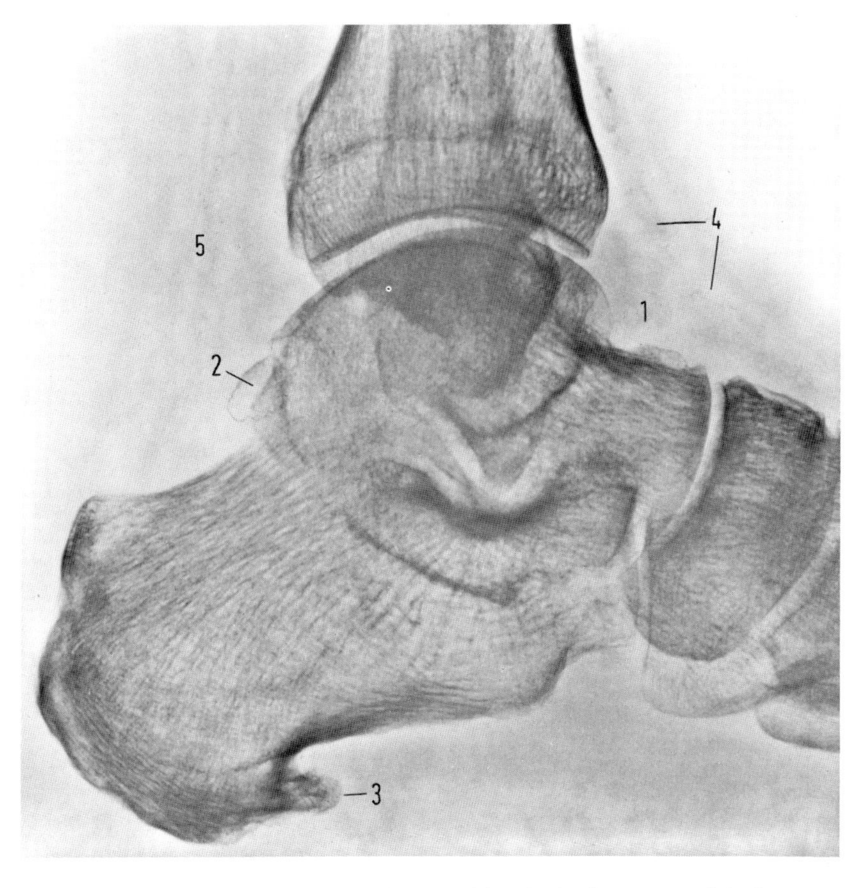

The radiographs (Figs. 867–871) show manifold appearances of the posterior process of the talus. In Fig. 868 it forms a longish, tail-like protuberance. Above it, in Fig. 867, an os trigonum is placed. The posterior process of the talus may be preformed independently and can fuse with an os trigonum. The centers of ossification of the posterior talar process and in the os trigonum appear between the 6th and 12th years of life. Therefore, it is often difficult to determine in a juvenile patient (Fig. 869) whether one is dealing with an os trigonum, an independent, unfused posterior process of the talus or an avulsion fragment.

1 Spur of talus
2 Os trigonum
3 Spur below calcaneus
4 Calcification in the wall of the anterior and posterior tibial arteries
5 Beginning calciferous deposit within the Achilles tendon

Fig. 867. Talocrural joint, lateral, of a 78-year-old female. Senile **atrophy of the bones.**

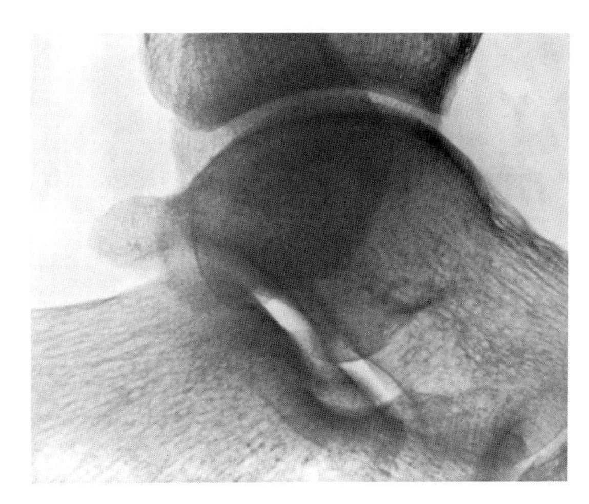

Fig. 868. Query **large posterior process of talus** or a bulge of the lateral tuberosity of the posterior talar process raised by a **coalescing os trigonum.** Layers of ground-off arthrotic material are also a possibility.

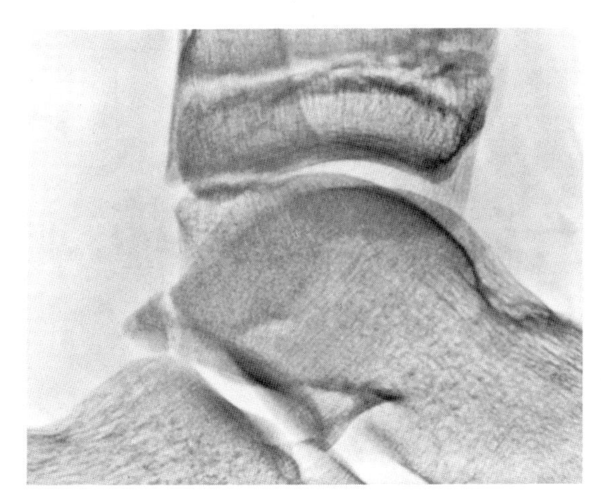

Fig. 869. Os trigonum in a juvenile (13 years old)? A non-fused posterior process of the talus? Or avulsion fracture of the posterior talar process *(Shepheard)?*

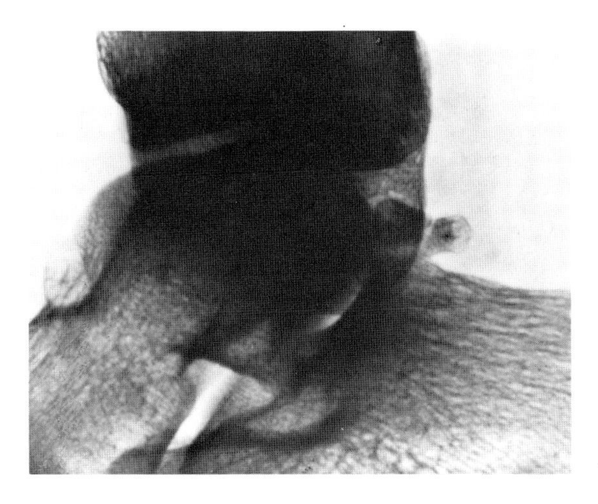

Fig. 870. Bipartite os trigonum, consisting of two nuclei of ossification which generally soon fuse with the talus. In this case fusion failed to occur (see also Fig. 823, No. 179).

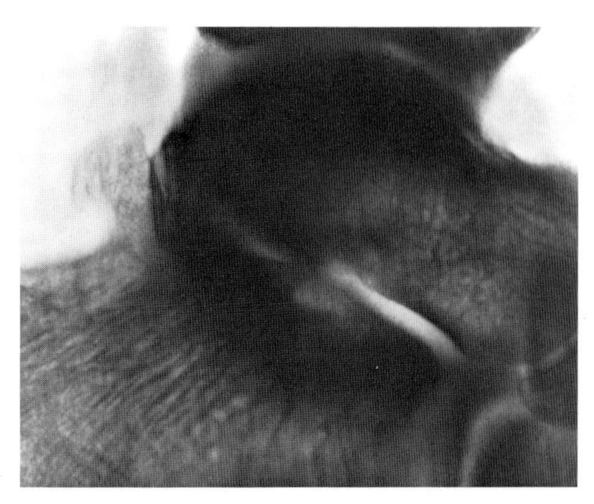

Fig. 871. Os trigonum, fused with calcaneus (tomographic view). *Maier* reported on the possibility of fusion of the os trigonum with the calcaneus.

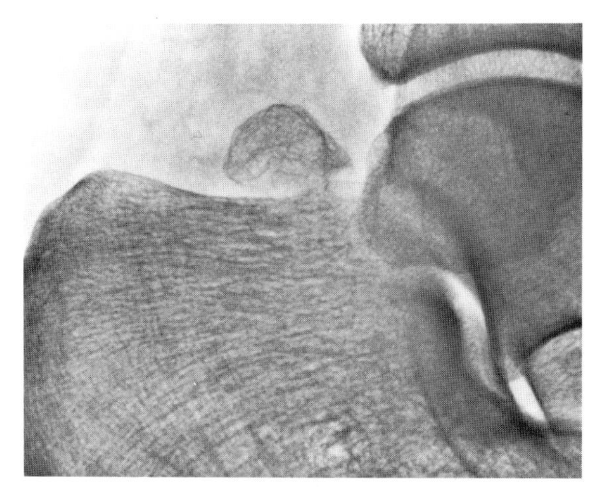

Fig. 872. So-called **os accessorium supracalcaneum.** According to *Ravelli,* it is a shifted os trigonum, which is often preformed in two parts (see Fig. 823, No. 179*).

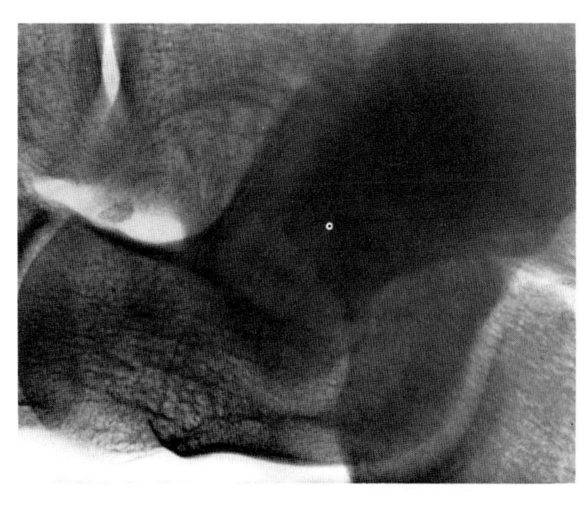

Fig. 873. Calcaneus secundarius, a round bone of match-head size. A triangular shape is more frequent (see Fig. 823, No. 180, and Fig. 874).

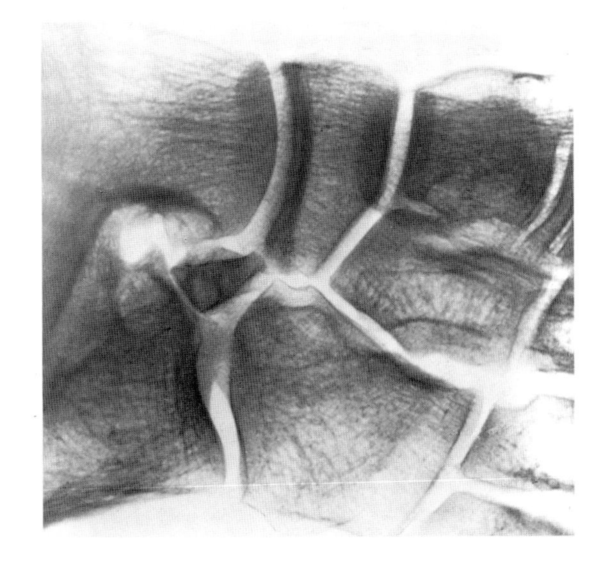

Fig. 874. Calcaneus secundarius. This is a large accessorium between calcaneus, talus, navicular and cuboid bone, which in this case has joint-like connections with four bones. It must be differentiated from a shearing-off fracture and from aseptic osteonecrosis.

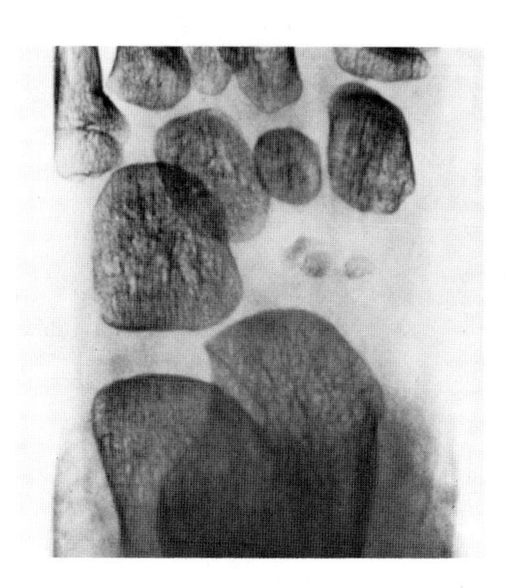

Fig. 875. Atypical preformation of the navicular bone, with three bony nuclei, in a $4^1/_2$-year-old boy. The ossification of this tarsal bone mainly occurs during the 4th year of life. In general, the navicular bone consists of a single nuclear preformation. Two preformations are more frequent than three. Five nuclear preformations have been described by *Schulte.* He presumed a connection of this atypical ossification with delay in the development of the skeleton. See also *Zimmer.*

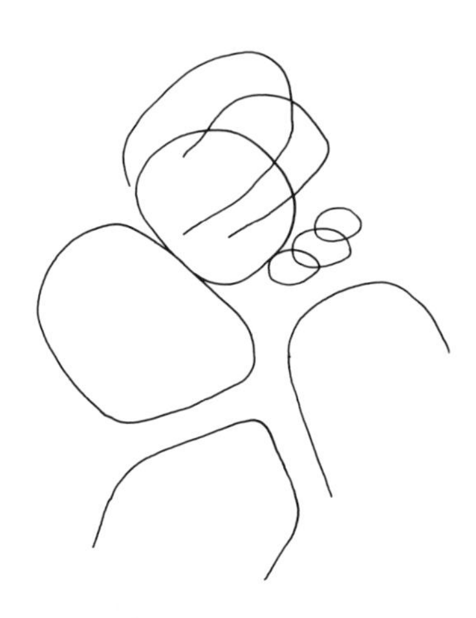

Fig. 876. Left tarsus in marked pronation (boy, 9 years old). The drawing shows the **navicular bone developing from three nuclei,** which will fuse later on. It should not be mistaken for *Köhler*'s disease of the navicular bone.

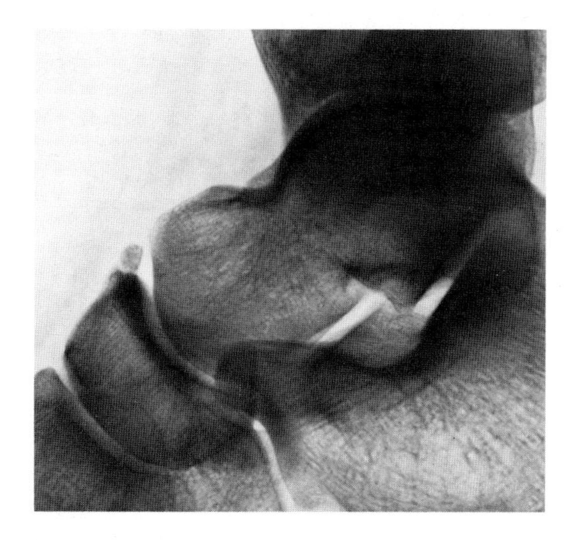

Fig. 877. Os supranaviculare (see Fig. 823, No. 175). This accessorium is found especially often in feet whose development has been disturbed; otherwise, it is rare. It is found dorsally, at the talonavicular joint, and is most often adjacent to the navicular bone but is sometimes also connected with the talus. Even in the adult, some expansion has been observed (see *Köhler-Zimmer).*

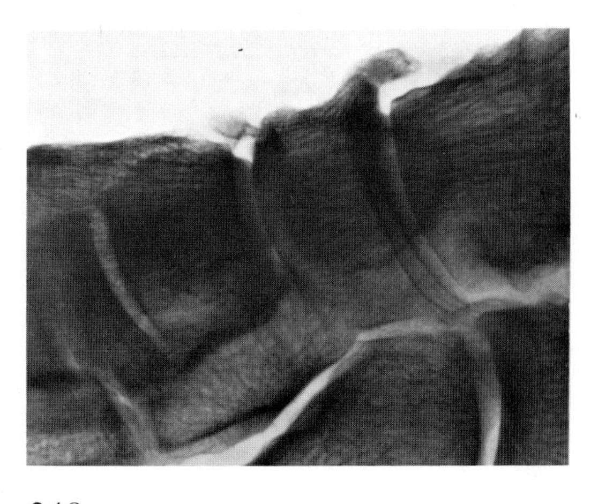

Fig. 878. Not a fused os supranaviculare or an os paracuneiforme. The navicular bone shows a considerable elongation beyond the talus. This distal growth is an isolated calcification of the articular capsule, like the beak-shaped formation above the calcaneonavicular joint; both are post-traumatic. As in the hand, split-off particles after minor traumata may simulate accessoria. For secondary centers of ossification and formation of accessory nuclei in the navicular bone, see also *Ueberschär.*

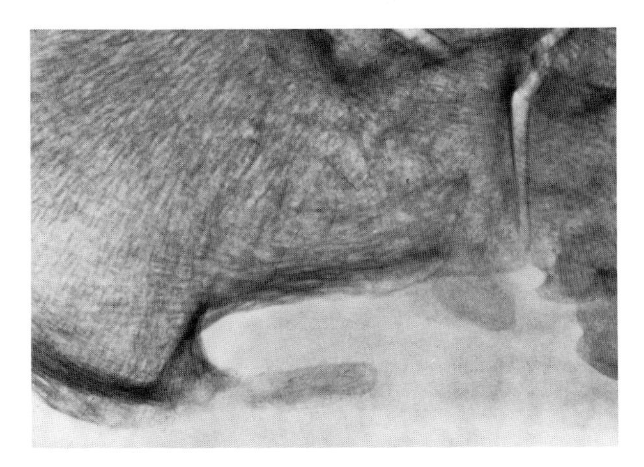

Fig. 879a

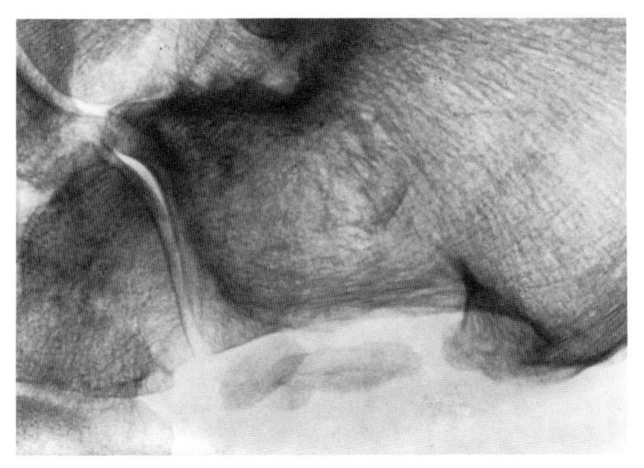

Fig. 879b

Fig. 879. Calcifications in the plantar aponeurosis of both feet in an elderly man, an incidental finding. See Fig. 823, No. 186. *Jaroschy* observed bone formation below the posterior half of the calcaneus. One has to differentiate it from a calcaneal spur, which shows a gap at its base and therefore simulates an isolated skeletal element. Bone formation below the calcaneal tuberosity has been described by *Niemann, Heimerzheim, Millikan,* as well as by *Köhler* (see *Köhler-Zimmer*): Os tuberis calcanei or os subcalcis (see Fig. 880).

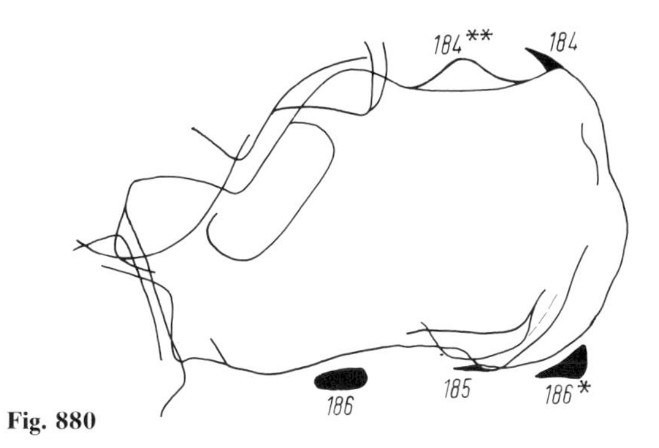

Fig. 880

184 Posterior spur of calcaneus. Ossification in the region of the insertion of the Achilles tendon. Spurs of advanced age occur bilaterally.
184** *Haglund* exostosis, a hump-like elevation on the upper posterior surface of the calcaneus, caused by chronic traumata (see Fig. 792)
185 Inferior spur of calcaneus, calcification of insertion at the medial process or result of a subcutaneous bursitis. *Mohing* and *Polyzoides* provided a contribution on the etiology of the calcaneal spur.
186 Calcification of the plantar aponeurosis
186* Os subcalcis or os tuberis calcanei (accessorium!)

The sustentaculum tali of the calcaneus generally originates from its own apophysis. Occasionally, it happens that this apophysis persists and remains isolated as an os sustentaculi. The result is always discomfort in the foot, as the sustentaculum does not provide the normal support for the talus. This is the case of a 14-year-old girl whose sustentaculum consisted of three well-defined ossicles, a particular rarity. In such cases, union of the sustentaculum with the calcaneus may still occur later on. One may speak of an os sustentaculi really only after completion of ossification. In 1942 *Grashey* described a very large os sustentaculi.
As no sagittal radiograph had been taken, one could also think of osteochondrosis dissecans of the talus, with loose bodies in the sinus tarsi, but no traumata had occurred previously.

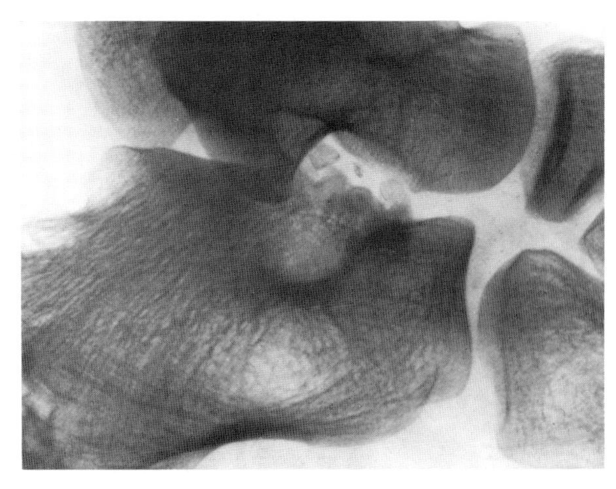

Fig. 881. Os sustentaculi tali, still consisting of several nuclei. Left foot, medial side.

V. Idiopathic Scolioses

One must differentiate between scolioses due to incorrect or faulty posture, which can be readjusted, and **structural scolioses,** which cannot be compensated, and whose main representatives are the **idiopathic scolioses** (90%). They are also called habitual, essential or genuine scolioses because, in contrast to other structural scolioses, no recognizable cause has been found for their occurrence. Only a limited number of scolioses show a single curvature (C-shaped scoliosis). S-shaped idiopathic scolioses are seen much more frequently. According to *Ponseti* and *Friedman,* there are four main types of idiopathic scolioses (Fig. 882):

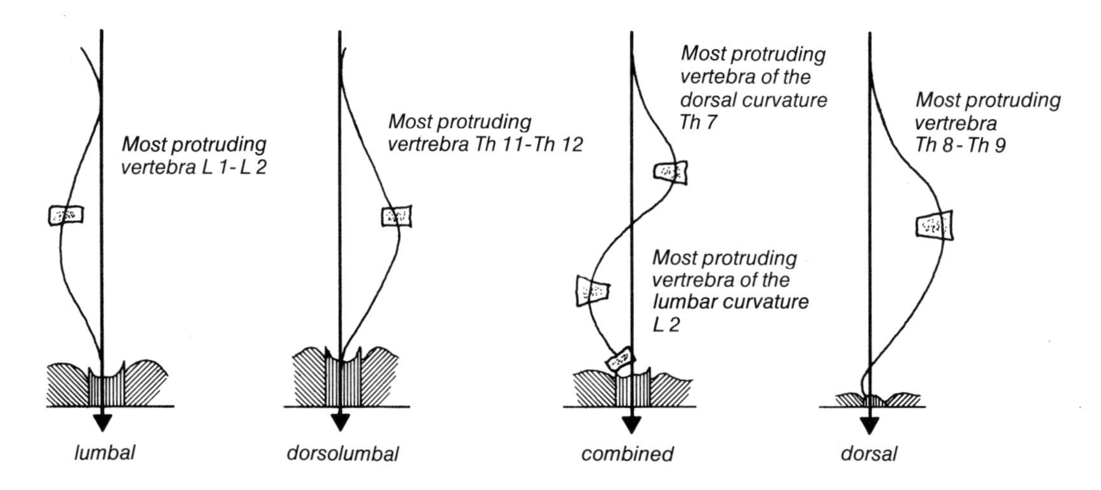

Fig. 882. The four main types of idiopathic scoliosis, after *Ponseti* and *Friedman.* For demonstration of scolioses one uses radiographs of the whole spinal column, which are distinguished from sectional radiographs by their comprehensiveness and clarity, and by the lesser load of rays. According to *Edinger,* one uses films 30 × 90 cm for these radiographs. The data for radiographs at a film–focus distance of 3 m are 80 – 110 kV and 300 – 500 mAs.

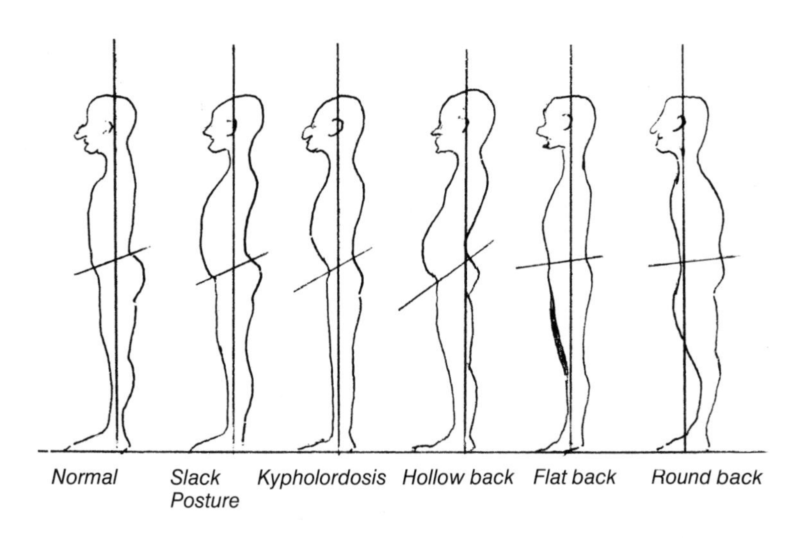

Fig. 883. Sagittal faulty postures. Best known is the asthenic, non-permanent round back (see Fig. 885). The most frequent sagittal faults of posture are schematically shown above, after *McMorris.*

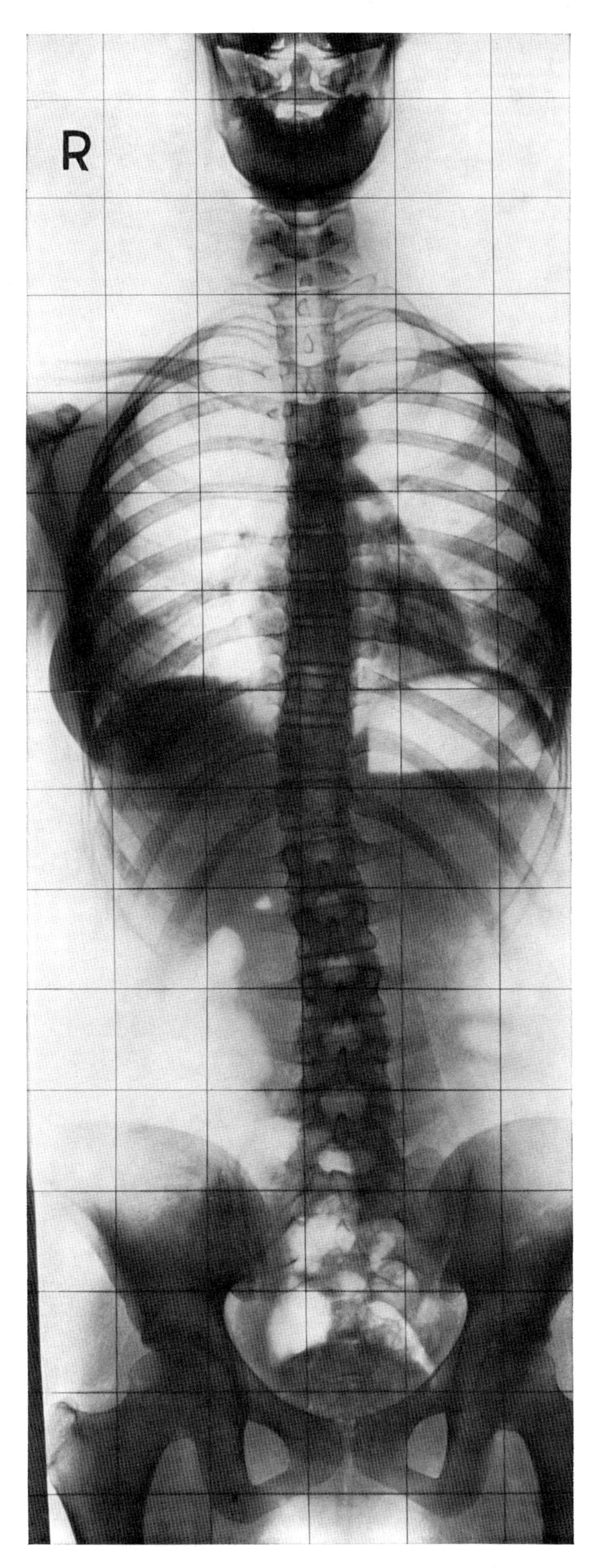

Fig. 884. Functional scoliosis in a 15-year-old girl, caused by the shifting of the body weight onto the right leg following an injury to the left foot.

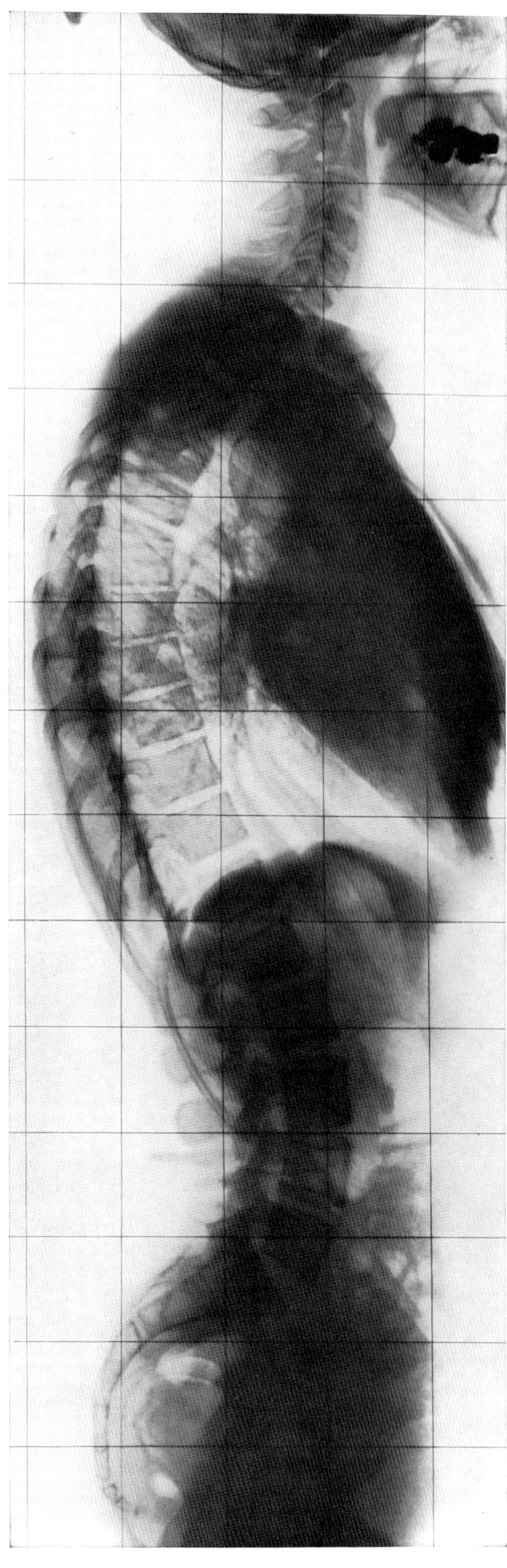

Fig. 885. Asthenic, not yet fixed, round back in a 23-year-old male.

C. Radiographic View of the Normal Infant and Adolescent Skeleton

I. General Introduction

Growth of bones and maturation of the skeleton proceed according to definite rules, which are in turn dependent on various conditions. First, hereditary factors, specific for different races, are responsible for development.

During the embryonic phase, influences of the surroundings may take effect within the fetus. Beyond that, in the postnatal period, there are many influences which may direct development, e.g., racial characteristics, climate, vitamin metabolism, surroundings, mode of life and especially hormonal controls, above all those by the anterior hypophyseal lobe (HVL), the thyroid gland, the adrenal cortex and the gonads (see also *Schreier*).

Of the hypophyseal hormones, the somatotropic hormone alone exerts direct influence on the growth of the skeleton.

The growth hormone, formed in the eosinophile cells of the anterior hypophyseal lobe, also called somatotropin, acts on the columnar cartilage and promotes its proliferation (and thereby the longitudinal growth of the bone) without acceleration of the closure of the epiphyses. Besides, it promotes the nuclear metabolism of the blown-up chondrocytes and, in addition, regulates the turnover of protein, carbohydrates and fat *(Matthiash)*.

The thyroid hormone exerts a favorable effect on the maturation of the skeleton and the longitudinal growth in the presence of somatotropic and gonadotropic hormones. During prepuberty the longitudinal growth is governed mainly by the somatotropic hormone of the anterior lobe of the hypophysis, while maturation of the skeleton occurs under the influence of the thyroid hormone. After puberty the sex hormones influence the acceleration of the maturation of the skeleton and, finally, the completion of the skeletal development.

The gonadotropic hormones and the steroids of the adrenal cortex, especially the glucocorticoids, regulate the protein metabolism and osteoblastic activity. Testosterone promotes formation of the bone matrix and calcification. In addition, it increases the growth of the epiphyseal cartilages. Estrogens act similarly to testosterone but do not promote longitudinal growth. ACTH impedes growth. Ever increasing importance is being accorded to the thymus with regard to immunological maturation and, further, for the calcium metabolism of the bones. There are also reciprocal effects with the gonads and connections to the growth of bones.

Disturbances of the hormonal metabolism can produce variable symptoms. A few especially characteristic ones will now be mentioned (see also Table 5).

Hypophyseal dwarfism is caused by a lack of the somatotropic hormone. The most important anatomical characteristic on the radiograph is the open epiphyseal clefts.

Persistence of the epiphyseal clefts may also be the result of insufficient production of gonadal hormones, leading to a retardation of skeletal maturation. The persistent epiphyseal clefts result, in many cases, in heightened growth, especially of the extremities, with development of eunuchoid proportions. Concurrent with this symptom, one almost always finds genital hypoplasia.

In the opposite case of precocious sexual maturity, one always finds accelerated maturation of the skeleton. Juvenile pregnancy, at the age of 15 years, results in premature cessation of longitudinal growth of the maternal body. During pregnancy or lactation the radiographs of these girls show a complete premature closure of the epiphyseal clefts. If the pregnancy occurs before the 15th year of life, longitudinal growth may be slightly resumed once more.

Figures 886 and 887 show two examples of opposite disturbances of body development, in a 12 and a 16-year-old girl, due to faulty or precocious hormonal activity. While the development of the 12 year old is advanced far beyond her age and shows the stage of maturity of a 16 to 17 year old, the girl of 16 has reached the approximate stage of development of a 12 year old. The views of the skeleton show a state of maturity corresponding to the stage of development. For instance, the view of the hand of the 12 year old already shows complete differentiation of the carpal bones and only narrow epiphyseal clefts at metacarpal bones and phalanges. A sesamoid has been formed at the metacarpophalangeal joint I. Likewise, the epiphyseal clefts at radius and ulna are quite narrow. In contrast, the radiograph of the hand of the 16-year-old girl shows carpal bones not fully developed, and broad epiphyseal clefts at the metacarpal and phalangeal bones as well as at the bones of the forearm. This is confirmation that the state of skeletal development mirrors the stage of maturity of the whole juvenile organism (see also *Kopczynska, Moll*). Normally, the development of the skeleton runs parallel to the degree of maturity of the organism as a whole. It proceeds according to a definite time table of relatively little variation, comprising appearance of centers of ossification, growth and formation of the outer shape. For the evaluation of growth governed by autonomous, genetic and endocrinologic factors, body height and weight, because of their physiological variability, are of little practical value; nevertheless, these criteria are often applied.

Often the somatic effects are a more delicate indicator of disturbances of hormonal homeostasis than the estimation of renal hormonal excretions (gonatropine, 17 – ketosteroids, estrogen). Therefore, in accordance with *Zeller*'s studies (quoted by *Matthiash)*, disturbances of puberty can be comprehensively differentiated as follows:

1. Premature or delayed appearance of the prepubertal phase
2. Hypopituitary stigmatization, with retarded normal growth in height and ample fat depots. The result is a pyknic constitution. If the gonadotropic impulses appear especially late, the body becomes shaped in the direction of eunuchoid increased height.
3. Hyperpituitary stigmatization shows pronounced growth in length, especially of the limbs, with sturdy musculature. The results are types of athletic constitution.

Table 5. Diminished growth and dwarfism (from *Swoboda*).

Designation of the diminished growth	*Type of heredity*	*Onset of disturbance or manifestation*	*Constitution, proportions*	*Physiognomy*	*Intelligence*	*Sexual development*	*Ossification of epiphyses*
I. Constitutional and genetically conditioned retarded growth							
A. Without enchondral dysplasia							
Primordial dwarfism *(Paltauf)*	dominant & recessive	congenital	in proportion	normal	normal	normal	normal
Hereditary degenerative dwarfism *(Hanhart)*	recessive	1st–4th year of life	in proportion	elderly	normal	much delayed	delayed
Infantine dwarfism	recessive	2nd–5th year of life	in proportion	elderly	retarded	much delayed	much delayed
Mongolism	recessive?	congenital	in proportion	mongoloid	reduced	delayed	varying
Progerie *(Hutchinson-Gilford)*		congenital	in proportion	senile	normal	delayed	accelerated
B. With enchondral dysplasia							
Fetal chondrodystrophy	dominant	congenital	muscular, micromelia	hydrocephalic	normal	normal or increased	normal or retarded
Dyostosis multiplex *(Pfaundler-Hurler)*	recessive	2nd–3rd year of life	squat, often micromelia	gargoylism	reduced	usually delayed	somewhat retarded
Enchondral dyostosis *(Morquio-Brailsford)*	recessive	1st–3rd year of life	dwarfism caused by vertebral column	usually normal	normal	normal	somewhat retarded
II. Retarded growth on endocrine basis							
Hypothyroidism	–	mostly congenital	in proportion	cretinoid	reduced	delayed	much retarded
Insufficient function of anterior hypophyseal lobe	–	mostly in infancy	in proportion	infantile	normal	much delayed	much retarded
Dyscerebral dwarfism *(Roessle)*	–	early infancy	in proportion	"cerebral"	usually disturbed	delayed	normal or retarded
III. Retarded growth due to disturbed bone metabolism							
Rickets of deficiency	–	2nd–8th year of life	slight disproportion	caput quadratum	normal	normal or delayed	normal
Renal-tubular rickets							
a) genuine vitamin -D-resistant rickets	dominant?	mainly 2nd year	genu varum, otherwise in proportion	normal	normal	normal	often delayed
b) *Fanconi*-syndrome	recessive?	mainly 1st year	in proportion	normal	normal	normal or delayed	usually delayed
Renal osteochondro-dystrophy	–	1st–8th year of life	in proportion	normal	normal	normal or delayed	normal or delayed

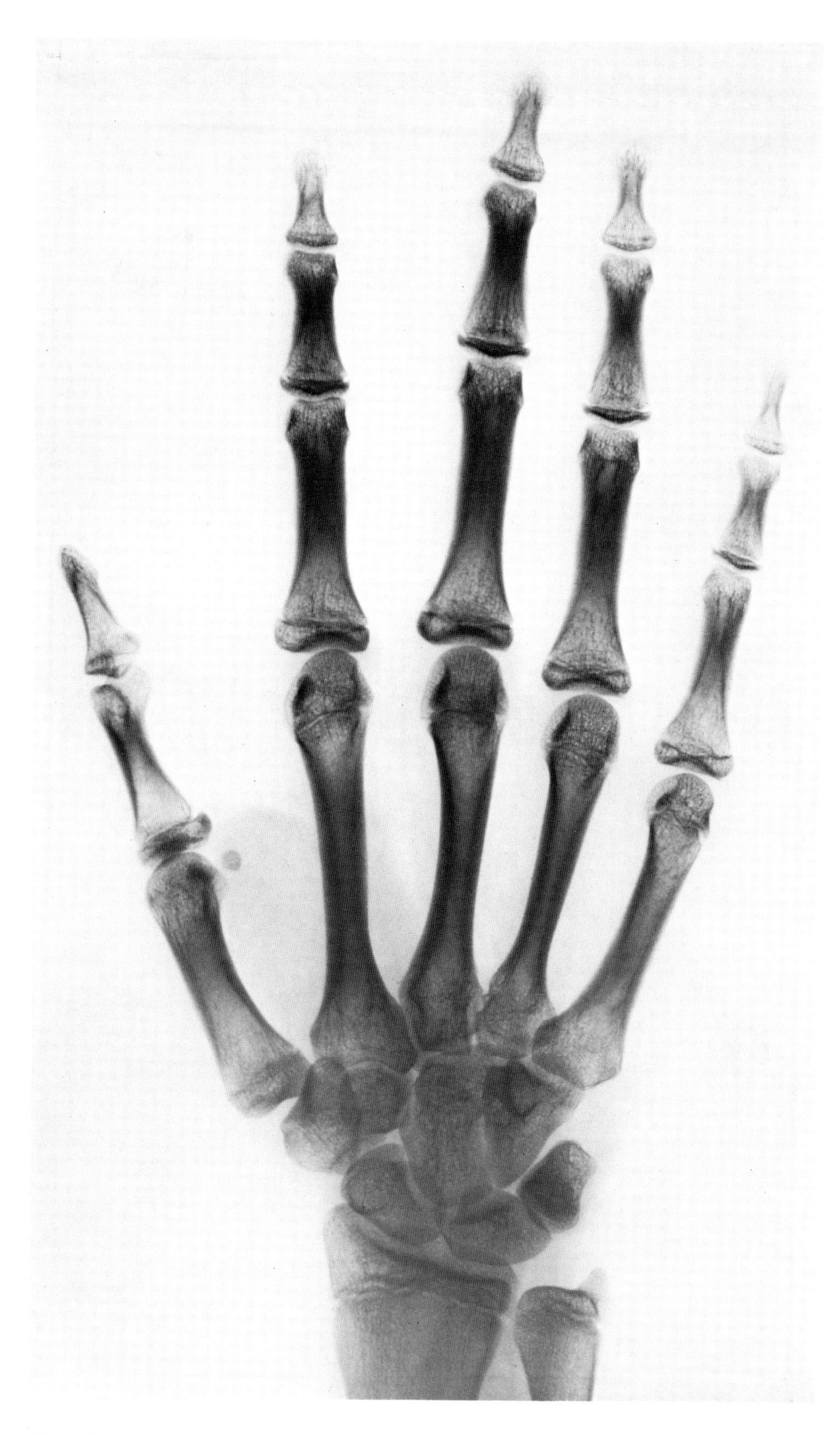

Fig. 886 a

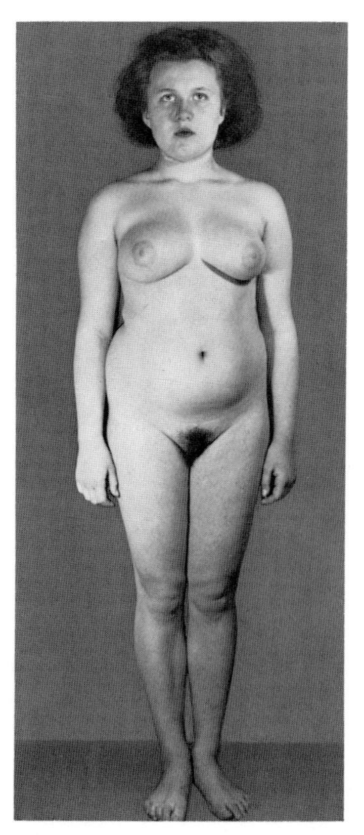

Fig. 886 b

Fig. 886. Girl, 12 years of age, at the stage of development of a 16-17 year old. Most epiphyses are closed. The appearance of sesamoids, especially of the ulnar sesamoid at the basal joint of the thumb, is considered as a sign of maturation. The sesamoids occur mostly together, with pronounced secondary sexual attributes. Deviation from the state of ossification at the ulnar sesamoid is being used for differential diagnosis of acceleration or retardation *(Rochlin* and *Zeitler)*.

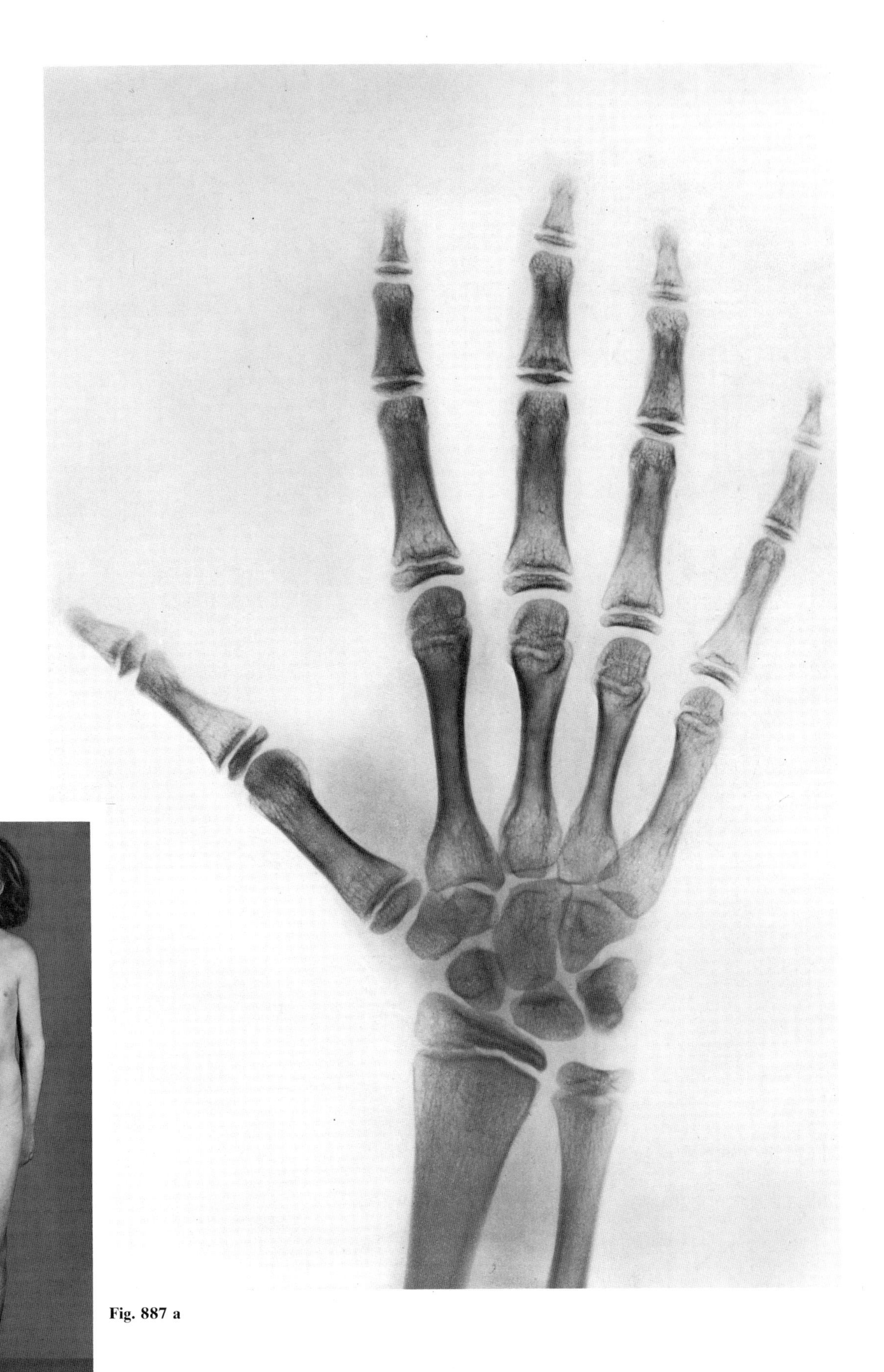

Fig. 887 a

Fig. 887 b

Fig. 887. Girl, 16 years of age, at the stage of development of a 12 year old. The skeleton, too, corresponded in development and maturity to that of a 12-year-old girl.
All epiphyses are still open. Nowhere can sesamoids be demonstrated. The retardation of development was also proven at the skeleton.

In hormonal derangement and longitudinal growth, exclusive promotion of hypogonadally stigmatized leptosome-eunuchoid forms of increased height develop.

Deviation from the norm in the growth of bones, due to faulty regulation of the gonads and of the function of the adrenal cortex, respectively, expresses itself, apart from the above mentioned examples, in certain forms of osteoporosis. This is a disturbance of bone metabolism which may result in retardation during the period of growth. The osteoporoses form certain groups of the halisteretic osteopathies (*Bartelheimer*). According to *Bartelheimer* and *Schmitt-Rhode,* the metabolic disturbances of bones can be divided clinically into six large groups:

In the first group belong osteoporoses, caused by insufficiency of the osteoblasts. These comprise osteoporoses of imperfect osteogenesis, of scleoderma with calcinosis, of inactivity, of senility and of post-menopausal and hypogonadal origin.

The second group is formed by osteoporoses from nutritional causes: osteoporoses of hunger, lack of vitamins and of minute traces of elements and of disturbances of resorption. The mixed forms of osteoporosis and osteomalacia belong in this group.

The third group comprises the osteoporoses of overproduction of hormones with antianabolic or catabolic action in cases of glucocorticoidism, acromegalia, *Morgagni* syndrome and hyperthyroidism.

The fourth group consists of primary and secondary hyperparathyroidism.

In the fifth group one finds the osteoporoses occurring in metabolic diseases: hyperthyroidism, diabetes mellitus, *Fanconi* syndrome, *Mauriac* syndrome, chronic liver diseases and alkaptonuria (*Cocchi, Boulet* and *Mirouze*).

In the sixth group one finds the osteoporoses in diseases of the blood (*Boll* and *Schmitt-Rohde*).

During pregnancy physiological hyperplasia of the parathyroids may occur. This may lead to mobilization of the maternal calcium deposits for the fetus. Hyperthyroidism leads to precipitate reconstruction of the bones in the growing skeleton where the osteoid tissue remains uncalcified at first.

Failure of menstruation may exert some influence promoting osteoporosis. Therefore, women often suffer from osteoporosis after menopause or after sterilization by irradiation or by total extirpation of uterus and ovaries. Lack of estrogen as its cause is being disputed today (*Krokowski,* 1976). In puerperal osteoporosis the pelvis is mainly affected; in the senile form, essentially the spinal column and, surprisingly, the neck of the femur in women. In *Cushing's* disease osteoporosis is especially pronounced. One may consider as its cause the excessive production of glucocorticoids by the adrenal cortex. Its result is a negative balance of calcium, phosphorus and nitrogen. After lengthy therapeutic administration of cortisone, hydrocortisone and ACTH, lasting demineralization of the skeleton occurs not infrequently, as proved by reports on spontaneous fractures after pro-

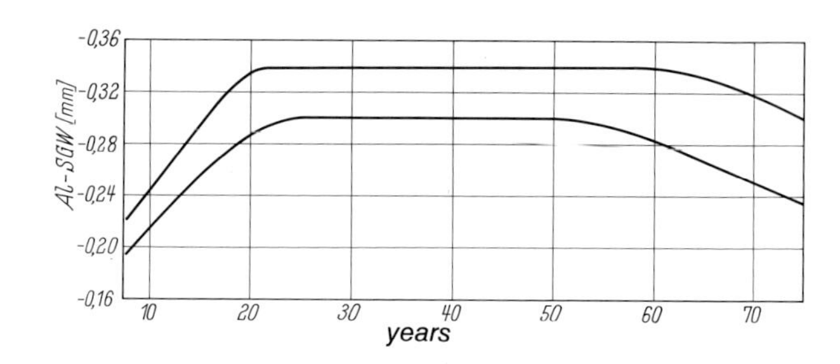

Fig. 888. Curve of the normal range of the content of mineral salts of the skeleton, expressed in mm Al–SGW (according to the method of *Balz* and *Birkner).*

longed ACTH and cortisone therapy. Pathological osteoporosis may also be the consequence of a preponderantly acidotic state. In this connection, one should especially note the osteoporosis based on rickets, with its characteristic disturbances of growth, and further the renal osteopathy occurring during chronic treatment with hemodialysis.

Apart from the pathological osteoporosis of the skeleton which is preponderant in adults, there occurs a "physiological" osteoporosis. *Stettner* found it in 50% of boys, slightly more frequently than in girls (41%), until the 13th year of life.

The peak of frequency of osteoporosis is reached during the 2nd year of life. Until the 8th year, osteoporosis is again less frequent. Thereafter, a certain instability seems to take place, occurring as an attendant phenomenon to the period of prepuberty, somewhat earlier in girls than in boys. Damages of nutrition are of relatively slight effect; they only intensify the tendency to "physiological" osteoporosis and somewhat postpone its adjustment. In contrast, rickets causes intensification of osteoporosis and delays the return to normal calcium-containing bony tissue.

Quantitative radiologic demonstration of generalized osteoporosis is difficult. Following the method of *Balz* and *Birkner*, one can draw conclusions from the weakening of the rays by a test object – the basal phalanx of the thumb – on its relative content of mineral salts and, through it, on their content in the rest of the skeleton. For this test one photometrically compares the weakening of X-rays of a definite quality (50kV) by an aluminous set of steps (height of step 0.5 mm), with a wedge of plexiglass placed in front of it (coefficient of weakening equals that of water), with the weakening by the bone and its covering soft tissues (the thumb in a water phantom – Wasserphantom). The resulting graduated value (so-called equivalent of weakening by aluminum Al-SGW) is to be reduced by calculation to the comparative value of 1 mm thickness of bone (see curve of normal range in Fig. 888).

The usefulness and value of this method have been confirmed by numerous clinical examinations (*Balz* and *Birkner; Balz, Birkner* and *Schmitt-Rohde; Hölscher; Lutterbeck; Jobstvogt*). From the curve of the equivalent of weakening by aluminum, one can read an increase of the content of mineral salts of the bones during the age of growth until adulthood, and from there a distinct decrease, corresponding to the decrease of production of gonadal hormones.

Disturbances of growth due to changes of the enchondral process of ossification, once they are healed, leave transverse lines on the radiograph in the metaphyses of growing bones, the so-called intermediary bands (Figs. 769 and 1163). Correspondingly, one finds histologically a dense network containing remnants of calcified basic cartilaginous substance beyond its physiological amount *(Hamperl)*. Besides resulting from disturbances of growth in rickets, transverse lines also occur after infectious diseases, phosphorous intake of small doses and lead poisoning *(Chobot* and *Merrill)*. *Harris* also found transverse lines in the metaphyses under seasonal influences on the amount of growth. Lines of growth may occur in very young children, more frequently in older children, but also in adults. They are especially frequent in weakly children after a lengthy illness.

Wolf and *Psenner* found in newborns transverse zones of increased density at the epiphyseal borders of the long bones; only in isolated cases were they able to demonstrate pathologic-anatomically that syphilis had been a possible cause.

Preferred localizations of transverse lines on roentgenograms are the distal end of the femur, the proximal and distal ends of tibia and fibula, the distal ends of radius and ulna and the proximal end of the humerus. *Péhu* and *Policard* found transverse lines in 2–3% of their examined cases. These transverse lines must be differentiated from epiphyseal scars (Figs. 768, 1176, 1177 and 1179) of the human skeleton which may occur in all kinds of bones which contain genuine epiphyses, from the firm transverse lamella to the most delicate spongy bone.

The reaction of the epiphyses to mechanical and other irritations is of special importance for clinical medicine *(Kühne)*. It is known from experimental examinations that formation of bony nuclei and ossification of epiphyses can be impeded by strong, continuous pressure. In contrast, inflammatory irritations may greatly stimulate longitudinal growth.

From these arguments follows the importance of the humoral substances of the organism, as well as other factors for the growth, maturation and metabolism of the skeleton. They represent only isolated links in the wide functional sphere of the organism as a whole, inserted into the regulating central and peripheral nervous system. To explain the significance of the nervous system for skeletal growth, one has only to mention the trophic disturbances with underdevelopment of the affected limbs in poliomyelitis.

Ken Kuré and his assistants demonstrated by their research special trophic nerve fibers which take an efferent course via the posterior roots. Studying organic nervous diseases with trophic disturbances, e.g., tabes dorsalis, syringomyelia and leprosy, *Ken Kuré* found degeneration of these efferent fibers of the posterior roots and of their respective ganglionic cells in the spinal cord. Furthermore, *F. Schmid* described disturbances of development of skeletal growth in early infantile affections of the central nervous system. These results have been confirmed by *Geisler* and *Bannes*.

Normal maturation of the skeleton differs early between males and females. These sexual differences constantly become more pronounced with further development. One may expect, for instance, completion of ossification in the female generally about four years earlier than in the male, while the order of appearance of nuclei is almost the same in both sexes.

The first appearances of ossification of the skeleton become perceptible in the clavicle. They can already be demonstrated in its middle part during the 3rd embryonal week as an outer bone formation. General development of bones starts only during the 2nd embryonal month.

Normally, the development and maturation of the skeleton proceed in four stages of ossification. These are interrupted by periods of longitudinal growth, the development of the child progressing, as in any organic development, not continuously but periodically:

1. *Intrauterine stage of ossification:*
   Development of the basic skeleton,
   Development of the diaphyses of the long and short tubular bones,
   Development of the epiphyseal nuclei at the distal end of the femur and the proximal end of the tibia. Preformation of the nuclei of calcaneus and talus.
2. *Stage of ossification in the infant:*
   Development of the nuclei of the bone in the epiphyses of the short and long tubular bones,
   Development of carpal and tarsal bones.
3. *Stage of ossification during puberty:*
   Development of the apophyseal nuclei.
4. *Stage of ossification in the adult:*
   Bony closure of the epiphyses and, therewith, completion of development of the skeleton and of growth in height.

The embryonic skeleton is mainly preformed as cartilage, apart from the covering bones of the skull which are preformed by connective tissue (almost all facial bones, the flat bones of the cranium and the flat parts of several cranial bones). The ossification which starts soon after the middle of the 2nd embryonal month (about the 6th

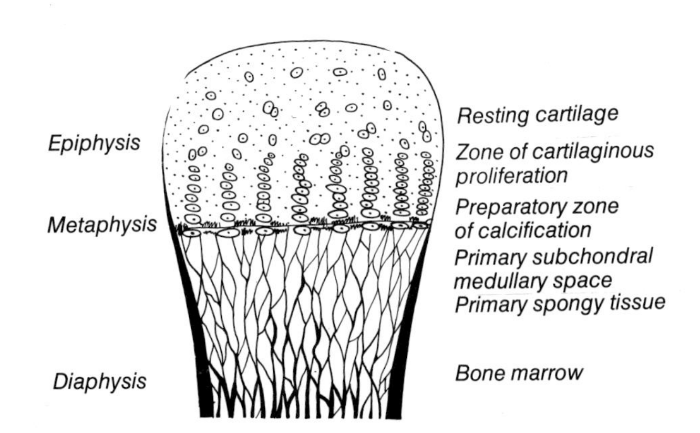

Fig. 889. Schema of enchondral ossification (from *F. Schmid* and *H. Moll*).

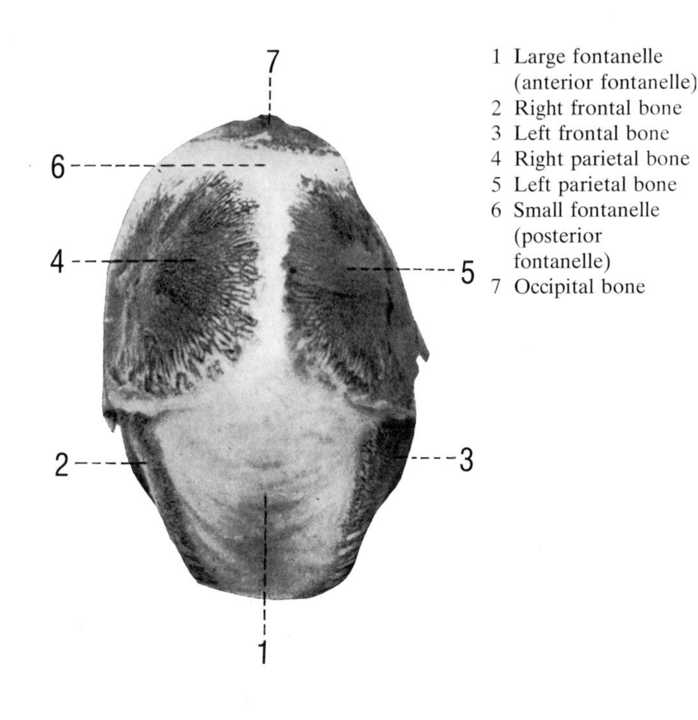

1 Large fontanelle (anterior fontanelle)
2 Right frontal bone
3 Left frontal bone
4 Right parietal bone
5 Left parietal bone
6 Small fontanelle (posterior fontanelle)
7 Occipital bone

Fig. 890. Cranium of a fetus, 11 cm long. Seen from above (after *Broman*).

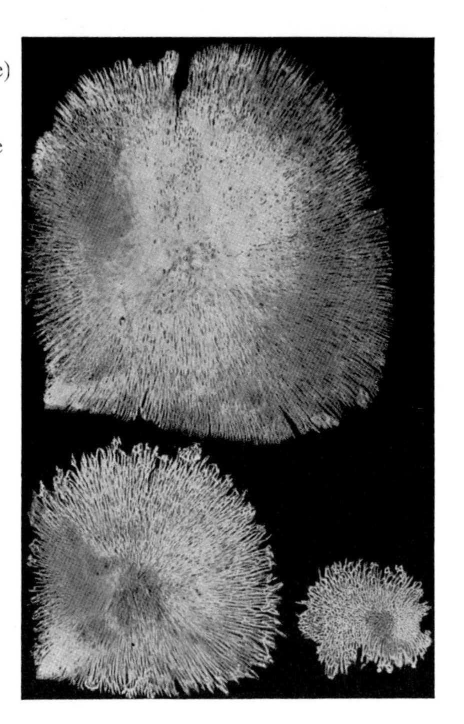

Fig. 892. Three stages of development of a covering bone, the parietal bone (1/1). Bottom right, of a fetus in the 3rd month; bottom left, in the 5th month; above, of a newborn (from *Sobotta-Becher).*

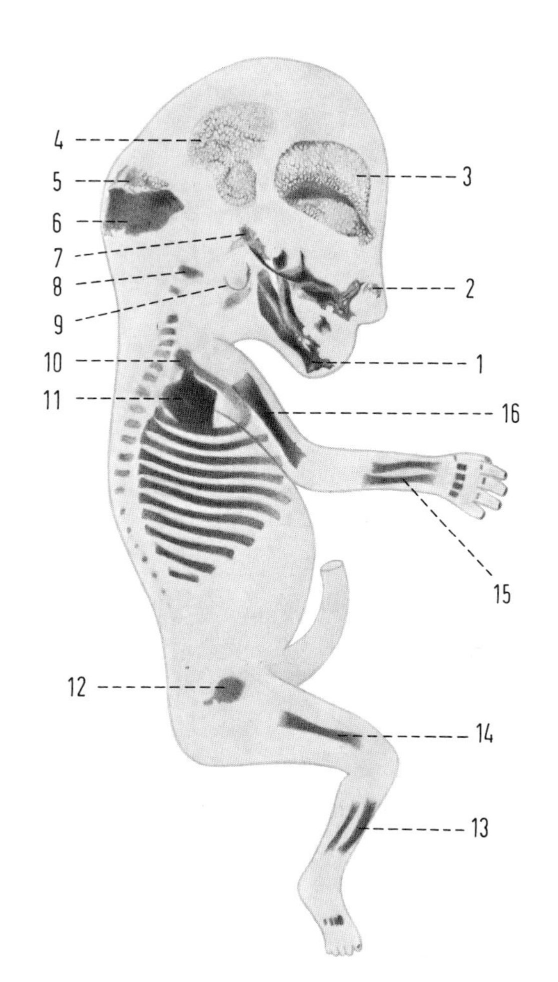

Fig. 891. Bony skeleton, stained dark, of a **fetus about 7 cm long** (after *Broman*).

week) is completed after the 17th year in girls and the 21st year in boys with the fusion of the last epiphyseal clefts in the long tubular bones. For details of onto- and phylogenesis, see *Theiler.*

In chondral and connective tissue, preformed section of the skeletal ossification starts from a nucleus of the bone. This ossification proceeds basically differently in parts of the skeleton preformed by cartilage or by connective tissue.

The cartilaginous preformed bone becomes ossified only after dissolution of the cartilage, arising from the ventrally placed bony nucleus (enchondral ossification, schematic view = Fig. 889) as well as from the periphery in the shape of a bony cuff (perichondral ossification).

In the covering bones which are preformed by connective tissue, ossification also starts from a center, but this is only a bone development out of connective tissue. The clavicle occupies a certain in-between position. It is the only tubular bone preformed by connective tissue, while its two ends are preformed purely cartilaginously *(Benninghoff-Goerttler, Pernkopf).* The first indications of ossification can be demonstrated earlier on some covering bones than on the chondrally preformed skeleton. Maxilla and mandible ossify between the 6th and 7th em-

1 Mandible
2 Nasal bone
3 Frontal bone
4 Parietal bone
5 Superior squama of occipital bone
6 Inferior squama of occipital bone
7 Temporal bone
8 Occipital bone
9 Annulus tympanicus
10 Clavicle
11 Scapula
12 Ilium
13 Tibia
14 Femur
15 Ulna
16 Humerus

	At birth	%
Head of humerus		5
Distal epiphysis of femur		95
Proximal epiphysis of femur		60
Calcaneus		100
Cuboid bone		60
Ribs 3, 4, 5, 6, 7		100
Ribs 8, 9, 10, 11, 12		100
Ribs 1 and 2		100

Table 6 shows the **time of appearance of various nuclei of ossification** and, simultaneously, gives the percentages of probability of their being demonstrable at the end of a normal pregnancy (from *Pschyrembel*).

bryonal weeks. The ossification of most of the remaining, chondrally preformed parts of the skeleton starts in the 3rd fetal month. By the end of the 3rd fetal month, the bony skeleton is already present, with the exception of a few short component parts of hands and feet (see Figs. 890–892).

Through radiographic study of the fetus, one can determine its age with comparative certainty as time and sequence of the appearance of the individual nuclei of the bones are constant. This is of special forensic importance. The radiograph can testify the following about *Béclard*'s point (i.e., about the distal epiphyseal nucleus of the femur which, according to *Lahm,* was a sure forensic indicator of the maturity of the fetus for the early anatomists; see also Table 6): The distal epiphyseal nucleus of the femur can be recognized et the beginning of the 9th month (limits: 9th fetal to 3rd postnatal months) and is always present in mature infants. The proximal nucleus of the tibial head appears later; *Tatafiore* found it at birth in only 80% of all cases. The appearance of the nuclei of distal epiphysis of the femur and of the head of the tibia are connected to the weight and length of the fetus. In addition, at birth most segments of skull, spine, ribs and diaphyses of the long tubular bones show bony differentiation. Then there are about 270 individual bones.

Knowledge of the normal development of the skeleton is of great clinical significance, as its age provides more information on the effective state of development of the examined subject than body height or weight and, furthermore, as illnesses greatly influence the formation of the nuclei of the bones and, thereby, the development of the skeleton.

Table 6 shows the time of appearance of the nuclei of the bones and of bone synostoses, as do Tables 7–10, taken from the textbook of radiologic diagnostics by *Schinz, Baensch, Friedl* and *Uehlinger.* The dates represent average values. As mentioned before, the nuclei appear somewhat earlier in females than in males. The dots show the appearance of the nuclei, the transverse beams the period of synostoses. As a supplement, the table of ossification taken from *Schmid* and *Halden* has been added.

Acceleration of Development

The acceleration of development observed in civilized countries since the turn of the century has led to a shift of the norms of ossification. Therefore, some older tables of norms (as reprinted in this chapter) are of only limited value.

This change in development denotes, according to *de Rudder,* "the comprehensive phenomenon of growth, sexual and intellectual acceleration as the answer of the human organism to living in an urban milieu, where masses of somatic and psychic stimuli and subsequent stimulation axquire central importance." On the other hand, high-quality and protein-rich diets, as well as improvement of social-hygienic conditions, are cited as essential factors. Thus, today's school children, due to earlier development of puberty, are 15–20 cm and adults about 10 cm taller than three generations ago.

For a long time, the main significance for the processes of development and maturation has been apportioned to the hormones, obviously under the impact of their discovery, including the effects of their deficiency and overproduction. Today, however, we know that the decisive role is played by hereditary, constitutional factors which are then activated by the hormones *(Bennholdt-Thomsen* and *Freund).*

Because of questions connected with acceleration of possible early hormonal therapy, especially in girls, *Greulich* and *Pyle* approached the possibility of a final determination of height in juveniles by producing an atlas of the growth and development of the hand and wrist. According to the state of ossification (i.e., the degree of development of epiphyses and nuclei of the bones, compared to age and already attained height), one is able to make a prognosis, which will be exact within a few centimeters, of final height.

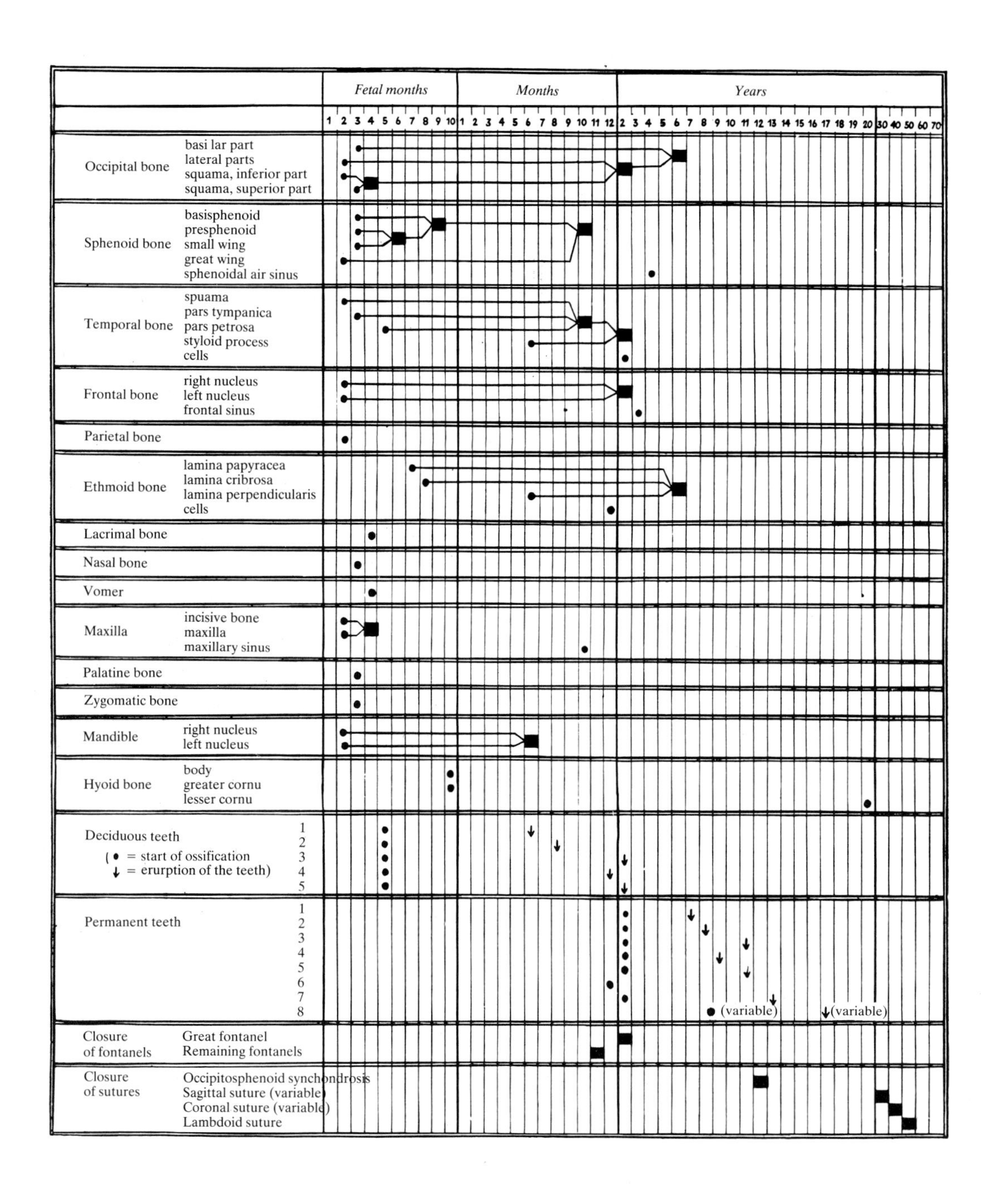

Table 7. Appearance of bony nuclei and synostosis: skull, including teeth (from *Schinz, Baensch, Friedl* and *Uehlinger*). Lamina papyracea of the ethmoid bone = lamina orbitalis (PNA).

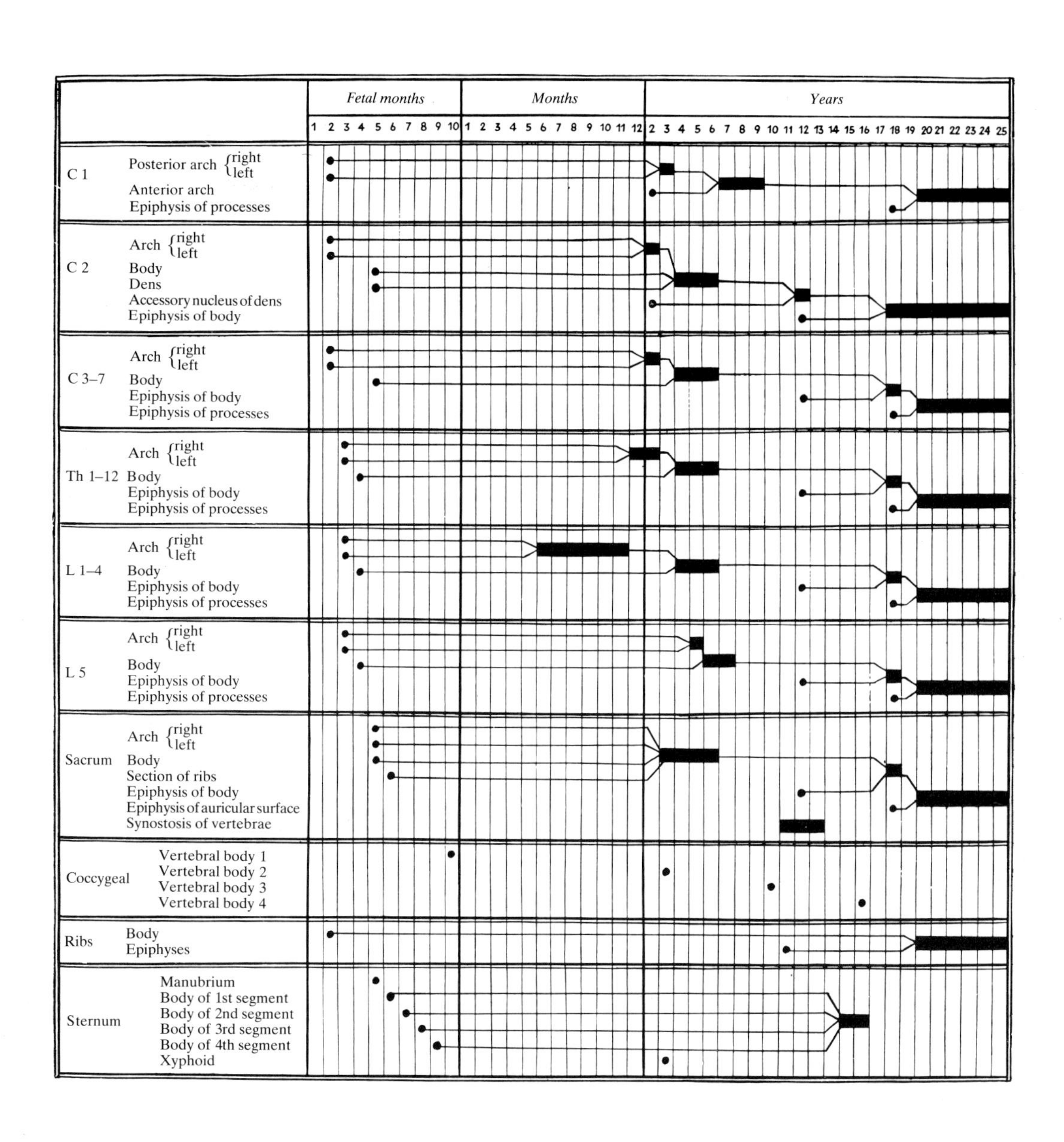

Table 8. Appearance of bony nuclei and synostosis: spine, ribs, sternum (from *Schinz, Baensch, Friedl* and *Uehlinger*).

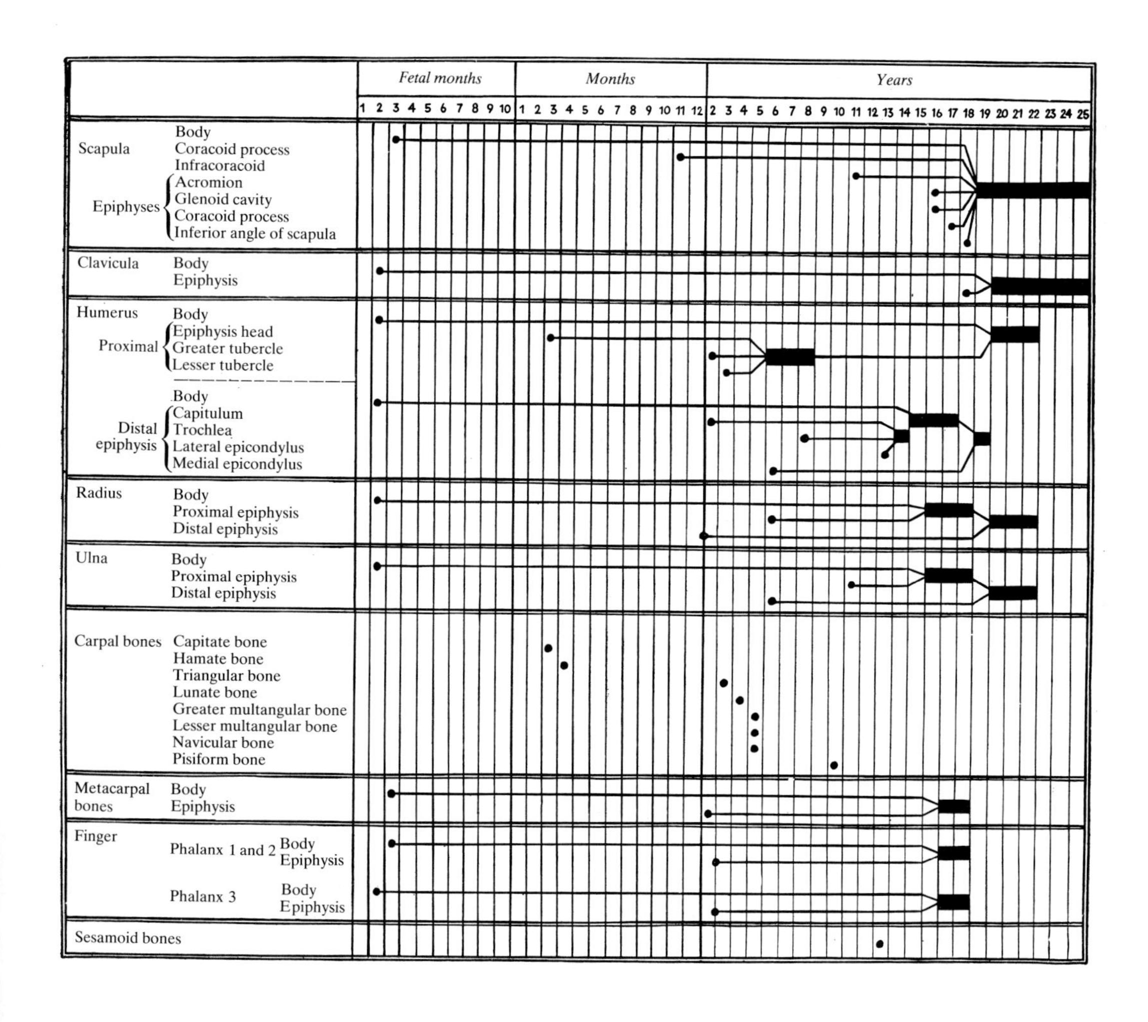

Table 9. Appearance of bony nuclei and synostosis: shoulder girdle and upper extremities (from *Schinz, Baensch, Friedl* and *Uehlinger*).

Os multangulum majus = Os trapezium (PNA) = greater multangular bone
Os multangulum minus = Os trapezoidum (PNA) = lesser multangular bone
Os naviculare = Os scaphoideum (PNA) = navicular bone

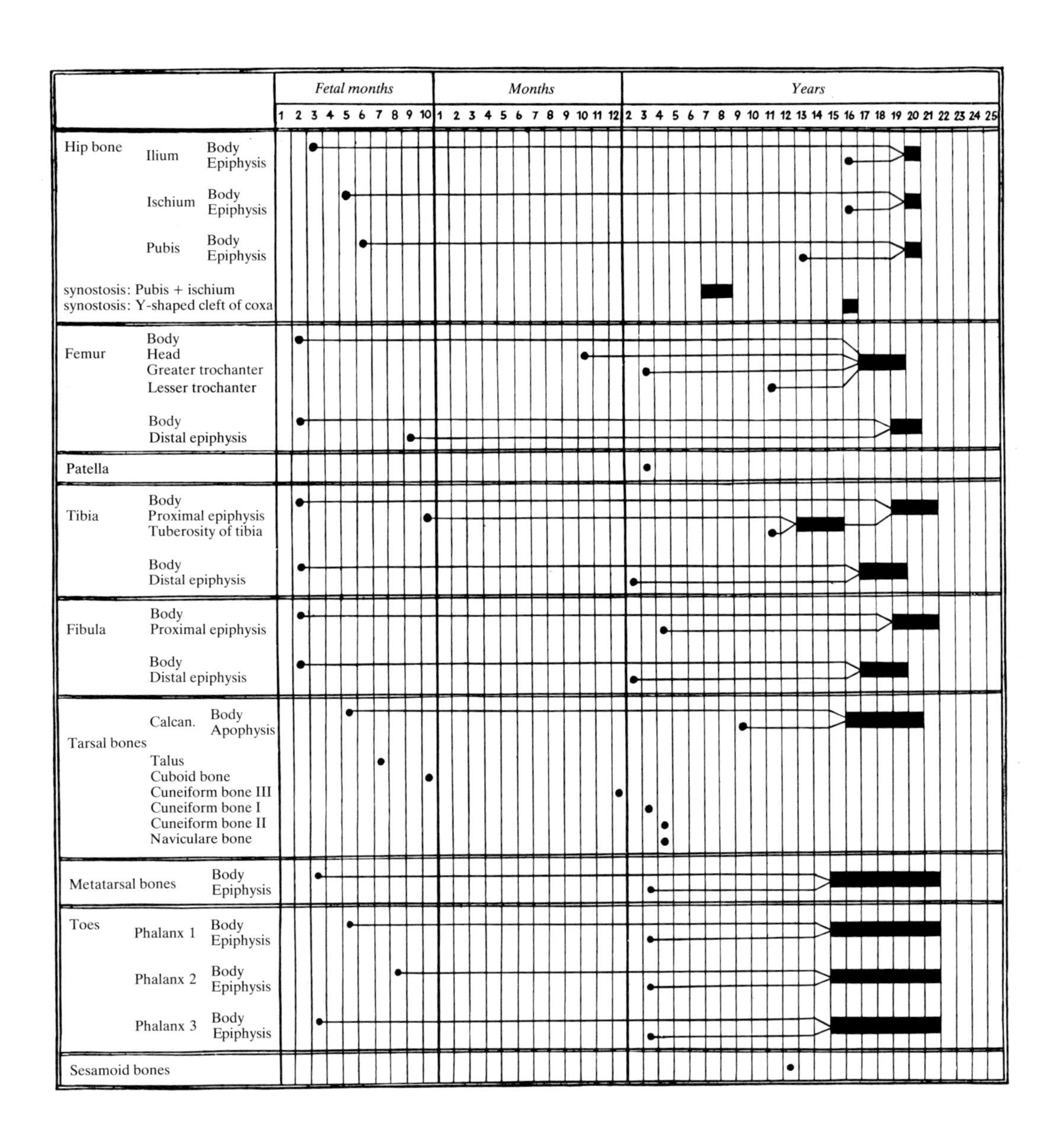

Table 10. Appearance of bony nuclei and synostosis: pelvis and lower extremities (from *Schinz, Baenesch, Friedl* and *Uehlinger*).

Os cuneiforme III = Os cuneiforme laterale (PNA) = third cuneiform bone
Os cuneiforme I = Os cuneiforme mediale (PNA) = first cuneiform bone
Os cuneiforme II = Os cuneiforme intermedium (PNA) = second cuneiform bone

Table 11. **Table of ossification** (after *Schmid* and *Halden)*.

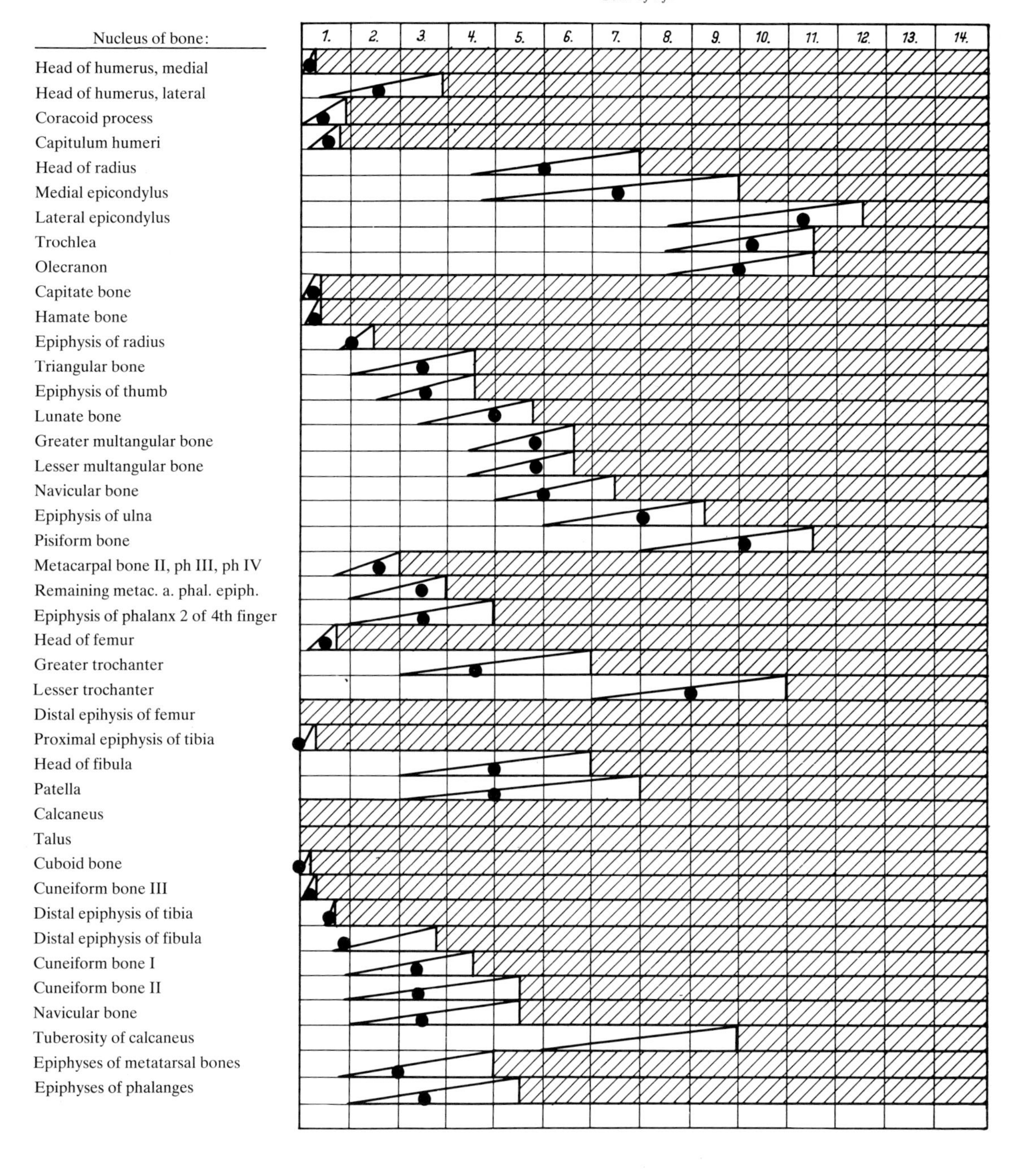

Inconstant nucleus — Time of most frequent appearance — Nucleus, constantly present

II. The Skull

The bones of the skull are mainly preformed as membranous bones, i.e., most of the facial bones and the flat bones of the cranium. Among them are included the parietal, frontal, nasal, lacrimal and zygomatic bones, maxilla, palatine bone and vomer. One cranial bone, the ethmoid bone, is preformed purely cartilaginously, as a replacement bone. Other cranial bones are preformed partly by connective tissue, partly by cartilage (temporal, occipital and sphenoid bones).

Ossification of the cranial bones, which occurs about the 7th embryonal week, begins with the occipital bone. Then follow the petrous part, the zygomatic bone, the mandible and the squamous portion. The sphenoid bone becomes ossified about the 9th week and the nasal bone about the 10th *(Broman)*. Against this opinion, the mandible is the first ossifying cranial bone according to *Theiler*. Almost simultaneously, the maxilla becomes ossified. In the cranium, too, the first minute beams can be demonstrated in the covering bones. There, they appear first in the frontal and parietal bones.

The first radiographic demonstration of ossifications in the skeleton of the skull succeeds after the 3rd fetal month *(Markovits)*; see Fig. 893.

Certain signs on the fetal skeleton are of clinical importance, among others the shape of the skull, as roof-tile-like shifts of the cranial bones, so called *Spalding's* sign, together with relaxation of the tone of the spine with extension, denote intrauterine embryonal death (Figure 903). For comparison, Fig. 904 shows a live fetus in the 9th – 10th month in normal right occipital presentation. But normally, roof-tile-like shifts of the cranial bones may occur before the beginning of labor and rupture of the amniotic sac during the 10th lunar month; they may also be caused by distortion due to projection.

Therefore, we distinguish between physiologic and pathologic step formation at the fetal skull.

Physiological step formation of the fetal skull is considered to be a prepartum configuration of the infantile skull as it arises during the last weeks of pregnancy due to premature labor pains and pressure of the surroundings, especially with cephalic presentation *(Wichtl, Borell* and *Fernström)*. They arise before the start of labor, before rupture of the amniotic sac and the entry of the skull into the maternal pelvis. In these cases the parietal bones almost always project outward at the great or small fontanelle or in both places. In isolated cases, a physiological shift of the cranial bones has been observed with breech presentation.

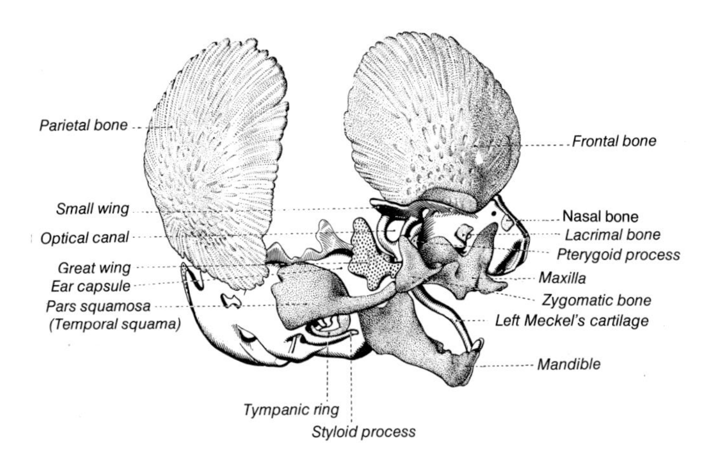

Fig. 893. Oblique lateral view of a model of the primordial cranium of a human fetus in the 3rd month, with the appertaining covering bones made prominent by punctation. The cartilage is white and only slightly prominent (from *Benninghoff-Goerttler)*.

Physiological step-shaped and (due to unfavorable projection) roof-tile-like shifts of the fetal cranial bones make the diagnosis of "intrauterine embryonal death" far more difficult during the 10th lunar month than before that time *(Wichtl)*. Physiological step formations before the onset of labor occur, according to *Borell* and *Fernström,* in about 5% of cephalic presentations.

Pathological step formations on the fetal skull usually appear much earlier. Such step formation after fetal death usually occurs by outward shift of the parietal bones, and leads after some time to the well-known *Spalding-Horner* symptom.

Only the height of the step and the time of its appearance are of differential diagnostic significance.

A pathological step at the fetal skull may occur at any stage of pregnancy after fetal death and may even appear a few hours thereafter. A fully developed *Spalding* symptom, i.e., roof-tile steps of 2–3 cm after the 36th week of pregnancy, occurs only after several days, sometimes even after weeks. Before the 34th–36th weeks of pregnancy, each roof-tile shift of the cranial bones, be it ever so minute, must be considered a *Spalding* symptom (see p. 379). *Fochen* has presented a survey on obstetric radiographic diagnostics.

It is difficult to radiographically demonstrate the exact prenatal development of the individual bone segments *(Baensch)*. Knowledge of the normal development of the cranial bones in postnatal life is of clinical importance, however, as significant deviations from the norm may provide important indications of developmental disturbances or anomalies *(Theiler, Ebel)*.

It must be taken into account that the growth of the skull depends on the development of the brain. In the newborn the weight of the brain amounts to about 350 gr. At the end of the first year the brain has reached almost 50% and at the end of the 7th year 90% of its final size. The infantile skull shows disproportion between cranium and facial skull: the facial skull forms only 1/8 of the surface of the entire skull, while in the adult it comprises 5%.

Growth of the skull is most intense during the 1st and 2nd years of life *(Bergerhoff)*. Further growth of the skull until puberty proceeds slowly; its final size is reached about the age of 20 in many cases. Therefore, one can infer the development of the brain from radiographs of the skull.

Fontanels

At birth the skull has six fontanels, of which only the two larger ones – the anterior (frontal) and the posterior (occipital) fontanels – are of practical importance (Figs. 940–942).

The frontal fontanel closes at about the 18th month of life, while the occipital one is often closed at birth or closes until the end of the 3rd month of life. The two anterior lateral fontanels, the anterolateral fonticuli (sphenoid fontanels), close within the first three months of life, while the two posterior lateral fontanels, the posterolateral fonticuli (mastoid fontanels), close only during the 1st to 2nd years of life.

In the sutures of the medial plane (frontal and sagittal sutures), accessory fontanels may be the cause of meningoceles or encephaloceles, though such an occurrence is relatively rare. They are found at the root of the nose as a glabellar fontanel (nasofrontal fontanel), in the frontal suture as a metopic fontanel, in or next to the sagittal suture as parietal fontanel, and in the inferior squama of the occipital bone as cerebellar fontanel. Occasionally, very large accessory fontanels occur from birth symmetrically in the parietal bones. Such lacunae in the parietal bones have been designated by *Zarfl* and *Voigt* as fenestrae parietales symmetricae. They are usually found together with other disturbances of development.

These accessory fontanels must be differentiated from the parietal foramina, also symmetrically arranged near the median line of the cranium. They result from incomplete ossification of the parietal bones *(Markovits)*. Normally, they are of pin-head size and roundish. If these bone defects are bean-sized, they are called foramina parietalia permagna. They lie about 2–3 cm above the lambdoid suture, adjacent to the sagittal suture, a dominantly hereditary but clinically insignificant anomaly.

One has to separate from these cranial gap formations pathological bone defects in cases of meningoceles, syphilis or tuberculosis of the skull, *Hand-Schüller-Christian's* disease, eosinophile granuloma and neoplasms. Sometimes one can demonstrate a rare, usually bilateral anomaly, a symmetrical thinning of the parietal bones which is seen on lateral exposure as a zone of increased radiolucency.

Based on his theory of cranial centers of bone formation, *Frassetto* has enumerated 22 possible fontanels. The number of fontanels depends on the number of centers of bone formation. At any point of the skull where three or more centers of ossification touch one another, a fontanel may be formed and persist. In addition, within the fontanel an intercalary bone may be formed. Generally, only six constant fontanels are observed at birth.

Delay of closure of the fontanels may point to disturbance of skeletal development in rickets; it can also be found in mongolism *(Schiffer* and *Strubel)*.

Synchondroses

For the longitudinal growth of the skull, two of the six synchondroses of the cranial skeleton are of practical importance:

a) Intersphenoidal synchondrosis. The sphenoid bone consists of several nuclei which form a unified posterior sphenoidal body in the 3rd lunar month. This sphenoidal body is separated from the orbitosphenoidal section by a cartilaginous junction, the so-called intersphenoidal synchondrosis. It runs transversely through the body of the bone in the region of the tuberculum sellae. It is of special significance as it shares responsibility for the longitudinal growth of the skull. Normally, it is present only until the end of the 7th fetal month, but it may also be visible into the 1st year of life.
b) Synchondrosis spheno-occipitalis. This is a suture between the sphenoid and the occipital bone. This junction, too, has practical significance for the longitudinal growth of the skull. It is seen on lateral exposures of the skull of children at the clivus of the sella. This junction closes with puberty until the 20th year of life, and changes into a synostosis. This completes the longitudinal growth of the skull (Figs. 920, 921, 923, and 925).

Cranial Sutures

The sutures of the cranium are of a different morphologic structure than the sutures of the facial skull. These run smoothly, while the sutures of the cranium are jagged and bridged outside and inside by periost.

There are no proper sutures in the newborn. In their place one finds broad clefts (Fig. 944), bordered by linear edges of bone, which during the course of the 1st year of life become more and more narrow, until they are 1 to 2 mm wide at the end of the 1st year. From then on, the sutural edges of the external lamina become more and more jagged and, finally, deeply cogged. The cog formation of the external lamina reaches its final shape about the 3rd year of life. It is remarkable that the cogs are limited to the external lamina, while the internal lamina retains the normal shape of the clefts. This can be seen occasionally on radiographs.

The radiographic conception of a suture, therefore, does not include the whole suture – only that part which corresponds to the external lamina *(Haas)*. With suitable projection, the smooth suture line of the internal lamina may be seen and should not be confused with a fracture line running along the suture.

After completion of the growth of the skull, ossification of the sutures begins in the diploë and the internal lamina, while the external lamina ossifies very much later.

Premature closure of fontanels and sutures (premature craniostosis or craniosyntosis with the symptoms of craniostenosis) may be the result of deficient development of the brain. In cases of such microcephaly, symptoms of increased intracranial pressure are absent. In cases of primary craniostosis with normal development of the brain, increase of intracranial pressure may occur, with augmented digital impressions after long duration. With premature closure of sutures, the skull expands parallel to the axis of the closed suture. In cases of a closed sagittal suture, scaphocephaly develops; with closed coronal suture, a high dome (tower skull, see Figs. 929, 956 and 958).

Examining the principles governing the order of obliteration of the cranial sutures, *Gremjazky* found that each of the two main sutures (coronal and sagittal) starts to obliterate at a definite spot, the sagittal suture in the region of the obelion (crown of the head) and the coronal suture in its temporal section.

Crocellà studied this problem radiographically. Accordingly, the union of the sutures starts earlier at the internal than at the external lamina, while at the base and in the face it occurs simultaneously.

During the 15th to 16th years of life, the spheno-occipital synchondrosis begins to close, followed slightly later by closure of the petro-occipital synchondrosis, the occipito mastoid and the sphenoethmoidal suture. Between the 20th and 30th years of life follow in the male the squamosal, parietomastoid and sphenosquamosal sutures and often also the outer part of the zygomaticofrontal, sphenozygomatic and zygomaticomaxillary sutures.

In the female the sutures close in the following order: zygomaticofrontal, zygomaticotemporal and zygomaticomaxillary sutures; further, the sphenozygomatic, frontonasal, frontomaxillary, ethmomaxillary and transverse palatine sutures.

The remaining sutures ossify between the 30th and 50th years of life. The times of ossification vary considerably.

The sutura mendosa can be seen most clearly and distinctly and with remarkable regularity on the radiograph of the infantile skull (Figs. 940, 941 and 944). For its localization, one uses the connecting line between the posterior end of the upper ridge of the petrous bone and the external occipital protuberance.

In the infant, the sutures and clefts appear considerably narrower but more sharply designed lines of increased radiolucency. In sutures formed by connective tissue, especially in the region of the lambdoid suture, the development of the sutural spikes becomes more and more distinct with advancing age. At the place of termination of the sutura mendosa, a suture which *Grob* found in 93% of all cases during the 1st year of life, one often recognizes a so-called intercalary bone. From the 5th year on, this suture is found rarely (4%). The so-called transverse occipital suture results from the union of the right and left sutura mendosa.

In the infant, the synchondrosis intraoccipitalis anterior (basilateralis ossis occipitalis) is only faintly recognizable on lateral exposure. The extent of the synchondrosis intraoccipitalis posterior (squamolateralis ossis occipitalis) provides the occipital bone of newborns and young infants with characteristic radiographic features. Later on, it becomes reduced to a suture-like line (visible until the 5th year of life). Confusion with a fracture is not infrequent (see Figs. 940–942).

Occasionally, variants of sutures in the region of the occipital squama can be observed (Fig. 944). See also the section on variants in the chapter on the adult skull: os interparietale (interparietal bone) and os praeinterparietale. These may complicate considerably the interpretation of the lateral view of the sutures.

Caffey found in 0.4% of 3800 examined newborns preformed accessory ossicles in the synchondrosis between the lateral parts and the occipital squama. In lateral views, they were often covered by denser adjacent bones. They are better visible with the modified technique of *Towne* (quoted by *Caffey*), a forward-tilted anteroposterior exposure of the skull. One to four round ossicles appear; the medially placed ones are usually larger. They often protrude beyond the outer surface of the squama, in contrast to the so-called *Kerckring* bone which, on lateral view, is mostly projected above the inner surface of the squama. *Kerckring's* bone appears during the 4th to 5th fetal months and fuses with the squama a few weeks before birth. Rarely, it remains isolated for a long period; usually it appears as a bony process at the inferior margin of the squama, above the foramen magnum. According to *Caffey,* one has to separate most definitely *Kerckring's* bone from the accessory ossicles. The accessory ossicles originate from the segmented cartilaginous arch of the occipital bone and may be precursors of bony thickenings of the edges of the foramen magnum at the adult skull. Anatomists and anthropologists speak of an occipital vertebra or a proatlas. The segment in question is the third one of the spondylocranium. These differentiations, which remind one of a vertebra, are considered a regressive variant (manifestation of an occipital vertebra), or they are considered a progressive variant (the partial or complete fusion of the atlas with the occipital bone), the so-called atlas-assimilation *(Brocher).*

The most frequent intercalary bones (ossa suturarum) are found in the lambdoid suture. They must not be mistaken for comminuted fractures.

As a sign of an acutely starting increase of intracranial pressure in the infantile skull, one finds bulging of the fontanels and early dehiscences of the sutures, which must be differentiated diagnostically from persistent open sutures, e.g., in rickets *(Hünermann).* With slow increase of intracranial pressure, changes at the base of the skull and at the sella are typical. Furthermore, an increase of the size of the skull and elongation of the saw-like shape of the sutures, but no gaping sutures, are found. The separation of sutures in infants due to increased intracranial pressure lasts, according to *Markovits,* about 4 months. *Hoen* and *Kaiser* examined views of skulls of 589 children. Out of 21 cases of "pressure damage" and "borderline cases," only 5 showed clinically unequivocal signs of increased intracranial pressure. Two cases were completely free of symptoms. The radiographic diagnostic of increased intracranial pressure becomes much more certain by observation of the cranial sutures.

Constant cranial sutures (after *Lassrich, Prévôt* and *Schäfer):*

(Data on times of ossification vary a great deal in the literature; see also Figs. 246 and 953.)

1. Frontal suture (Figs. 946 and 947), between right

and left halves of the frontal bone. Ossification begins in the 2nd year of life, and only during the 8th year will a unified frontal bone have formed. This suture, as persistent frontal suture (metopic suture), may remain open for decades. *Torgersen* found a metopic suture in 7.2% of cases. It probably occurs even more often if one considers that a slightly incomplete persistence will become invisible on the radiograph as soon as the internal lamina has closed. Closure of the persistent frontal suture begins in men at the age of 20 to 30 years, in women somewhat later *(Hiltemann).*

2. Sagittal suture, between the two parietal bones. It disappears between the 20th and 30th years of life.
3. Coronal suture, between the frontal and parietal bones. It disappears between the 30th and 40th years of life. The last suture to disappear is the lambdoid suture, which may still be open in about 35% of males between the 70th and 80th years.
4. Sphenofrontal suture, between the great wings of the sphenoid bone and the frontal bone. It starts from the anterior lateral fontanel.
5. Squamosal suture (squamoparietal suture), between the parietal bone and the squamous portion of the temporal bone.
6. Parietomastoid suture, between the parietal bone and the petrous portion of the temporal bone.
7. Occipitomastoid suture, between the lateral part of the occipital bone and the petrous portion of the temporal bone.
8. Sutura mendosa (transverse occipital suture), between the superior and inferior parts of the occipital squama (see Figs. 940 and 941). In this connection, compare the legend to Figure 237.
9. Posterior intraoccipital synchondrosis, between the lateral part of the occipital bone and the squama.
10. Spheno-occipital synchondrosis, between the sphenoid bone and the basilar part of the occipital bone.

Digital Impressions and Cerebral Juga, Diploic Veins and Vascular Canals

During the period of active growth of the child, as an expression of adaptation of two adjacent tissues, digital impressions develop due to alternation between bony ledges (juga cerebralia) and zones of diminished bony thickness (*Friedmann* and *Seiferth*). In the adult they are usually marked so little that they hardly appear on the radiograph. On the skull of the newborn such impressions of the cerebral convolutions into the cranial bones cannot be recognized on the radiograph. Their development begins with the continuous differentiation of the cerebral surface, starting in infancy about the 4th month of life. During the first 3 to 4 years of life one can observe a quick rise in the formation of the impressions *(Macaulay),* while the situation between the 4th and 10th years remains fairly unchanged, with a certain regression from then on. Beyond the 5th decade of life, they hardly occur. If they persist beyond the 15th year, one ought to assume a general increase of intracranial pressure, usually of obstructive hydrocephalus (*v. Lengerke;* see also *Tönnis* and *Friedmann*). The impressions especially develop in the region of the parietal and occipital bones. Reduced formation of the impressions may run parallel with a delay of mental development. However, extreme care must be taken with diagnostic evaluation, even with much pronounced digital impressions (Figs. 956, 958).

Deepening and increased formation of the impressions of the skull of the child are physiological to a certain degree *(Macaulay, K. H. Schäfer* and *Hünermann),* and only together with gaping sutures can they be taken as a diagnostic sign of increased intracranial pressure. On the one hand, their augmentation may be missing in some cases of chronic intracranial pressure; on the other hand, they are found not infrequently in clinically healthy children *(Davidoff* and *Gass).*

Increase of digital impression can be evaluated as a radiologic sign of augmented intracranial pressure only in connection with further symptoms, e.g., dehiscence of sutures, changes at the sella *(Hoen* and *Kaiser).* According to *Marcovits,* their development in cases of chronic increased intracranial pressure takes about four months. Pronounced increase within a short period is also significant. In infancy and the toddler stage, early disruption of the sutures occurs frequently and prevents a noticeable deepening of the impressions (premature synostosis of sutures is an exception). While in young children the cranial sutures gape easily with increased intracranial pressure, their dehiscence is rendered more difficult from the 10th year on *(Markovits). Mayer* writes: "Only in the region of the bregma may the gaping of the suture be better recognizable on lateral view. In children dehiscence of the sutures may reach considerable proportions. The first sign of beginning sutural dehiscence in childhood may consist in the cogs of the sutures developing more regular borders and becoming elongated by the effect of the pull. The degree of sutural dehiscence is not only dependent on the state of the sutures and the intensity of pressure but also on the period during which the increase in pressure developed. Therefore, we sometimes see an infant with considerable hydrocephalus without dehiscence of sutures, in rare cases even with sutures narrower than in conformity with age." Inversely, flattening of the roof of the skull, thickening of the homolateral diploë with smoothing out of the digitate impressions in the region of the homolateral internal lamina and asymmetry around the base are important radiographic signs for cerebral hemiatrophy. A remarkable feature of these changes is their relatively quick appearance, according to the results of research by *Lefebvre, Guy* and *Metzger.*

Outlines of the diploic veins in the skull of the child appear on the radiograph at the earliest during the 3rd year of life. Until then, they are completely absent. Between the 10th and the 15th years, the venous design increases considerably and is demonstrable in about half the examined cases *(Kuhnhenn);* between the 15th and 20th

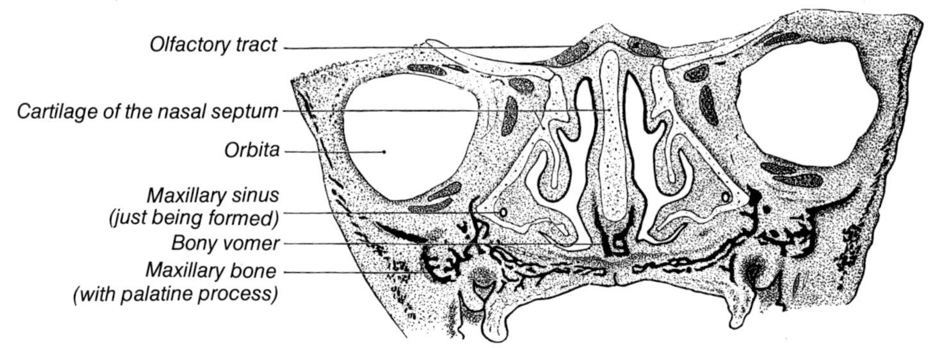

Fig. 894. Frontal section through the face of an approximately 15-week-old fetus. Enlargement 7 times (from *Broman*, after *Kallius*).

years, it is shown in more than 50%. After the 30th to 40th years, the findings become less. In the 7th decade of life, *Kuhnhenn* could recognize venous outlines in only 20% of the cases. These facts are connected with the development of the diploë, which develops most strongly in early childhood, preponderantly in the parietal bone, becoming reduced again with advancing age, together with the disappearance of the sutures and the approximation of both laminae, until their fusion into one bony plate. The diploic veins may show reticular, tree- or antler-like or star-shaped ramifications. Most frequently, large venous stars are found in the parietal bone which has the best developed diploë (*Breschet's* venous star). Occasionally, they occur in the infant *(K. H. Schäfer)*. By means of their localization and shape, one can distinguish the diploic veins from the sulci of the medial meningeal artery with their antler-shaped terminal ramifications and from the sinuses. In this connection, it must be kept in mind that the course of arteries is narrower and straighter than the venous course (Fig. 234).

The dilatation of veins may sometimes be used for localization and diagnosis of an outflow obstruction, e.g., due to tumor *(Mayer)*. They serve, in such cases, as collaterals to the intracranial venous sinuses, comparable to the caput medusae in the abdominal wall *(Kuhnhenn)*. In addition, knowledge of the diploic veins enables distinction between defects of the skull, fissures and arterial sulci in cases of racemose aneurysm.

Arterial sulci are to be found in typical places (Fig. 108); on the frontal view the sulci of the adjacent and the film-distant sides are projected parallel to each other, and their course is straighter than that of venous sulci. They taper towards the periphery and erode only the internal lamina. Their differentiation from traumatic fissures is important. As those spread through the whole roof of the skull, they appear brighter than vascular furrows and show narrowing only near the end of their frequently straight course. They can only be demonstrated by vertical entry of the central ray into the fissural cleft. Sutures are to be found in typical places and often show a toothed course.

Paranasal Sinuses

The paranasal sinuses arise from invagination of the epithelium of the sulci or furrows bordering the conchae into the connective tissue which lies below.

The maxillary sinuses (sinus maxillares) invaginate from the middle meatus during the middle of the 3rd fetal month (Fig. 894). In the newborn, they are roughly pea-sized and are difficult to differentiate on radiographs. The upper jaw as a whole is a flat disk *(Knutsson)*. At the end of the 1st year of life the maxillary sinuses can be demonstrated radiographically. Their development proceeds relatively fast until the 5th year of life.

Only during the 5th to 6th year do the maxillary sinuses assume their pyramidal shape. Thereafter, their development slows somewhat *(Majer)*. They reach their maximal width at the age of about 15 years. *Moczkowa* found in most cases of tomographically examined children, distinctly developed maxillary sinuses from the 2nd year on, while beginning pneumatization could occasionally be demonstrated before the end of the 1st year. She could also ascertain bulging of the dental alveoli into the maxillary sinuses during the 6th year of life. *Stern* and *Majer* found the maxillary sinuses relatively larger in the male than in the female, and the left larger than the right. They attain their final size between the 15th and 18th years of life *(Haas, Sedwick, Schwarz, Johnson;* also *Köhler-Zimmer)*.

The frontal sinuses (sinus frontales) develop, as the maxillary sinuses, from hollow invaginations of epithelium which arise from roughly the same region the maxillary sinuses originate. In general, the first radiologic demonstration of the frontal sinuses succeeds between the 4th and 12th years of life *(Tanew, Knutsson, Stern)*, rarely soon after the 1st year. Height and width reach their almost final dimensions at the age of 15 to 20 years, though the maximum is attained only in the 40th year of life.

Like the maxillary sinuses, the frontal sinuses are generally larger in males than in females; again, the left is larger than the right. Hypoplasias and aplasias occur more often on the right than on the left. There is no connection between the height of the frontal sinuses and their distance from the orbita, nor could any connection be found between the size of the frontal sinuses and deviation of the nasal septum or pneumatization of the mastoid process. In the infant and toddler, the paranasal sinuses cannot always be distinctly defined due to the relatively slight contrasts. The fluctuation of the time of appearance in pneumatization of the paranasal sinuses is greatest in the frontal sinuses *(Moczkowa)*; Fig. 911.

Development of one or both frontal sinuses in the adult is often absent, or one finds only rudimentary, preformed, small cavities as continuation of the ethmoidal cells from which they must be differentiated. Shadows of the paranasal sinuses may be simulated by their slight extension in depth; therefore, a lateral view should be taken in any case and, if needed, an additional axial exposure (Figs. 57 and 60).

Weickmann reported comprehensively on vicarious hyperplasia of the paranasal sinuses in hypoplastic cerebral processes (cf. Figs. 271 and 272).

"The finding of unilateral vicarious hyperplasia of the paranasal sinuses is characteristically and constantly combined with cerebral hemiatrophy, to such a degree that the changes in the skull alone permit diagnosis of cerebral hemiatrophy, without the aid of encephalography" *(Epstein* and *Davidoff).* Typical for such cases is the pneumatization of the roof of the orbita which, according to *Haas,* may develop on the basis of a supraorbital recess of the frontal sinus, as well as by greater expansion of the ethmoidal cells. After the 10th year of life, during the period of their main development, very asymmetrical frontal sinuses with pronounced hyperplasia are almost pathognomonic for a homolateral hypoplastic cerebral process *(Weickmann).*

The ethmoidal cells (cellulae ethmoidales) develop, as the maxillary and frontal sinuses, from hollow invaginations of epithelium, which start from the same region as the previously mentioned paranasal sinuses. After the end of the 1st year, the anterior ethmoidal cells can be demonstrated, the posterior ones only during the 3rd to 4th years. Their origin can already be found at birth, while their development will be completed with the 16th year of life *(Moczkowa).*

They reach from the frontal to the sphenoidal sinus and are recognizable on radiographs next to the orbita.

Sphenoidal sinuses (sinus sphenoidales) develop from a recess in the region of the posterior upper corner of the nasal cavities but penetrate only later, during the first years after birth, into the sphenoid bone. Formation of a cavity can generally be recognized only by about the 4th year of life. Their greatest expansion is reached about the 10th year *(Jakob).* The extension of the sphenoidal sinuses varies extraordinarily, from a very small sinus in each side of the anterior section of the sphenoid bone to cavity formation into the dorsum sellae. The sphenoidal sinuses are often asymmetrical.

When evaluating paranasal sinuses of children, it is important to remember that pneumatization of the paranasal sinuses may proceed asymmetrically; therefore, differences in transparency of the paranasal sinuses may be of limited value.

Sella Turcica

In contrast to the adult with a fully developed skeleton, the sella turcica of the newborn is constructed comparatively simply. The nuclei of the bones are separated fairly far from each other by cartilage, and they are also covered by cartilage at the protruding edges. Therefore, the

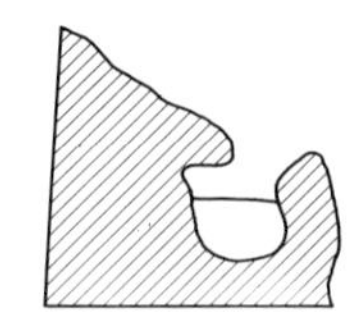

Fig. 895 (from *Sartorius*). **Measuring the sella turcica.** Upper limit: a connecting line between the lowest point of the roundness of the tuberculum sellae and the innermost point of the tip of the dorsum. The surface of the space below the border line is taken as the surface of the sella.

sella of the infant appears as a flat, tiny dish whose anterior border, through the already developed anterior clinoid processes, stands higher than the dorsum sellae whose bony nucleus appears shortly after birth but whose posterior clinoid processes are being developed only in the 3rd to 4th years of life. By that time, the sella has already acquired its customary shape. In the newborn, one can demonstrate the intersphenoidal synchondrosis between the basisphenoid and the presphenoid as a small cleft in the most anterior part of the sella. Generally, however, bony union takes place in the 7th fetal month *(Haas).* In hydrocephaly and in premature infants the synchondrosis appears especially distinctly.

According to *Gefferth,* one can distinguish four types of shapes of the sella: round, ellipsoid, compressed and flat sellae turcica.

The size of the sella is subject to great individual variation. According to *Bergerhoff* and *Höbler,* the growth of the cranium of children and juveniles proceeds in exactly determinable periods. The size of the sellar profile increases quickly up to the 3rd year of life. *Bergerhoff* and *Martin,* in their research on the growth of the skull in infants and toddlers up to 3 years of age, were able to measure a sellar profile growing in proportion to the cranium. Between the 3rd to 12th years of life, the size of the sellar profile remains fairly constant. During puberty a new spurt of growth occurs, whereby the sella reaches its final size. In girls, this development proceeds somewhat faster. There are no unequivocal connections between the shape and size of the sella turcica and the size of the skull, body weight and age *(Gefferth, Klöppner).*

Different methods for determination of the size of the sella have been devised by *Sartorius, Unterberg* and

Table 12 shows the normal values of the size of the sella during various periods of life (from *Grundler* and *Seige*).

Age	*Size of sella in mm²*	*Age*	*Size of sella in mm²*
1 Month	15	1 Year	24
2 Months	17	2 Years	37
3 Months	18	3 Years	45
4 Months	19	4 Years	50
5 Months	22	5 Years	56
6 Months	22	6 Years	58
7 Months	23	7 Years	61
8 Months	23	8 Years	63
9 Months	23	9 Years	66
10 Months	23	10 Years	69
11 Months	24		
		Male	Female
12 – 15 Years		69	69.8
16 – 19 Years		79	78.5
20 – 50 Years		96.3	88.1

others. The size of the surface (see Fig. 895) amounts in the 1st month to 10 to 17 mm². Using *Haas'* method, *Sartorius* found ± 5 mm² to be a normal deviation based on average values of the 1-to-10-year age group. Differences from ± 5 mm² to ± 10 mm² are to be regarded as conditionally normal, and those of more than ± 10 mm² as definitely pathological.

Measurements based on *Haas'* method show considerable deviation; besides, they do not relate to the shape and size of the cranium as a whole. These parameters are included in the calculation of the angle after *Bergerhoff* (see also *Bergerhoff* and *Höbler, Bergerhoff* and *Martin*).

Changes of size and shape of the sella are found in the following endocrinological disturbances, in changes of intracranial pressure and in certain anomalies:

Preponderantly enlarged sella in oxycephaly (Figs. 929, 956 and 958), hypothyroidism and athyrosis, goiter, adiposogenital dystrophy and congenital soft skull.

Reduced sellar surfaces have been determined in lipodystrophy, progressive muscular dystrophy and proportioned dwarfism.

In adiposity, no unequivocal changes at the sella could be found. *Nobécourt* and *Haguenau* stress that no conclusion can be drawn from radiologic changes of the sella to the hypophyseal origin of adiposity. *Wieser* found the sella conspicuously large in hypothyroidism and remarkably small in hyperthyroidism, but stresses that from the size of the sella alone no conclusions as to size and function of the hypophysis can ever be drawn without simultaneous consideration of the state of function of other glands with internal secretion, especially the thyroid gland. In genuine epilepsy, thickenings at the anterior clinoid processes, the dorsum sella or at both have been found almost regularly. In cases of imbecility, no peculiarities of shape or size of the sella have been observed. According to *Klöppner,* many more variants of its shape can be seen in the adult than in the newborn. The demonstrable changes of the sella caused by internal hydrocephaly in the adult cannot be ascertained in congenital hydrocephalus. However, one finds in the newborn considerable variants of the sellar shape in malformations of the central nervous system, especially in microcephaly.

Petrous Part (Tympanic Cavity, Tympanic Antrum and Semicircular Canals)

The bony development of the petrous bone shows several peculiarities. During the 5th fetal month, when the fetus is 20–25 cm long, the cartilaginous capsula of the labyrinth changes, by means of enchondral ossification, into spongy bone substance. In addition, direct ossification takes place at the outer walls of the perilymphatic space, which consists of fibrous connective tissue; this process leads to the development of the ivory-hard, bony labyrinth. In the newborn and toddler the relative size of the petrous bone is conspicuous. With further development of the skull the size of the petrous bone increases relatively little. The organs within the petrous bone, cochlea, semicircular canals and tympanic cavity with the auditory ossicles are embryonally preformed at their final size and show very little further growth until old age. Therefore, the fetal skull and skull of the newborn show the well-recognizable semicircular canals, i.e., the superior and posterior semicircular canals (Fig. 943). The third, the lateral semicircular canal, appears much shortened by such a projection. The tympanic cavity proper, the entrance to the antrum and the tympanic antrum have almost reached their definite size with the maturity of the fetus *(Broman).* As has been stated before, the auditory ossicles are the only bones of the human body which at birth have acquired their final size and shape. But at that time, mastoid cells have not yet been formed. This seems self-evident if one considers that the mastoid process which includes these cells in the adult is not yet present in the fetus. The mastoid cells may be observed in isolated cases 6 months or even earlier postpartum. Complete pneumatization of the mastoid process is usually demonstrated only towards the end of the 5th to 6th year of life *(Schillinger).*

Complete symmetry of structure of the two mastoid processes can almost never be found. Pneumatization of the petrous bone begins after the 3rd year of life and may proceed until the most advanced age. Even with completely normal pneumatization of the mastoid process, cell formation within the whole petrous part is not usual.

Pathological changes are best recognized on comparable exposures, according to the method of *Schüller* and *Sonnenkalb* (Figs. 936, 937). Bilateral processes may make interpretation more difficult, as usually one can only draw conclusions from the difference between the two sides.

The external acoustic meatus is preformed at first as a bony ring, the tympanic ring (Figs. 940, 941), above the tympanic cavity, and only later grows in a lateral direction, whereby fusion between temporal bone and squamous part will take place. In the newborn, the position of the tympanic membrane is more horizontal than in the adult. Roof and floor of the medial part of the acoustic canal therefore still lie very near to each other, and the anterior and posterior walls are still absent. On lateral view, the tympanic ring appears in the newborn more or less below the occiput.

Radiographic presentation of the mastoid antrum:

Rossmann described a simple technique for a better method of projection of the small and difficult-to-recognize antrum of the newborn. The infant is placed prone, with the head turned to the side, with the pinna of the ear to be examined turned forward and upward and taped to the skin of the forehead. The thus-produced "tip of the ear" lies one finger's breadth from the upper edge of the cassette; the posterior edge of the turned-over pinna touches the middle line of the cassette. With a tube inclined craniocaudally by 15°, the pneumatic system is projected into the center of the film (see Figs. 129 and 130).

(Continue on page 412).

Figs. 897-902 (from *W. Meyer*).

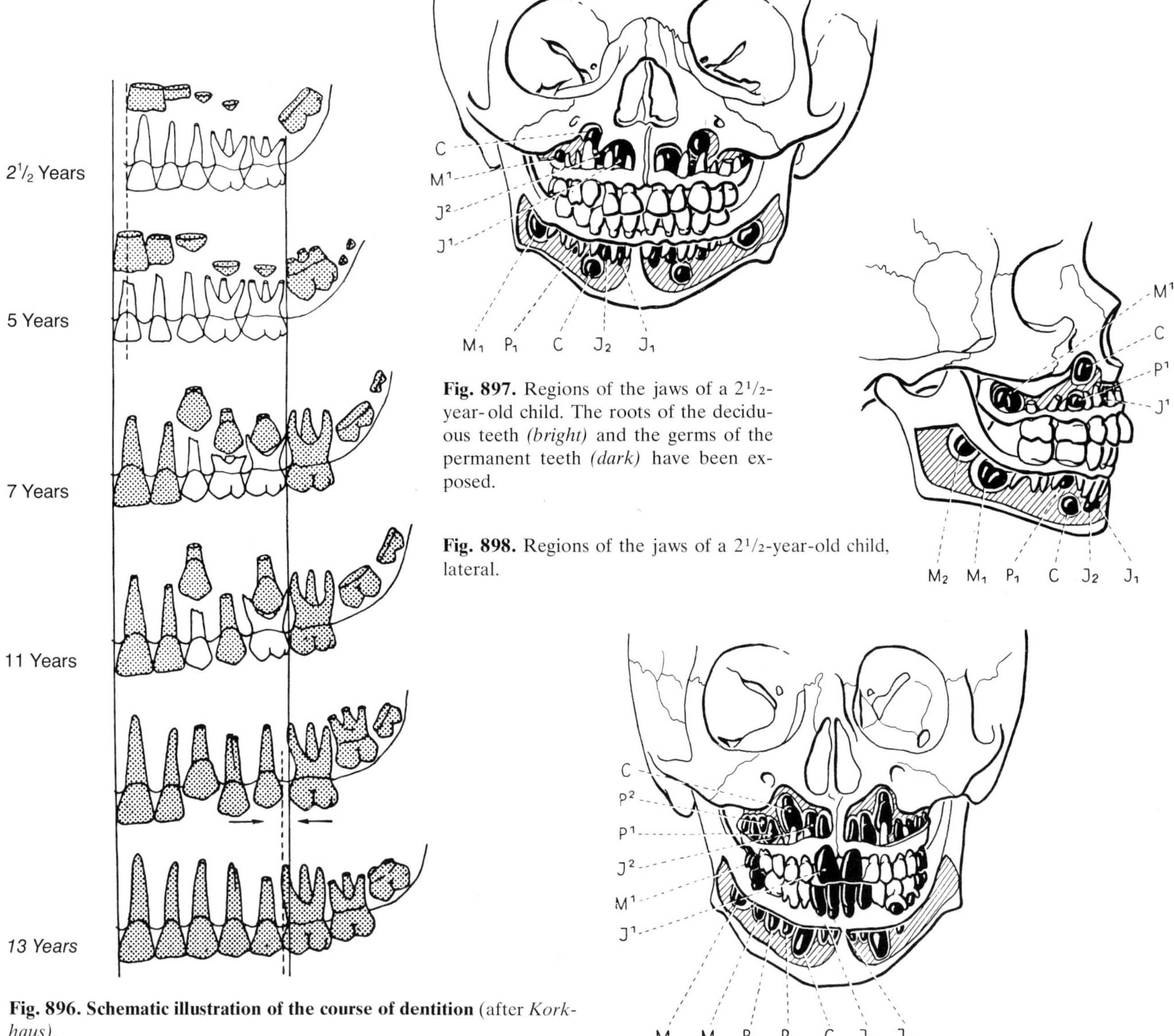

Fig. 896. Schematic illustration of the course of dentition (after *Korkhaus)*.

Fig. 897. Regions of the jaws of a 2½-year-old child. The roots of the deciduous teeth *(bright)* and the germs of the permanent teeth *(dark)* have been exposed.

Fig. 898. Regions of the jaws of a 2½-year-old child, lateral.

Fig. 899. Regions of the jaws of an 8-year-old child. Deciduous teeth shown *bright*, permanent teeth *dark*.

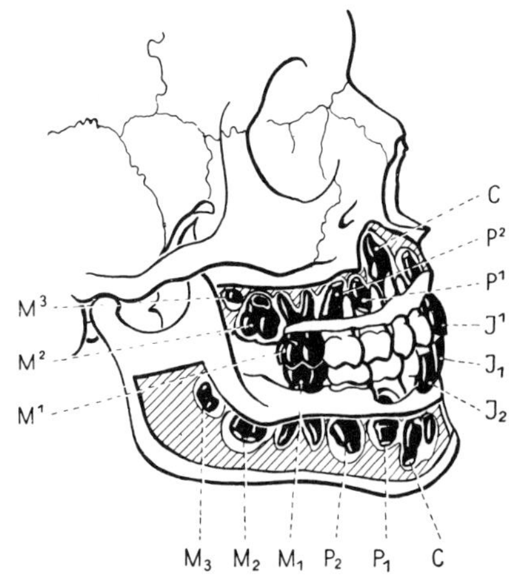

Fig. 900. Regions of the jaws of an 8-year-old child, lateral.

		Eruption of deciduous teeth	Order of appearance
i	1	6th–8th month	1
i	2	8th–12th month	2
c		15th–20th month	4
m	1	12th–16th month	3
m	2	20th–40th month	5

		Eruption of permanent teeth	Order of appearance
I	1	6th– 9th year	2
I	2	7th–10th year	3
C		9th–14th year	6
P	1	9th–13th year	4
P	2	11th–14th year	5
M	1	6th– 8th year	1
M	2	10th–14th year	7
M	3	16th–30th year	8

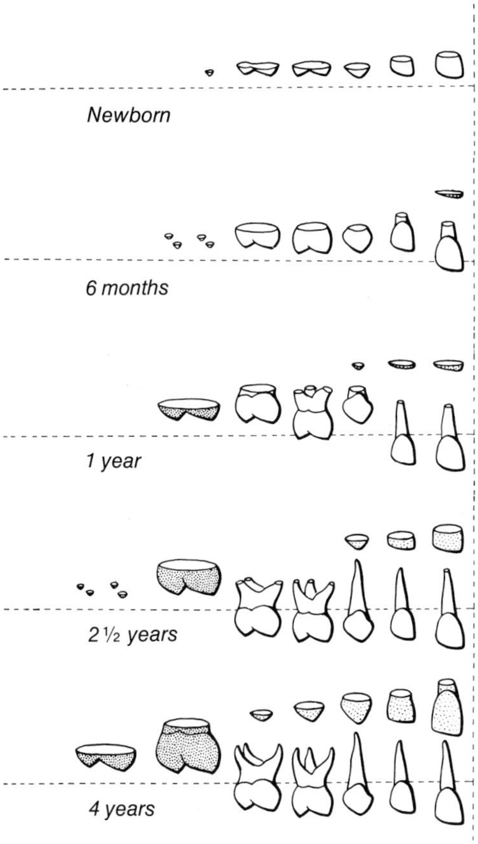

Fig. 901. Schematic illustration of the course of dentition of the deciduous teeth (from *W. Meyer*).

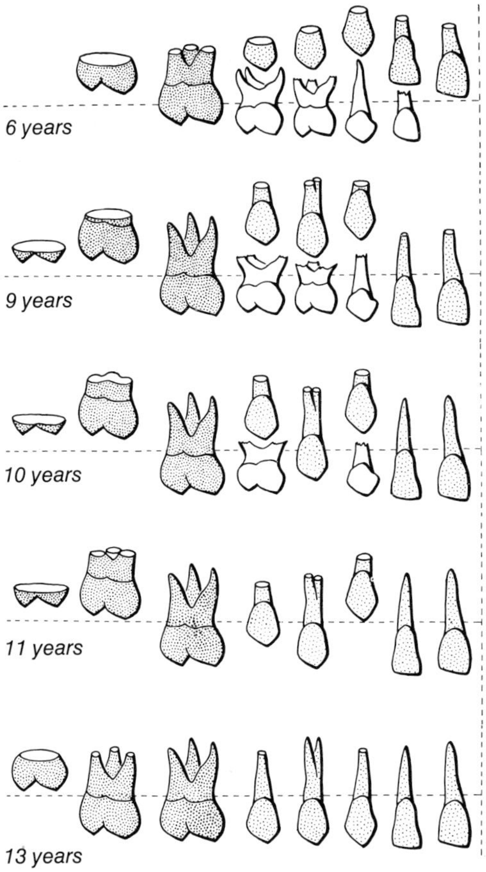

Fig. 902. Schematic illustration of the course of dentition of the permanent teeth (from *W. Meyer*).

Teeth white = deciduous teeth.
Teeth dotted = permanent teeth, of which 6–8 are dotted more densely as they are embryologically deciduous.

Fig. 903. Fetus which died towards the end of pregnancy, with *Spalding*'s sign and hyperextended spine.

1 Positive *Spalding*'s sign, with roof-tile-like overlapping of the parietal bone over the occipital squama ▷
2 Overextended section of the cervical spine
3 Humerus
4 Ulna and radius
5 Femur
6 Tibia with fibula
7 Calcified mesenteric lymph nodes
8 Articular space of hip joint
9 Sacroiliac articulation

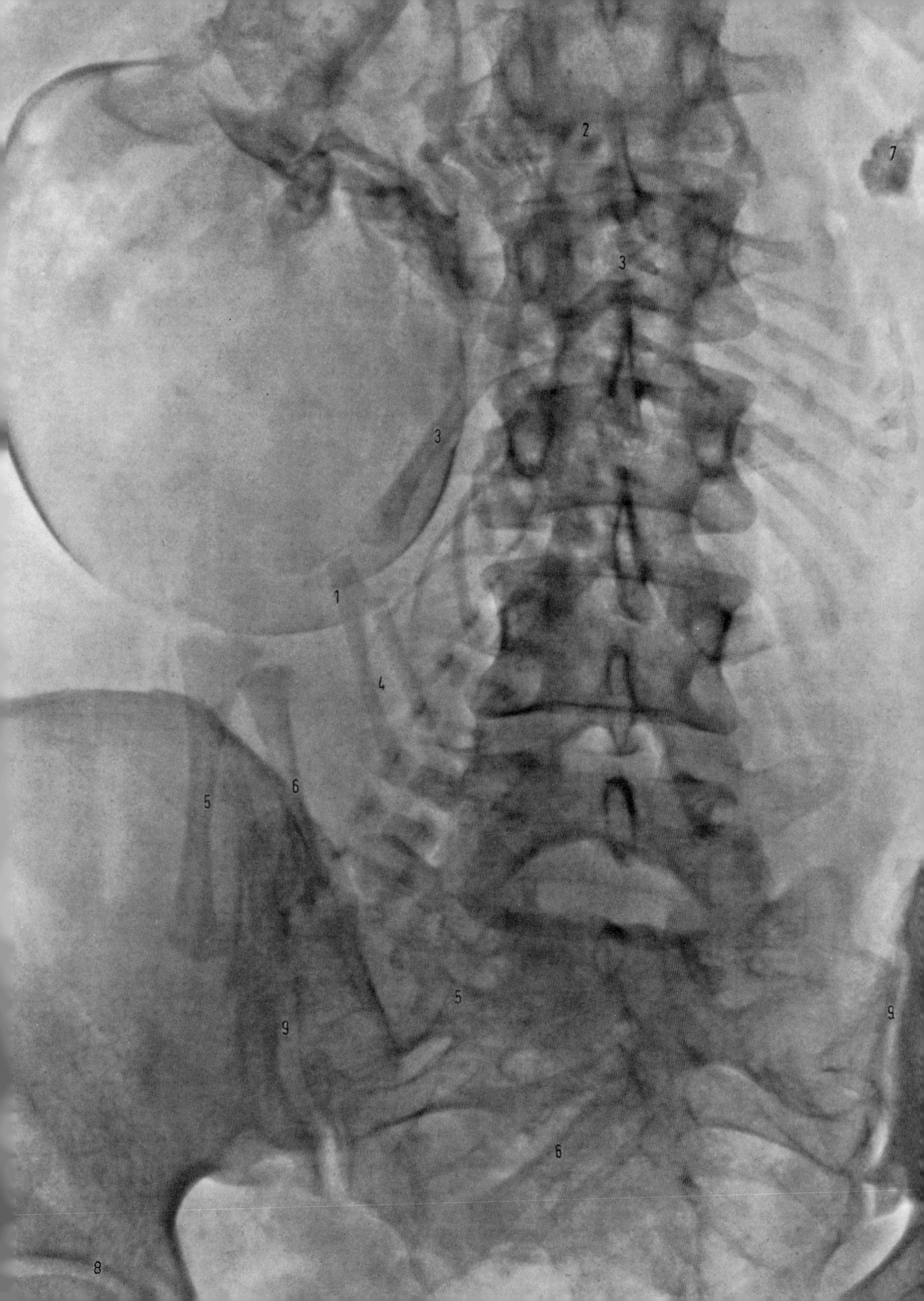
2
7
3
3
1
4
6
5
5
9
9
6
8

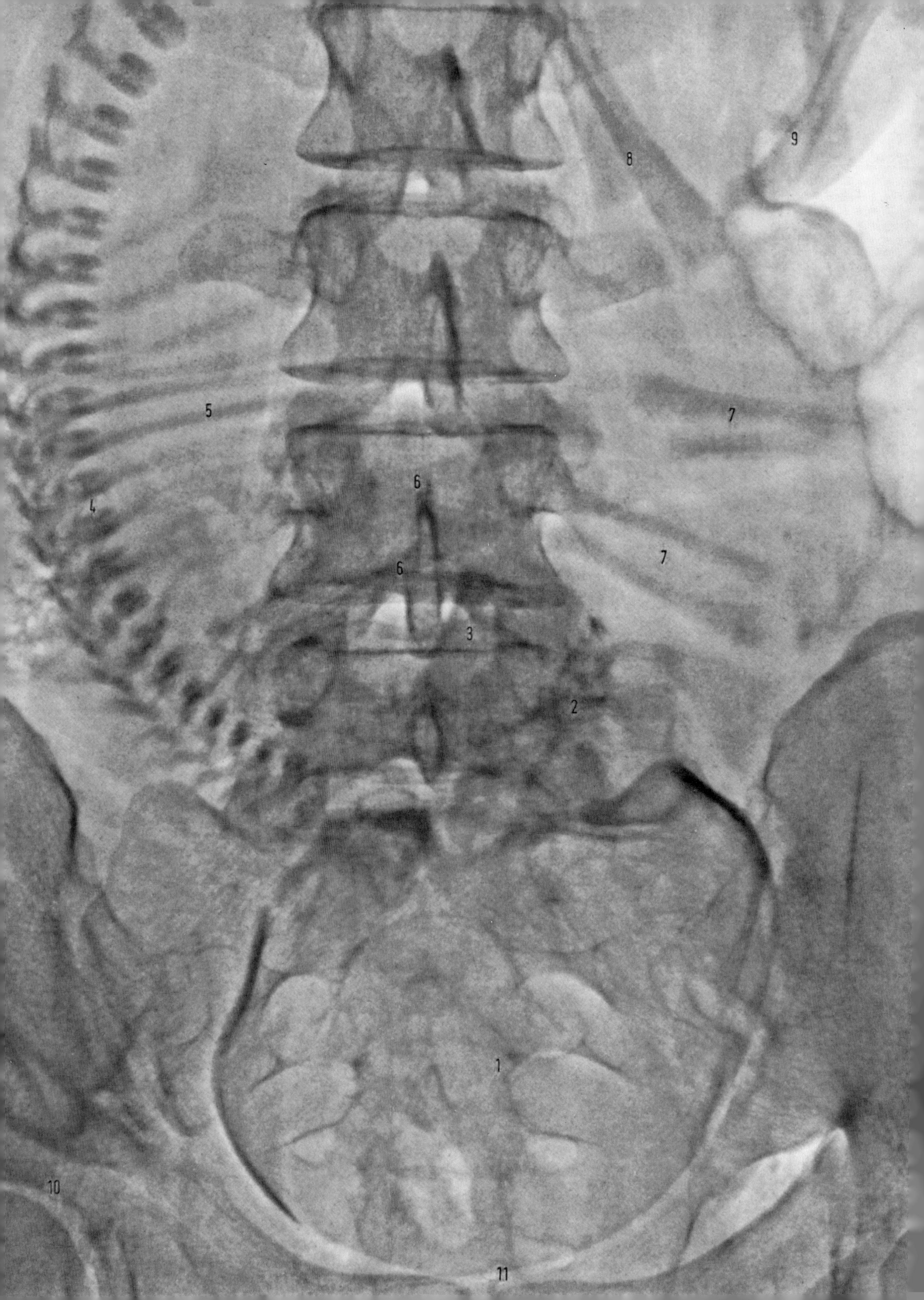
9
8
7
5
6
4
7
6
3
2
1
10
11

A Series of Radiographs of the Development of the Paranasal Sinuses and the Maxilla Denture from Infancy to Age 20

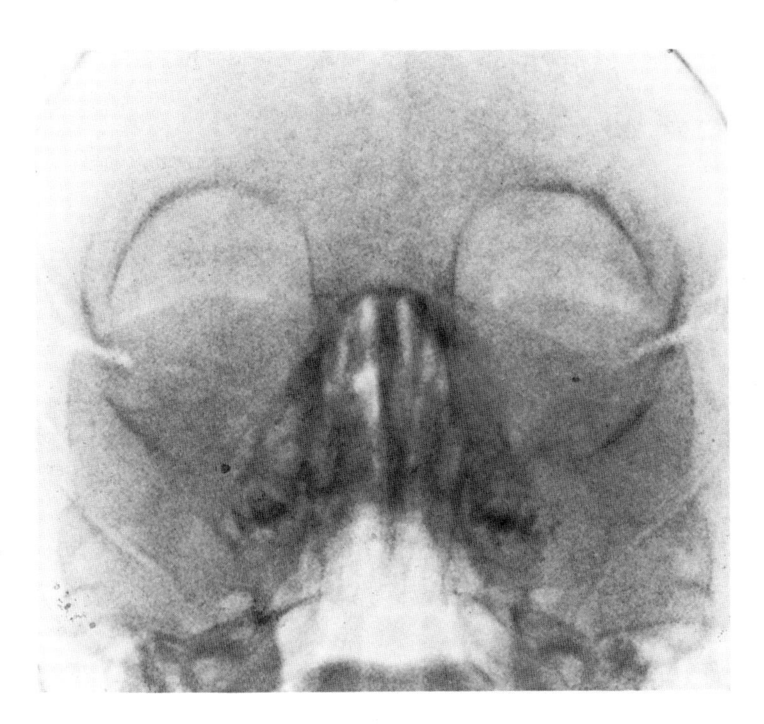

Fig. 905. 5 month old. The paranasal sinuses are not yet noticeable. A broad span of development. The frontal sinuses are arranged like a recess, but it is only between the 4th and 12th years of life that they may be regularly observed in radiographs.

◀ **Fig. 904. A living fetus with a low-standing cranium in the right occiput position.**

1 Cranium
2 Maxilla with discernible dental arrangements
3 Mandible
4 Spinal column with typical horizontal lighter lines in the vertebral bodies. Disk ligament height similar to vertebral height.
5 Ribs
6 Humerus
7 Ulna and radius
8 Femur
9 Tibia with fibula
10 Coxa articulation
11 Pubic symphysis

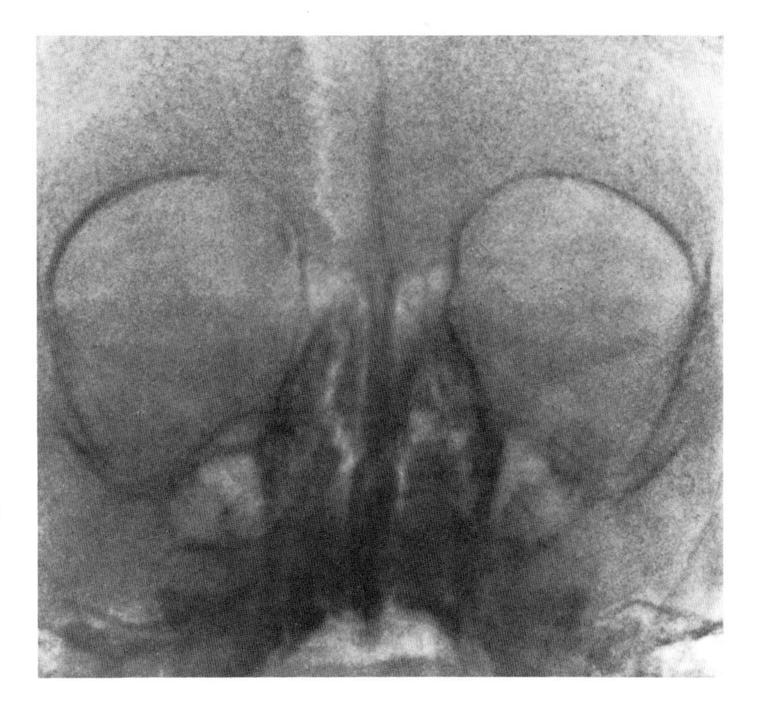

Fig. 906. 2 year old. Here is the beginning of pneumatization in the region of the maxillar sinuses. The frontal sinuses are not yet set. By tilting right paramedially, the frontal suture to the apparently lower continuation through an interconchal light cleft is traceable. It should be noted that during development the extension of the pneumatization is not always identical to the osseous rims of the said sinuses. A non-pneumatic "shaded" sinus therefore should not necessarily be regarded as pathological.

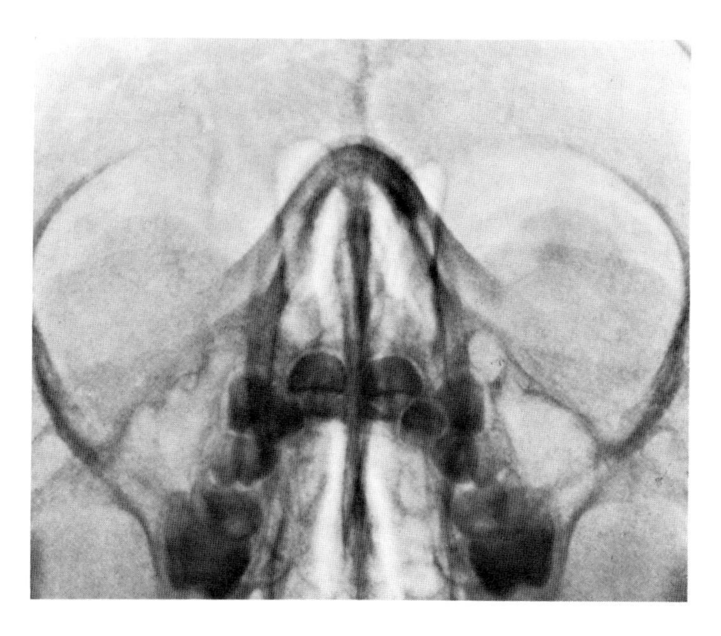

Fig. 907. $4^1/_2$ year old. Both maxillary sinuses are already clearly developed and almost completely pneumatic. The frontal sinus arrangements are discernible as well. In the region of the frontal teeth, above the deciduous teeth, the development of the permanent teeth can be seen. There is an asymmetric form of the maxillary sinuses with a cystic vesicular separate chamber in the superior medial left angle.

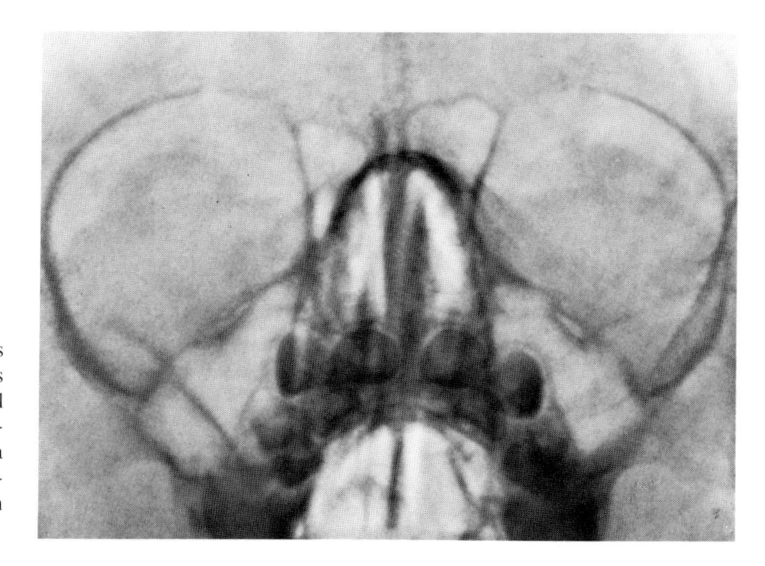

Fig. 908. $5^1/_4$ year old. Besides the maxillary sinuses, there is also a growth of the frontal sinuses. Now, as in Fig. 907, there is already an asymmetric growth in the development of the frontal sinuses. This may be seen very often in adults, too. Most frequently, the right frontal sinus is underdeveloped. In the maxilla denture a resorption of the roots of the deciduous teeth is beginning because of the development of the permanent teeth, which are crowding out the former.

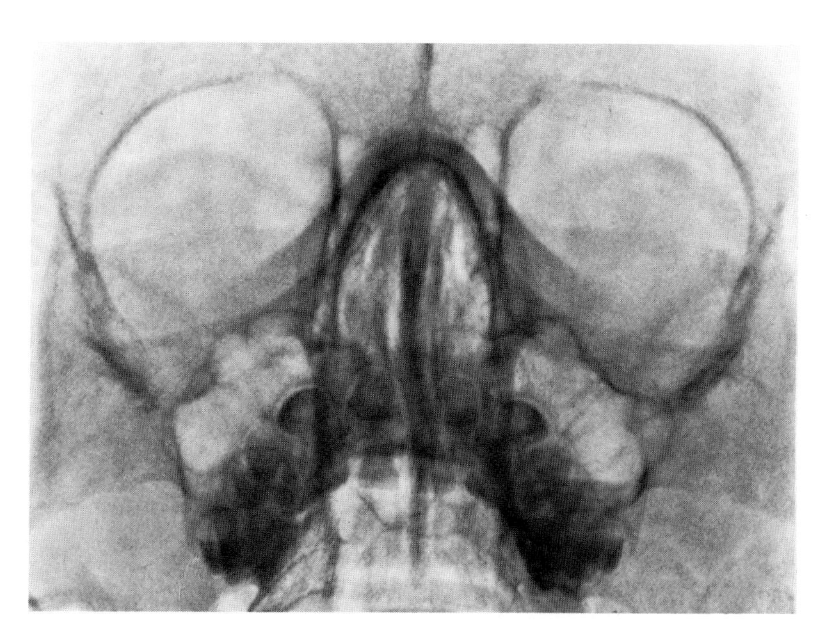

Fig. 909. 6 year old. Whereas, the maxillary sinuses are relatively well developed, the development of the frontal sinuses with respect to the width variation is rather retarded. The arrangement of the permanent teeth causes the base of the maxillary sinuses to curve.The sinuses themselves are frequently infected.

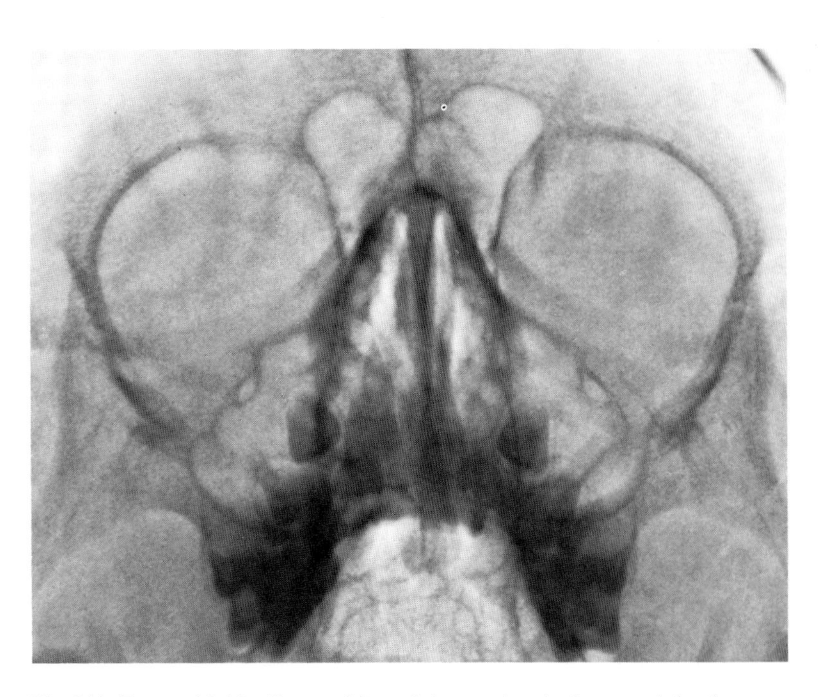

Fig. 910. 7 year old. Maxillary and frontal sinuses already show good development. Large infraorbital recesses. However, to the right there is an incomplete development of the alveolar inlet, which is filled with spongiosa. The progressive substitution of the deciduous teeth by the permanent teeth is very clear, especially in the area of the incisors. Only in the 2nd incisors are there still milk teeth residues, whereas the 1st is already completely substituted.

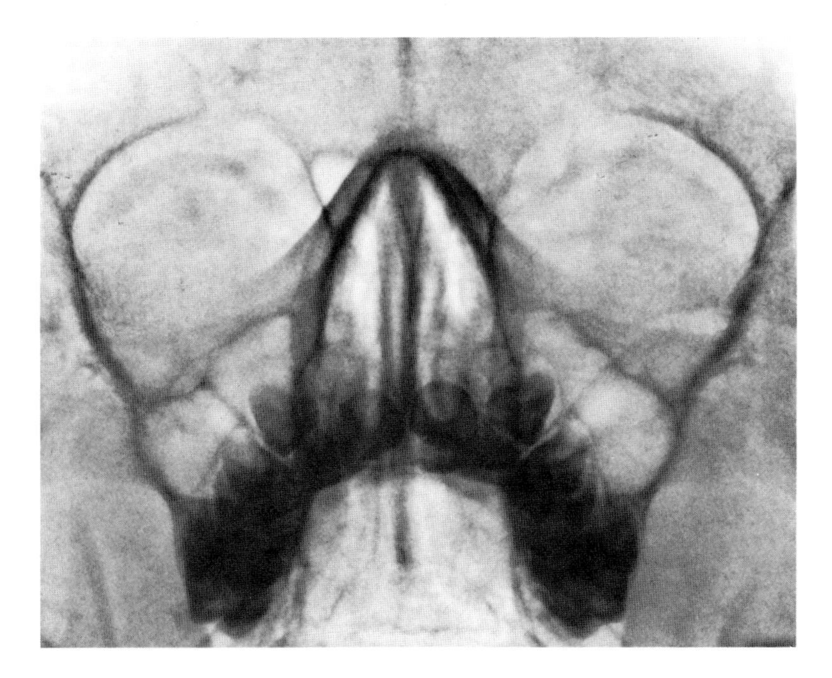

Fig. 911. 8 year old. Asymmetric, underdeveloped frontal sinuses, only slightly indicated on the left. The right maxilla is septic; the recess alveolar is still filled with spongiosa. The shading to the right due to the narrow sinus depth is simulated. Here, residues of the milk denture can still be seen in the region of the front teeth, while the molars of the milk denture are still present. The 1st molar of the remaining denture, which genetically is a milk tooth, is already noticeable.

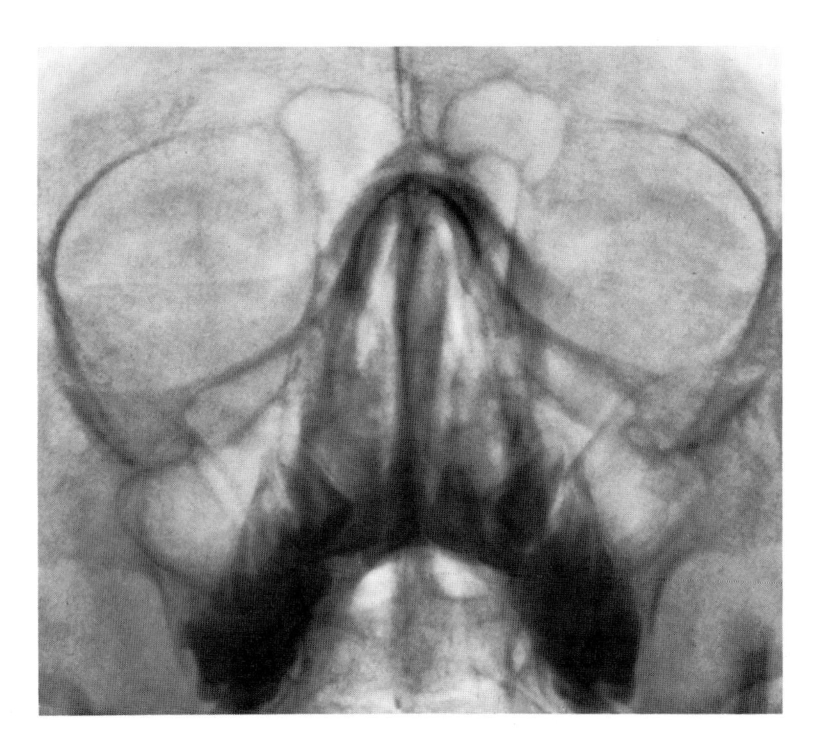

Fig. 912. 12 year old. Besides the maxillary and frontal sinuses, the ethmoidal cells are noticeable as well. Left: arrangement of a dilated pneumosinus of the orbital ethmoidal cells. The milk denture is now completely substituted by the permanent teeth; only the canine has not grown in completely in the inlet of the corresponding milk tooth.

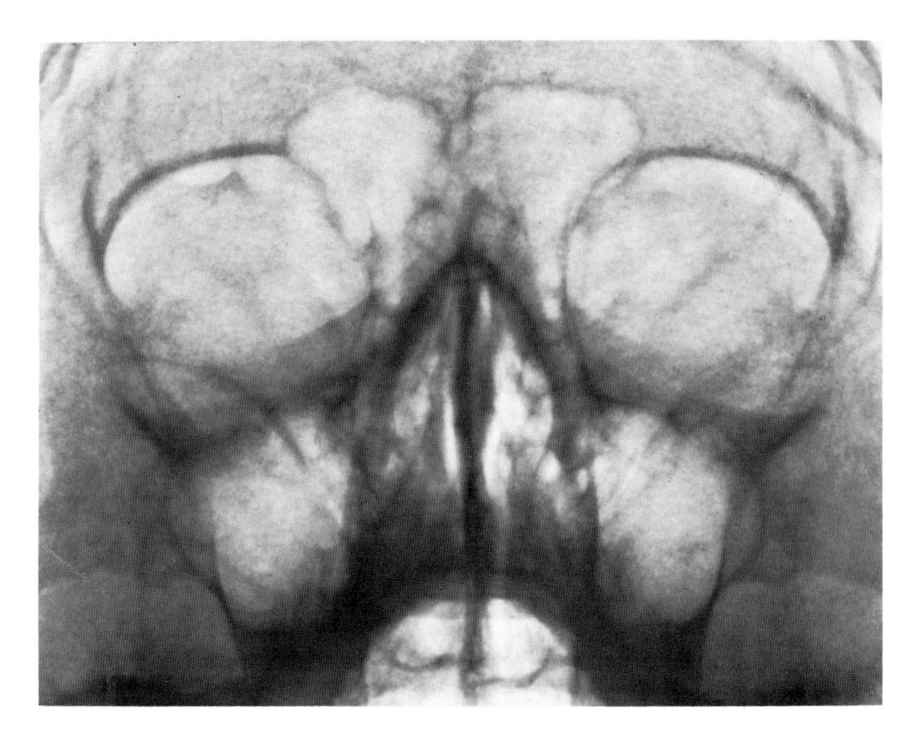

Fig. 913. 14 year old. All paranasal sinuses are well formed. Dense, horizontal terminating base; shading of the alveolar recess on both sides. An infectious secretion. The deciduous teeth are completely substituted by the permanent teeth.

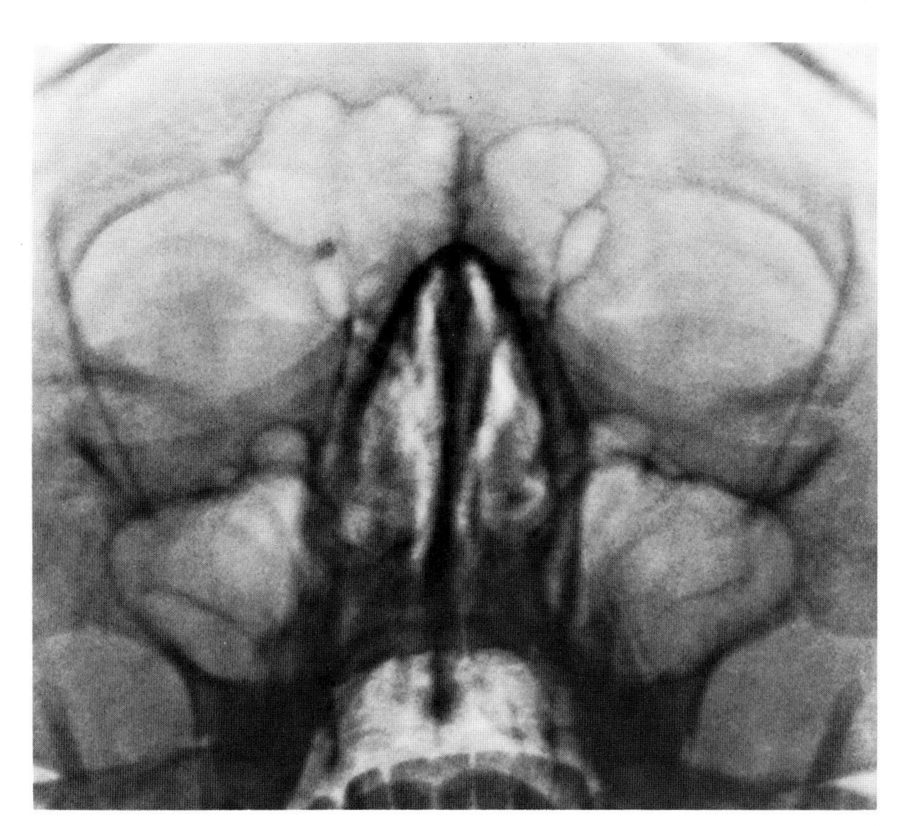

Fig. 914. 16 year old. The extending growth of the paranasal sinuses has proceeded. The frontal sinuses, here too, are distinguished by size and are, as usual, asymmetrically arranged.

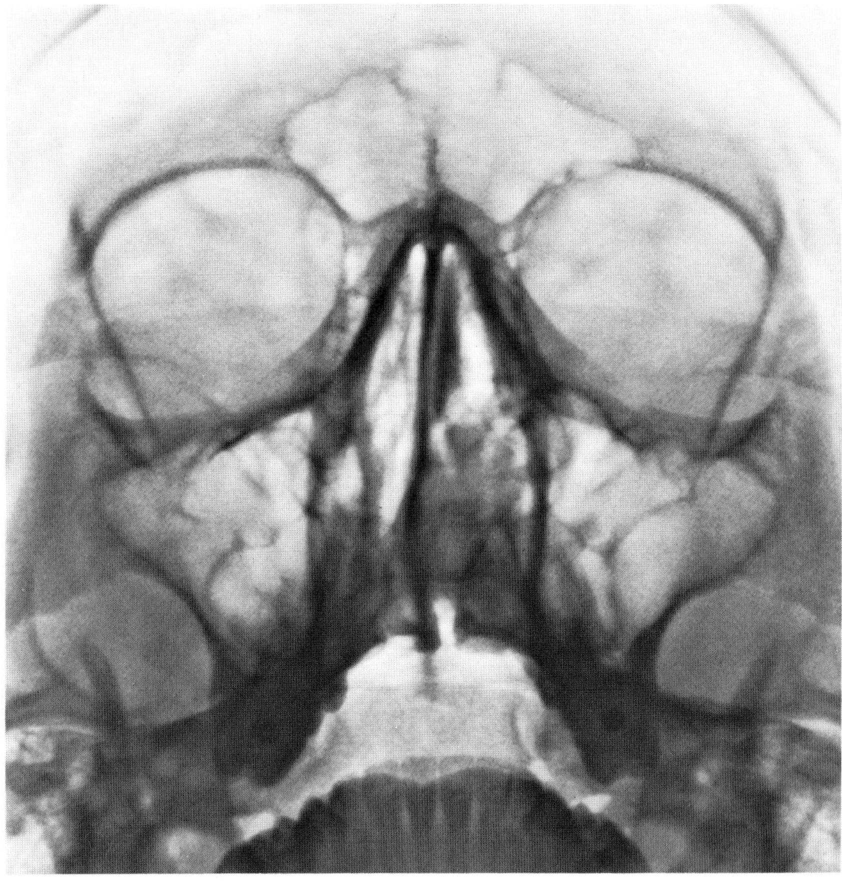

Fig. 915. 18 year old. Almost all nasal sinuses are well formed, symmetrical and have good pneumatization. Only in the region of the frontal sinuses is it possible to see a lesser asymmetry in development, which may progress so far that it causes formation of the frontal sinus on one side only. When the completely formed frontal sinus meets the other frontal sinuses, a one-sided aplasia of the frontal sinus may be ignored. The absence of the osseous septum shows the error immediately.

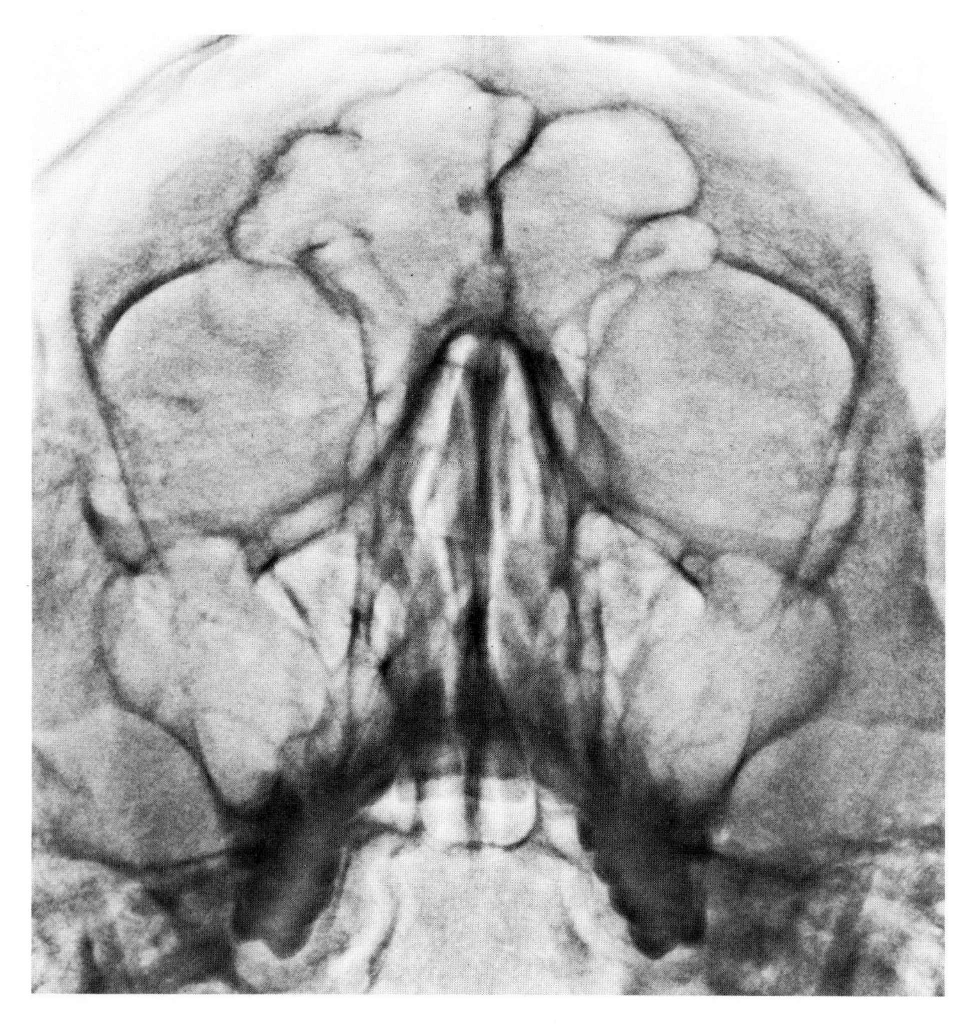

Fig. 916. 20 year old. Near the well-formed paranasal sinuses, it is possible to recognize the ethmoidal cells up to the orbit's vault. In extreme cases, a complete pneumatization of the orbital vault thus occurs, and in a dilated pneumosinus of the rear ethmoidal cells (Figs. 55, 56, 271 and 272). In such cases, a frontal picture explains the extension of the pneumatization.

After a control process of both sides, such a dilated pneumosinus is found. It is associated with septicity of the very large sinus.

The causes of the dilated sinuses have not been thoroughly researched. It may be related in part to hemiatrophic hypoplastic brain processes following brain damage during infancy, e.g., after meningoencephalitis *(Weickmann)*. The concurrence of dilated pneumosinuses and meningeoma is also unclear. Similarly, according to *Psenner,* the cause of the partial dilatation of the pneumosinus of the parasinus is unclear, e.g., an ethmoidal cell (see also Fig. 271).

In the usual hypoplasia of the paranasal sinuses, it is very often possible to note a catarrhal infection. This is related to a certain "mucous membrane weakness." The same observation can be made in the regions of the middle ear and the papillary process (see Figs. 131 and 132).

A Series of Radiographs of the Development of the Sella Turcica and the Sphenoidal Sinus from Infancy to Age 17

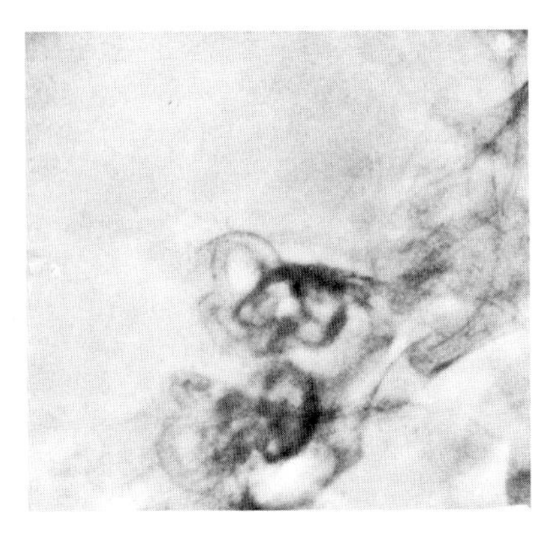

Fig. 917. 3 month old. The sella turcica is projected forward somewhat; therefore, it is easy to see the inner ear on both sides, especially the arcades, vestibule and cochlea, as well as the annulus tympanicus (cf. Figs. 129, 130, 940 and 941). Here, there is not yet pneumatization in the temporal bone, which can be proven and, according to *Rossmann,* is usually expected during the 3rd month of life.

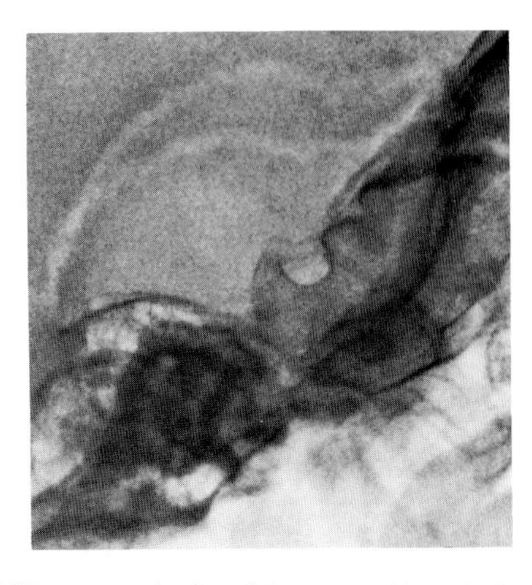

Fig. 918. 5 month old. The pneumatization of the temporal bone is already well developed. The sphenoidal sinuses are not yet established. The sutures are still present as relatively wide fissures.

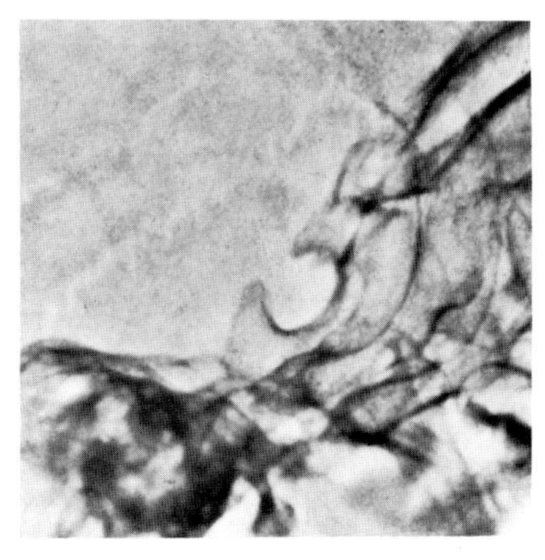

Fig. 919. 9 month old. The sella turcica has increased in size; it grows very quickly during the 1st year of life. Seen only from the scattered lateral radiograph, it is therefore not certain that it indicates a pathological sella growth because it may appear long and narrow as well as short and wide. The sella volume in both cases is within normal limits.

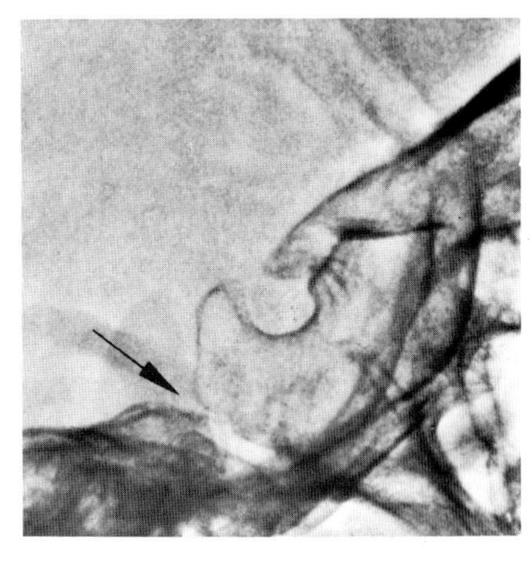

Fig. 920. 2 year old. The spheno-occipital synchondrosis (↘) is recognized here, as in Figs. 921, 923, 925, especially well as an oblique, lighter stripe behind the dorsum sella in the clivus. Its ossification takes place between the 16th and 18th years of life.

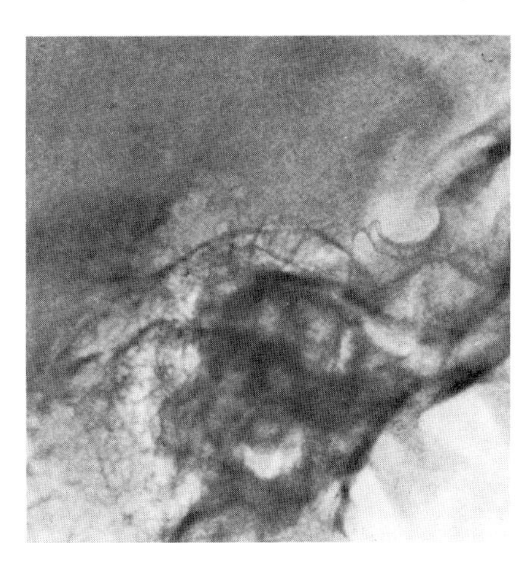

Fig. 921. 3 year old. As a secondary finding, the already well-advanced pneumatization of the papillary process region is seen. An arrangement of the sphenoidal sinuses does not yet show in radiographs, though it may already be seen in the 3rd year of life (see also Fig. 169).

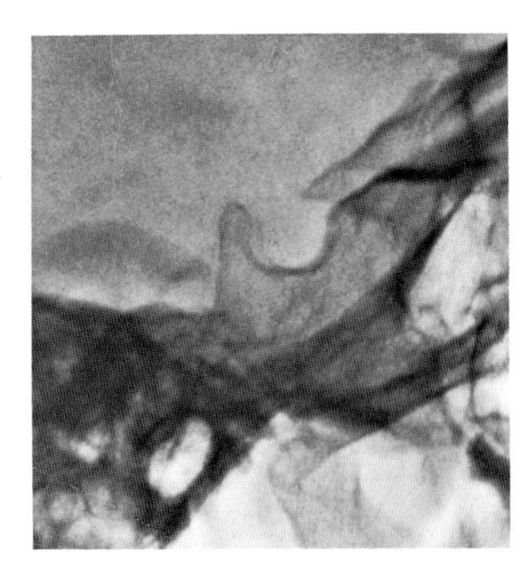

Fig. 922. 6 year old. The sphenoid begins to pneumatize from the front. The width variation, however, is extremely great since the pneumatization of this bone differs individually.

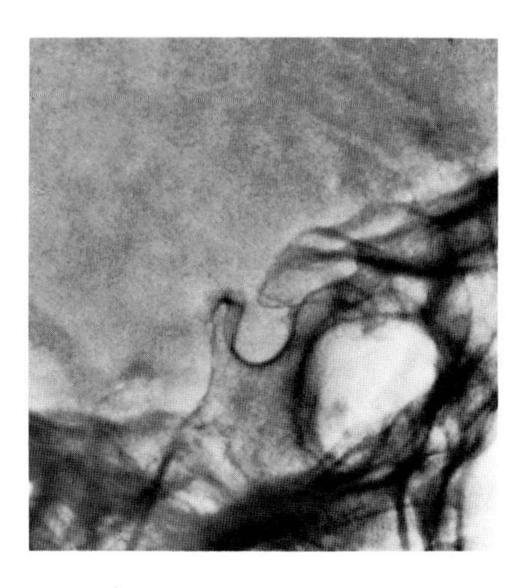

Fig. 923. 7 year old. The sphenoidal sinuses are already well formed. In many cases the pneumatization remains in this phase of development, or it may progress and lead to the pneumatization of the dorsum sella.

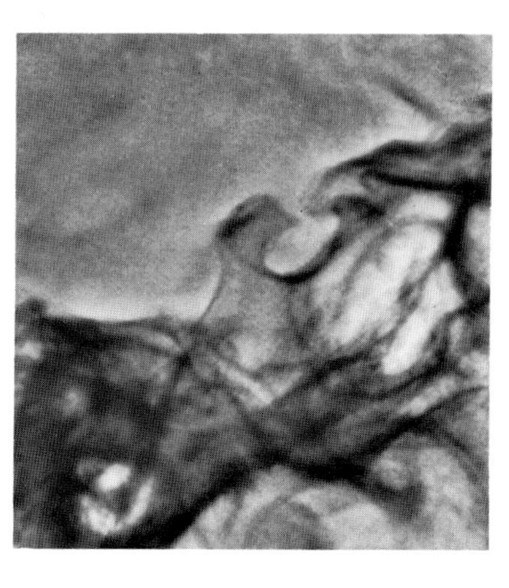

Fig. 924. 9 year old. Simulation of a massive swollen dorsum sella by means of an overturned (verkippt) radiograph in which the clinoid posterior processes project themselves under one another.

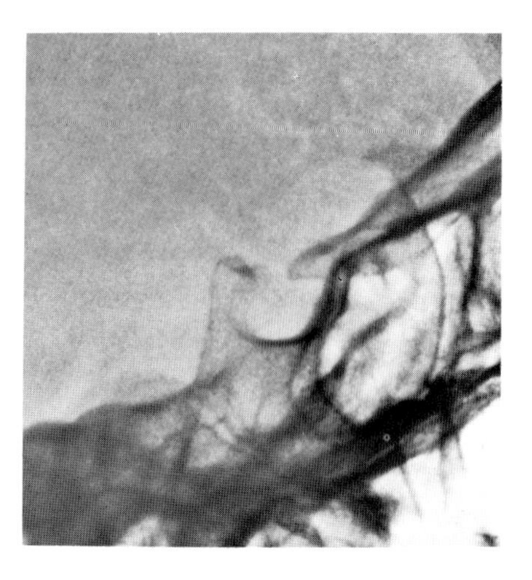

Fig. 925. 10 year old. The profile of the sella turcica has generally reached its final size at this age. Clearly visible spheno-occipital synchondrosis. The ossification of the bones can continue up to the 21st year of life.

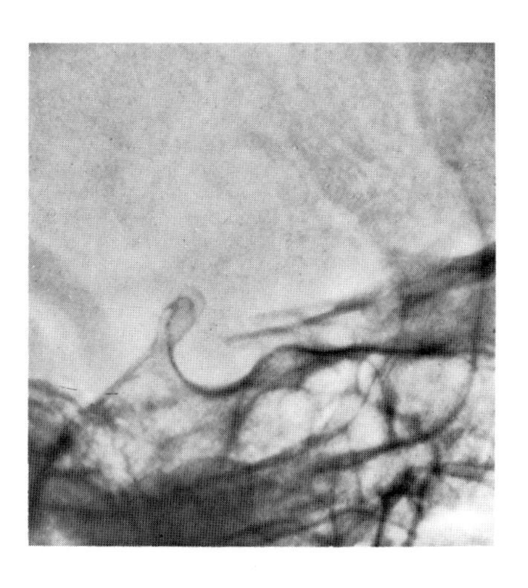

Fig. 926. 12 year old. No substantial increase in size takes place in the following years of development, except for individual variations. Remarkably deep-rooted sphenoidal planum in a case of small sphenoidal sinus (see also Fig. 162).

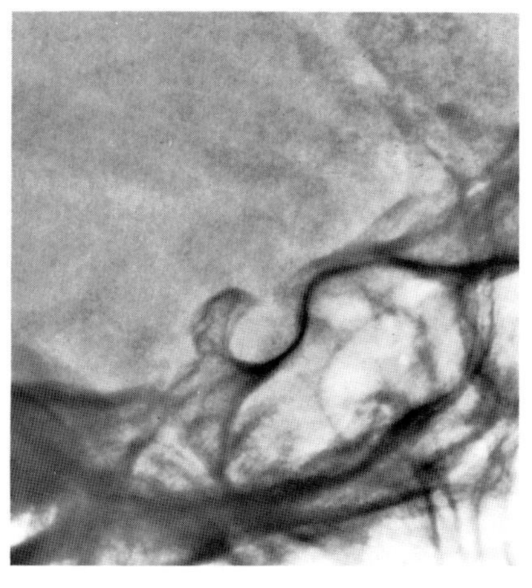

Fig. 927. 14 year old. The formation of the sphenoidal sinuses is well advanced. Their size development depends on genetic factors; total absence is not necessarily pathological.

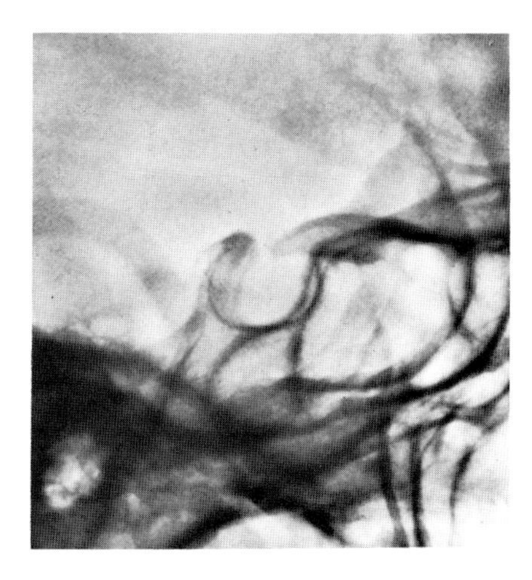

Fig. 928. 17 year old. Through the large extension in depth of the sphenoidal sinuses, the entire base of the sella is pneumatized. This is one reason for the high position of the sphenoidal planum (see also Fig. 156).

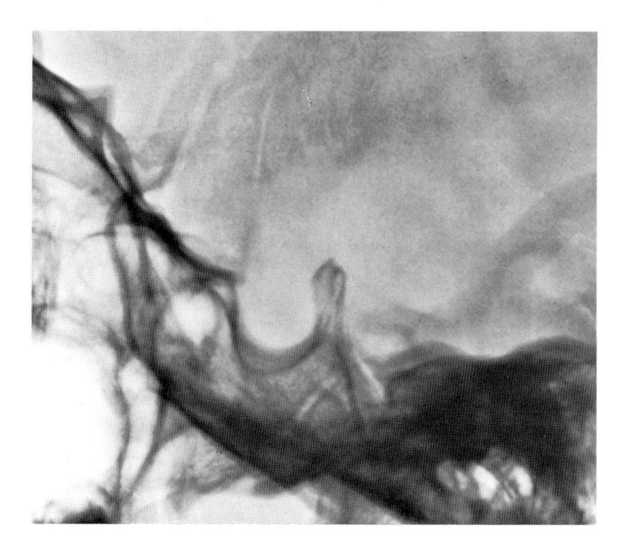

Fig. 929. Form of the sella turcica in an 11-year-old girl with turricephalic cranium. Premature termination of the coronal suture; otherwise, no further anomalies. The sella turcica is set remarkably deep and, contrary to pictures of hypophysis tumors, shows no erosion or atrophy. This form of arrangement of the sella is typical for turricephaly, which is not very intensely noticeable in this girl. The spheno-occipital synchondrosis and another one not yet named, sometimes behind the clivus and parallel to the fissures, are open. These, according to *Zimmer,* correspond to the fissure dividing the clivus and the petrous bone apex. Since the lambdoid suture is still visible (Fig. 956), it is possible for this turricephalic cranium to develop in the length axes instead and to bend the occiput.

A Series of Radiographs of the Development of Pneumatization of the Petrous Bone and Papillary Process from Infancy to Age 14

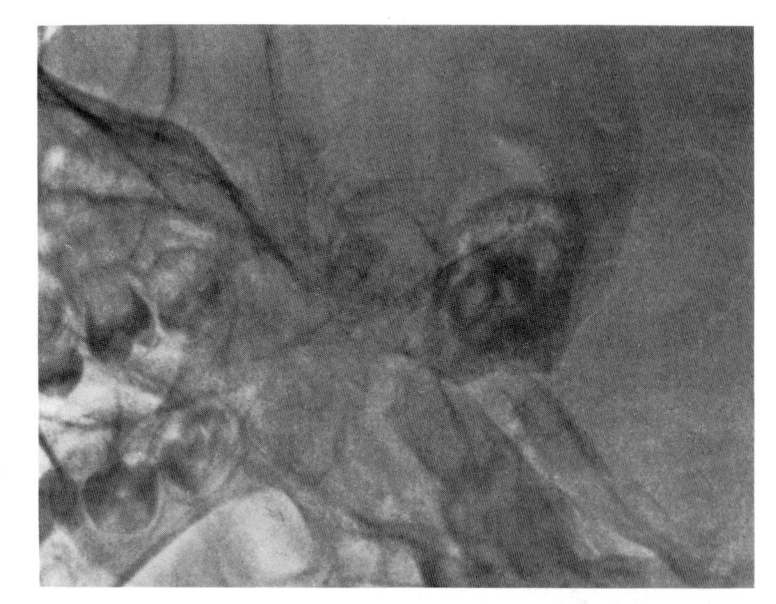

Fig. 930. *Schüller* radiograph, left, **6 month old.** The papillary process is not yet formed. The beginning of pneumatization of the temporal bone, which can set in during the 4th month of life, can already be seen. The temporal bones of healthy children are clearly distinguishable in their arrangement from the point of view of pneumatization. There are all sorts of transitions, from hypo- to hyper- to apneumatization, but in the arrangement and set-up of the cells there are large differences.

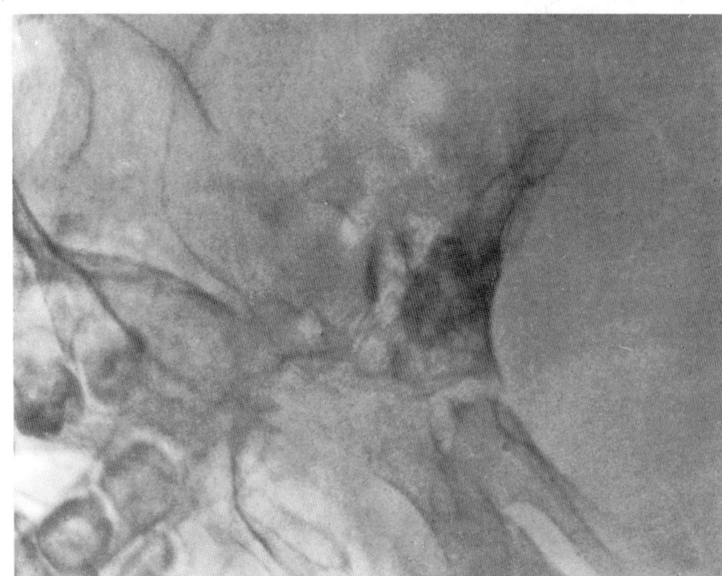

Fig. 931. *Schüller* radiograph, left, **1¾ year old.** Here, there is no pneumatization and large variations in width can be seen. Only from the 5th year of life onwards is it possible to refer to disorders in cases of absence of pneumatization. According to *Mayer,* the normal pneumatization is recognizable as follows:

1. The pneumatic system of the petrous bone from the 5th year of life onwards is well-developed and well-defined with respect to its surroundings.
2. The cells lie well away from the bone because of their uniformly equal air content. They are arranged evenly and are larger in the periphery than in the central regions.
3. The callous cells are delicate; the wall of the peripheral cells of the adjacent bone is slightly thickened, as a cortex of the bone (Kortikalis).

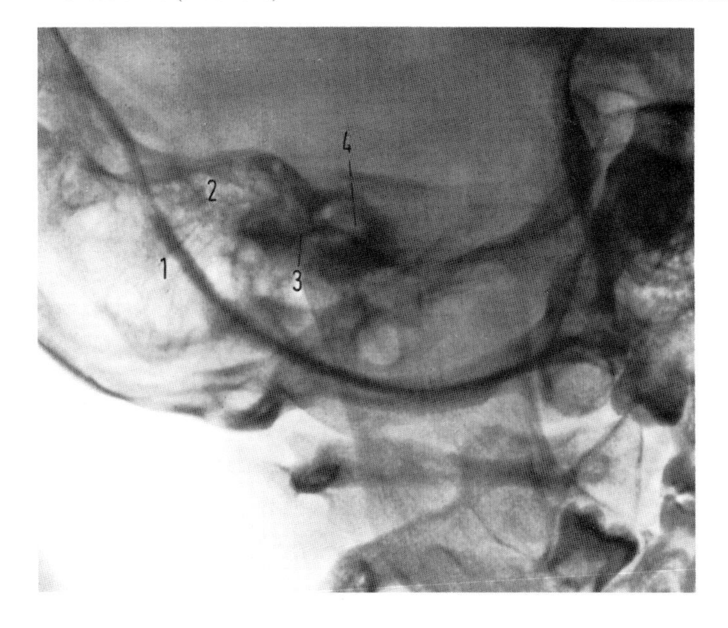

Fig. 932. *Stenvers* radiograph, right, **5 year old.** Here, the pneumatization is already well developed; the papillary process especially is completely pneumatized in contrast to the one in Fig. 933.

1 Mastoid cells
2 Mastoid antrum
3 Vestibule with arcade
4 Cochlea

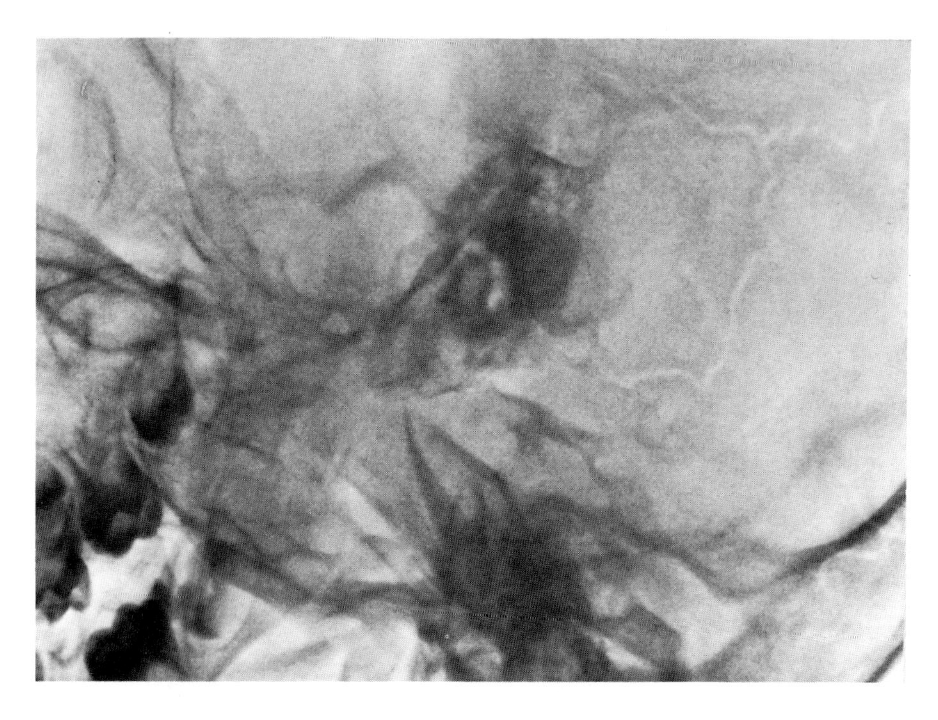

Fig. 933. *Schüller* radiograph, left, **5 year old.** The complete pneumatization of the papillary process can be shown during the 5th year of life and, in many cases, even earlier. In this radiograph, there is not yet pneumatization. Large width variations exist.

According to *Link* and *Handl,* noise damage occurs less frequently in well-pneumatized papillary processes than in cases of arrested pneumatization. The development of a pneumatization arrest or a complete sclerosis should be followed radiographically.

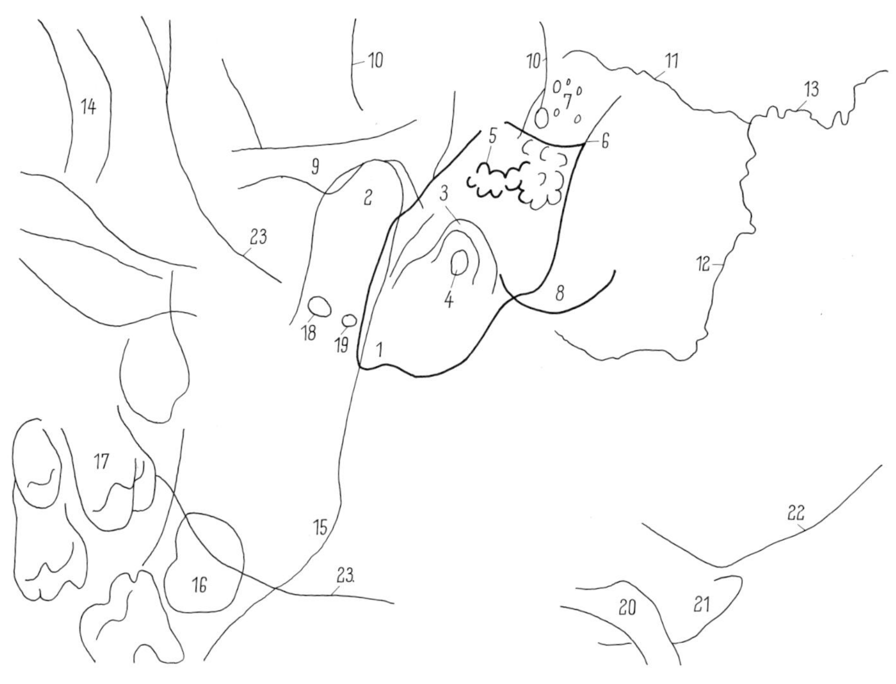

1 Apex of the petrous part
2 Mandible head
3 External auditory canal
4 Internal auditory canal
5 Mastoid antrum
6 Sigmoid sinus
7 Cells in the sinus dura angle
8 Mastoid process
9 Zygomatic arch
10 Ear conch
11 Parietomastoid suture
12 Occipital mastoid suture
13 Lambdoid suture
14 External edge of the adjacent orbit
15 Adjacent jaw angle
16 Adjacent mandible molars
17 Adjacent maxillar molars
18 Oval foramen
20 Dorsal atlas arc
21 Magnum foramen
22 Occipital external crest
23 Middle cranial fossa, limited in upper adjacent part and in lower part film-distant

Fig. 934. Sketch of Fig. 933.

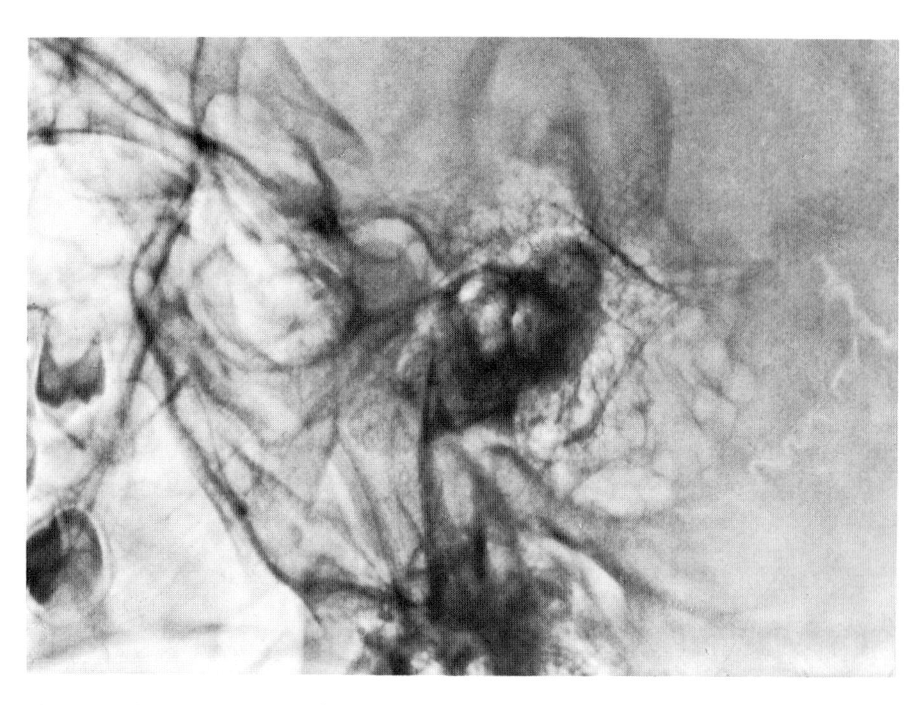

Fig. 935. *Schüller* radiograph, left, **8 year old.** A very dilated pneumatization of the petrous bone. The hyperpneumatization should develop out of a mucous membrane hyperplasia; the inhibition of pneumatization should be connected with a mucous membrane aplasia. In cases of a multiform normally pneumatized system, there are probably many other factors that play an important role in the development of the bones.

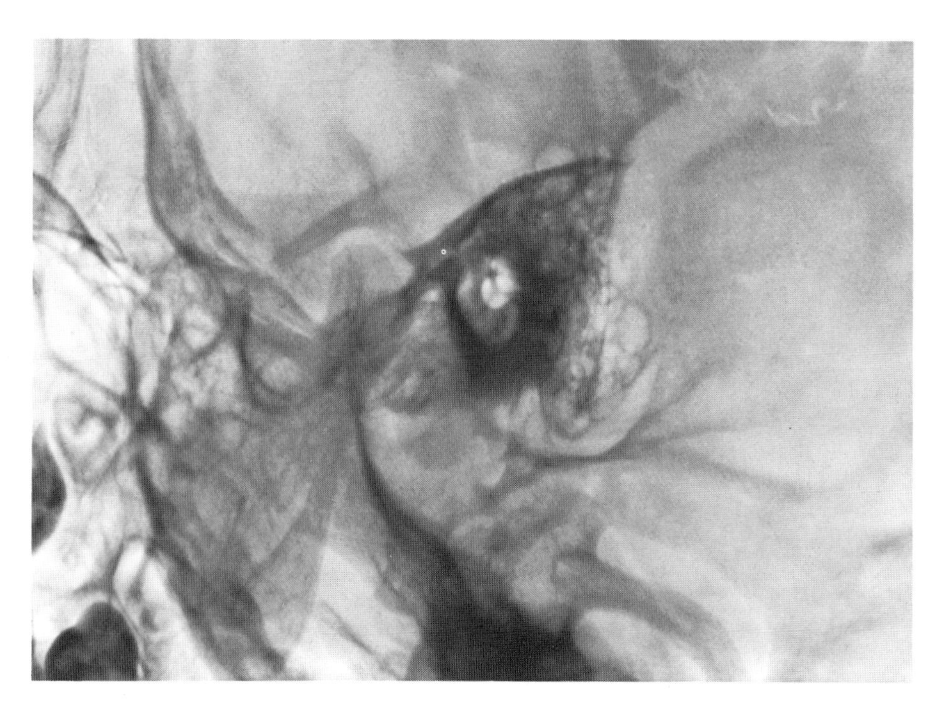

Fig. 936. *Schüller* radiograph, left, **11 year old.** The mastoid cells, as well as the pneumatization in the parietal region are clearly recognizable. According to *Sonnenkalb,* these are seen particularly well in the tangential radiograph of the papillary process (cf. also with Figs. 131, 132). Here, there is a wider sigmoid sinus sulcus with an arched emissary mastoid vein coming out of its lower third to pass through the mastoid foramen, where there is unification with external cranium veins (occipital, postauricular, jugular). The mastoid emissary *(Santorini)* is the largest and most constant of all the numerous and various emissaries.

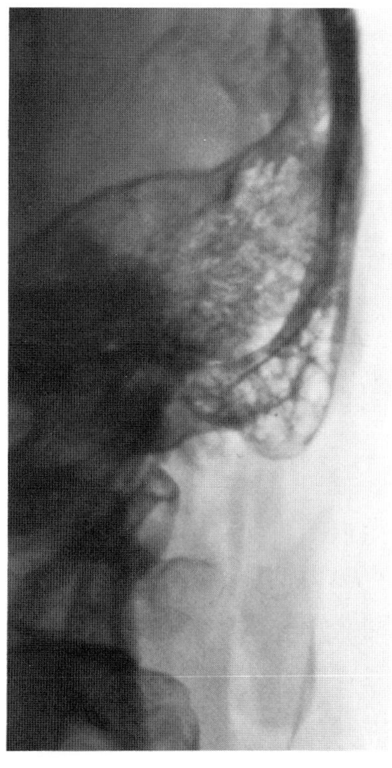

Fig. 937. The same mastoid process according to *Sonnenkalb.*

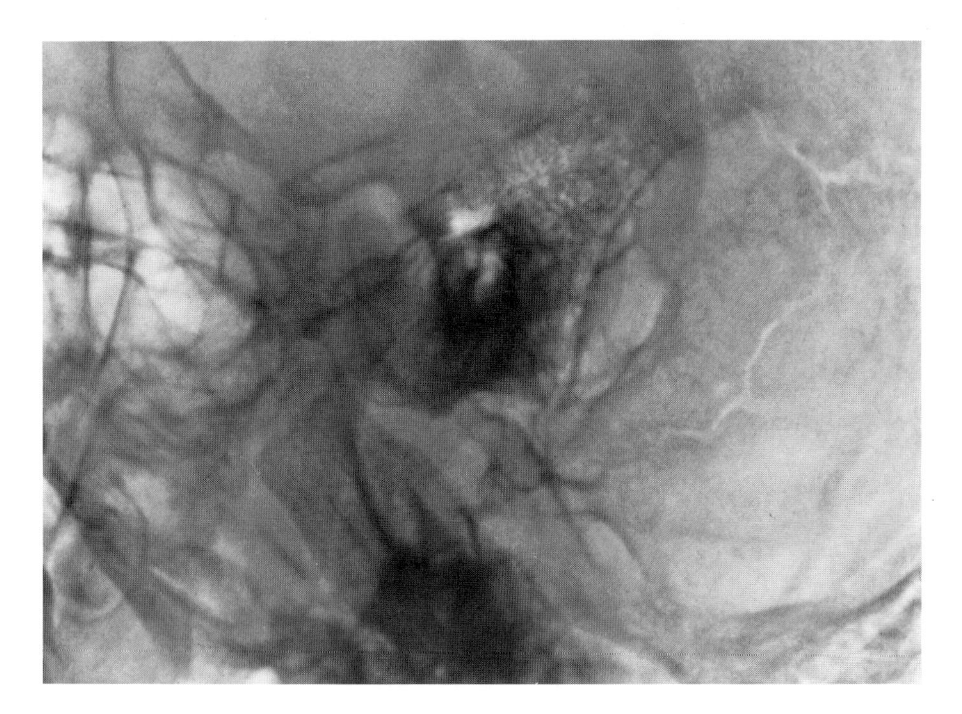

Fig. 938. 12 year old. *Schüller* radiograph, left. Next to a small-vesicle pneumatization, in a projection on the sigmoid sinus, there is a big-vesicle formation which could be considered as an old fusion. In this case, since there is no clinical pathological finding, it is just a large vesicle cell. In children and juveniles, distinguishing between harmless hyperpneumatization and fusion is rather difficult.

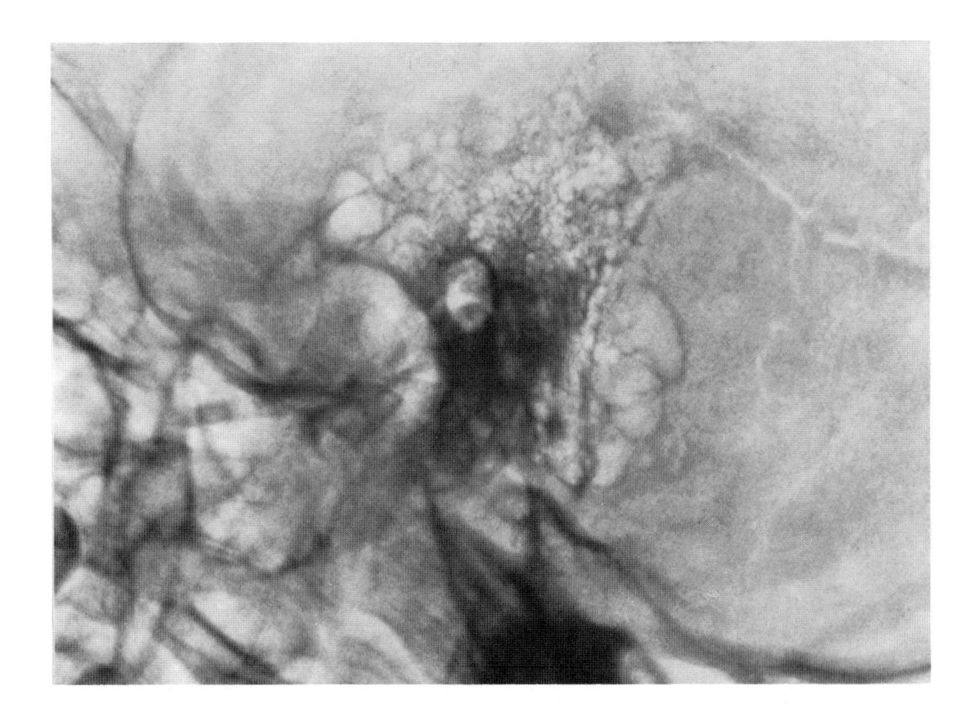

Fig. 939. 14 year old. *Schüller* radiograph, left. In addition to the age differences in Figs. 938 and 939, the difference in the size of the cells of both papillary processes is rather remarkable. The cells shown in Fig. 939 have somewhat large vesicles; here, the pneumatization of the temporal bone is very extended and reaches almost up to the beginning of the zygomatic process (temporal bone). The variability of the system pneumatization is therefore further emphasized since it does not stop throughout the life span. Even in old age, changes such as formation of cells or sclerosis of cells are still possible.

Figs. 940–942. Cranium of a newborn *(from Sobotta-Becher,* 17th Edition).

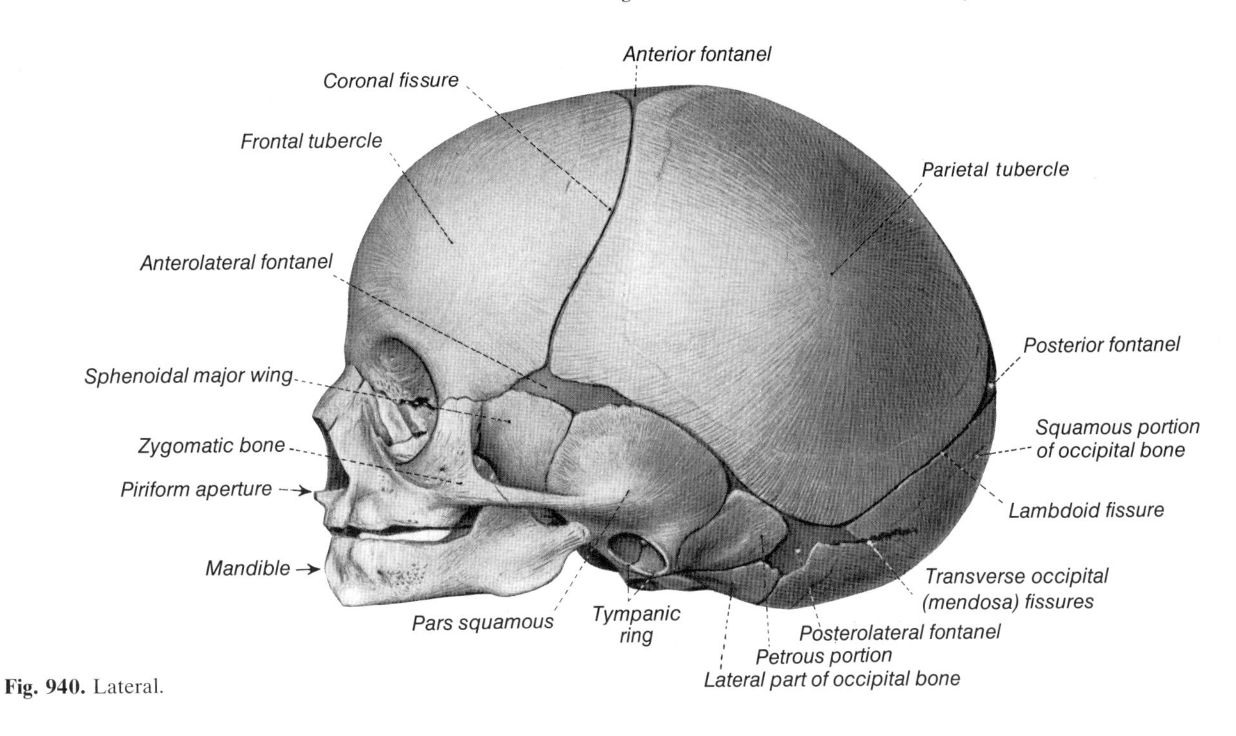

Fig. 940. Lateral.

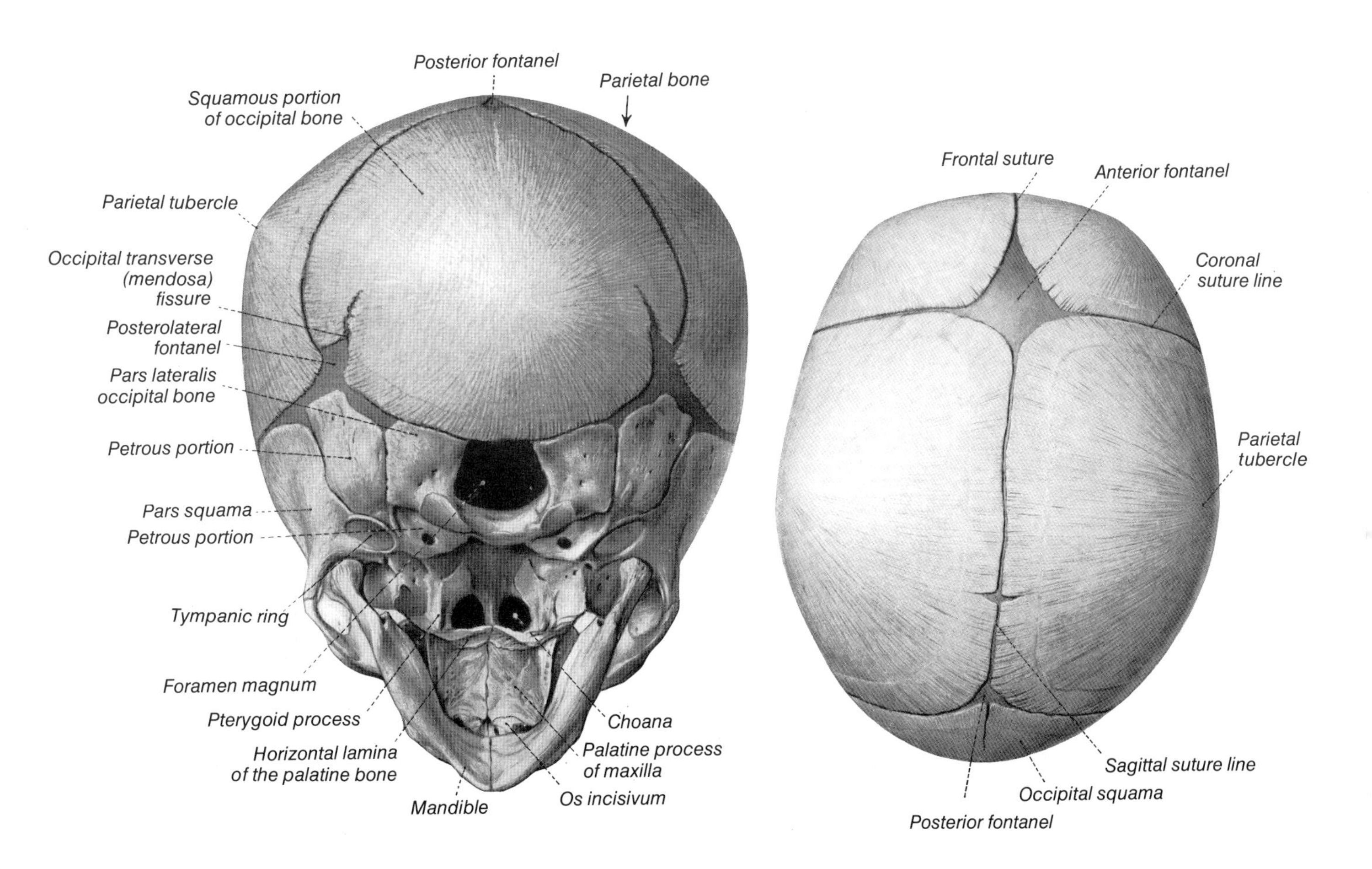

Fig. 941. Dorsal and cranial.

Fig. 942. Cranial.

A Series of Radiographs of the Development of the Skull and Its Sutures, the Digital Impressions and Denture from Infancy to Age 16

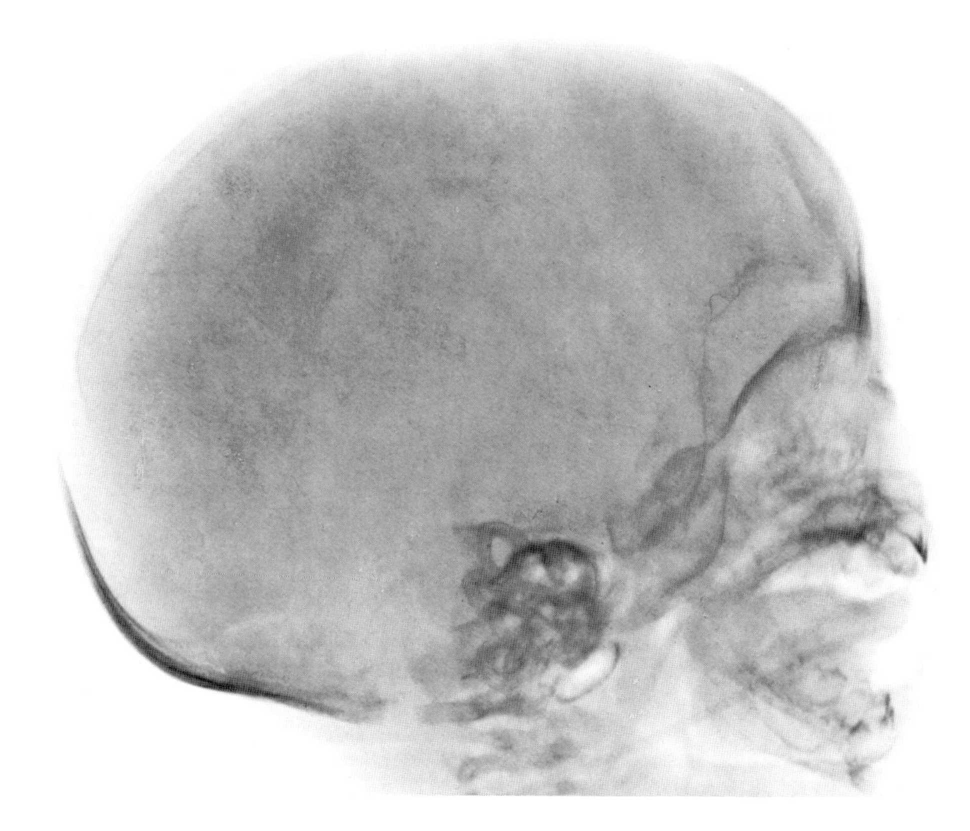

Fig. 943. 40-day-old infant after premature birth. The internal organs of the ear, which are projected onto each other, are very clearly seen, especially the arcade (cf. also with Fig. 917). Caudally and to the front, an oval ring appears as a result of the slanting direction of the tympanic ring (see Figs. 940, 941). A bone structure in the thin bones in lateral radiographs of the cranium is not yet recognizable. The arcades were only slightly retouched. They appear to be aconsequence to a lack of calcium deposit of the sella turcica and are seen rather clearly. Above the orbit, a curved double contour is marked. This is a vein course which flows into an emissary frontal vein. Of the denture, only small fragments are demonstrable. Suture grooves do not yet appear in the very thin bones of the cranial cap. Because of the early stage of development, the sutures and lateral fontanels are not visible. Indications of digital impressions or cerebral juga are also absent.

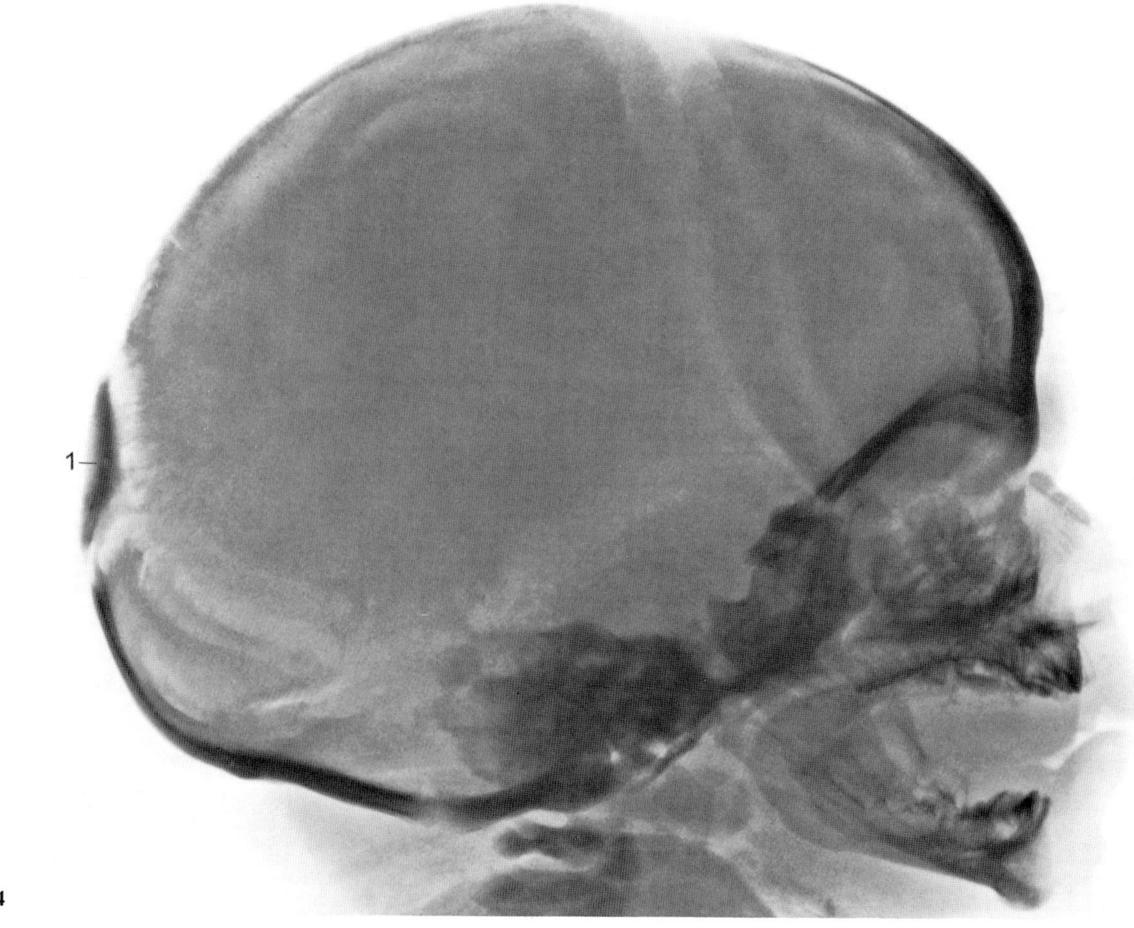

Fig. 944

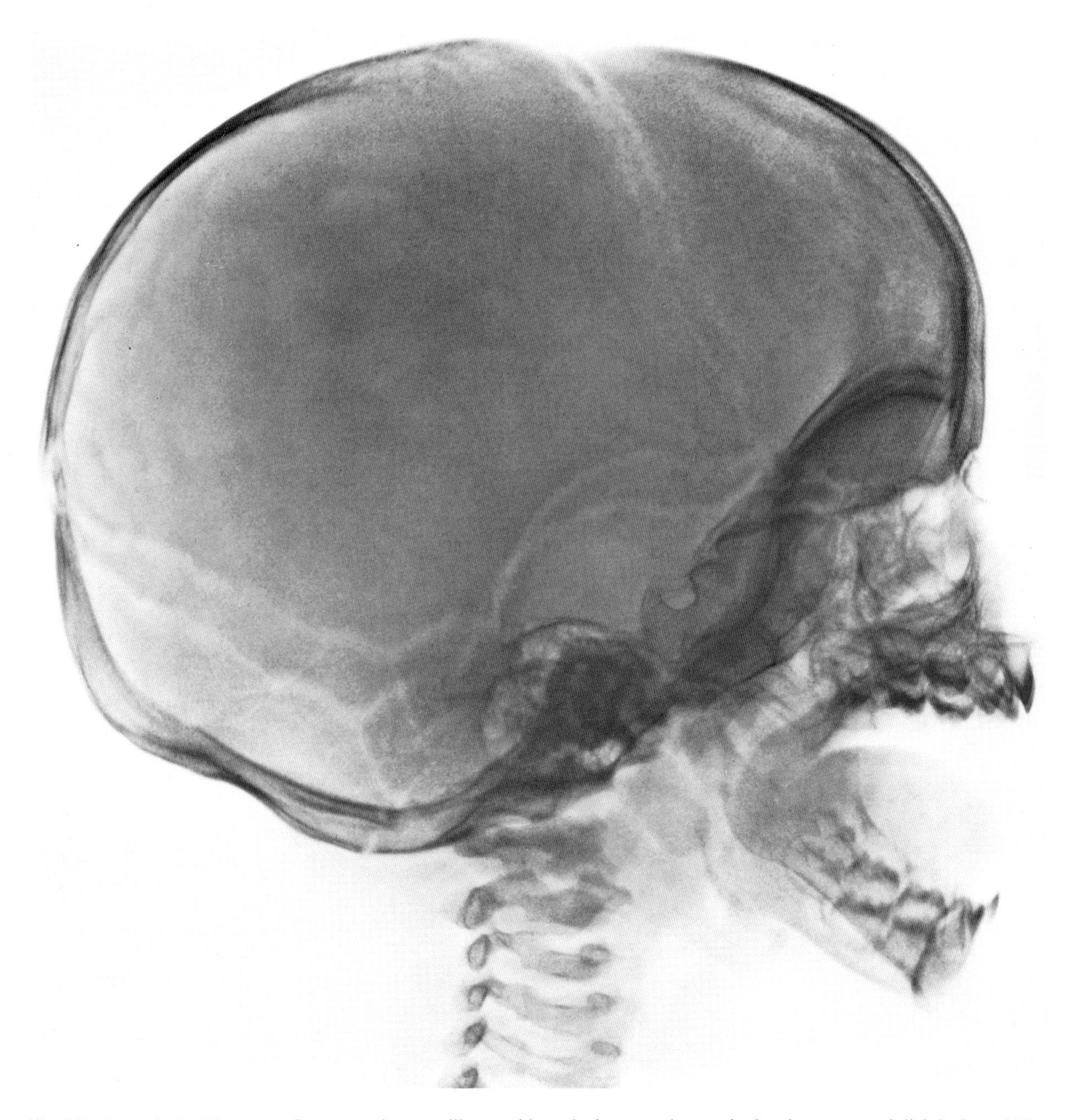

Fig. 945. 5 month old. The suture fissures are in part still very wide; only the coronal suture is already narrow and slightly dented. The posterior main sutures from osseous lacuna in the occipital and in the cranial base appear but should not be confused with fractures. The pneumatization of the sella turcica proceeds, while the sinuses of the petrous bone are not yet visible. The denture arrangement is easily recognizable.

◀ **Fig. 944. 3-day-old infant** (delivered). 1 (variation): segment bones at the lambdoid suture (cf. Fig. 275). The suture mendosa, which is not yet closed, is clearly visible (Figs. 940, 941). As indicators of future sutures, there are still smooth-edged, wide fissures at this age. The radiograph was made with soft radiation so as to make the suture fissures more evident, as the presentation of the soft tissues of the mouth section. The arrangement of the nasal bone is seen very clearly. It is still separated from the frontal bone by a wide fissure. The skull is much larger than the facial cranium. The ratio of the length of the head to the height of the body is 1 : 4 (in adults about 1 : 7). The orbits are remarkably large; the cranial base is flat. The mastoid process is not yet developed. The vessel canals in digital impressions are not yet formed. Tooth cells are visible in the mandible.

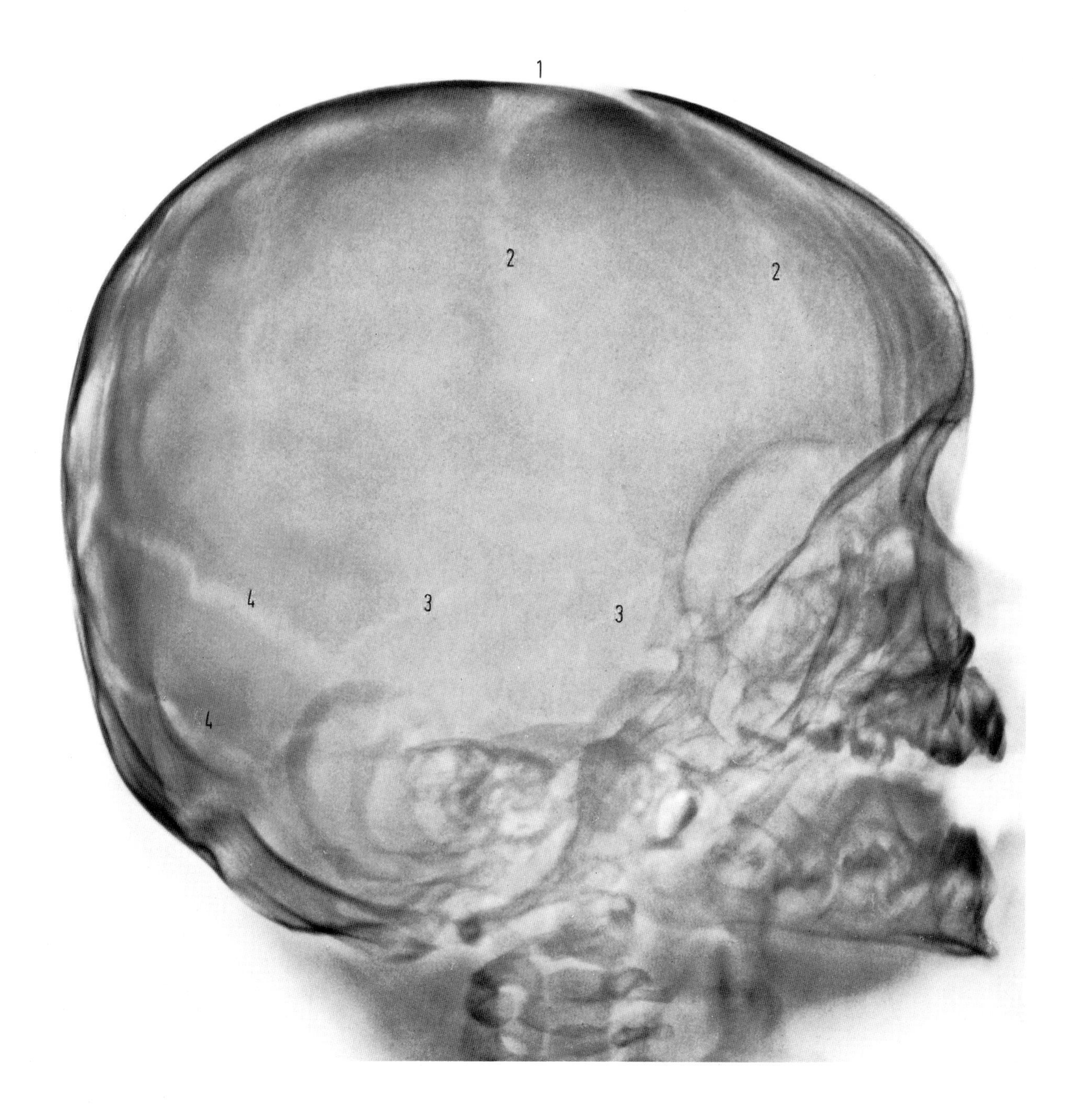

Fig. 946. 8 month old. Figs. 946 and 947, with the head in a somewhat rotated position, show the course of the projected sutures in an exactly focused normal radiograph. This way, it is possible to recognize in Fig. 947 the frontal suture, which still exists at this age and is usually covered by the end of the 9th year of life, but can in some cases persist (metopic suture). There are clearly recognizable tooth nuclei in the maxilla and the mandible.

1 Anterior fontanel
2 Coronal suture
3 Squamous suture
4 Lambdoid suture

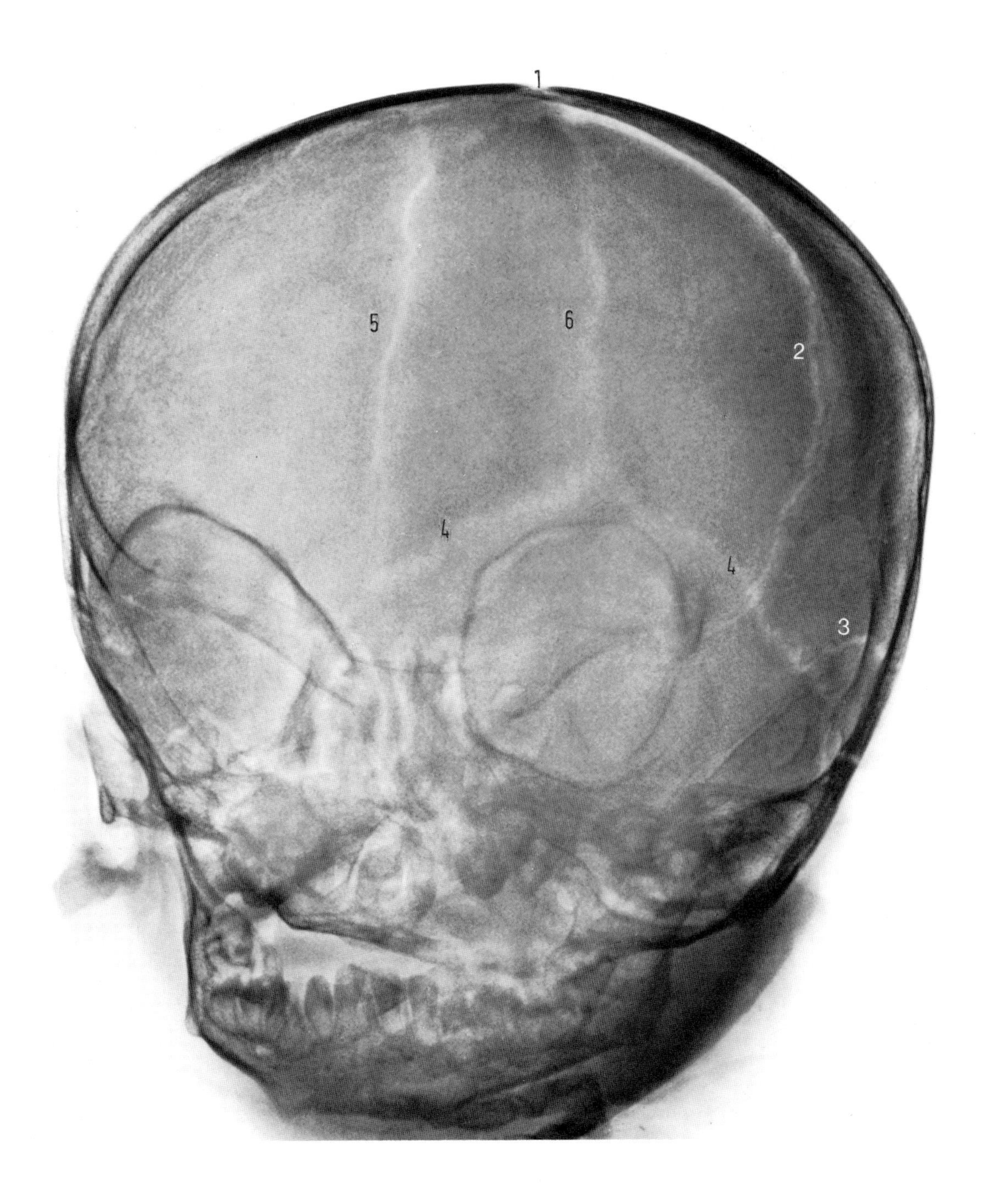

Fig. 947. 8 month old. The orbit of a newborn is still completely flat and therefore hardly covers the eye. It grows very quickly in infants and only then encloses the bulbus. In the 2nd year of life, it attains 75% of its final size. First, the width of the aditus is larger than its height. The eye cavity exit still has a square-oval form instead of the later round form. The final form of the superior edge of the orbit is not yet present after birth; the extension towards the front occurs later. The causes of this lie in embryonic development.

1 Anterior fontanel
2 Coronal suture
3 Squamous suture
4 Lambdoid suture
5 Frontal suture
6 Sagittal suture

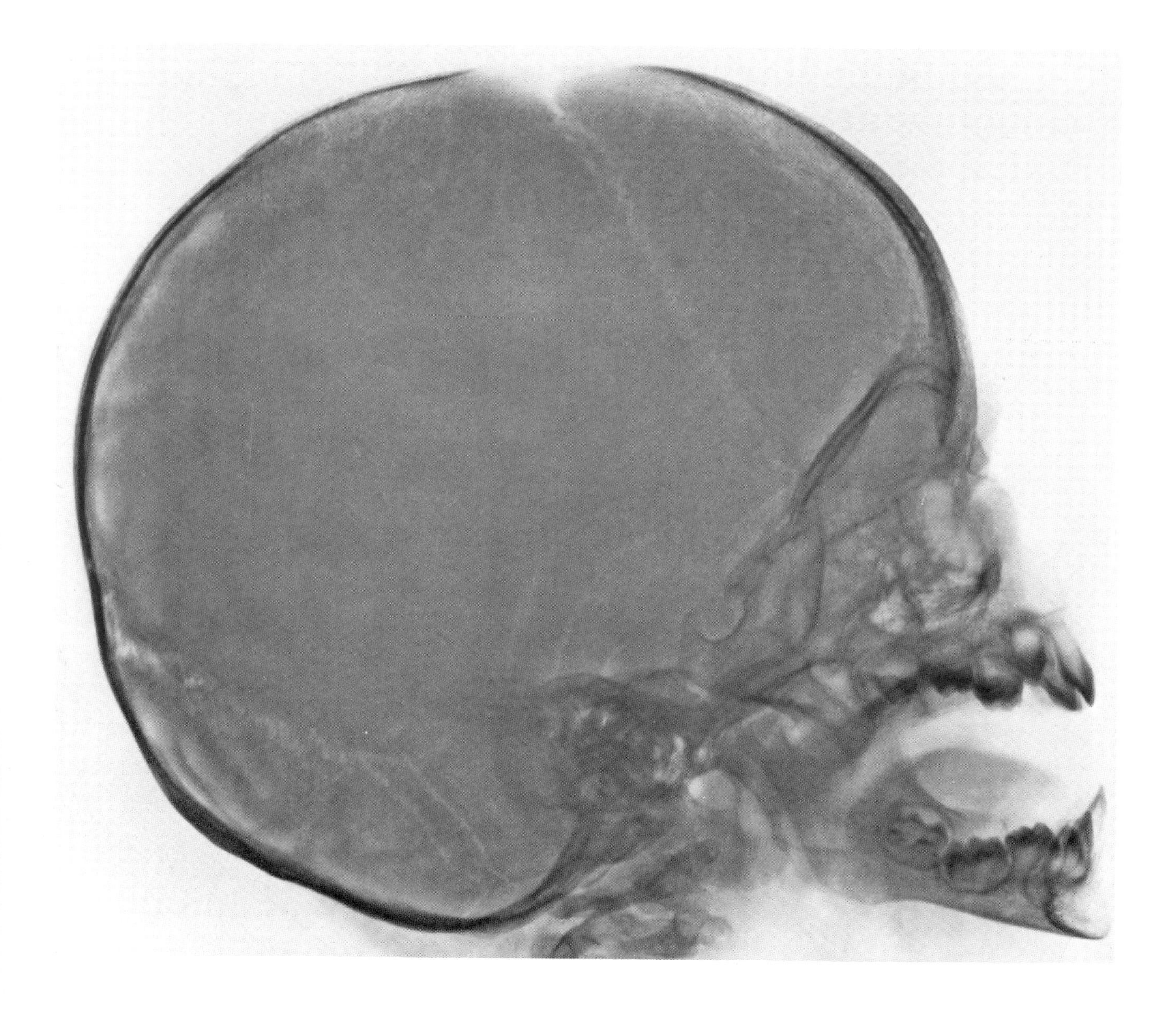

Fig. 948. 8 month old. The cranium cap still shows a very uniform image. The digital impressions develop only during the 2nd year of life; the cerebral juga appear just as small as the arterial grooves, veins and sinuses because of scanty bone calcium. The suture lines have become narrower and begin to become dented. This dentation emerges only from the lamina externa. The fissures of the lamina interna close through simple osseous apposition, smoothly edged and never dented. The big fontanels are still wide open. There is a well-developed arrangement of the teeth of the maxilla, of which the milk incisor teeth have already emerged. The next tooth chronologically (4) is about to emerge, whereas tooth 3 still remains deeper inside (cf. Fig. 901).

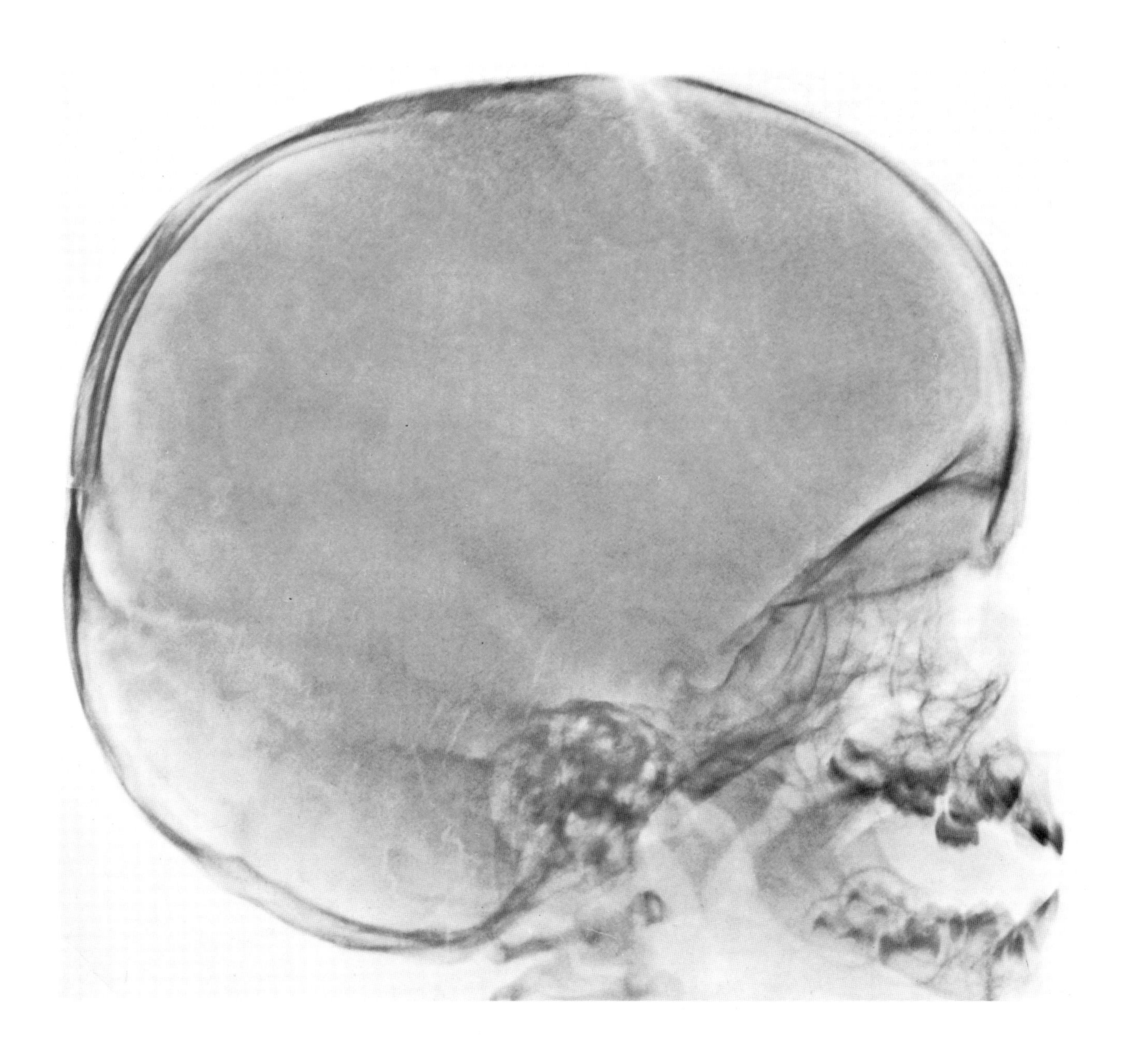

Fig. 949. 1 year old. The large fontanel has clearly become smaller. The digital impressions slowly begin to appear but are still barely recognizable. The fissures of the vault bones become narrower through appositional osseous formation. After the 1st year of life, the width of the fissure is still about 0.5 mm, which means that they disappear partly in the radiograph. The intensive development of the brain – 15% of the total body weight in the newborn as against only 3% in adults – has caused a remarkable enlargement of the cranium cap. In comparison, the facial cranium is very small. The 1st, 2nd and 4th teeth of the maxilla milk dentures have broken through. The 3rd tooth appears much later (sometime around the 15th to 20th month).

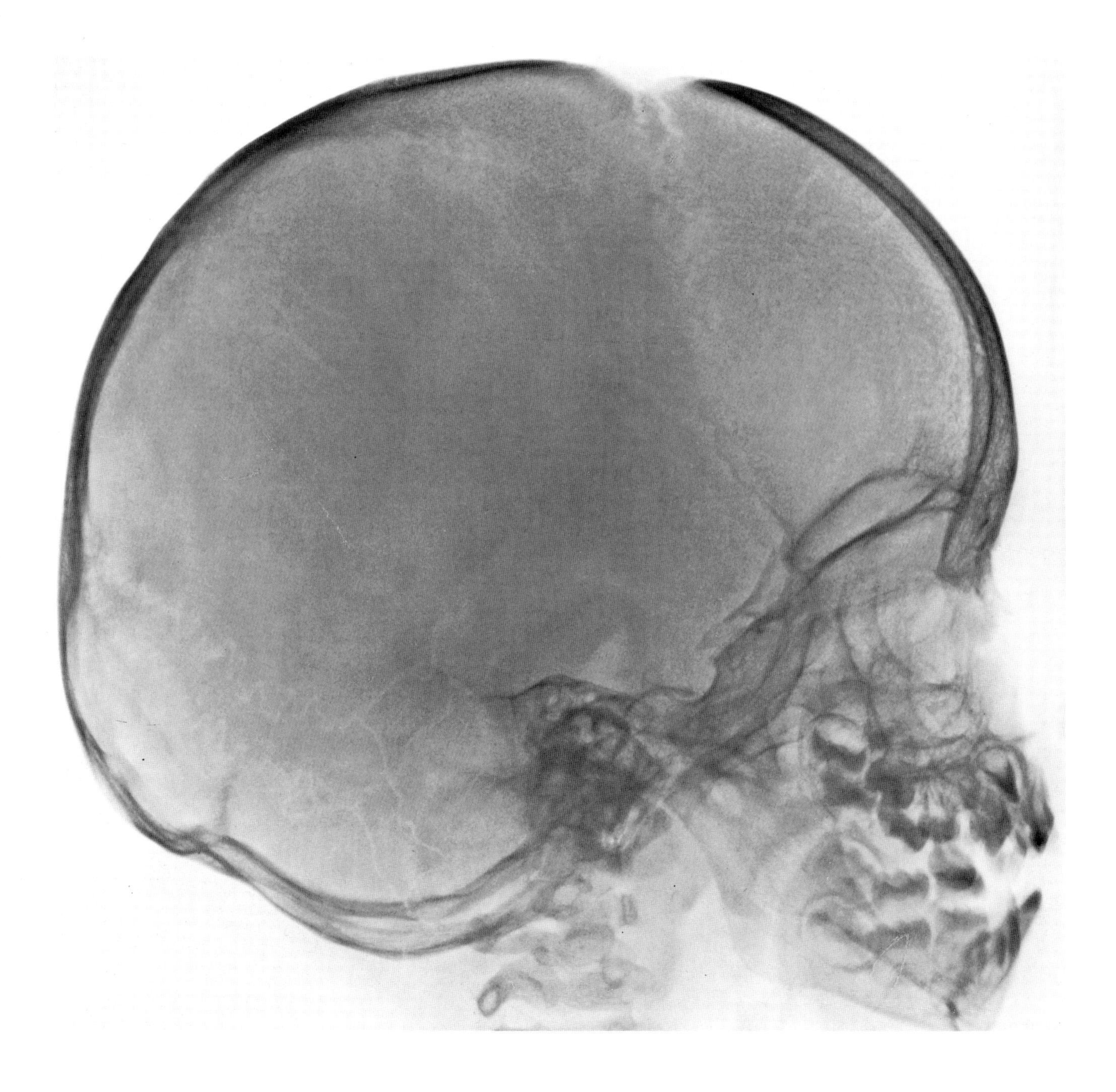

Fig. 950. 1 1/2 year old. Here, it is possible to recognize the still-open large fontanel, which appears even a little larger than in Fig. 949. The perforation of the sutures becomes very clear. It is possible to recognize the well-advanced situation of the milk molars, of which the lower rear molar is still surrounded by a cyst-like alveolus. According to *Merkel,* the first period of growth is both fast and regular up to the 7th year of life. Between the 2nd and 5th years of life, the parietal bones and the occiput curving (Hinterhauptwölbung) are formed. The cranium cap and the facial cranium become broader in the 6th and 7th years of life, followed by the lengthening of the base of the cranium. After this first period of growth, the growth in length of the cranium base with the sella turcica, the foramen magnum and the horizontal ethmoidal plate has developed to final size.

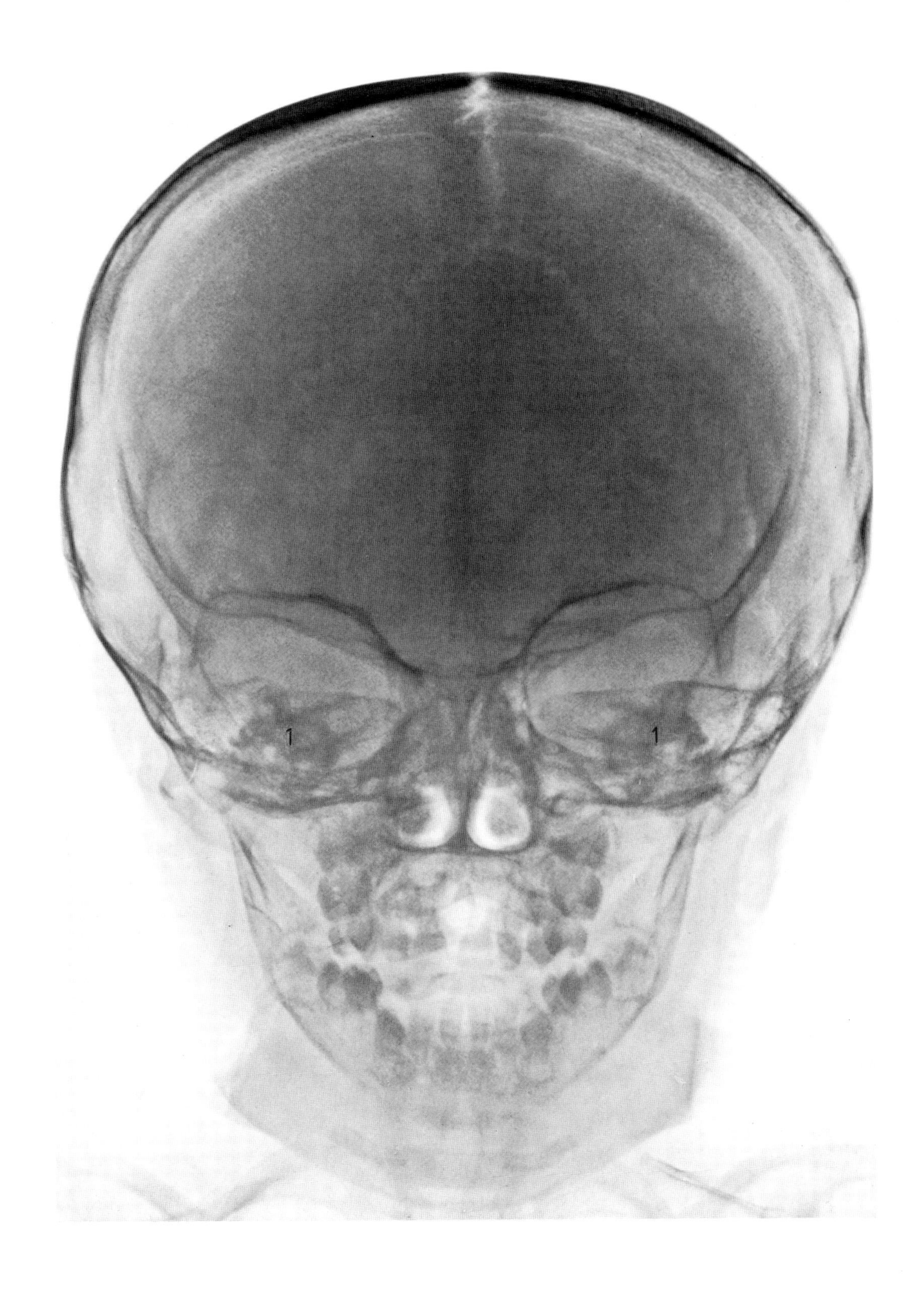

Fig. 951. 1½ year old. In this radiograph, according to the transorbital comparable radiograph of both petrous bones according to *Schüller,* the internal ear (1) with arcades and cochlea projects itself on both sides into the orbit (cf. Fig. 122). The course of the superior edge of the petrous bone is well exposed here. While on the right an arched eminence appears clearly for the superior arcades, on the left the edge of the superior petrous bone is regular and smooth. A slight difference in height between the two petrous bones can be seen, which is also a frequent finding in adults.

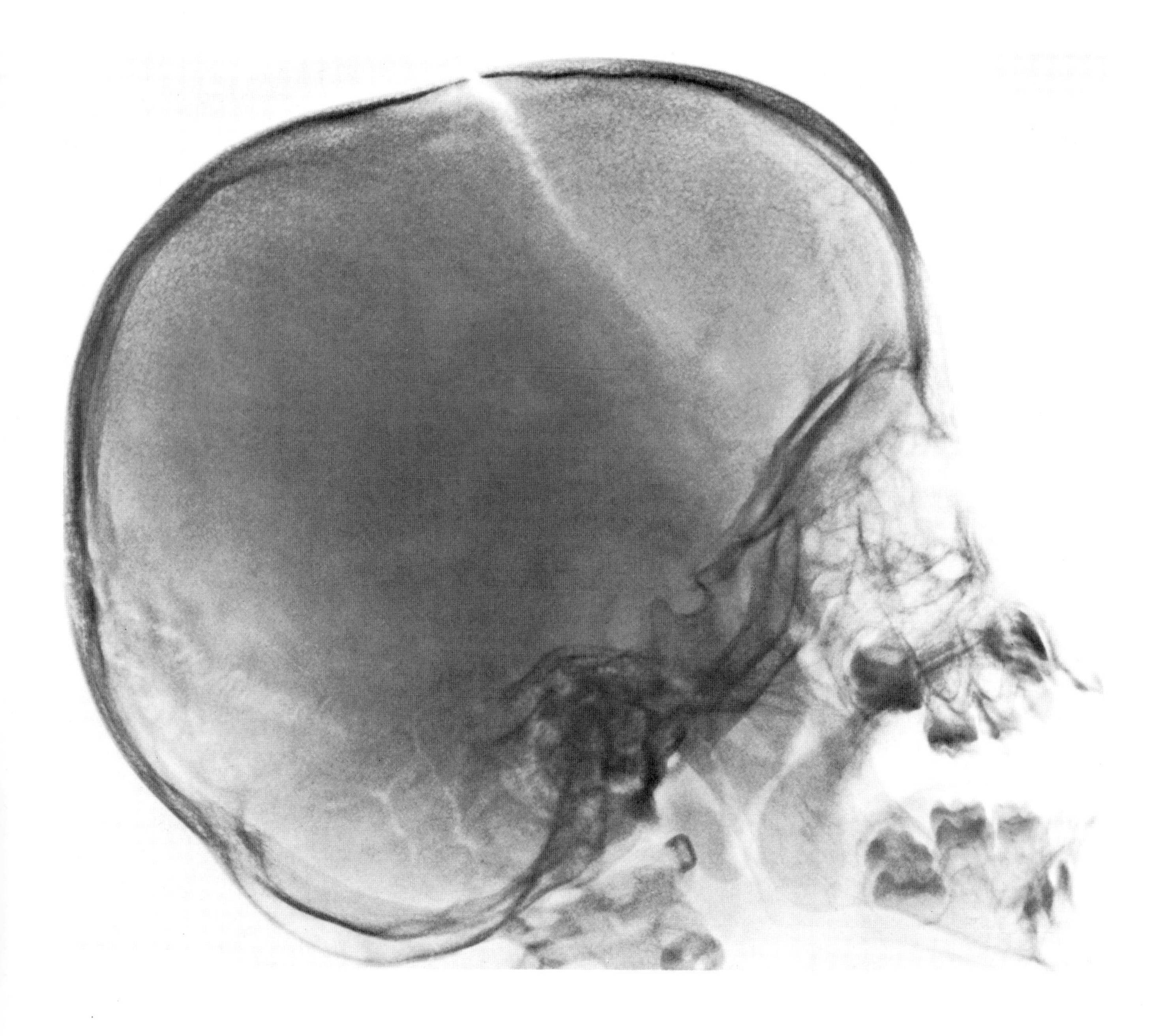

Fig. 952. 2 year old. The large fontanel is about to close. The digital impressions are becoming clearer. There are still remarkable gaping sutures and an arched frontal bone. Suspicion of internal hydrocephalus. This presumption may be suggested only on the basis of the width of the suture. According to *Loepp-Lorenz,* normal suture ratios are present if:

1. after the end of the first year the suture is no wider than 0.75-1 mm,
2. the lamina externa is well formed after the 2nd year of life,
3. the suture becomes narrower with age, or
4. in adults up to the end of life the sutures are still traceable but become more compact and more calcified.

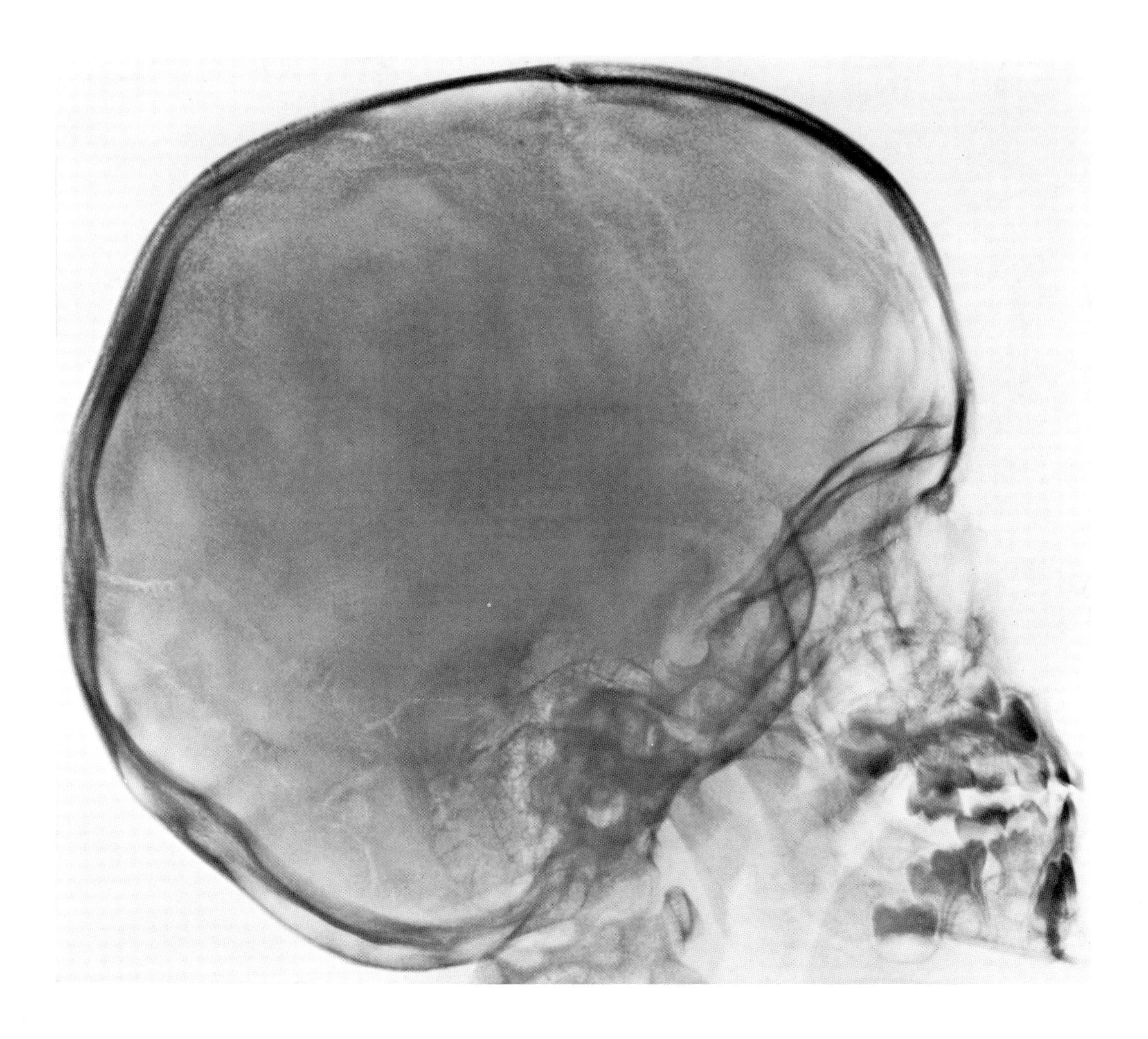

Fig. 953. 3 year old. The formation of the digital impressions has proceeded further. Around the 4th and up to the 10th year of life, it reaches a certain standstill. The milk denture is completely developed. The first remaining molar is shown in the maxilla and the mandible. The cavities in both jaws are already pneumatized. The clinoid processes are still underdeveloped since they ossify only during the 4th year of life. The lamina externa is now well formed. The ossification of the sutures continues throughout the whole life span. The coronal suture may ossify as early as between the 10th and 20th years of life; in the adult it is usually ossified. The sagittal suture is usually occluded in men between the ages of 50 and 70, and in women between the ages of 50 and 60. The lambdoid suture is visible for a longer period; it is still visible in about 35% of those aged 60–80. The visible perforation in the radiographs up to old age is no criterion for the "persistence" of the suture line as it is only the lamina externa which becomes perforated. The lamina interna and diploë can thus form continuous cranial layers. The union of the sutures of the diploë and lamina interna appears shortly after completion of cranial growth.

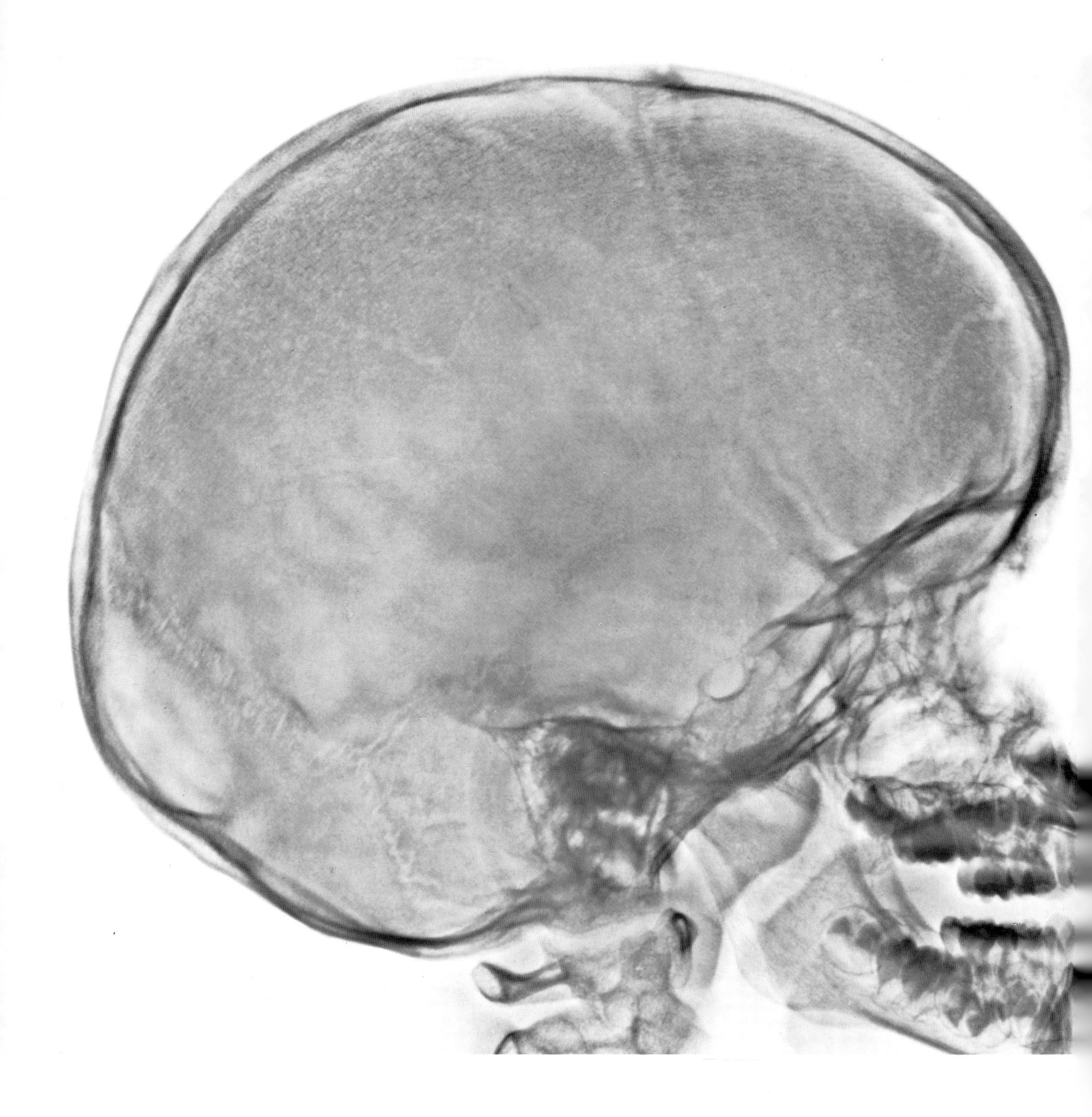

Fig. 954. 5 year old. Readily visible frontal diploic vein; behind it, the strongly perforated lamina externa of the coronal suture. Deep digital impressions. Suture bones in the lambdoid region with unblended sutures. Embedded arrangements of milk teeth and remaining teeth.
The diploë is formed through resorption processes of the lamina externa and interna, and the substitution of the compact bones by lamellas. In the newborn the blood flows freely in these diploic spaces. It is only from the 3rd to 5th years of life and onward that the blood gathers in four canal systems: the diploic, frontal temporal anterior and posterior, and occipital veins. Sometimes there is also a parietal diploic vein. The diploic veins are limited by the neighboring osseous substance. They extend through the lamina externa or interna or through emissary veins. They are easily visible between the 20th and 30th years of life. Afterwards, they become less visible; in old age they are no longer visible due to involution.
In this picture there is another remarkable lengthening of the posterior clinoid process almost up to the anterior clinoid process: variant form.

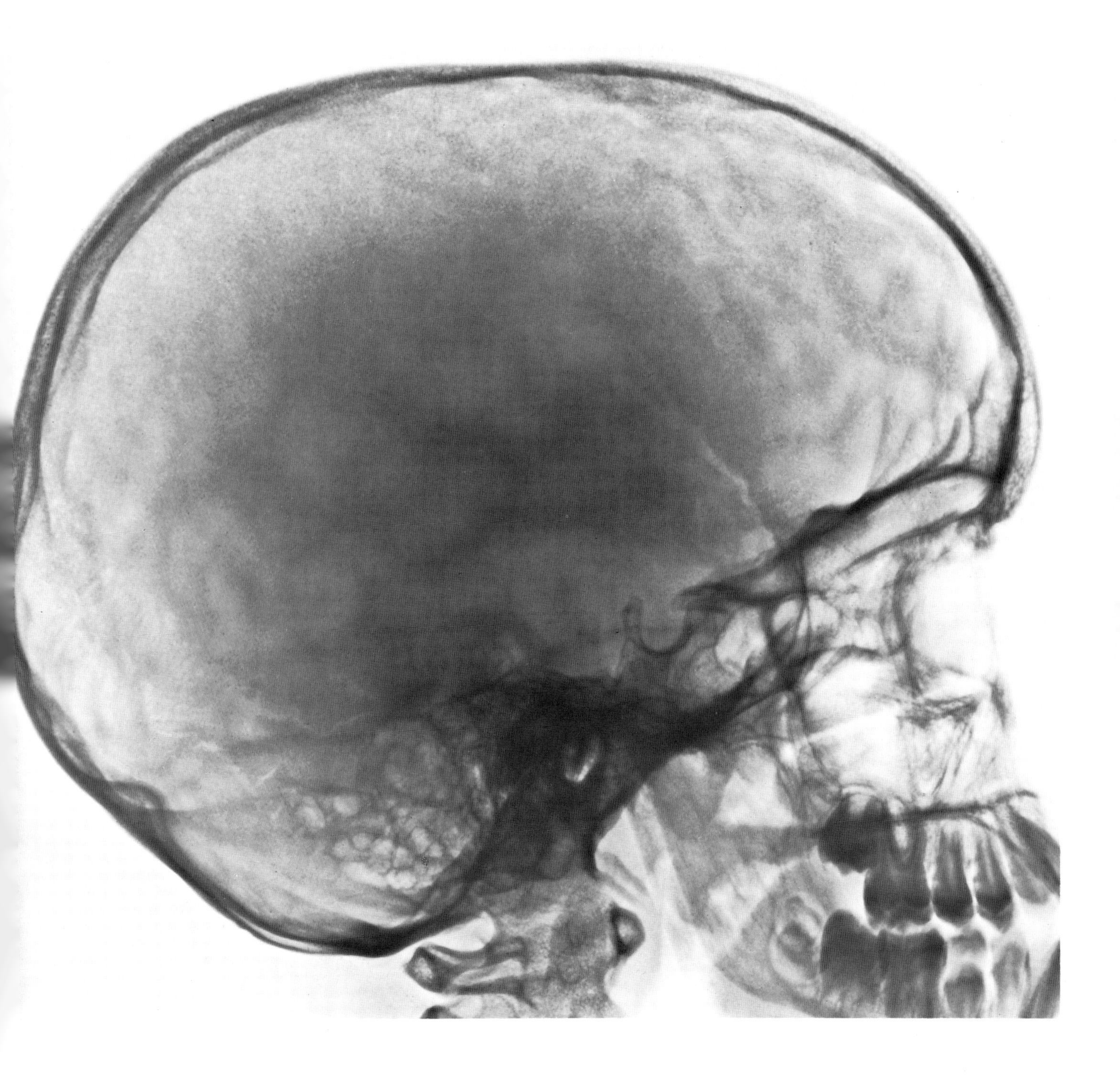

Fig. 955. 8 year old. Well-formed impressions, physiologically. The coronal suture is no longer perforated, while the lamina externa is extensively fused. There is a strong pneumatization of the pyramid and the papillary process, as well as of the frontal and sphenoidal sinuses. Altogether, the radiograph is similar to the cranium of an adult.
The second period of growth, which begins between the 8th year of life and puberty, is characterized by the development of the facial cranium, its lengthening and widening, as well as the intensification of the development of the frontal bone.
In this picture the double contour of the squamous portion of the occipital bone is clearly visible (pseudo-impression fracture).

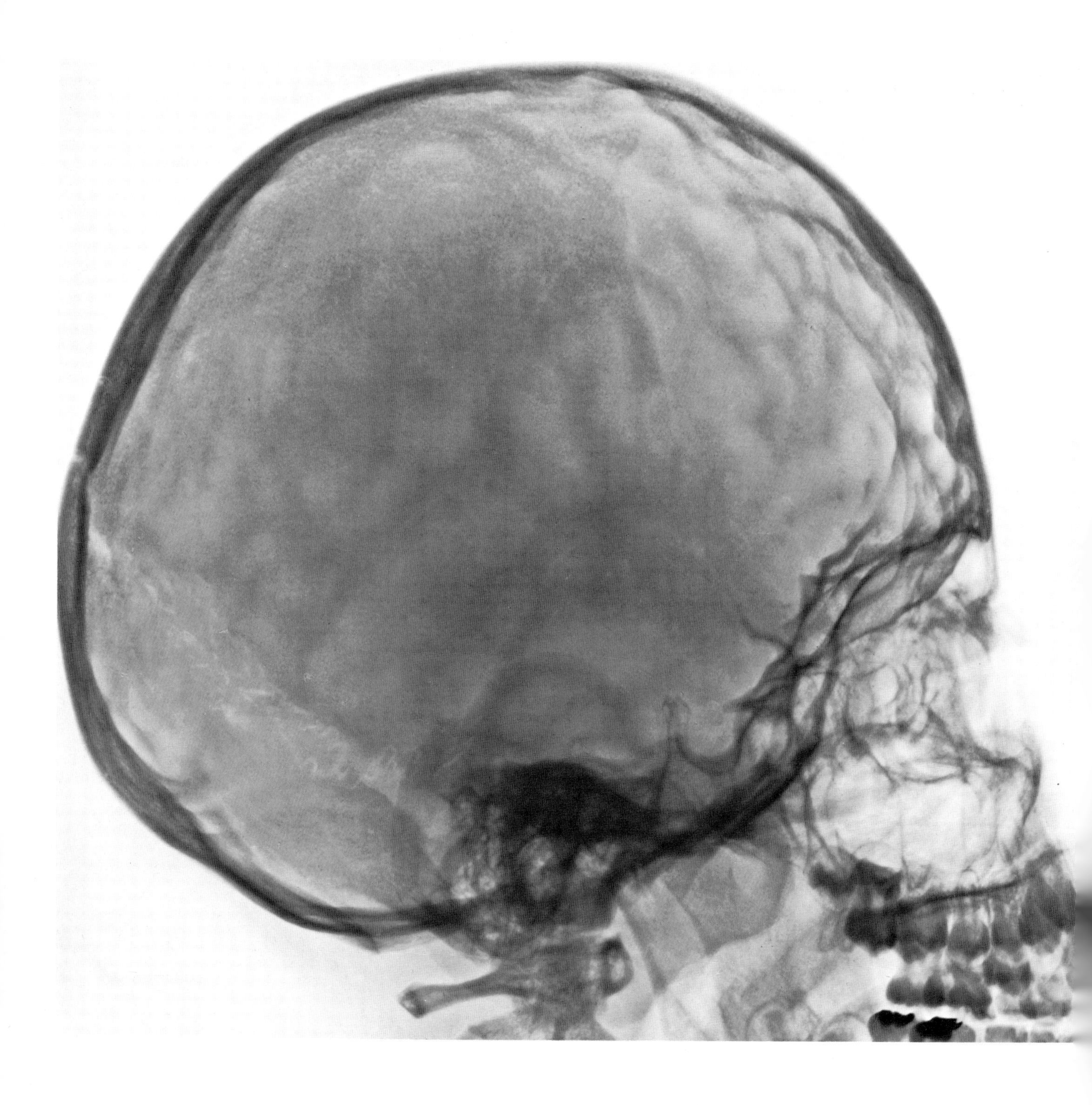

Fig. 956. 11 year old. Turricephalic cranium. The strong digital impressions are a consequence of an increased brain pressure due to early closure of the coronal suture.
The turricephaly originates from a congenital or premature synostosis of the coronal suture. The lambdoid suture, which is still visible, and the still-open synchondroses can cause the rearward deviation of the further development of the cranium. It seems doubtful that the stronger frontal digital impressions are symptomatic of increased brain pressure since other symptoms of such a disorder are absent.

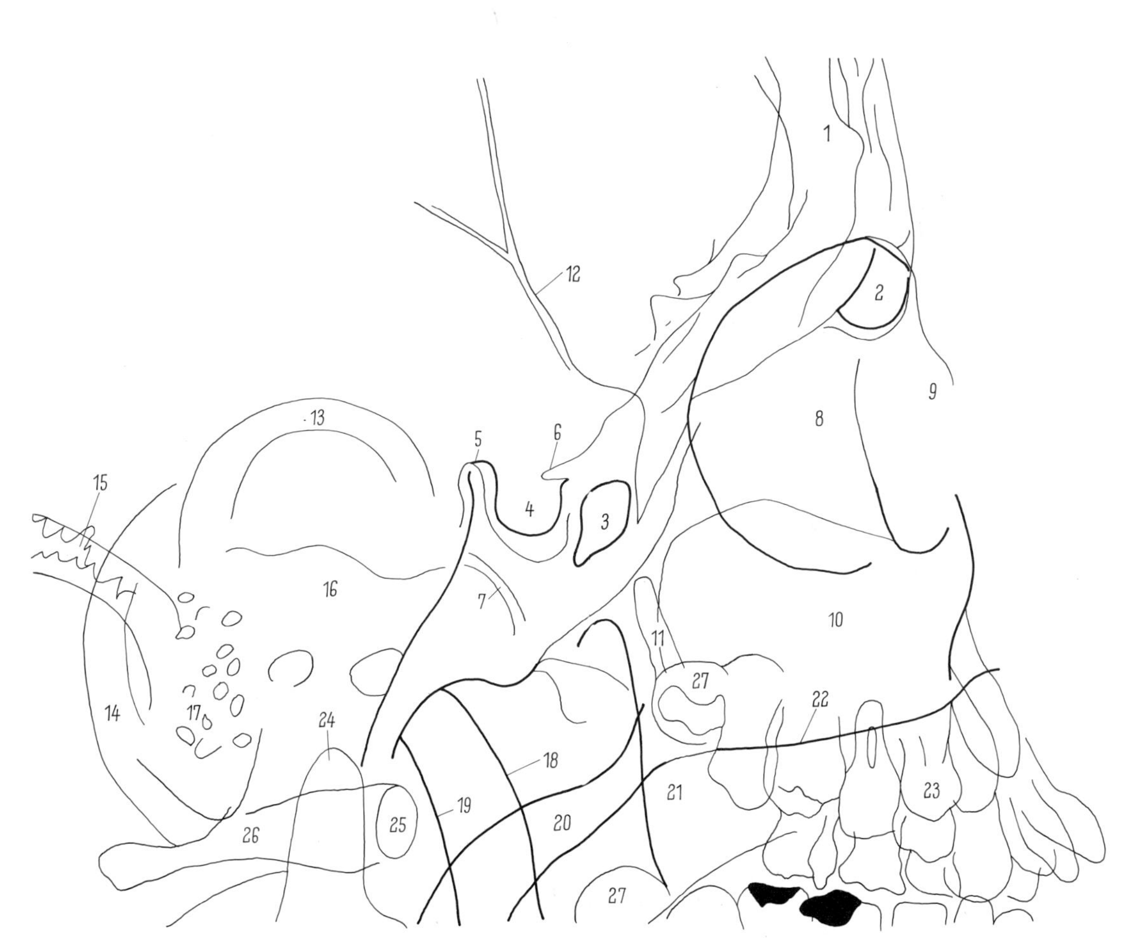

Fig. 957. Sketch of Fig. 956.

1 Intensified digital impressions
2 Frontal sinus
3 Sphenoidal sinus
4 Sella turcica
5 Dorsum sella
6 Anterior clinoid process
7 Spheno-occipital synchondrosis
8 Orbit
9 Nasal bone
10 Maxillary sinus
11 Pterygopalatine sinus
12 Medial meningeal artery
13 Ear conch of the film-near ear
14 Ear conch of the film-distant ear
15 Lambdoid suture, projects itself into the sigmoid sinus
16 Petrous portion
17 Mastoid cells
18 Rear edge of the film-near condylar process
19 Rear edge of the film-distant condylar process
20 Pharynx
21 Soft palate
22 Hard palate
23 Maxillary teeth
24 Dens (axis)
25 Anterior arch (atlantis)
26 Posterior arch (atlantis)
27 Molar arrangement in the maxilla

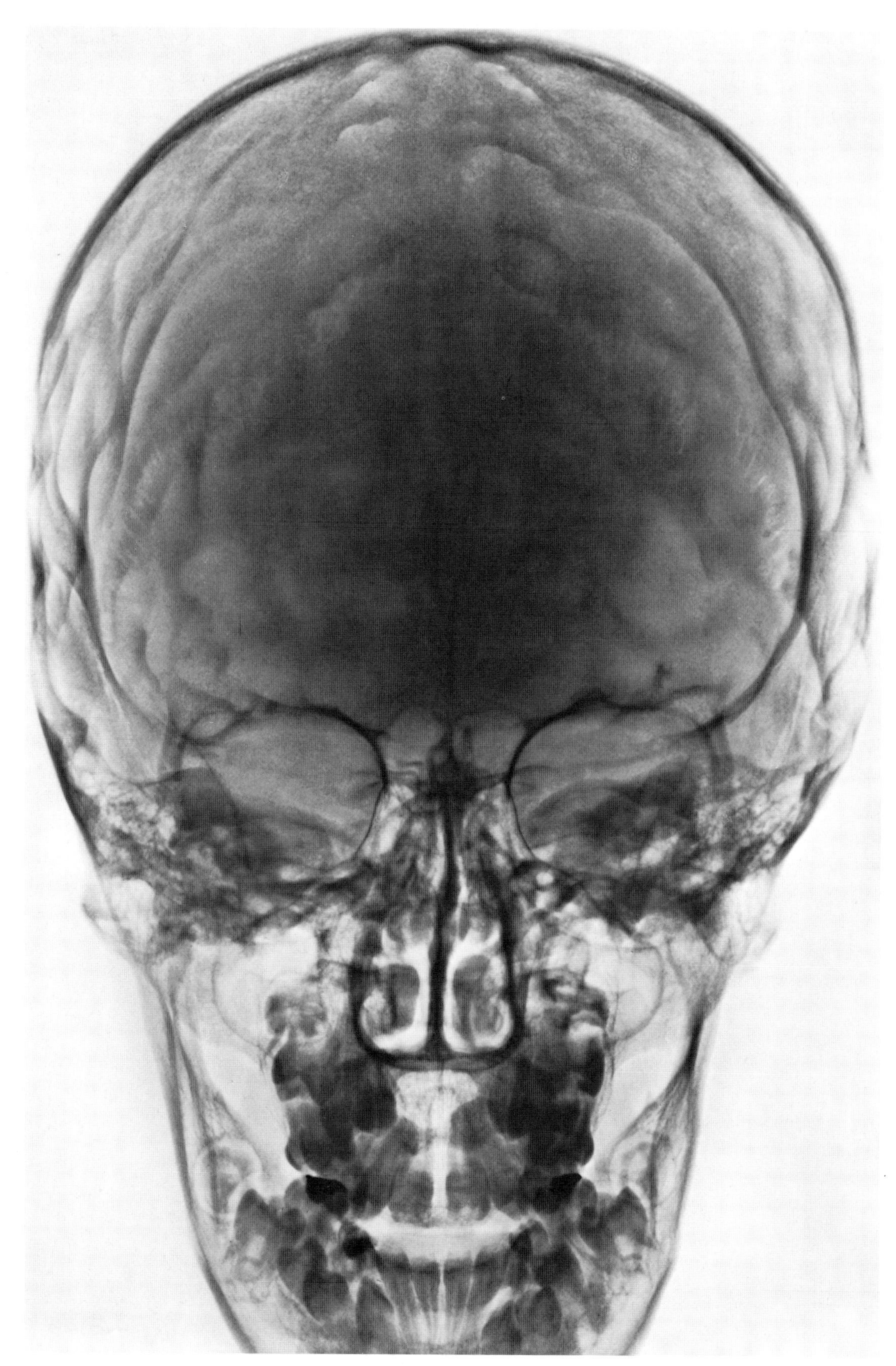

Fig. 958. 11 year old, turricephalic cranium (sagittal radiograph of Fig. 956). The posteroanterior radiograph shows the deep film-near digital impressions especially well. The left pyramid is somewhat higher than the right one. The internal acoustic canals are slightly wide, probably as a consequence of the compression of the pyramid in a longitudinal direction. This form of cranial stenosis is also called frontal dysphasia because of the effect of the base malformation which causes the anomaly in the frontal fossa.

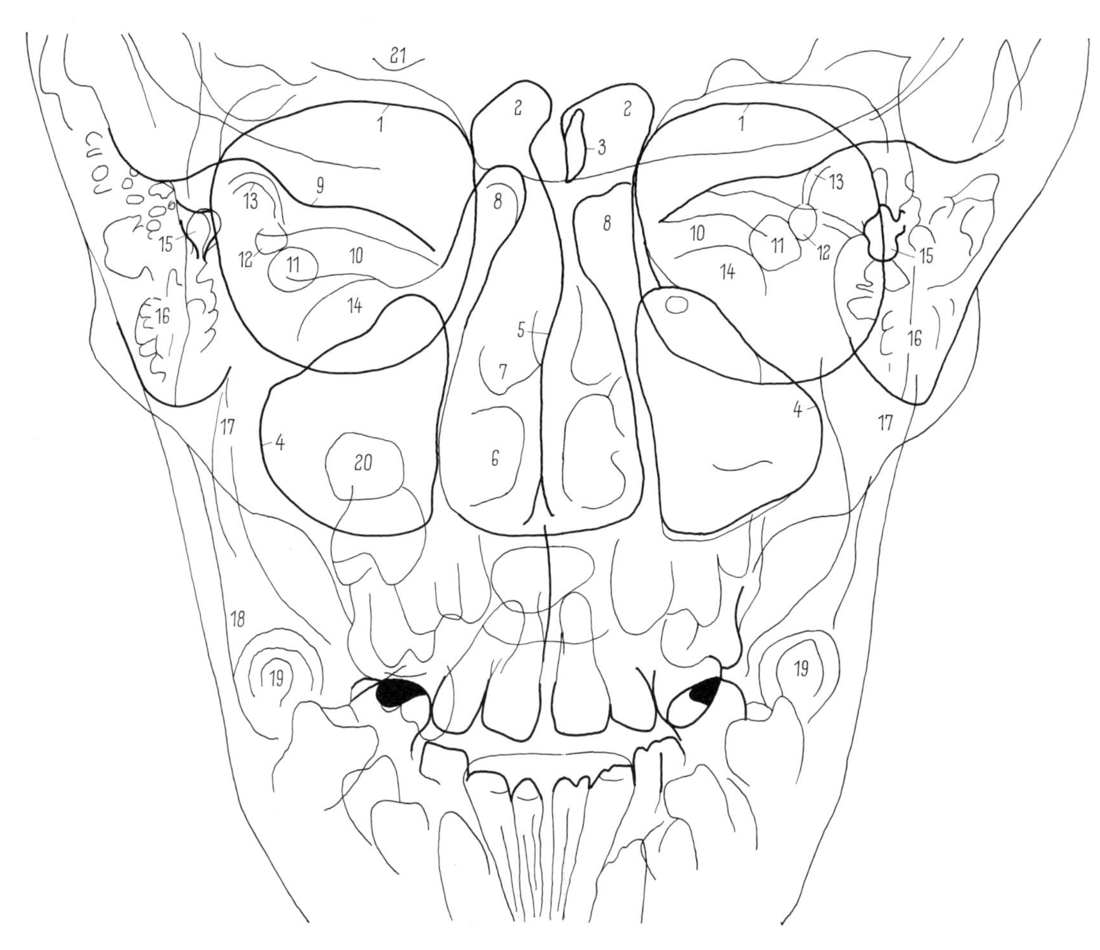

Fig. 959. Sketch of Fig. 958.

1 Superior orbit edge
2 Frontal sinus
3 Crista galli
4 Maxillary sinus
5 Nasal bone septum
6 Inferior nasal concha
7 Medial nasal concha
8 Ethmoidal cells (ethmoidal sinus)
9 Petrous portion
10 Internal acoustic meatus
11 Cochlea
12 Vestibule
13 Semicircular anterior canal
14 Carotic canal
15 Mastoid antrum
16 Mastoid cells
17 Condylar process
18 Mandible
19 Molar teeth arrangement, still in tooth cysts in the mandible
20 Molar teeth arrangement in the maxilla
21 Strengthened digital impressions

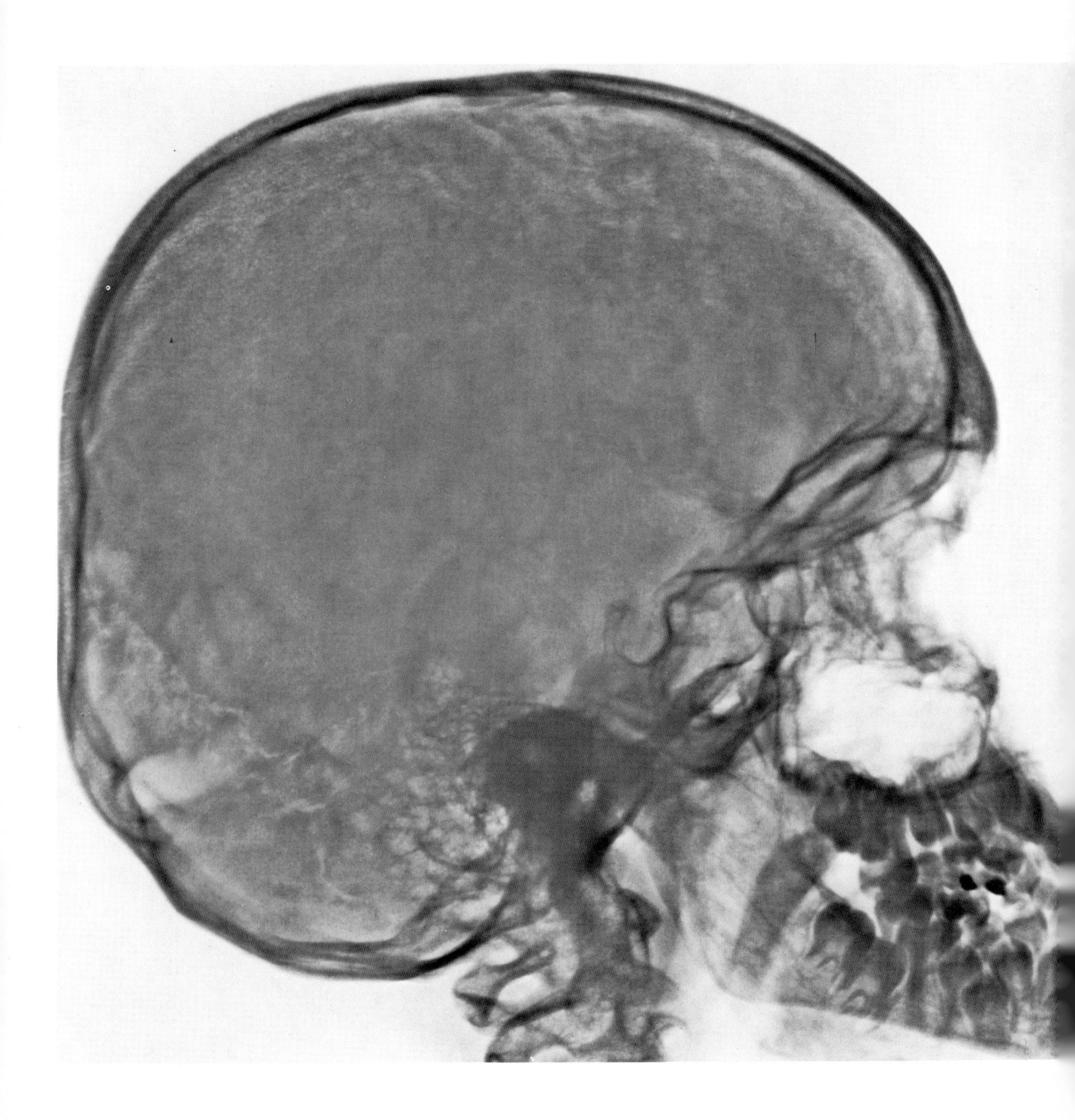

Fig. 960. 11 year old. The spheno-occipital synchondrosis is still clearly visible, and the noticeably deeply set sella is in front of it. In the temporal bone and in the squamous portion of the occipital bone, there are still many sutures, deeper and wider transverse sinus sulcus, and confluent sinus, as well as wide sulci of the frontal diploic veins. There are especially well-formed granular foveola *(Pacchioni),* which usually appear only after the 10th year of life. They are dispersed here on the whole lamina interna and more intensely in the frontal bone. A connection with an intracranial increase in pressure may be erroneously assumed. The *Pacchionian* sulci originate through the sinking of the arachnoidal villus into the osseous substance, where they disappear and cause resorption.

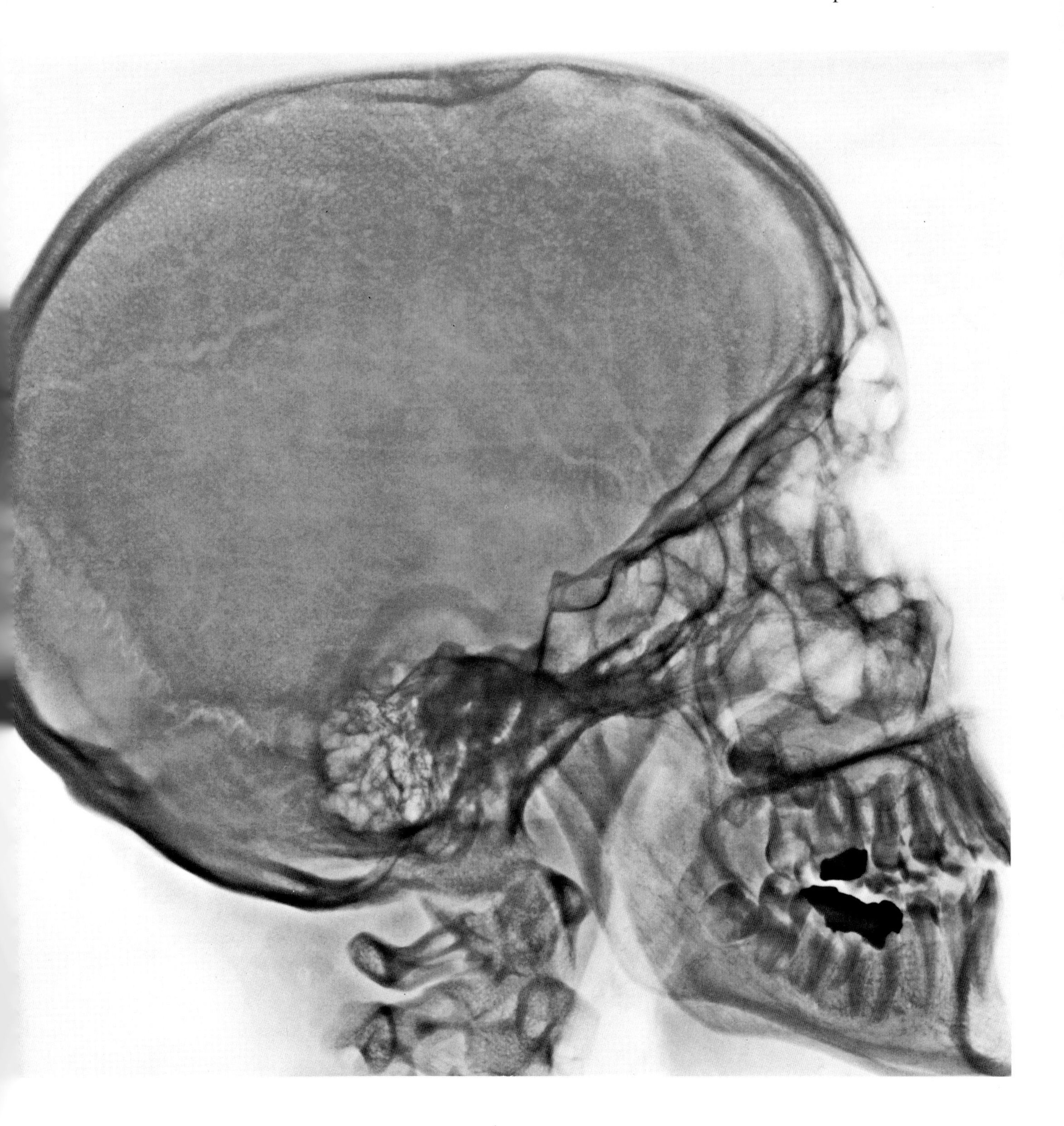

Fig. 961. 16 year old. The development of the cranial cap is almost completed. The development of the facial cranium continues up to the 22nd year of life. The paranasal sinuses as well as the pneumatic system in the papillary processes of the pyramids are well developed; the sphenoidal sinus even reaches up to the rear edge of the sphenoidal body. The individual size variation of the exposed sella turcica is here somewhat small and flat, but still normal. A typical sella bridge is seen, although it has no clinical significance. The veins are better marked and the arterial sulci, especially that of the medial meningeal artery, are more visible. The lamina interna of the cranial cap has more indentations. These are *Pacchionian* sulci, which lead to the localized thinning of the cranial bones, especially in the parietal region. Their development begins only after the 10th year of life. Above the pyramid, it is possible to see the shadow of the soft tissues of the ear conch as a curved contour. Of the teeth, only the wisdom teeth (dentes serotini) and the four 3rd molars of the denture are still deep in the tooth cyst. They usually emerge in the 16th year of life but often much later and, in certain cases, only in the third decade.

Development of the Teeth

The development of the deciduous and permanent teeth shows a wide range of deviation. This may be due to the fact that those factors which take part in general development have little influence on the specific development of the teeth *(Schmid* and *Moll).* But for medical practice, knowledge of the approximate time table of dentition is of importance (see Figs. 896–902).

Deciduous Teeth

Formation of dentin starts at the same time as the formation of the dental papilla, with the germinal crown of the tooth, and proceeds from there gradually into the root. At first a plate of dentin appears ("little dental shard") at the orally directed tip of the papilla.

The formation of enamel starts simultaneously and in the same places as the dentin formation. The root is never covered with enamel. Instead, it receives a cover of dental cement, a modified bony substance which is produced by the periost of the alveolus.

At the time of eruption of a tooth, its root has reached its full length but the apical parts of the root are not yet calcified. The end of dental development is reached only some time after the eruption of the teeth into the oral cavity. Only rarely does eruption of isolated teeth, e.g., of the middle incisors of the mandible, take place before birth. In the maxillary region of the newborn, the germinal domes of the 1st and 2nd teeth and the pointed small shard of the 3rd tooth are visible. On lateral views of the skull of the child, one can accurately follow the development of the deciduous teeth from the origin of the first five dental germs (cf. Figs. 943–956, 960 and 961 of the skull, taken with frontal path of rays). Onset of ossification and eruption of deciduous teeth can be seen in Figures 896 and 901.

During the first three months, the mass of the upper front teeth increases and calcification proceeds. The growth of the canine teeth and the longitudinal growth of the lower incisors are especially pronounced *(Mannkopf).* There are no permanent teeth as yet. During the second 3-month-period of life one can perceive the growth in width of the mandible through the moving apart of the germs of the incisor teeth.

During the third 3-month-period of life, the further longitudinal growth of the front teeth corresponds to the growth in height of the skeleton and expresses itself in the eruption of these teeth between the 7th and 9th months. The germs of the first three permanent teeth become visible on the radiograph.

During the fourth 3-month-period of life, the roots of the already erupted teeth are developing. The teeth of the mandible appear to mineralize more rapidly.

Permanent Teeth

During the 5th and 6th fetal months, anterior molars, as well as the incisor and canine teeth of the permanent set of teeth, are being preformed.

During the 2nd year of life, slow growth of the germs of the permanent teeth takes place, repeating the processes of development of the germs of the deciduous teeth. With the expansion of the origin of a replacement tooth, the root of the milk tooth which lies above it is being resorbed. Finally, only the crown of the deciduous tooth remains, which is shed with the eruption of the permanent tooth (see Figs. 896, 902, 943–956, 960 and 961 of the skull, taken with frontal path of rays).

III. Spine, Ribs and Sternum

Spine

The differentiation of the primitive vertebral arrangement begins in the cervical region and continues in a caudal direction, reaching the caudal spinal column end only in the 2nd embryonic month.

The ossification of the spinal column begins at the end of the 2nd embryonic month. It starts at the arch of the atlas (Fig. 962) and from there extends along the spinal arch caudally *(Rickenbacher, Denisch, Müller et al.).*

The first radiographically demonstrable ossification signs appear in the vertebral body during the 3nd fetal month and, as a matter of fact, the first nucleus of the vertebral body appears in the 12th thoracic vertebra. The ossification of the vertebral body extends from there in both the cranial and caudal directions (*Alexander, Broman, Hartmann*). However, development in the cranial direction is somewhat more rapid than in the caudal direction.

From the end of the 4th fetal month onwards, there are osseous nuclei in every vertebral body (Fig. 963).

While in the adult the longest transverse diameter of the spinal column is at the level of the 1st sacral vertebra, the next in order of length is in the atlas, and the 5th lumbar vertebra; in the fetus the longest transverse diameter is at the level of the atlas, the next in order of length at the level of the 7th cervical vertebra, and the 2nd lumbar vertebra.

The development of the bones of the vertebrae begins in three ossification centers: in two nucleus arrangements in the region of the spinal arch and one nuclear arrangement in the vertebral body (Figs. 964, 965). In this case, only the atlas and the axis are exceptions.

Page 142 gives a detailed report on the development of dens based on new opinions *(Töndury).* The atlas develops in the first place only from the 2nd arch in the posterior arch (Fig. 962), and it is only in the course of the 1st year of life that a 3rd nucleus develops in the anterior arch. The anterior arch originates in the hypercordal clip. The ossification can start from a medial or from two paramedial nuclei. In rare cases, the arrangement of the ossification nucleus may be lacking in the anterior arch; the ossification in the anterior of the arch atlas begins in the massa lateralis. A medial permanent fissure originates due to the absence of fusion with the frontal half of the arch (Fig. 308).

In 20.6% of 500 newborns, *Tompsett* and *Donaldson* found an anterior tuberculum of the 1st cervical vertebra. Besides two arched arrangements and a nucleus arrangement, the axis contains the nucleus arrangement of the dens (axis), which is markedly larger than the nucleus of the body.

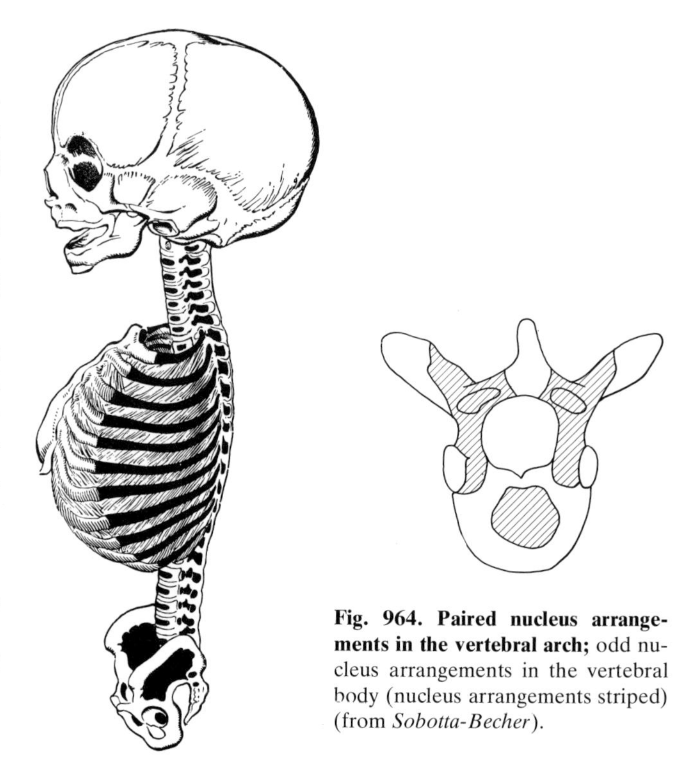

Fig. 964. Paired nucleus arrangements in the vertebral arch; odd nucleus arrangements in the vertebral body (nucleus arrangements striped) (from *Sobotta-Becher*).

Fig. 963. Human fetus in the 7th fetal month. Osseous nuclei black, drawn from a transparent slide (according to *Spanner,* from *Benninghoff-Goerttler*).

During the 2nd and 3rd years of life, an additional bone nucleus originates at the apex of the dens in the form of a plate-like epiphysis, the origin of which is not completely clear. It is probably a residue of a rudimentary vertebra in the last occipital segment. This bone nucleus unites with the dens during the 12th year of life. For views on the development of the dens, see *Jenkins.*

According to *Probst,* there are two contradictory opinions regarding the form of the ossification of the vertebral arches; both enchondral and perichondral ossifications are possible. *Töndury* is of the opinion that there is only an enchondral nucleus, namely, in the vertebral body. The vertebral arches ossify in the perichondral. According to *Töndury,* an open fossa may already appear in the mesenchymal stage in the vertebral arch. If there is a mesenchymal gap, the tensile stress necessary for the os-

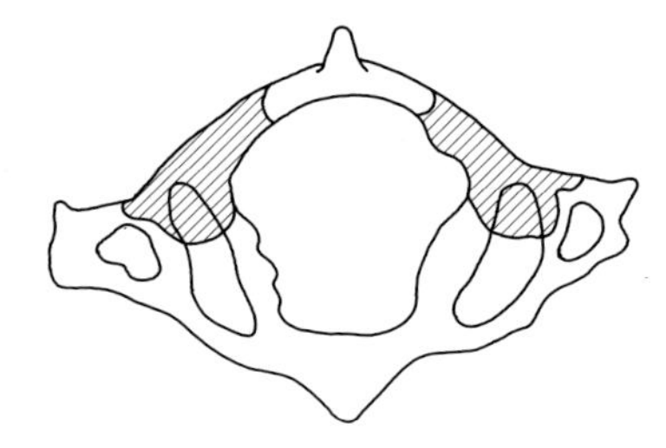

Fig. 962. Paired nucleus arrangements in the posterior arch of the atlas (nucleus arrangements striped).

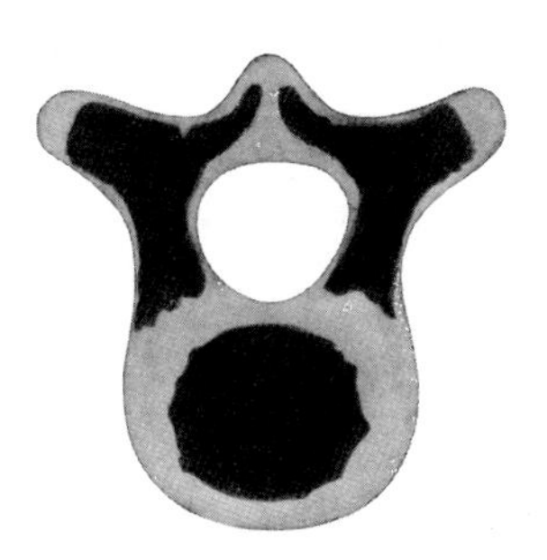

Fig. 965. Glycerine potassium slide (bone dark, cartilage light; 1/1). **Lumbar vertebra of a child, at the end of the 1st year of life** (from *Sobotta-Becher*).

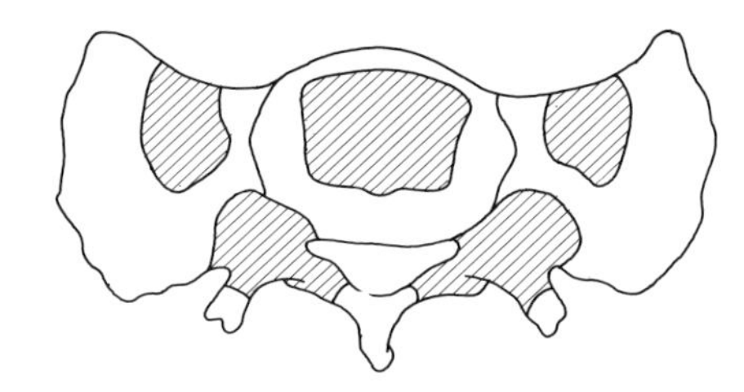

Fig. 966. Nucleus anlage (hatched) **in the region of the sacral vertebra.** Near the paired nucleus anlage in the arch region and the single nucleus anlage in the vertebrae body, a paired nucleus anlage in the lateral part (sacral vertebral) is found.

sification becomes ineffectual and therefore the ossification may not occur.

The arched spinal column is bridged, not by bones, but by a tense ligature (see also *Diethelm, Schinz* and *Töndury, Junghanns* and *Schmorl-Junghanns).*

In about the 5th lunar month, the development of the spinal column is very well advanced and a further differentiation of the single vertebral sections, especially the formation of the transverse process, begins to take place.

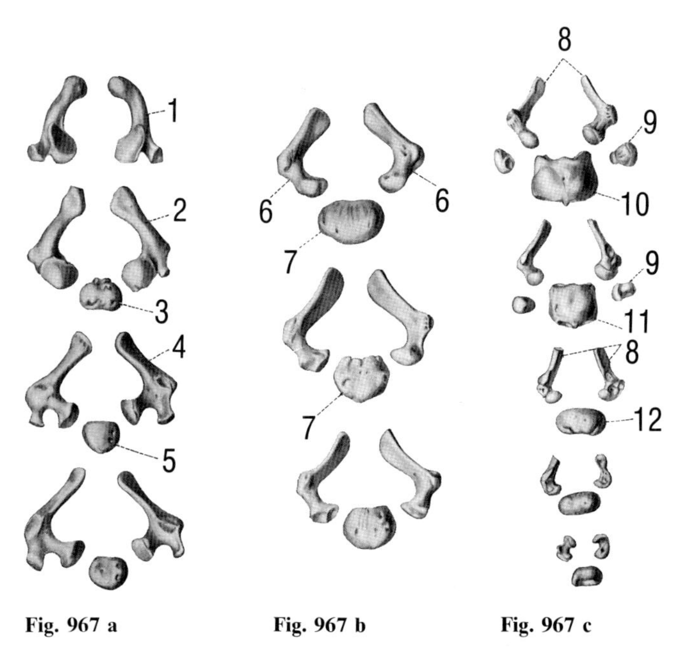

Fig. 967. Segment (bones) of the macerated spinal column of a newborn (from *Sobotta-Becher*).

a) First four cervical vertebrae
   1 Posterior arch (atlantis)
   2 Arch of the axis
   3 Axial body
   4 Arch
   5 3rd cervical vertebral body
b) Three lumbar vertebrae
   6 Six arched vertebrae (lumbar)
   7 Seven vertebral bodies (lumbar)
c) Five sacral vertebrae
   8 Eight arches
   9 Nine rudimentary ribs
   10 1st sacral vertebral body
   11 2nd sacral vertebral body
   12 3rd sacral vertebral body

In the second half of pregnancy, the formation of the nucleus arrangement occurs in the sacral vertebra in the lateral parts; the individual sacral vertebrae are formed out of five osseous nuclei (Fig. 966).

As early as the end of the 3rd fetal month, *Köhler* (in *Köhler-Zimmer)* found three osseous nuclei in the sacral vertebrae parallel to the nucleus arrangement in the lumbar vertebrae. In newborns, the bodies of all five, the arches of the first four and the rudimentary ribs of the first two sacral vertebrae are ossified (Fig. 967).

About the 12th year of life, the superior and inferior peripheral inguinal annular nuclei appear on radiographs (Fig. 968). The osseous fusion of the bodies of the sacral vertebrae begins about the 6th year of life towards the caudal vertebra, and terminates with a synostosis of the first two sacral vertebrae between the 25th and 30th years of life. The fusion of the arch of the sacral vertebrae takes place between the 15th and 18th years of life.

The coccyx shows only one ossification nucleus for each segment (4–6), of which the 1st segment appears during the 1st year of life, and in some cases even shortly before birth. Then, during the 4th and 9th years of life, the 9th and 13th years and the 14th and 18th years, the 2nd, 3rd and 4th (up to the 6th) coccygeal vertebrae ossify. They may undergo a synostosis.

The **Spinal Column of a Newborn** (Fig. 967) in the frontal radiograph (Fig. 974) shows only one frontal concave curving. Cervical and lumbar curvings follow only later, according to actual weight-bearing. The intervertebral spaces at first appear almost as high as the vertebral bodies. In a side view, they show an explicit oviduct configuration (Fig. 974). During growth, the length of the distance between the nuclei of the vertebral bodies is constantly reduced. In this way, a more nearly square profile of the vertebra, usually reached in the 1st or 2nd year of life, develops gradually from the oviform vertebra.

The **Fillet of the Vertebral Body and the Apophysis of the Vertebral Processes.** The fillet of the vertebral body, which is at first cartilagenous, develops between the 6th and 9th years of life. At the vertebral edge, a step-like space exists, which is filled in from the 10th year of life onwards by the ossified fillet. It occurs in all the vertebral bodies except for the atlas, axis and coccyx. In addition, during puberty a secondary formation of apophyses on the spinal process in the region of the vertebral bodies takes place, as well as on the superior and inferior articular processes (Fig. 968).

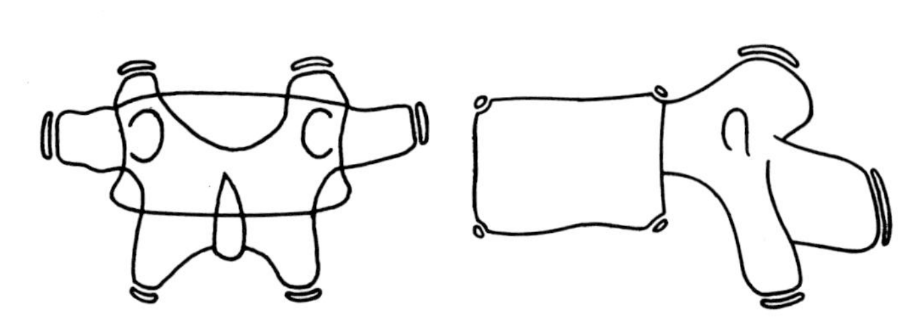

Fig. 968. Vertebral apophyses.

Around the 15th to 17th year of life, the ossified unification of the vertebral body fillet and the apophysis of the vertebral processes take place. Usually, it terminates around the 25th year of life. *Junghanns* proved the early frequent indication of "epiphysis of vertebral bodies" to be incorrect. That is, it is a question not of epiphyseal disks but of annular fillets, which have a cartilagenous consistency in the young; later on, they ossify and unite with the vertebral bodies. In females, the synostosis of the fillet and the apophyseal vertebral process begins a bit earlier than in males. The annular fillet has no relationship to the growth of the vertebral bodies. This begins from the end-plates of the intervertebral disk *(Köhler-Zimmer).* The apophysis of the vertebra or vertebral arched processes, which are also called sesamoid bone nucleus, have a chronologically anticipated and a more irregular development than the fillets of the vertebral bodies *(Schmorl-Junghanns).*

Arches End. The fusion of the two separate half arches continues in the second half of the 1st year of life in the region of the lumbar spine and proceeds towards the cranium. By the end of the 2nd year, the vertebral arches are fused up to the atlas; the osseous fusion of the posterior arches takes place only during the 3rd year of life.

The fusion of the vertebral arches with the vertebral bodies begins between the 4th and 6th years of life. At the same time, the osseous fusion of the dens (axis) with the body of the 2nd cervical vertebra takes place. Likewise during this time span, the lateral parts fuse with the sacral vertebral bodies. The frontal arch termination in the atlas then follows from the 7th to 9th years of life.

The Connecting Vessels of the Vertebral Bodies. In lateral and, less frequently, in sagittal radiographs, vertebral bodies of children and adolescents show a characteristic lightened ligament, which passes horizontally through the center of the vertebra. *Hahn,* who first described this fissure-like inlet in the frontal edge of the vertebral body, with its ligament progress, thought it to be a nutrient foramen. In fact, they are communicating vessel canals known as *"Hahn's* fissures." These canals are traceable in adults, too. This finding has no pathological implication in adults *(Lyon).* In a check using the *Balz* and *Birkner* method, there was no connection between *Hahn's* fissures in the adult and osteoporosis. *Hanson* found the canal formations most roomy in those vertebrae which were most frequently tuberculosis-ridden; however, he does not attribute any pathogenic meaning to these vertebrae.

The Hyoid Bone. The ossification of the hyoid bone is found in some 75.2% of newborns, according to *Tompsett* and *Donaldson*'s studies of lateral radiographs of the cervical spinal column.

Form Variations. Modifications in the shadow density of the intervertebral space may occur through masses outside the spinal column which are projected by chance in the spinal column and simulate the intervertebral disk calcification (lung shadow mass). Pure calcification of intervertebral disks in children has been described by *Marx, Walker, Silverman* and others. These calcifications may either persist or disappear.

Regarding their etiology, birth traumas, other traumas which lead to bleeding, infections, D-hypervitaminosis, neurological affection, etc. are discussed.

Various form variations of the vertebrae can be attributed to early phases of childhood or even fetal life, according to *Seyss.* Inhibitory malformations may occur, depending on pathological processes and pre- and postnatal influences. These are traceable by means of ventral vertebral sides. Through the joint influence of further complications, the formation of the beak-like form takes place as observed in chondrodystrophy dysostosis multiplex *(Pfaundler-Hurler),* osteochondrodystrophy *(Morquio-Brailsford)* and myxedema. Without pathological etiology, it is possible to see in the progressive growth of a child's vertebral body, a cone deformation caused by the fact that every layer of the vertebral body stimulates the development of another. In a further follow-up of the growth, these deformed vertebrae later showed a normal configuration (Figs. 969, 970, 974–996 and 998–1000).

An extraordinary anomaly in the middle of the vertebral body appears as a cylinder-like running stripe of residual chorda tissues connected to the two neighboring intervertebral disks *(Lossen).*

Since the spinal column shows no original fusion but is composed of the vertebral body line and the vertebral arch line, which usually fuse by the 14th week of fetal life *(Rowley),* a distinction must be made between anomalies, variations of form and malformations of the vertebral bodies and the vertebral arches *(Kirchhoff* and *Rohwedder).* Teratological modifications originate in the earliest termination period. Since these malformations can remain formless during the developmental process, frequently unclear and complex images are created (see *Murczynski* and *Uniecka, Burrows).*

Likewise, for the measurement of malformations the termination period is of major significance. It is early applied and occurs in the period between gastrulation and neurulation. The articulation of the segmentation material is under the control of the chorda, where the influence of the form originates from two "guide rails," chorda dorsalis and neural tube *(Kirchhoff* and *Rohwedder).*

Block vertebrae with only a partial fusion in the frontal sections or with totally extended fusion of several vertebrae (Fig. 467), fissure vertebrae *(Swoboda, Rowley),* hemivertebrae *(Rosenkranz)* and single aplasia of vertebrae are due to malformations of the vertebral bodies.

Sagittal spinal process fissures (spina bifida; *Curtius, Cook),* lateral spinal process fissures, fissures of the interarticulated portion and fissures of the arch root *(Runge)* are due to malformations of the vertebral arches; see also Fig. 384.

Partial ventral synostosis of some thoracic and lumbar vertebral bodies, according to *Schuknecht,* is the final phase of an adolescent kyphosis. He presumes this to be an infectious rheumatic condition. Corresponding observations were made by *Knutsson.* It is rather difficult to

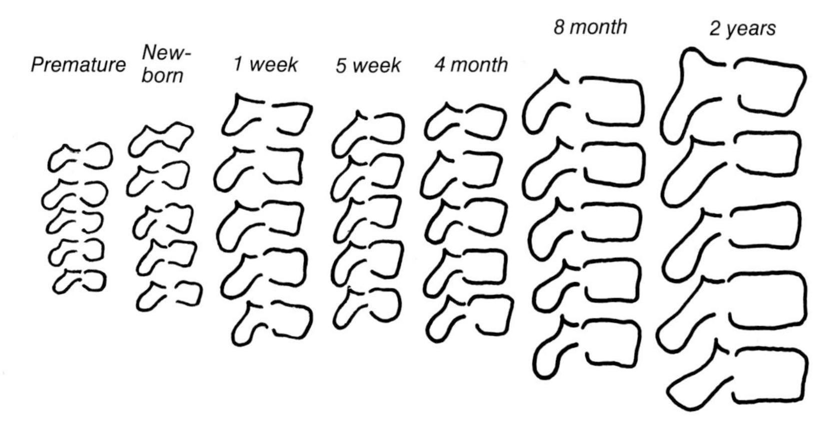

Fig. 969. Development of the spinal column of a premature infant (8-month pregnancy) up to the age of 2 years (from *Seyss*).

fix a limit for the primary malformations. There must be a distinction between congenital block vertebrae and the malformations seen after an illness. Characteristic indications of synostosis are a series of factors, which combined with other vertebral malformations or multiple variations, should be considered as the most important ones.

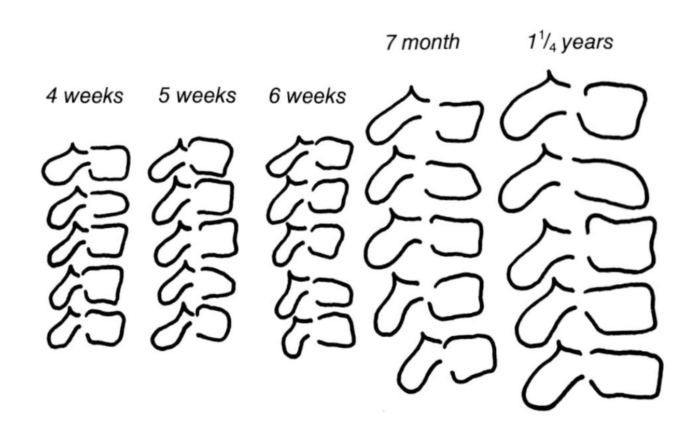

Fig. 970. Conic and parallelogram formation of vertebral bodies through irregular growth. The finding is still to be regarded as normal (from *Seyss)*.

Ribs

The ribs are arranged in pairs and show an osseous nucleus at the vertebral extremity of the rib as early as the end of the 2nd fetal month. The enchondral ossification proceeds rapidly towards the sternum, though without reaching it. In the 4th month, the permanent ratio between the ribs and the cartilage has already been reached. The sternal extremities of the ribs remain as rib cartilage. During puberty the ribs have two ossification nuclei, i.e., an apophysis on the rib head and an apophysis on the costal tubercle (Fig. 997). The fusion of these two nuclei occurs between the 20th and 24th years of life. Rather frequently the 12th rib presents a different formation of the apophysis nucleus. Therefore, the nuclei can be absent in either one or both sides. Very frequently an asymmetric formation of the length of the rib is present in the 12th rib. For further rib anomalies and variations, see Figures 355, 364, 365, and 368 and Figures 335 a, b, 361–363, 366 a, b, 367, 369, 371, 372, 374 and 375.

The costal cartilage edge is clinically rather meaningful because it shows especially clearly a rachitic swelling (rachitic "rosary") *(Gersten* and *Lecomte-Ramioul)*.

Sternum

The development of the cartilagenous preformed sternum originates out of numerous nuclei, in which the superior nuclei appear first and the inferior ones later. Before the 6th fetal month only one osseous nucleus appears, while all the others, with the exception of the nucleus of the xiphoid, appear later (between the 6th fetal month and birth, and only then as an exception). The osseous nucleus in the sternal manubrium appears at the beginning of the 6th fetal month fairly regularly. Sometimes two to three smaller nuclei appear in addition. The sternal body ossifies from numerous, frequently paired nuclei (6–13 nuclei); in Figure 972 this even occurs in a 6-year-old child. These first fuse among themselves, and in the young form a segmented sternum, consisting of 3 to 5 osseous segments (Figs. 971, 972).

The osseous nuclei are frequently arranged asymmetrically. About the 12th (and more often about the 16th) year of life, the segments fuse to form a sternum, which every now and then shows transverse grooves up to the 25th or 26th year of life. It is only after the 30th year of life that the segments of the body grow and fuse completely.

No fusion of the sternal body and the manubrium occurs. These two parts remain connected only by means of cartilage throughout the life span. Synchondrosis becomes synostosis in only some 10% of the cases, and only after the 50th year of life. This synostosis superior lies at the level of the 2nd rib ring. Around the 6th year of life, an osseous nucleus originates in the region of the xiphoid process. The fusion of the xiphoid process with the sternal body takes place a long time after puberty, in about the 3rd or 4th decade. Therefore, the formation of the xiphoid process is subject to an extraordinarily large number of forms. For variations and anomalies, see Figures 336 and 341 and *Pfeiffer*.

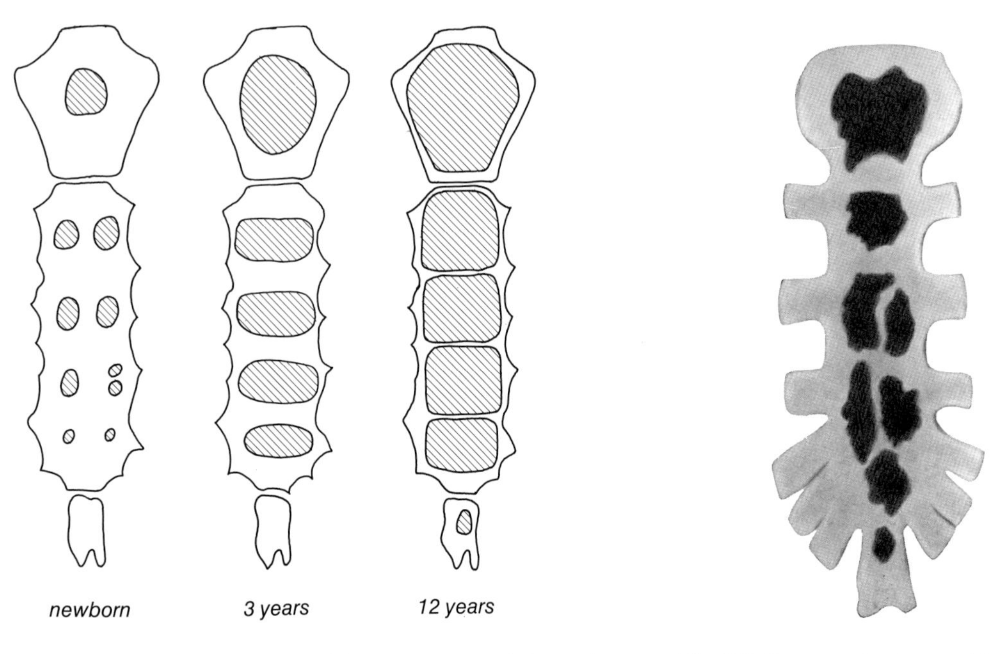

Fig. 971. The usual development of the sternum from birth to puberty.

Fig. 972. Sternum of a 6-year-old child. Potassium glycerine prepared slide (bones dark, cartilage light; from *Sobotta-Becher*).

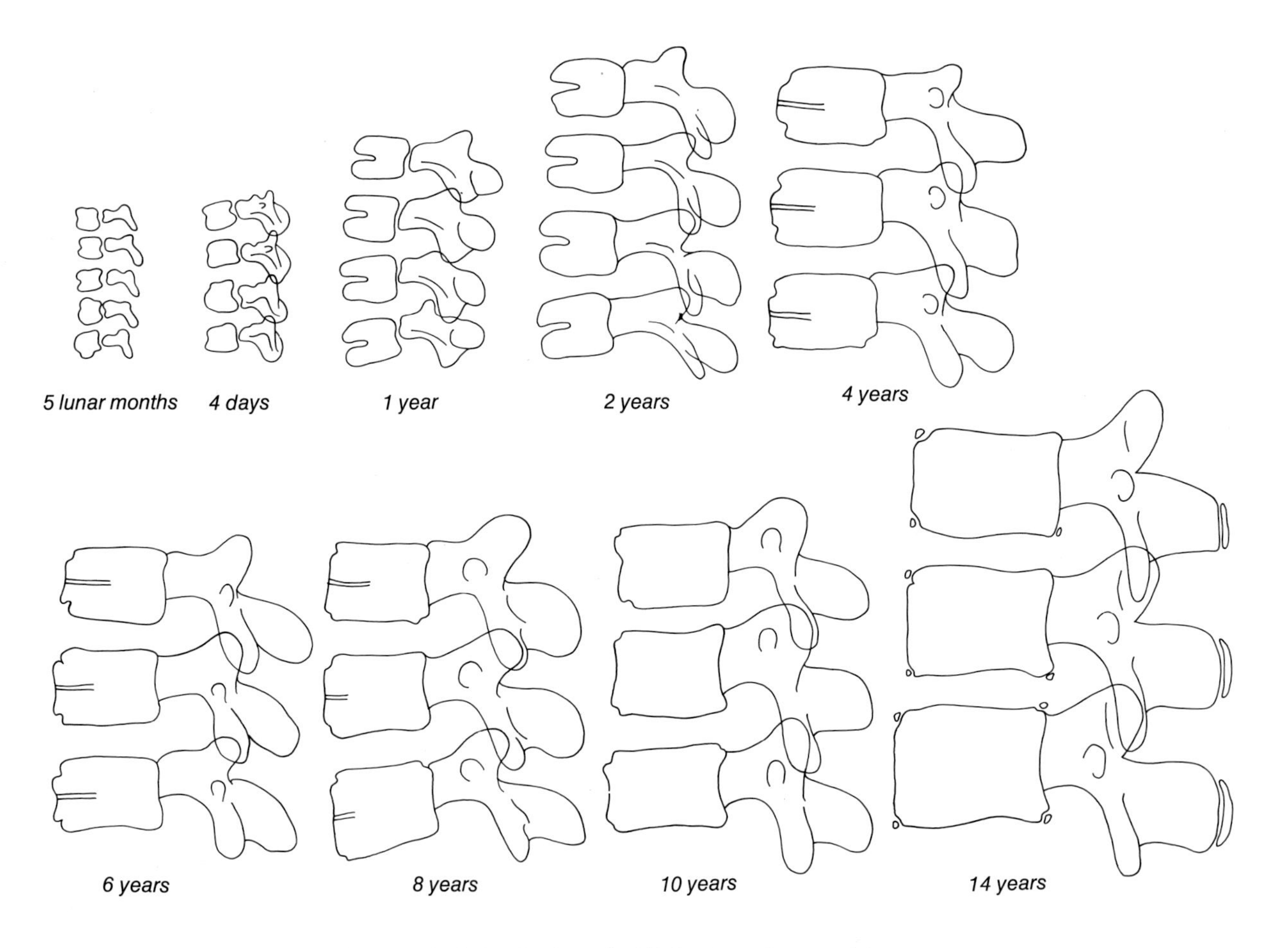

Fig. 973. Spinal column sections in chronological order from the 5th fetal month to age 14.

A Series of Radiographs of the Development of the Spinal Column from Infancy to Age 19

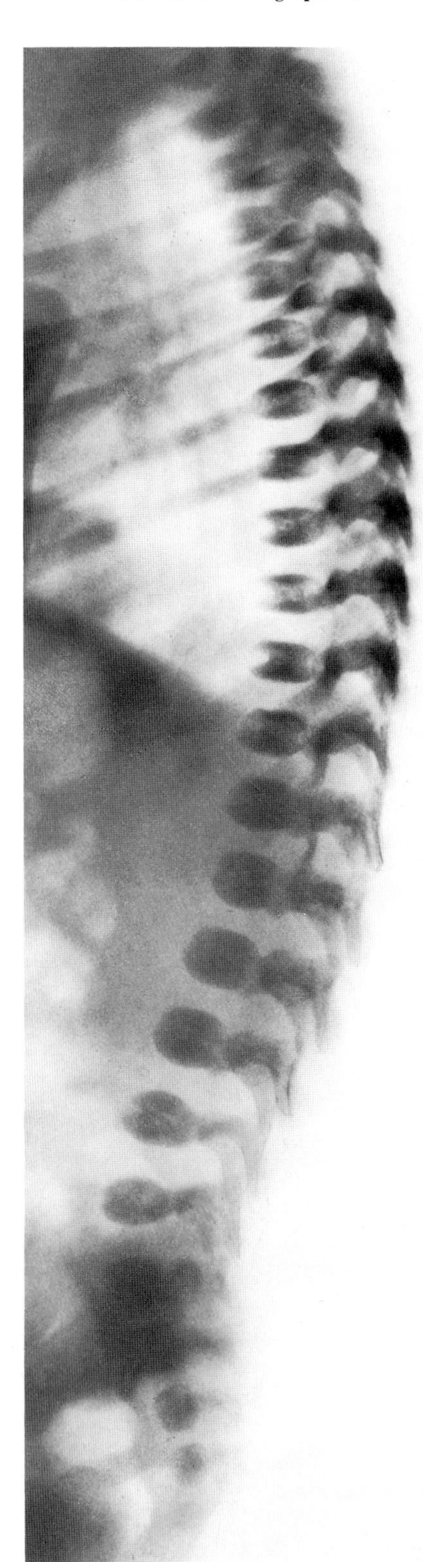

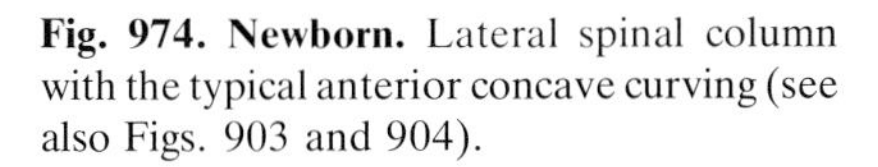

Fig. 974. Newborn. Lateral spinal column with the typical anterior concave curving (see also Figs. 903 and 904).

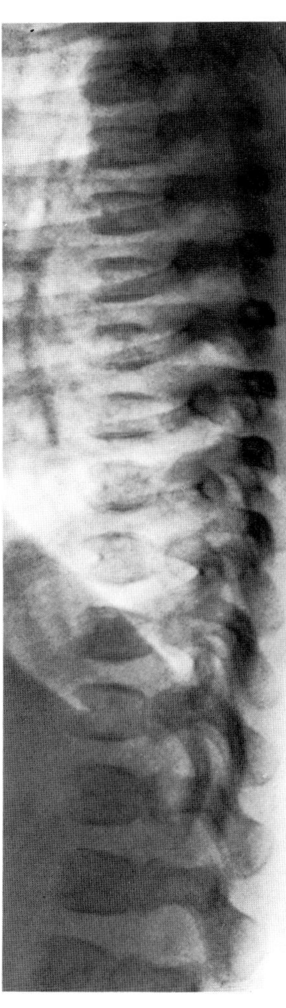

Fig. 975. 3 ½ month old. Figs. 974 and 975 show the characteristic oviferous form with the horizontal opaque stripe in the middle of the vertebral body and the cartilagenous articulation at the vertebral arch root. The wide intervertebral spaces here are filled with dense intervertebral disks. In the center of the disk lies the disk-like, gelatinous nucleus cavity, which replaces the chorda dorsalis with its segments of the fetal period *(Töndury)*.

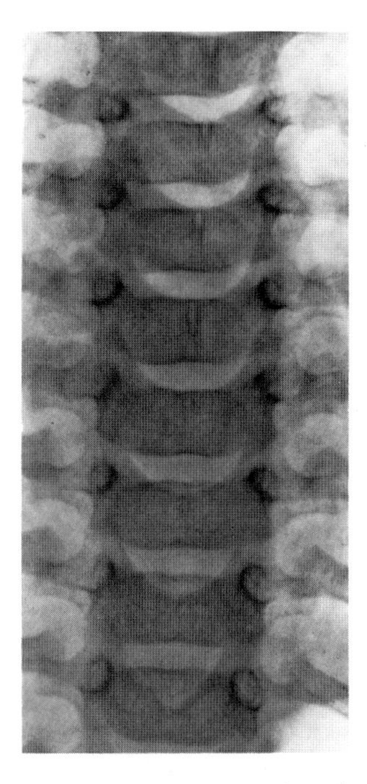

Fig. 976. 7 month old. Thoracic spinal column, anteroposterior.

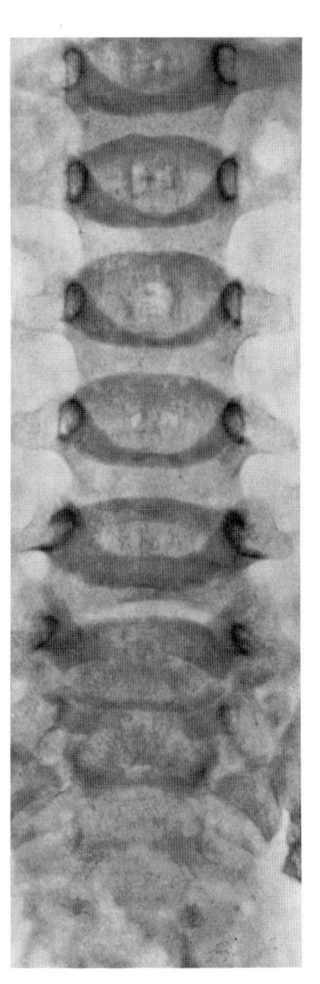

Fig. 977. 7 month old. Lumbar spinal column, anteroposterior.

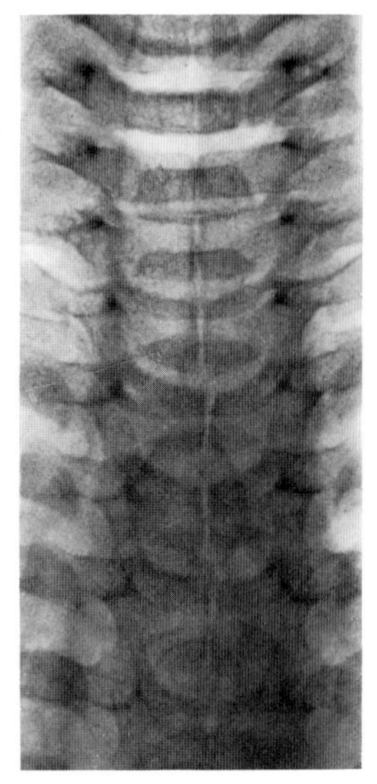

Fig. 978. 1 year old. Medial opaque stripe in the arches (see also Fig. 1030).
Since *Töndury* rejects the accepted theory of two symmetrical osseous nuclei in both halves of the arch and asserts that the ossification of the curving is not endochondral but perichondral, a medial fissure formation in incomplete arch termination is only optional. The fissure formations lie paramedially in the posterior or anterior arch section; this cannot be explained by means of enchondral or perichondral ossification *(Wolfers* and *Hoeffken)*.

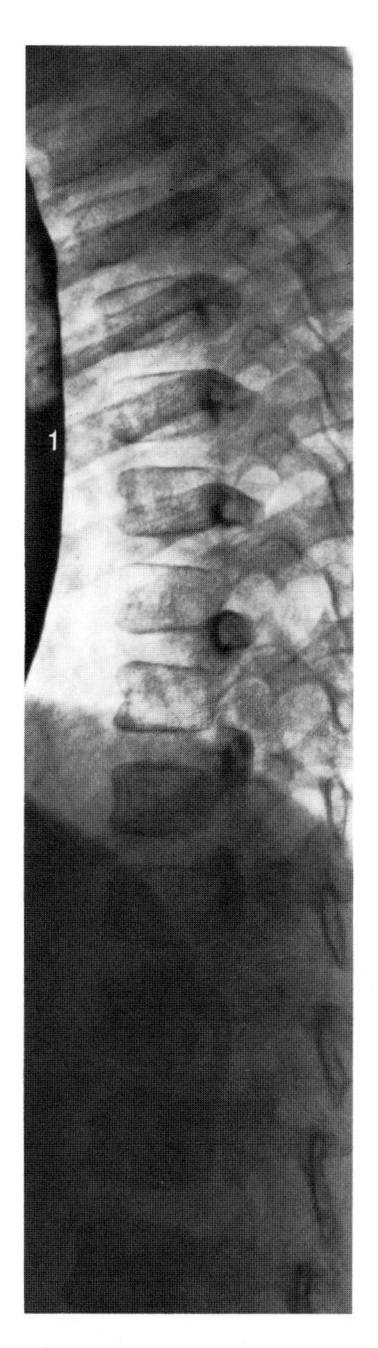

Fig. 979. 18 month old. Thoracic spine, lateral. 1 = esophagus *(Breischluck)*.

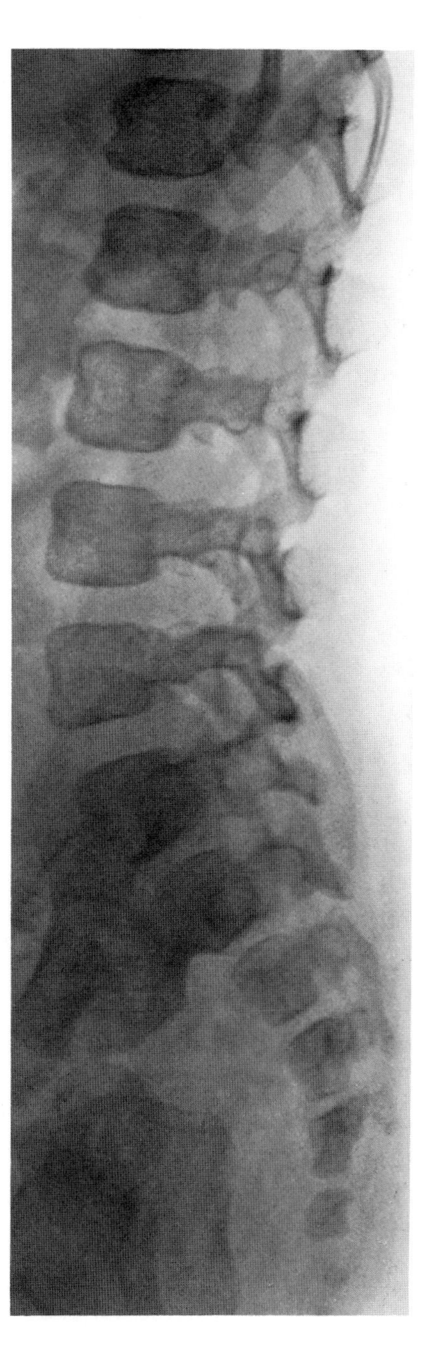

Fig. 980. 18 month old. Lumbar spine with sacral and coccygeal vertebrae, lateral.

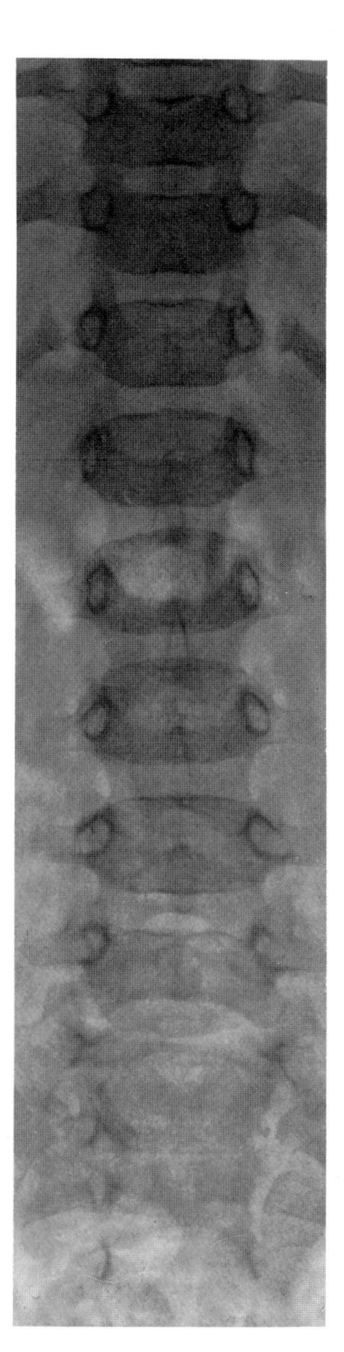

Fig. 981. 18 month old. Lumbar spine, anteroposterior.

Thoracic vertebrae are still partly oviferous; lumbar vertebrae are already in a box-like form. In Fig. 980 it is still possible to see a cartilagenous articulation in the vertebrae arch root on a few lumbar vertebrae. Some inferior thoracic and superior lumbar vertebrae very clearly show a ventral notch of *Hahn*'s communicating vascular grooves. The very slightly curved, almost straight spinal column with the limited lordotic curving in the lumbosacral angle is still normal in children. The erect position forces the spinal column into two S-like curves (see pp. 352–353). Later, there is a stretching only in the region of the lumbar spine pathologically; in the cervical region the erect position in juveniles is normal *(Buetti)* and present in almost every other case.

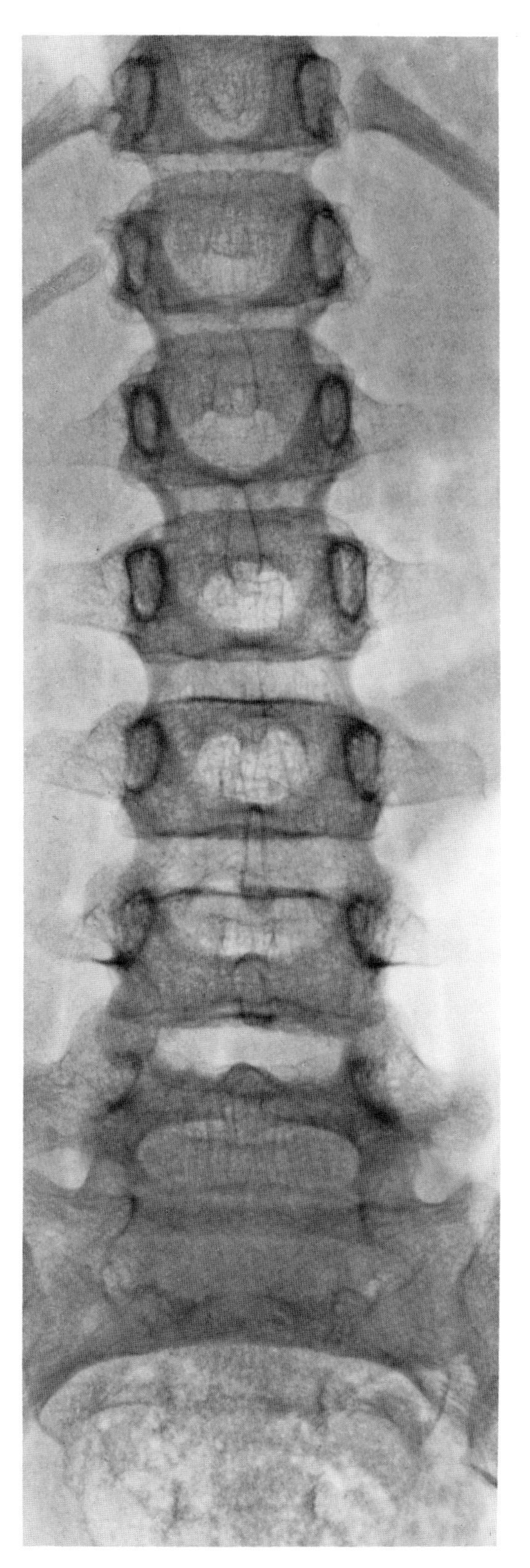

Fig. 982

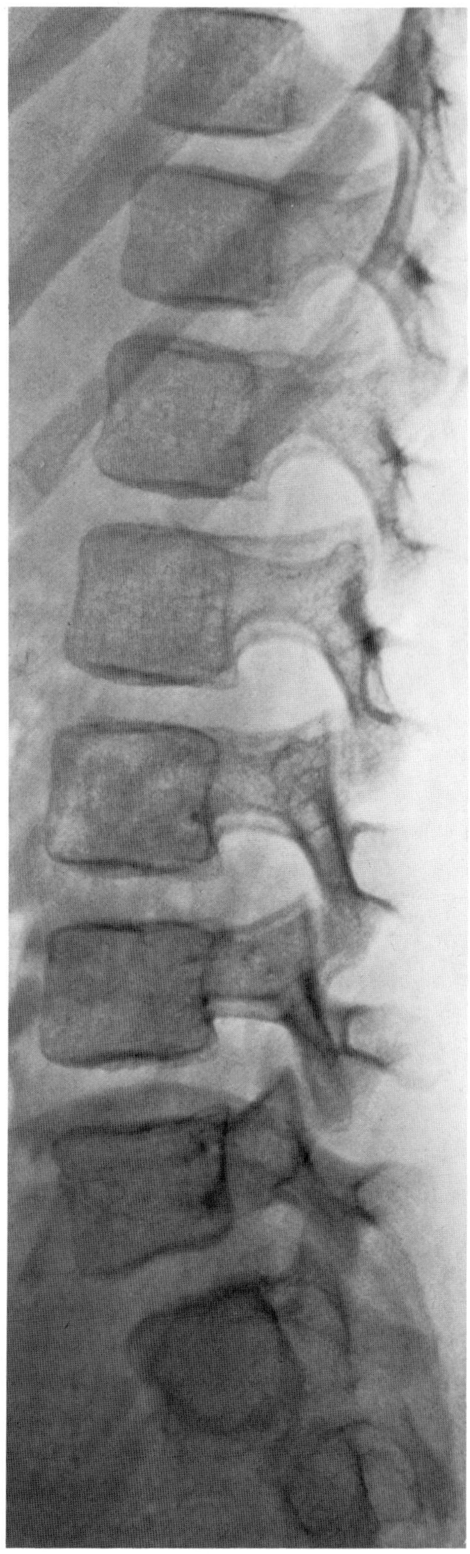

Fig. 983

Fig. 982 and 983. 4 year old. Lumbar spine and superior sacral vertebrae, anteroposterior and lateral. Only the right rib is connected to the 12th thoracic vertebra, though hypoplastic. Instead of the rib, only a bud-like transverse process is seen. In addition, there is a fissure formation in S-1, probably with a complete arch aplasia: may be an inherited inhibited malformation of the whole arch or only a retarded arch development in the lumbosacral passage, where the arch development occurs in the last phase. In this region, there are open fissures or wide breaches: "fontanella lumbosacralis" *(Hintze)* in up to 81% of cases during the 5th year of life and up to 44% during the 15th year.

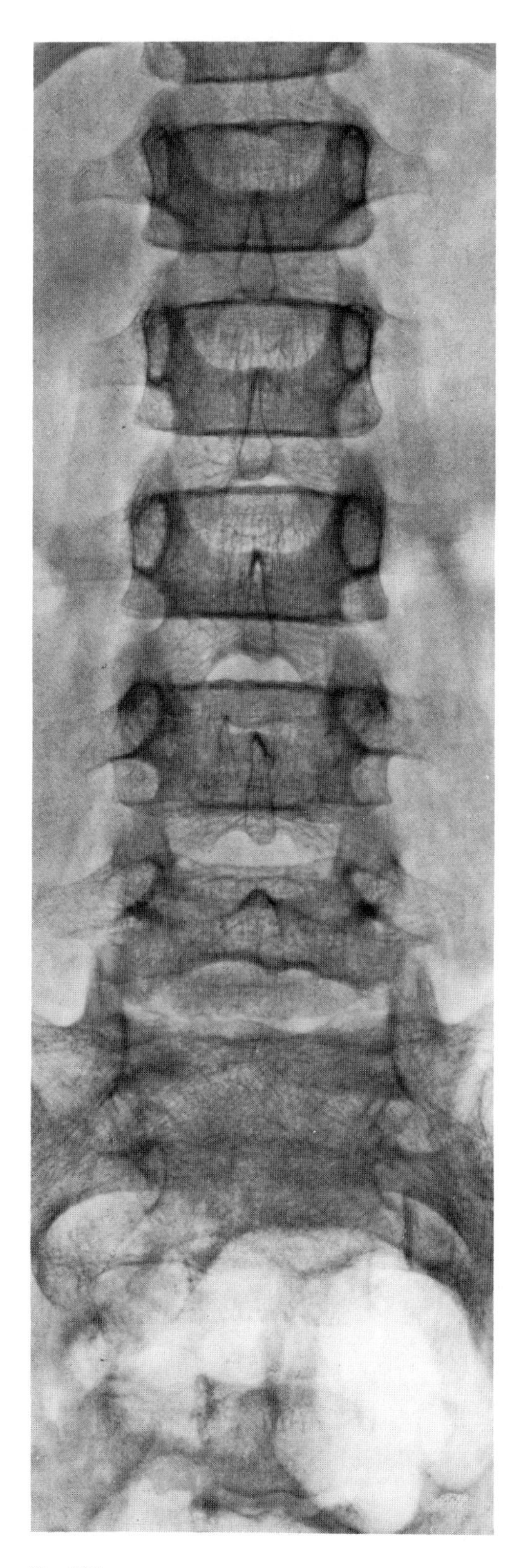

Fig. 984

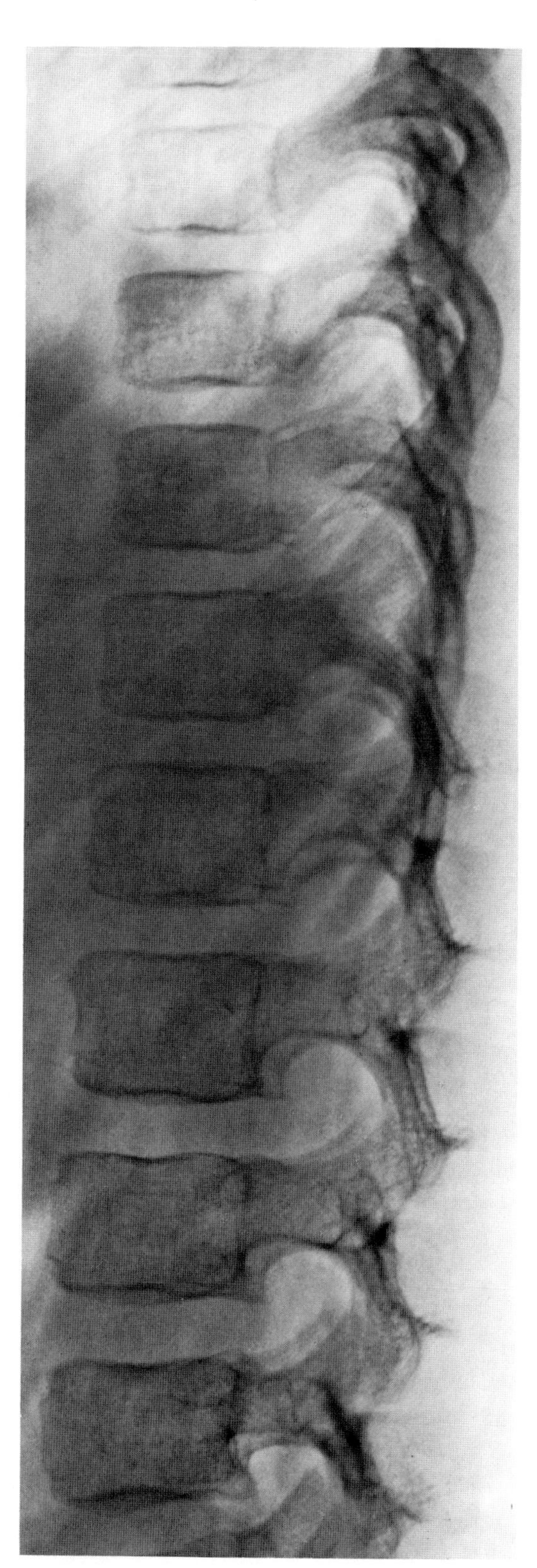

Fig. 985

Figs. 984 and 985. 5 year old. Lumbar spine, anteroposterior; inferior thoracic vertebrae and lumbar spine lateral. In the forefront, the step formation in the front vertebral body edges may be seen like the beginning of the vertebral body fillet (around the 6th to 8th years of life, final termination at age 15). While the spinal processes of the five lumbar vertebrae stand out clearly, there are not even rudimentary sacral vertebrae. From S-2 onwards, there is an open arch.

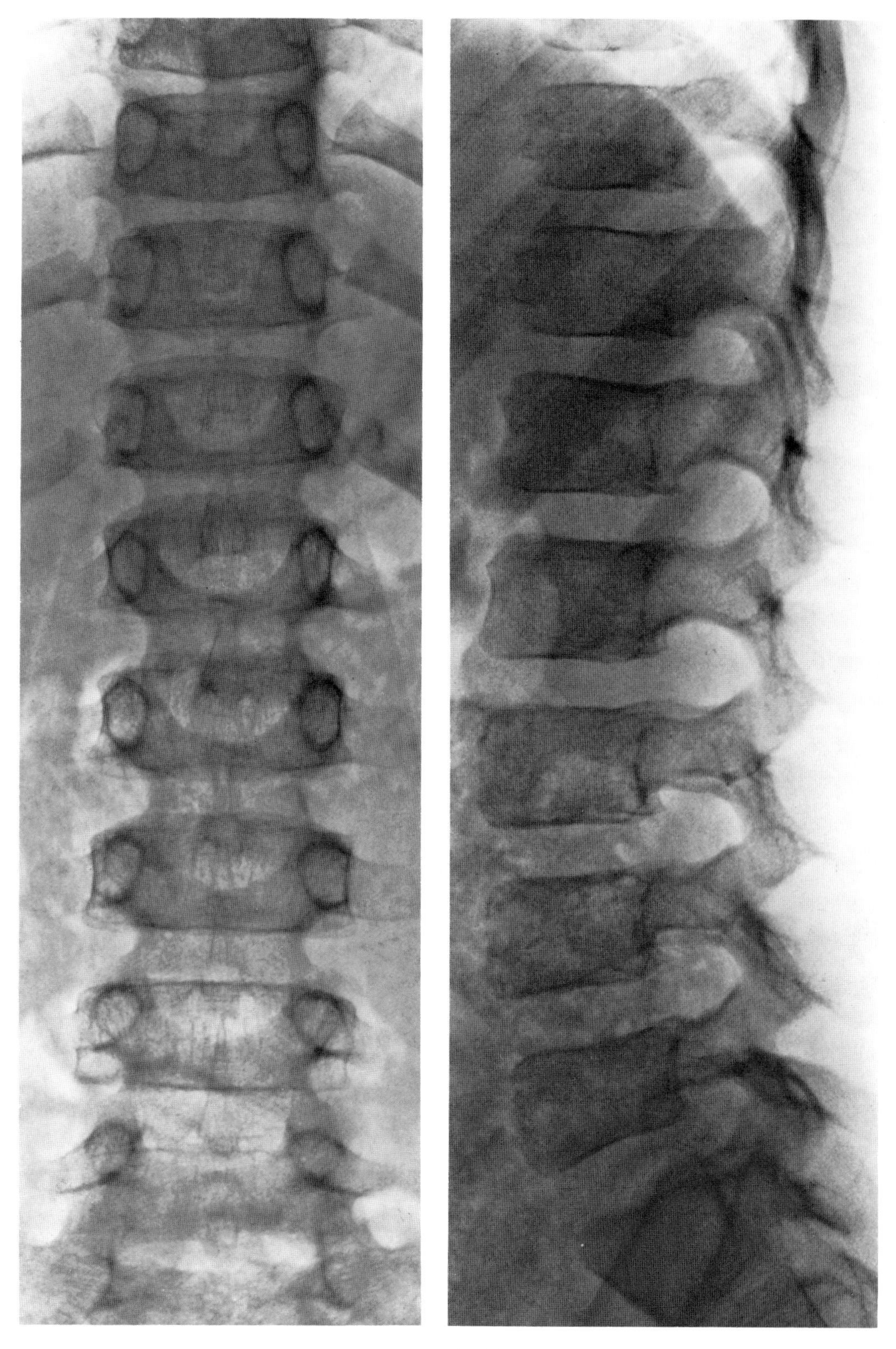

Fig. 986

Fig. 987

Figs. 986 and 987. 6 year old. Inferior thoracic spine and lumbar vertebra, anteroposterior and lateral. The vertebral bodies' fillet arrangement has become clearer; the steps on the vertebral bodies are deepened. The root of the edge is still cartilagenous. Probably strand-like (osteoporotic) structure of the lumbar vertebrae simulated through overloaded contents of intestine.

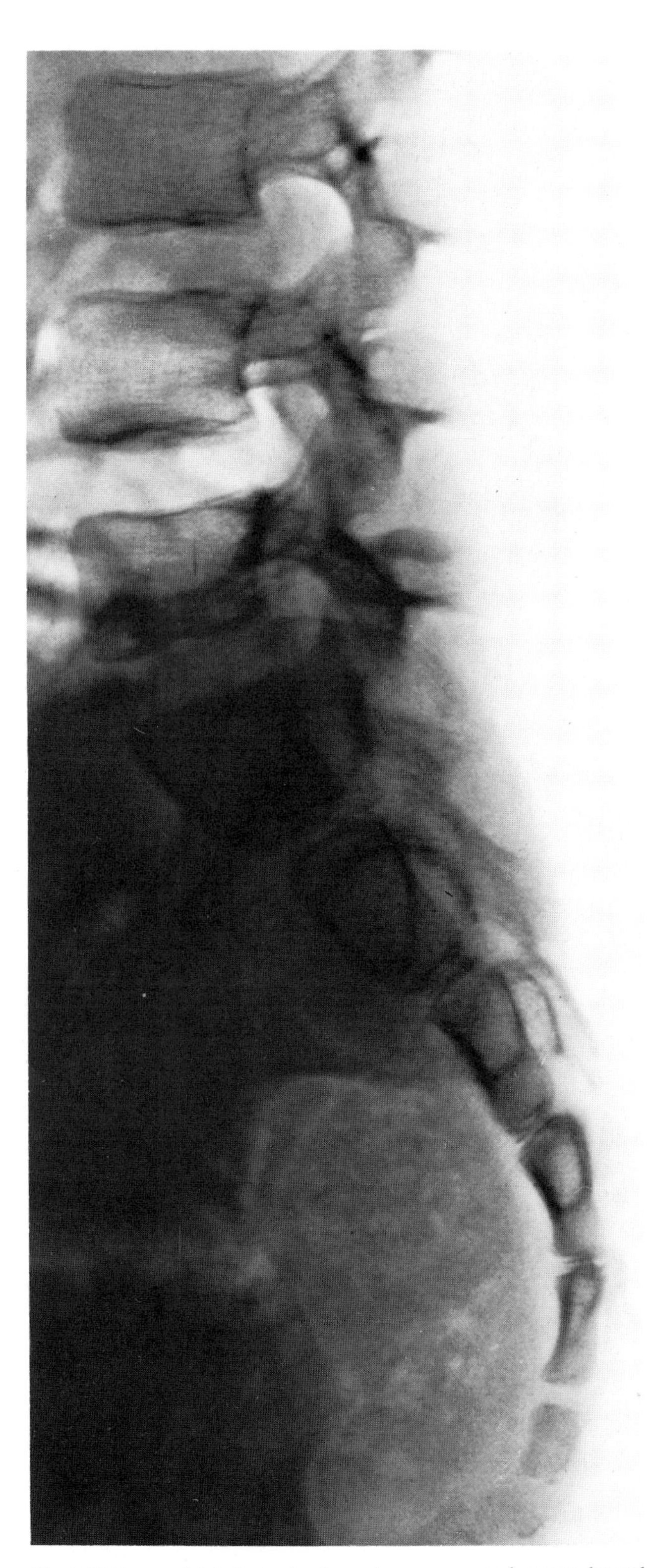

Fig. 988. 7 year old. Inferior lumbar spine, sacrum and coccyx, lateral. The sacrum and coccyx are still separately recognizable.

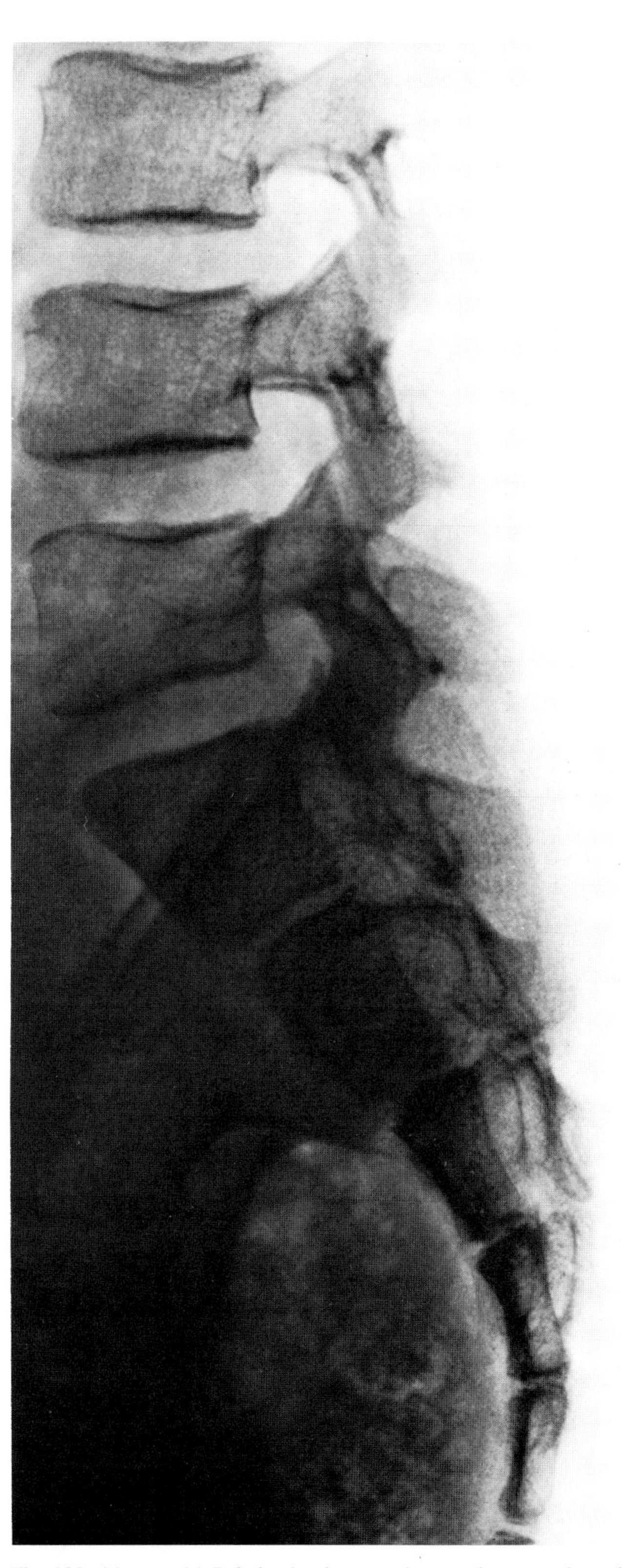

Fig. 989. 14 year old. Inferior lumbar vertebrae and sacrum, lateral. Corresponding to the variations in width, no osseous nuclei can yet be seen in the fillets of the lumbar vertebral bodies (they are usually missing at the coccygeal vertebrae).

If the sacral and coccygeal vertebrae have not ossified (synostosis) but are sometimes cartilagenously connected (synchondrosis), it is still possible to identify them separately in the adult.
Around the 10th to 15th year of life, the sacral fusion begins in a craniocaudal direction, first with the synostosis of the arch and rib processes, then the spinal processes and finally the vertebral bodies. This fusion process ends only around the 30th year of life.

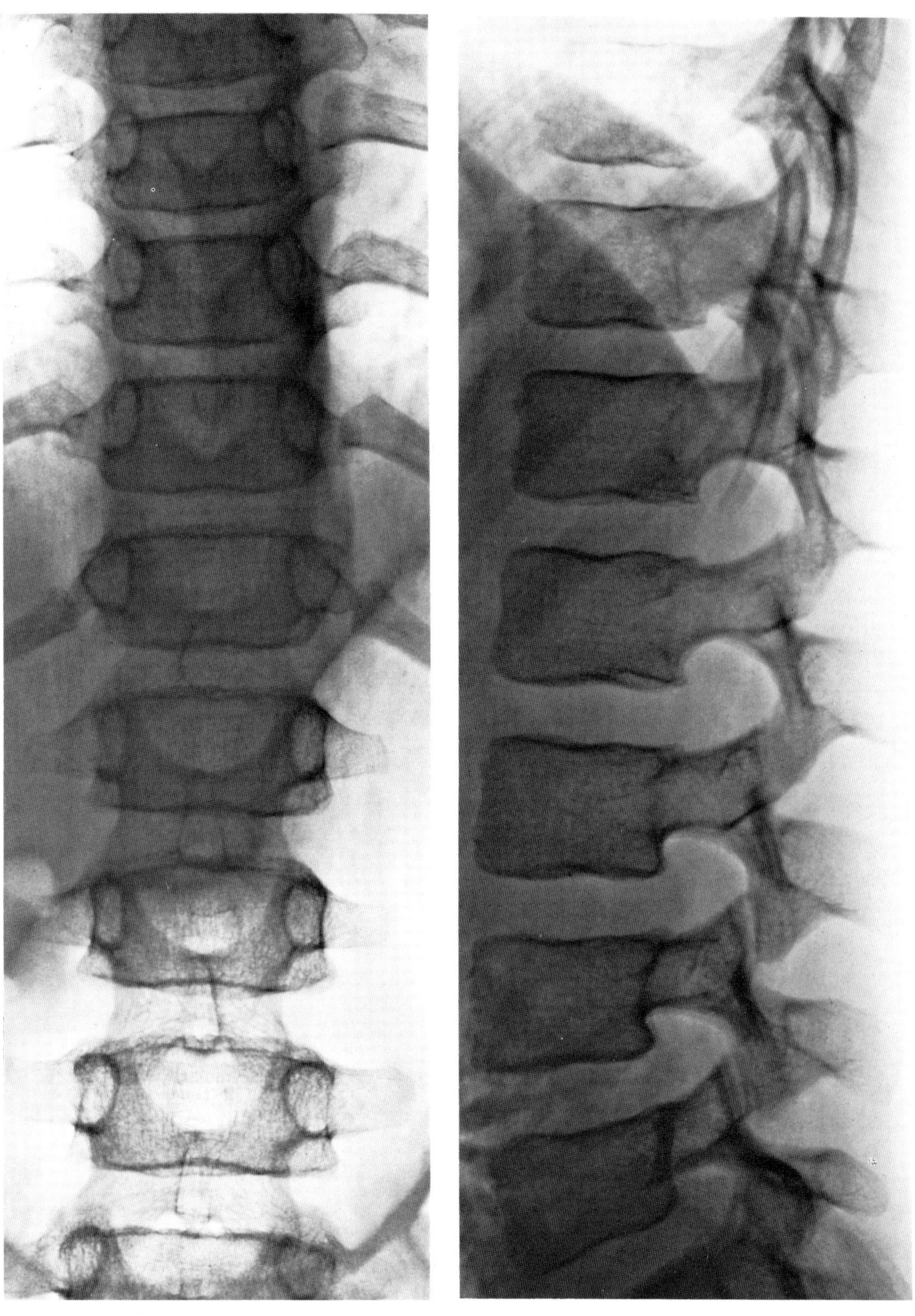

Fig. 990

Fig. 991

Figs. 990 and 991. 8 year old. Inferior thoracic spine and lumbar spine, anteroposterior and lateral. Compared with the adult skeleton, the intervertebral spaces are still high, as the growth in height of the vertebral body begins from the cartilagenous end disk of the intervertebral disk. The fillet arrangement varies in formation; here, it is less clear.

The involution of the blood vessels of the intervertebral disks begins in the small child, so that, in 5 year olds there frequently are no blood vessels in the intervertebral disks. From the early involution of vascularization, one can draw the conclusion of early degeneration processes. Frequently, even in juveniles, there are insufficient intervertebral disks, especially in the thoracic spine.

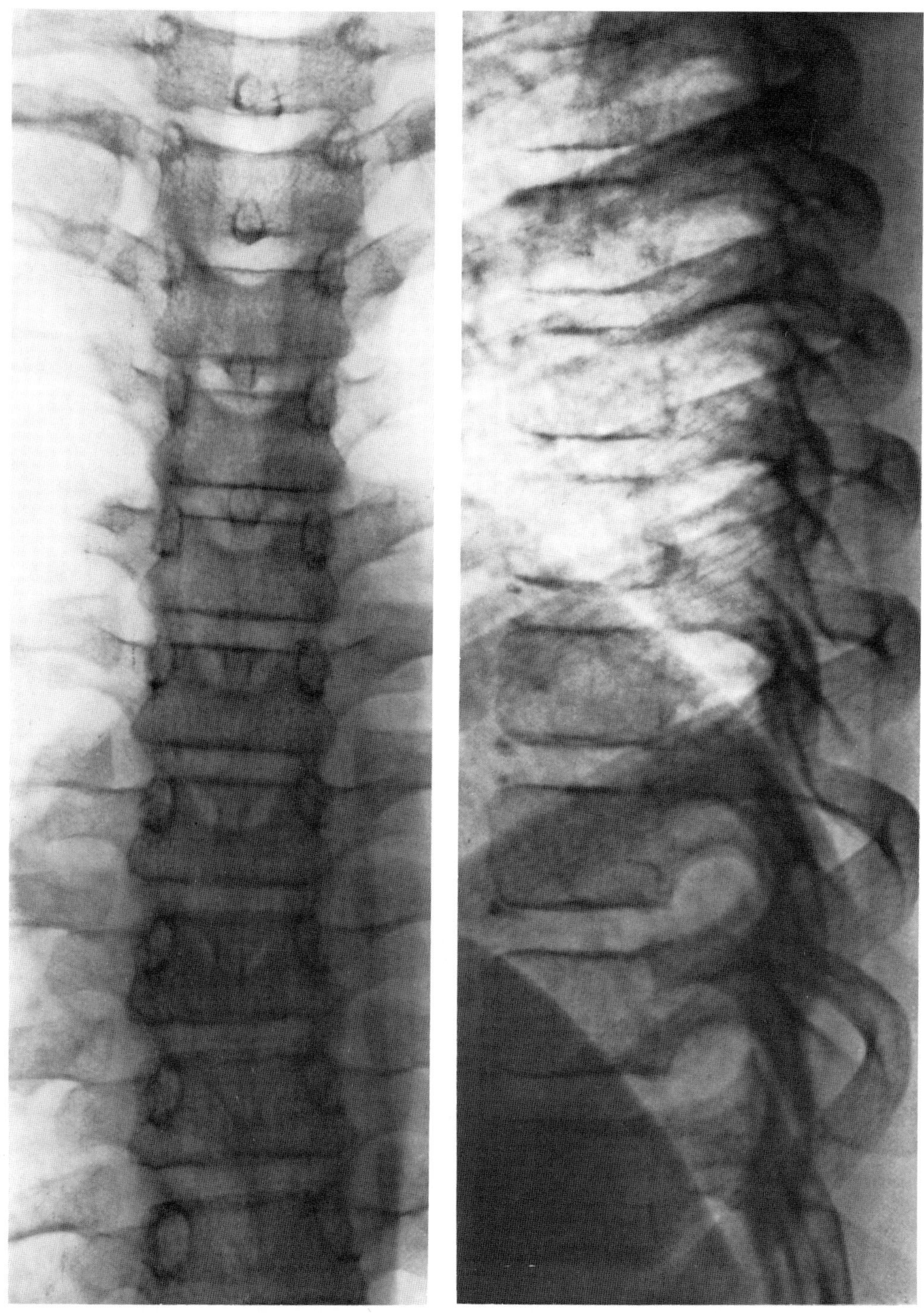

Fig. 992

Fig. 993

Figs. 992 and 993. 11 year old. Thoracic spines, anteroposterior and lateral. The vertebral fillets are easily traceable because ossification has already started; width variations. On a radiograph this can be seen around the 10th and 11th years, and sometimes even later.

The fusion of the osseous edge with the vertebral body ends at age 25. The later appearance of a dented edge formation comes through degenerative processes in the fibrous ring of the intervertebral disk, which is dented with the fillet.

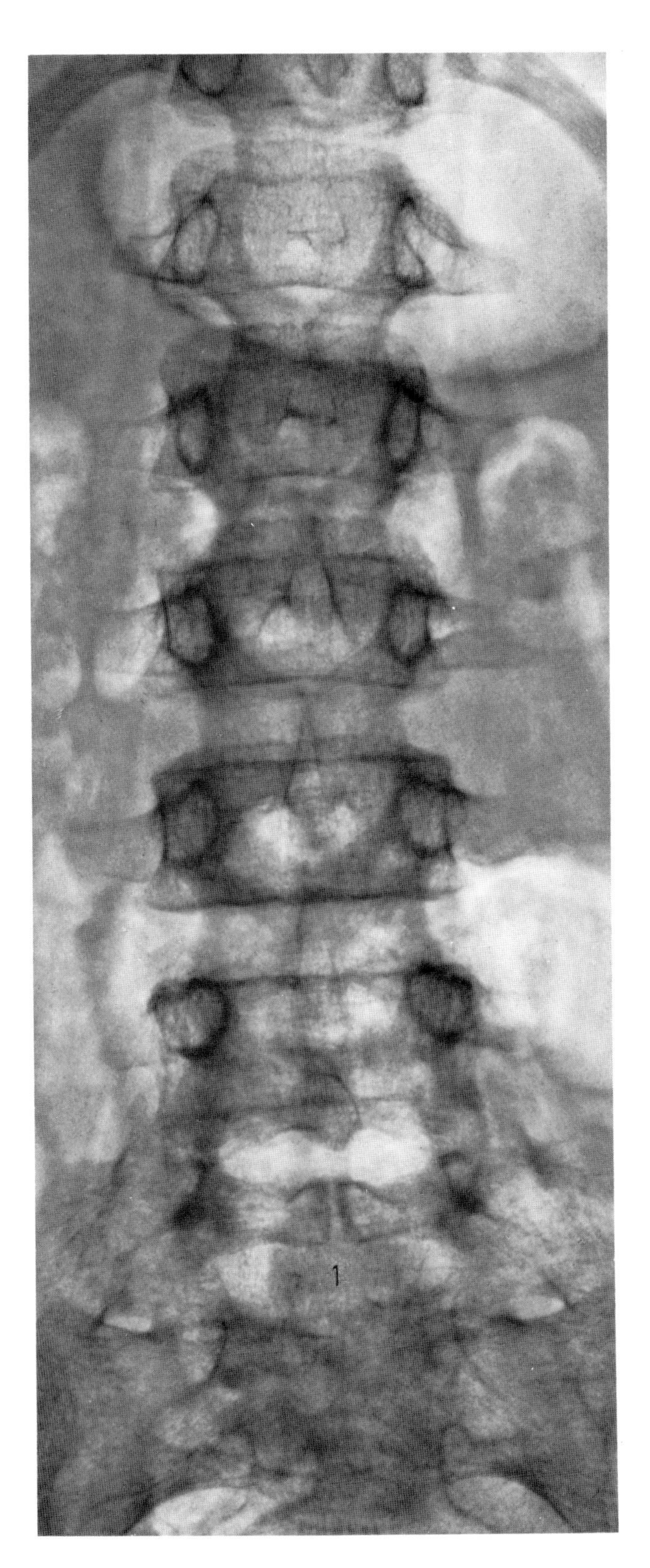

Fig. 994. 11 year old. Lumbar spine, anteroposterior. 1 = still wider curving arch than in S-1. Here, there is a corresponding vertical fissure formation of a so-called "spina bifida occulta," a "harmless variation of the norm." Almost 65% of all healthy children up to the age of 10 have such a "spina bifida occulta" (quoted in Selecta 36, [1971], 2749).

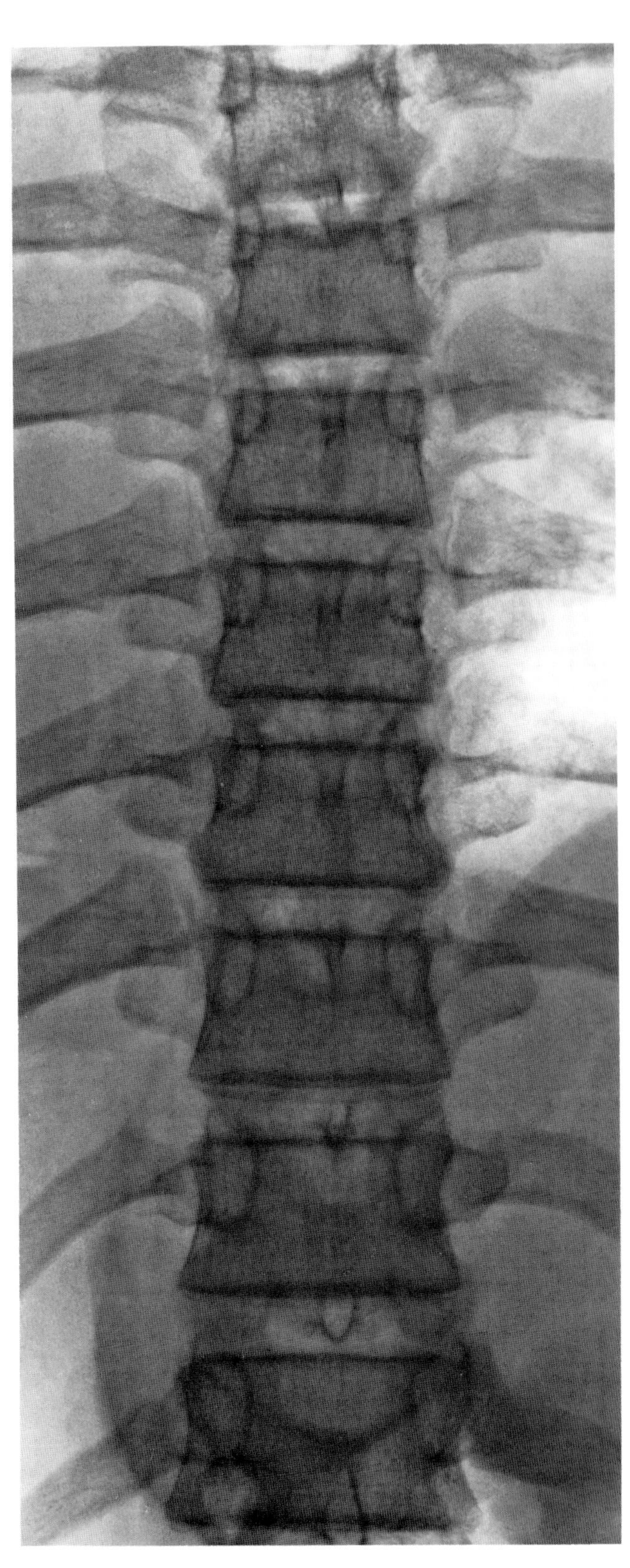

Fig. 995. 13 year old. Thoracic spine, anteroposterior. The vertebral fillets are recognizable as fine rims.

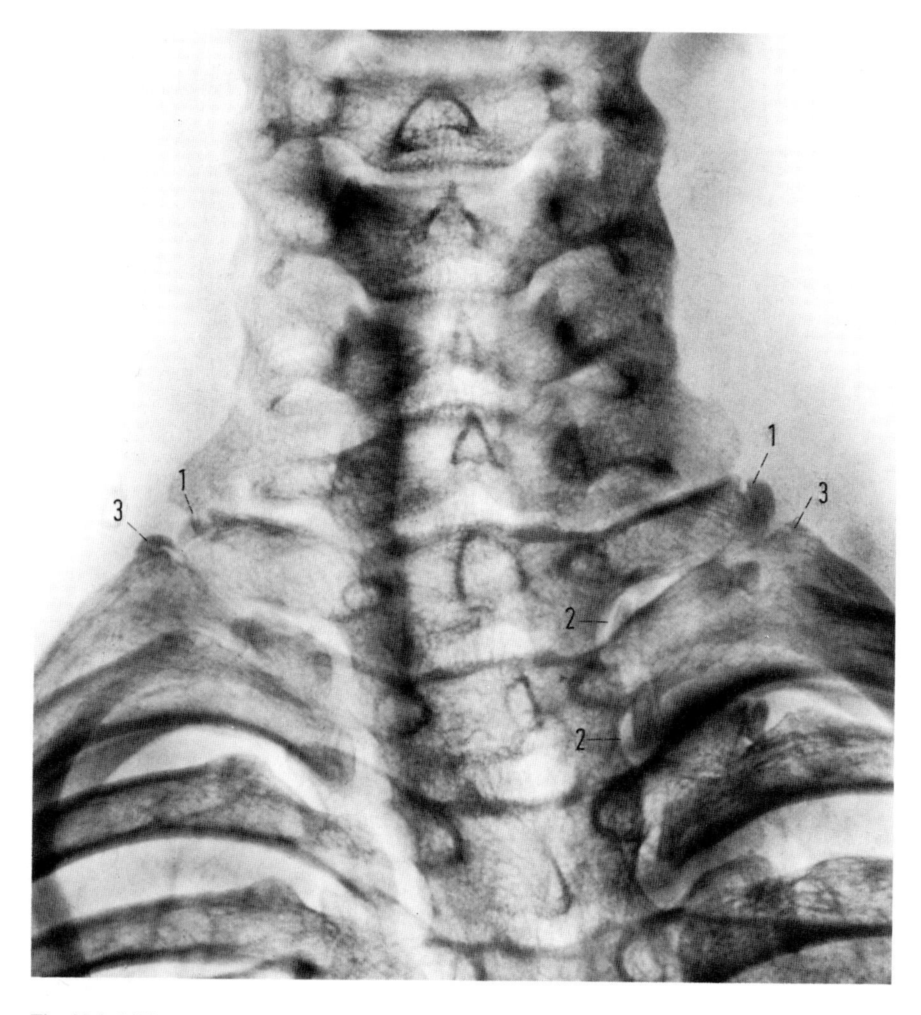

Fig. 996. 14 1/2 year old. Passage of the cervical spine to the thoracic spine, anteroposterior, without apophysis nuclei. Scoliotic softening of the superior thoracic spine. The opaque stripe above originates because of the air rim of the trachea (effect of subtraction). Laterally: the transverse processes of the cervical spine.

1 Apophyseal nucleus of the vertebral transverse processes
2 Apophyseal nucleus of the rib head
3 Apophyseal nucleus of the costal tubercule I

1 Apophysis of the transverse processes of the 1st thoracic vertebra
2 Apophysis of the rib head of the 1st rib
3 Apophysis of the costal tubercule of the 1st rib
4 Apophysis of the transverse process of the 2nd thoracic vertebra
5 Apophysis of the rib head of the 2nd rib
6 Apophysis of the costal tubercule of the 2nd rib

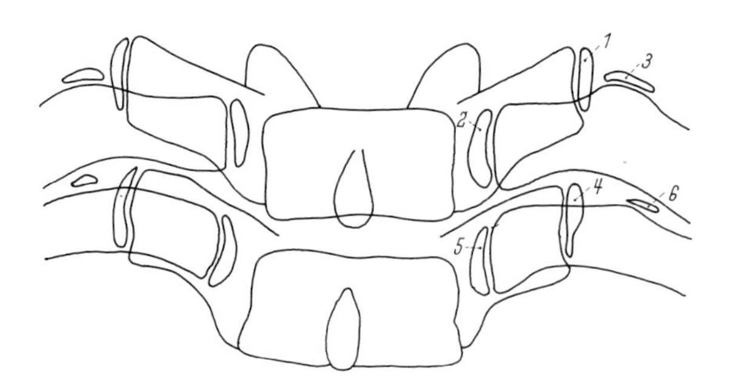

Fig. 997. 1st and 2nd thoracic vertebrae, with the 1st and 2nd pair of ribs.

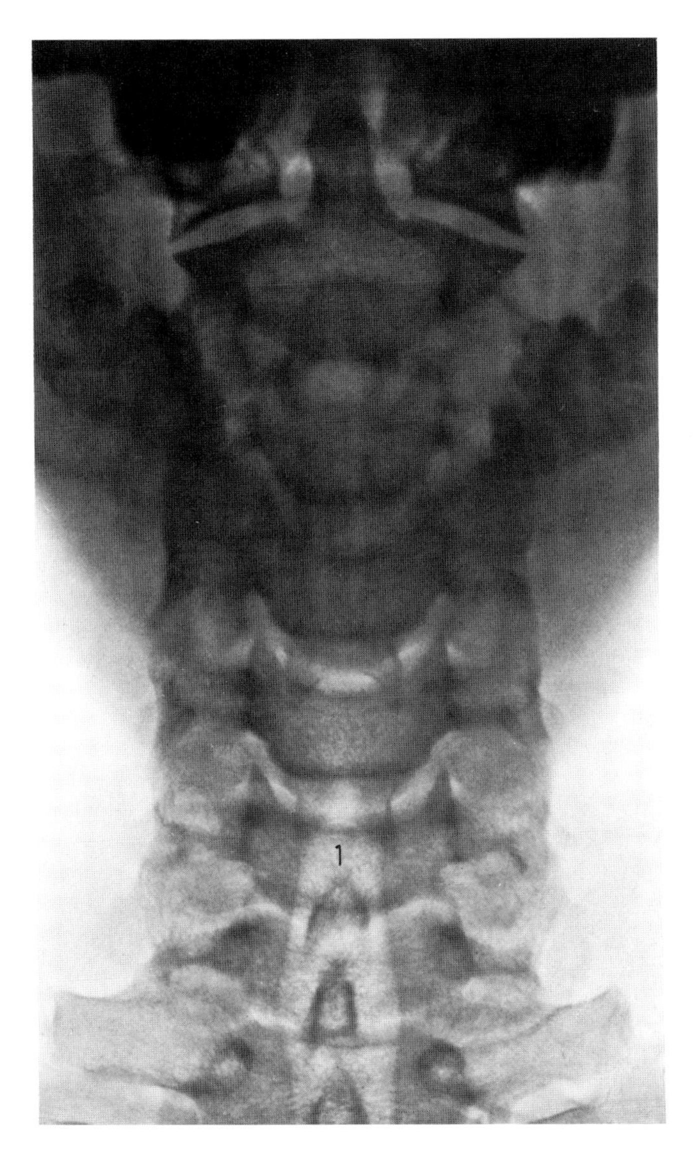

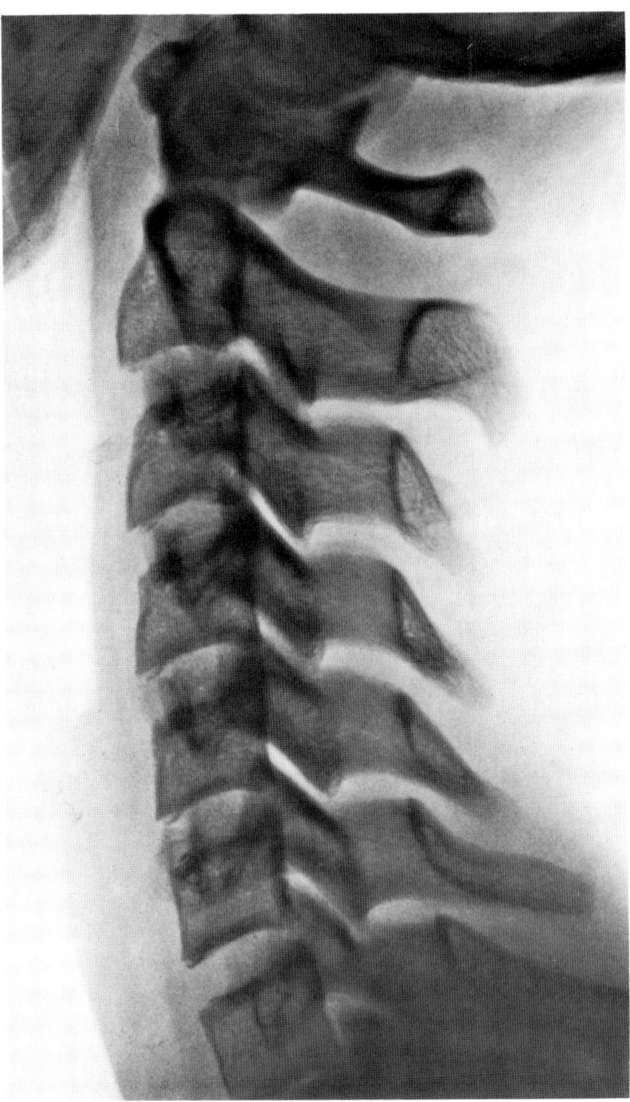

Figs. 998 and 999. 16 year old. Cervical spine, anteroposterior and lateral.

On the anteroposterior radiograph, the lower jaw has been blurred because of movement during the exposure so as to better present the superior cervical spine. 1 = opaque stripe of the trachea. In the space between the superior and inferior jaw, it is possible to see the dens and the atlantoaxial articulation rather well. The narrowing towards the lateral parts and the probable stretching of articulation edges are normal. In the lateral image, it is still possible to see the vertebral fillet, though they are shortly to fuse with the vertebral bodies. The anterior tubercule of the transverse processes is effected axially and projected into the vertebral bodies.

The unciform process is visible. During the period of growth, horizontal laceration formations originate in the early loosening and narrowing intervertebral disks of the cervical spine. Thus, the unciform processes link themselves directly to the nearest vertebral bone. Through the continuous pressure on the apexes of the processes, reactive osseous sclerosis occurs in the uncovertebral links, up to a so-called uncovertebral arthrosis (see Fig. 232, No. 40*), similar to the interspinal pseudoarthritis.

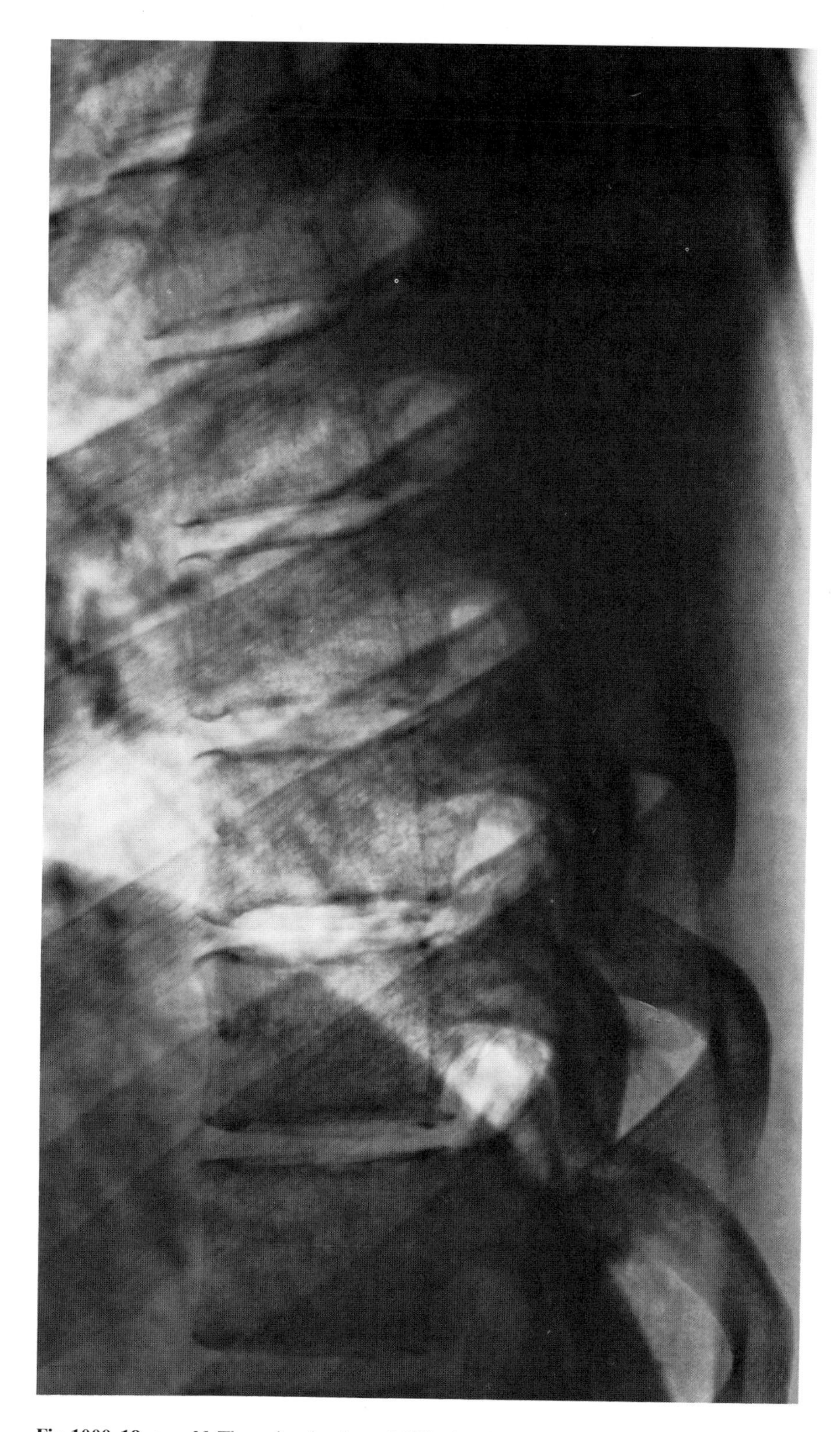

Fig. 1000. 19 year old. Thoracic spine, lateral. Fillet fused. The start of fusion is usually sometime in the 15th year of life, with termination occurring at the latest during the 25th year. The overloaded lung sections with their vessels indicated render judgment of the vertebral structure more difficult (cf. Fig. 332).

Here, there is already a height decrease of the intervertebral disks of the superior thoracic spine, which may be attributed to the early articulation involution of the turgor loss. The insufficiency is due to the aging of the intervertebral disks which takes place during youth, and may be explained by the lack of proportion between load and load capacity of the disks. Thus, there are secondary degenerative variations of the bones and articulation of the spine. So all its structure modifications begin in the intervertebral disks.

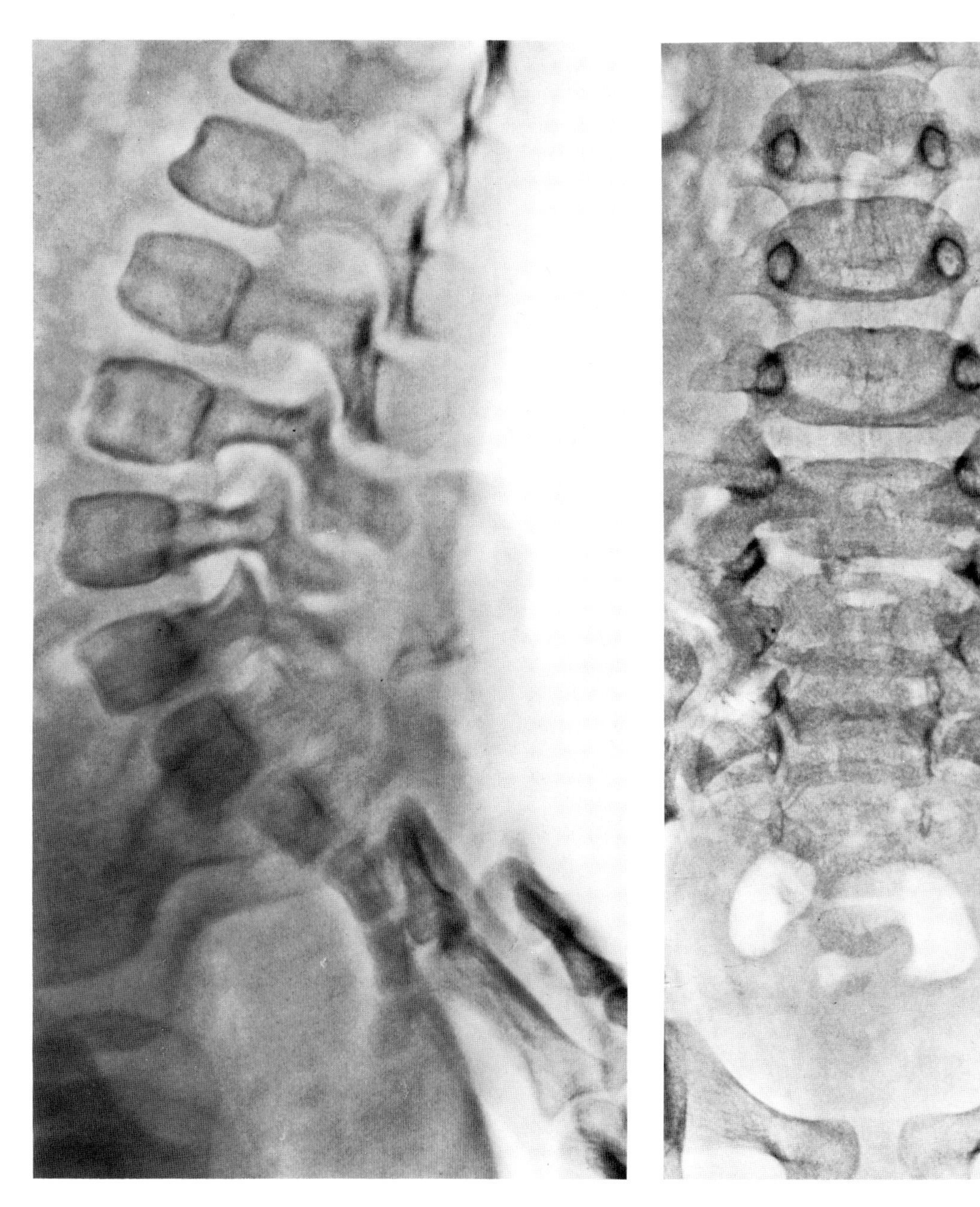

Fig. 1001 Fig. 1002

Figs. 1001 and 1002. 1 1/3 year old. Extended vertebral arch malformations. Aplasia of the sacral arch. Spina bifida with swollen vertebral line of root arches. Isolated spinal processes behind suspended myelomeningocystocele in S-1. The occurrence of malformations of vertebral arches, together with dysplasia of the neural tubes in this region of the shoulder skeleton, may indicate that these malformations originated at the same time in the early fetal period. *De Cuveland* reports an undeveloped system of spinal processes that remained isolated. One must distinguish between the very rare diastematomyelia (diplomyelis) and this condition. It is characterized by a bone spur which develops at the expense of a vertebra and sticks out in the vertebral canal *(Lefebvre et al., Chambers).*

A Series of Radiographs of the Development of the Sternum from Infancy to Age 25

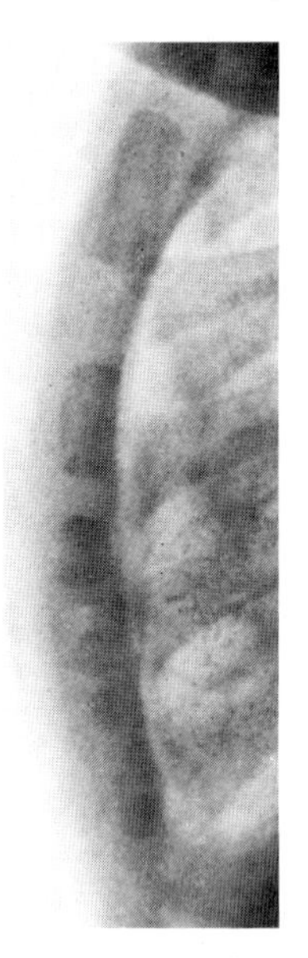

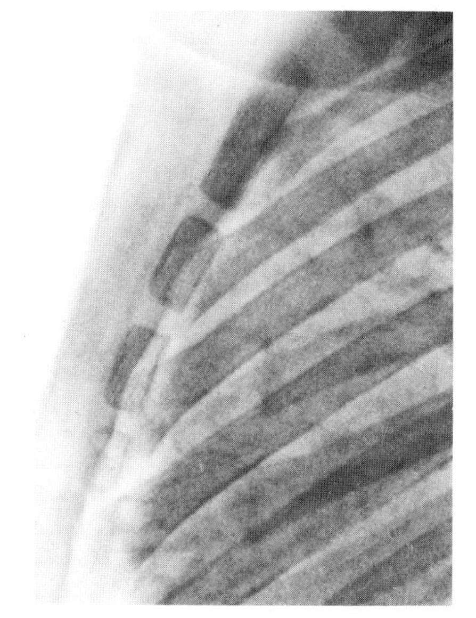

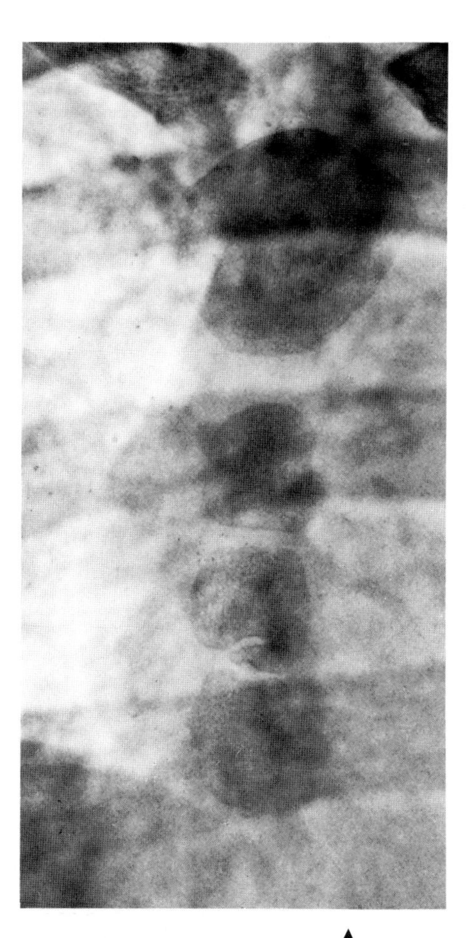

▲ **Fig. 1007. 5 year old** (Close-up).

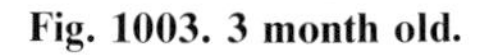

Fig. 1003. 3 month old.

Fig. 1004. 10 month old.

Figs. 1003 and 1004. Osseous nuclei of an infant's sternum in the lateral picture, free of distracting overloading.

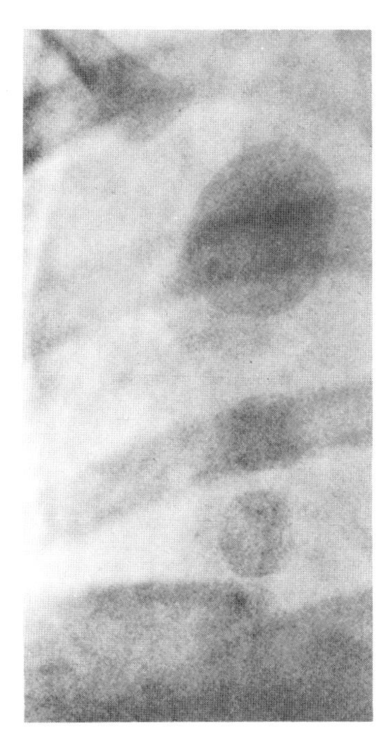

Fig. 1005 (Close-up).

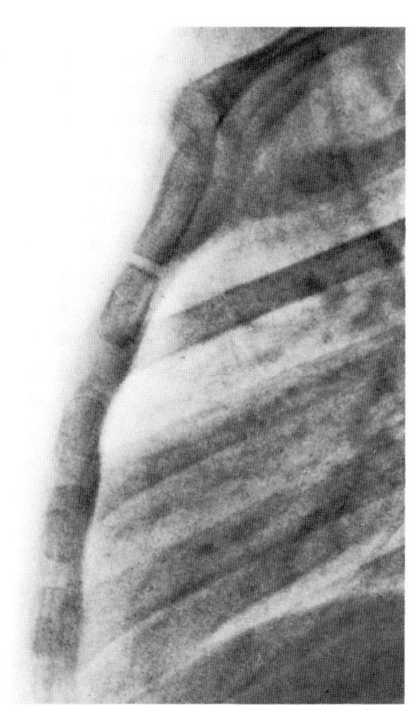

Fig. 1006

Figs. 1005 and 1006. 1 year, 10 months of age. In the lateral picture, the osseous nuclei are clearly seen. On an anteroposterior radiograph at a normal distance, the lung vessels obscure the still relatively weak calcium layers of osseous nuclei. The lung vessels can be shown by a close-up and can thus be completely eliminated.

At this age, the big increase in osseous nuclei is indicated by a narrowing of the cartilagenous interspaces which occur simultaneously. These may be compared with the intervertebral spaces of the spinal column. As a matter of fact, we could in one case prove a so-called *Schmorl*'s node of the synchondrosis in the manubrium and sternal body (Fig. 338).

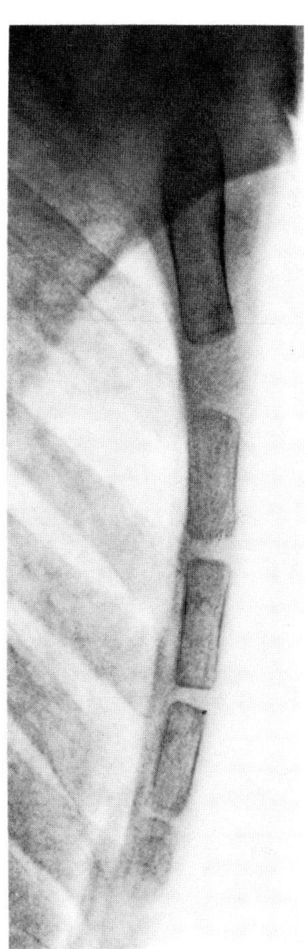

Fig. 1008. $5^1/_2$ year old.

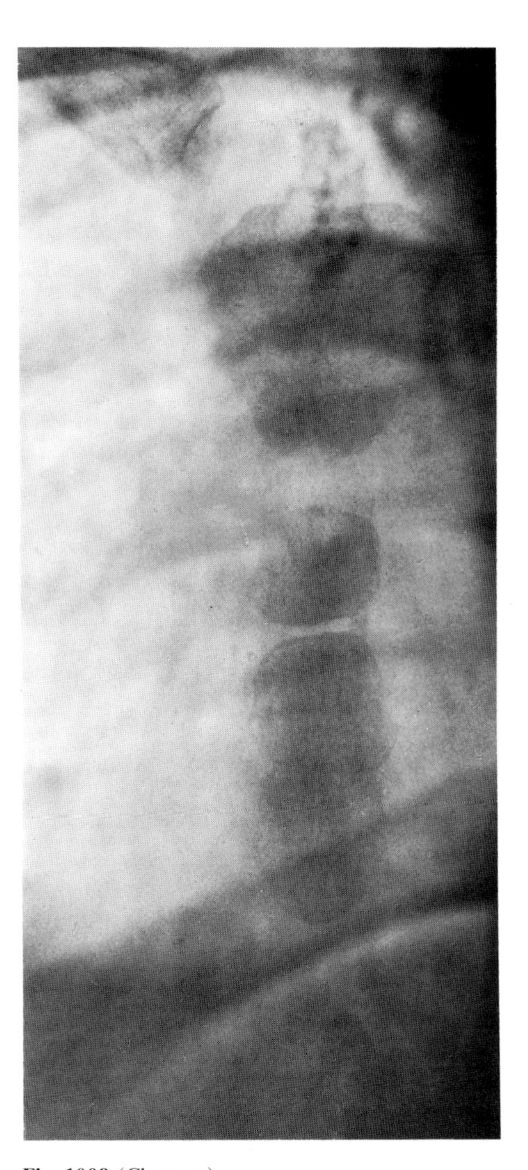

Fig. 1009 (Close-up).

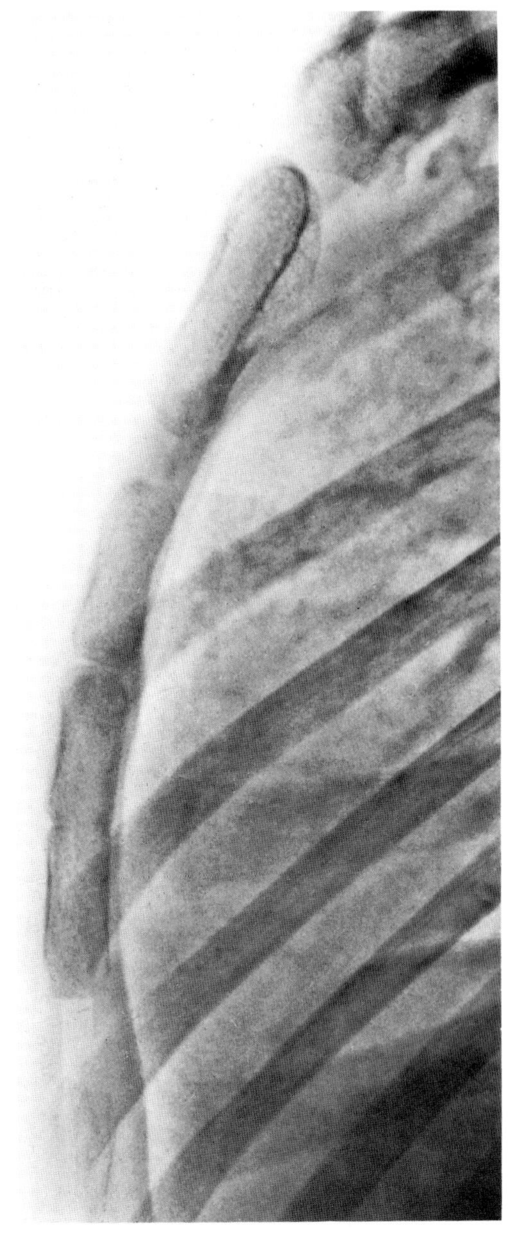

Fig. 1010

Figs. 1009 and 1010. 11 year old. Meanwhile, the fusion of both inferior osseous nuclei of the sternal body has taken place. The osseous nuclei system in the xiphoid process is also readily traceable on the anteroposterior view.

On the basis of comprehensive phylo- and ontogenetic examinations, it is the present author's opinion that sternal development according to the costal theory is the most likely. According to this theory, two sternal rims develop and fuse continuously from the front extremities of the still mesenchymal ribs 1–7 to form the body and the xiphoid process. The manubrium has two generating tissues:

1. The superior sternal rim for the lateral part,
2. A separate interclavicular blastema (*Reiter,* who quotes from *Bánki)* for the middle and superior parts of the sternal manubrium with the sternoclavicular joint and the sternosuperior masses.

The different widths of the manubrium, hole formations and other multiple variations of the sternum can be explained on the basis of this development (see also Figs. 378 and 379).

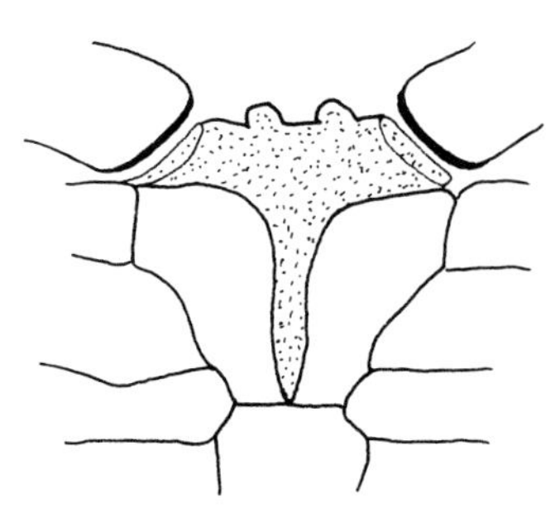

Fig. 1011. Sternal development (from *E. Fischer).*

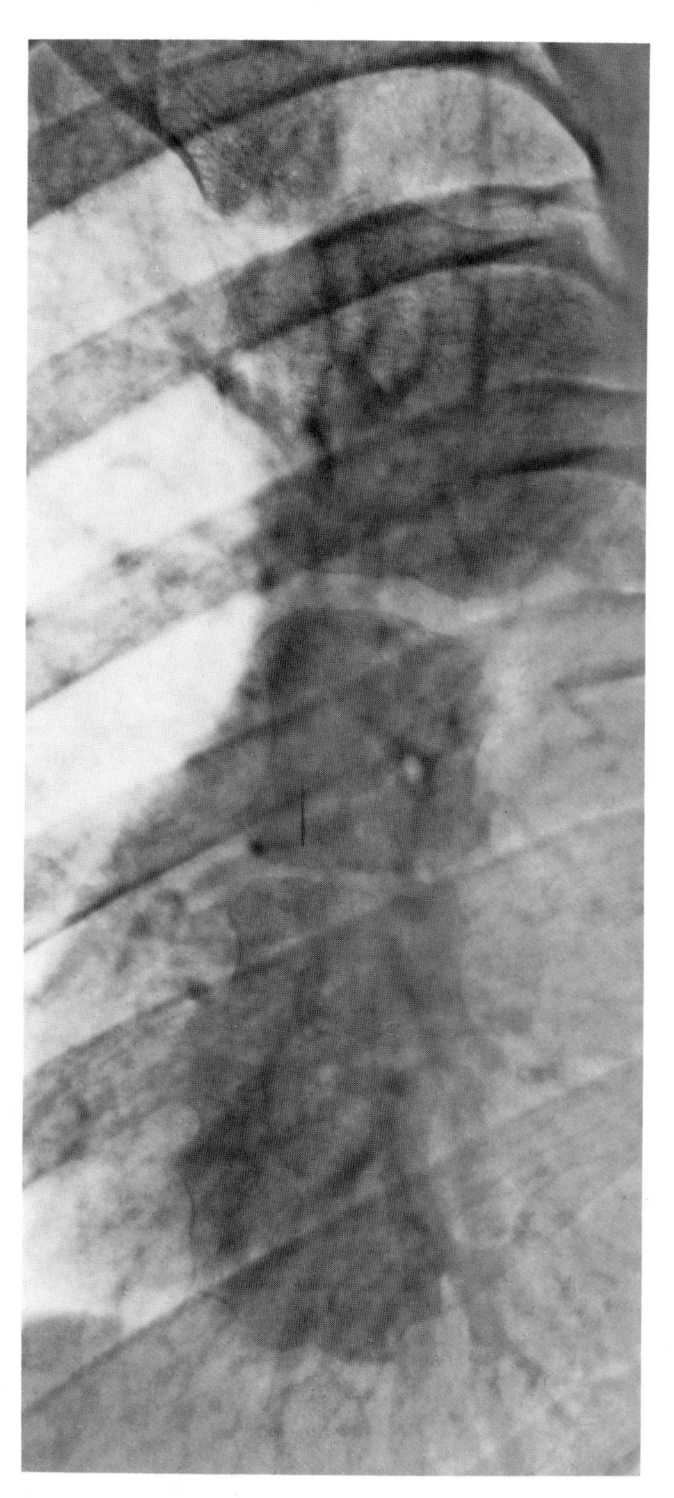

Fig. 1012. 15 year old. In the female, the sternum is short and wide, as is the case here. In this case, the cranial and caudal synchondrosis and a sternal cartilagenous articulation are visible; for this age, they represent a normal finding and appear with a frequency of 20%. The prominent pulmonary vessels obscure the underlying structures.

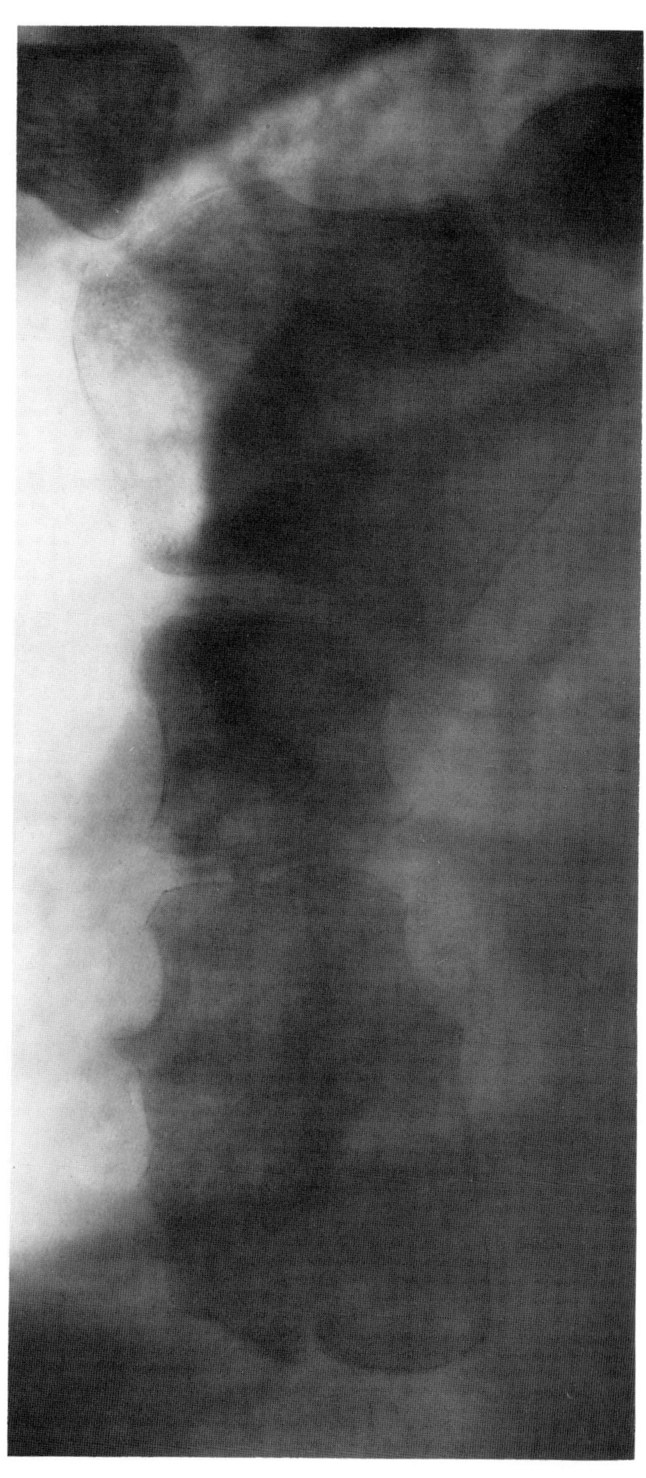

Fig. 1013. 15 year old. In the same patient, the close-up no longer shows the shadows of the pulmonary vascular structures. The xiphoid process is very small and lies hypoplastically. This is one of the large number of possibilities of variation in this sternal section, which range from complete absence of the process to its bi- and trifurcation on to an extreme length, e.g., to the navel.

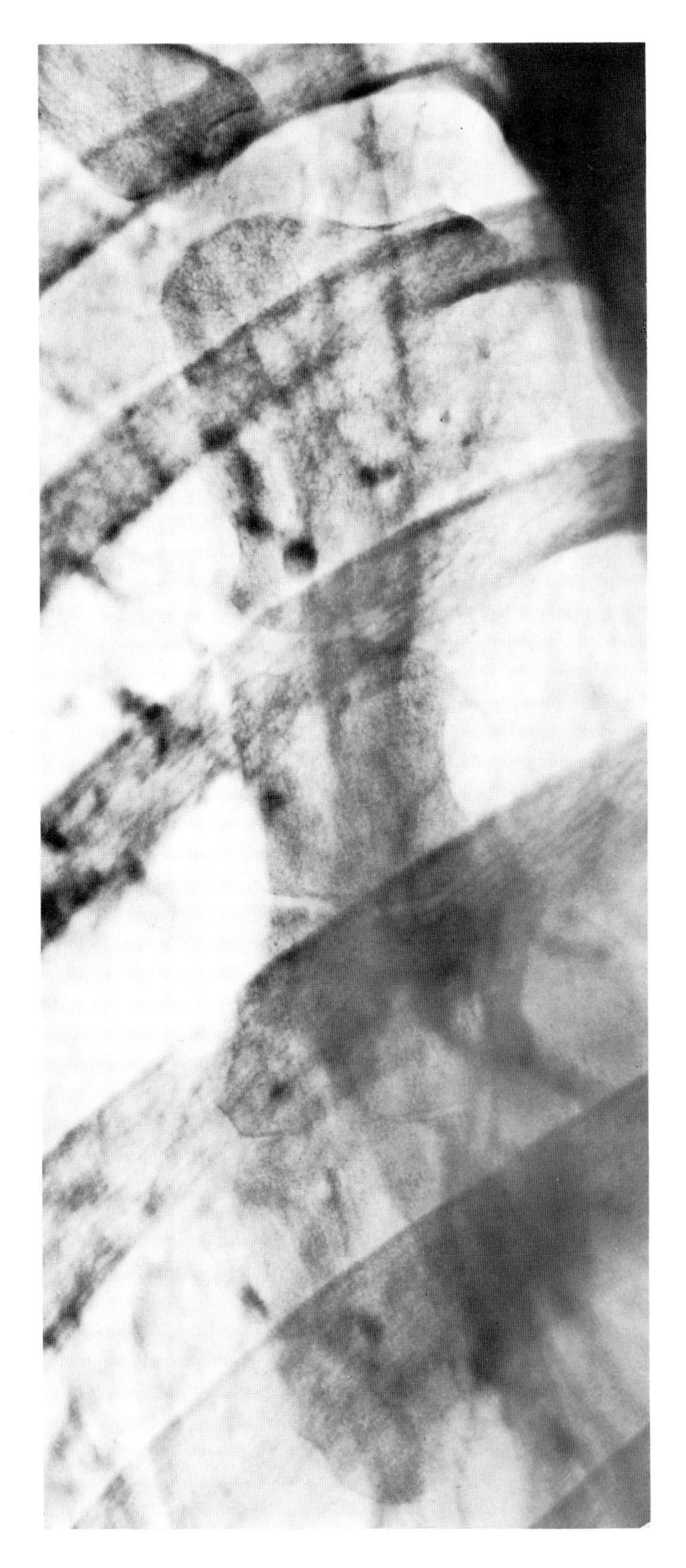

Fig. 1014. 20 year old. In contrast to Fig. 1012, the sternal body in the male is narrow and long. Here, too, we find the cranial and caudal synchondrosis and a cartilagenous articulation in the body. Frequency according to age is approximately 34% *(Pässler)*.

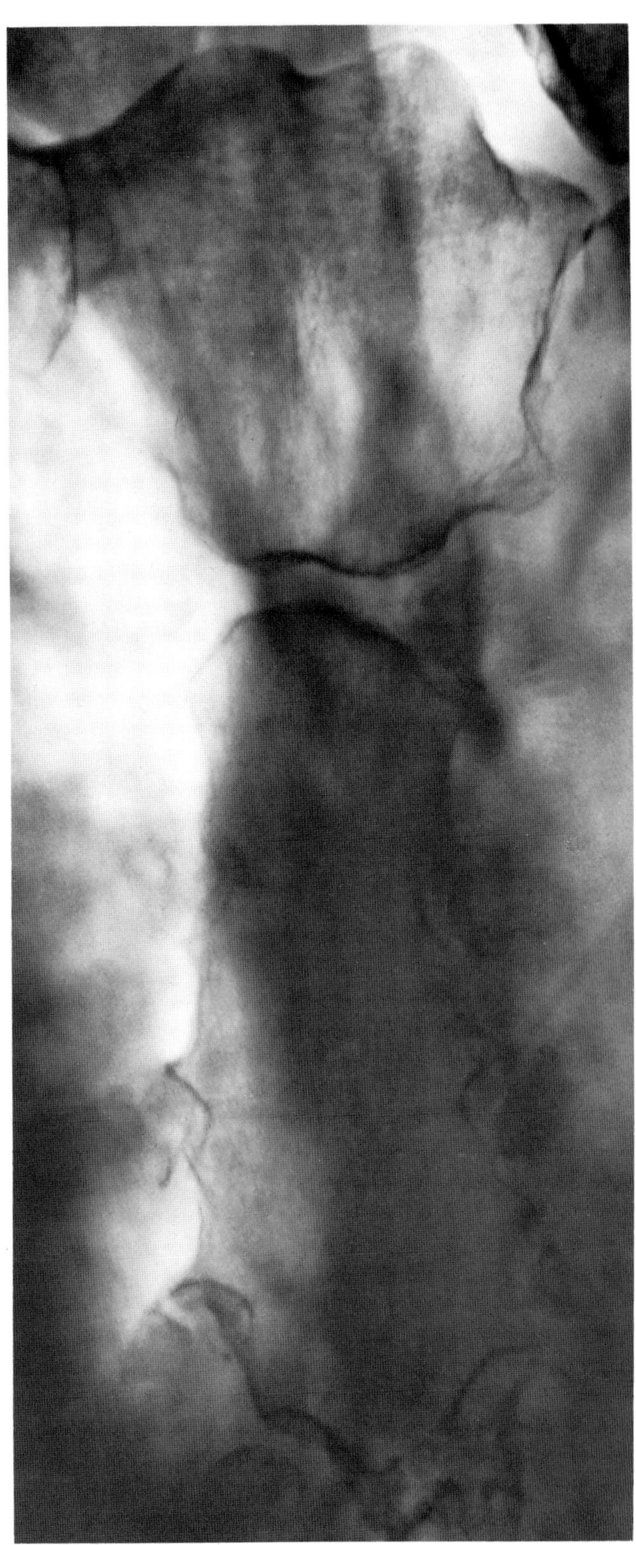

Fig. 1015. 25 year old. The sternal body forms one bone after the closing of all the transverse articulations (often after the 30th year of life). The similarity of the long, open synchondrosis superior with intervertebral disks originates from the existence of the cartilagenous knot (see Fig. 338), as *Schmorl* described them in the intervertebral disks. There is an early deposition of lime in the rib cartilage (short focal distance exposure).

IV. Shoulder Girdle and Upper Extremities

Prenatal Development

The ossification of the arm skeleton (cf. Fig. 1016) begins with the formation of an osseous nucleus in the central part of the clavicle in a 15-mm-long embryo (7th embryonic week and earlier). This is the first osseous nucleus in the human skeleton. Slightly later, during the 8th embryonic week, the large bone arrangements in the upper extremities begin with one osseous nucleus, each in the central section *(Broman, Wolf)*.

The formation of the main osseous nuclei of the phalangeal and the metacarpal bones begins with the terminal phalanx of the thumb in 30-mm-long embryos (8th to 9th embryonic week).

Postnatal Development

The carpal bone anlage remains cartilagenous during the entire embryonic and fetal period. All the epiphyseal nuclei of the arm skeleton also appear only during the extrauterine developmental period. The long tubular bones have osseous epiphyses at both their extremities, while the short bones have them at only one extremity. The existence of one epiphyseal nucleus only, according to *Retterer,* is not a principle but a gradual difference in the development of the tubular bones as compared with the epiphyseal nuclei.

This is also supported by the appearance of interim forms, or so-called pseudoepiphyses (see Figs. 1091, 1103, 1111).

According to *Siegert,* pseudoepiphyses indicate independent osseous nuclei in an epiphyseal cartilage, which normally starts to ossify from the diaphysis. These are accessory epiphyses in the metacarpus, metatarsus and, occasionally, in the phalanges, which usually have only one epiphysis. Most frequently, the pseudoepiphyses appear near the metacarpus I and II and metatarsus I. The development starts rather early (around the 2nd to 3rd year of life) from an originating accessory nucleus, which grows more rapidly than the other nuclei and unites (after the 6th to 7th year of life) with the diaphysis. As a remainder, for a certain period of time there is still a narrow groove where the pseudoepiphysis is most frequently recognizable.

Disorders of epiphyseal development may occur during the ossification of the tubular bones.

Shoulder Girdle

Clavicle. During ossification this bone has a special characteristic: the partial ossification as a coated bone in the central part, as is already known from the neurocranium. Both extremities are first formed of cartilage. The clavicle is the only bone in the region of the upper extremity that originates from a connective tissue basis and in which the growth in length starts first without epiphysis formation. Phylogenetically, it is therefore an integument bone. The ossification begins in the central part and is the first in all our body. Only after puberty (ages 18 to 21 in males, and ages 14½ to about 20 in females) can a disk-shaped epiphysis be found in the sternal extremity of the clavicle (Fig. 1018). The former fuses with the clavicle during the first half of the 3rd decade of life (ages 23–25).

Because of the limited morphologic and histogenetic differences between the hyaline cartilage in the epiphyses and the onset cartilage in the apophyses *(Knese* and *Biermann, Knese),* it is also possible to refer to a clavicular apophysis.

In the acromial extremity of the clavicle, no osseous nucleus of its own is ever found. In general, in the 2nd decade of life the sternal clavicular extremities show a hint of a cup form which, finally, in the 3rd decade, becomes like a hallmark. A rare ossification disorder, which should not be confused with the results of an injury, is the persisting epiphysis at the sternal extremity of the clavicle *(E. Fischer). Ravelli* has undertaken some interesting research on the genetic significance of some definite properties of the clavicle and its ligaments.

Scapula. The perichondral ossification of this trilateral, flat bone begins with the appearance of an osseous nucleus in the vicinity of the collum in the 7th to 8th embryonic week. In the newborn, considerable parts of the skeleton are still cartilagenous (acromion, coracoid process, the three angles, the entire shoulder articulation glenoid cavity and the margo medialis).

As early as the 1st year, the **Coracoid process** (Figs. 1020–1024) develops out of its own osseous nucleus

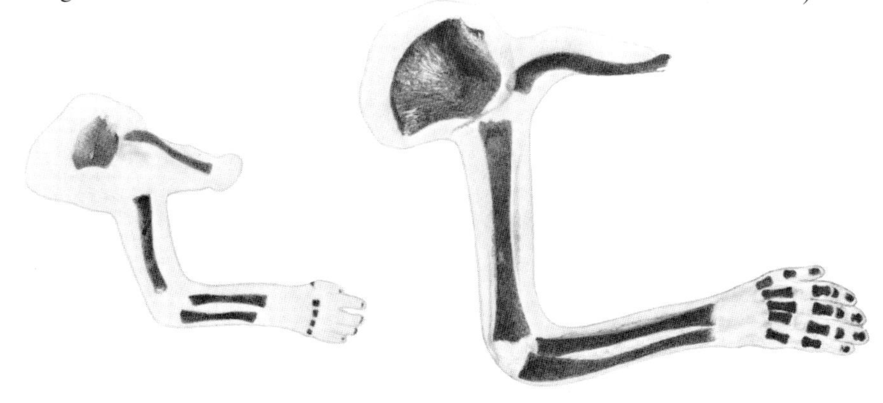

Fig. 1016 a **Fig. 1016 b**

Fig. 1016. Osseous nuclei of the arms, enlarged two times (according to *Broman*).
a) Fetus with a total length of 6 cm.
b) Fetus with a total length of 12 cm.

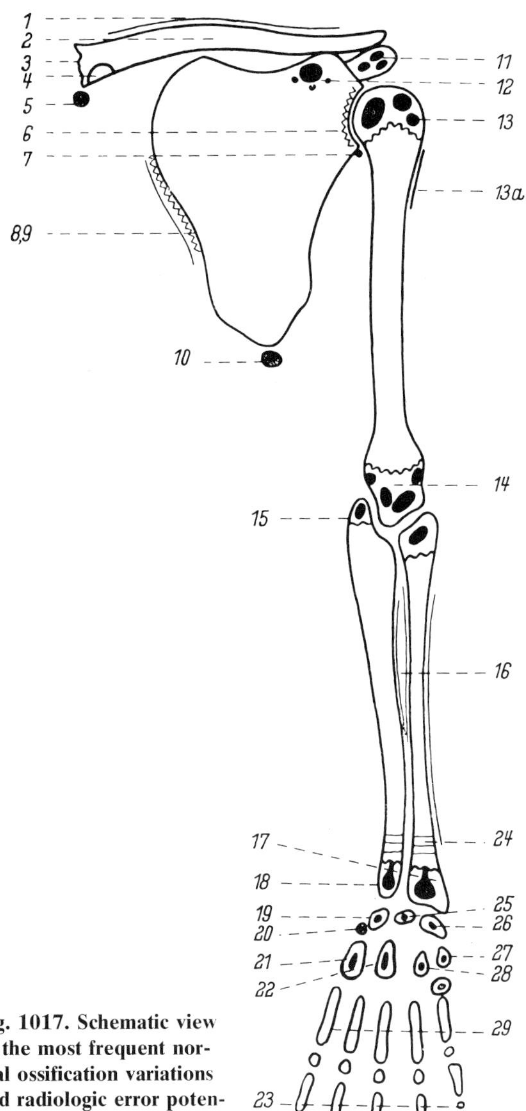

Fig. 1017. Schematic view of the most frequent normal ossification variations and radiologic error potential in the bones of the shoulder girdle and the upper limbs (according to *W. Swoboda:* Das Skelett des Kindes, 2nd Edition, Thieme, Stuttgart, 1969).

1 Accompanying shadow of clavicle
2 Changing curves
3 Irregular limits of the sternal extremity
4 "Defect" simulated by ligamental grooves (costoclavicular ligament)
5 Apophysis (after puberty)
6 Grooved socket rim
7 Socket rim apophysis (puberty)
8 Grooved medial rim
9 Apophyseal fillet (puberty); very controversial *(Neiss)*
10 Infrascapular bone (puberty)
11 Several acromial nuclei (puberty)
12 Coracoid nuclei (1st year of life) with nucleoli
13 Humeral caput with 3 osseous nuclei
13a Normal double contour
14 Distal humerus extremity with 4 osseous nuclei
15 Olecranon with 1 to 2 nuclei (before puberty)
16 Normal double contours
17 Bone bridges at the distal epiphyses of the ulna and radius, which interrupt the epiphysis fissures to the metaphysis
18 Distal ulnar epiphysis with 1–2 nuclei
19 Triquetrum bone: double nucleus
20 Pisiform bone: multicentered ossification
21 Hamate bone: compact isle, accessory nuclei, especially ulnar
22 Capate bone: accessory nuclei
23 Base phalanx: normal "shaft thickening"
24 Transverse striae "growth lines"
25 Lunate bone: double nucleus, "smallness"
26 Scaphoid bone: double nucleus
27 Trapezium bone: double nucleus? Bridge formation with scaphoid bone or the I metacarpal bone
28 Trapezoid bone: double nucleus? Bridge formation with scaphoid bone or the I–III metacarpus and capate bones
29 Metacarpus: normal "shaft thickening." Pseudoepiphyses, sesamoid bone at the distal extremities
30 Middle phalanx: brachiomeso- and cone-shaped (especially V, infrequently IV radiation). "Roof shaped" and "Zapfen-" epiphyses
31 Terminal phalanx: anomalous forms

(main nucleus) and fuses with the scapula, only long after puberty. Thus, the development of the coracoid process must be regarded as an independent bone development. This may be explained by the fact that, philogenetically, in reptiles and birds the "raven's beak" is considered to be a real bone.

The osseous nucleus of the coracoid process in the human body develops very quickly and becomes the characteristic raven-beak process. Until the 15th–20th years of life, it is clearly separated from the scapula on radiographs. The isolated raven-beak process in juveniles can be shown only in axial shoulder articulation or tangential scapula radiographs. It must not lead to the incorrect diagnosis of a fracture. *Günsel* reports a rare case of a persisting coracoid nucleus in a 68-year-old man. The same author calls this rare variation the coracoid bone.

The paranuclei in the coracoid process remain to be mentioned; they appear, however, only after the 10th year of life (Fig. 1058). Such a bow-shaped nucleolus is seen in the anteroposterior medial radiograph from the base in the "knee" of the coracoid process (ages 13–17); see Figs. 1043 and 1048. Another nucleolus is seen at the free extremity of the coracoid process (in an axial radiation process) as a coracoid apex nucleus (ages 13–15); see *Ravelli.*

Since the nucleoli serve only the local formation and not the growth in length, they are both to be regarded as apophyses.

Another nucleus is called the infracoracoid bone, be-

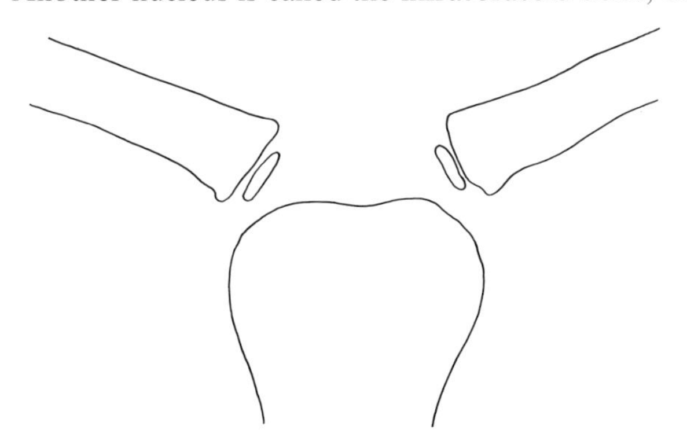

Fig. 1018. Sternoclavicular articulation of a 17 year old. Disk-shaped epiphysis at the sternoclavicular extremity.

tween the coracoid process and the glenoid cavity, which is thought to originate out of a secondary ossification center (Figs. 1022–1024). It is usually found in 10- to 14-year-old subjects and disappears about two years later *(Lossen* and *Wegner).* The infracoracoid bone can unite either with the scapula or, first, with the still isolated coracoid process; in rare cases the fusion does not take place (Figs. 543 and 1954).

Scapular Apophyses. In the scapular region, besides the apophyseal development in the acromion, an additional six secondary ossification centers occur, of which the infracoracoid bone already described between the coracoid process and the glenoid cavity appears only infrequently (Figs. 543 and 1022–1024). Two of these ossification centers may be found at the coracoid process (apophysis at the apex of the coracoid and another at the cranial curve of the raven-beak process: see coracoid process and Fig. 1058). Between the ages of 16 and 18, a further apophysis appears at the inferior angle of the scapula. This secondary ossification nucleus can occasionally persist. *Zimmer* (in *Köhler-Zimmer)* proposes the denomination of infrascapular bone for this ossification (Figs. 1057, 1059). Between the ages of 16 and 18, one apophysis should be present in the medial margin of the scapula *(Rittweger).* Its appearance, however, is not proved roentgenologically. *Aumann* and *Neiss* doubt its anatomic existence. A small osseous nucleus is described by *Zimmer* (in *Köhler-Zimmer)* in the superior angle, which again should appear between the ages of 16 and 18. Aside from *Ochs,* no one has shown this persistence (see Fig. 525).

Finally, corresponding to the acetabulum bone of the hip joint, we also find in the shoulder articulation, precisely in the glenoid cavity edge region, a ring-shaped apophysis. Its persistence as a glenoid bone in the inferior glenoid cavity is very rare (Fig. 532). For ossification of the shoulder-glenoid cavity articulation, see also *Ziegler.*

Acromion Apophysis. During puberty a broad apophysis forms in the acromion. This apophysis is developed out of two, three and at times even more separable ossification centers, the so-called pre-acromion, mesa-acromion and meta-acromion (see Fig. 1019). The fusion of this apophysis with the acromion occurs in about the 20th year of life, but in certain cases as early as age 17. If the joint termination has not occurred beyond the 25th year of life, the persisting apophysis is called the acromial bone. This variation is found in 7 to 15% of the cases examined; usually it is bilateral *(Köhler-Zimmer);* see Figs. 417 and 551. *Schär* and *Zweifel* report on the clinical significance of the acromial bone.

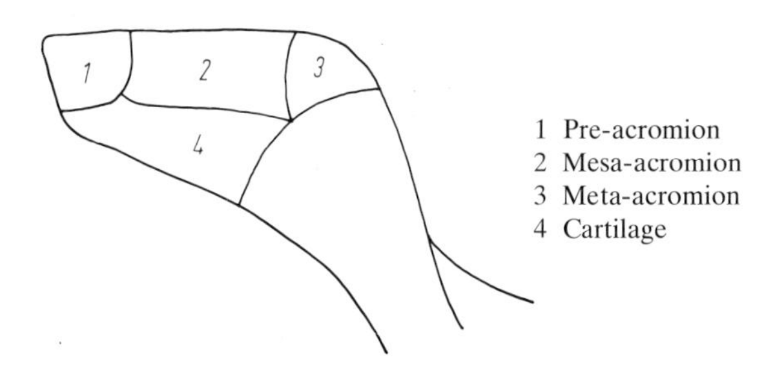

Fig. 1019. The ossification centers in the acromion (according to *Bernardeau).*

Ossification Disorders of the Scapula. These most frequently take place in the region of the secondary ossification centers in the form of persistence of the cartilaginous joints or modifications of the osseous nuclei. In younger subjects, there are rare variations of hole-like defects in the fossa infraspinata of the scapula; their genesis is not yet clear *(E. Fischer).* In older subjects, in differential diagnosis, one might consider a senile atrophy.

Humerus, Proximal Part. This is composed of three nuclei: the main nucleus (caput humeri), one nucleus in the major tubercle, and one in the minor tubercle. The osseous nuclei in the epiphysis always appear earlier in girls than in boys. This difference is so sharp that it is useful in diagnosis *(Davies* and *Parsons).*

Caput humeri: The beginning of the ossification of the turned caput humeri of the glenoid cavity of the scapula (medial nucleus) takes place about the 4th to 8th month of life. In rare cases, there is already a small ossification nucleus in the caput region in the newborn (Fig. 1027).

Tuberculum majus: This lateral nucleus appears about the second half of the 1st year of life (girls) and up to the 2nd year of life. Sometimes, however, it appears only in the 3rd year.

Tuberculum minus: This 3rd nucleus, which appears in the 2nd year of life and later (4th and 5th years) is very rarely discernible radiographically as it is usually covered by the tuberculum majus. *Cocchi* managed to find this 3rd nucleus with good projections in 3- to 4-year-old subjects.

Fusion to the Proximal Humerus Epiphysis. This fusion results from the unification of the three nuclei of the caput humeri, the tuberculum majus and the tuberculum minus. The fusion of these three nuclei into one epiphysis occurs between the ages of 3½ and 6. The roof-ridge-shaped, obliquely double proximal extremity of the humerus diaphysis, over which the proximal humerus epiphysis seems to ride, is characteristic. In radiographs, this leads to projections which erroneously can be taken for a fracture (Fig. 531). Fractures inside the epiphysis joint are rare. Spontaneous luxations of the epiphysis are seen in congenital lues, secondary hyperparathyroidism, inflamed articulation processes, scurvy and in *Möller-Barlow* syndrome.

The rather frequently discernible double contour in the lateral edge of the humerus metaphysis and in the remaining bone extremities is to be regarded as a normal finding in juveniles *(Köhler-Zimmer).* In addition, bowl-shaped epiphyses with spur formations are seen. These roentgenological growth signs appear relatively often in children between the 2nd and 6th months of life and then later disappear.

Termination of the Ossification in the Scapula. Between the ages of 15 and 20, the coracoid process unites with the scapula. No apophyses in the acromion and coracoid are present. In the 14 year old of Figure 1025, both apophyses are already present.

Figs. 1020–1024. Scapula, in chronological order from newborn to a 14 year old.

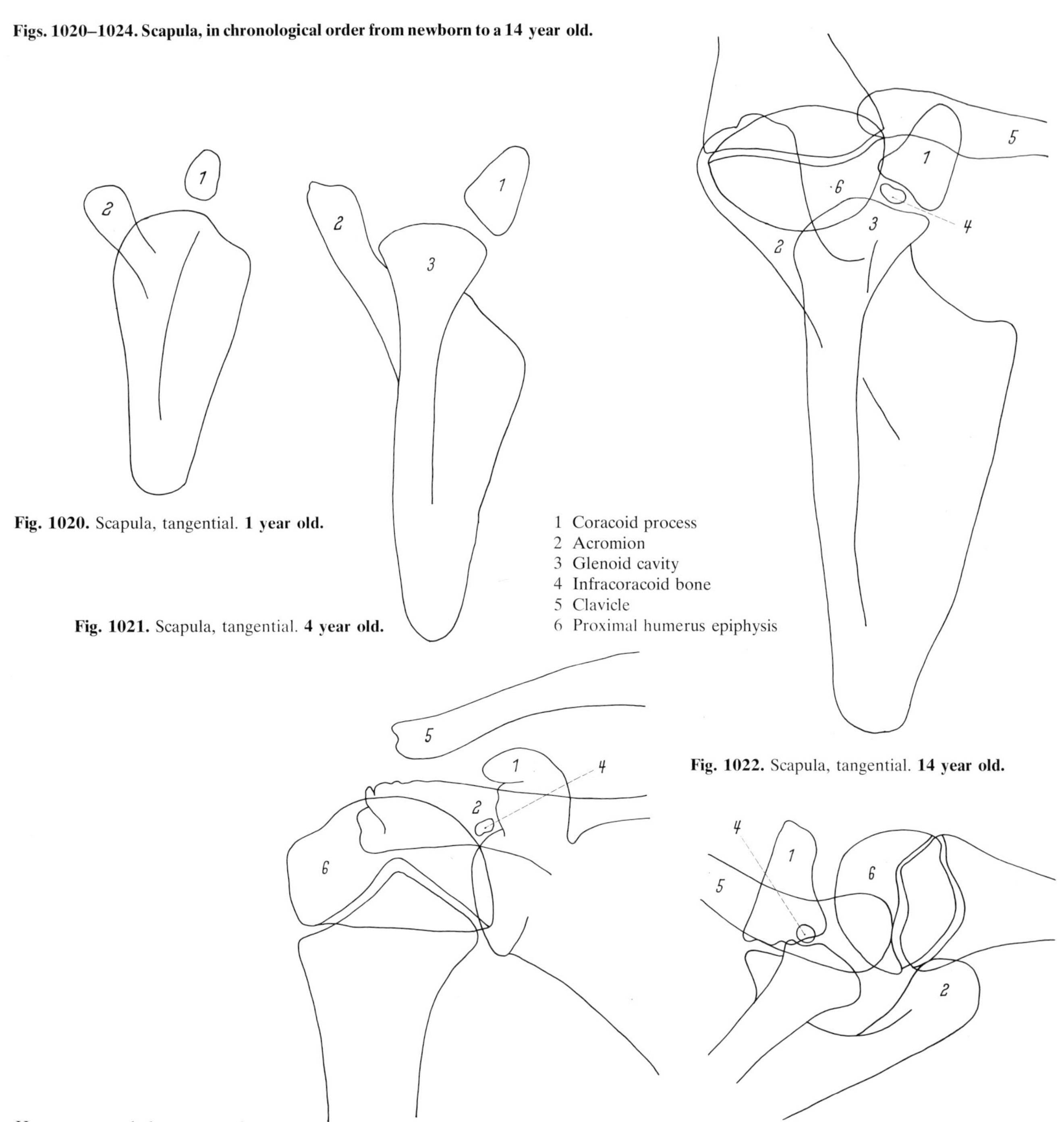

Fig. 1020. Scapula, tangential. **1 year old.**

Fig. 1021. Scapula, tangential. **4 year old.**

1 Coracoid process
2 Acromion
3 Glenoid cavity
4 Infracoracoid bone
5 Clavicle
6 Proximal humerus epiphysis

Fig. 1022. Scapula, tangential. **14 year old.**

Here no apohphyses at the eoracoid and acromium, but they exsist at a 14 year old in Fig. 1025.

Fig. 1023. Shoulder articulation, anteroposterior. **14 year old.**

Fig. 1024. Shoulder articulation, axial (craniocaudal). **14 year old.**

At the age of 20, the acromion apophysis fissure closes. The apophyses of the coracoids disappear at the age of 18 to 22. At the same time, the ossification at the caudoscapular angle and in the region of the glenoid bone is terminated. The epiphysis termination in the region of the proximal humerus extremity occurs during the 18th to 20th years of life.

The anatomically "real" articulation fissure is illustrated when the arm is elevated, especially during early infancy (vacuum phenomenon, according to *Magnusson's* or *Fick's* designations; see also *Ravelli* and Fig. 1030). *Fick* had already discovered the vacuum phenomenon of the proximal articulation of the fingers in 1897, and explained its existence as it is explained today. So far, it has been traced on almost all articulations.

Congenital anomalies of the caput humeri are rare. According to *Köhler,* the roentgenologic criteria of the humerus varus are the diminishing of the shaft-head angle below 140°, the elevation of the tuberculum majus over the superior edge of the anatomical cervix, as well as the diminishing of the distance of the articulation layer from the external layer of the humerus. Additional congenital malformations of the upper extremities are described by *Max.*

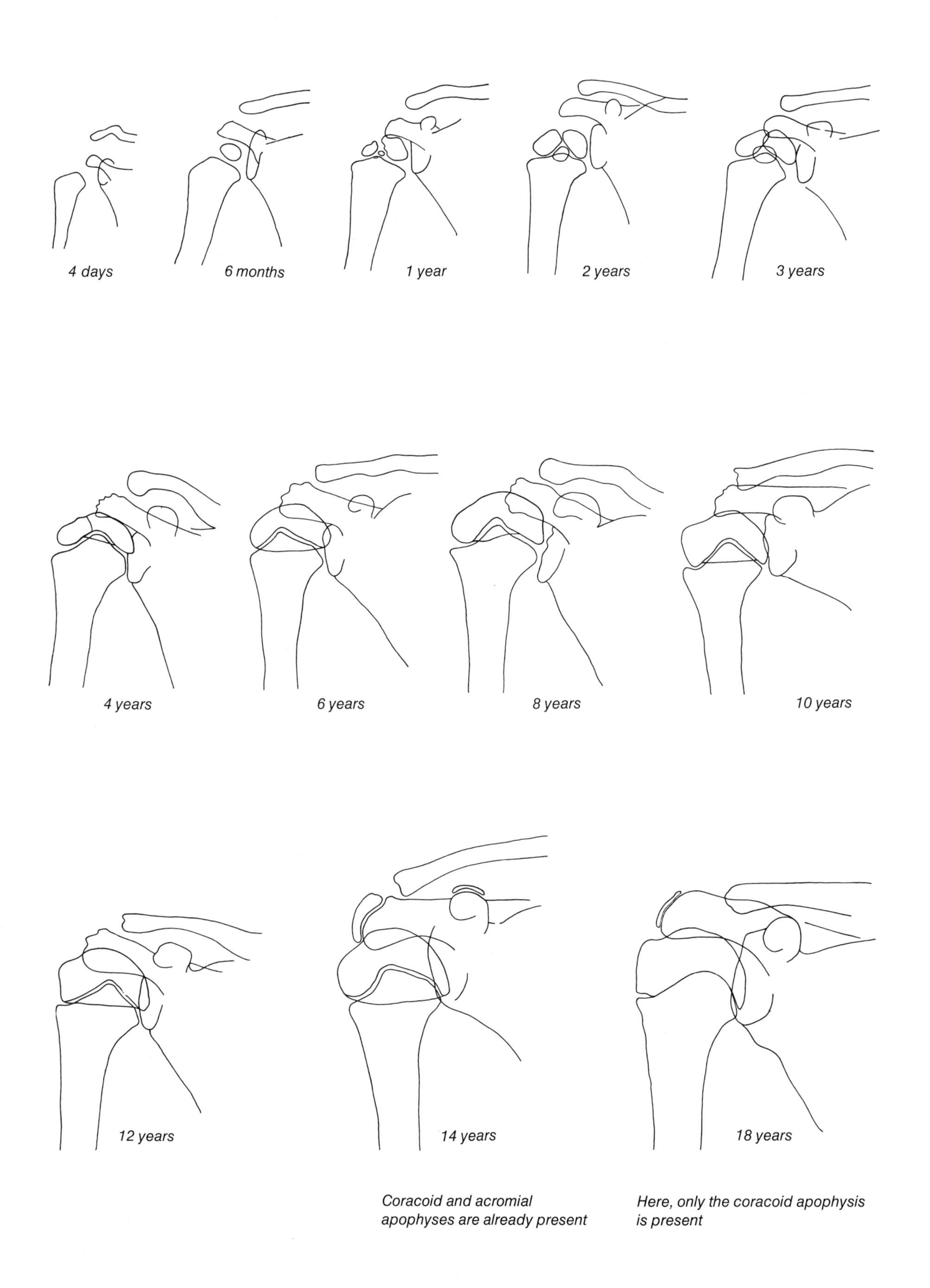

Fig. 1025. Shoulder articulation in chronological order from a newborn to an 18 year old.

A Series of Radiographs of the Development of the Shoulder Articulation Region from Infancy to Age 18

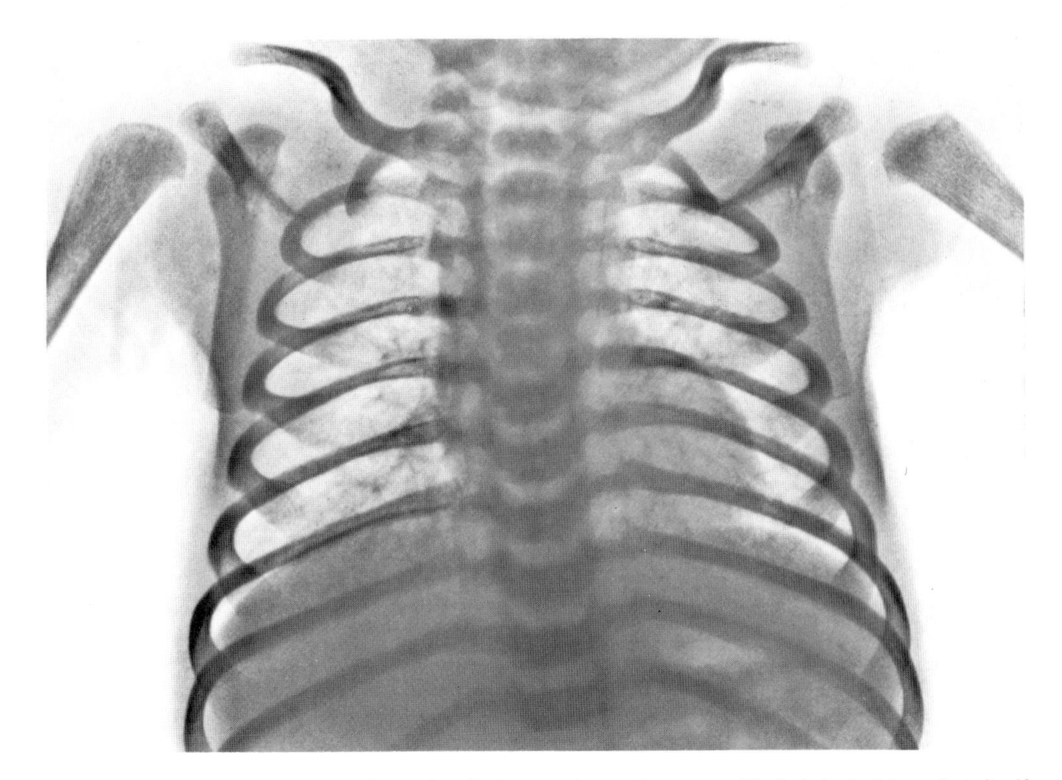

Fig. 1026. 14 day old. No osseous nucleus anlage in the caput humeri is yet seen. The baby's clavicle projects itself rather far beyond the first rib; it projects itself even more when the arm is raised. Here, the S-shaped arched course of the clavicle at this age is especially well recognized; the clavicle turns in the center dorsally almost at a right angle. If this clavicular arch is taken axially, a ring shadow caused by the cortical (Corticalis) may simulate a fracture. The lung hilus in a baby is covered by the broad middle shadow. The diaphragm is in an inspiration position; therefore, the otherwise broad middle shadow is not so evident. The bifurcation of the lung arteries and veins has an important role in the formation of the normal hilus shadow. The normal lymph nodes and the hilar connective tissue, like the main bronchi, have almost nothing to do with the formation of the hilus.

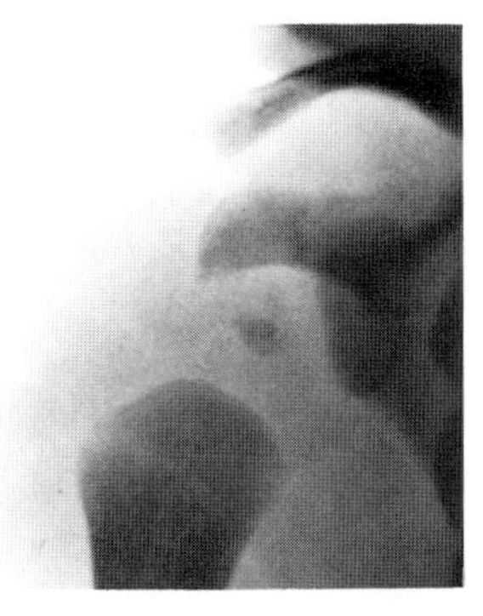

Fig. 1027. 15 day old. Very premature ossification nucleus in the caput humeri; usually it appears between the 4th and 8th months of life (example of the variation range).

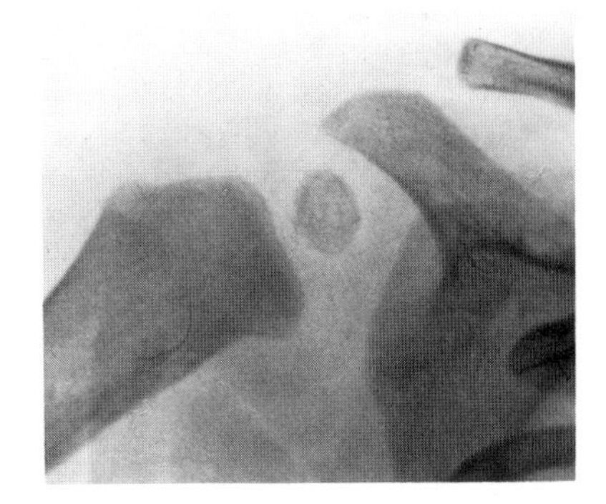

Fig. 1028. 6 month old. The roof-ridge-shaped structure of the proximal humerus diaphysis is recognizable near the osseous nucleus anlage in the caput humeri.

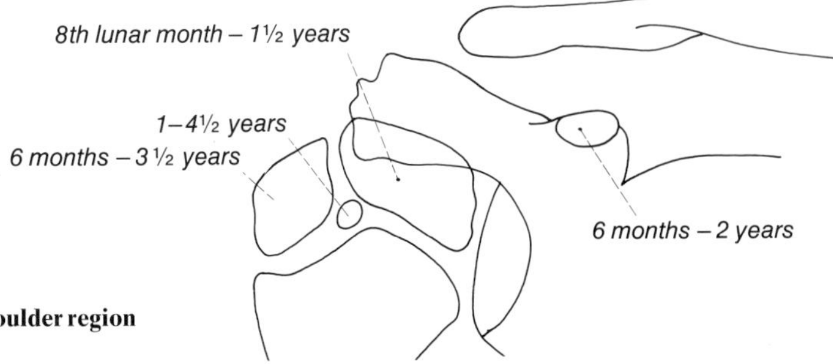

Fig. 1029. The time span during which the osseous nuclei of the shoulder region usually appear.

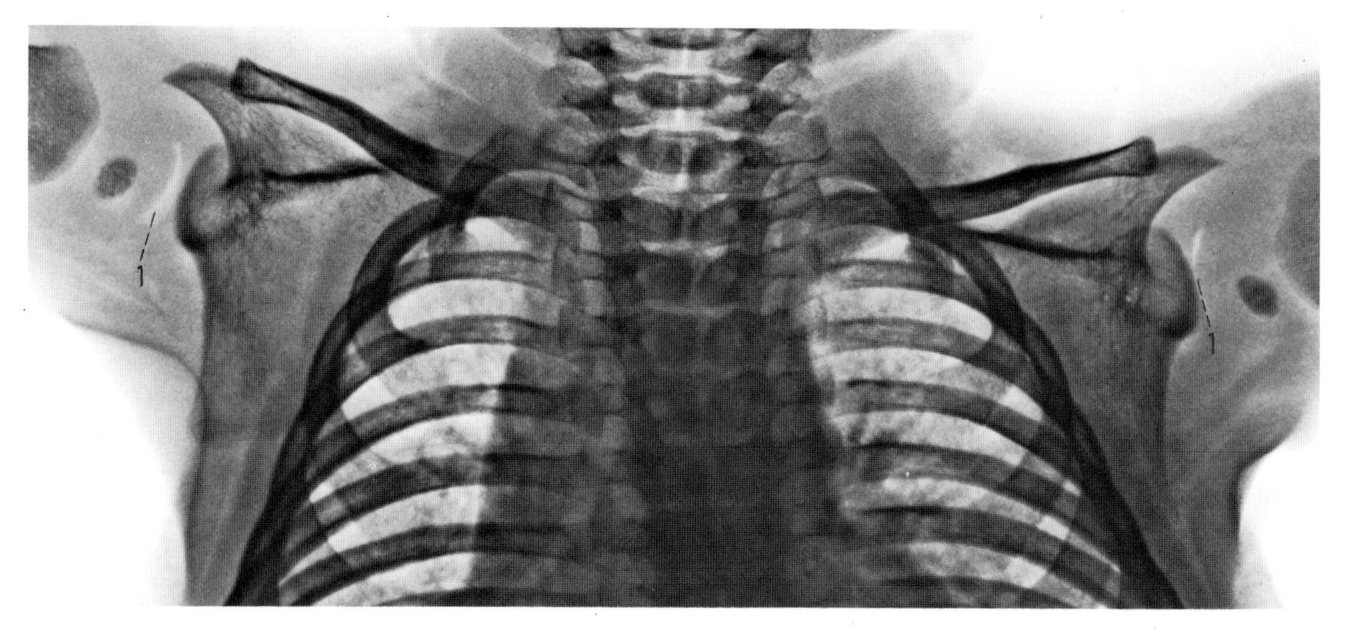

Fig. 1030. 6 month old. In this infant, the radiograph, with both arms raised, shows the "true shoulder articulation fissure" (1) as a "vacuum phenomenon." The middle shadow in the thorax is still typically broad; the vertebral arch fissure is not yet bridged with bones. Unlike Fig. 978, the fissure here due to the radiographic projection is limited only with respect to the arches and does not exceed them. In Fig. 978 the projection is such that the medial brightening strip extends over the contours of the arches and the vertebral bodies. The clavicles, which indicate as connective tissue bones the beginning of the ossification, are completely formed. Their extremities are covered by cartilaginous tissue. Between the 14th and 20th years of life, the medial clavicle obtains its own ossification center, the so-called sternoclavicular apophysis. The lateral cartilaginous cap very seldom has such an ossification zone. The suture of the medial clavicular apophysis closes between the 20th and 25th years, at the latest up to the 30th year of life.

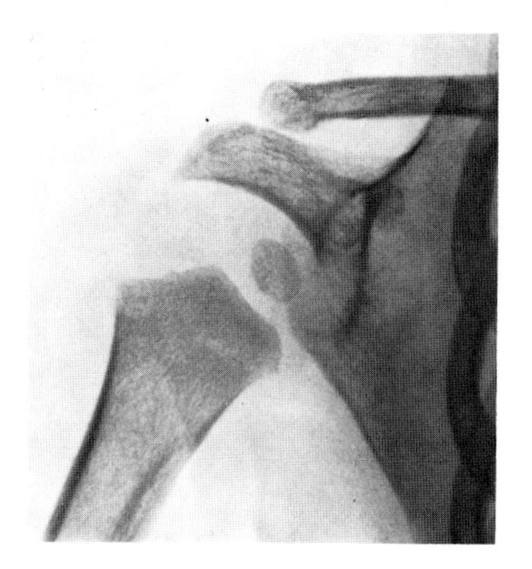

Fig. 1031. 9 month old. Additional bone anlagen not yet discernible.

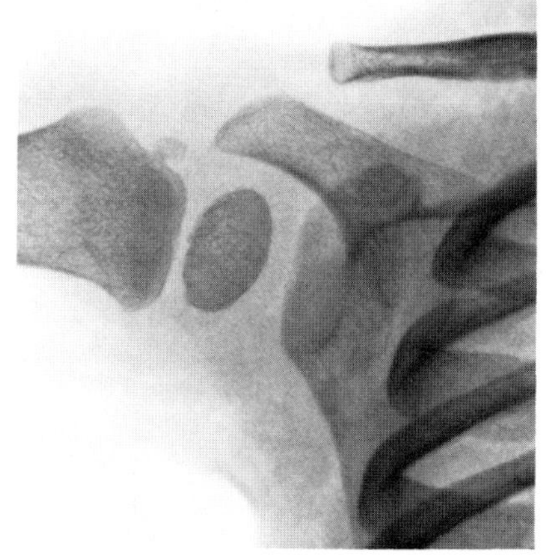

Fig. 1032. 11 month old. Besides the ossification nucleus in the caput humeri, the additional ossification nucleus, which appears around the second half of the 1st year of life, is already recognizable as the osseous nucleus of the tuberculum majus.

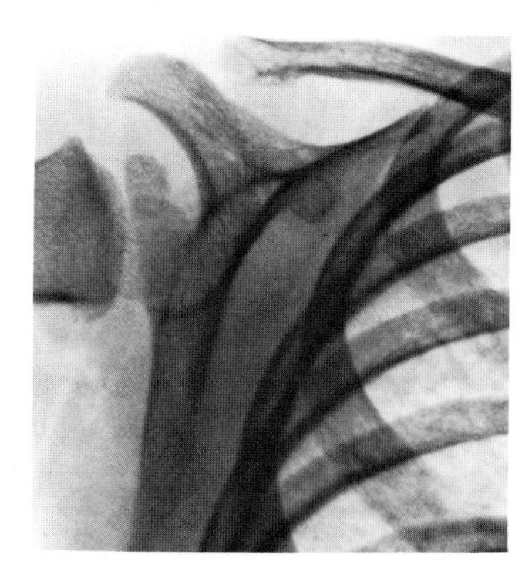

Fig. 1033. 1 year old. Here, additional bone anlagen are recognizable. In this projection the caput humeri nucleus looks remarkably spherical.

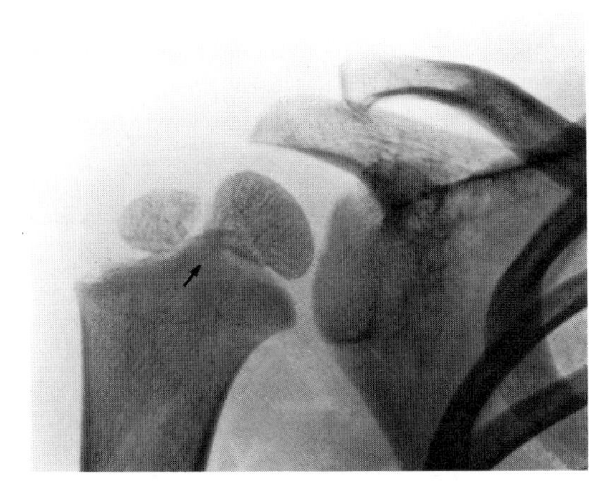

Fig. 1034. 2 year old. Another osseous nucleus belonging to the tuberculum minus has developed; it is covered by the nucleus anlage of the caput humeri in the caudal and lateral edge so that it shows itself in this nucleus anlage only as a compression zone (↗).

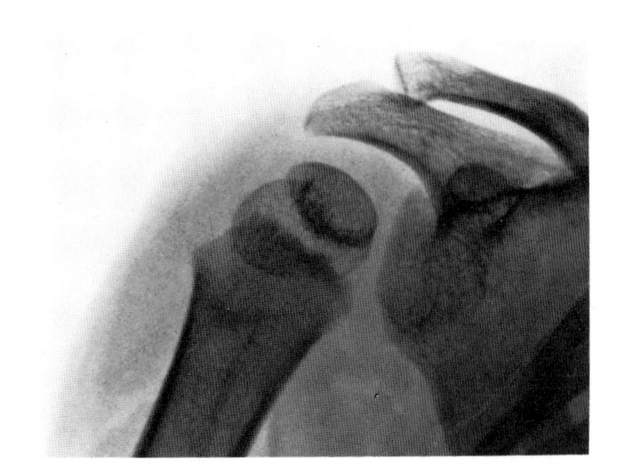

Fig. 1035. 3 year old. The growth increase of the osseous nucleus is easily recognizable, despite the somewhat different technical disposition. The nucleus of the tuberculum minus is not seen however, because it is covered by the tuberculum majus.

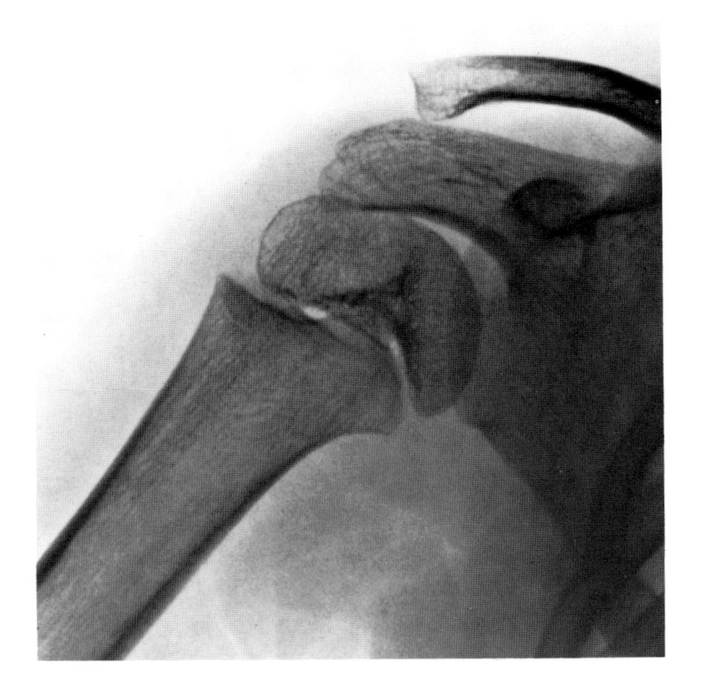

Fig. 1036. 4 year old. The fusion of the three nuclei into the proximal humerus epiphysis has taken place. The epiphysis fissure is still broad. The fusion occurs between the ages of 3$^{1}/_{2}$ and 6 years. The double oblique proximal humerus diaphysis extremity on which the proximal epiphysis seems to ride is well recognizable.

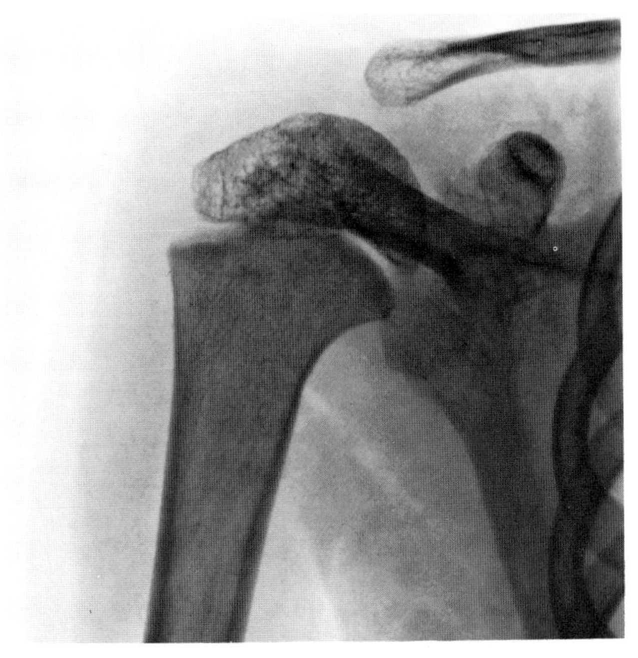

Fig. 1037. 5 year old. The acromion partly covers the epiphysis of the humerus and the epiphysis fissure.
The extremity of the acromion has a node-like bulge and its contours seem frayed. There is an ossification disorder here, which may be the beginning of a necrotic transformation. This occurs rather often in adults as a consequence of micro-traumas or a long time after an accident.

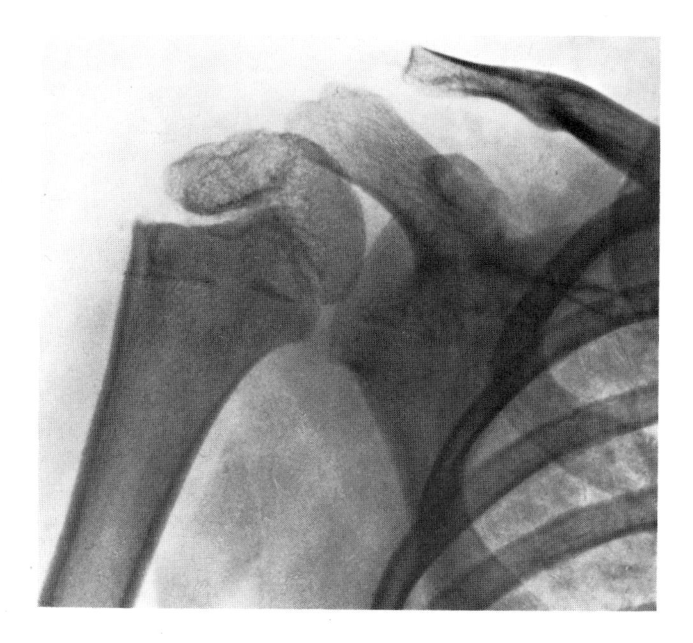

Fig. 1038. 6 year old. The proximal diaphysis limit appears clearly as a roof ridge on which the epiphysis rides. This is the beginning of dentation of the bone cartilage boundary of the glenoid fossa edges. Small coracoid. Already extraordinarily clear conoid tuberculum of the clavicle at the onset of the coracoclavicular ligament.

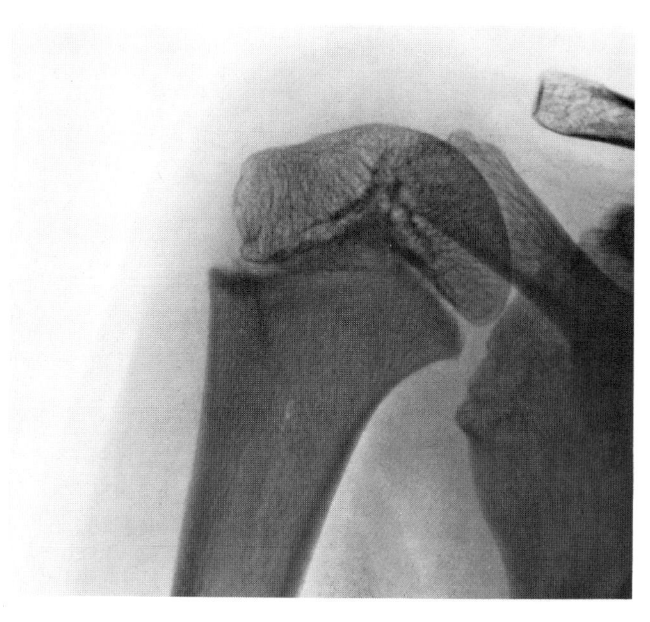

Fig. 1039. 8 year old. In this picture, an irregular edge of the glenoid cavity is recognizable. Here, it is a normal finding. A similar articulation limit may be observed in the glenoid cavity section of the hip joint in a growing skeleton, as well as in the covering plates of the vertebral bodies as so-called "growth notches."
The notched, wavy boundary of the pelvic apophysis may be understood similarly from the bone development (see Figs. 1150 and 1151).

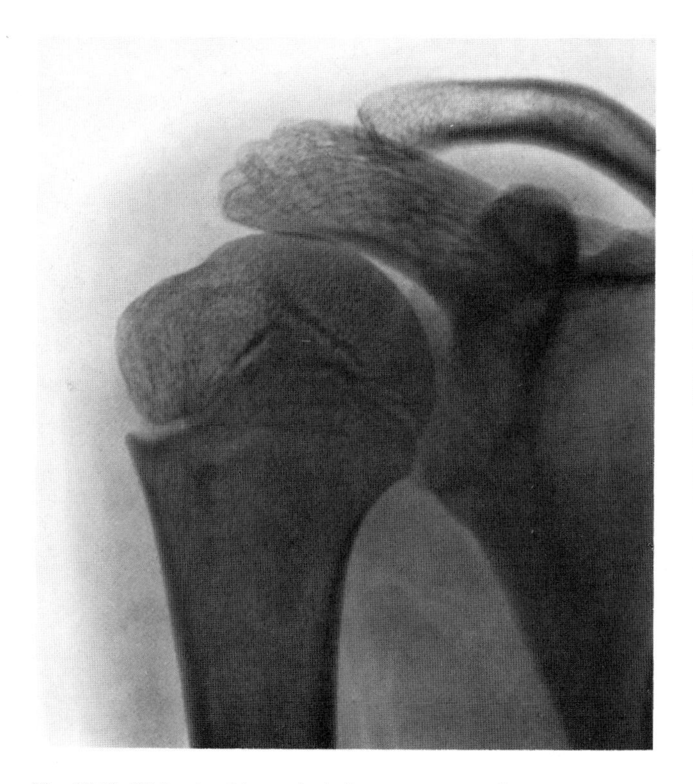

Fig. 1040. Right shoulder articulation, anteroposterior.

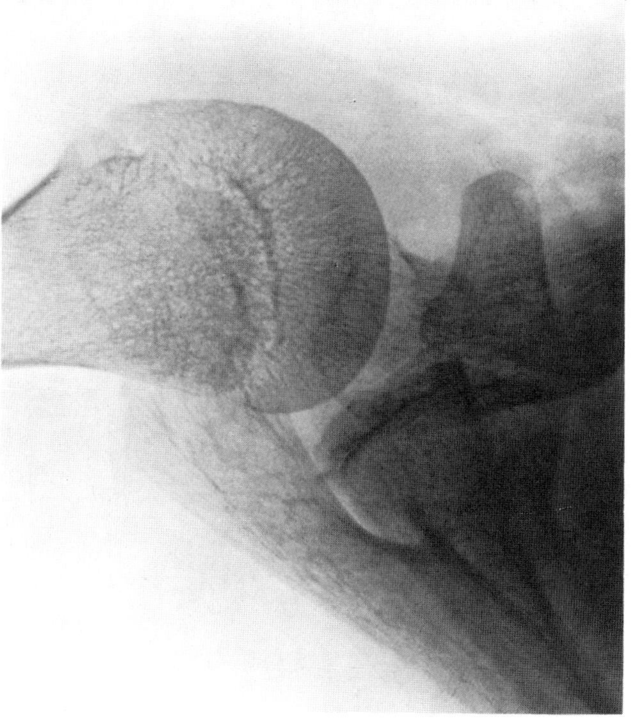

Fig. 1041. Right shoulder articulation, axial.

Figs. 1040 and 1041. 10 year old. Besides the continuous narrowing of the epiphysis fissure in the axial radiograph, the isolated development of the coracoid process is also recognizable.

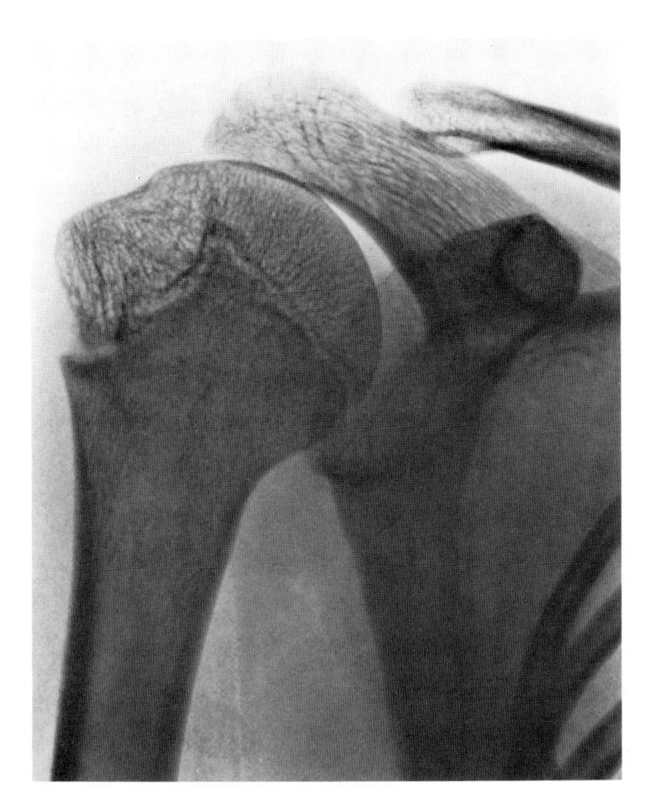

Fig. 1042. 12 year old. The beginning development of the apophysis of the acromion is already slightly marked. It takes place during puberty.

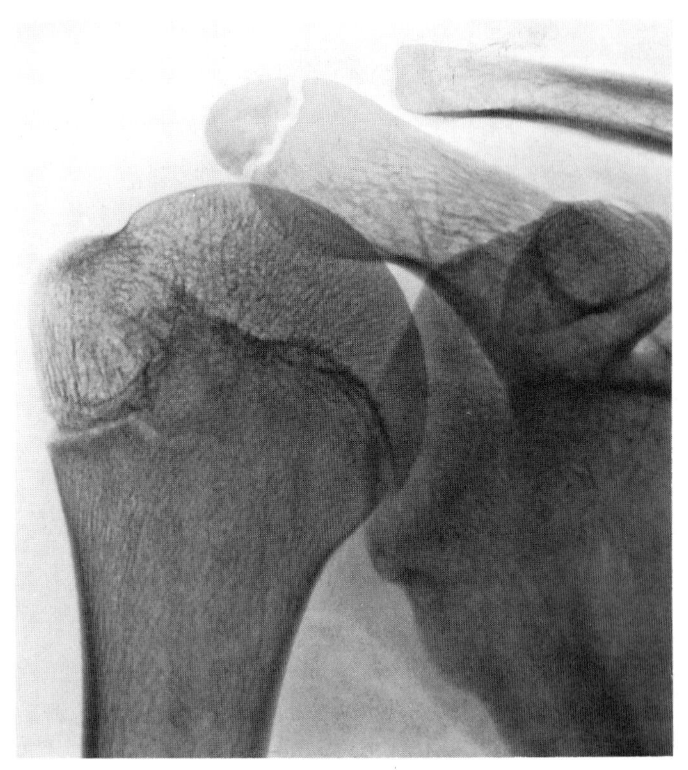

Fig. 1043. 13 year old. The apophysis of the acromion is already well formed. The coracoid apophysis at the "knee" of the coracoid process is also recognizable. It most frequently appears around the 15th to 17th year of life; however the time range may be longer.

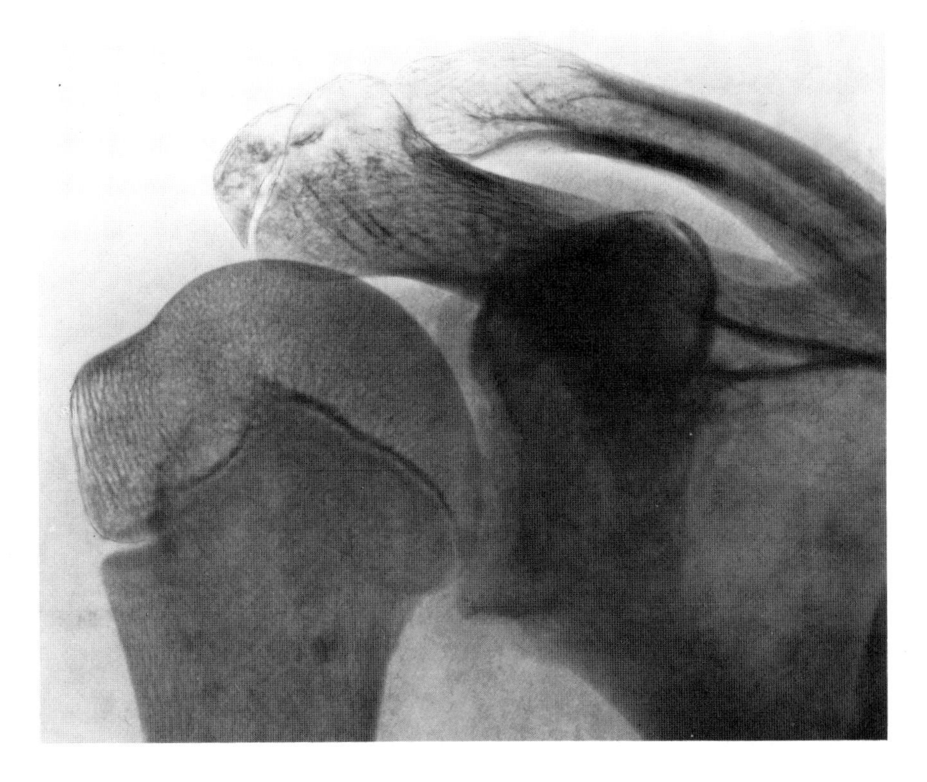

Fig. 1044. 14 1/2 year old. The apophysis of the acromion is formed; the apophysis fissure has slightly narrowed. The fusion of this apophysis nucleus with the acromion usually occurs around the 18th to 20th year of life. Also, the coracoid apophysis at the medial limit of the coracoid process is recognizable. The coracoid apophyses disappear around the 18th to 22nd year of life. The acromial clavicular extremity has here (as in most cases) no proper ossification center; it is smoothly and regularly edged. The smoothing of the edge of the glenoid cavity has advanced.

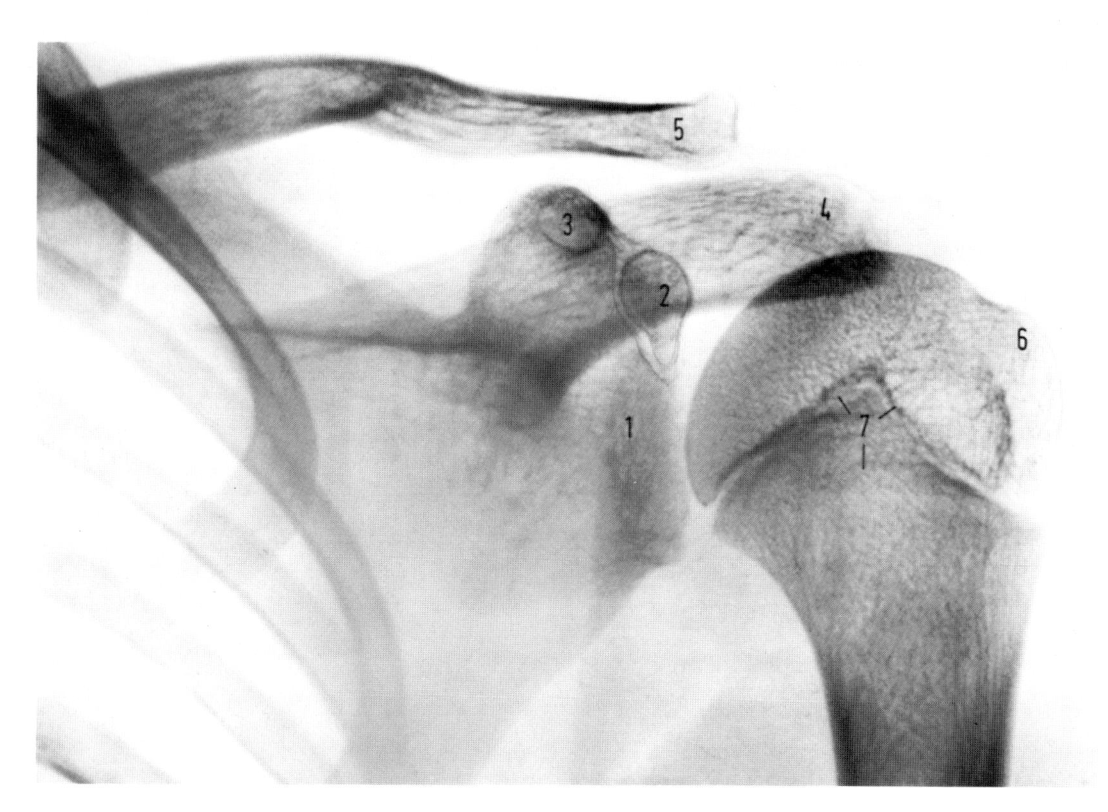

Fig. 1045. 14¹/₂ year old. Left shoulder articulation, cranioventrodorsal. The humerus is in a middle rotary position. The infracoracoid bone can be represented best in an axial radiograph. Here, it is readily recognizable, by means of a cranioventrodorsal radiation path, at the base of the coracoid as a superior glenoid cavity edge. The infracoracoid bone is still separated by a narrow cartilaginous suture from the scapula as well as from the coracoid process. The coracoid and acromial apophyses are not yet visible (variation).

1 Glenoid cavity edge
2 Infracoracoid bone (slightly retouched)
3 Coracoid
4 Acromion
5 Acromial extremity of the clavicle
6 Major tubercle
7 Epiphysis suture of the head of the humerus

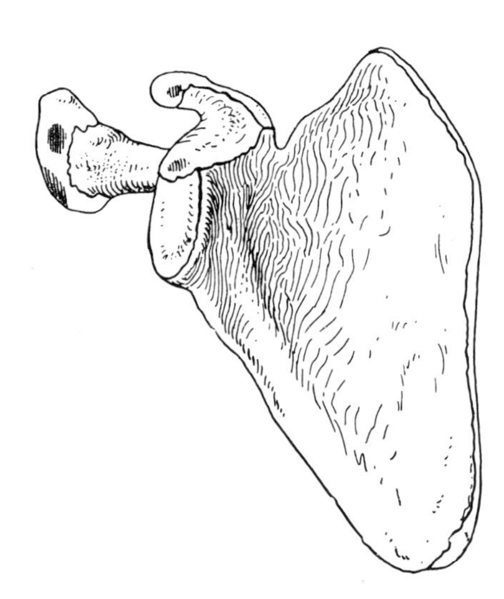

Fig. 1046 shows the secondary ossification centers (hatched), inside the still cartilaginous covered coracoid and acromial parts. The former appear only in the 2nd year of life. The cartilaginous rim at the scapular edge is also discernible. The acromial apophysis may persist up to an advanced age = acromial bone (from *Merkel*).

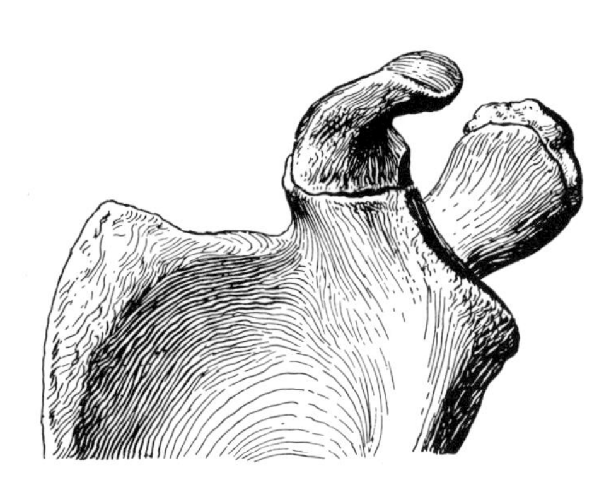

Fig. 1047 shows the **apophyseal fissures** in a favorable view for the correct reading of radiographs (from *Heitzmann*).

1 Coracoid apophysis at the knee of the coracoid process
2 Coracoid apophysis at the apex
3 Glenoid cavity
4 Superior angle (scapula)
5 Acromion
6 Clavicle

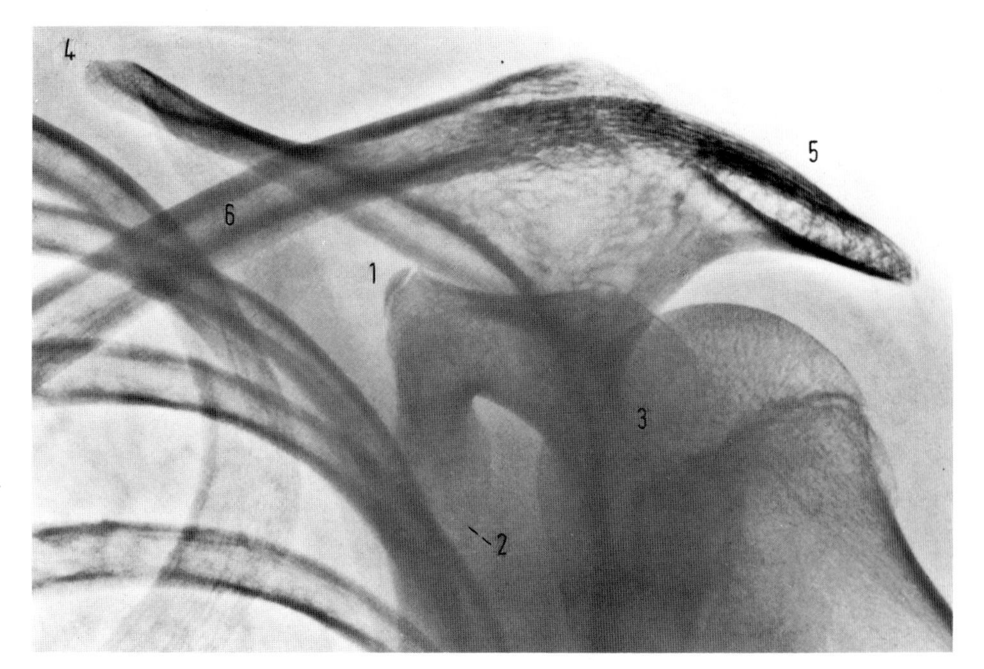

Fig. 1048. 16 year old. Left shoulder articulation, craniodorsal (for setting, see Fig. 517).

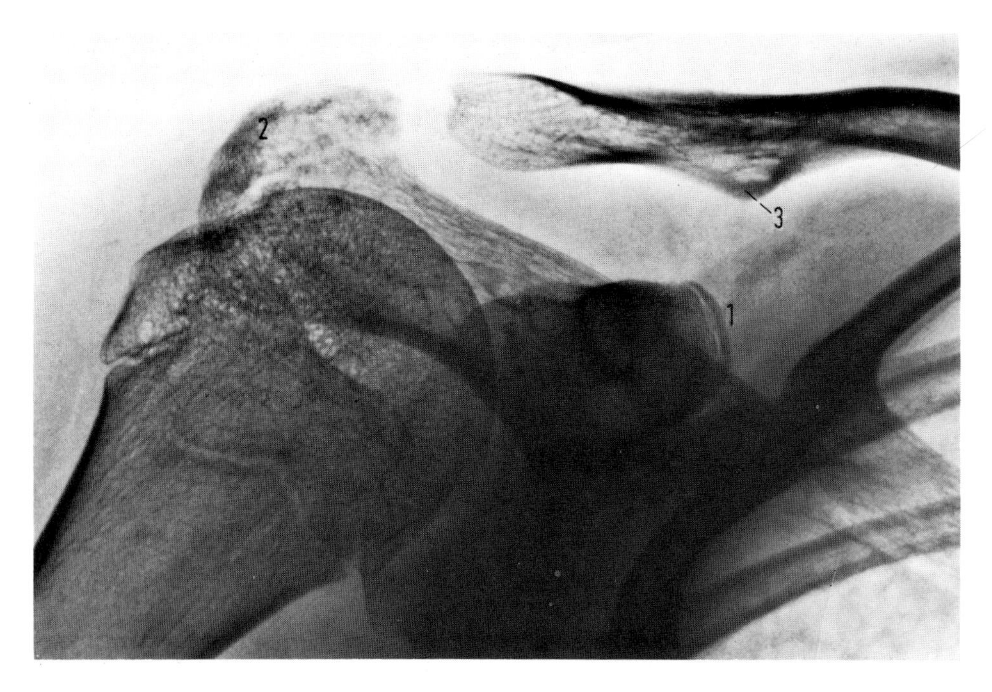

Fig. 1049. 16 year old. Right shoulder articulation, ventrodorsal (for setting, see Fig. 516). Here, one still sees denticulation and fibrillation of the sternal cup-shaped clavicular extremity.

1 Coracoid apophysis at the knee, taken axially
2 Acromial apophysis fused with the acromion around the 20th year of life, possibly even earlier
3 Conoidal tubercle, especially large here, with two oviferous cavities in the bone structure

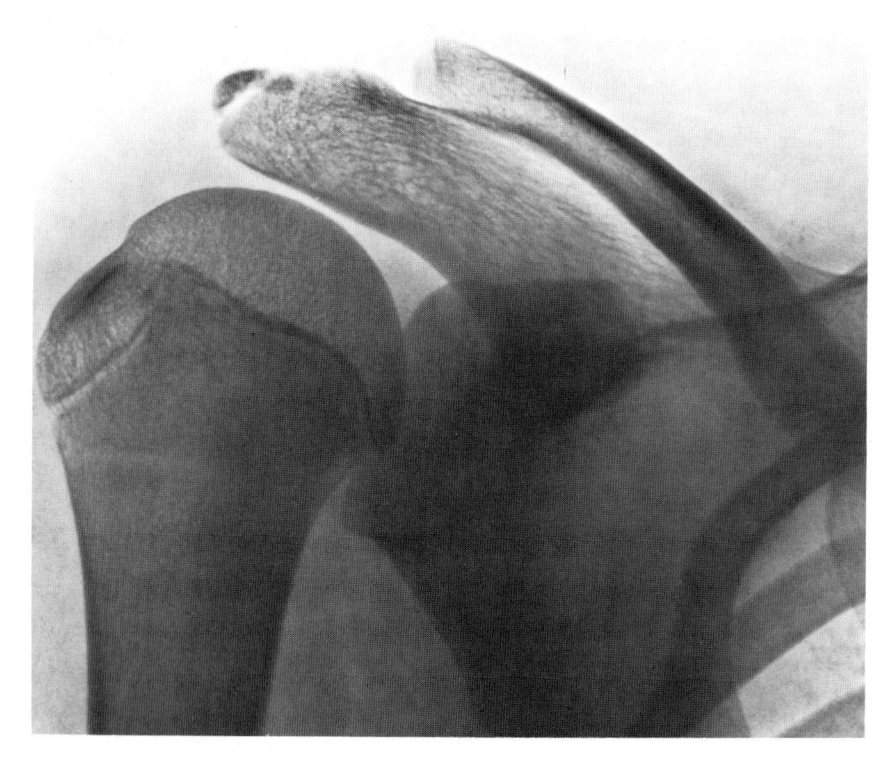

Fig. 1050. 16 year old. The epiphyseal fissure of the proximal humeral epiphysis has become narrower and is about to ossify. The coracoid process is taken axially and is therefore recognizable only as a dark disk. The acromial apophysis, in this case, is very slightly developed and shows a clear division into two parts. A fine lightened strip, in the proximal diaphysis section of the upper arm bone in the external part, may be erroneously taken for a fracture. Actually, this lightened strip is due to the radiograph; it conforms to a part of the epiphyseal fissure which develops in an oblique direction (see Figs. 531 and 1051). The contour of the acromial clavicular extremity is still slightly fissured.

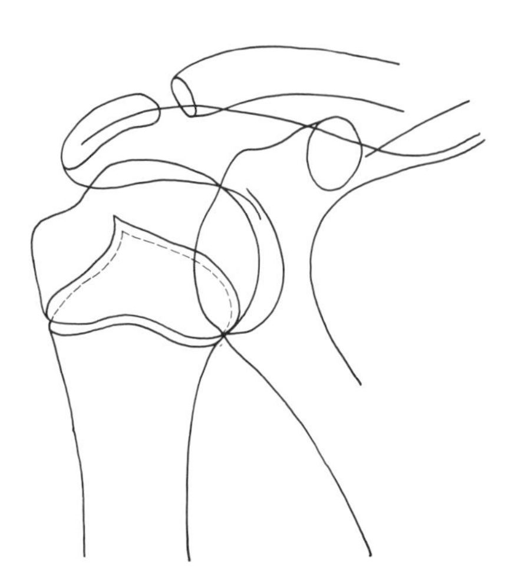

Fig. 1051. Shoulder articulation of an 18 year old. The figure shows the borders of the epiphysis corresponding to Fig. 1050. This projection of the epiphyseal fissure resembles an upside-down heart on a playing card. This is the way the roof ridge originates, over which the humeral epiphysis rides farther down the lightened strip, obliquely over the humerus. This may lead to an incorrect diagnosis of fracture.

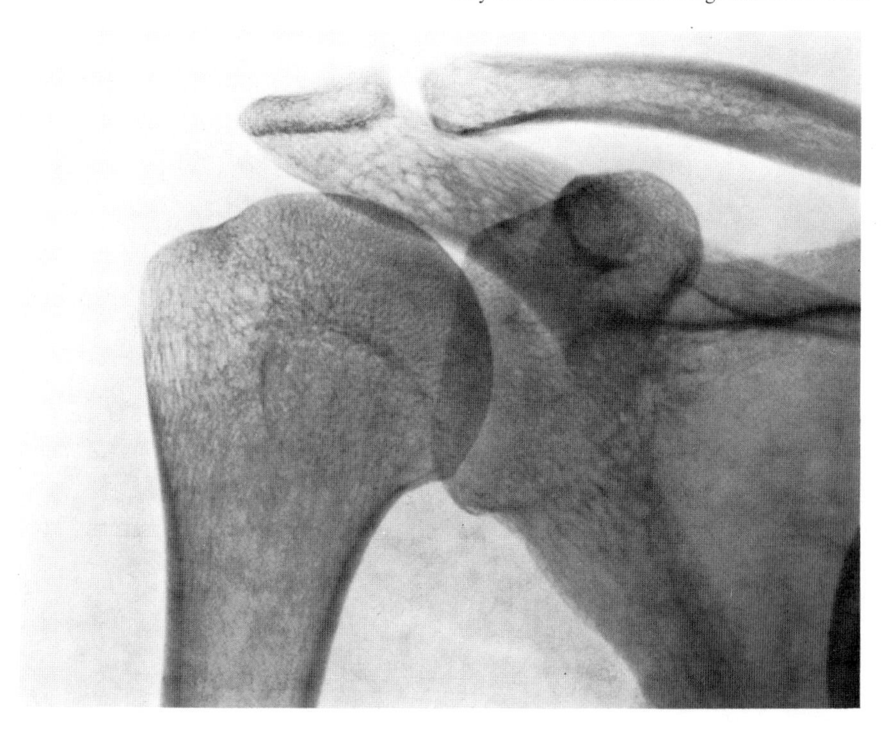

Fig. 1052. 18 year old. All apo- and epiphyseal sutures are already closed and thus, at this stage, growth has terminated. Below the proximal humeral epiphysis there is still a strip-like compression, a so-called epiphyseal scar, traces of which may remain throughout the life span (cf. Figs. 1179 and 768).
Also, the lateral part of the clavicle is smooth, rounded and with no completed osseous nucleus of its own.

A Series of Radiographs of the Development of the Scapula between Ages 5 to 18

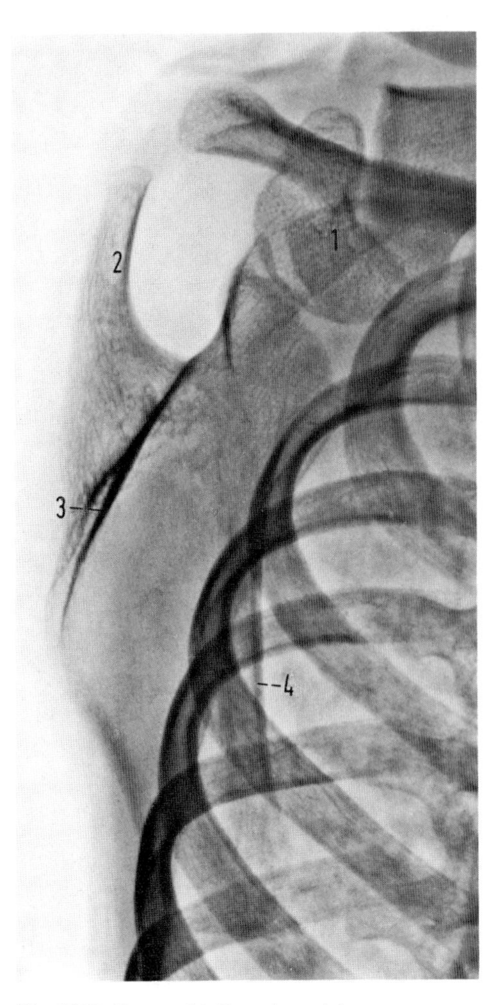

Fig. 1053. 5 year old. Scapula, axial.

It is possible to see the cartilaginous suture at the base of the coracoidal nucleus. The development of the coracoid process begins in the 1st year of life. The representation of the acromion is somewhat distorted due to the projection.

1 Coracoid nucleus
2 Acromion
3 Lateral margin (orthograde)
4 Medial margin

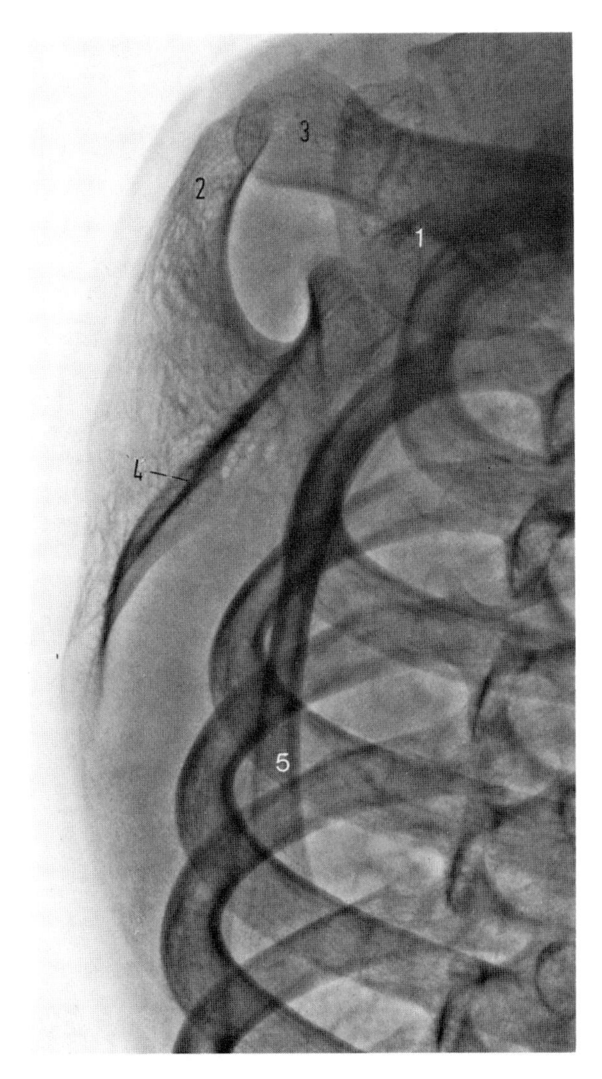

Fig. 1054. 8 year old. Scapula, axial.

1 Nucleus of the coracoid process superimposed by the proximal upper-arm epiphysis
2 Acromion
3 Clavicle
4 Lateral margin
5 Medial margin

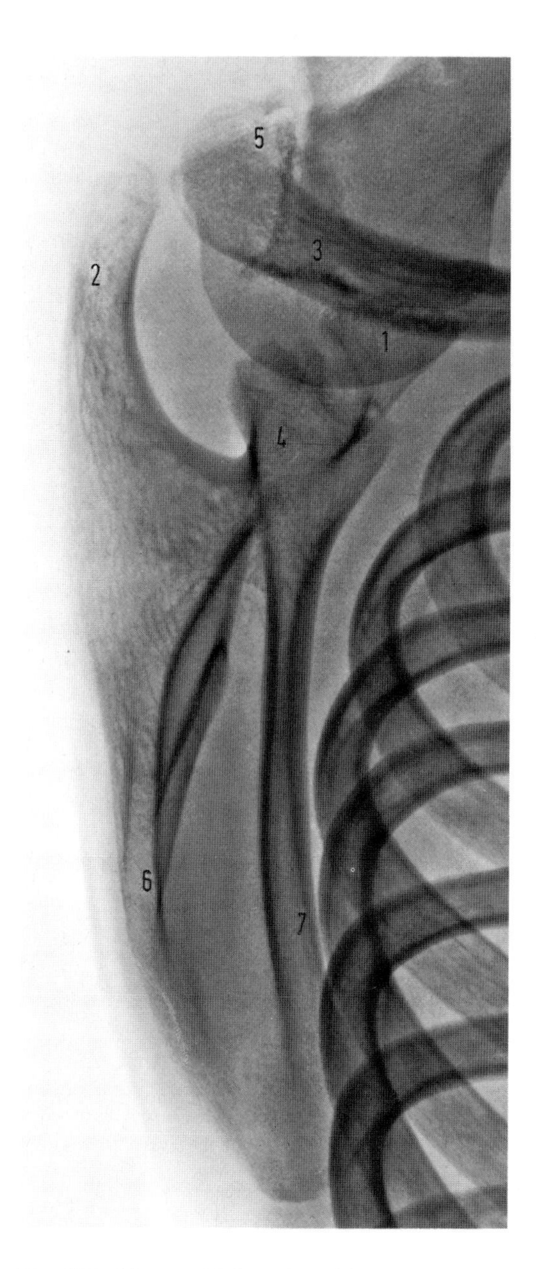

Fig. 1055. 12 year old. Scapula, axial.

1 Nucleus of the coracoid process
2 Acromion
3 Clavicle
4 Tangential projection of glenoid cavity, with typical growth notches
5 Nucleus of the major tubercle
6 Lateral margin
7 Medial margin

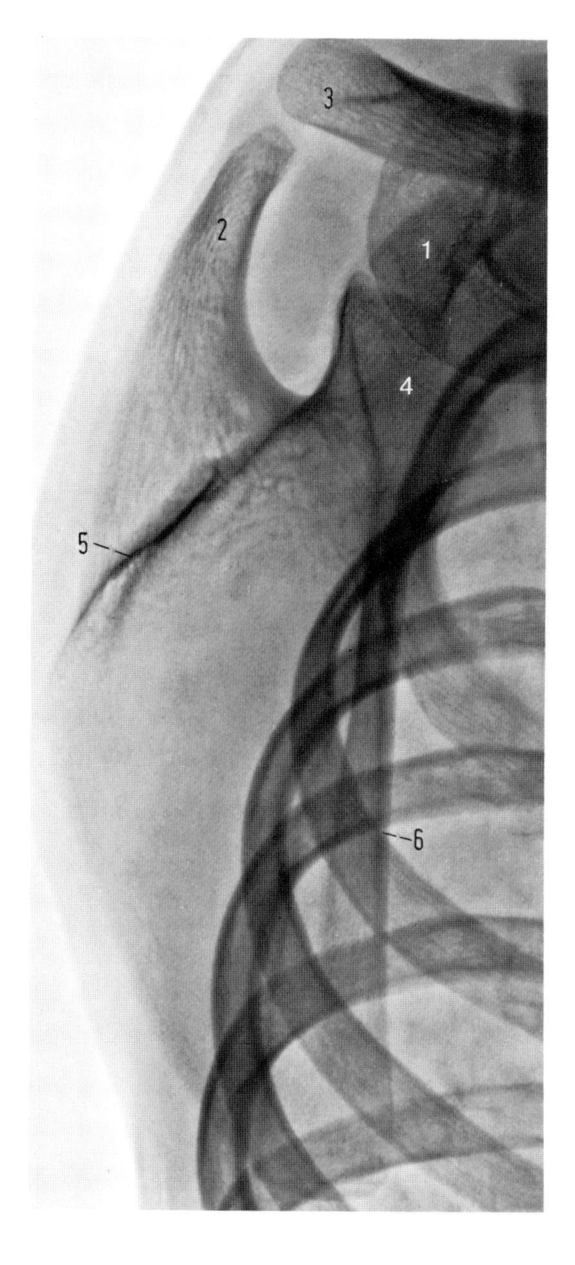

Fig. 1056. 14 year old. Scapula, axial. The osseous fusion of the coracoid nucleus with the scapula is not effected until age 15 to 20.

1 Here, too, the coracoid nucleus projects itself partly on the upper-arm apophysis
2 Acromion
3 Clavicle
4 Tangential projected glenoid cavity
5 Lateral margin
6 Medial margin

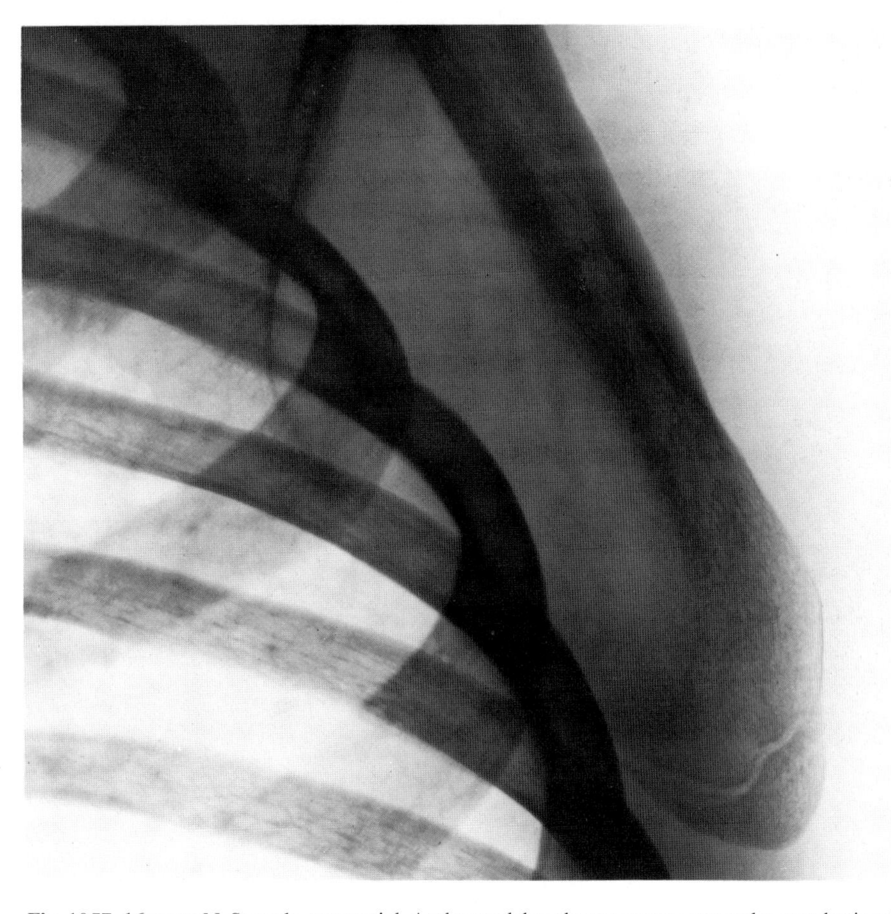

Fig. 1057. 16 year old. Scapula, tangential. At the caudal angle one can see a scapular apophysis, which may persist (see also Fig. 534).

The apophysis at the inferior scapular angle appears between the 16th and 18th years of life as an independent, secondary osseous nucleus, which is fused with the scapula in adults. The designation of a persisting apophysis at the inferior scapular angle, either as an infrascapular or a subscapular bone, is admissible, in the present author's opinion, only if it persists in adulthood.

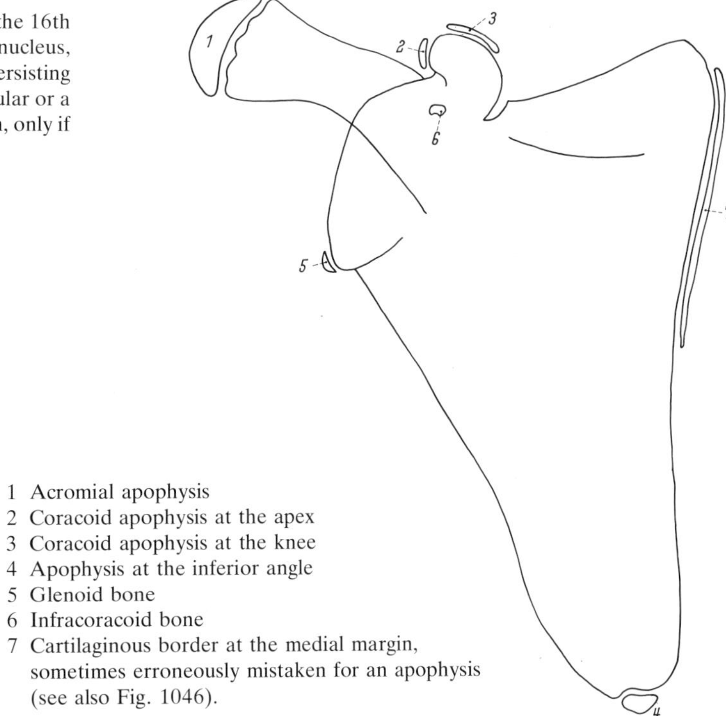

Fig. 1058. Radiographically discernible secondary ossification centers in the region of the scapula.

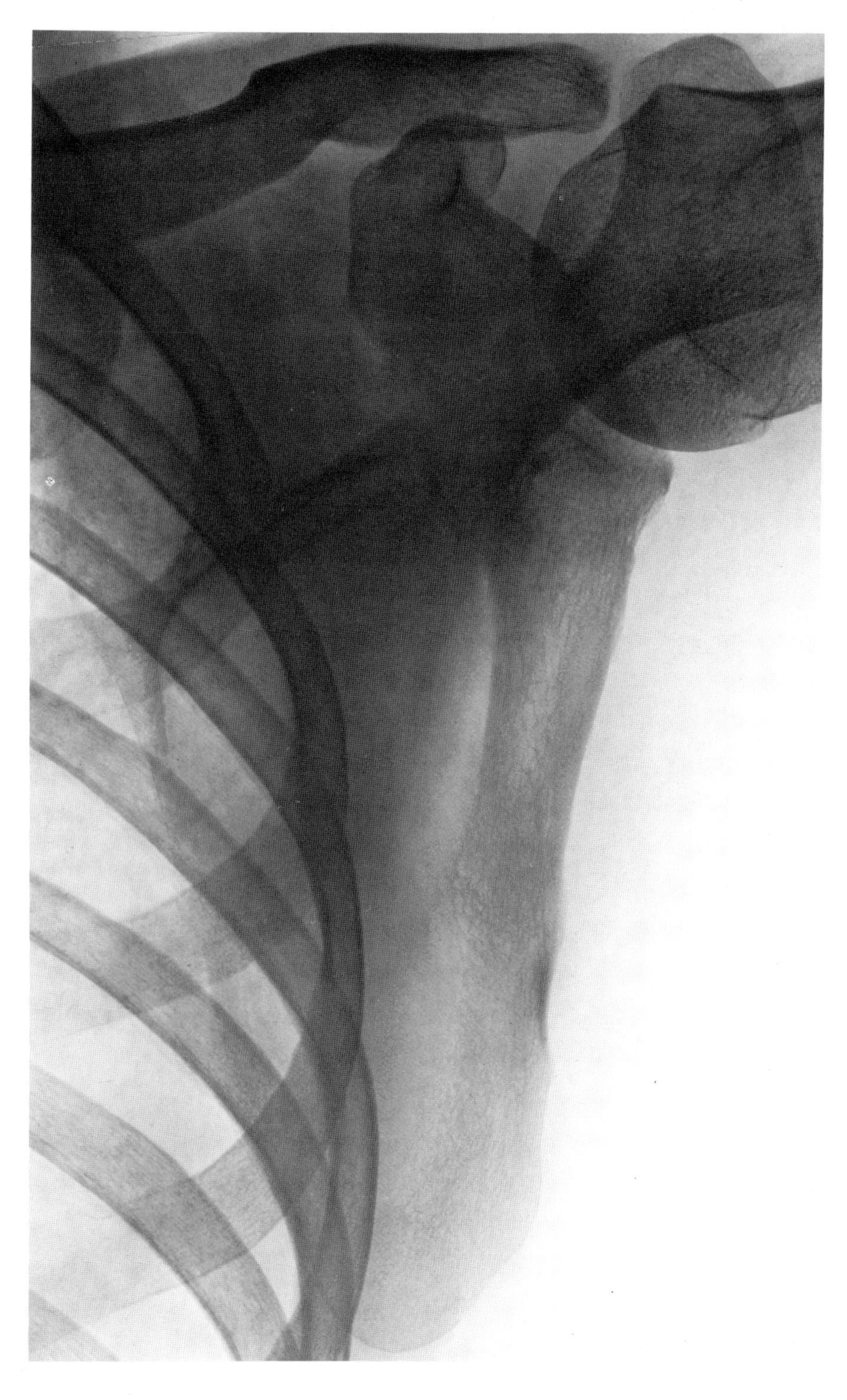

Fig. 1059. 18 year old. Scapula, lateroventrodorsal. For setting, see Fig. 512. The development of this bone is now terminated. The apophysis at the inferior angle is fused with the scapular bone. The acromial apophysis, which is already fused by about the 20th year of life, is no longer separately discernible. The glenoid cavity and its borders are well excavated and smooth.

Elbow Region

No epiphyseal nuclei are found in the elbow region of a newborn. The ossification course is complicated because the humeral epiphysis is composed of several separable nuclei. It is difficult to form an opinion, especially in cases of advanced age, because of the impossibility of projecting isolated sections of the elbow.

The distal epiphysis of the upper arm bone is formed out of four osseous nuclei, of which the capitulum humeri appear first; the nuclei of the epicondyles and the trochleas appear much later *(Banki)*.

Capitulum humeri. The nucleus of the capitulum humeri is always the first nucleus to be found in the elbow region. Its appearance occurs, according to the usual concept, around the 2nd year of life *(Davies* and *Parsons)*. However, we noted its appearance in an earlier developmental phase (Figs. 1066 and 1067), probably around the end of the 1st year of life. This discrepancy can be attributed to routing prophylactic treatment with vitamin D against rickets, possibly causing a premature ossification of the nucleus.

Medial epicondyle. According to the literature, it appears around the 6th to 9th year of life. But according to our observations, this nucleus, too, appears much earlier (Figs. 1068, 1069). During this development, a small groove forms at the distal humeral extremity at the level of the medial epicondyle, and the epicondyle anlage nestles against this groove. From time to time, a division of this nucleus into two is found.

Trochlea. The trochlea appears almost together with the olecranon, i.e., between the 8th and 10th years of life. A nucleus that is irregularly split and very frequently divided into various ossification centers is characteristic here.

Lateral epicondyle. This scale-shaped nucleus is the last to appear in the elbow region. It usually appears at the beginning of puberty. It is seen as an isolated osseous nucleus for a short period only. One or $1^1/_2$ years later it fuses with the capitulum humeri into one nucleus.

Fusion into the distal humerus apophysis. One or $1^1/_2$ years after the appearance of the lateral epicondyle, during puberty, it fuses with the capitulum humeri into one nucleus. Somewhat later, the capitulum and the trochlea fuse so that the distal humerus epiphysis is composed of a fusion of the trochlea, the capitulum humeri and the lateral epicondyle (Fig. 1061).

Lower arm bones with proximal epiphysis. The diaphysial nuclei of the ulna and the radius are discernible at almost the same period as the humerus (8th embryonic week). Still, the ossification of the proximal epiphysis is slower in relation to the ossification of the distal, while the proximal epiphyseal nucleus of the radius appears before that of the ulna.

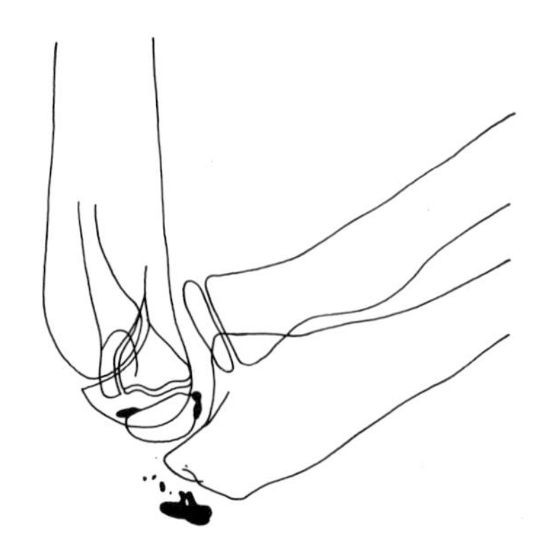

Fig. 1060 shows how split the **ossification anlage of the olecranon** can be (a $12^1/_4$-year-old child).

Radius head. This nucleus appears over a very long time span. It usually occurs during the 4th to 7th years of life, and somewhat earlier in girls than in boys. The nucleus quickly forms an osseous disk, which occupies the entire diaphysial breadth of the radius.

Olecranon. Between the 9th and 12th years of life, numerous fissured ossification centers appear in the region of the olecranon, and out of these one or two osseous centers are built up (Fig. 1060). The time span required for the fusion of these two nuclei is relatively long. A wavy and segmented epiphyseal glenoid cavity at the olecranon, which can measure up to 5 mm at first, is always striking. The fusion occurs during the 16th to 20th years of life, first in the volar side, while on the dorsal side a deep groove remains at first. Luxation of the olecranon epiphysis can frequently be excluded only through comparison with a similar radiograph.

Termination of the ossification. The closure of the distal humerus epiphysis occurs around the 14th to 17th years of life, occurring earlier (14 years) in girls and strong individuals and later (16–17 years) in boys. Shortly afterwards, the suture between the medial condyle and the humerus shaft closes. The epiphyseal closure of the caput radii and the olecranon occurs one year earlier than the closure of the epiphysis at the distal humerus extremity.

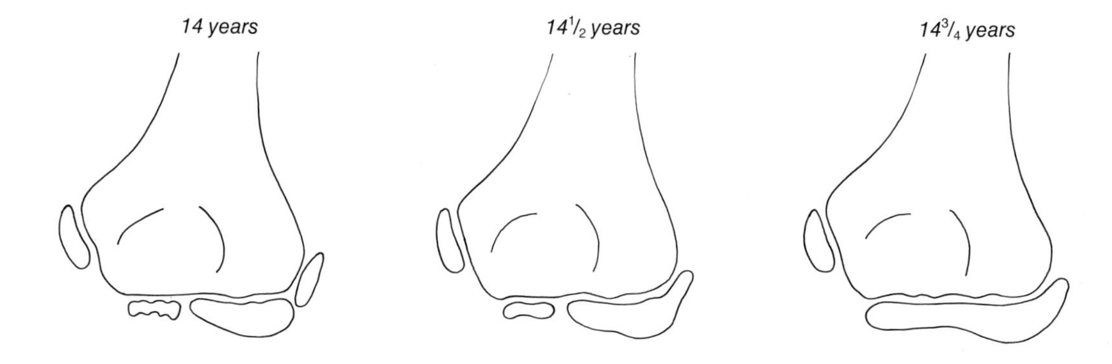

Fig. 1061. Formation of the distal humeral epiphysis.

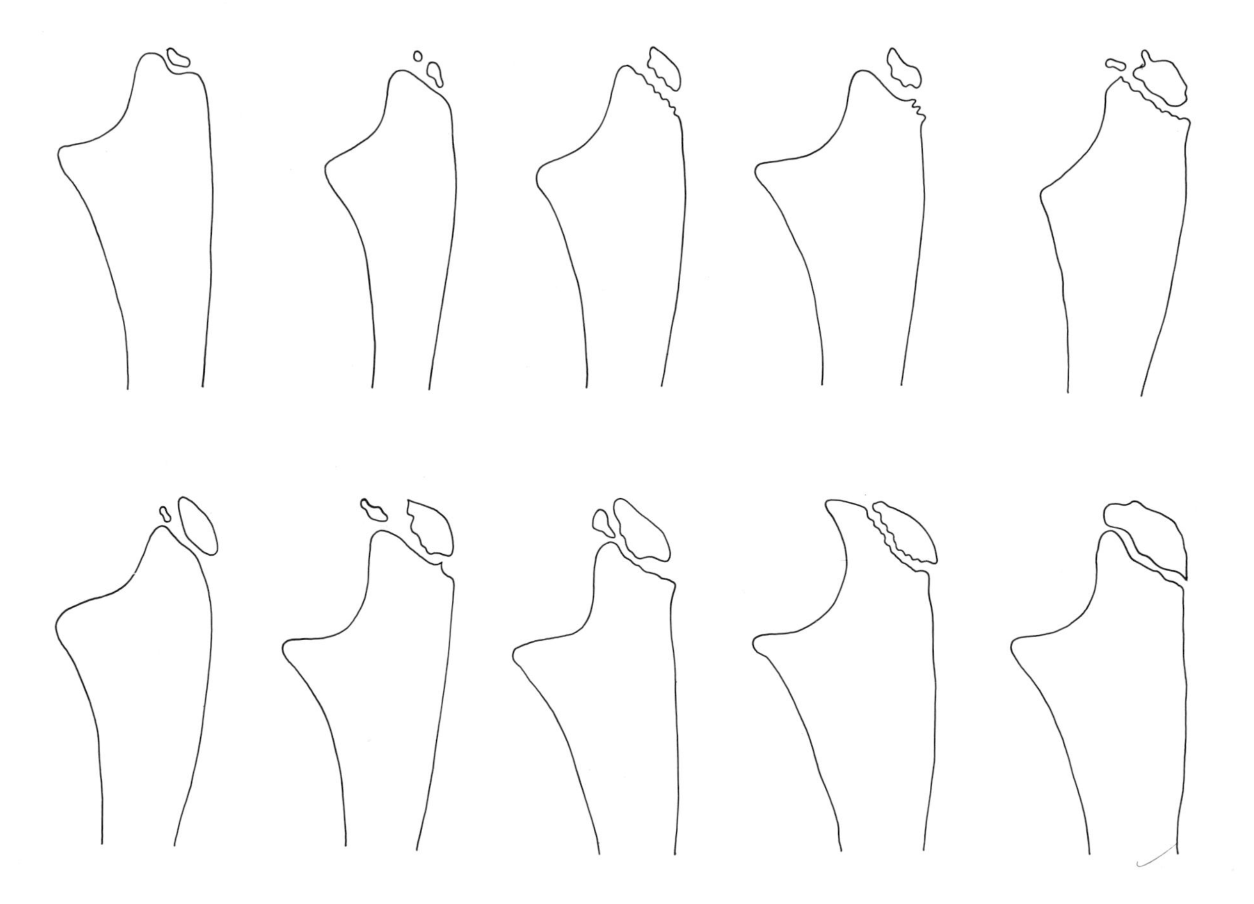

Fig. 1062. Various ossification forms of the olecranian epiphysis in 8- to 10-year-old children.

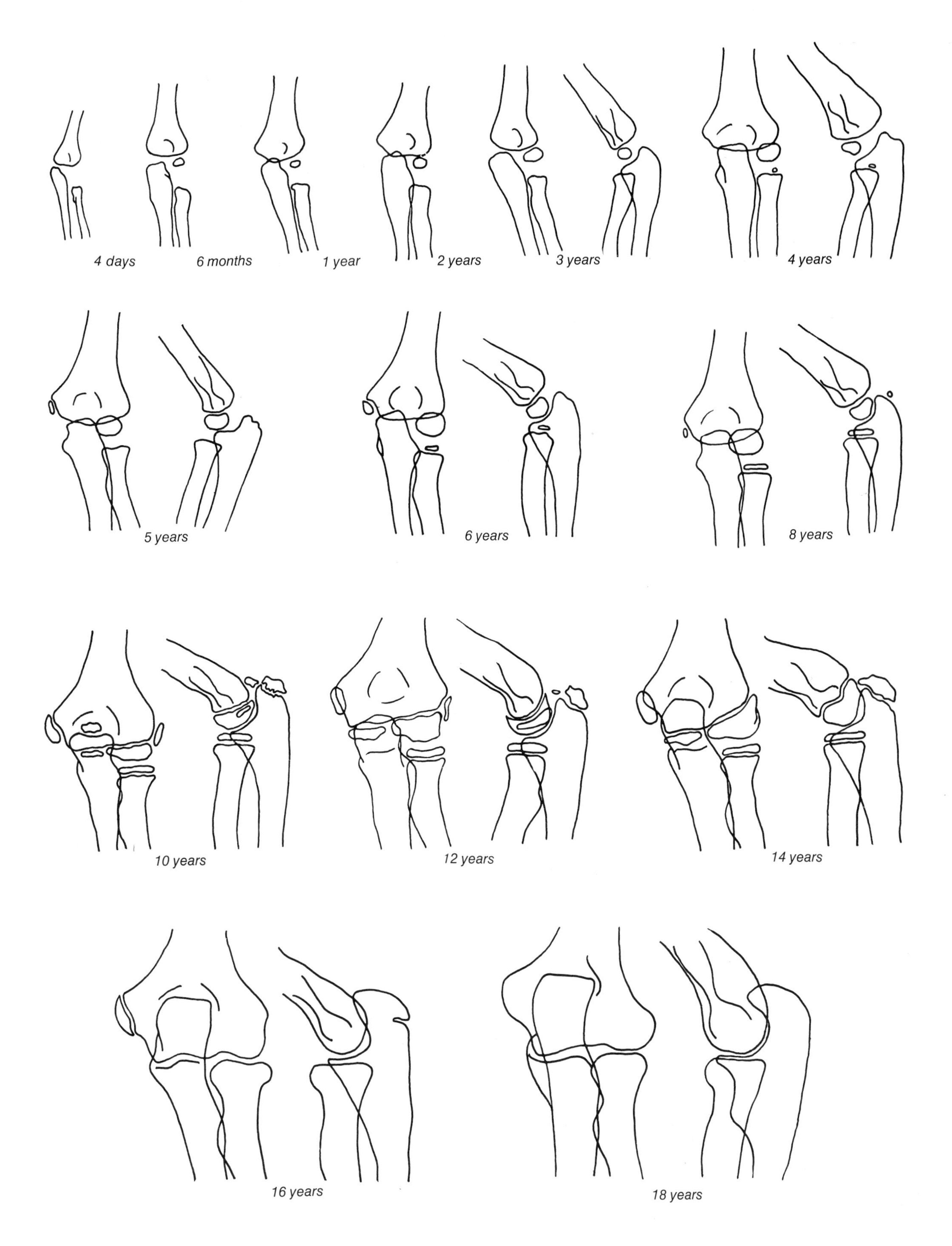

Fig. 1063. Elbow articulation in chronological order from early infancy to age 18.

A Series of Radiographs of the Development of the Elbow Region and Its Articulations from Infancy to Age 18

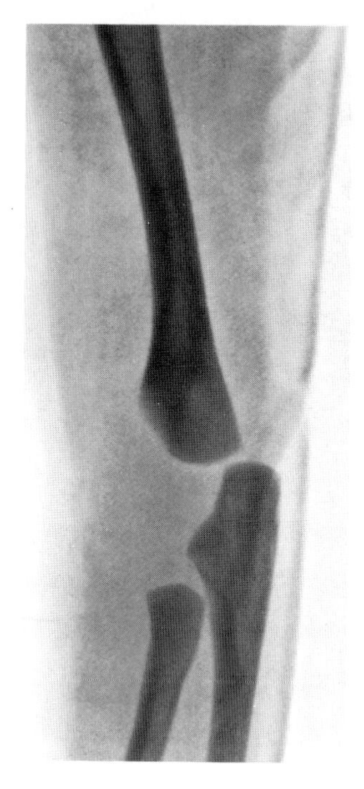

Fig. 1064. 1 day old. No bone anlage.

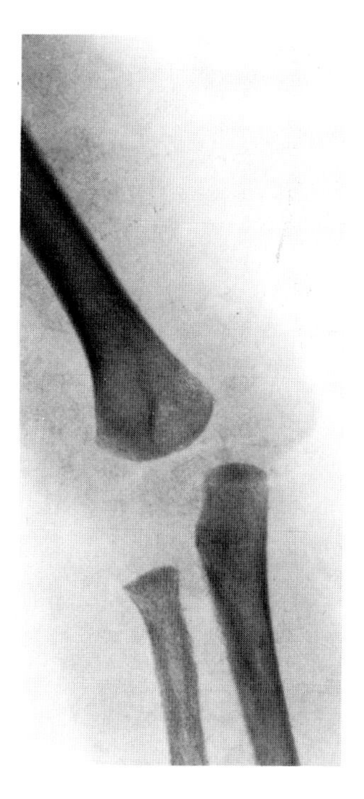

Fig. 1065. 2 month old. No bone anlage.

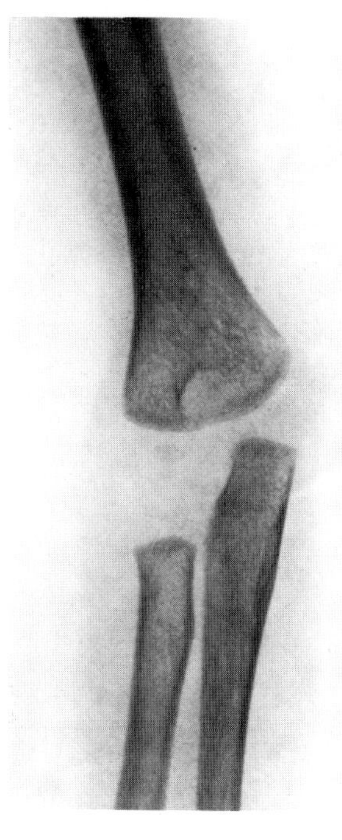

Fig. 1066. 9 month old. 1st osseous nucleus in the capitulum humeri.

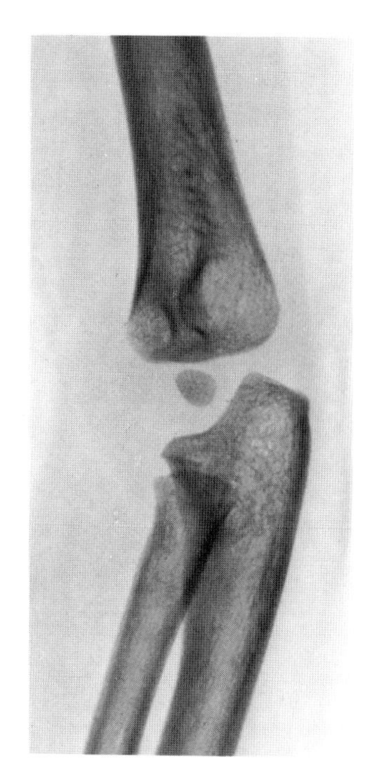

Fig. 1067. 1$^{1}/_{2}$ year old. Distinct increase of the osseous nucleus in the capitulum humeri.

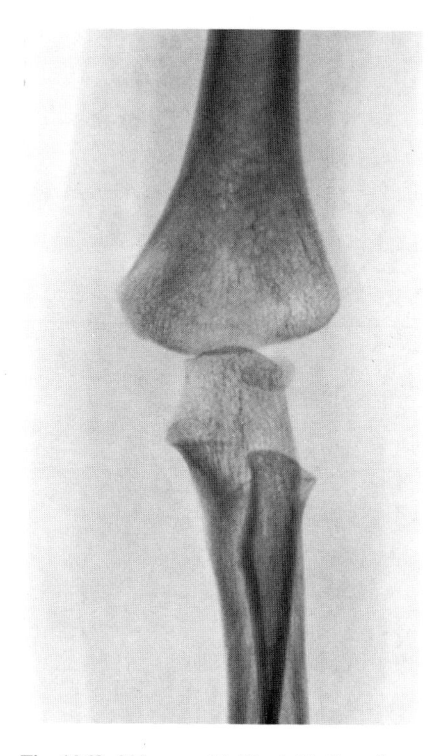

Fig. 1068. 2$^{1}/_{2}$ year old. The initiation of ossification of the next osseous nucleus is faintly discernible in the medial epicondyle. Its appearance usually occurs in the 6th year of life. However, it can occur much earlier (as a consequence of rickets prophylaxis?).

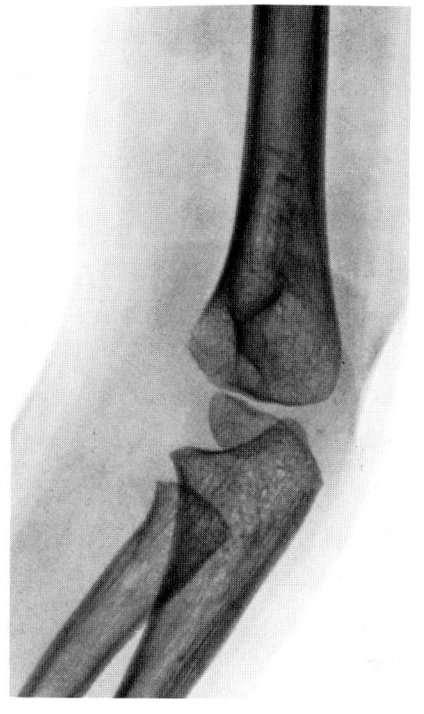

Fig. 1069 a

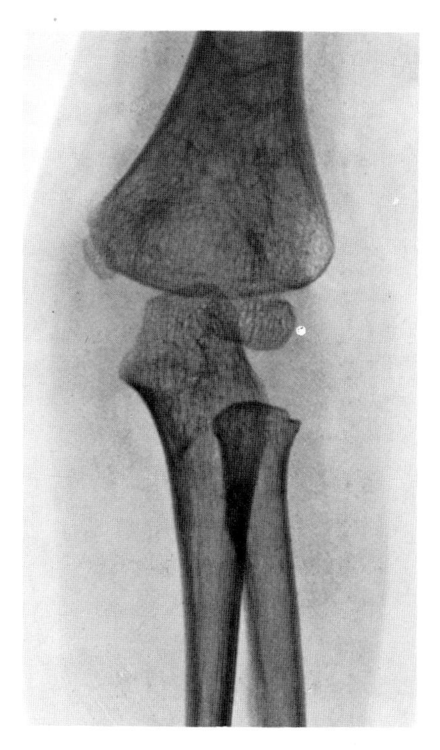

Fig. 1069 b

Fig. 1069. 4 year old. The nucleus of the capitulum humeri has grown, and the nucleus anlage in the medial epicondyle is now clearly discernible.

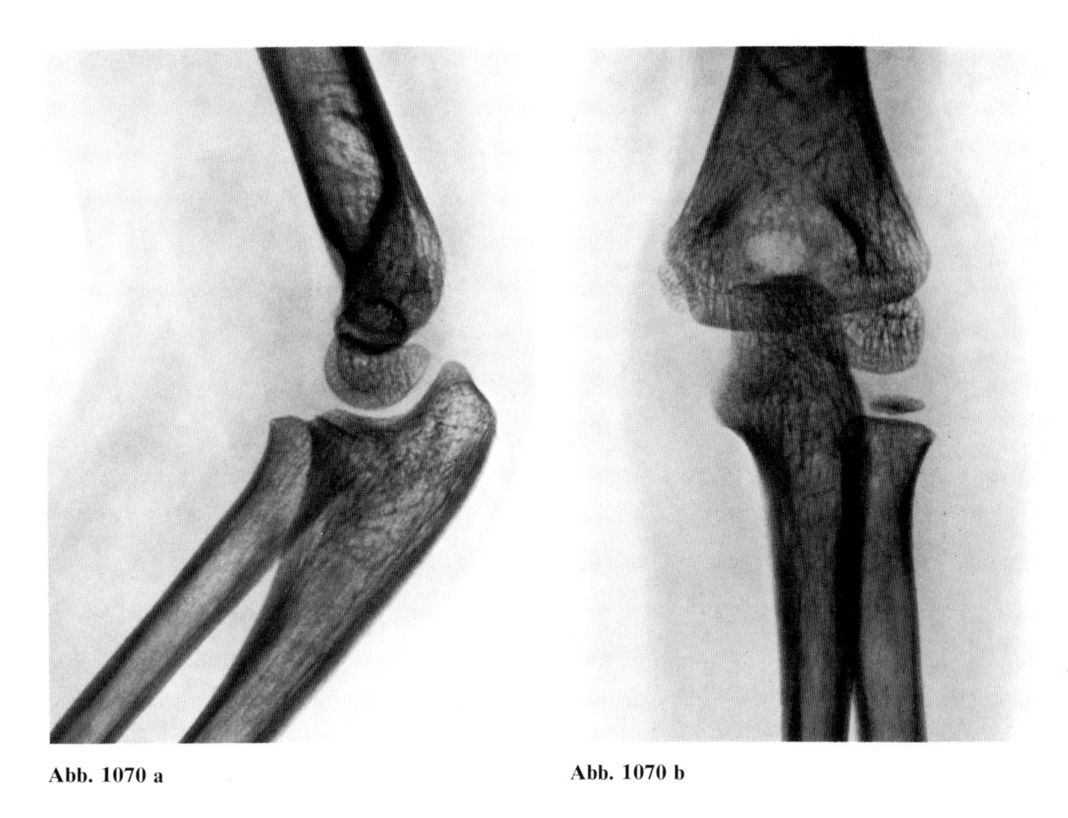

Abb. 1070 a **Abb. 1070 b**

Fig. 1070. 6 year old. Apart from the nuclei of the capitulum humeri and the medial epicondyle, the bony nucleus in the caput radii can be recognized as the 3rd nucleus (4th to 7th year).

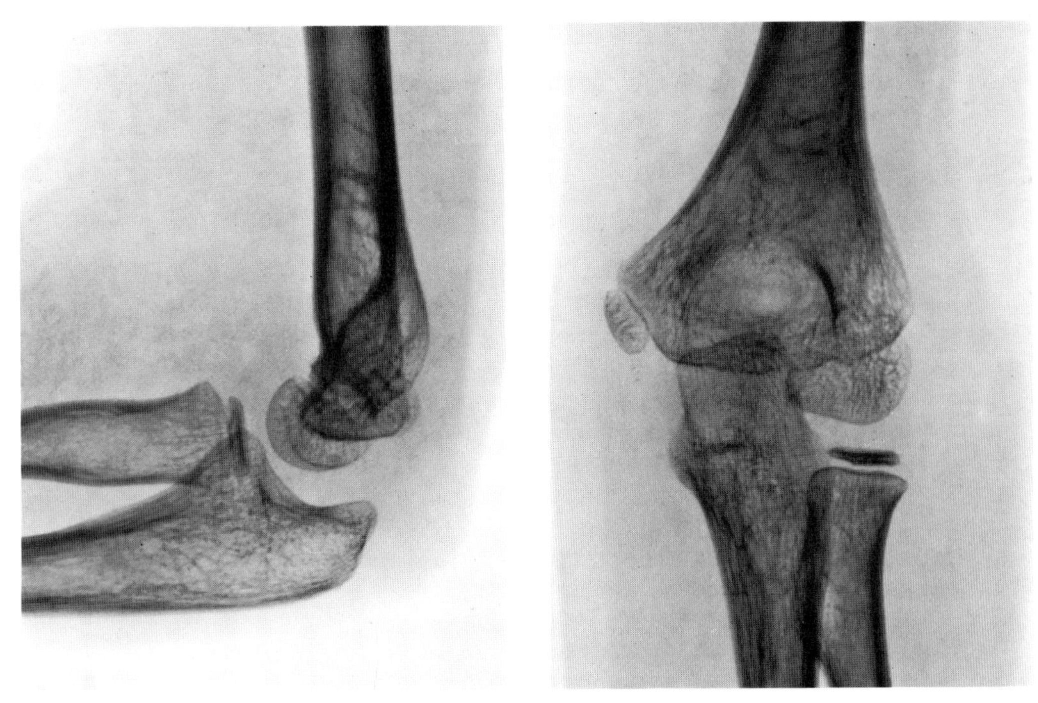

Fig. 1071 a **Fig. 1071 b**

Fig. 1071. 8 year old. New nuclei are not yet recognizable but the ossification of the olecranon, which starts at this age, may already be proved (9th to 12th year).

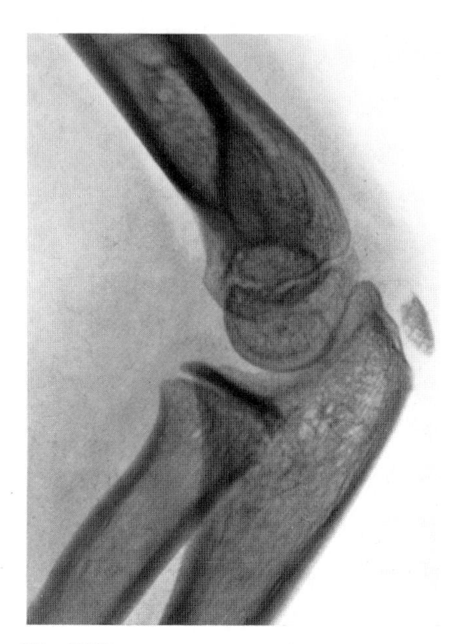

Fig. 1072 a

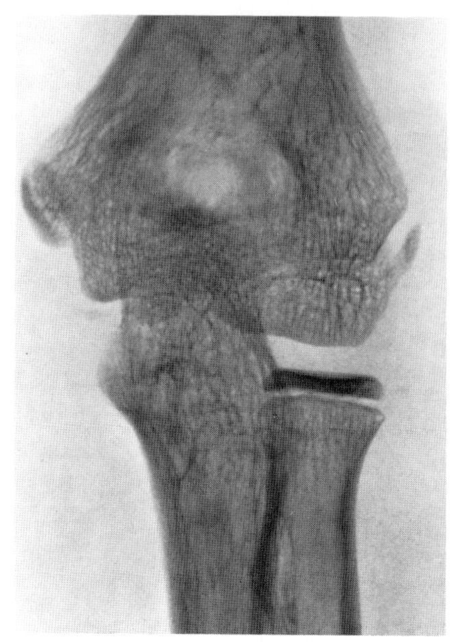

Fig. 1072 b

Fig. 1072. 10 year old. While the olecranon nucleus is visible in the lateral picture, the nucleus of the epicondyle, which appears isolated for only a short time, is recognizable in an anteroposterior picture. It usually appears as the last nucleus in the elbow region. The nucleus of the trochlea is already discernible; it usually develops at the same time as the nucleus of the olecranon, and the nuclei are completely discernible. The strong compression of the disk-shaped caput radii epiphysis indicates a healing phase of a juvenile chondro-osteonecrosis or a chondrocalcinosis, which is limited only to the epiphysis of the radius.

Fig. 1073. Sketch of Fig. 1072b.
1 Humeral diaphysis
2 Ulnar diaphysis
3 Epiphyseal suture of the caput radii
4 Epiphyseal suture of the capitulum humeri
5 Epiphyseal suture of the trochlea humeri
6 Osseous nucleus of the olecranon
7 Osseous nuclei of the trochlea humeri
8 Osseous nucleus of the capitulum humeri
9 Proximal extremity of the ulnar diaphysis
10 Fossa olecrani
11 Nucleus of the medial epicondyle (humerus)
12 Nucleus of the lateral epicondyle (humerus)
13 Tuberositas radii
14 Coronoid process (ulna)

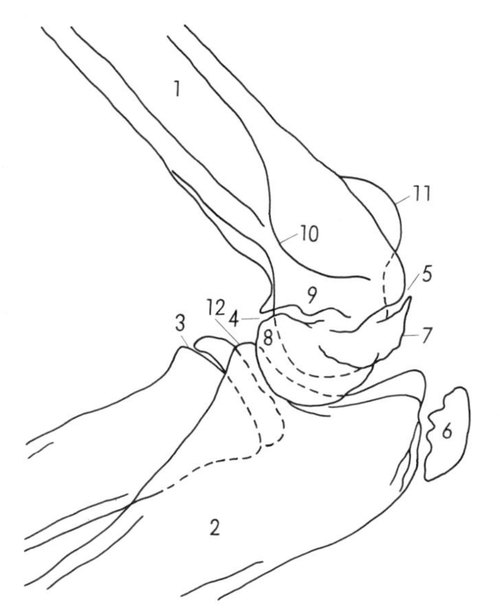

Fig. 1074. Sketch of Fig. 1075a.
1 Humeral diaphysis
2 Ulnar diaphysis
3 Epiphyseal suture of the caput radii
4 Epiphyseal suture of the capitulum humeri
5 Epiphyseal suture of the trochlea humeri
6 Osseous nucleus of the olecranon
7 Osseous nucleus of the trochlea humeri
8 Osseous nucleus of the capitulum humeri
9 Humerus metaphysis
10 Fossa olecrani
11 Medial epicondyle (humeri)
12 Coronoid process (ulna)

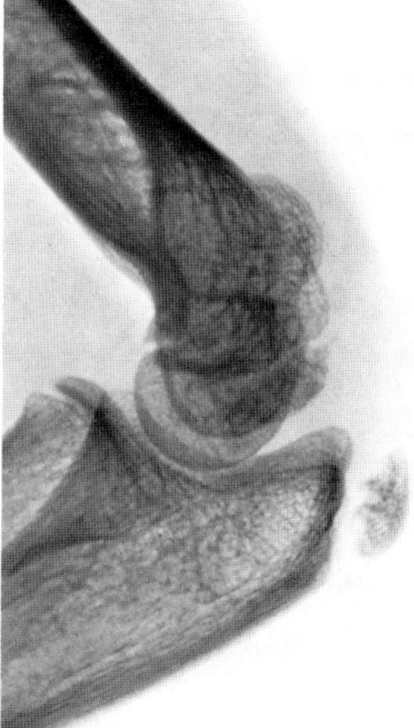

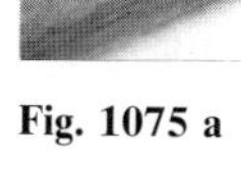

Fig. 1075 a

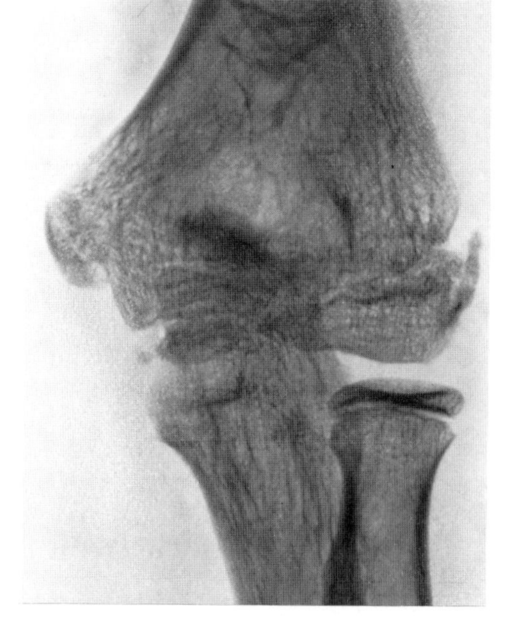

Fig. 1075 b

Fig. 1075. 12 year old. The nucleus of the lateral epicondyle begins to fuse with the nucleus of the capitulum humeri. All other nuclei have increased considerably in size. The splitting of the trochlea and olecranon nuclei and their frequent multinuclear anlagen often render the differential diagnosis for results of trauma difficult. The osteochondrosis of the capitulum humeri (Morbus *Panner*) appears between the 4th and 12th years of life.

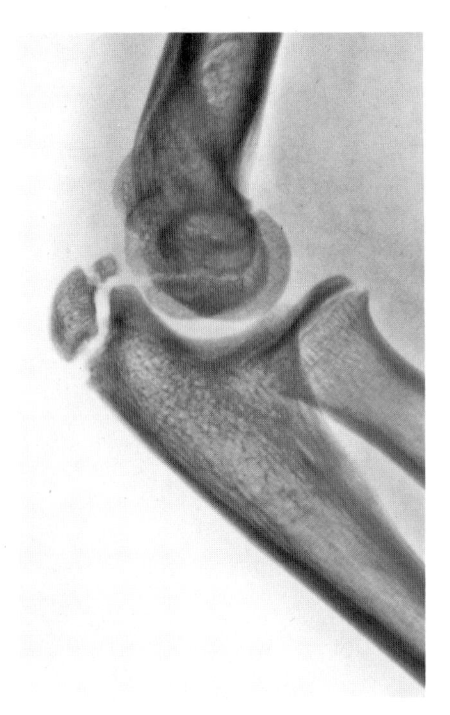

Fig. 1076 a

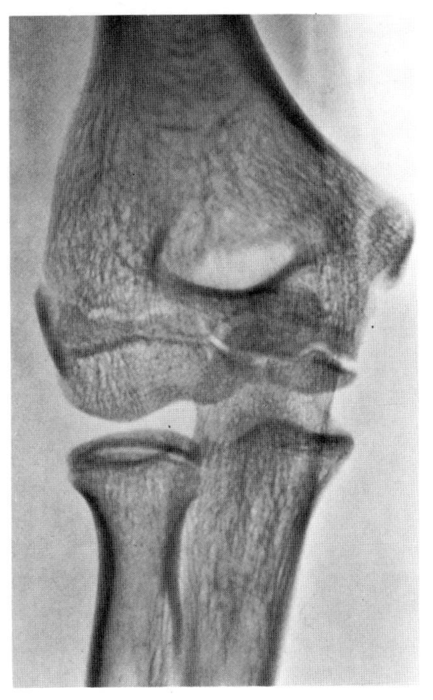

Fig. 1076 b

Fig. 1076. 14 year old. Here, in the lateral picture, there is a splitting of the olecranal nucleus; this splitting may occur to an even greater extent. The olecranal nucleus may originate from one, two or more osseous nuclei, which fuse into one nucleus. In the anteroposterior picture, fusion of the capitulum humeri and the trochlea is about to occur.

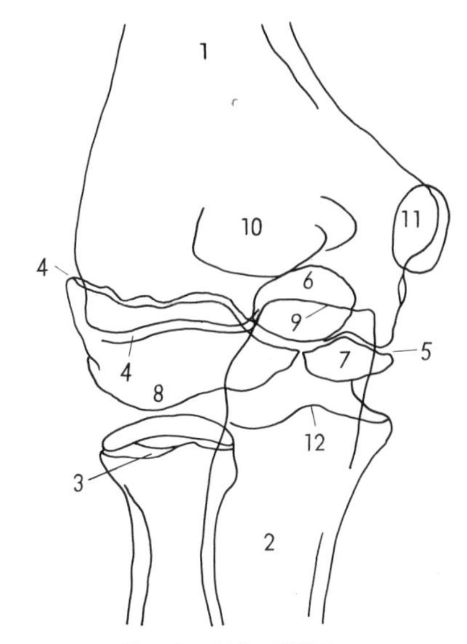

Fig. 1077. Sketch of Fig. 1076b.

1 Humeral diaphysis
2 Ulnar diaphysis
3 Epiphyseal suture of the caput radii
4 Epiphyseal suture of the capitulum humeri
5 Epiphyseal suture of the trochlea humeri
6 Osseous nucleus of the olecranon
7 Osseous nucleus of the trochlea humeri
8 Osseous nucleus of the capitulum humeri
9 Proximal extremity of the ulnar diaphysis
10 Olecranic fossa
11 Osseous nucleus of the medial epicondyle
12 Coronoid process (ulna)

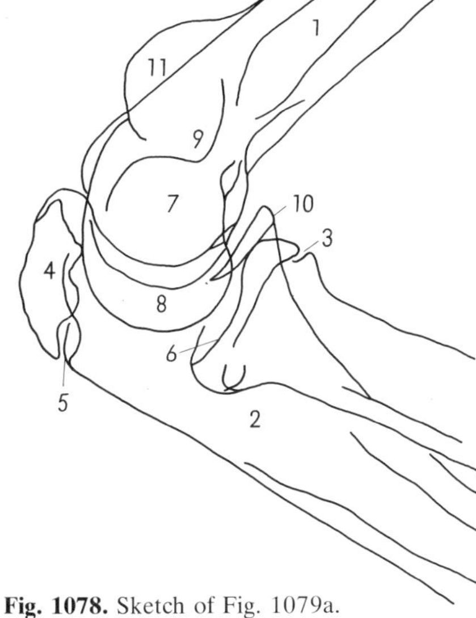

Fig. 1078. Sketch of Fig. 1079a.

1 Humeral diaphysis
2 Ulnar diaphysis
3 Epiphyseal fissure of the caput radii
4 Osseous nucleus of the olecranon
5 Epiphyseal fissure of the olecranon
6 Caput radii
7 Trochlea humeri
8 Capitulum humeri
9 Fossa olecrani
10 Coronoid process (ulna)
11 Medial epicondyle (humeri)

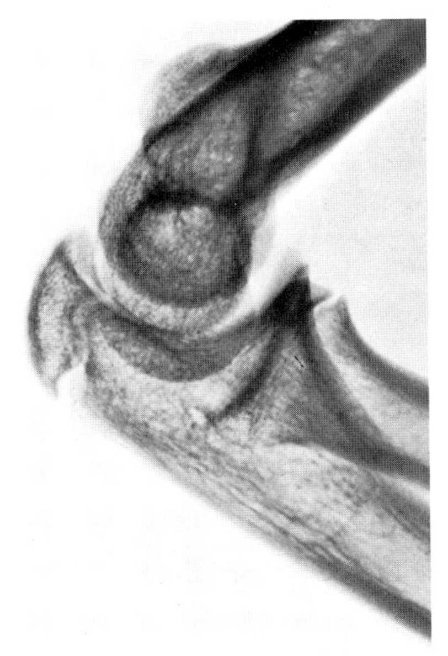

Fig. 1079 a

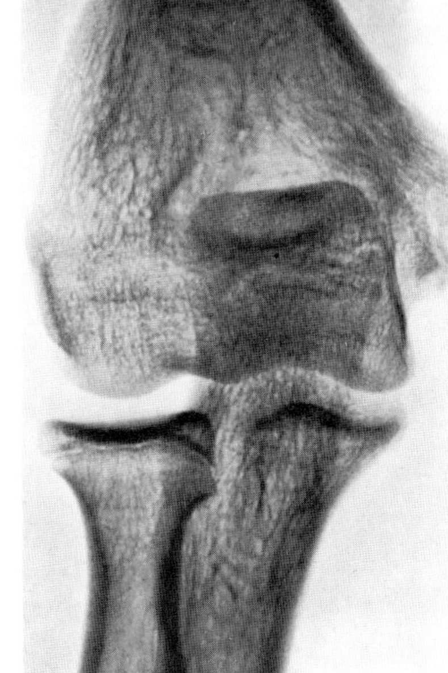

Fig. 1079 b

Fig. 1079. 15 year old. The capitulum humeri, trochlea and lateral epicondyle are fused together and to the humeral shaft (14th to 17th years of life). The fusion of the medial epicondyle with the humeral shaft has begun (a short while after the fusion of the distal humeral epiphysis with the humeral shaft). There is a calcium compression of the cartilaginous disk of the radius and of the articulation cartilage of the ulnar semilunar face; this is probably caused by a D-hypervitaminosis.

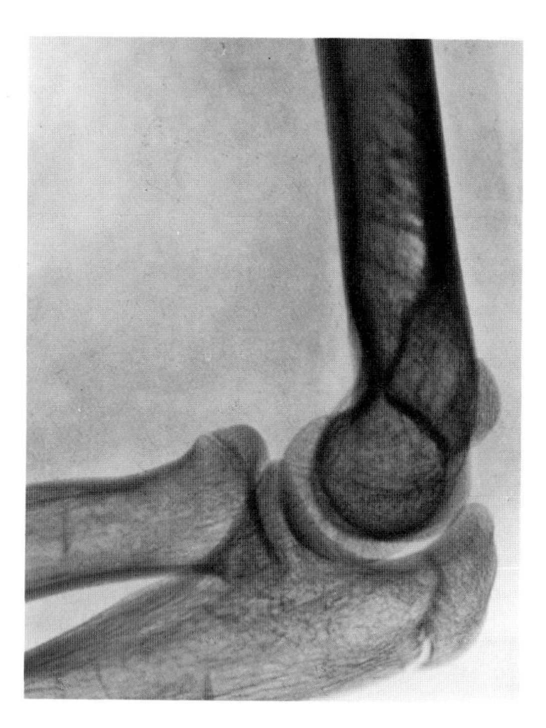

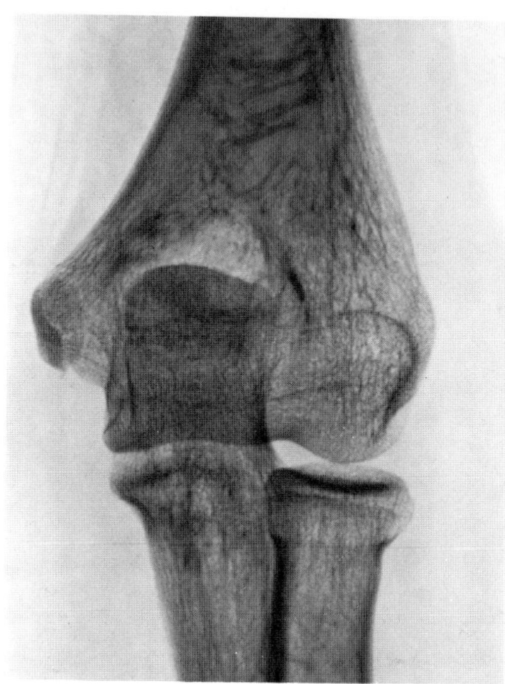

Fig. 1080 a **Fig. 1080 b**

Fig. 1080. 16 year old. The remaining epiphyseal sutures have become still narrower and in part are traceable only as lines. The fusion of the epiphysis of the caput radii and the olecranon occurs about one year earlier than the epiphyseal closure at the distal humeral extremity (see also Fig. 593).

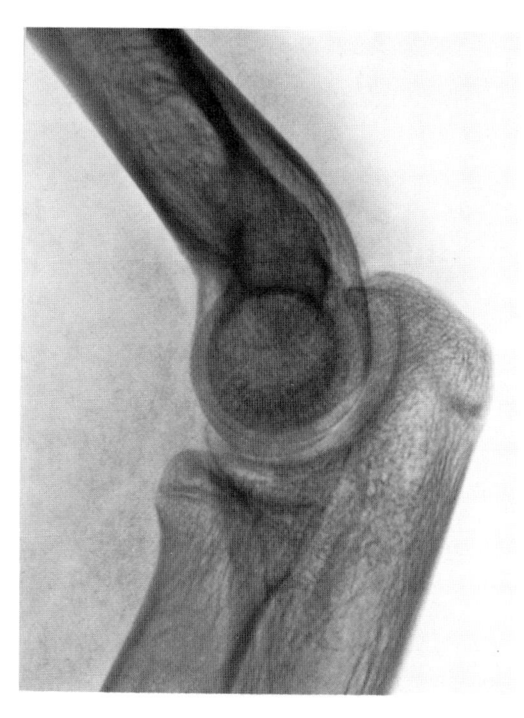

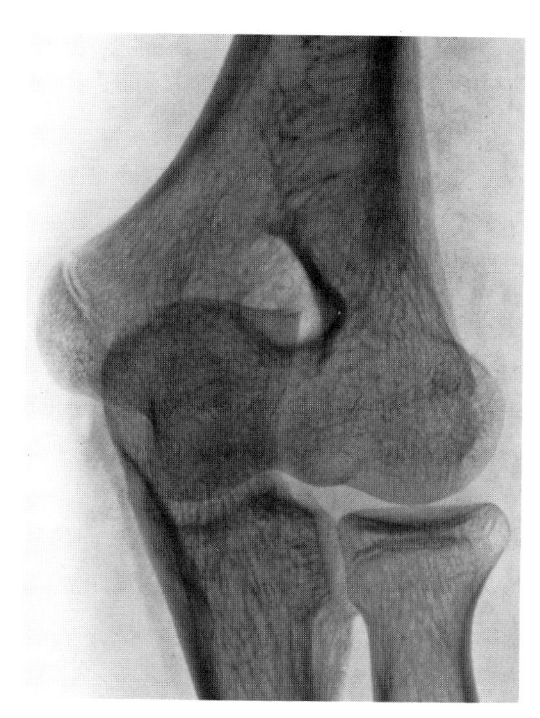

Fig. 1081 a **Fig. 1081 b**

Fig. 1081. 17 year old. The epiphyseal sutures are visible almost as "epiphyseal scars," only the suture of the medial epicondyle is still clearly seen. Their "persistence" beyond the normal fusion period (around the 26th year of life) sometimes occurs. Since the ligament root ossifications of the ulnar collateral ligament may also appear later (see Fig. 592), the differential diagnosis is especially difficult in cases of accidents. The contour of the lateral olecranal apex is noticeably angular.

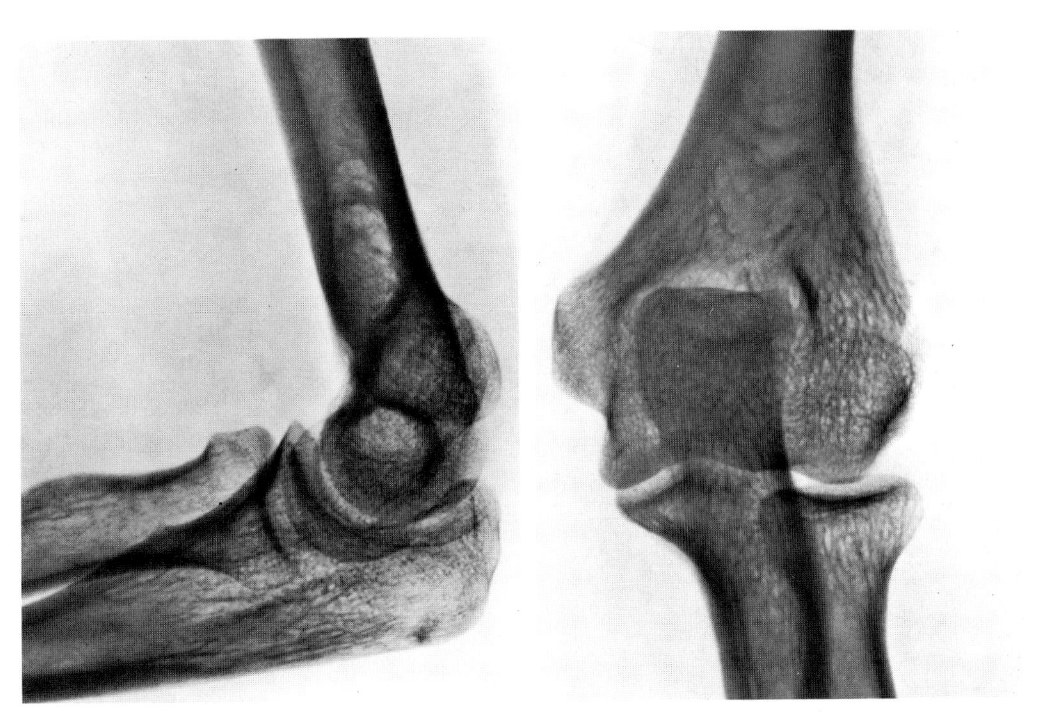

Fig. 1082 a **Fig. 1082 b**

Fig. 1082. 18 year old. The ossification is complete. With the disappearance of the epiphyseal sutures, the growth in length of the long tubular bones also comes to a close.

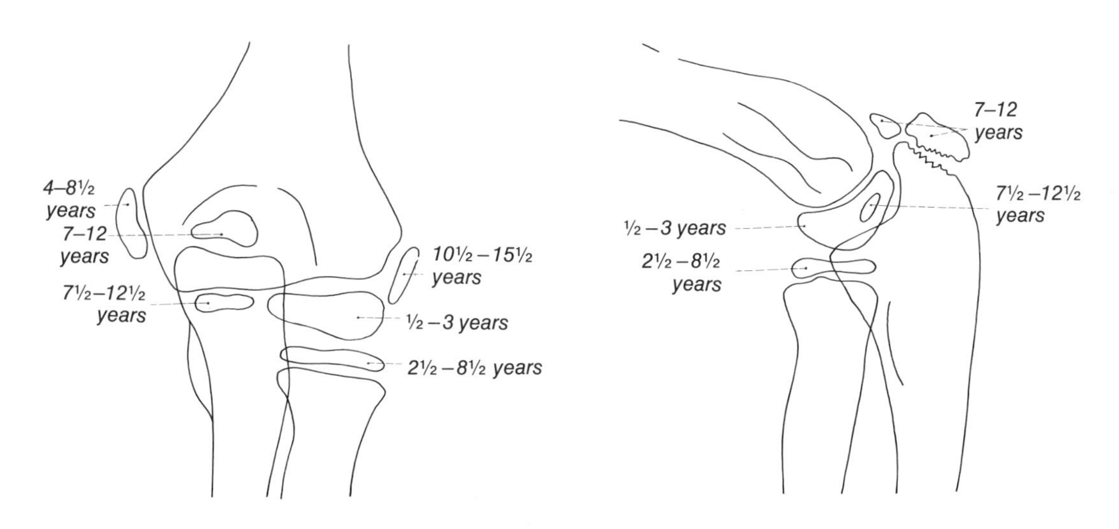

Fig. 1083. Time span in which the osseous nuclei in the region of the elbow usually appears.

Hand

It has been shown that the development of the skeleton provides important information on the process of physical maturation. There are many methods for exactly determining the stage of development of the bones in a radiograph and relating it to the age of the child, the size of the body and sexual development. A distinction can be made between the polysegmental and monosegmental methods:

1. In the polysegmental method, the age of the bone is determined by a radiograph of a part of the skeleton together with a determined articulation.
2. In the monosegmental method, the age of the bone is determined by a radiograph of one skeletal part only, i.e., the hand with the hand articulation.

Since the polysegmental method is associated with a radiation that is too strong and therefore cannot become a routine method, we must limit its use to unclear individual cases and attempt to proceed with the monosegmental method. The polysegmental method of *Sontag* and collaborators (extremities of one side without a foot with 56–61 osseous nuclei), as compared to the monosegmental method according to *Schmid* and *Moll* (a hand of a 5-year-old child with 40 osseous nuclei), does not offer any noteworthy advantage.

In the monosegmental method, attention must be given to the appearance of the ossification centers and, later, to the disappearance of the epiphyseal sutures. This method has the disadvantage that possible concordance disorders in the maturation process of the various sections of the skeleton are not discovered.

It is of historical interest that in 1898, after the discovery of X-rays in 1895, *H. V. Ranke* was the first to note the significance of the radiographically detectable ossification of the hand root for the determination of age in medicolegal jurisdiction.

The radiograph of the skeleton of the hand of the child is an important diagnostic means for determining the state and rate of development.

A comprehensive presentation by *Graser* of the influence of rickets on the development of the hand root explains which pathological disorders of the normal osseous metabolism may occur. In this case, it is possible to see that the growth of the hand root decreases or even stops due to rickets. In the recovery process, there may be an accelerated ossification process so that there is an above-average monthly growth rate. Therefore, the layer of the already-started hand root nucleus can grow so quickly in a few weeks or months that the appearance of additional osseous nuclei must directly follow. *Wimberger* indicates that in Florida rickets, the growth in length of the long tubular bones decreases but evens out during the phase of healing by an above-average growth in a very short period of time. *Stettner's* experiments have indicated that there are a number of illnesses which may bring about the acceleration or slackening of the differentiation (Table 13).

Siegert adds to these illnesses additional cerebral disorders and mongolism. The seasons of the year play an important role in growth. According to *Wimberger,* growth proceeds in a wave-like pattern, with the peak occurring in the spring. *Schmid, Geisler* and *Bannes* point out, on the basis of corresponding experiments, the regulating influence of the central nervous system on the differentiation process of the hand skeleton. They found brain damage, a slackened as well as an accelerated development, form modifications, an irregular succession in the appearance of the hand root nuclei, pseudoepiphyses and asymmetries in the fetus and in early infancy. According to *Geisler* and *Bannes,* in 71% of cerebral-damaged children there was a pathological hand skeleton finding, which seemed to appear more frequently than pathological neurologic findings, while pathological EEG modifications appeared with the same frequency. Cerebral damage was traced more frequently only through the pneumoencephalogram. Retardation was found in 82% of the cases, acceleration of development in 18%; the delayed ossification was therefore the most frequent deviation. *Schulte-Brinkmann et al.* report on the role of cardiac disorders with respect to the developmental process of the hand and foot root skeleton.

Schmid and *Hoffmann* concluded that during the developmental period the metric aberrations should be taken into account in the following disorders:

"Excessive length of the hand is to be found in arachnodactyly, achromegalia, adiposogigantism, primary chronic arthritis, early puberty.

Deficiency in the length of hand is frequently or regularly to be found in chondrodysplasia, dysostosis enchondralis, brachydactyly, mesenchymomasis, mongolism, athyreosis, hypophyseal dwarfism, *Cushing* syndrome and certain forms of the cerebral poliomyelitis."

In view of X-ray and radiation protection laws, there is great importance in the findings of *Schmid* and *Moll;* that in the hand skeleton there is "a region that by evaluation

Table 13. **View of the important differentiation disorders:** o = optional, i. e., not regular (from *Schmid* and *Moll*).

Delay	*Acceleration*
Athyreosis	Arachnodactyly
Chondrodystrophia (-plasia)	Rheumatoid arthritis
Insipid diabetes	Dyscerebral growth disorders (o)
Diabetes mellitis (o)	Calcinosis (o)
Clidocranial dysostosis	Exudative diathesis (o)
Dysostosis *Morquio*	Gigantism, adipose gigantism
Dysostosis multiple	Myositis ossificans
Glycogen accumulation disease	Hyperthyreosis
Hypothyreosis	Progeria
Infantilism	Early puberty
Imperfect ostiogenesis (o)	Healing rickets (o)
Niemann-Pick	Hypophysial gigantism
Leukosis (o)	Genital gigantism
Florid rickets (o)	
Hypophysial dwarfism	
Paltauf's dwarfism	
Cardiac dwarfism	
Renal dwarfism	
Cystindiathesis	

Table 14. **Relationship between length of body and hand** (from *Schmid* and *Hoffmann*). The mean value shows the arithmetic average; the lower and upper limit values represent the actual measured limit values. Data are given in millimeters. For orientation, body length is presented with corresponding age.

Body length cm	*Age*	*Lower Limit*	*Mean Value*	*Upper Limit*
50–54		67	71	75
55–59	2–4 Months	69	76	81
60–64	3–5 Months	75	80	84
65–69	6–8 Months	81	87	92
70–74	9–12 Months	85	93	100
75–79	12–15 Months	95	98	102
80–84	15–20 Months	97	103	108
85–89	1½–2½ Years	105	110	115
90–94	2–3 Years	112	117	121
95–99	2½–3½ Years	113	118	123
100–104	3–4½ Years	119	125	130
105–109	3½–5 Years	127	131	136
110–114	4–6 Years	135	138	142
115–119	5–7 Years	136	140	144
120–124	6–7½ Years	145	149	152
125–129	7–8½ Years	147	153	157
130–134	7½–9½ Years	154	161	168
135–139	8½–10½ Years	158	167	175
140–144	9½–11½ Years	168	173	180
145–149	10–13 Years	170	176	182
150–159	11½–14½ Years	177	186	194

of all given possibilities can be representative for the entire skeleton and a sure indicator for the entire development from birth up to the end of sexual development."

This concept agrees with the fact that in the hand skeleton there are together 11 osseous nuclei and the phalanges, whose 11 nuclei in the hand root skeleton region appear in the first 10 years of life. In the course of their research, *Schmid, Homma* and *Hoffmann* could therefore determine not only the already known relationship between body length and the development of the hand root nucleus, but *Schmid* and *Hoffmann* also determined the relationship between body length and hand length based on considerations of metric aberrations during the age of development. *Swoboda* and *Wimberger* also determined radiographic hand length measurements as a criterion for the growth in body length. It was found that the hands of girls were usually smaller than those of boys. The smallest deviation involving the measurement was found to be in the distance between the proximal extremity of the 3rd metacarpal and the distal extremity of the terminal phalanx of the same finger, with the shadow of the soft tissues not taken into account.

The findings concerning development corresponding to age frequently deviate from one other, including a larger physiological range of variation. *Schmid, Homma* and *Hoffmann* speak of a much closer relationship between the appearance and the differentiation of the osseous nucleus and the body length. Their experiments were based on observations and measurements of 569 hand skeletons, and their results gave rise to their statement that "the body length must be taken as a starting point especially in measuring the size of the hand root bones, because in this case age offers no measurement corresponding to the size values." During their investigations on the relationship between the growth of body length and hand length, *Schmid* and *Hoffmann* concluded that "the hand of the baby is relatively longer than that of a small child or even of a child of school age. This change in proportion begins to occur during early infancy."

In newborns, the metacarpals and phalanges are usually already formed in the hand region, similar to the bones of a 5-month-old fetus, as in Figure 1084. Osseous nuclei in the carpal region are an exception.

Figures 1108 and 1109 show the differentiation of the hand root and the epiphyseal nuclei, as well as data regarding variations. In this connection, see also Figs. 1085 and 1096, as well as Table 15. Regarding the most frequent and normal ossification variations and erroneous radiographic diagnosis, see Fig. 1017.

Capitatum (os magnum) and the hamatum. The nuclei of these two bones are to be expected as the first nuclei in the carpal region. They appear almost at the same time, usually in the 3rd or 4th month of life; in very rare cases they may appear as early as the 10th lunar month. However, at the latest they are developed by the end of the 1st year of life. The nucleus of the capitatum is usually larger than that of the hamatum. *Ross* even described a division of the capitatum into two parts.

Distal radial epiphysis. Towards the end of the 1st year of life – slightly earlier in girls than in boys – we first find a round nucleus, which extends laterally and increases its diameter at the radial edge. Thus, it keeps the typical wedge-shaped form at the distal radial epiphysis. A division of the nucleus into two parts is found occasionally. In a number of cases, the styloid process may have its own divided nucleus.

Triquetrum. The nucleus takes form about the 2nd to 3rd year of life *(Siegert)*. The end of the ossification of this

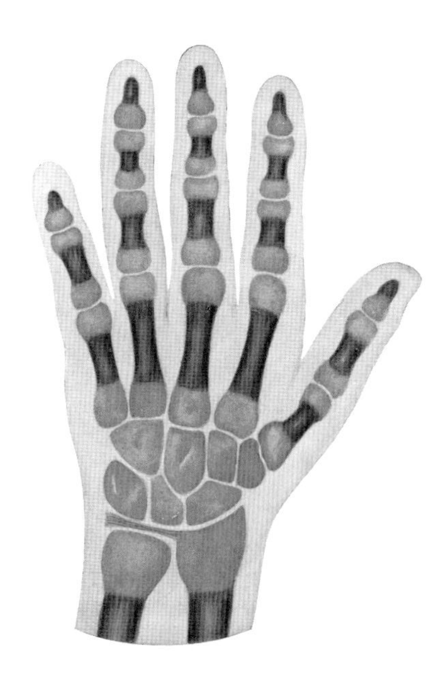

Fig. 1084. Hand of a 5-month-old fetus; potassium glycerine slide (bones dark, cartilage bright, from *Sobotta-Becher*).

bone has a rather large range of variation *(Graser)*. According to *Pfitzner,* the nucleus will usually be divided.

Lunatum. Ossification is normally expected during the 4th or 5th month of life; however, there are quite a number of variations. The lunatum may appear earlier than the triquetrum, but it may also appear much later, even around the 7th year of life. The lunatum lies opposite the apex of the hamatum, and if this positioning is taken into consideration, it will never be confused with the triquetrum. *Eggimann,* inter alia, indicated a possibility of a double-nucleus anlage in the lunatum. We were also able to observe such an anlage (Fig. 701). Anlagen with a double nucleus were further described by *Ravelli,* who in the course of an experiment was able to observe the fusion of the two anlagen. *Turpin* and collaborators showed a one-sided lunatum, which was divided into monozygotic twins.

Trapezium and Trapezoideum (greater and lesser multangulum). The two nuclei appear at almost the same time, the trapezium sometimes a few months earlier, around the 5th year of life. In this case, too, the appearance of the nuclei is expected somewhat earlier in girls than in boys. Fusion of the trapezium with neighboring bones has been repeatedly described between the trapezium and the scaphoid bone *(Marti)*. Next to the single nucleus ossification of the multangular bone, bicentral ossifications with two nuclei were described. They are, however, very rare *(Ravelli, Ruckensteiner)*.

Scaphoid bone (navicular). Its appearance can be expected at the same time as that of the trapezium and the trapezoideum, but most frequently it precedes them somewhat. A division into two is occasionally discernible; both nuclei, however, fuse very soon and become one bone. As is the case with the lunatum, there is also clear evidence of a remaining congenital scaphoid bone divided into two parts, which should not be confused with a pseudoarthrosis (see Fig. 694a and b).

Distal ulnar epiphysis. This nucleus appears about the 7th year of life. Quite often it is formed at the beginning of two independent ossification centers, which fuse very soon into one nucleus. An isolated nucleus may be occasionally found in the styloid process, which may persist as an ulnar styloid bone *(Viehweger)*.

Pisiform bone. This nucleus forms as the last nucleus in the carpal region. Its appearance is subject to great oscillations in breadth; it usually appears in the 10th year of life. The nucleus is frequently overlooked at first because the triquetrum is superimposed on it. A disintegrated, non-linear nucleus is often found in the pisiform bone in several ossification centers.

Epiphyseal development in the hand region. The first epiphyses in the metacarpal and phalanx region are the epiphyses of the basic phalanx, which are found around the 1st to 3rd years of life. The 5th finger, unlike the other fingers, has a very slow epiphyseal development. Shortly afterward, the epiphyses of the 2nd to 5th metacarpals appear. Half a year later, the epiphyses of the first metacarpal as well as those of the middle and terminal phalanges follow.

Termination of ossification. The metacarpal bones have attained their final form at puberty; thus, ossification is terminated.

The epiphyses of the metacarpal bones and the phalanges close themselves between the 15th and 20th years of life; the epiphyses of the metacarpal bones, however, close a year earlier than the epiphyses of the phalanges. The epiphyseal termination at the radial and ulnar extremity occurs very late, i.e., in the 18th to 24th years of life. It is usually the last epiphyseal termination.

Sesamoid bones. The osseous formation of the sesamoid bones takes place at the beginning of puberty (see Fig. 659).

Ossification variations in the carpal region. The nuclei of the lunatum, scaphoid, trapezium and trapezoid usually appear in that order, the trapezium preceding trapezoideum. This succession is to be regarded as a normal type of ossification. In one variation, which is still normal however, the trapezoideum seems to precede the trapezium (see Fig. 1098). In radiographs of children's hands, two divided osseous nuclei may be found rather frequently in the region of the lunatum (see also lunatum).

Anomalies. As an anomaly, one finds, with varying degrees of frequency, numerous epiphyses (pseudoepiphyses; see Figs. 1091 and 1100) at the proximal extremity of the 2nd metacarpal, more rarely at the same time at the 4th and 5th metacarpal bones. These epiphyses last for a short time. Mostly at the same time, the 1st metacarpal and likewise an extra epiphysis appear at the distal extremity. All these epiphyses appear earlier than the normal nuclei and evidence a rapid growth process. They also fuse with the shaft, rather earlier than the normal epiphyseal nuclei, usually in the 6th or 7th year of life instead of the 17th *(Weinert, Snodgrasse* and others). The pseudoepiphyses are ossification anomalies in healthy subjects; they are found more frequently in cases of endocrine disorders, cerebral damage and malformed children.

The so-called *Friedreich* hand may also be attributed to cerebral damage: excessive extension of the finger base and the hand articulation upon bending the distal articulations *(Pschyrembel)*.

Posener, Walker and *Weddell* found pseudoepiphyses in 96% of the 100 children between the ages of 4 and 8 whom they examined. *Stettner* found them most frequently between the 7th and 10th years of life in 23% of the males and 21% of the females of a total of 1,843 subjects. *Schäfer* attributes no clinical significance to these findings. *Maas* observed multiple pseudoepiphyses in cases of clidocranial dysostosis, and *Stettner,* also, found that two thirds of the subjects he examined were suffering from various developmental disorders due to pseudoepiphyses, constitutional malformations and internal secretion disorders. The frequency according to *Weinert* is: 33.3%, 2nd metacarpal; 29.4%, 5th metacarpal; 20.7%, 1st metacarpal; 12.4%, 3rd metacarpal and 9.9%, 4th metacarpal.

Table 15. **Age upon appearance of the nuclei of the carpal bones and the epiphyses, with details on variations** (according to *Stuart* and *Stevenson*).

	Boys		*Girls*	
	Mean	*Standard deviation*	*Mean*	*Standard deviation*
Capitatum	2 Months	2 Months	2 Months	2 Months
Hamatum	3 Months	2 Months	2 Months	2 Months
Radial epiphysis	1 Year, 1 Month	5 Months	10 Months	4 Months
Prox. 2nd phalanx	1 Year, 4 Months	4 Months	11 Months	3 Months
Prox. 3rd phalanx	1 Year, 4 Months	4 Months	10 Months	3 Months
Prox. 4th phalanx	1 Year, 5 Months	5 Months	11 Months	3 Months
Distal 1st phalanx	1 Year, 7 Months	7 Months	1 Year	4 Months
2nd metacarpal	1 Year, 6 Months	5 Months	1 Year	3 Months
3rd metacarpal	1 Year, 8 Months	5 Months	1 Year, 1 Month	3 Months
Prox. 5th phalanx	1 Year, 9 Months	5 Months	1 Year, 2 Months	4 Months
4th metacarpal	1 Year, 11 Months	6 Months	1 Year, 3 Months	4 Months
4th middle phalanx	2 Years	6 Months	1 Year, 3 Months	5 Months
3rd middle phalanx	2 Years	6 Months	1 Year, 3 Months	5 Months
2nd middle phalanx	2 Years, 2 Months	6 Months	1 Year, 4 Months	5 Months
5th metacarpal	2 Years, 2 Months	7 Months	1 Year, 4 Months	5 Months
4th dist. phalanx	2 Years, 4 Months	6 Months	1 Year, 6 Months	1 Year, 3 Months
3rd dist. phalanx	2 Years, 4 Months	6 Months	1 Year, 6 Months	4 Months
Triquetrum	2 Years, 6 Months	1 Year, 4 Months	1 Year, 9 Months	1 Year, 2 Months
Thumb epiphysis	2 Years, 8 Months	9 Months	1 Year, 6 Months	5 Months
1st prox. phalanx	2 Years, 8 Months	7 Months	1 Year, 8 Months	5 Months
Distal 2nd phalanx	3 Years, 1 Month	8 Months	1 Year, 11 Months	6 Months
Distal 5th phalanx	3 Years, 1 Month	9 Months	1 Year, 11 Months	6 Months
5th middle phalanx	3 Years, 3 Months	10 Months	1 Year, 10 Months	7 Months
Lunatum	3 Years, 6 Months	1 Year, 7 Months	2 Years, 2 Months	1 Year, 1 Month
Trapezium	5 Years, 7 Months	1 Year, 7 Months	3 Years, 11 Months	1 Year, 2 Months
Trapezoideum	5 Years, 9 Months	1 Year, 3 Months	4 Years, 1 Month	1 Year
Scaphoid	5 Years, 6 Months	1 Year, 3 Months	4 Years, 3 Months	1 Year
Ulnar epiphysis	6 Years, 10 Months	1 Year, 2 Months	5 Years, 9 Months	1 Year, 1 Month
Pisiform	–	–	–	–
1st sesamoid	12 Years, 8 Months	1 Year, 6 Months	10 Years, 1 Month	1 Year, 1 Month

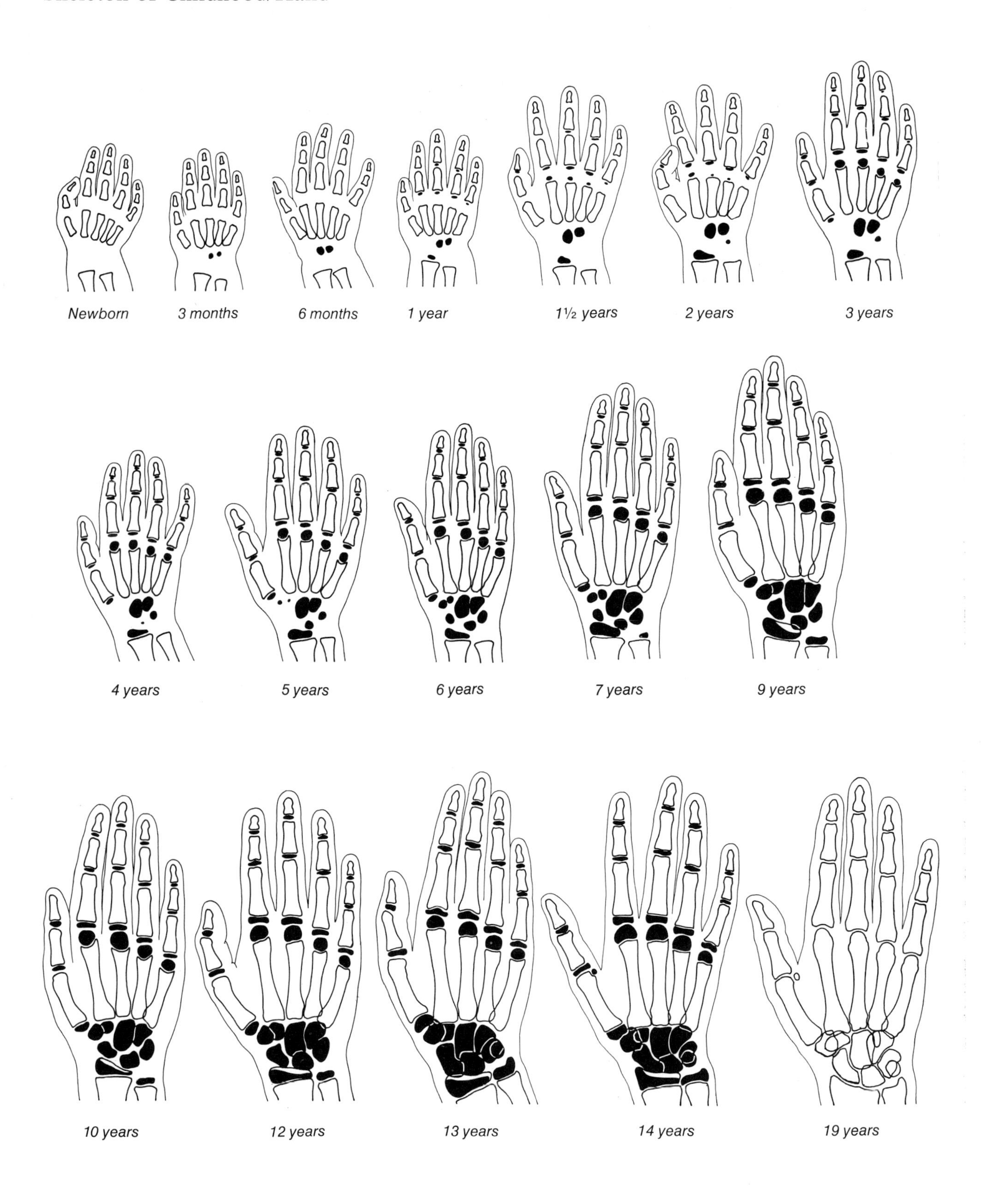

Fig. 1085. Scheme of the development of the hand skeleton. The size and deviation of the proportions in the process of growth (from *Schmid* and *Moll*).

Fig. 1089. 6 month old. These hands are those of two different babies. Left, there are no osseous nuclei yet; right, there are already the nuclei of the hamatum and capitatum, shown in Figs. 1088 and 1089 b as normal, while Fig. 1089 a is at the lower level of normality. Left, there was suspicion of rickets; however, no unequivocal findings were obtained in the examinations of the skeletal sections. ▶

A Series of Radiographs of the Hand and the Hand Root from Infancy to Age 18

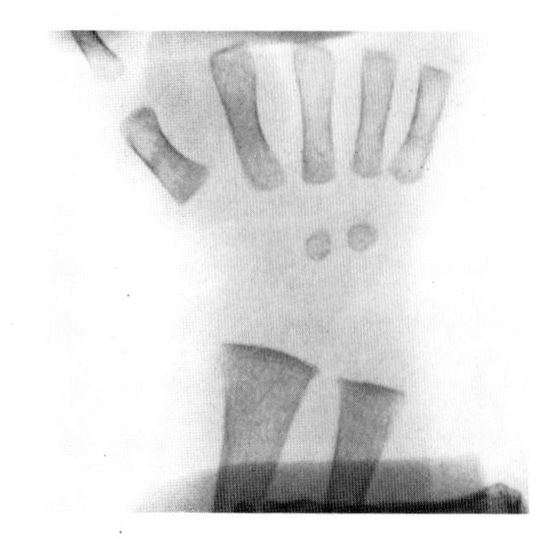

Fig. 1086. 3 day old. The hamatum and capitatum are already arranged in the carpal region. This finding was obtained in both hands. It is rather unusual to find these two nuclei formed in a newborn; however, it is within the normal limits of ossification, which in this case has already begun in the 10th lunar month.

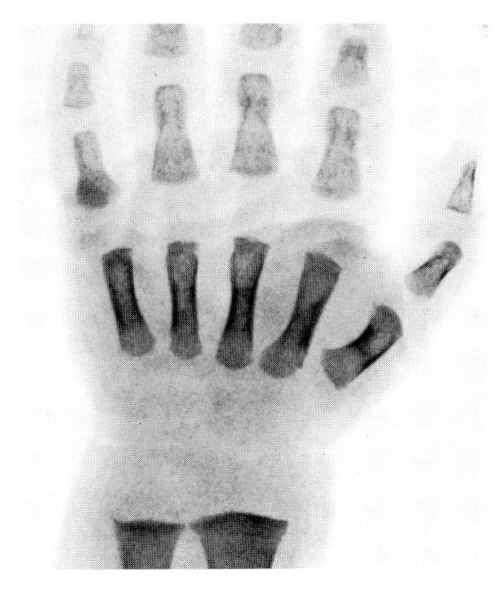

Fig. 1087. 2 month old. Average norm: no nucleus formed yet.

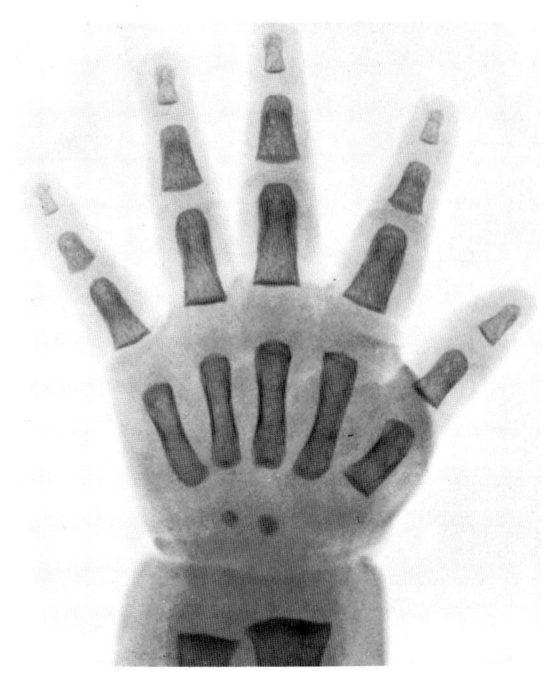

Fig. 1088. 3 month old. The nuclei of the hamatum and capitatum are already formed. Average standard.

Fig. 1088

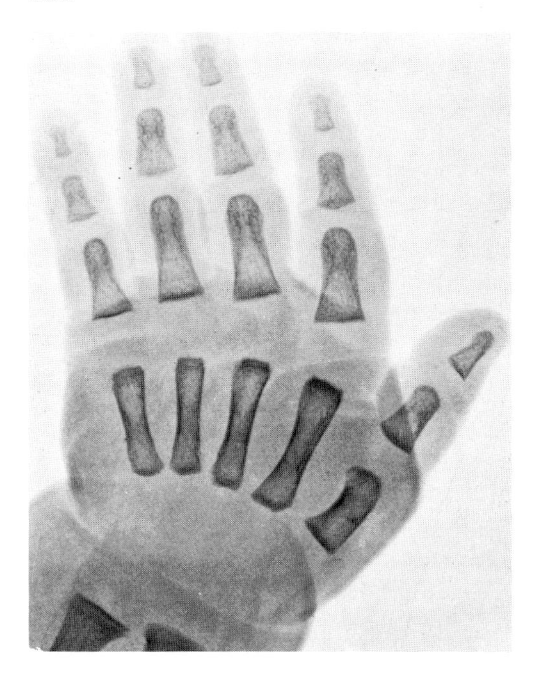

Fig. 1089 a

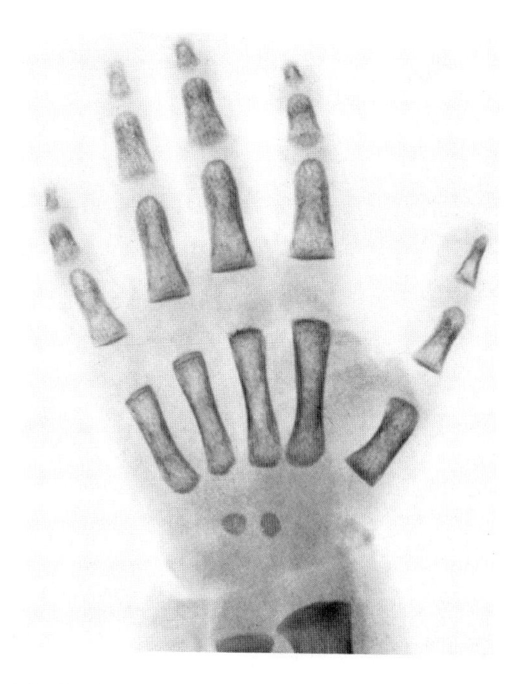

Fig. 1089 b

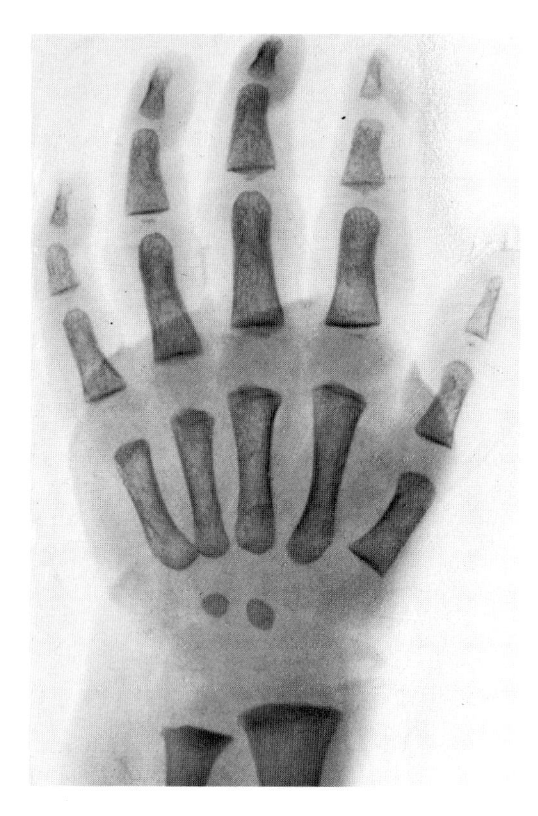

Fig. 1090. 7 month old. Average norm.

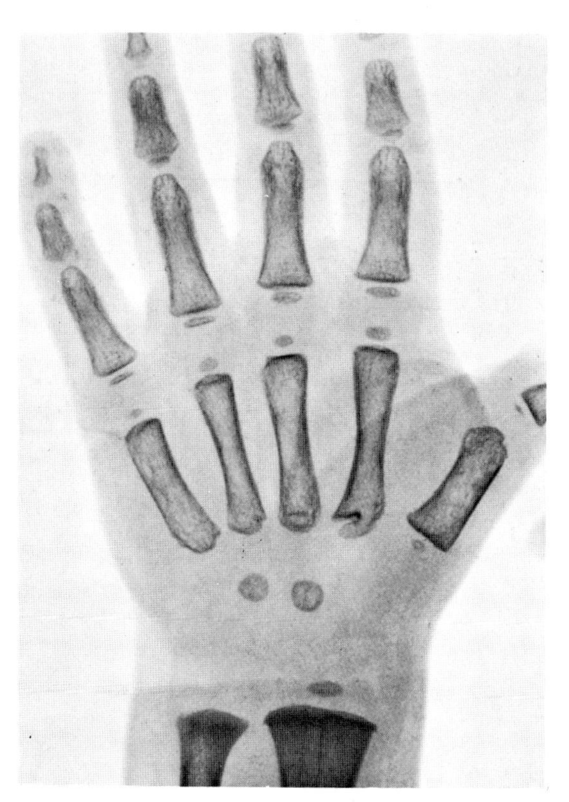

Fig. 1091. $1^1/_2$ year old. In this hand the development of the osseous nuclei does not seem to have progressed in numbers, but the square dimension as compared with the finding in Fig. 1092 has progressed. The picture corresponds to the lower limit. The appearance of a pseudoepiphysis at the base of the 2nd metacarpal (see text page 466) is rather interesting. Here also is found the proximal epiphysis in the 1st metacarpal.

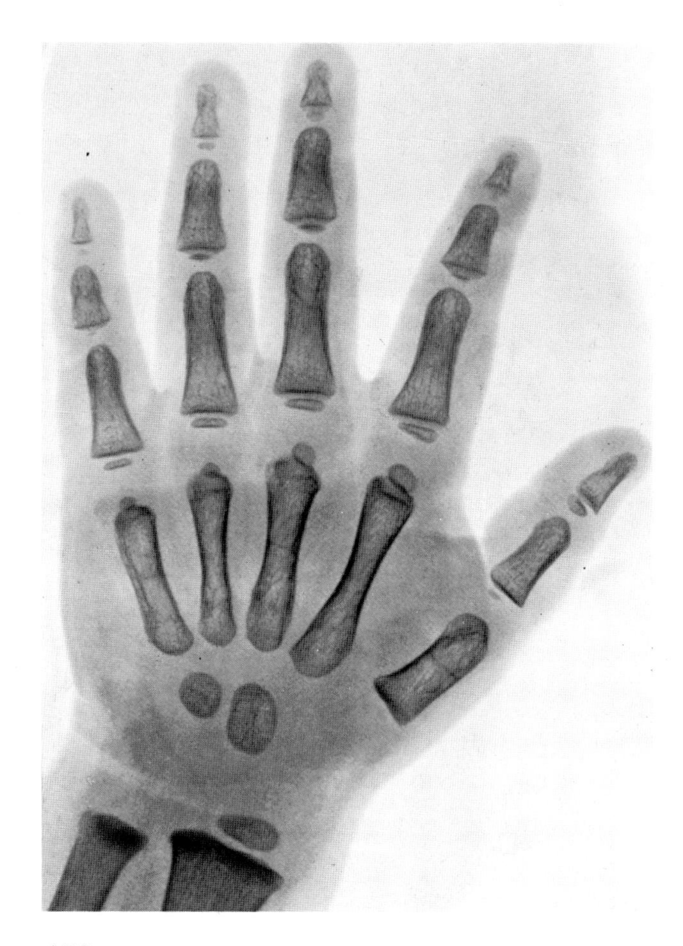

Fig 1092. $1^1/_2$ year old. In the region of the hand root, the nuclei of the hamatum and capitatum are well developed with respect to their square measurement. In addition, the osseous nuclei of the radial epiphysis (appearing around the end of the 1st year of life) as well as the epiphyses of the 2nd – 5th metacarpal and the epiphyses of the phalanges are discernible.

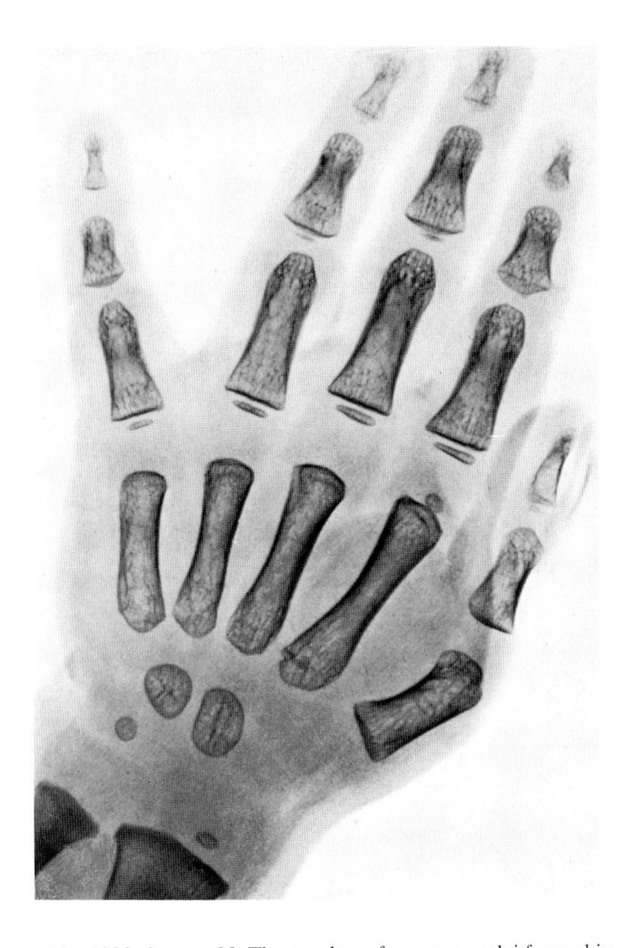

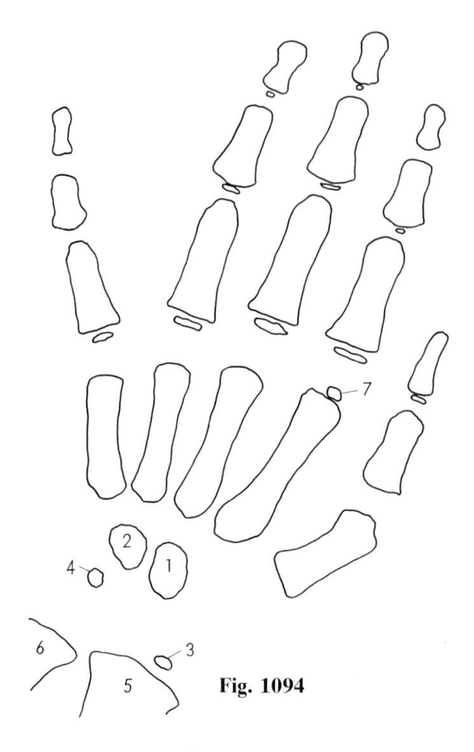

1 Capitatum
2 Hamatum
3 Distal radial epiphysis
4 Triquetrum
5 Radial epiphysis
6 Ulnar diaphysis
7 Epiphysis of the 2nd metacarpal bone

Fig. 1093. 2 year old. The number of osseous nuclei formed in the region of the hand root (hamatum, capitatum and triquetrum bones) corresponds to the upper norm. The surface of the nucleus in the distal radial epiphysis is approximately that of the lower limit of a 1 1/2-year-old child (cf. with Fig. 1091). The variation possibilities within the limits of development are also shown.

Fig. 1094. Sketch to Fig. 1093. The osseous nuclei of the hand root are numbered according to their order of appearance.

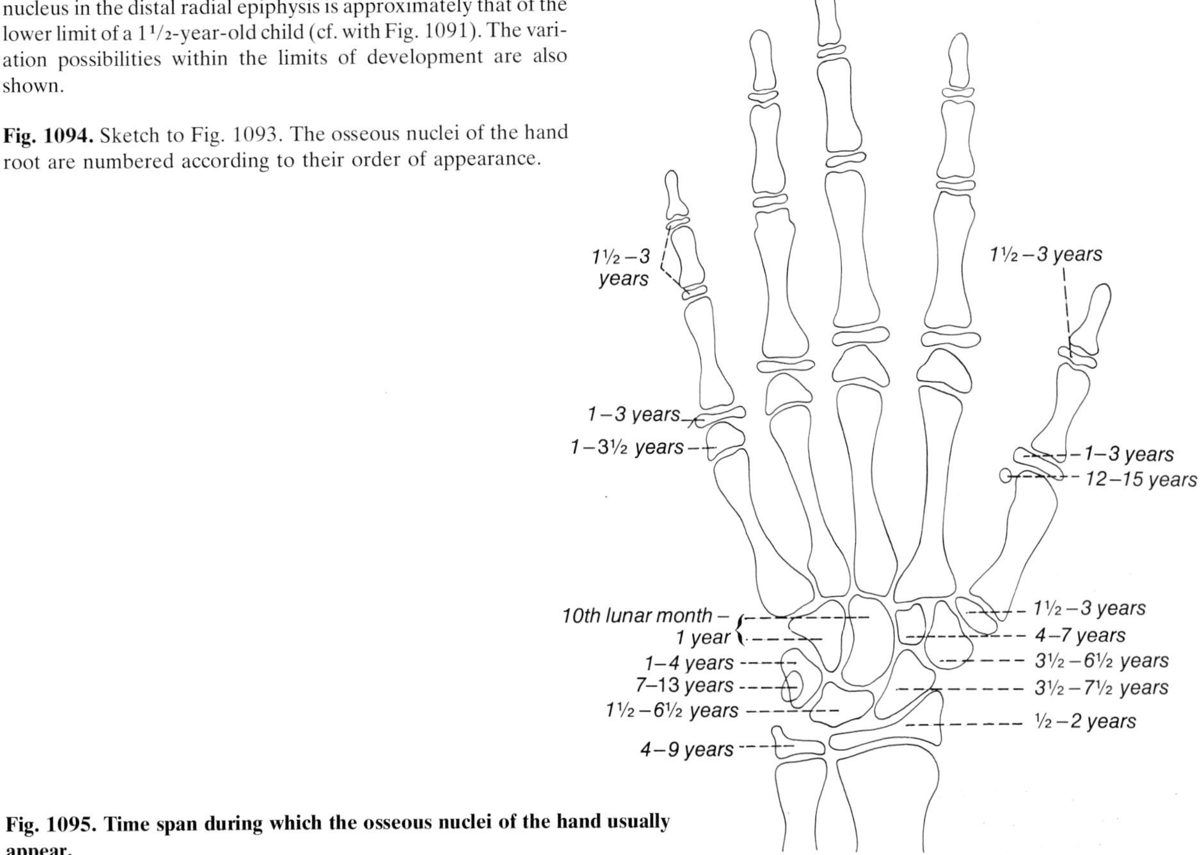

Fig. 1095. Time span during which the osseous nuclei of the hand usually appear.

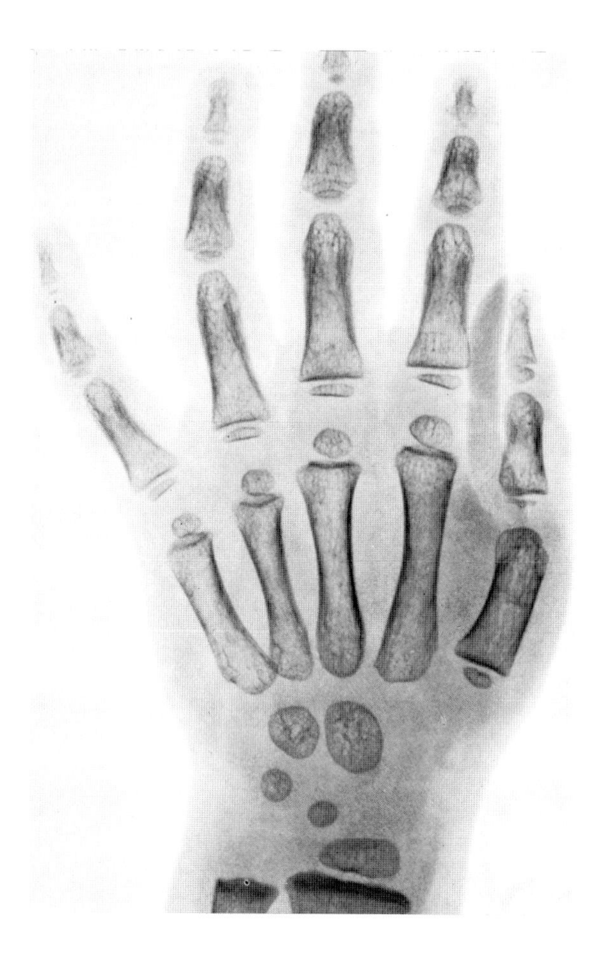

Figs. 1096 and 1097. 3 year old. In Fig. 1096 the nuclei of the hand root bones such as the capitatum, hamatum, triquetrum and lunatum are already arranged. This corresponds to the age of 3½. On the other hand, in Fig. 1097 only the nuclei of the hamatum and capitatum bones are already arranged. This corresponds to the development of a 2-year-old child. In this example, there was a previous light case of rickets which explains the irregular development. Both radiographs present extreme cases. The finding in Fig. 1096 may be explained by "rickets prophylaxis," while in Fig. 1097 the subject has recovered from rickets. Using vitamin D for the prophylaxis and treatment of rickets, fairly frequently, leads to a rapid ossification.

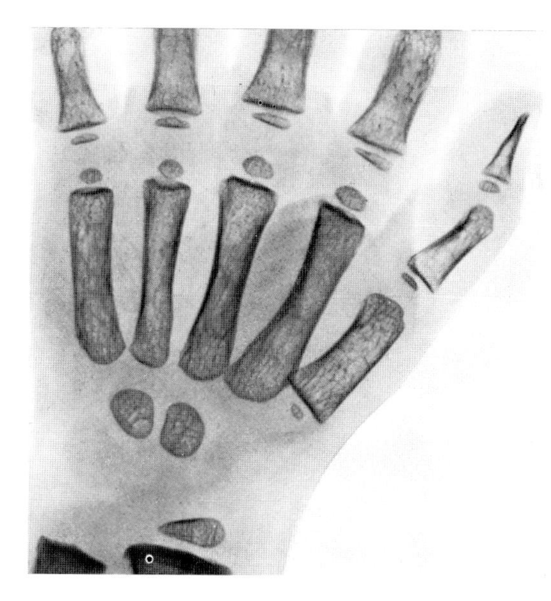

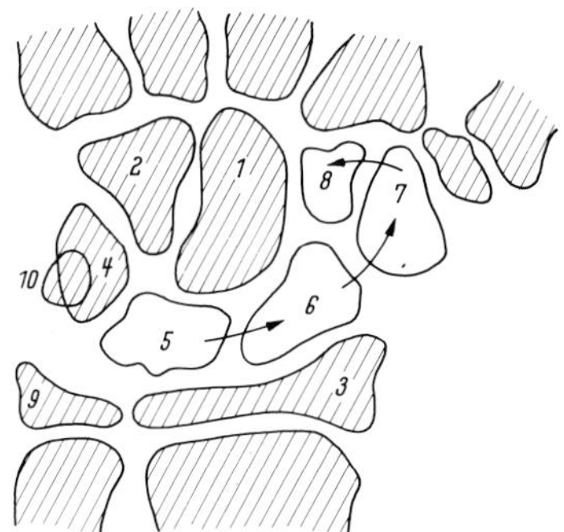

a) Normal type

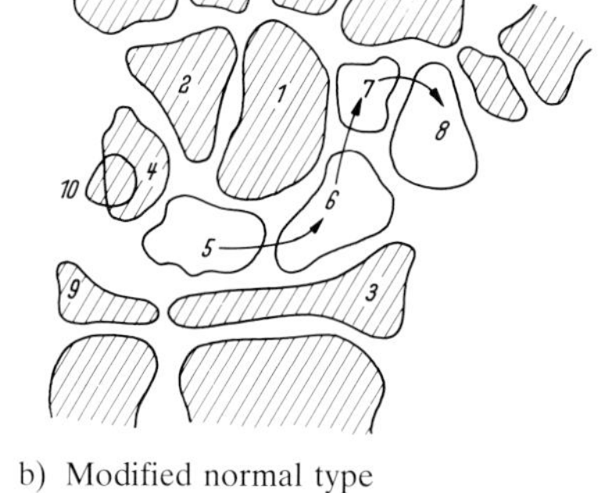

b) Modified normal type

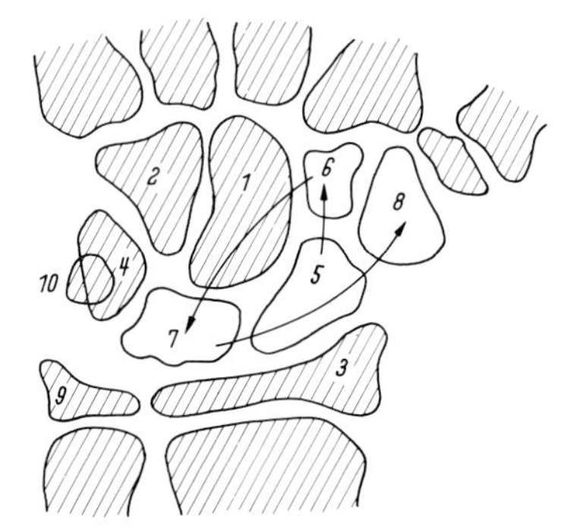

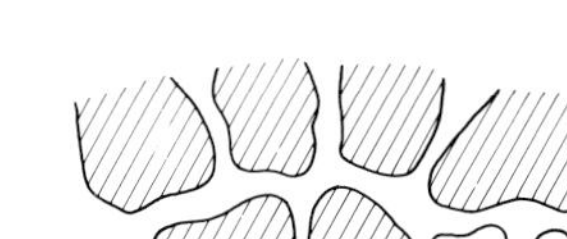

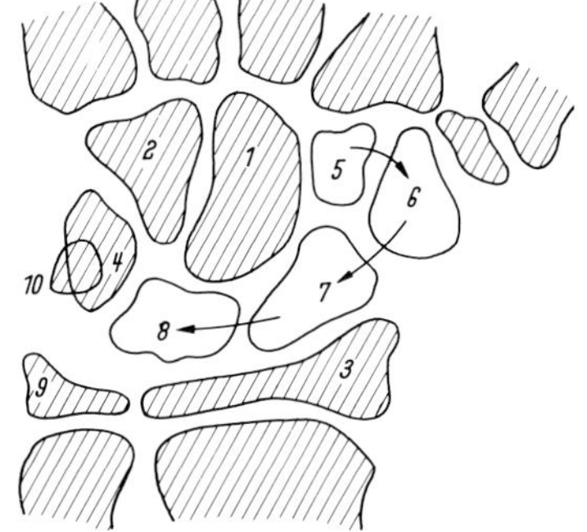

c) and d) Rare variations

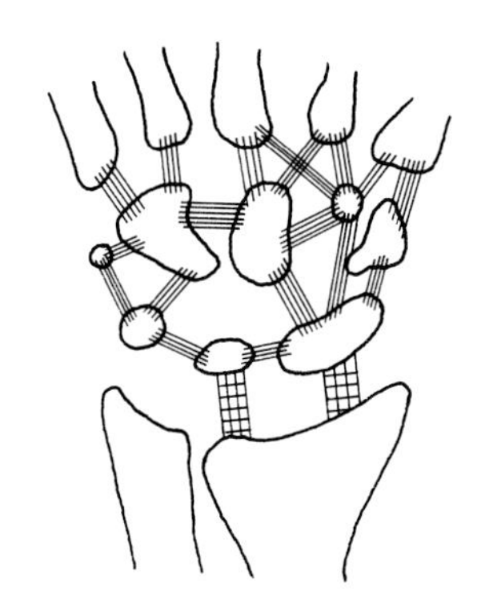

Fig. 1099. Localization of coalescence (according to *Rochlin* and *Zeitler*).

Fig. 1098. Variations in the chronological order of the appearance of the osseous nuclei in the carpal region. The above figures indicate the succession of the individual osseous nucleus. Progression is constant in the hatched bones and inconstant in those shown as white.

|||| probably innate

♯ suspected to be congenital

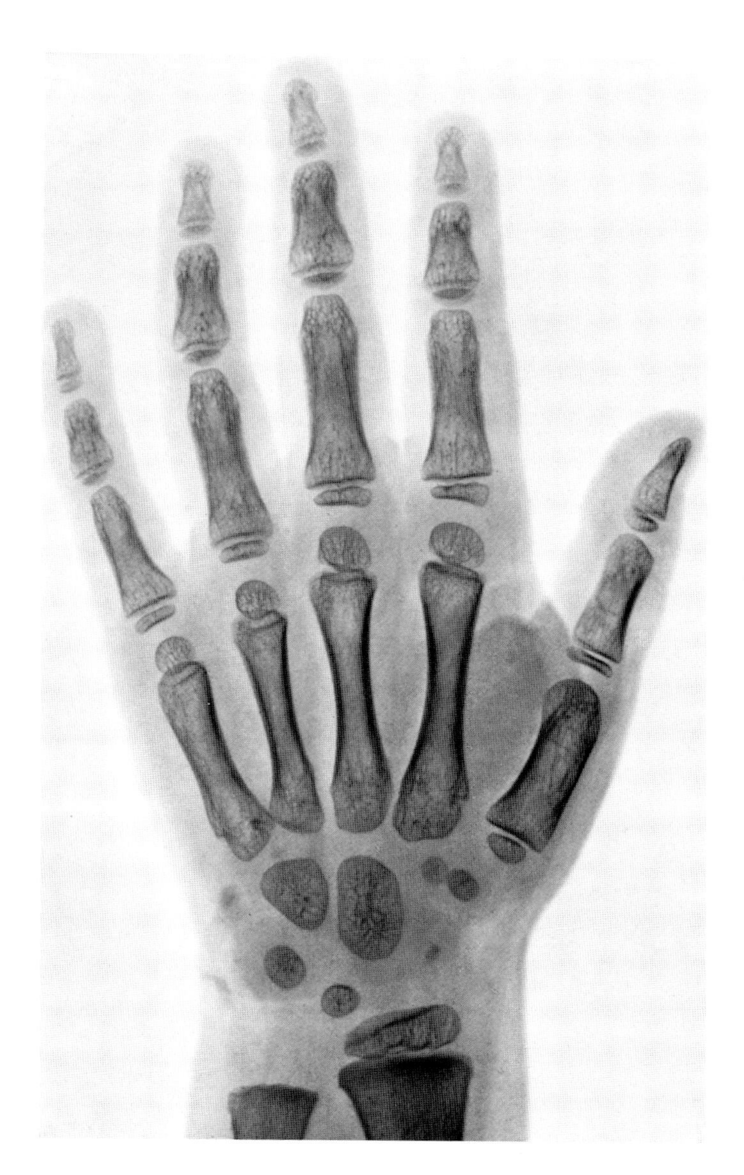

Fig. 1100. 4 year old. The nuclei of all the hand root bones, except for the pisiform, are already arranged. This corresponds, considering the square dimension of the ossification nuclei, to the upper norms of a 5-year-old child. The smallest and youngest nucleus in the picture is the nucleus of the scaphoid bone, which appears simultaneously with the nuclei of the trapezium and trapezoideum. There is a pseudoepiphysis in the 5th metacarpal bone and an indication of a pseudoepiphysis in the 2nd metacarpal. The accelerated development may be attributed to the normal rickets prophylaxis of inoculation with high doses of vitamin D.

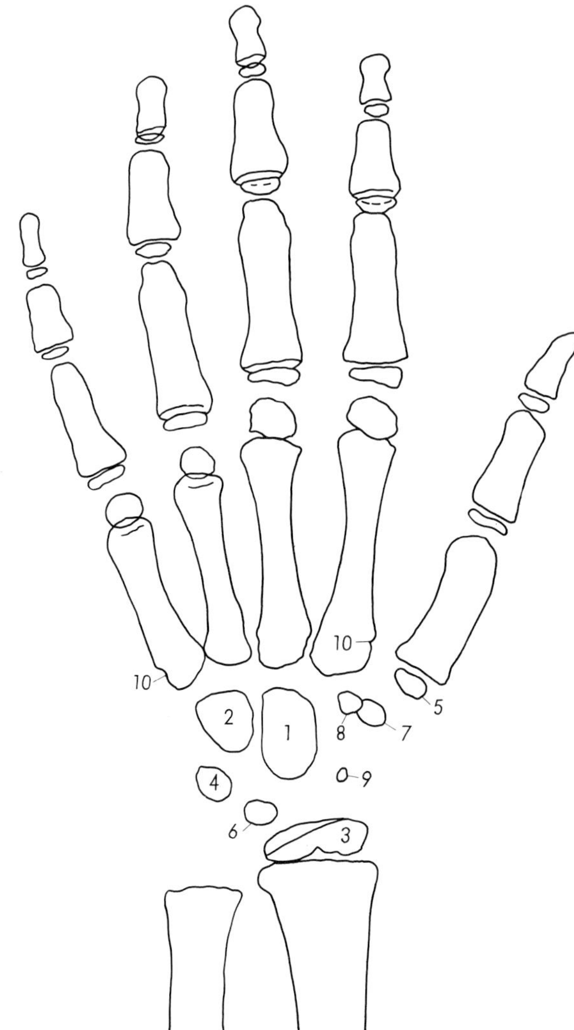

Fig. 1101. Sketch to Fig. 1100. The osseous nuclei of the hand root are numbered according to their order of appearance.

1 Capitatum
2 Hamatum
3 Distal radial epiphysis
4 Triquetrum
5 Epiphysis of the 1st metacarpal
6 Lunatum
7 Trapezium
8 Trapezoideum
9 Scaphoid
10 Pseudoepiphyses

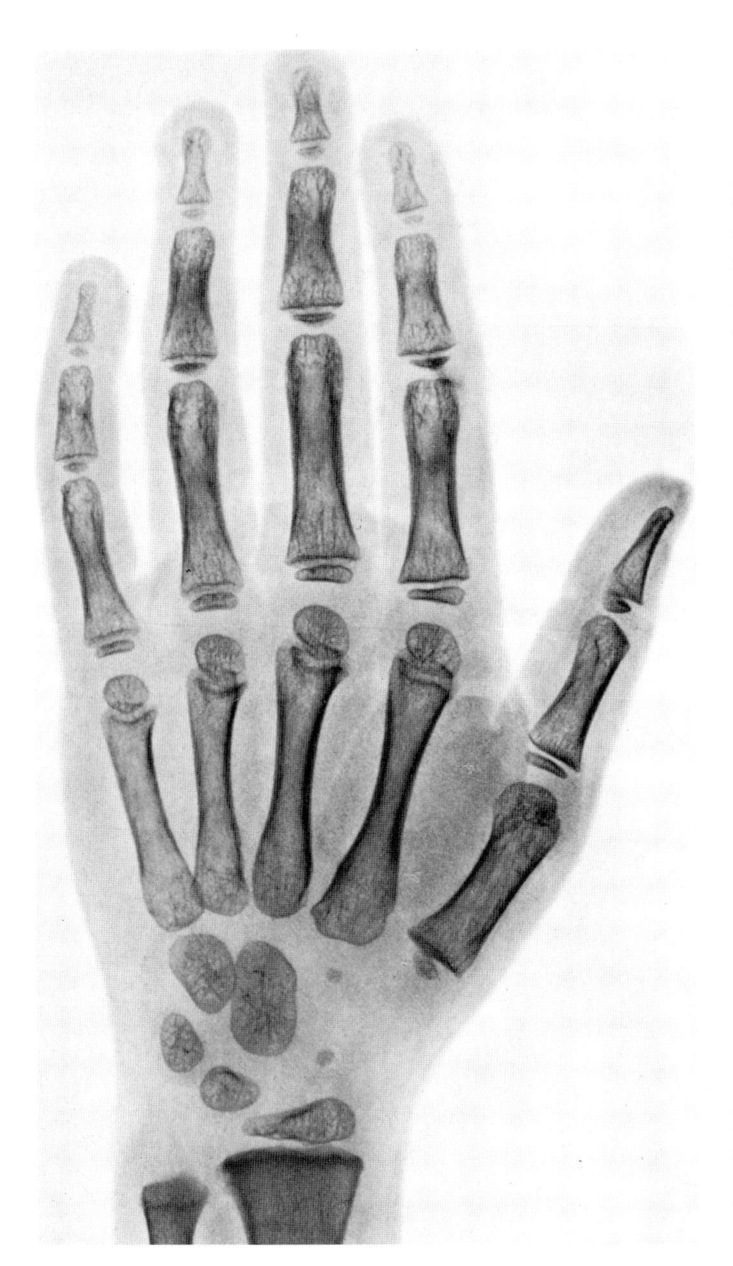

Fig. 1102. 5 year old. All hand root bones, including the nuclei of the trapezium and the pisiform, are arranged in accordance with the age norm. Since the nucleus of the scaphoid appears simultaneously with the trapezium and the trapezoideum, in this case it is not necessarily a variation of a premature ossification process. The picture corresponds to median or high norms.
The thickness of the corticalis of the finger joints in the middle phalanx seems to have the same compactness as the metacarpal diaphysis. The further development causes the compacta of the metacarpal bones and the metaphyses of the long tubular bones to become thick sclerotic layers, while the finger joints remain almost with no compact corticalis layer.

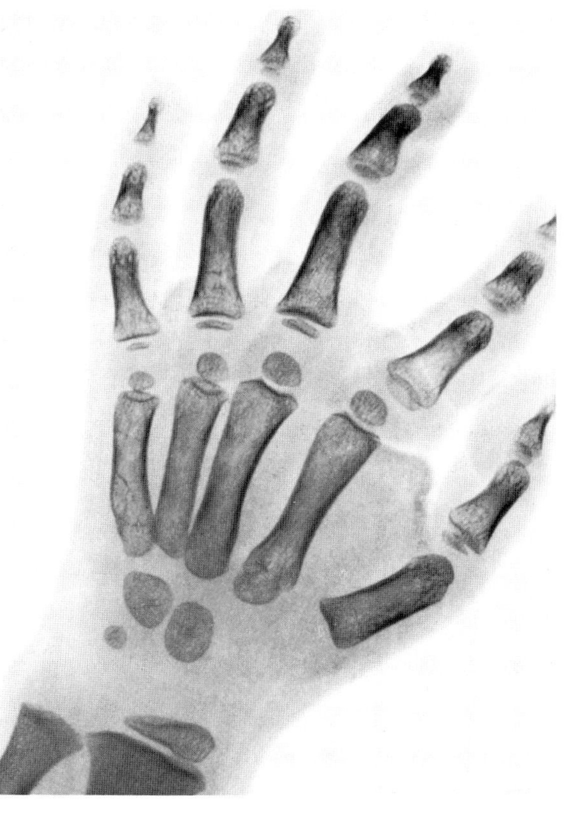

Fig. 1103. 5 year old. Hand of a mongoloid child of the same age. Besides the low number of arranged osseous nuclei, the shapelessness and relative shortness of the fingers are rather striking. The hand is also very small. In addition, the basis of the 2nd metacarpal shows a pseudoepiphysis.

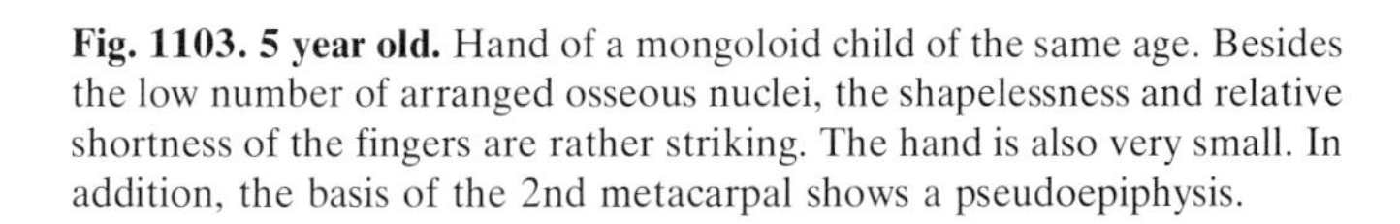

The sequence of appearance of the osseous nuclei in the carpal bones has been maintained (capitatum-hamatum-triquetrum); the appearance, however, is very retarded, corresponding to the hand of a 2 year old. The cup-shaped hand indicates a rudimentary formation of the middle phalanx of the 5th finger.

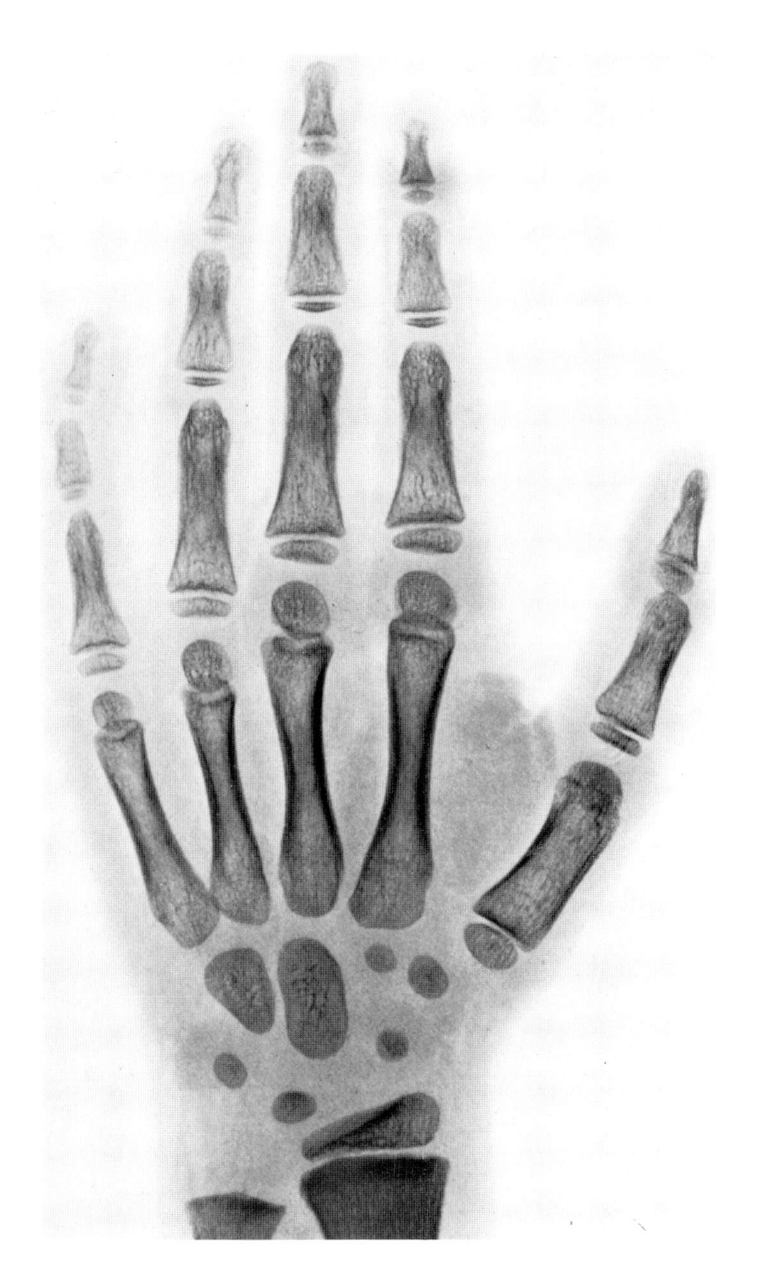

Fig. 1104. 6 year old. Besides the nucleus of the pisiform (it appears in about the 10th year of life as the last nucleus) and the distal ulnar epiphysis (appears about the 7th year of life), the other osseous nuclei are all arranged. The square dimension of the hand root nuclei corresponds to the lower norm. It can be clearly seen that the phalanges have very little or no compacta, and that the metacarpal bones in the middle diaphysial third develop a thick compacta.

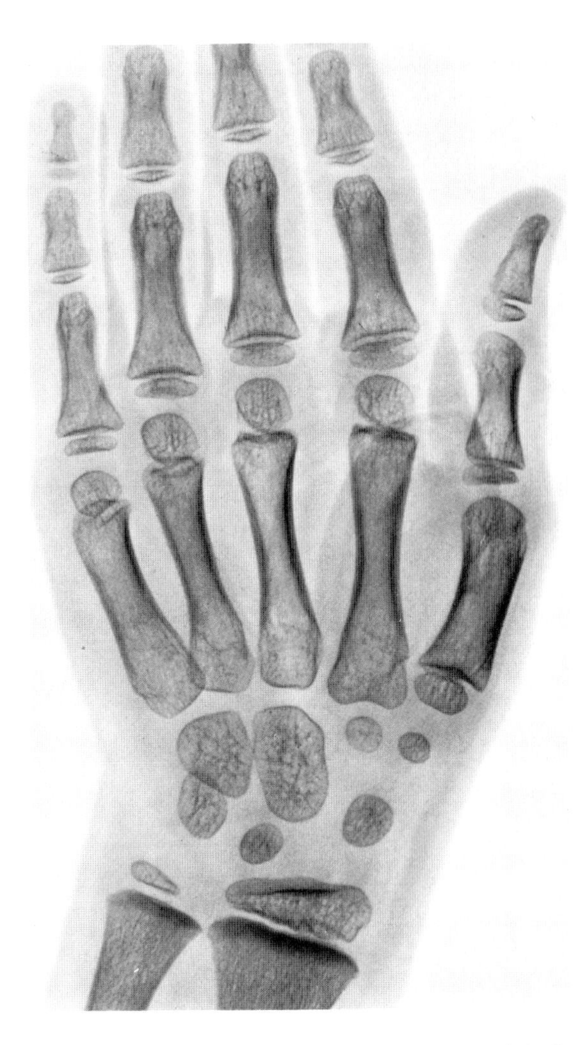

Fig. 1105. 7 year old. The nucleus of the distal ulnar epiphysis is already arranged. It can be divided. The picture corresponds to the lower norm.

1 Capitatum
2 Hamatum
3 Distal radial epiphysis
4 Triquetrum
5 Epiphysis of the 1st metacarpal
6 Lunatum
7 Trapezium
8 Trapezoideum
9 Scaphoid
10 Distal ulnar epiphysis

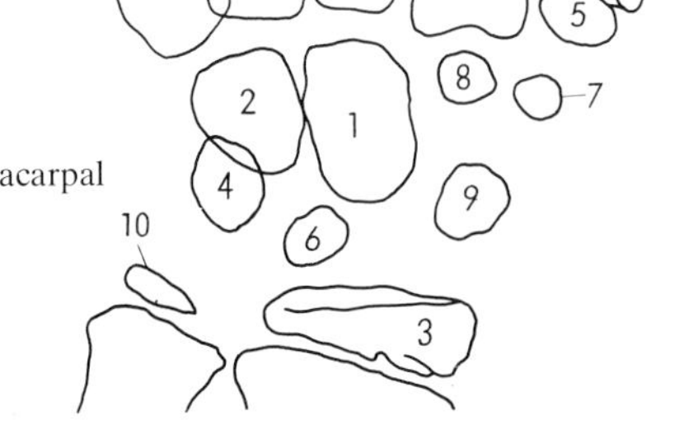

Fig. 1106. Sketch to Fig. 1105. The osseous nuclei of the hand root are numbered according to their order of appearance.

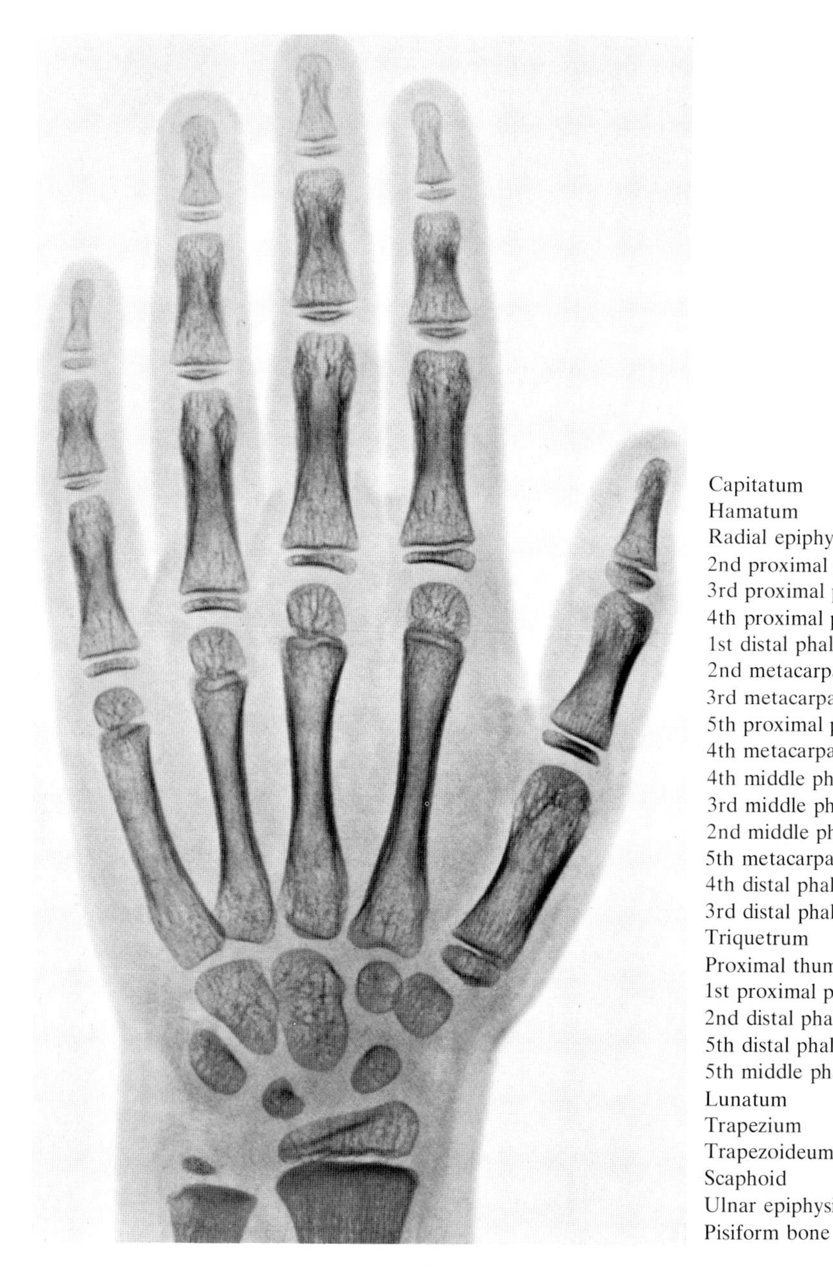

Fig. 1107. **8 year old.** In comparison with Fig. 1105, the only difference that appears here is the enlarged square dimension, especially of the trapezium and the trapezoideum.

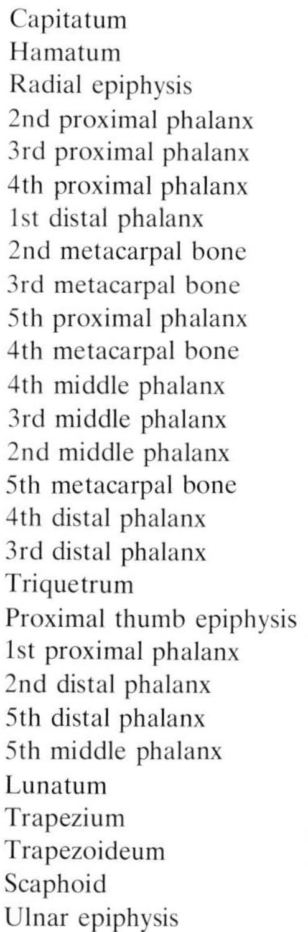

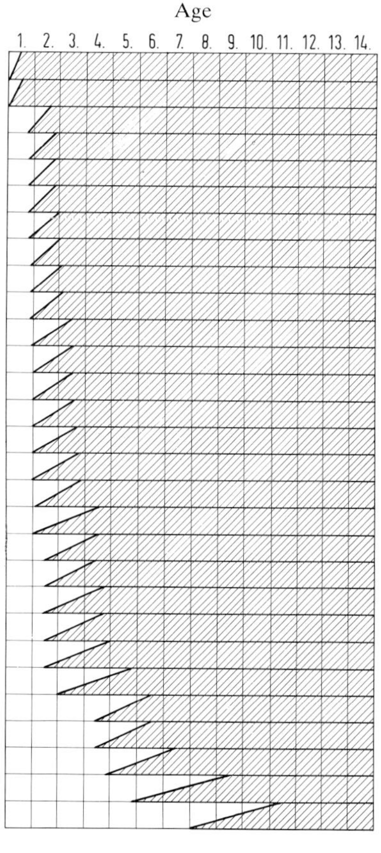

Fig. 1108. Differentiation of the hand root and the epiphyseal nuclei, with details of variations (oblique surface), according to *Schmid* and *Moll* (1960). Its comparison with the ossification table in Fig. 1109 according to *Gött* (1925) clearly shows the acceleration in between.

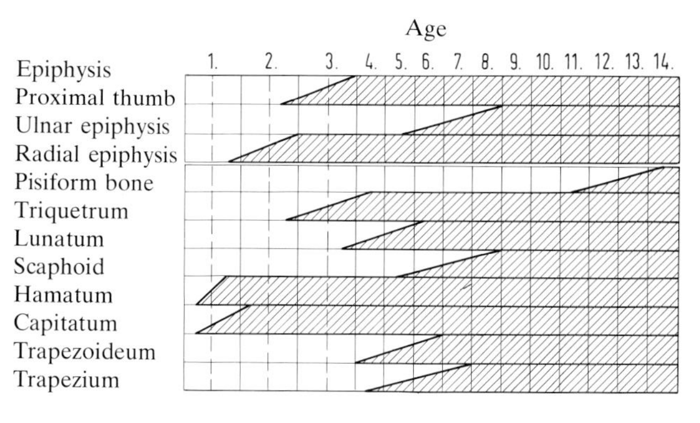

Fig. 1109. Ossification scheme of the hand root osseous nuclei (according to *Gött,* 1925).

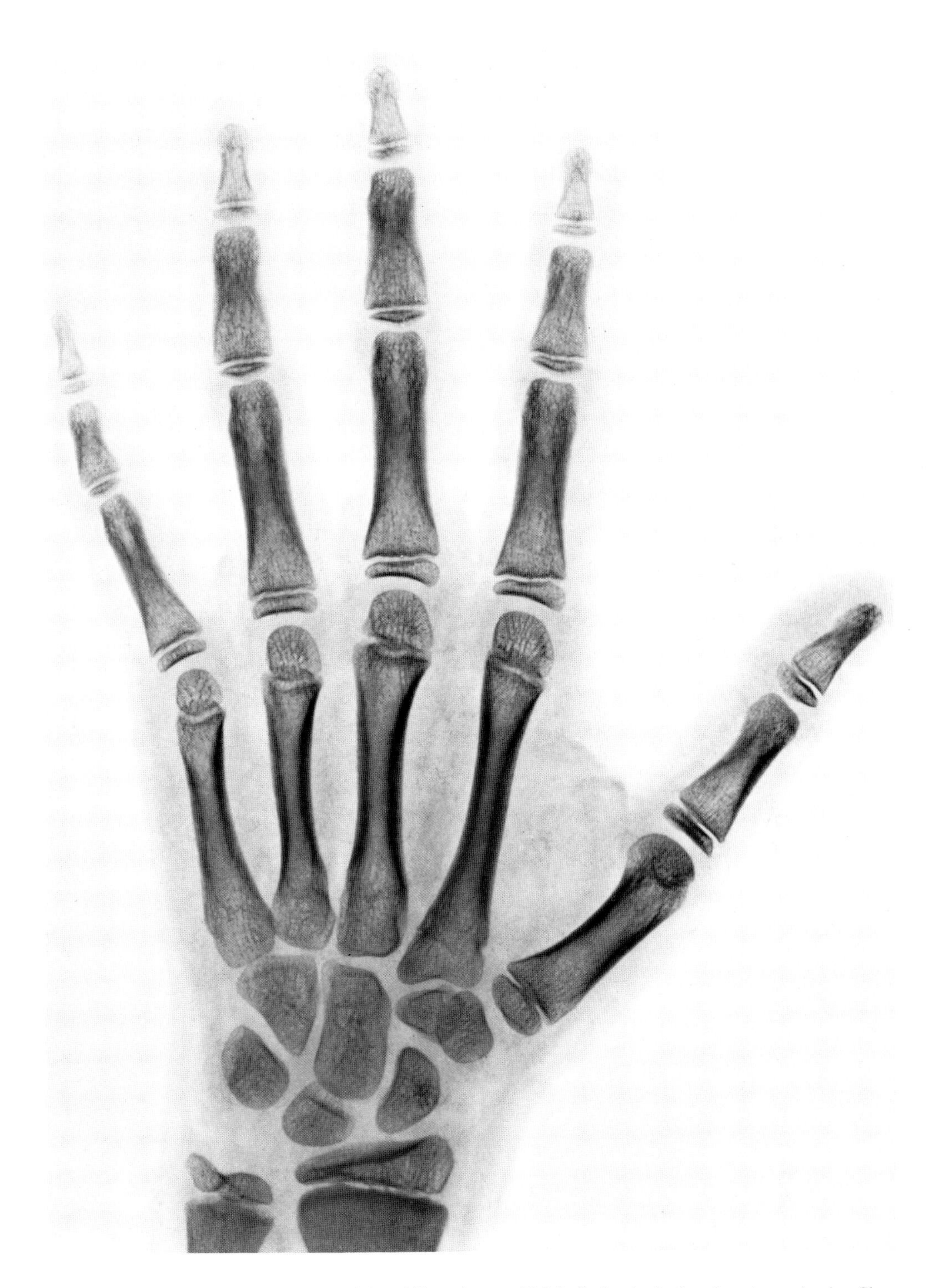

Fig. 1110. 10 year old. The ossification of the pisiform bone, which is the last in the hand root, now begins. Since the pisiform is not freely projected and the triquetrum is superimposed on it, it is rather difficult to detect its borders in this radiograph. The picture corresponds to the average norm.

The ulnar epiphysis consists of two nuclei. So-called pseudoepiphyses are seen at the heads of the 1st metacarpal and the basis of the 2nd metacarpal (notch). Pseudoepiphyses are accessory epiphyses *(Siegert)* with premature appearance of accessory osseous nuclei, which usually fuse prematurely (6th–7th year of life) with the diaphysis. They are usually linked with developmental disorders of all kinds (see page 466).

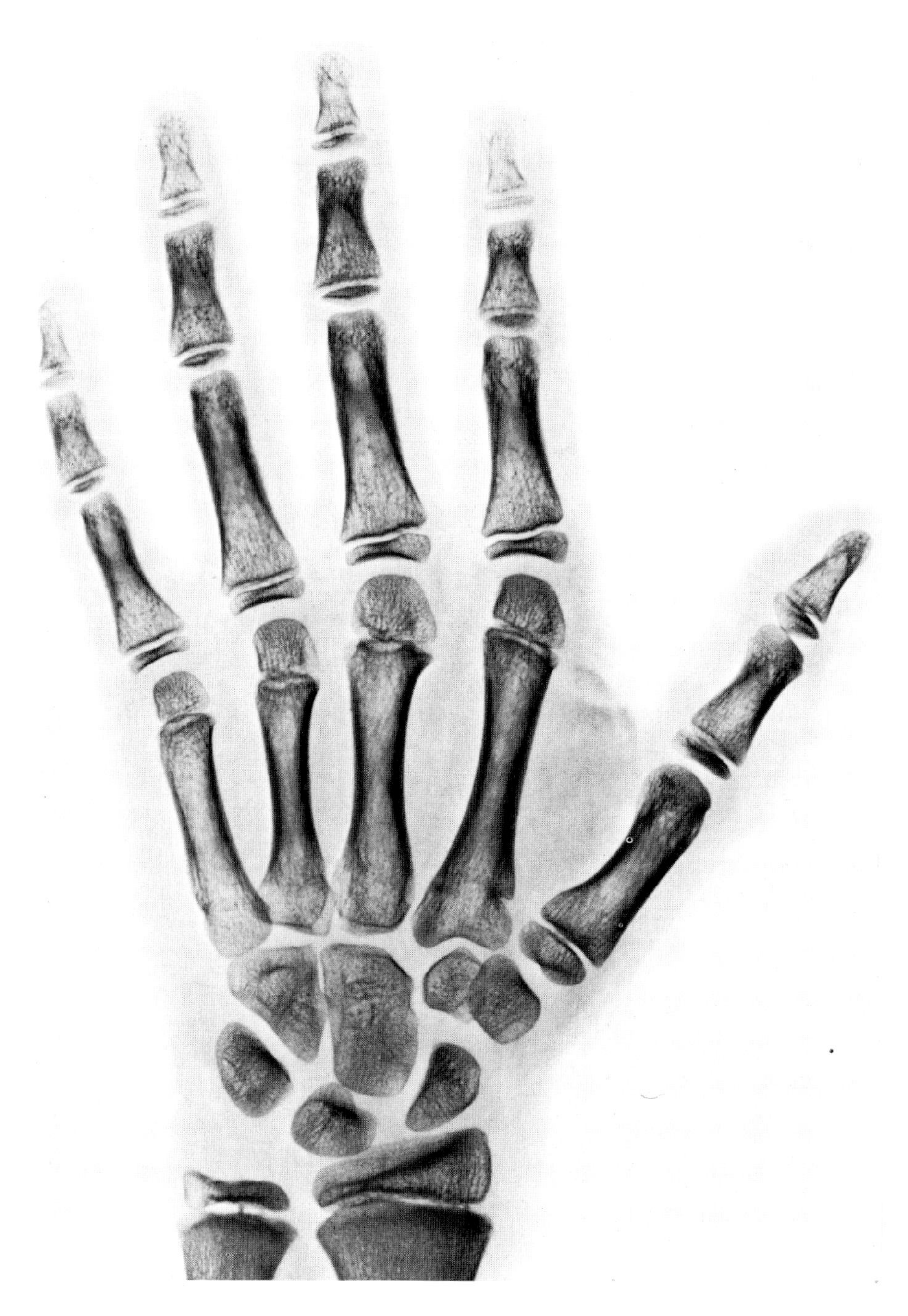

Fig. 1111. 11 year old. Average norm. Further increase of the square dimension of the hand root bones, the contours of which are progressively taking on their final form. In this picture, we again have a pseudoepiphysis in the 2nd proximal metacarpal bone. The epiphyseal fissure of the 2nd metacarpal begins to disappear.

In this period the first sesamoid bones are visible, especially in girls.
Physiological sclerosis is noticeable in the concavity of the articulation. It may be detectable in the concavities of the hamatum and scaphoid bones and in the proximal phalanges. Physiological sclerosis plays an important role in the formation of the hand. Pseudoepiphyses indicate an ossification anomaly.

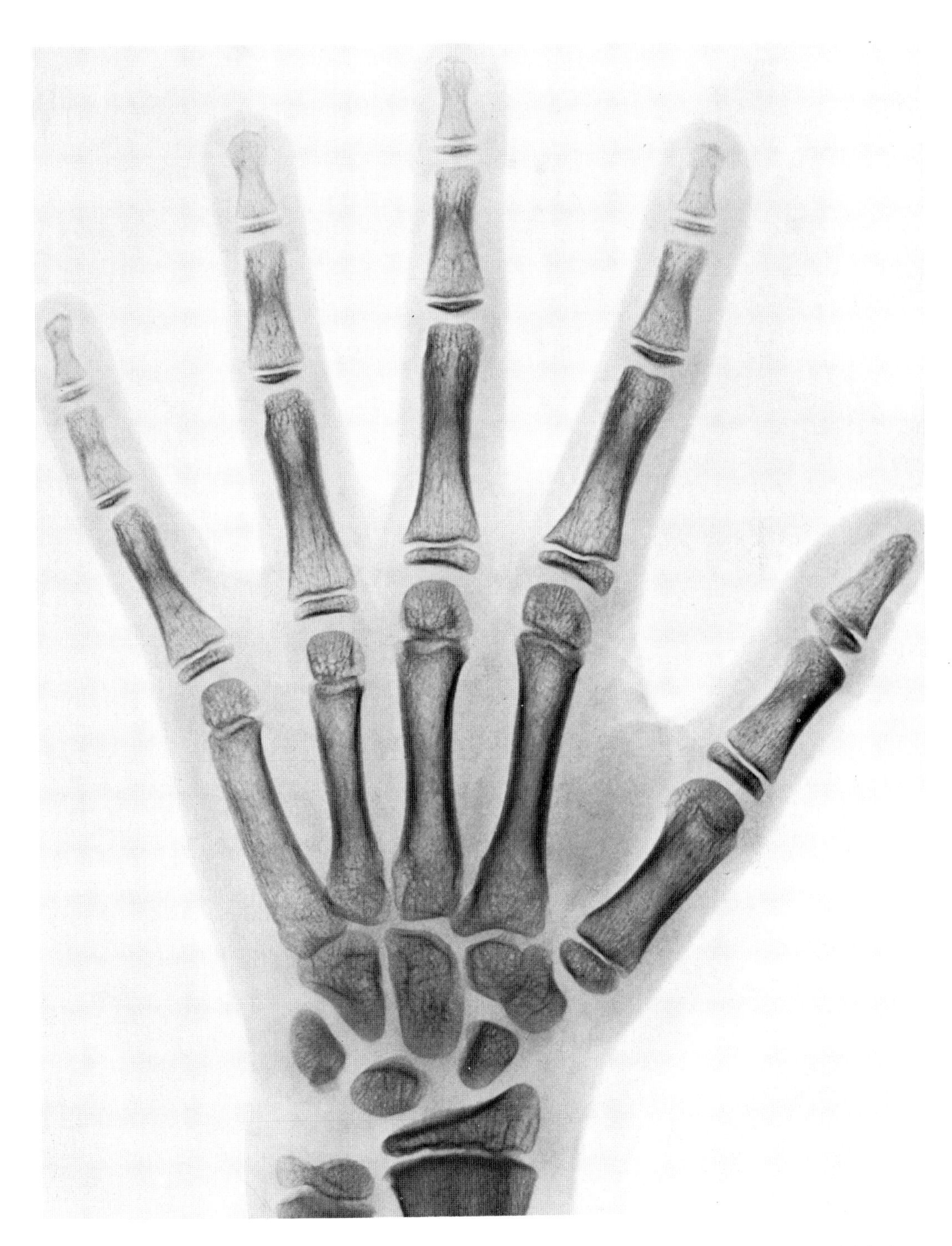

Fig. 1112. 12 year old. The picture corresponds to the average norm. The pisiform bone is clearly seen with its borders. In addition, radial sesamoid bones are projected in the head of the 2nd and 3rd metacarpal. In this case, there is a *Hulten*'s deficiency variation (shortening) of the distal ulnar extremity, with a possible development of manus vara. The deformity of the ulnar epiphysis indicates a developmental disorder as a cause of deficiency variation. The *Hulten*'s excessive variation (lengthening) of the distal ulnar extremity may lead, due to developmental disorders or trauma, to manus valga.

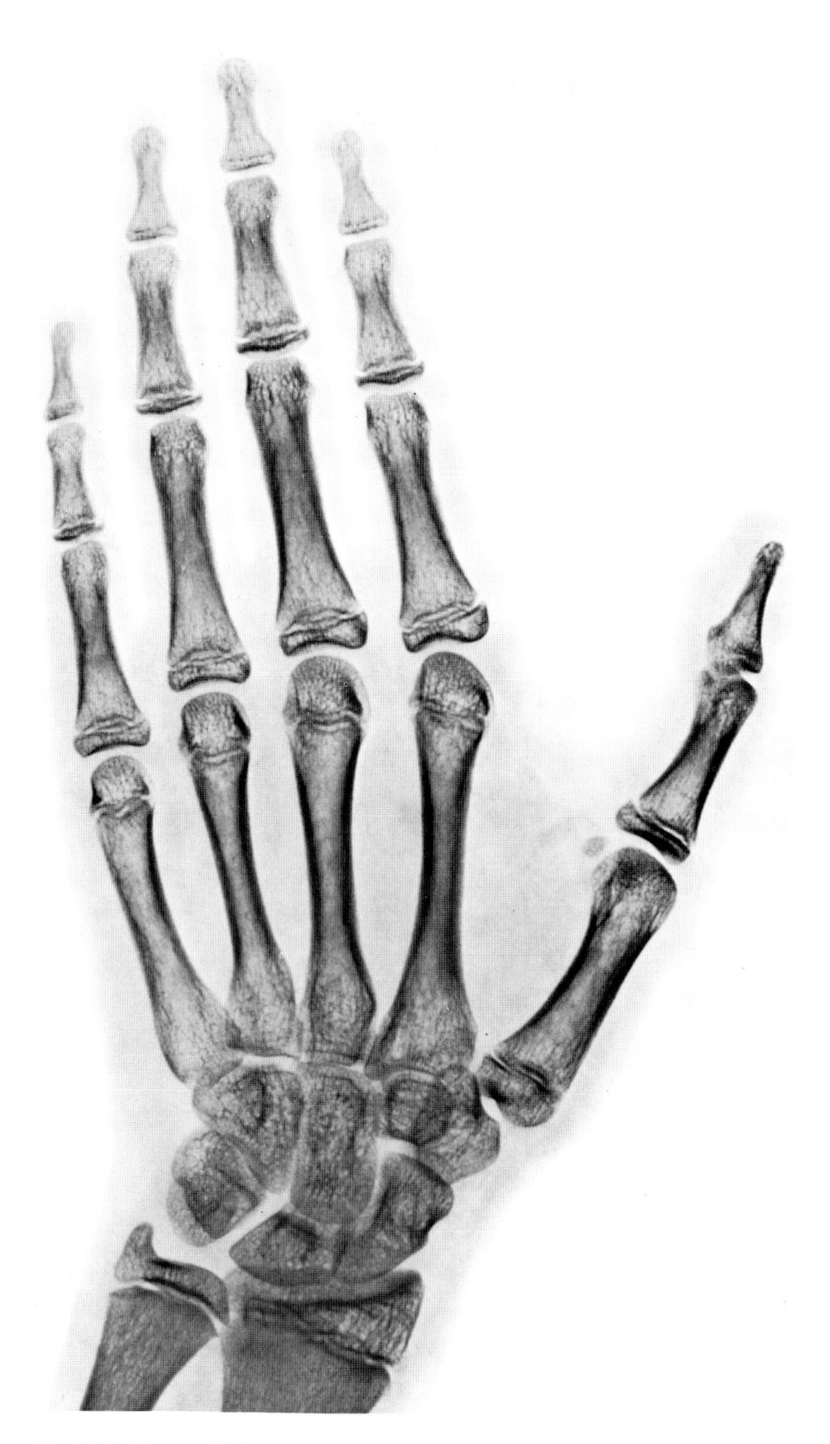

Fig. 1113. 14 year old. Average norm. All hand root bones, including the pisiform, are well formed; the glenoid cavity is only slightly broader than the adult's. A sesamoid bone is discernible in front of the 1st metacarpal bone. The styloid process (ulnar) is normally shaped. The radial and ulnar sutures have become markedly narrower; the sutures of the metacarpal bones begin to close.

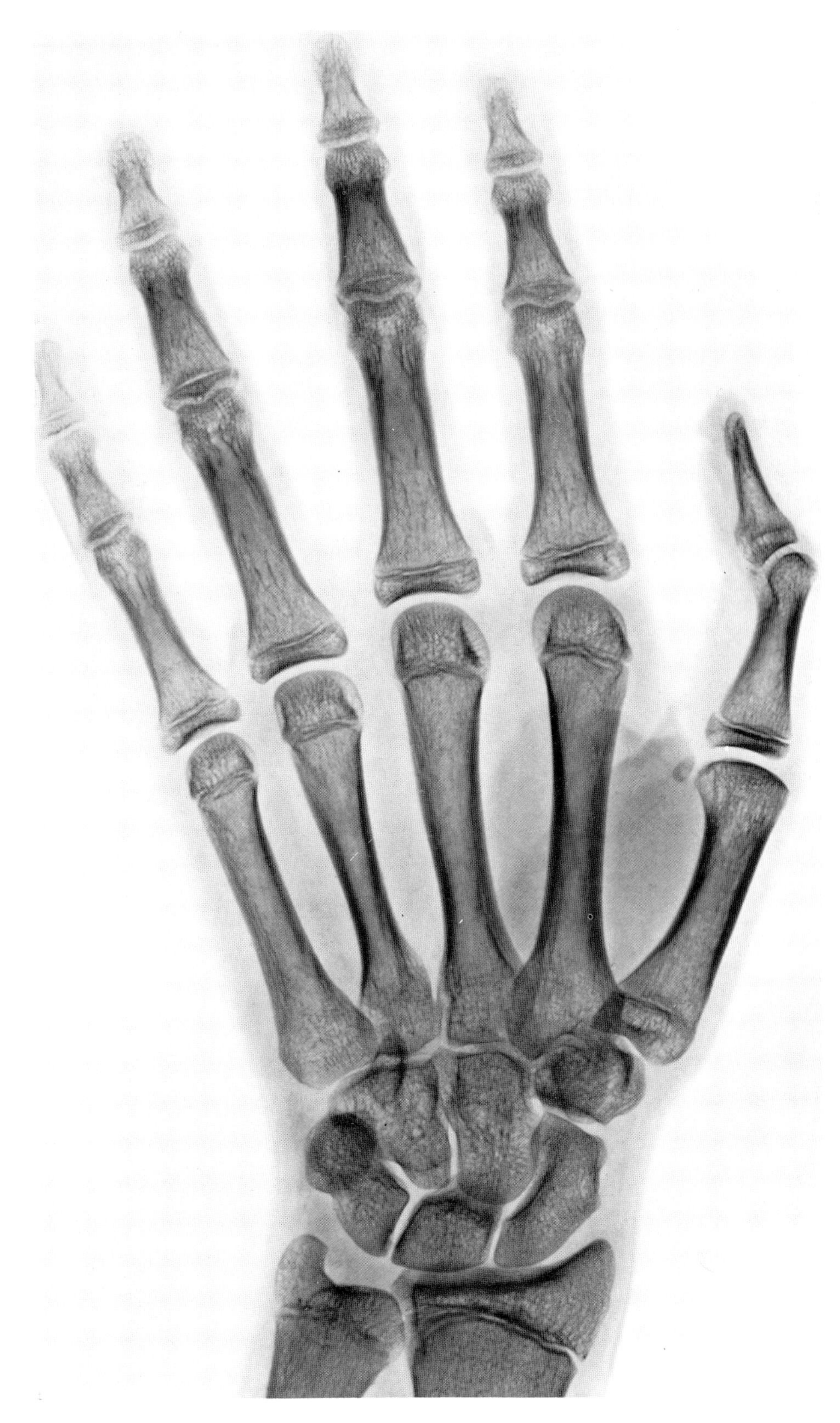

Fig. 1114. 15 year old. Average norm. The process of closure of all the epiphyseal sutures is continuing. The suture of the 1st metacarpal is already closed and discernible at the "epiphyseal scar."

The numerous cystic brightenings in the metacarpal bones, the hand root bones and the radial epiphyses should be regarded as a normal intermediate state of development. These bones, however, are preferred sites for the formation of small cysts throughout life.

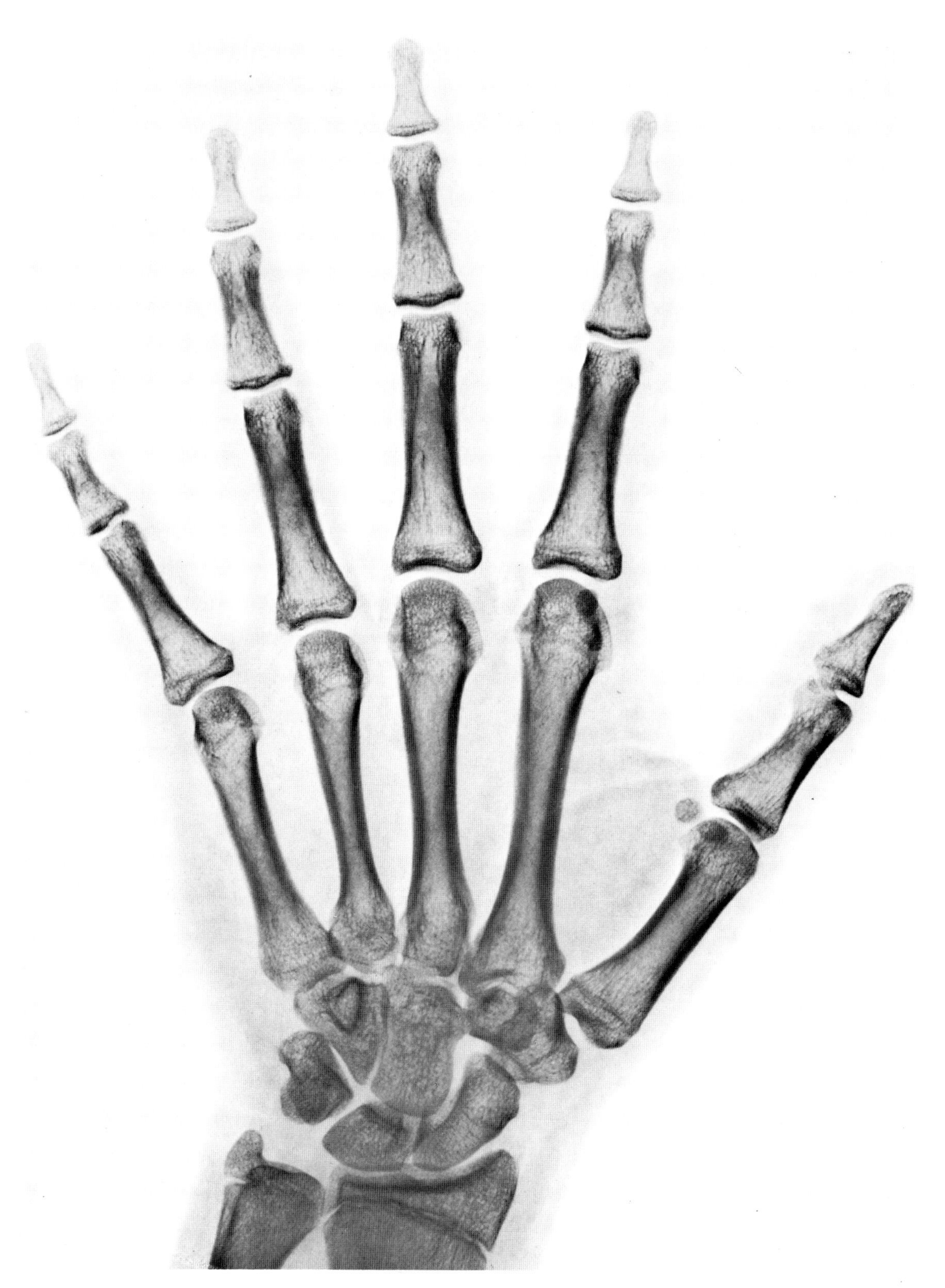

Fig. 1115. 16 year old. Average norm. The closure of the epiphyseal sutures of the metacarpal bones and phalanges is already completed. There are only fine strips, so-called epiphyseal scars, which indicate their former existence.

In many metacarpal heads and the respective metacarpophalangeal articulations, there are sesamoid bones. They are regarded as indications of maturity after puberty and appear simultaneously with developed secondary sexual characteristics. A deviation of the ossification of the sesamoid bones at the ulnar side of the thumb base articulation can be used for the diagnosis of an accelerated or retarded development compared with normal development (*Rochlin* and *Zeitler*).

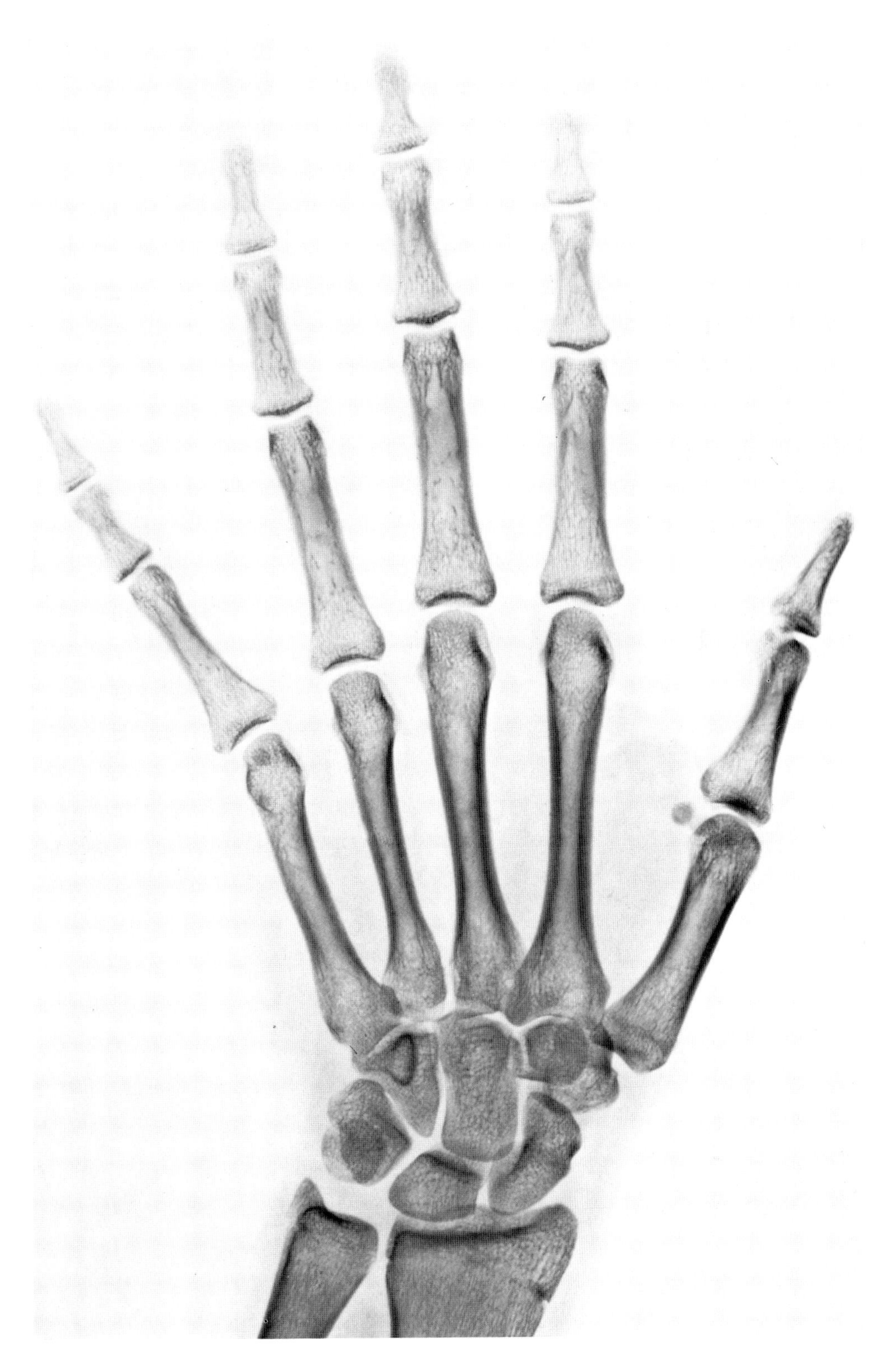

Fig. 1116. 17 year old. Average norm. There are still small notches in the ulna and radius, precisely where the epiphyseal sutures were, while no "epiphyseal scars" are to be seen in the metacarpal bones and the phalanges. The maturation sign, i.e., the sesamoid bone in the thumb base articulation, is also discernible.

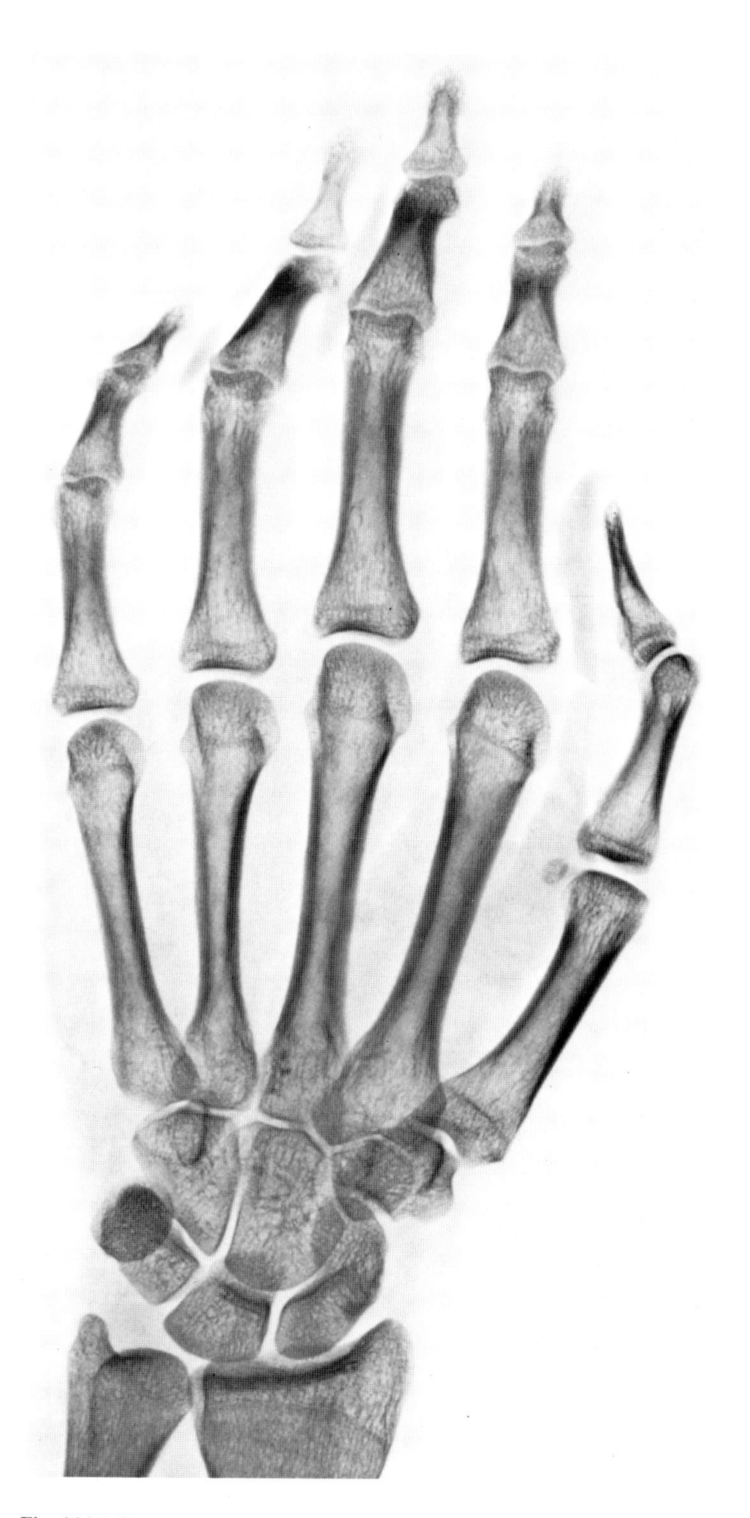

Fig. 1117. 18 year old. All epiphyseal sutures are closed. There is only a compressed zone discernible in the radius where the epiphyseal development site was. All the articulation layers have their final contours. In the distal diaphyses of medius and ulna, as well as in the epiphyses several compact isles are to be found in the same region as the small cysts.

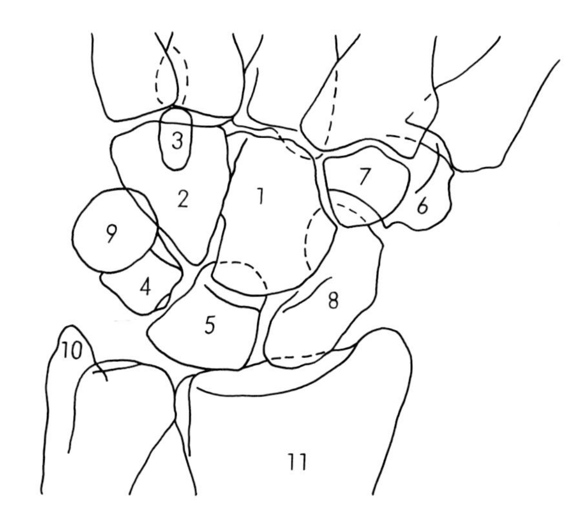

Fig. 1118. Sketch to Fig. 1117.

1 Capitatum
2 Hamatum with
3 Hamulus ossis hamati
4 Triquetrum
5 Lunatum
6 Trapezium
7 Trapezoideum
8 Scaphoid
9 Pisiform
10 Styloid process
11 Distal radial extremity

The hand root bones are numbered according to their order of appearance.

V. Pelvis – Hip Articulation and Lower Extremities

Prenatal Development

Ossification in the femur and the tibia (see also Fig. 691) begins in embryos 18 to 20 mm long (around the end of the 2nd embryonic month). The diaphysial nucleus of the femur is rather large at birth, whereas, of the two epiphyses, only one main epiphyseal nucleus, usually at the distal epiphysis, is discernible shortly before birth. Of all the epiphyseal nuclei of the extremities of the skeleton, the main epiphyseal nucleus is the first to appear in the body; however, it fuses later than the nucleus of the proximal epiphysis, only after the 20th year of life.

The ossification nuclei in the bone appear in the following order: in the ilium, in the 3rd-4th fetal month; in the ischium, in the 4th–5th fetal month; and in the pubic bone, in the 6th–7th fetal month.

The kneecap remains cartilagenous throughout prenatal development. It is noteworthy, that the knee articulation of a 10–12-mm-long embryo is composed of two parts, which are separated from each other by a dividing wall. This is important because of variations which occur.

The ossification of the foot skeleton begins with the formation of the main osseous nuclei of the phalanges and the metatarsal bones, whereby the terminal phalanges of the big toe and the second metatarsal bone of a 35-mm-long fetus begin to show the first signs of ossification *(Broman)*. Prenatal ossification is completed in the 8th or 9th fetal month with the middle phalange of the 5th toe. There is a considerable time difference with respect to the development of the foot skeleton as compared to the hand skeleton; at birth the ossification of the tarsus has already begun. The calcaneus as well as the talus and (but not regularly), also the cuboid bone show osseous nuclei. In the calcaneus the ossification begins as early as the 5th or 6th fetal month, and in the talus in the 7th or 8th fetal month, whereas the first ossification signs in the cuboid bone appear shortly before or after birth.

Postnatal Development

As in the upper limbs, the lower limbs present a number of peculiarities and variations in their course of ossification. The following three chapters on the postnatal development of the lower limbs are compared with Figure 1122, which supplements Figure 1017.

In a radiograph, the pelvic blade of the newborn looks like a design radiating out from the center; at this phase, this may still be attributed to the plexus bone structure (Fig. 1129).

Hip Bone with Hip Articulation and Thigh

Coxae bone. The coxae bone is formed from three nuclei which are arranged separately and develop individually: the ilius bone, the ischium bone and the pubic bone. At birth all three anlagen are already osseous. In the radiograph, however, they can be separated through extended zones of soft compressions of cartilage (Figs. 1119 and 1133). This is best seen through an oblique projection of half the pelvis (Fig. 1120).

The broad cartilagenous sutures between the ilium, ischium, and pubic bones meet each other in the region of the pelvic articulation in a Y-shaped form. This region, therefore, is also called the Y-cartilage or the Y-suture (Figs. 1121 and 1134).

With a proper setting, such as in Figure 434, it is possible to present the Y-suture through a surface projection of the pelvic glenoid cavity. The Y-suture shows a varia-

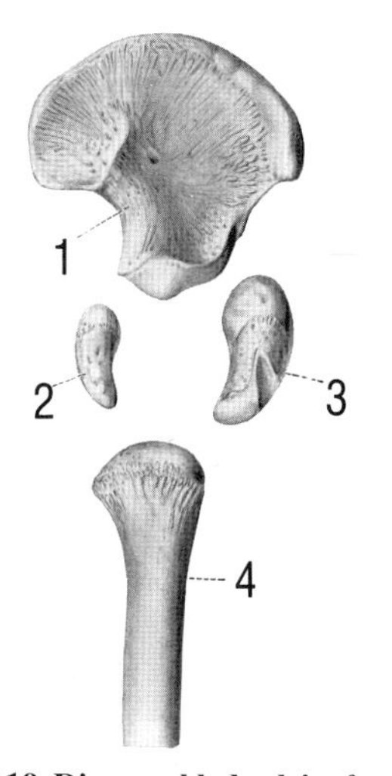

Fig. 1119. Disassembled pelvis of a newborn. (1/1: from *Sobotta-Becher,* 17th edition).

1 Ilium bone
2 Pubic bone
3 Ischium bone
4 Femoral body

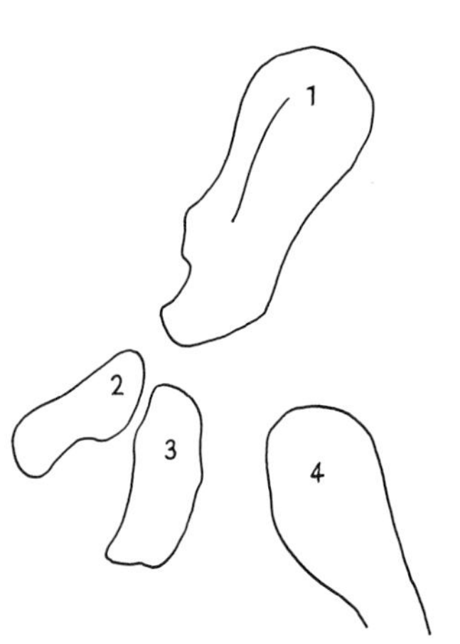

Fig. 1120. 3-day-old baby. Oblique projection of the pelvis.

1 Ilium bone
2 Pubic bone
3 Ischium bone
4 Femur

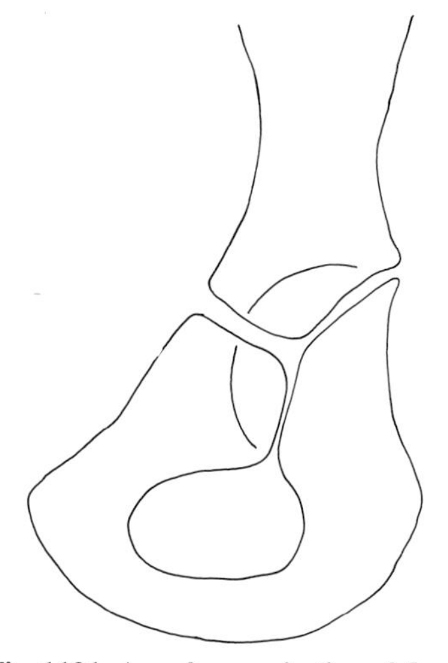

Fig. 1121. A surface projection of the pelvic glenoid cavity to show the Y-suture.

tion in its direction in the course of development. The synostosis of the three osseous parts (ilium, pubic and ischium bones), which become the coxae bone, occurs with the closure of the Y-suture and lasts many years.

The cartilagenous suture between the lateral extremities of the ischium and the pubic bone is usually invisible in radiographs, because these two bones are projected onto each other in a sagittal projection.

The closure of the Y-suture occurs with the beginning of puberty. However, there are individual variations regarding the closure of the Y-suture since, rather frequently, a narrow fissure in the glenoid cavity of 17- to 18-year-old males sometimes still remains.

A broad fissure opens between the inferior branch of the ischium and the pubic bone, whose closure occurs between the 4th and 8th years of life. At this site (synchondrosis ischiopubic), an irregular ossification with a broadening of the bone extremities is discernible *(Junge* and *Heuck);* see Figs. 1146 and 1147. The bone cavity may be confused with aseptic bone necrosis!

Acetabulum. It is noteworthy, that at birth no other articulation is so slow in its development as the pelvic articulation. Later on, enchondral dyostoses are discernible due to endocrinal disorders, as well as aseptic bone necroses and local inflammation processes in the pelvic articulation. The radiograph of the hip is therefore taken

1 Vascular canals
2 Split glenoid roof (normal)!
3 Irregular symphysis border, small apophyses
4 Thickened ischiopubic fusion
5 Apophysis in the ischiadic tuber (puberty)
6 Nucleolus in the minor trochanter
7 Pelvic crest apophysis (puberty) (Beckenkammapophyse)
8 Osseous nucleus in the anterior inferior ilius spine (puberty)
9 Acetabulum bone in the glenoid roof (coxae quartum bone)
10 Undular epiphyseal suture
11 Greater trochanter: unclear contours and nucleolei
12 Collum shaft angle about 140° (errors due to poor arrangement of subject)
13 Nonspecific periosteum apposition
14 Pointed metaphyseal edges
15 Large ossification variations of the kneecap (divided kneecap)
16 Proximal tibial nucleus: double nucleus, unclear borders
17 Pointed metaphyseal edges and undular epiphyseal lines
18 Horizontal lines (growth lines)
19 Horizontal lines (growth lines)
20 Unclear border of the epiphyseal nucleus, normal in early childhood
21 Proximal fibular epiphysis: nucleolus
22 Tibial apophysis: irregular ossification
23 Tibial tuberosity (see Fig. 739, No. 166)
24 Nonspecific "periosteum apposition" and normal double contours
25 Horizontal lines (growth lines)
26 Distal tibial epiphysis: nucleolus (10th–12th years of life)
27 Talus: double nucleus
28 Trigonum bone (dorsal)
29 Navicular bone: double nucleus, unclear borders
30 External tibial bone
31 Cuboid bone: multicentralized ossification
32 Intermetatarsal bone
33 Distal fibular epiphysis: nucleolus
34 Sustentaculum bone
35 Calcaneus: most frequently double nucleus (calcaneus bifidus), compacta isles, irregular ossification of the tuber calcanei
36 Cuneiform bones: numerous nucleolei, especially medial
37 Metatarsal bone V: basal apophysis
38 Metatarsal apophysis: sesamoid bones, pseudoepiphyses and irregular ossification at the proximal extremity, double nucleus in the heads
39 Basic and middle phalanges: "thick" and "split" epiphyses, missing epiphyses (especially 5th radiation), double nucleus (especially 1st radiation)
40 Terminal phalanges: hypoplastic or lacking

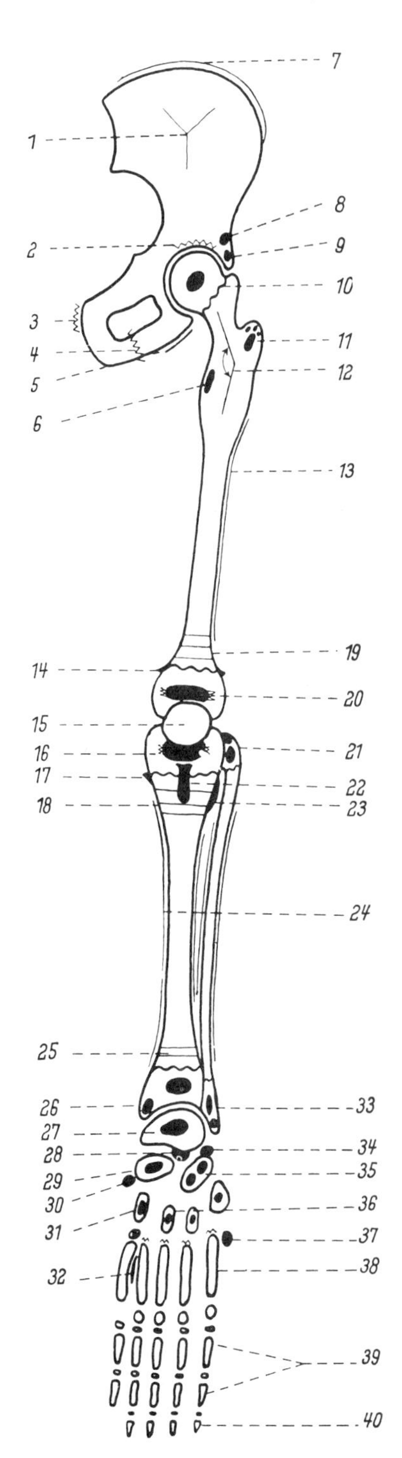

Fig. 1122. Schematic view of the most frequent normal ossification variations and possibilities of radiologic error in the bones of the pelvic girdle and the lower limb masses (from *Swoboda:* Das Skelett des Kindes, 2nd edition, Thieme, Stuttgart, 1969).

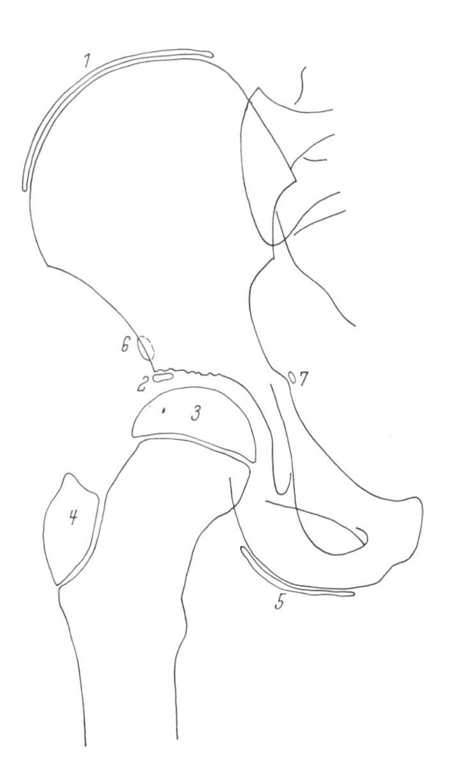

Fig. 1123. Osseous nuclei and apophyses in the pelvic region.

1 Apophysis of the ilium crest (Figs. 1150 and 1151): appears in the 12th to 15th years of life and between the 21st and 25th years and fuses with the ilium bone
2 Glenoid edge apophysis of the acetabulum bone, not to be confused with the bone ad acetabulum of the radiologists; appears in the 9th to 11th years of life and fuses around the 15th to 17th years of life; it may persist
3 Femoral head epiphysis
4 Major trochanter
5 Apophysis of the ischiadicum tuber; appearance and fusion occur simultaneously like the ilium blade
6 Nucleus of the anterior inferior ilium spine; appears around the 13th to 15th years of life and fuses relatively quickly in the 16th to 18th years
7 Apophysis of the ischiadica spine; appears around the 13th to 15th years of life and fuses around the 20th to 25th years

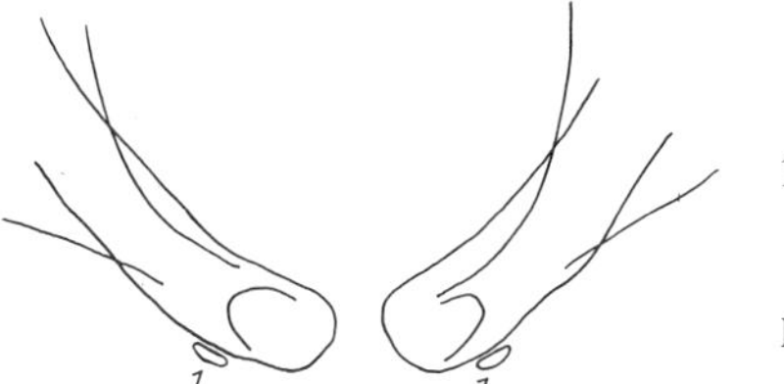

1=apophysis in the pubic tubercle.

Fig. 1124. Axial radiograph of the symphysis.

several times so that the femoral collum, shaft and angle may be better seen.

The acetabulum of the newborn has only a flat cavity. It is only in the 5th year of life that the glenoid cavity takes on its semispherical form. *Imhäuser* indicates an interpelvic rise of the base of the pelvic glenoid cavity between the 7th year of life and puberty as a typical and physiological developmental phase. According to his examinations, this physiological protrusion disappears with the closure of the growth region. There is no connection with the idiopathic acetabulum protrusion in the adult (see also Fig. 490).

Acetabuli bone. As an introduction to the synostosis in the acetabulum, the ossification of the acetabuli bone of the anatomists (coxae quartum bone, cotyloid bone) takes place around the 9th to 12th years of life as a multinuclear *Schaltknochen* in the Y-suture between the ilium and the public bone. This glenoid bone should not be confused with the bone (skeleton element?) of the radiologist bearing the same name *(Schaltknochen)*. For a long period it is discernible as an independent bone, although it changes its form and size. It forms the front external part of the glenoid base and edge, and fuses with the other bones of the hip glenoid cavity around the 18th to 20th years of life *(Morrison)*; it can remain independent. Sometimes one side ossifies earlier.

H. Schmid signifies that part of the intercalary bone, which forms the glenoid cavitiy edge (acetabuli bone), as a glenoid edge epiphysis (better apophysis). It should occasionally persist. This bone fits eventually into the joint of the glenoid roof and never lies near the glenoid base (Figs. 1147 and 1148).

The isolated bone, with changing form and size near the glenoid roof, in the adult has a special but insufficiently explained origin.

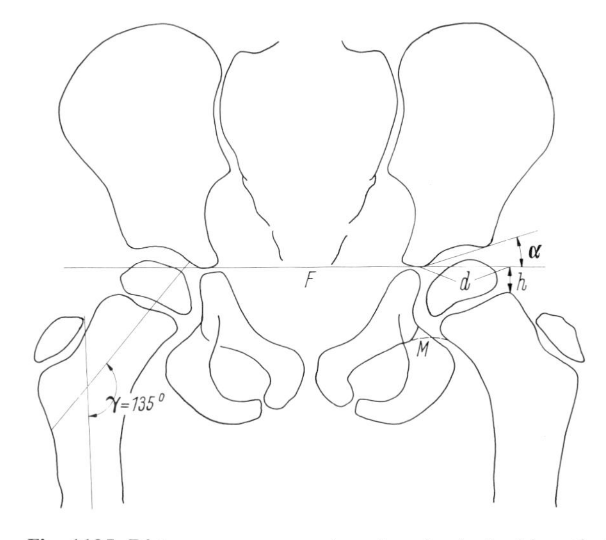

Fig. 1125. Distance measurements and angles in the hip articulation (see also Fig. 1153).

F Horizontal suture, joins the two sides of the Y-suture
α Glenoid cavity angle (at birth ca. 30°, after growth termination 12–20°)
h Distance between the highest point of the femoral diaphysis and horizontal suture (7–10 mm)
d Distance between section point F/h and the Y-suture (10–15 mm)
M *Menard*'s or *Shenton*'s line
The distance measurements h and d, as well as *Ménard*'s line, serve to determine a possible craniolateral displacement of the femur in cases of hip dysplasia.
γ Femoral collum angle (at birth 140°, after growth termination 120–130°). Radiograph to be carried out in a normal position.
120° = coxa vara;
$\gamma >$ 135° = coxa valga.
For further information on the diagnosis of coxa vara in juveniles, see *Jacobs*.

This bone, which so far has been called acetabuli bone, would better be called ad acetabulum bone or glenoid edge bone (see also Figs. 441, 442, 485, 487 and 488). In later years an extended dented formation is found in the glenoid roof. This formation may occasionally lead to peculiar borders in the radiographs. This is a case of ossification notches with no pathological significance (Figs. 1136, 1137, 1139 and 1141).

Apophyses in the pelvic region. As in all other flat bones, apophyseal ossifications occur in the pelvic region during puberty (Figs. 1123 and 1124). At the end of the second or the beginning of the third decade, they fuse with the pelvic bone.

These are the striped apophyses at the ilium crest, which reaches up to the anterior inferior ilium spine, further a similarly striped apophysis at the ischiadic tuber and an osseous nucleus in the pubic tubercle (Fig. 1124). The striped apophyseal nucleus at the ilium crest, which appears in the 12th to 15th years of life, can show a spiral growth dens similar to the apophyseal fissure in the border line of the glenoid roof (Figs. 1150 and 1151), which fissure later becomes smooth. Between the 21st and 25th years of life, the fusion of this nucleus with the ilium takes place. In rare cases the complete fusion does not occur and the apophysis persists *(J. Petersen)*.

One nucleus, which was first discovered by *Janker,* located on the anterior inferior ilium spine, is radiographically discernible through a slight external rotation of the pelvis. A further apophysis during synostosis in the 3rd decade of life is found in the ischiadic spine. For ossification variants and ossification disorders in the ischisicum tuber (tuber ossis ischii), see *Teichert.*

Femoral head. The osseous nucleus in the femoral head does not appear before the second half of the 1st year of life; its form is spherical or oval. Up to the 3rd year of life, the proximal diaphysial extremity grows towards the formation of a femoral collum. The epiphyseal cartilage becomes narrower. The epiphyseal nucleus on the proximal extremity gradually attains its semispherical form. For a topographical judgment of the proximal femur section two guidelines are important: the middle point of the epiphyseal nucleus should be located in the lengthened visible suture of the Y-cartilage, and the medial apex of the femoral collum should be located at the level of the lower glenoid edge.

To judge whether the femoral head is in a normal or a pathological position in a radiograph, the *Shenton* line is also used. It is identical with the *Ménard* line, which forms an arched joint of the femoral collum edge with the obturator crest of the pubic bone (Fig. 1125).

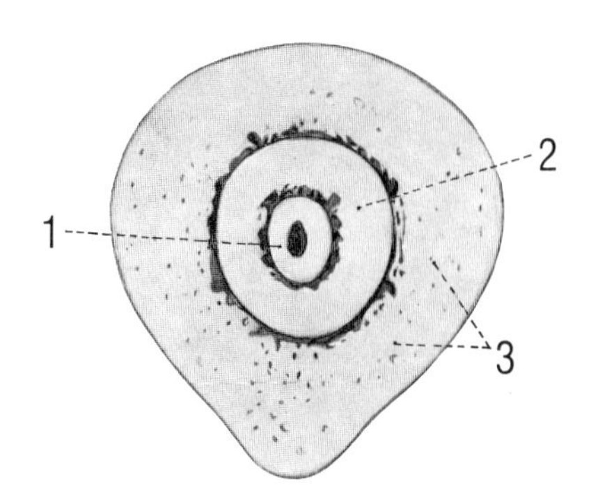

Fig. 1126. Cross-sectional slice of the femoral head of an adult (3 = external), of a 4-year-old child (2=middle) and of a newborn (1=internal). The youngest bone is inlaid in the medullar space (Markraum) of the next oldest (from *Sobotta-Becher,* 17th edition).

To judge the femoral collum, especially the collum-shaft angle, the child must be placed carefully with his legs rotated slightly inwards; with an external rotation, a coxa valga may be erroneously diagnosed. The right position can be controlled by the method of the radiograph of the trochanter.

See *Ravelli* and *Dihlmann* on the subjects of measurements of the glenoid angle, the disposition of the femoral collum (especially in newborns) as well as the line of direction of the Y-suture as a guideline for an early diagnosis of congenital pelvic luxation, and radiographic indications and measurement methods for the diagnosis of the congenital dysplasia of the pelvis.

In addition, see *Fiedler*'s X-ray research on the pelvis in newborns and the studies of *Glauner* and *Marquardt.*

Greater trochanter. Around the 3rd year of life, several ossification centers appear in this bone; these centers fuse and become a single nucleus in the course of development. Later, this nucleus is located on the femoral diaphysis with a notch-like form.

Lesser trochanter. Around the 10th to 14th years of life, but also later or earlier (the variation range is rather broad), a flat squamous apophysis is formed in this region.

Closure of the ossification. The first nucleus to fuse is the apophysis of the lesser trochanter toward the end of puberty, while the sutures of the femoral collum and of the greater trochanter close at the age of 17 to 19; in males this occurs slightly later.

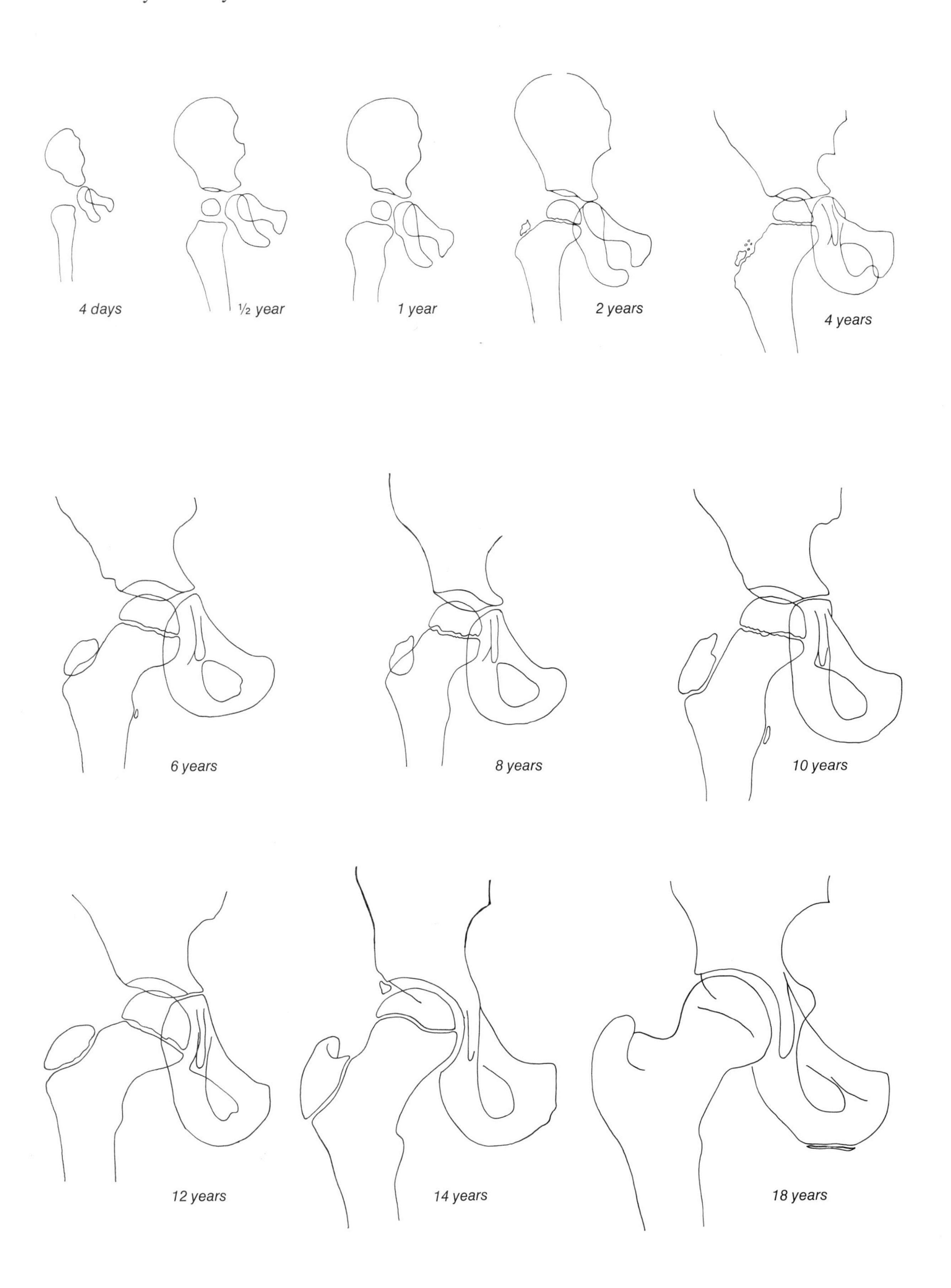

Fig. 1127. Hip articulations in chronological succession from early infancy to age 18.

A Series of Radiographs of the Development of the Pelvis and Hip Articulation from Infancy to Puberty

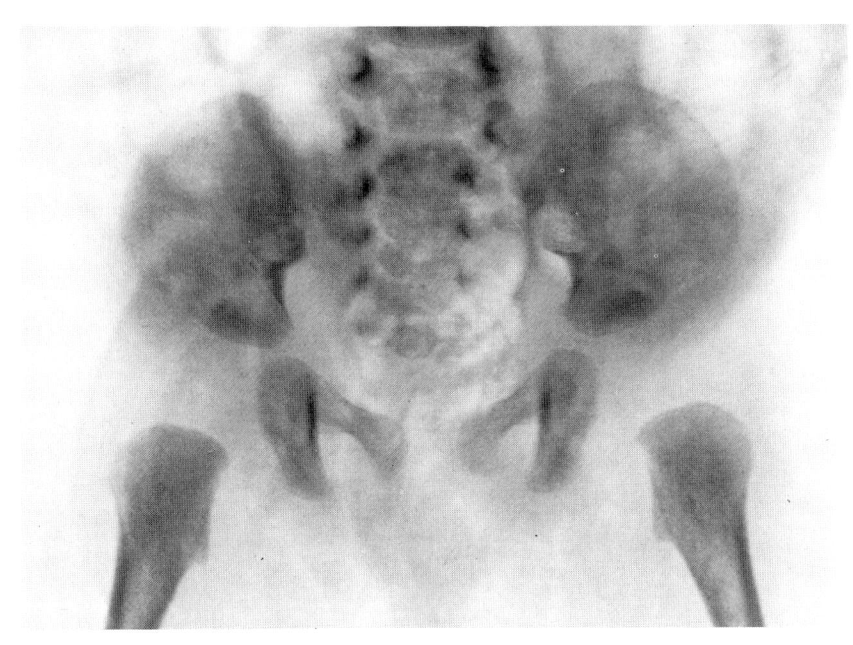

Fig. 1128. 22 day old. Pelvic radiograph.

The determination of sex in newborns is unimportant because sexual differences of radiographic determination do not exist at this age *(Zseböck)*. Likewise, it is difficult to determine sexual differences anatomically in the pelvis of a newborn in the 1st year of life. Only later and in the pathological case of congenital pelvic dysplasia do these differences play a definite role in metric and angular determinations (see angle measurements, p. 505). In this case, there are normal proportions with slight "neonatal distance" of the femur. The osseous nuclei of the sacral vertebra are also discernible. The Y-suture, which is still very broad between the three parts of what later becomes the coxae bone, is not completely visible due to the overlapping projection of each of the ossification nuclei of the pubic bone and the ischium. The Y-suture of the newborn plays a special role in the early diagnosis of congenital hip luxation. The higher half-shaft (Halbachse) of the collum diaphysial angle of 125° must meet the Y-suture vertically. If the angle is larger (pre-luxation), the half-shaft meets the pelvis above this place.

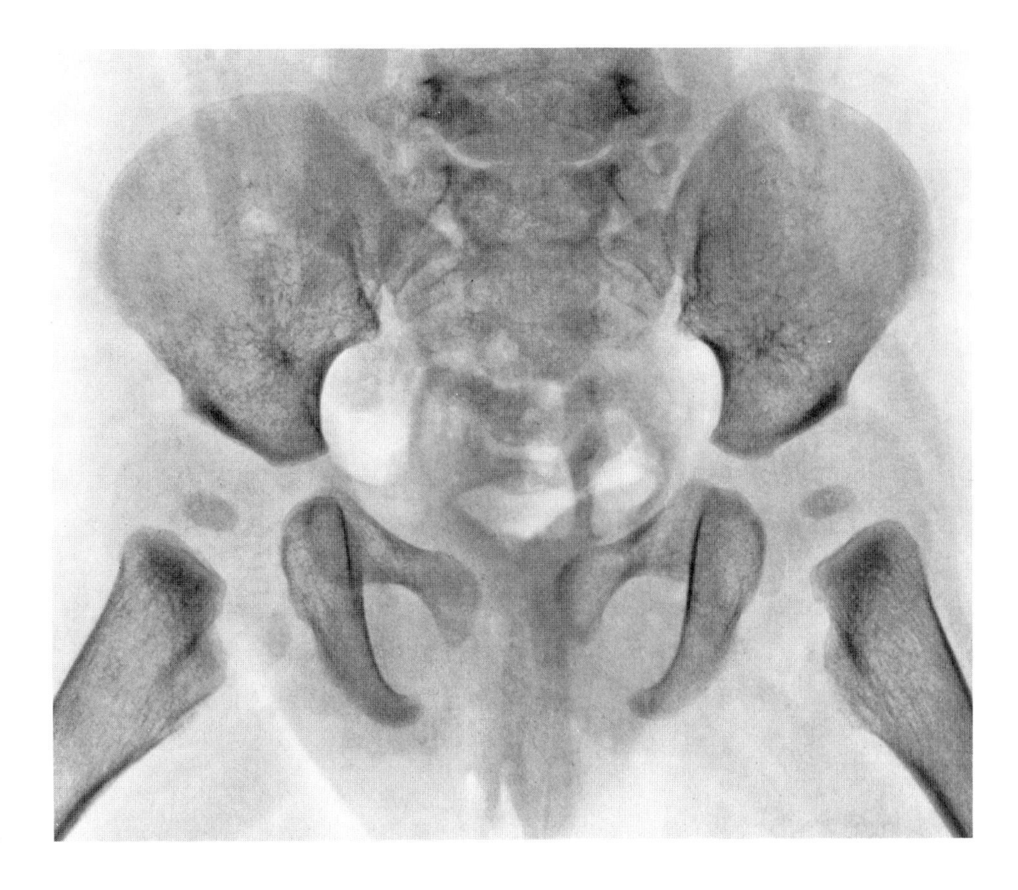

Fig. 1129. 1 year old. Pelvic radiograph.

The ossification nucleus in the femoral head is visible as a lateral oval bone shadow; it appears around the age of 6–18 months. In the pelvic blades, the original ossification center of both sides, which are symmetrical, is still discernible. The ray-like bone structure that extends from here causes this peculiar star-shaped design in the radiograph of the ilium in the newborn and small child.

The relationship between the size of the sacral bone and the other bones is quite impressive. In a baby it is the most extended. Later, sexual differences appear in the breadth of the sacral bone. The sacral bone of the female increases more in breadth.

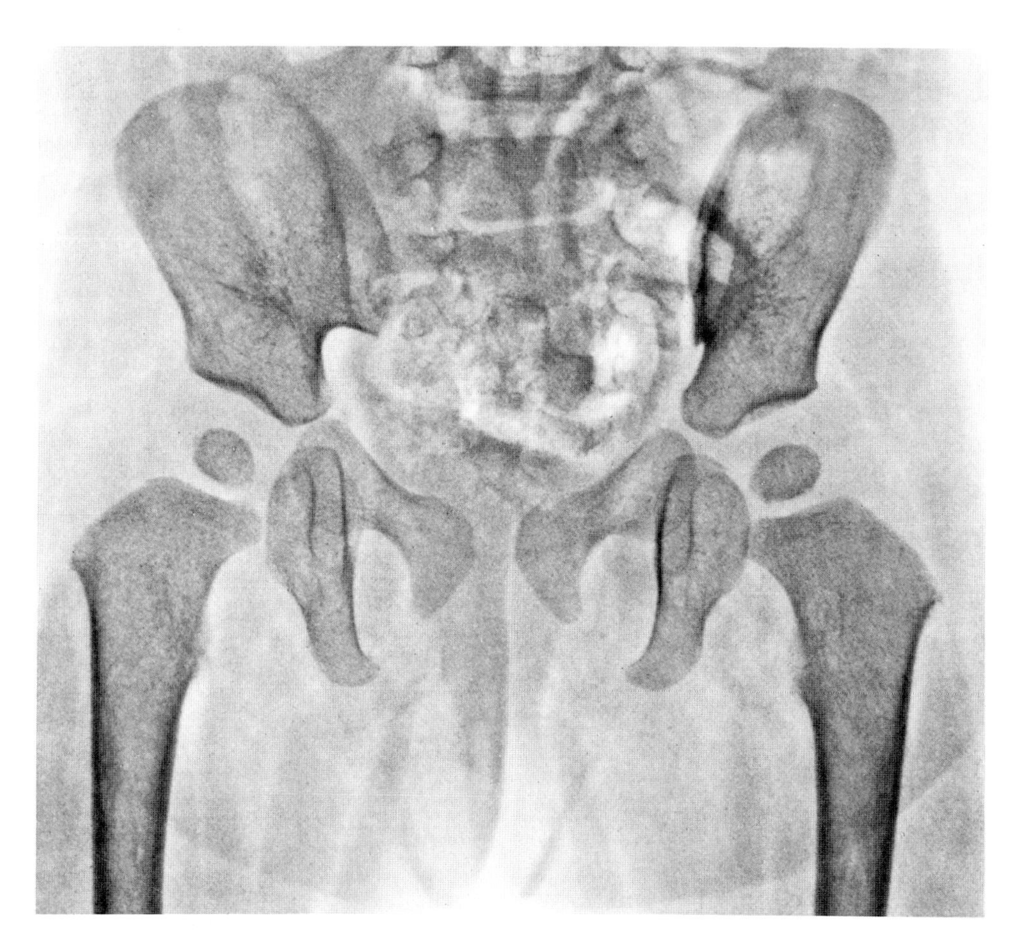

Fig. 1130. 15 month old. Pelvic radiograph. Further extension of the surface of the femoral head nucleus. The cavity of the glenoid begins to be marked in the glenoid roof. Left, the Y-suture is in perspective, seen slightly changed and shortened.

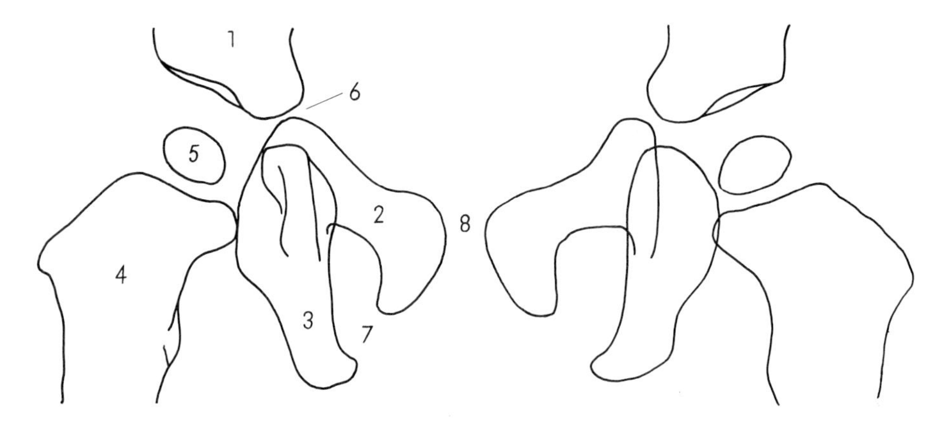

1 Ilium bone
2 Pubic bone
3 Ischium bone
4 Femoral diaphysis
5 Femoral head nucleus
6 Y-suture
7 Ischiopubic synchondrosis
8 Symphysis

Fig. 1131. Sketch of Fig. 1130.

Until the end of the 1st year of life, there is especially rapid growth of the pelvis. Afterwards, it slows down to a more even yearly rate.

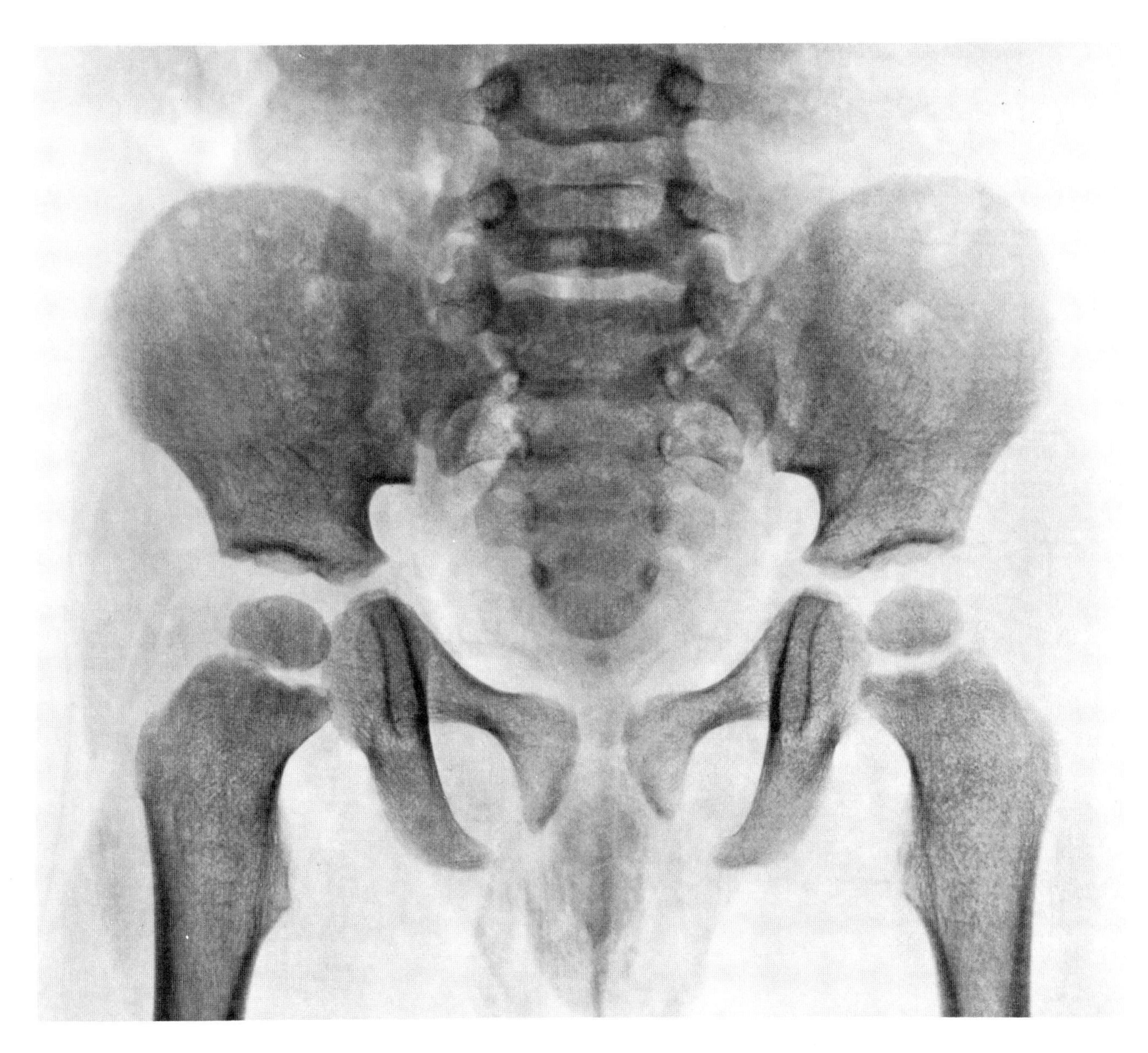

Fig. 1132. 2 year old. Pelvic radiograph. The contour of the glenoid roof, the femoral head nucleus and the proximal border of the femoral diaphysis present an undulation which is typical and characteristic for the stage of development. No pathological significance is to be attributed to this contour. The cartilaginous sutures between the three bone anlagen of the coxae bone become narrower, and also the fissure between the lower bough of the ischium and pubic bone has become smaller. In the lower sacral vertebra, the fusion with the lateral part of the lower vertebral bodies has already taken place. Usually, the lateral part fuses with the sacral vertebral bodies around the 4th to 6th years of life, at the time of the fusion of the vertebral arch with the vertebral body.

In the higher sacral vertebrae the corresponding suture between the vertebral body and the lateral part is still easily discernible.

Additional growth and ossification continue steadily and regularly until puberty, and no noteworthy variations occur during this period. Special attention should be given to the ischiopubic synchondrosis, which still presents a broad suture. Its closure can occur before the 4th year of life. Ossification does not occur at the same time in the left and right sides. The variation range may be seen in the radiograph series in Figs. 1135 and 1147. Fig. 1135 shows the pelvis of a $5^1/_2$-year-old child with a complete synchondrosis ossification. In Fig. 1147 the ischiopubic synchondrosis is still visible in a 14 year old. Its susceptibility is noticeable in ossification disorders and in the numerous infectious and non-infectious specific and non-specific illnesses.

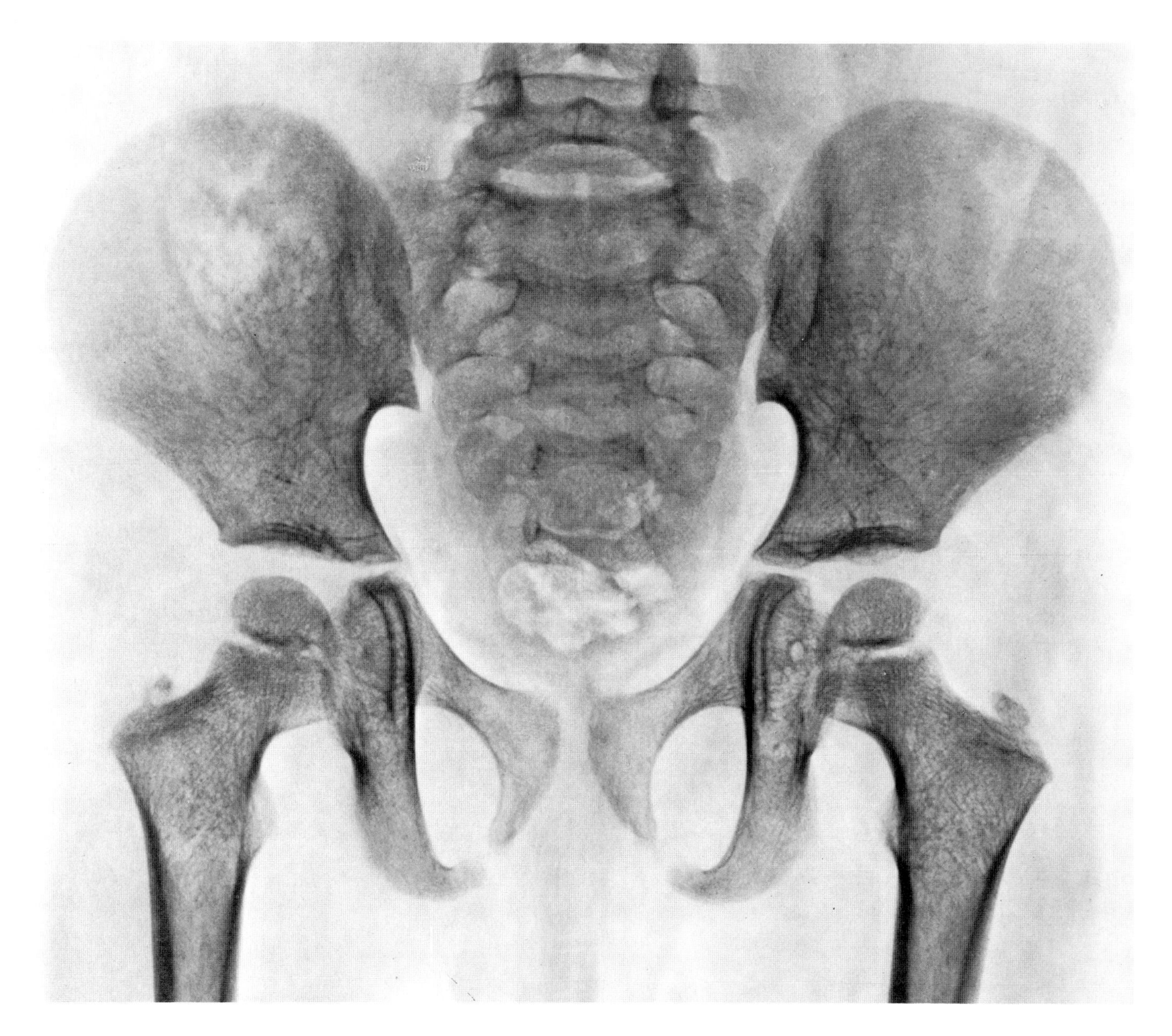

Fig. 1133. 5 year old. Mongolism. General hypoplasia of the pelvic skeleton and the proximal femor part. The femoral head nucleus is relatively well formed, but the nucleus of the greater trochanter (appearing in the 3rd year of life) is still remarkably small and the suture between the lower pubic and ischium boughs is still rather broad. Here, the pelvis of a mongoloid shows the typical wing-shaped projection of the pelvic blades. The slow formation of the nucleus as compared to normal subjects of the same age (Fig. 1135) is very clear. Even more impressive in mongoloids is the deviations of the skull. There are brachycephalies and also tussicephalies with the radiographic signs of the underdevelopment of the middle cranial groove, disorders of the suture synostosis with persisting frontal suture, and a Schaltknochen formation. Further, there is a slowed dentation *(Gött)*.

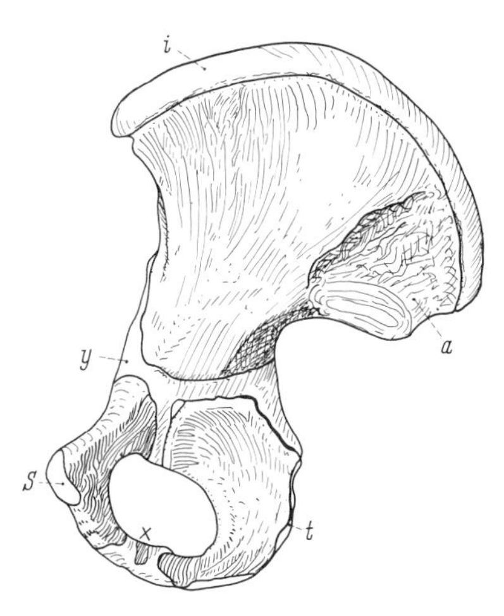

Fig. 1134. Pelvis, general view. Compare with Fig. 1138 (from *Heitzmann*).

a Articulation layers of the sacroiliac articulation
i Cartilaginous margin of the ilium
s Symphysis
t Ischiadic tuber
y Y-cartilage
X Symphysis between the pubic bone and the ischium (=ischiopubic synchondrosis)

In i, t and the superior glenoid edge, apophysial osseous nuclei appear during adolescence; they also appear in the pubic tubercle, the anterior superior ilium spine and in the ischiadic spine (see *Schinz*).

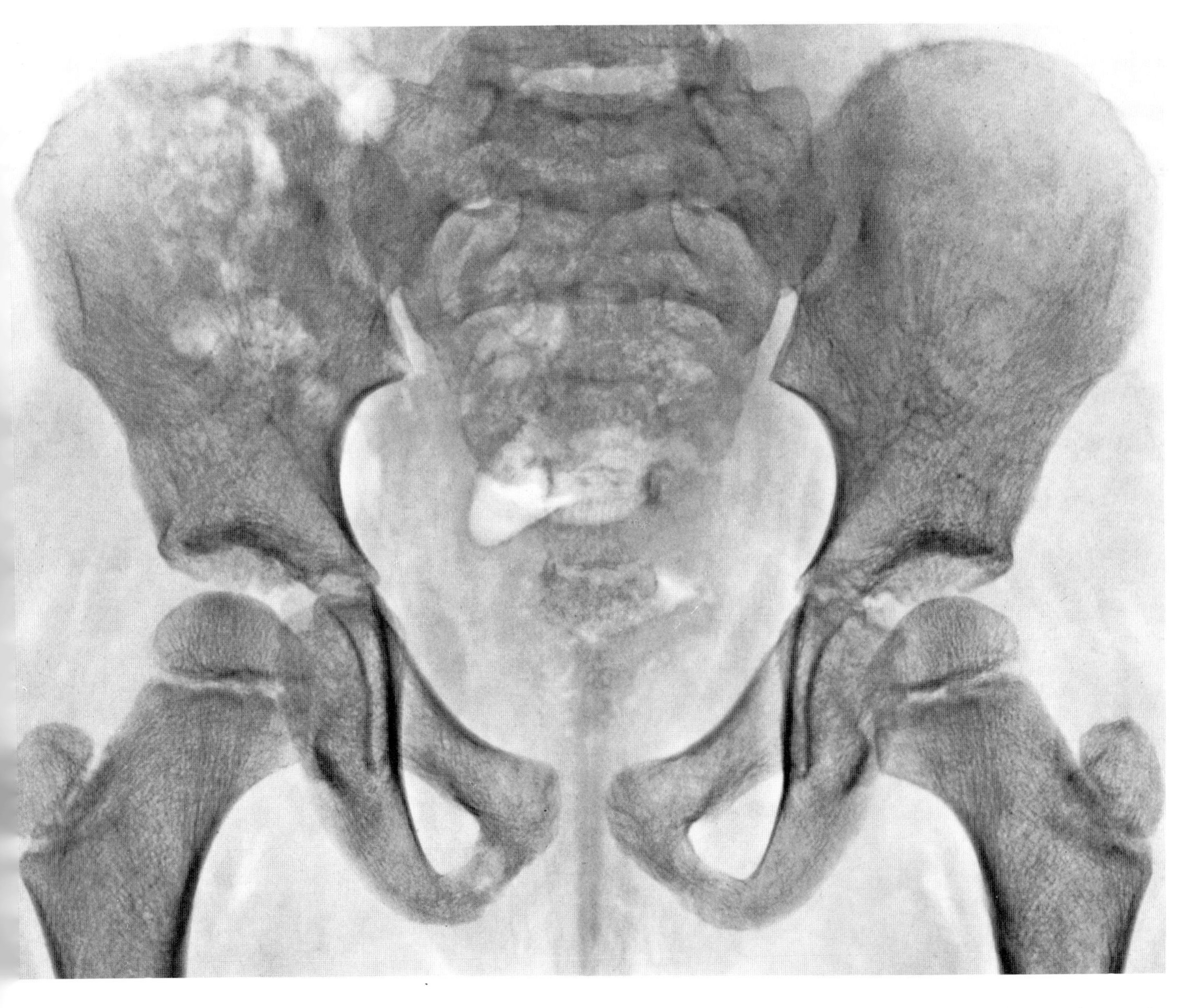

Fig. 1135. 5 1/2 year old. Average standard. The cartilaginous suture between the three hip bone sections becomes narrower; the suture between the inferior ischiatic and pubic bone boughs is already bridged. The site where it joined is discernible as a lightened strip (fusion around the 4th to 12th years of life). The growth notches in the glenoid roof have become clearer. The lateral part of the sacral bone is in the meantime completely fused with the sacral vertebra.

In the medial pelvic glenoid there is a clear *Koehler*'s tear-drop configuration. It plays a special role in juvenile osteochondrosis deformans (= M. *Perthes*). The distance from the lateral tear-drop formation to the medial edge of the proxial femoral metaphysis (= distance of the tear-drop formation) becomes larger in this and other disorders as compared to the healthy side.

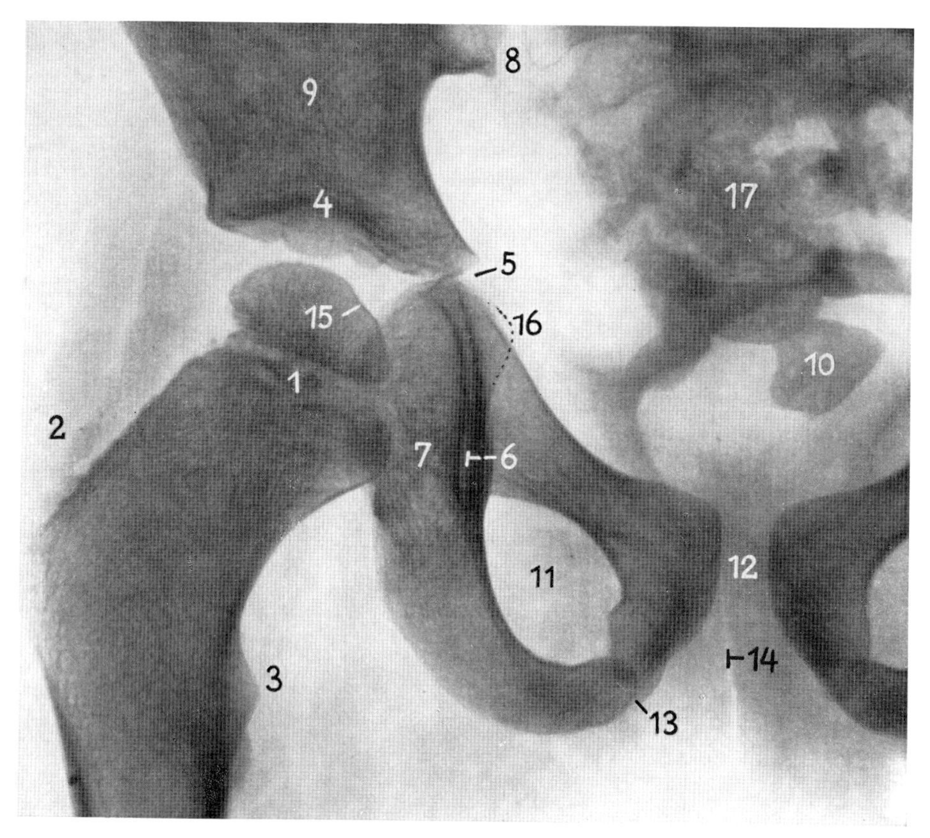

1 Epiphyseal cartilaginous disk, undulated edge, therefore numerous intertwined light lines
2 Nucleus of the greater trochanter, often curved, not ossified as a whole
3 Lesser trochanter
4 The glenoid roof; the glenoid border is undular or notched
5 Part of the Y-cartilage
6 Tear-drop formation (cf. Fig. 430, No. 4)
7 Lower glenoid border; the ischial tuber overlies this border
8 Sacroiliac articulation
9 Ilium bone
10 Coccyx, deviation to the left
11 Obturator foramen
12 Symphysis
13 Osseous fissure between the ischium and pubic bone (= ischiopubic synchondrosis) is about to synostose; taken obliquely, therefore it does not appear as a light fissure
14 Bright vertical line: buttock cleft
15 Flat cavity: femoral head fovea
16 Ischiatic spine
17 Sacral bone, covered by the contents of the colon mixed with gas

Fig. 1136. 5 1/2 year old. Hip articulation, ventrodorsal, with leg extended. Variation in the osseous nucleus anlage of the greater trochanter, which is seen more clearly in Fig. 1137. The coccyx (10) – in the adult formed by 4 to 6 vertebrae – originates here from a not yet differentiated anlage which deviates to the left. There are frequent sacral and coccyx bone variations. The sacral coccyx synchondrosis may ossify. The coccyx may be rudimentary or even completely absent.

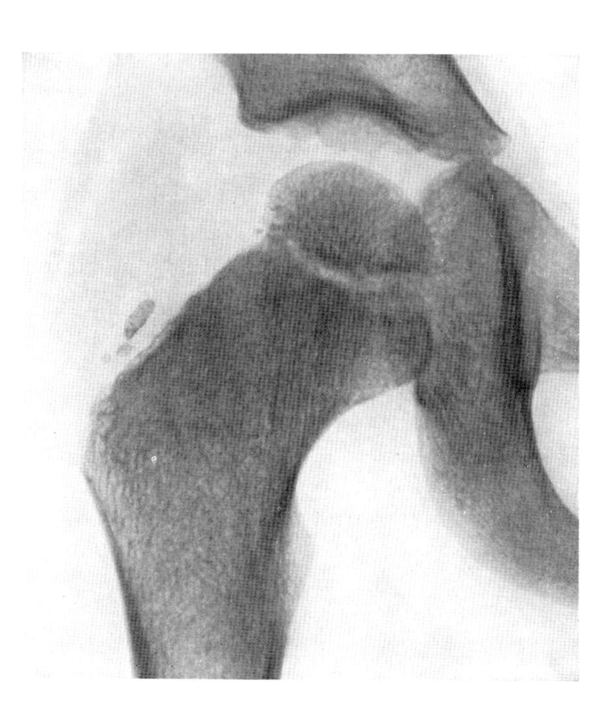

Fig. 1137. 5 1/2 year old. Ventrodorsal radiograph of the hip bone while the leg is bent. The femoral collum seems shorter owing to the bent position of the leg; the epiphyseal suture border of the femoral collum is still very split.

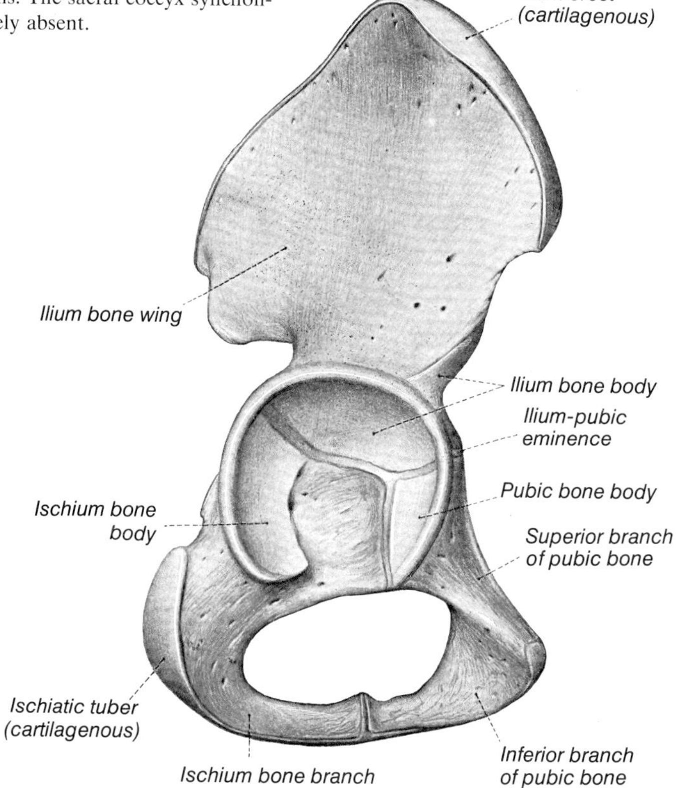

Fig. 1138. Hip bone radiograph of a 5 or 6-year-old child. External view to show the Y-suture in the acetabulum (cf. Fig. 1134, from *Sobotta-Becher,* 17th Edition).

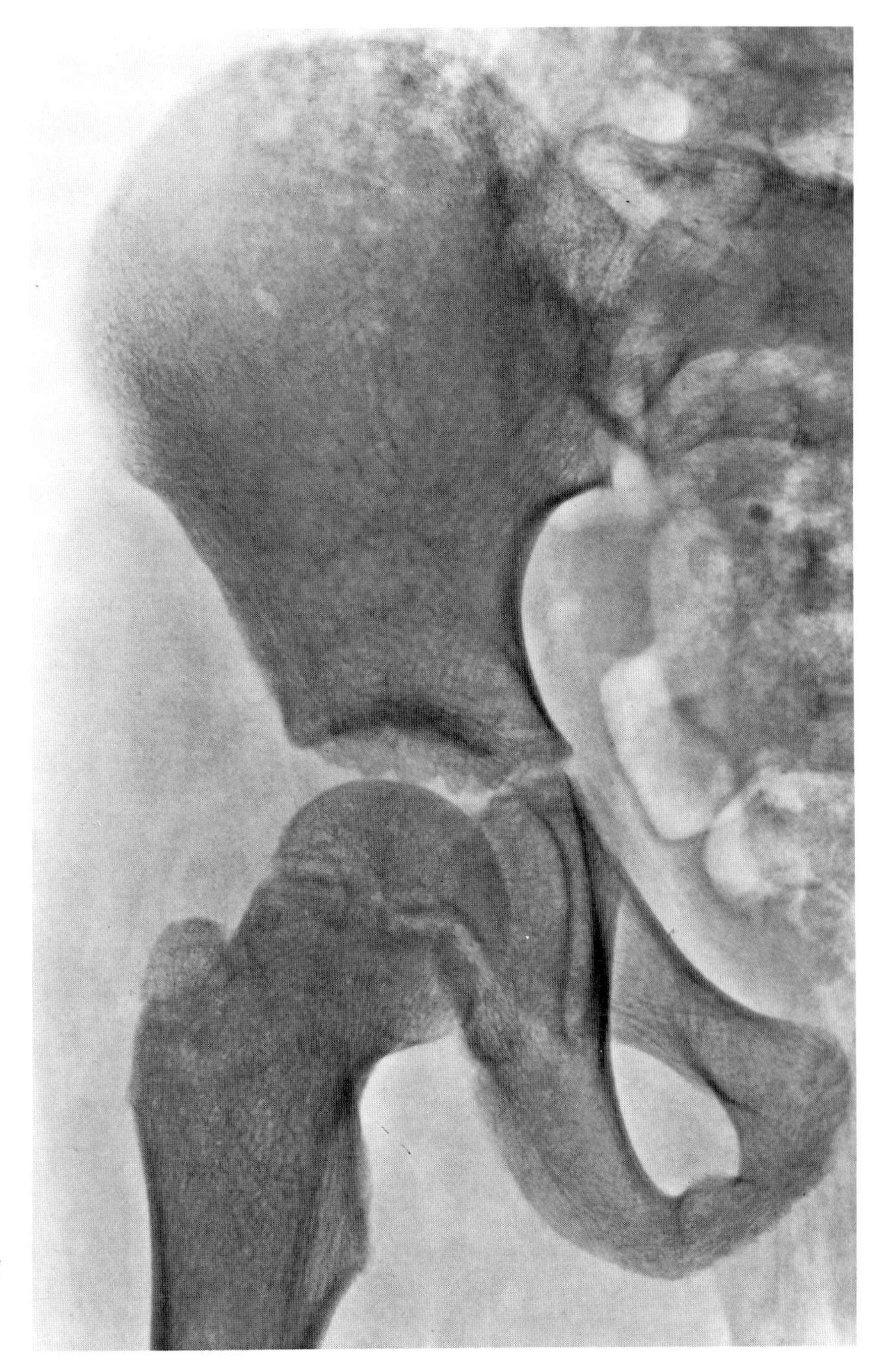

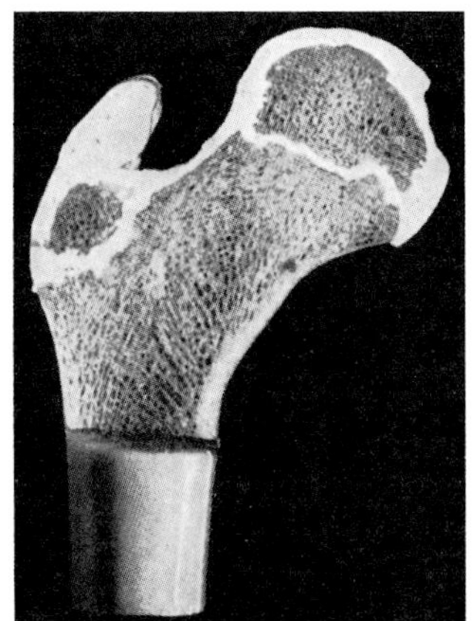

Fig. 1140. Frontal view through the epiphysis of the proximal femoral extremity of a 6 1/2-year-old child (from *Benninghoff-Goerttler,* 10th Edition).

Collum-diaphysial angle
(according to *Lanz* and *Wachsmuth*):

3 weeks:	150°
1 year:	148°
3 years:	145°
5 years:	142°
9 years:	138°
15 years:	133°
60 years:	120°

Fig. 1139. 6 1/2 year old. Right hip articulation. Average norm. The femoral collum seems slightly shortened; the femoral collum angle (see Fig. 1125) is enlarged because of coxa valga. In fact, the right femur is only slightly rotated externally, which is discernible from the appearance of the lesser trochanter. Here, the fissure between the inferior pubic and ischium bone is already ossified. The glenoid edge is very split. The osseous "articulation fissure" due to the thick cartilaginous coating is relatively much broader than in adults. Very undulated, almost torn epiphyseal edge. *Koehler*'s tear-drop formation is very clearly seen; its medial ridge is tangentially touched by the pelvic wall edge of the ischium bone body. Like the bones and the articulations of the pelvis, the angles too undergo development. There is the collum-diaphysial angle (γ) and the glenoid roof angle (α); the latter is formed of the ligature of the inferior ilium angle with the Y-suture *(Hilgenreiner's* line) and the line extending from the glenoid roof and the external inferior ilium angle in the Y-suture (see p. 505).

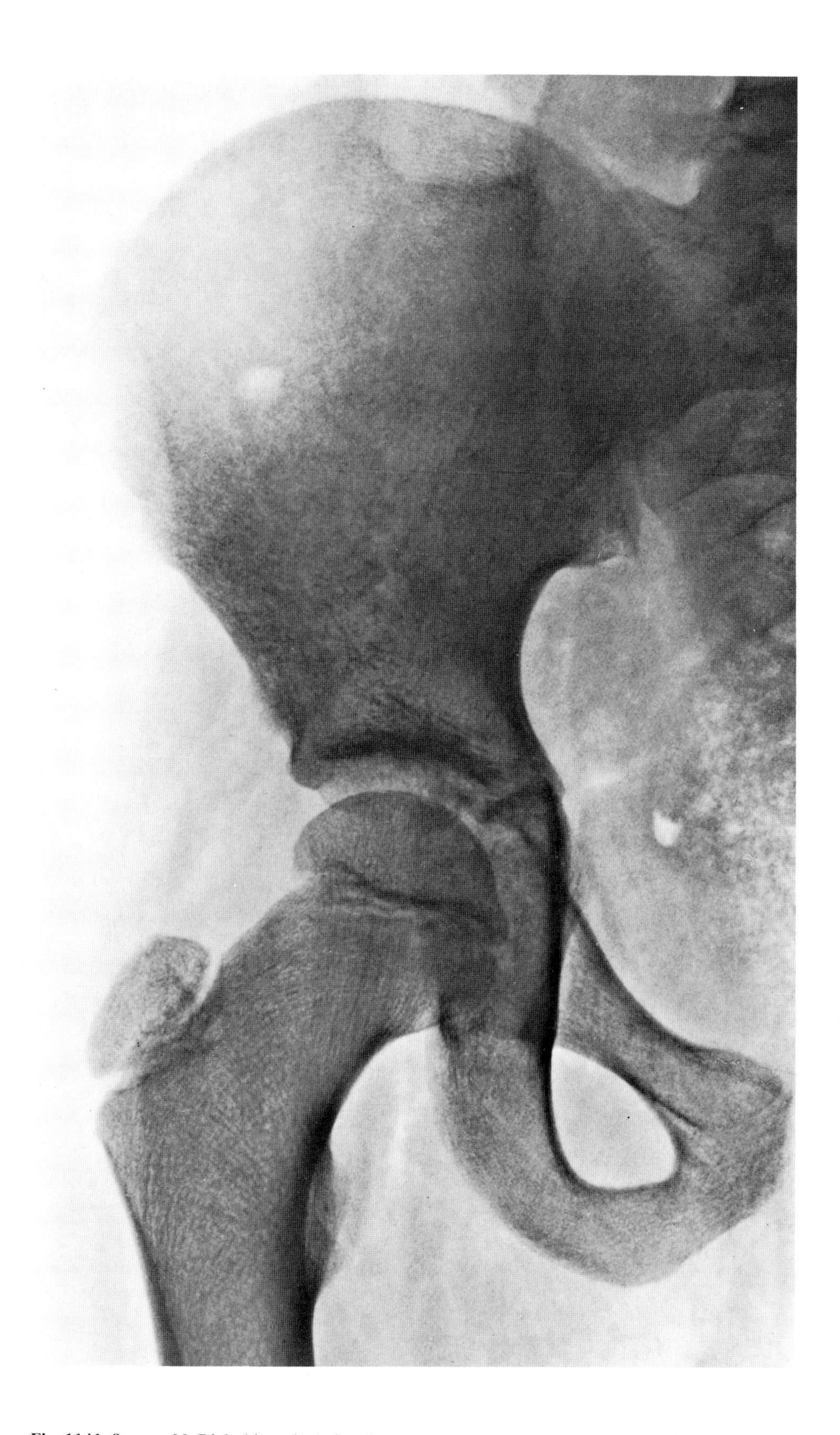

Fig. 1141. 8 year old. Right hip articulation. Low to average norm. The synostosis between the lower pubic and ischium boughs is complete. No signs of the suture are discernible. The tear-drop formation, which meets the pelvic wall at its edge (ischium bone body) and proceeds into the lower border of the obturator foramen, is covered.

The size of the osseous nucleus of the greater trochanter changes in the radiograph series because there is a normal range of variation. The narrowing of the Y-suture (which closes during puberty) and the epiphyseal cartilaginous disks is clearly visible.

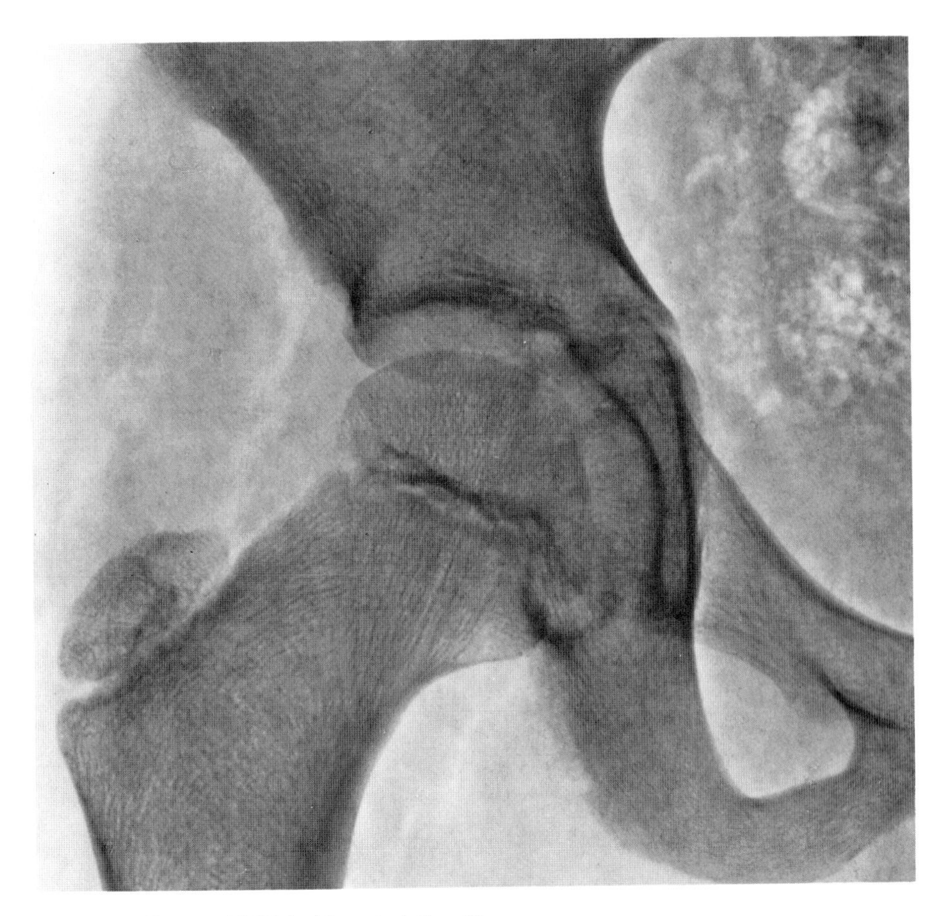

Fig. 1142. 10 year old. Right hip articulation. Mean norm.

The lesser trochanter shows no apophyses yet, which at this stage could already be discernible as they are formed between the 10th and 14th years of life. The glenoid edge is well levelled and is no longer undular. The epiphyseal suture of the femoral head is narrower and levelled. The tear-drop formation is cut across the length by the pectes pubic bone.

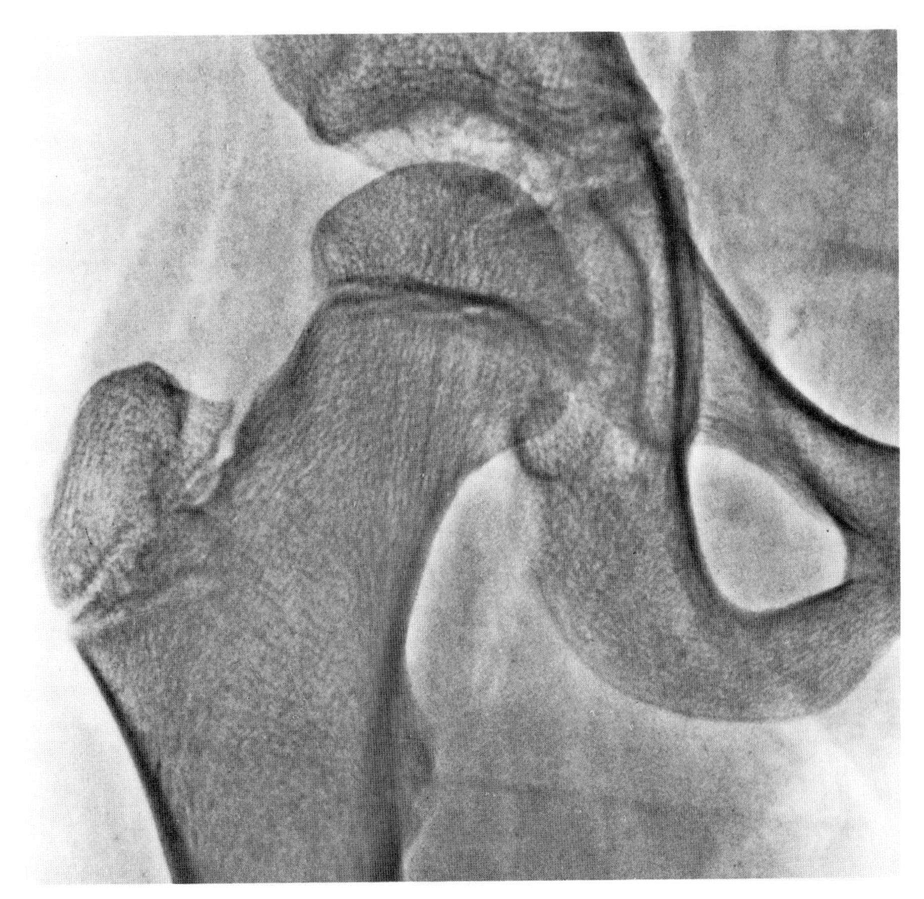

Fig. 1143. 11 year old. Right hip articulation. Mean norm.

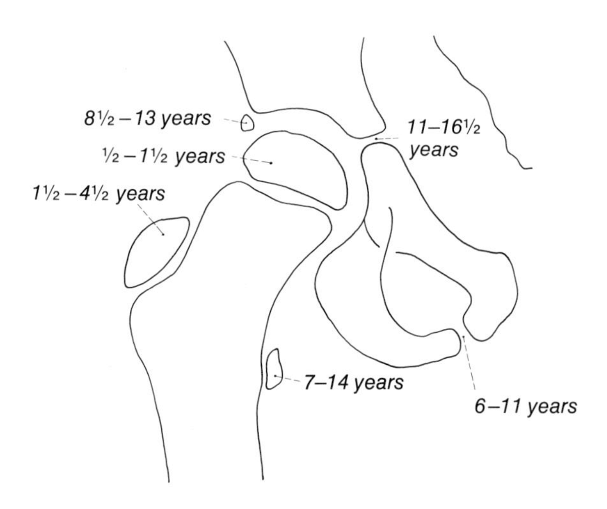

Fig. 1144. Time span during which the osseous nuclei of the pelvic region may normally appear, and synostosis times of the Y-suture and the ischiopubic synchondrosis.

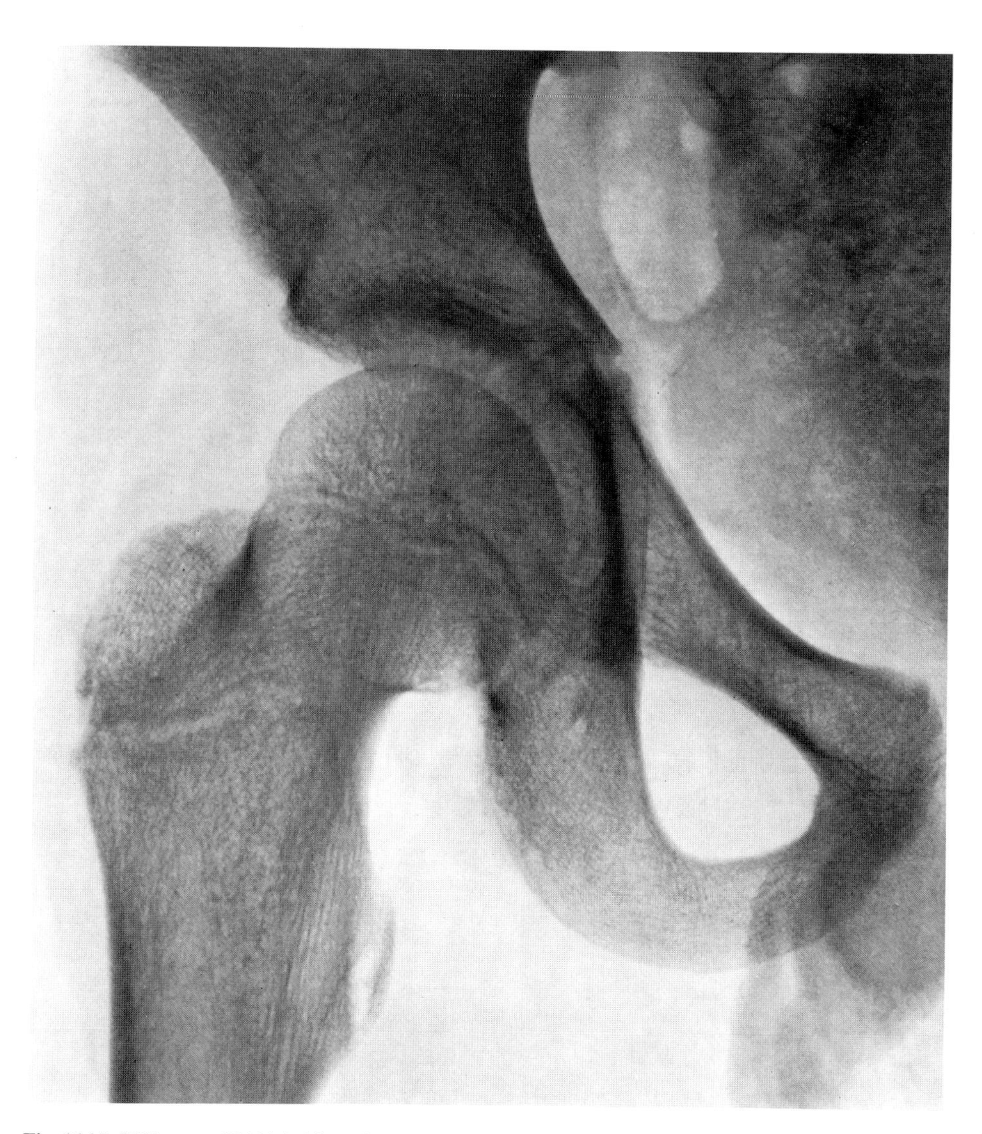

Fig. 1145. 11¼ year old. Right hip articulation. Average norm. The femur is rotated more to the left to better show the lesser trochanter. The cartilaginous sutures are very much narrowed. Through the external rotation, the epiphyseal suture of the greater trochanter is also projected on the femoral shaft and appears in its lateral section as a transverse brightened band.

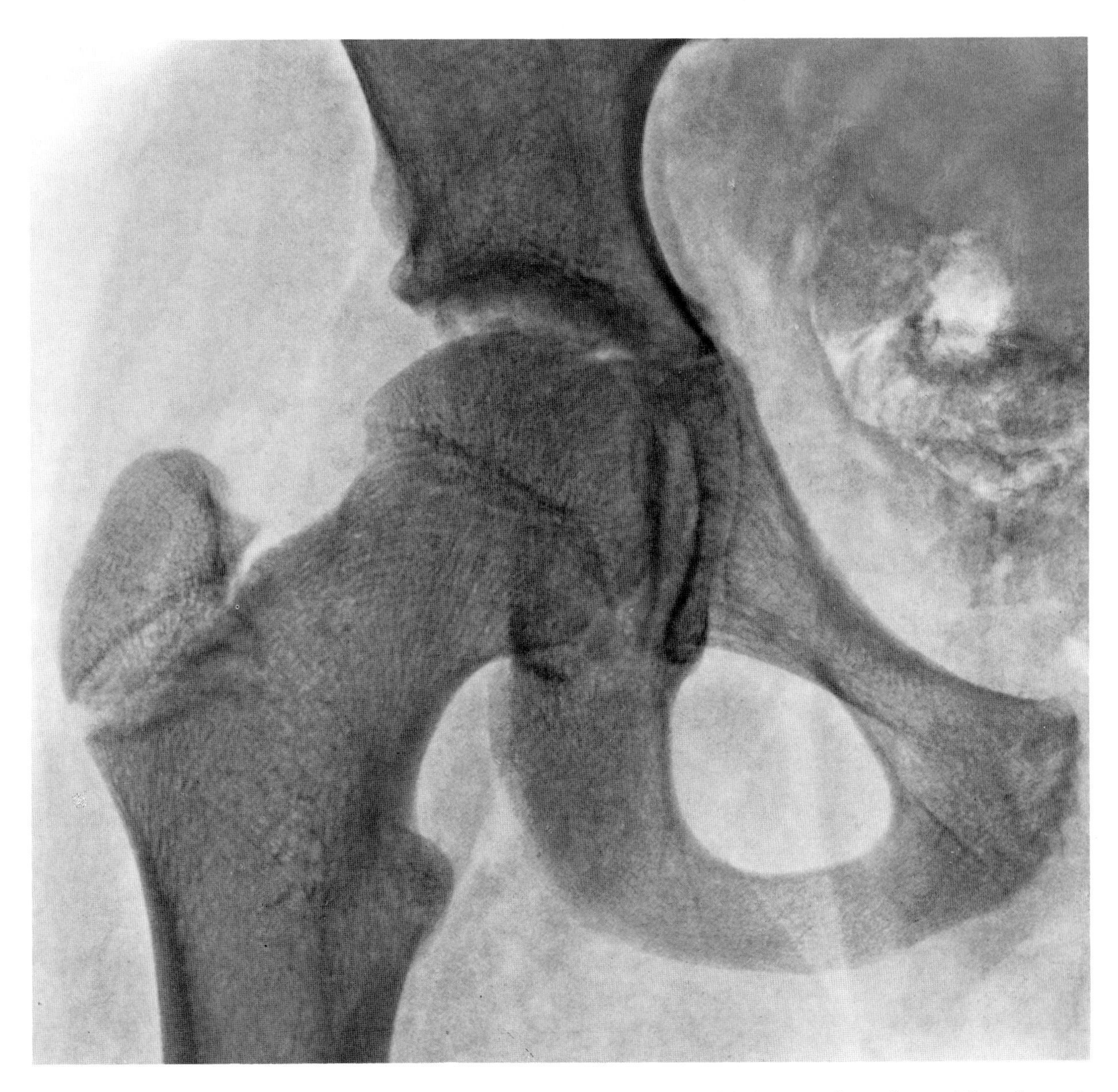

Fig. 1146. 12 year old. Right hip articulation. Mean norm. The apophyseal nucleus of the lesser trochanter is especially well seen. Its extended size leads one to determine, that in this case, it has probably appeared much earlier. Its apophyseal fissure is seen only as a narrow osseous lightened zone because the suture is not taken axially. The glenoid edge limit is again undular; the pubic bone edge at the symphysis is also still toothed.

Between the 12th and 16th years of life (earlier in girls than in boys and bilateral in 50% of cases), an epiphyseal insufficiency develops due to slow displacement of the head cap, which becomes loosened. This insufficiency may later lead to adolescent coxa vara. A well-known occurrence. All stages of the juvenile epiphyseolysis up to epiphyseal necrosis derive from a slow pre-epiphyseolysis.

The sudden slipping off due to traumas, which has symptoms similar to femoral collum fracture, leads to separation of tissues between the epiphysis and metaphysis, and often causes non-formation of nails.

Figs. 1147 and 1148. 14 year old. Right hip articulation. In both radiographs the glenoid edge apophysis is seen very clearly; the apophyseal nucleus in the lesser trochanter is also discernible. The remaining cartilaginous sutures are about to ossify and are correspondingly narrow. The limit of the symphysis fissure is just slightly indicated and is undular; this is a normal finding.

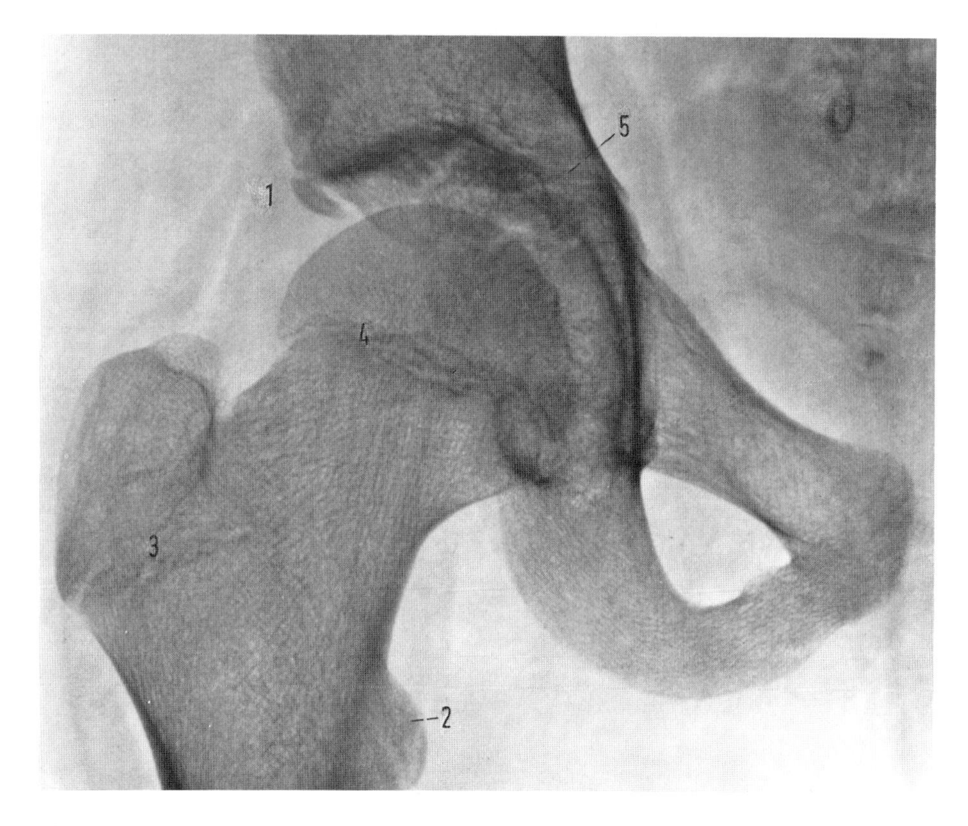

Fig. 1147. Ventrodorsal. Mean norm.

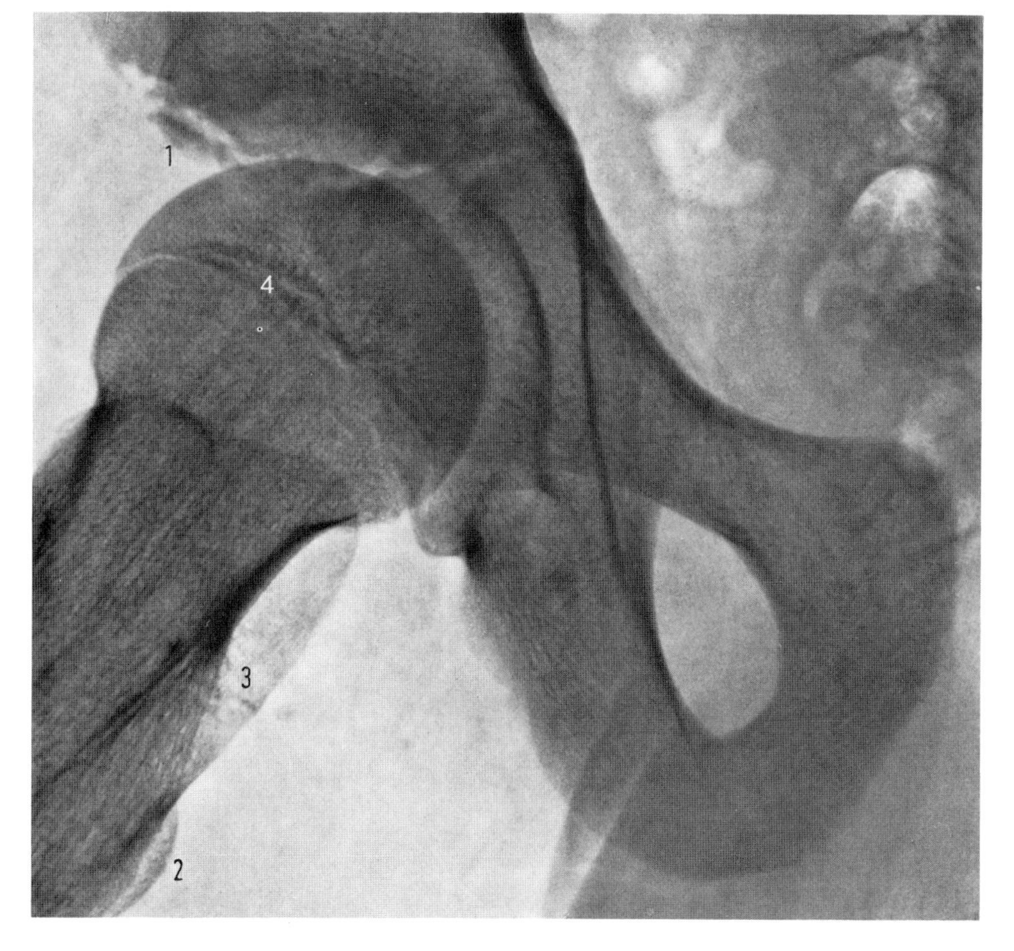

1 Glenoid edge apophysis of the acetabulum bone; it can persist
2 Apophyseal nucleus of the lesser trochanter
3 Epiphyseal fissure of the greater trochanter
4 Epiphyseal fissure of the femoral head
5 Remainder of the Y-suture

Fig. 1148. Hip articulation the same as in Fig. 1147, according to *Lauenstein*.

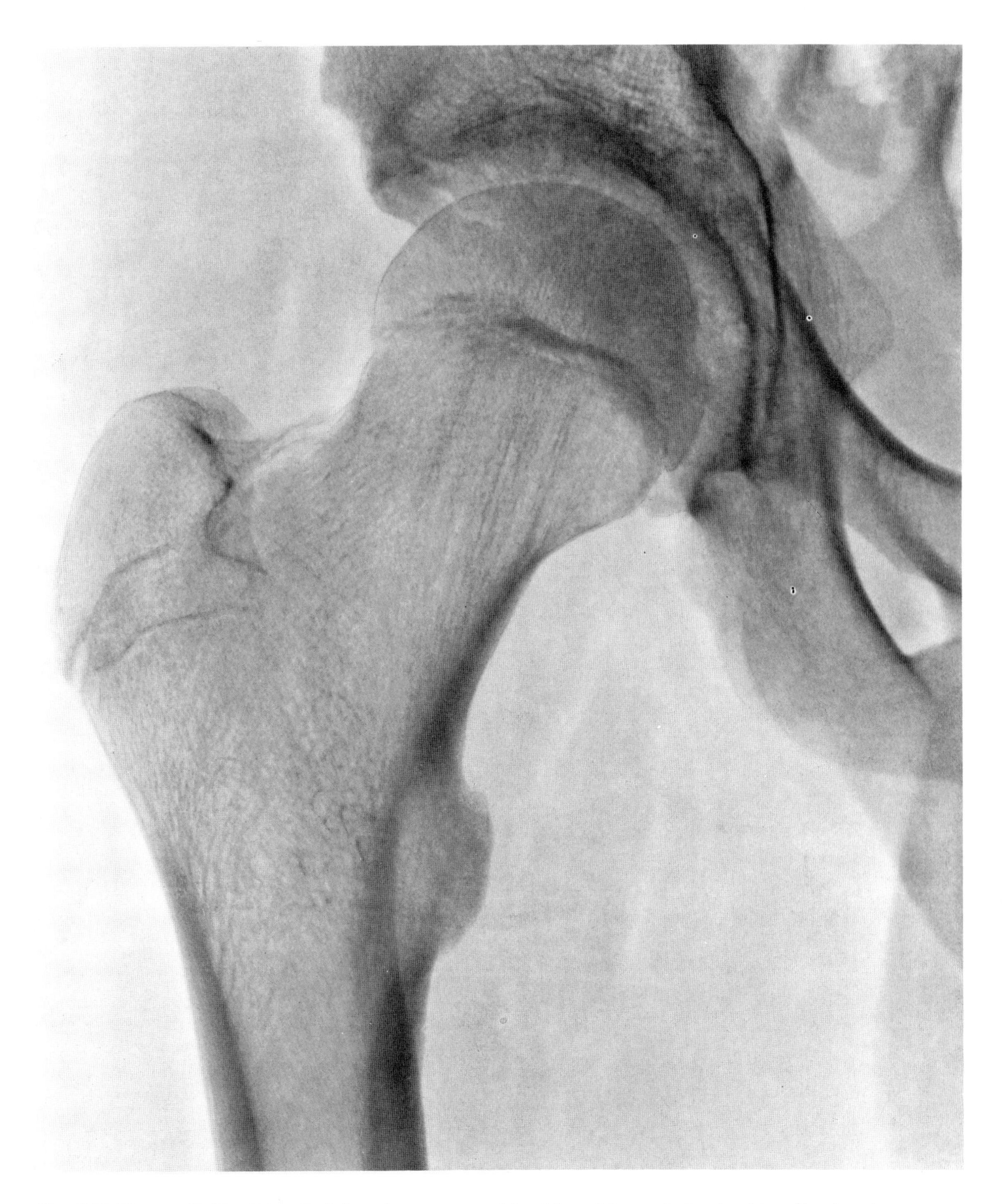

Fig. 1149. 15 year old. Right hip articulation. Average norm. All epiphyseal fissures in the glenoid roof too have become very narrow and are about to fuse. The moment of synostosis, i.e., the moment of growth termination, is subject to individual variations of many years.

Every juvenile can suffer from epiphyseal insufficiency, which leads to epiphyseolysis. A chronic damage of the bones and cartilage in the vicinity of the epiphysis can also occur, e.g., due to occupational overexertion. In this radiograph, however, there is no indication of epiphyseolysis, but there is an ossification of the iliofemoral ligament, which may be an indication of a previous trauma.

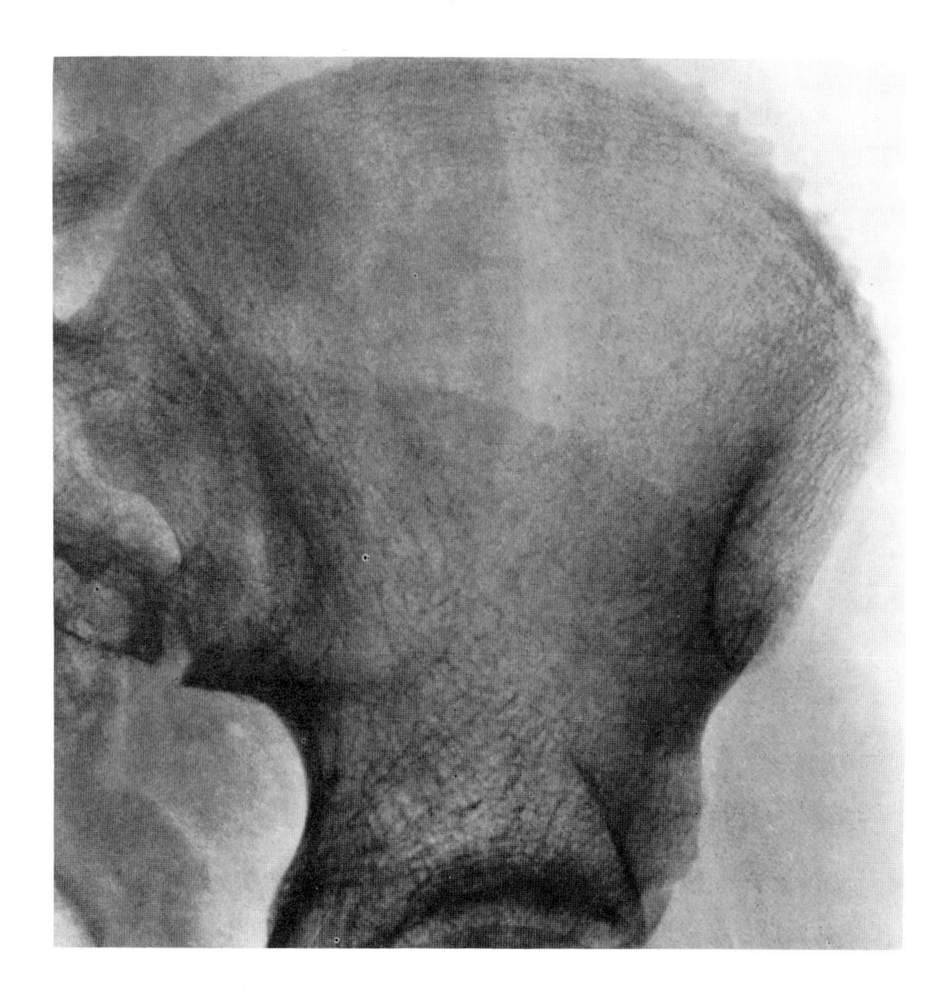

Fig. 1150. 12-year-old girl. Left ilium. The pelvic crest apophysis has not yet ossified, but an undular toothed ilium crest is already discernible; this crest will be the caudal limit line of the apophyseal fissure.

There is some connection with puberty, as 6 months after the appearance of the pelvic crest apophysis in the radiograph, the menarche is expected to appear.

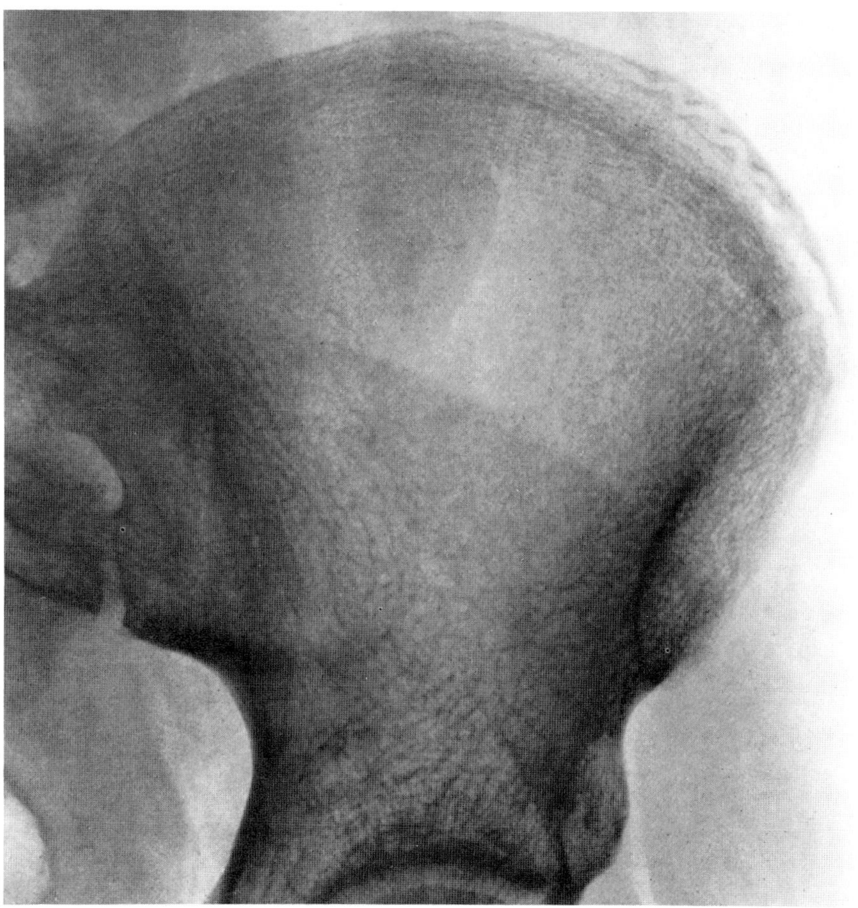

Fig. 1151. 1 1/2 years later. A striped apophysis is discernible with a characteristic undular apophyseal fissure. In later years the apophyseal line extends to become a straight fissure. It usually disappears with the fusion between the apophyseal nucleus and the ilium crest in the 21st to 25th years of life; it may also persist *(J. Petersen)*.

Congenital Hip Luxation

Hip luxation derives from a congenital dysplasia, the frequency of which is three times higher than that of congenital luxation.

Radiographic symptoms according to *Hilgenreiner* and *Putti* include:

1. Considerable delay in the appearance of the femoral head nucleus or a hypoplasia of that nucleus.
2. Flat glenoid cavity and a steep glenoid roof; the normal "glenoid angle" is almost 29° in the newborn.
3. Laterocranial shifting of the proximal femoral extremity.
4. Fracture of *Ménard*'s line, with its course shifting in a cranial direction.

Table 16. Normal glenoid roof angle (α) in the radiograph.

Age	*Boys*	*Girls*
1th Month of life	27 degrees	29.5 degrees
2nd Month of life	24.4	27.5
3rd Month of life	23.7	26.7
4th Month of life	22.4	25.7
5th Month of life	21.3	24.8
6th Month of life	20.7	24.2
7th Month of life	20	23
8th Month of life	19.2	21.4
9th Month of life	18.7	20.8
10th Month of life	18.5	20.5
11th Month of life	18.4	20.2
12th Month of life	18.4	20
2nd Year of life	18	19–20
3rd Year of life	16–18	17.2–19.3
4th Year of life	14.4–16.3	14.8–17.2
5th Year of life	below 15	below 15

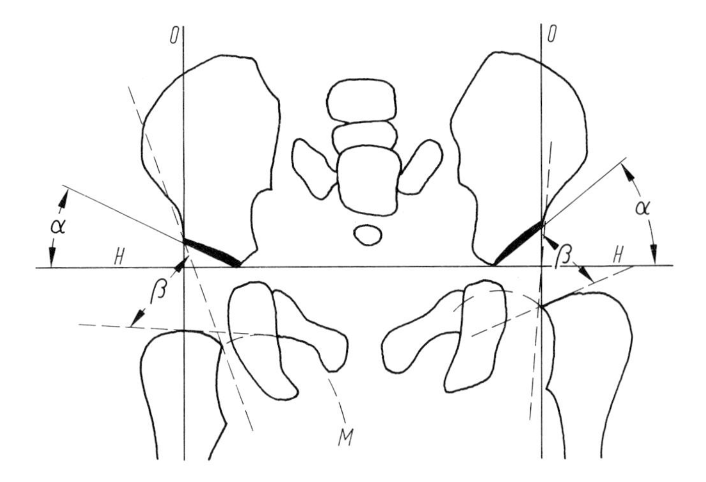

Fig. 1152. Symptoms of congenital hip luxation.

- *α* Glenoid angle
- H *Hilgenreiner*'s line (horizontal through the Y-suture)
- O *Ombredanne*'s line (perpendicular to the glenoid arch H-H)
- M *Ménard-Shenton*'s line (the internal limit of the femoral collum contour meets the superior limit of the obturator foramen)
- *β* Angle between the proximal femoral extremity, the medial femoral spine and the glenoid bow *(Zsernaviczky* and *Türk).*

β ∢	Normal	Transition	Dysplasia	Subluxation Luxation
35-40°				
41-43°				
44-46°				
47-49°				
50-51°				
52°				
53°				
54-56°				
57-59°				
60-62°				
63-65°				
66-68°				
69-72°				
73-75°				
over 75°				
number	752	116	201	105

Fig. 1153. Values of the β-angle in the various forms of hip dysplasia (graphic presentation according to *Zsernaviczky* and *Türk).* The first fissure shows the relatively good limitation of the normal values. Between 50° and 56° there is an abrupt physiological transition.

Congenital hip luxation in an 18-year-old girl

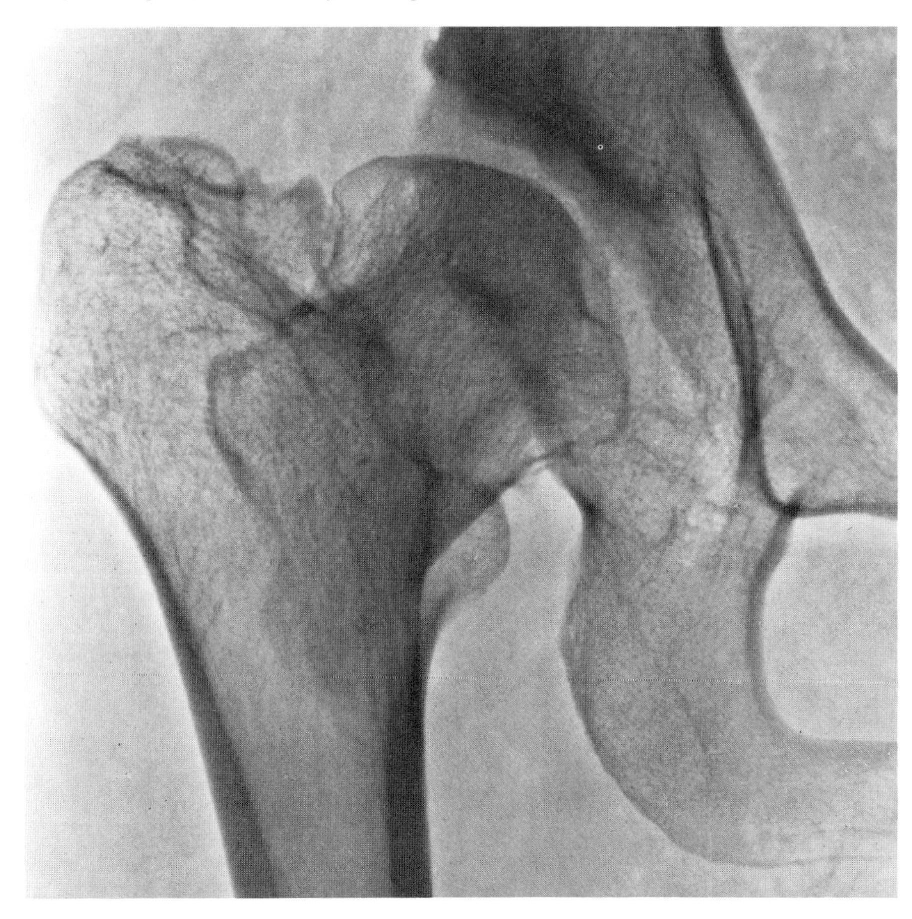

Fig. 1154. Congenital hip luxation. A condition after a transposition operation, with shifting of the femoral collum in the previously luxated hip articulation. A good functional result. A strong flattening of the dysplastic femoral cap and a shallow cavity of the hip articulation glenoid. The trochanter mass is located at a high level.
The dislocation of the hip bone head epiphysis due to damage of the growth zone and the results of hip luxation are described by *Imhäuser*.

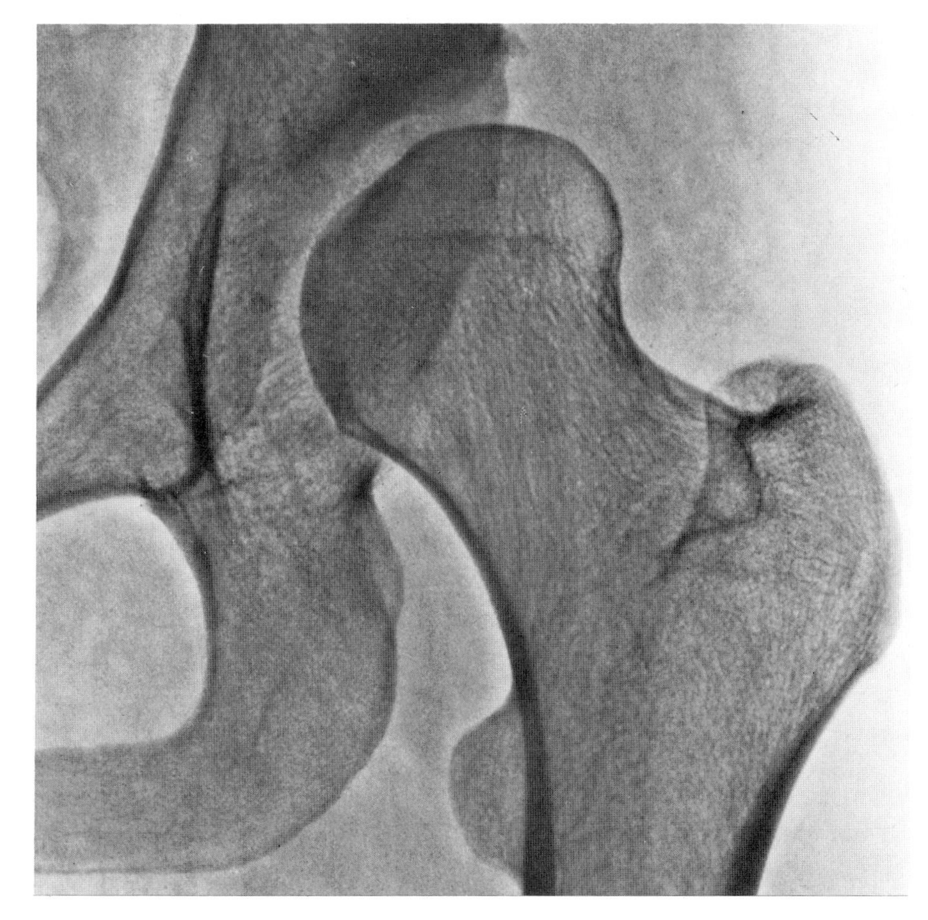

Fig. 1155. Left hip articulation. The articulation still gives a nearly normal impression. The femoral head is less flattened, although it is slightly "dysplastic". Remarkable (and arranged for the hip) are the steeply located articulation luxation, slightly filled flat acetabulum and the enlarged femoral collum angle. Because of this, there is already an indication of coxa valga (cf. Fig. 1125). The development is altogether slowed and persists finally in a hypoplastic state when the cartilaginous sutures are closed *(Schinz)*. *Ueda et al.* indicate in the radiographs, the so-called spontaneous healing of the congenital hip luxation.

Knee Area

Distal femoral epiphysis. The so-called *Béclard* nucleus begins to form around the 10th lunar month; in most cases it is well formed at birth. It is an important indicator of maturity in forensic medicine (see also Table 6). This nucleus undergoes a rapid extension and differentiation. Around the 5th year of life, the diaphysial extremity reaches its full width and, at the latest around the 10th year of life, the distal femoral epiphysis attains its final form (Fig. 1161).

It is important to know that the blurred image of the radiograph in the medial and, less strongly, in the lateral limit of the distal epiphyseal nucleus of the femur, appearing after the 2nd year of life, is a normal finding (Figs. 1157–1180). Likewise, similar roughenings may be noted in the proximal tibial epiphysis, although far less frequently.

Titze reported the occurrence of a triangular accessorial bone shadow in the medial femoral condyle excluding a previous trauma or other developmental disorder.

Proximal tibial epiphysis. The formation of this nucleus usually occurs about the time of birth. In many cases the nucleus is developed in its first form in the newborn. In this case too, the final form of the epiphysis is reached up to the 10th year of life.

Tibial diaphysis. Of the diaphyses of the long tubular bones of the lower limbs, the diaphysis of the tibia tends to curve (varus form) due to stress and faulty torsions *(Consentius)*. The fibula is also involved. In the radiograph the corticalis, on the internal and lateral side, usually indicates a thickening, which may appear in the external part through an external rotation of the femur. The external side of the femur and the internal side of the tibia are favored sites for "periosteal appositions" in babies; they are mostly of a benign nature. *Swoboda,* too, does not attribute this periosteal apposition to syphilis. On bone development of syphilitic fetuses and newborns in radiographs, see especially *Rumphorst.* He was able to show that the specific infection in the region of the ossification centers of the long tubular bones could lead to an underdevelopment of the bones.

Tibial apophysis. In the site of what will later be the tibial tuberosity, we find in 8 to 10 year olds a step-like recess in the frontal edge of the proximal diaphysial extremity. Around the 9th to 14th years of life, an apophyseal nucleus forms in this place; it may have different forms, e.g., it may be divided into two or have numerous nucleolei (Fig. 1171b). It is not unusual for the left and right tibial apophysis nuclei to have nonidentical forms. At the same time in which this apophyseal nucleus forms, a tongue-shaped process moves from the frontal side of the tibial epiphysis to reach the apophysis and to fuse with it soon afterwards. The proximal tibial epiphysis then shows the characteristic beak-shaped process in the region of the tibial tuberosity (see Figs. 1167, 1172, 1173, 1174b and 1175). The irregularities of the ossification of the tibial tuberosity often render the radiographic definition of an aseptic bone necrosis difficult or even impossible *(Osgood-Schlatter)*.

The **patella,** which is actually a sesamoid bone in the quadriceps, is usually formed in the 3rd to 4th years of life. It may (especially in boys) appear slightly later, but never after the 6th year of life. *Hellmer's* radiographic observations of the ossification of the patella should be mentioned here. The patella usually forms from a large quantity of ossification sites which very soon fuse into one nucleus, out of which the normal patella develops (Fig. 1162). The cause of bi- or multipartitions *(Grothe)* should be sought in this frequent anlagen of the patella with numerous nuclei.

Even in later years, up to puberty, small, non-fused ossification nuclei can be found in the patella edge, and they are not a pathological symptom. Most often, there is an osseous fusion of these nucleolei with the patella (Figs. 758a, b, 957 and 761).

Likewise, an irregular, roughened contour of the patella up to puberty has no pathological significance. The absence or underdevelopment of the patella is described in cases of "hereditary osteo-onchyodysplasia" *(Roeckerath)*.

The **fibular head** is established in the same period as the patella, or sometimes a half year later. The nucleus of the fibular head can also occasionally be divided, however, the single nuclei fuse into one epiphysis very soon.

The **fabella** is a sesamoid bone, which originates in the tendon of lateral gastrocnemius head (Fig. 774a and b). Its appearance is very irregular. Ossification occurs during puberty. A bipartition may occasionally occur.

Completion of ossification. The epiphyseal closure in the distal femoral, proximal tibial and fibular regions occurs around the 17th to 22nd years of life, first in the femur and the tibia and then slightly later in the fibula.

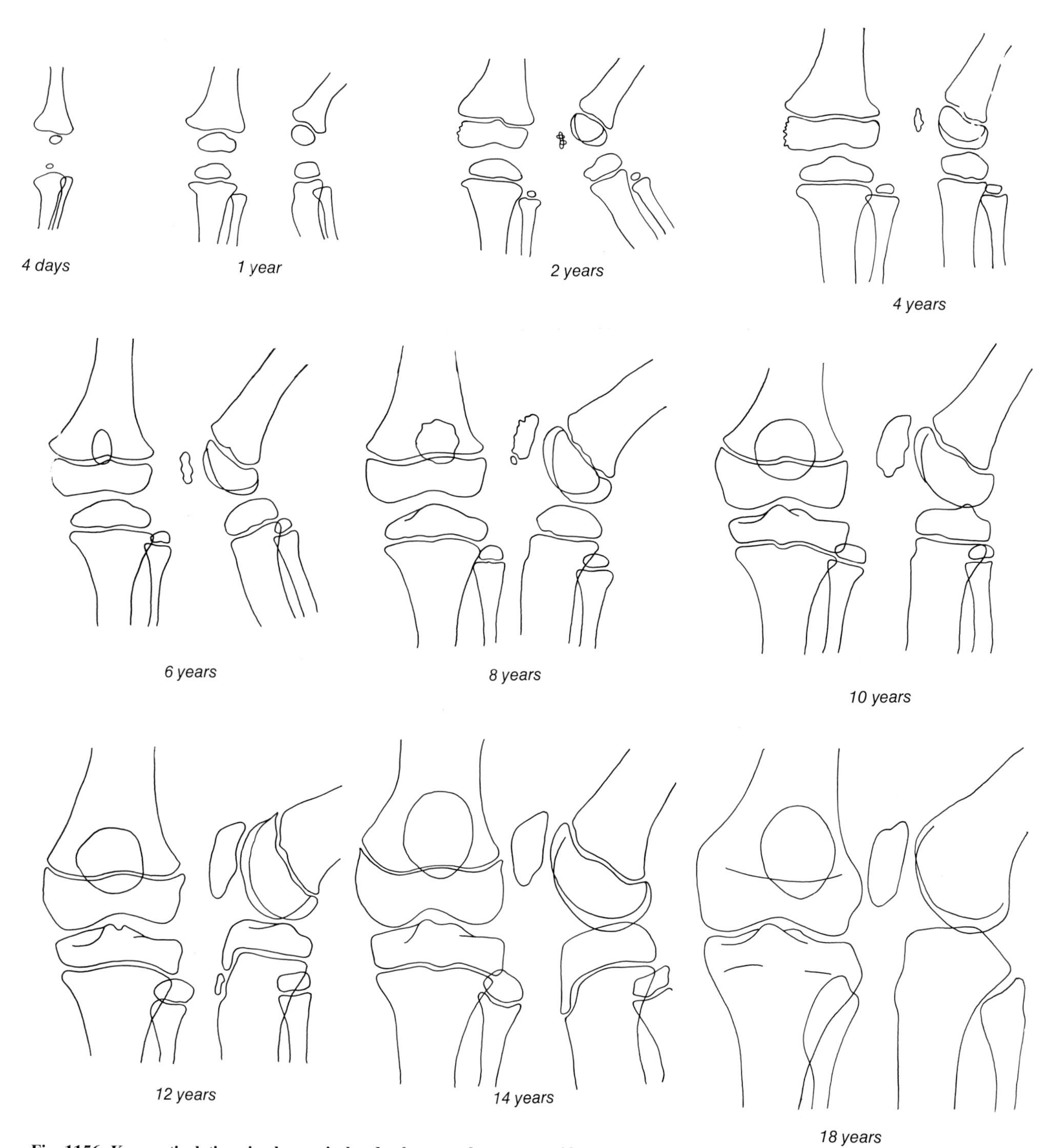

Fig. 1156. Knee articulations in chronogical order from newborn to age 18.

A Series of Radiographs of the Development of the Knee Articulation from Infancy to Age 25

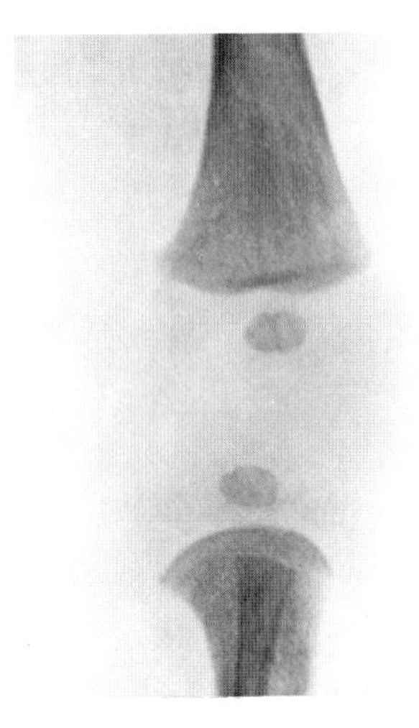

Fig. 1157. 22 days. The distal femoral epiphysis ossifies from about the 10th lunar month *(Béclard's* nucleus); the proximal tibial epiphysis ossifies at about the time of birth.

Fig. 1158. 5 month old. Knee articulation, lateral (very soft radiograph). The cartilage in the articulation is well separated from the adipose layer, which is very pervious to the radiation.

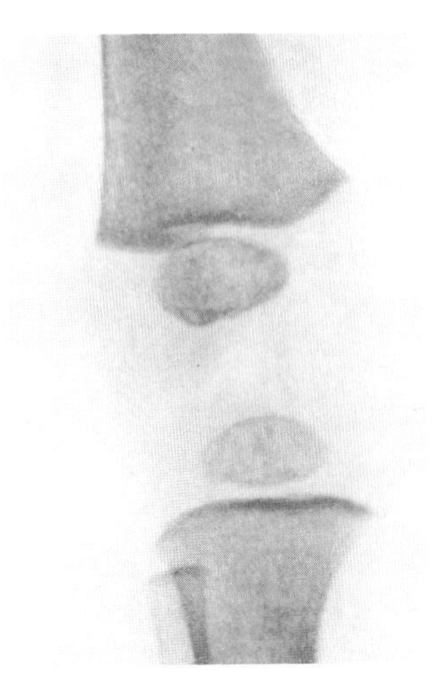

Fig. 1159. 7 month old. There is already a clear extension of the surface of both epiphyseal nuclei.

1 Cartilage of the nucleus in the inferior femoral extremity
2 Cartilage of the nucleus in the tibial head
3 Patella, still cartilaginous
4 (Light field) Pre-articulation adipose body, alary plica
5 Patellar ligament
6 Posterior muscular system (gastrocnemius)
7 Skin folds
8 Quadriceps tendon

Fig. 1160. 1 1/2 year old. Right knee, anteroposterior and lateral. The diaphyseal extremity, especially of the femur but also of the tibia, has extended through the formation of smaller protuberances in the edge. The already-noticeable blurring of the medial limit of the distal femoral epiphysis should be noted. This usually occurs, especially, clear after the 2nd year of life and is a normal finding. This blurred edge can at times be noted also in the medial edge of the proximal tibial epiphysis. In rare cases the blurred image is found in the lateral limit of both osseous nuclei.

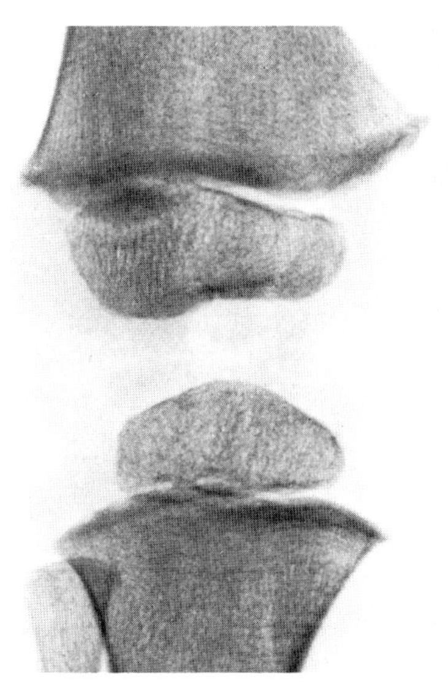

Fig. 1160 a

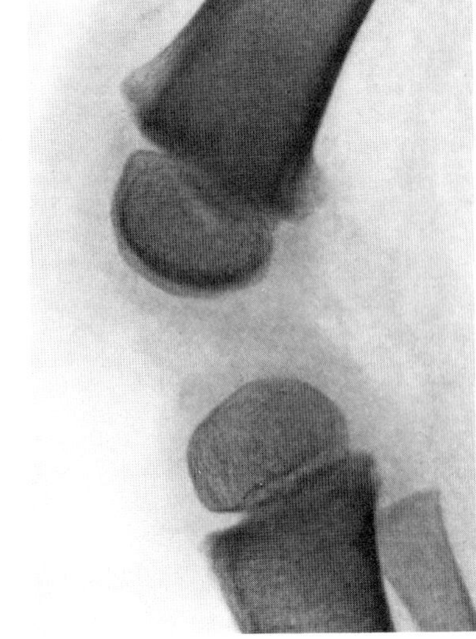

Fig. 1160 b

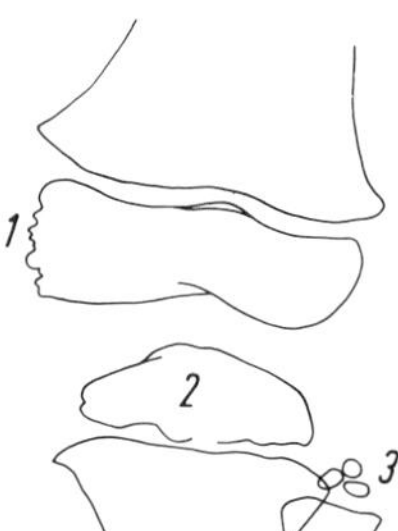

1 Femoral epiphysis (rough)
2 Tibial epiphysis
3 Multinuclear arrangement of fibular head

Fig. 1161. 3 year old. Radiograph of the knee right articulation.

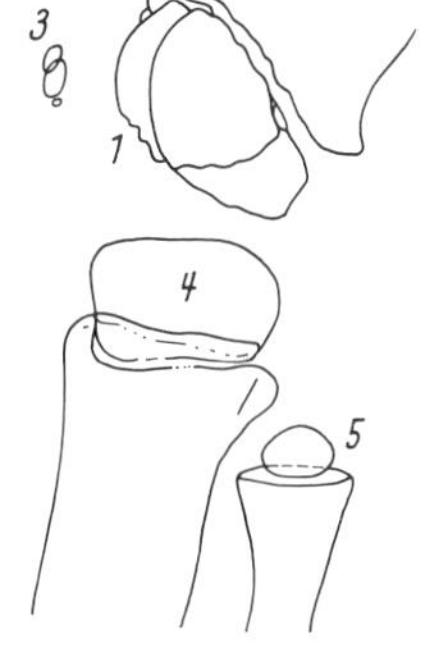

1 Femoral condyle (normal roughness)
2 Small nuclei in the epiphyseal edge
3 Split arranged patellar nucleus
4 Tibial epiphysis
5 Fibular epiphysis

Fig. 1162. 3 1/2 year old. Radiograph of the knee articulation, lateral.

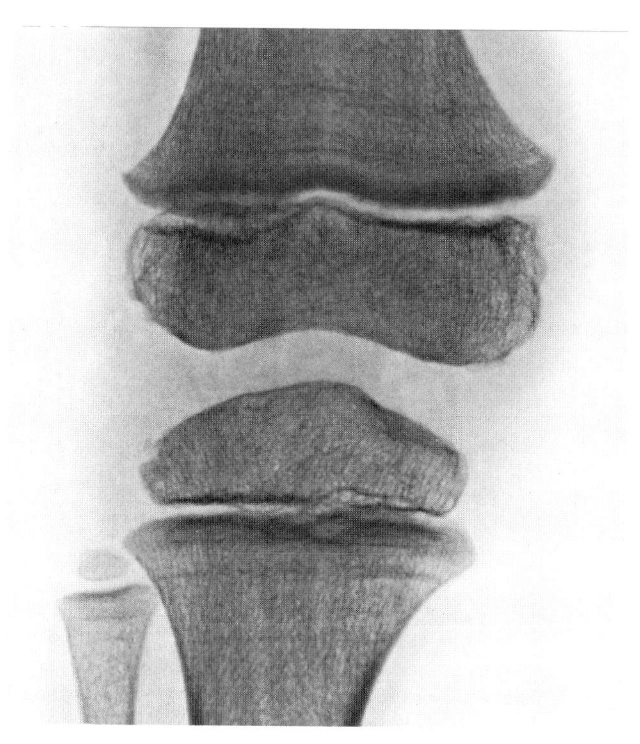

Fig. 1163 a

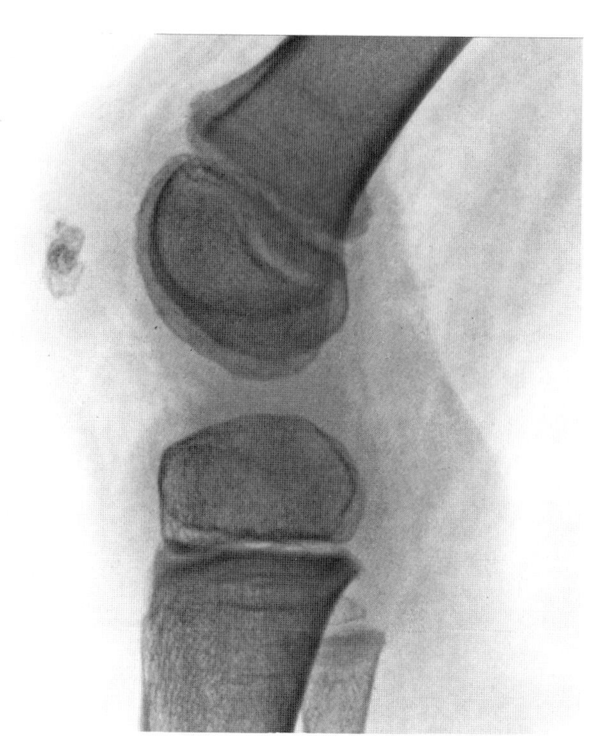

Fig. 1163 b

Fig. 1163. 4 year old. Right knee articulation, anteroposterior and lateral. The femoral and tibial epiphyses have reached their full extension. Further ossification nuclei are visible, e.g., the nucleus of the patella, which is still divided (3rd–4th years of life), as well as the nucleus of the fibular head (at the same time as the patella or 6 months later). The nucleus of the fibular head may first be divided. The medial and lateral boundaries of the femoral epiphysis as well as the lateral boundary of the tibial epiphysis are rough. There are also the typical vertical growth lines, the so-called intermediate lines, which are clearly seen, especially after rickets, chronic infectious diseases, juvenile rheumatism, *Möller-Barlow* disease and lead poisoning.

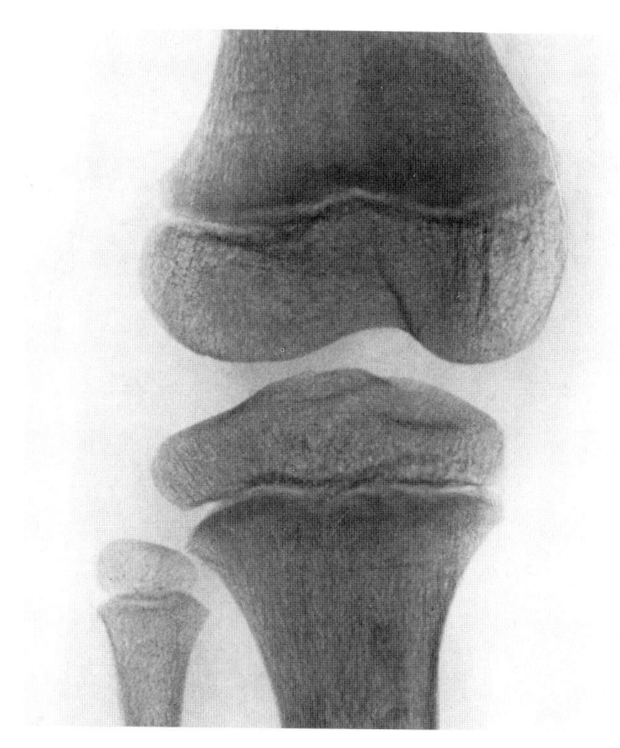

Fig. 1164 a

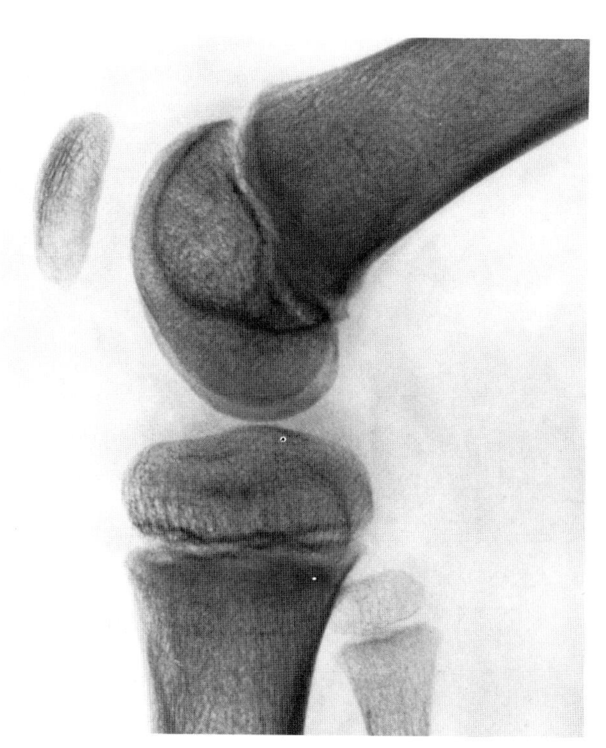

Fig. 1164 b

Fig. 1164. 8 year old. Right knee articulation, anteroposterior and lateral. Average norm. The osseous nucleus of the patella now shows clearly the form of this large sesamoid bone; the articulation fissure is seen through the still-thick cartilaginous layer. The humped plate of the cruciform ligament of the tibial epiphysis is indicated only through a flat convexity.

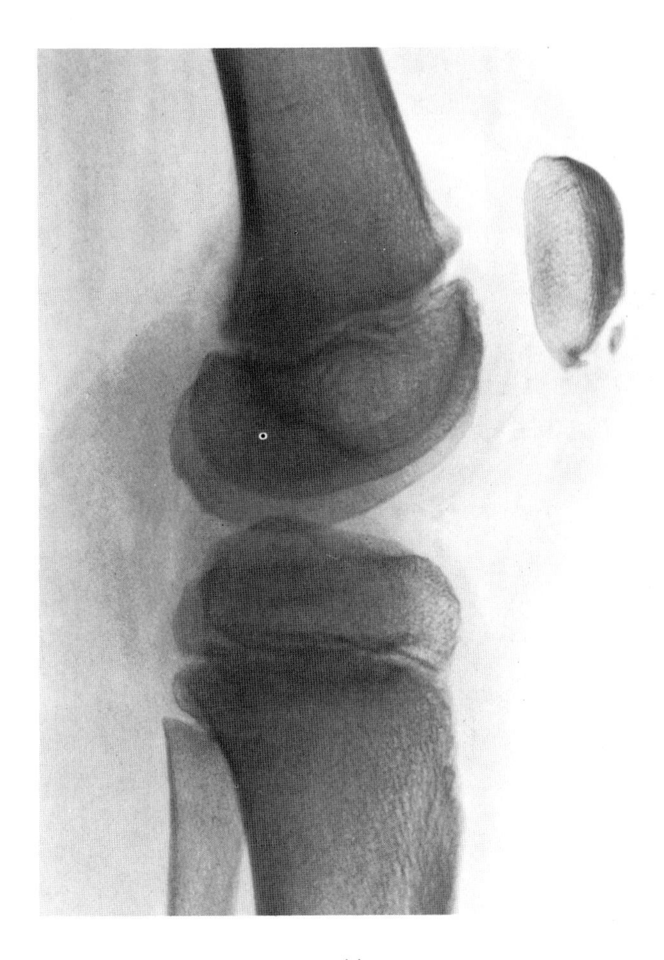

Fig. 1165. 9 year old. Left knee articulation, lateral. At the apex of the patella small nucleolei are visible; they can still fuse with the patella (cf. Fig. 761). The tibial tuberosity shows the beginning of roughness on the anterior surface.

1 Femoral diaphysis
2 Distal femoral epiphysis
3 Tibial diaphysis
4 Proximal tibial epiphysis
5 Intercondylar eminence
6 Fibular diaphysis
7 Patella
8 Nucleolei of the patella

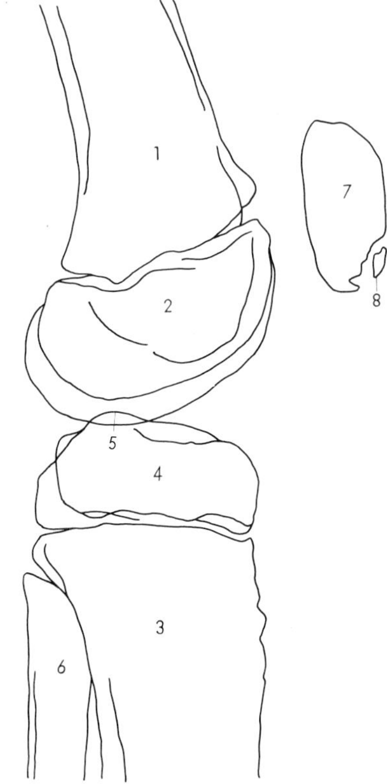

Fig. 1166. Sketch for Fig. 1165.

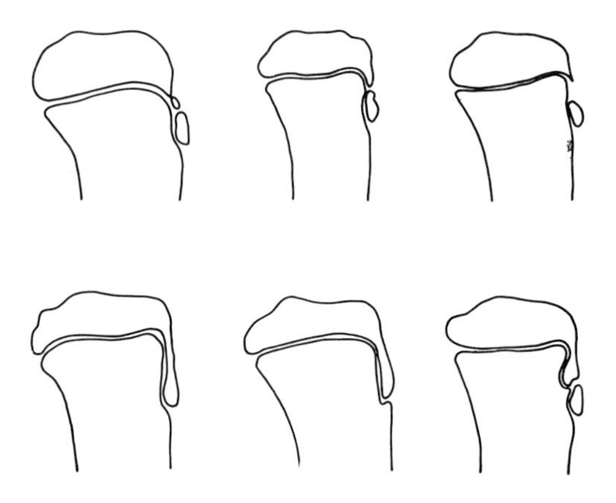

Fig. 1167. Various ossification forms of the tibial tuberosity in 10 to 12-year-old children.

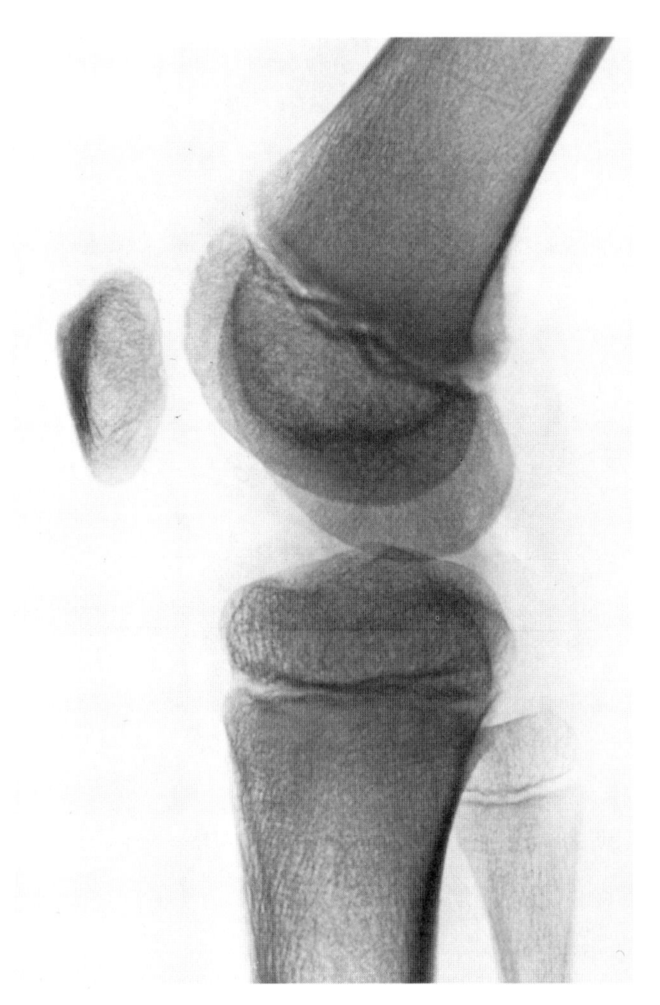

Fig. 1168 a

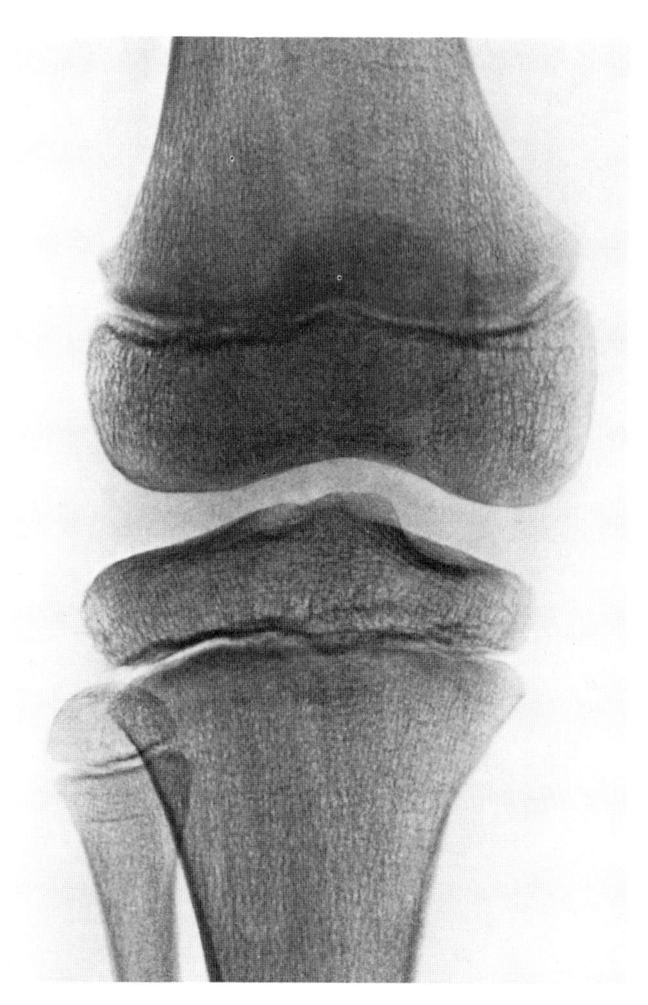

Fig. 1168 b

Fig. 1168. 10 year old. Right knee articulation, lateral and anteroposterior. The epiphyseal lines are undular and irregularly defined. In the lateral radiograph it is possible to note a slightly rough anterior contour of the femoral condyles and the articulation side of the patella. These irregularities at the borders of the growing bones are normal and may be seen in other sites in the skeleton, e. g., in the glenoid roof of the hip articulation (Figs. 1136, 1137, 1139, 1141, 1142, 1143, 1145, 1146, and 1160 b).

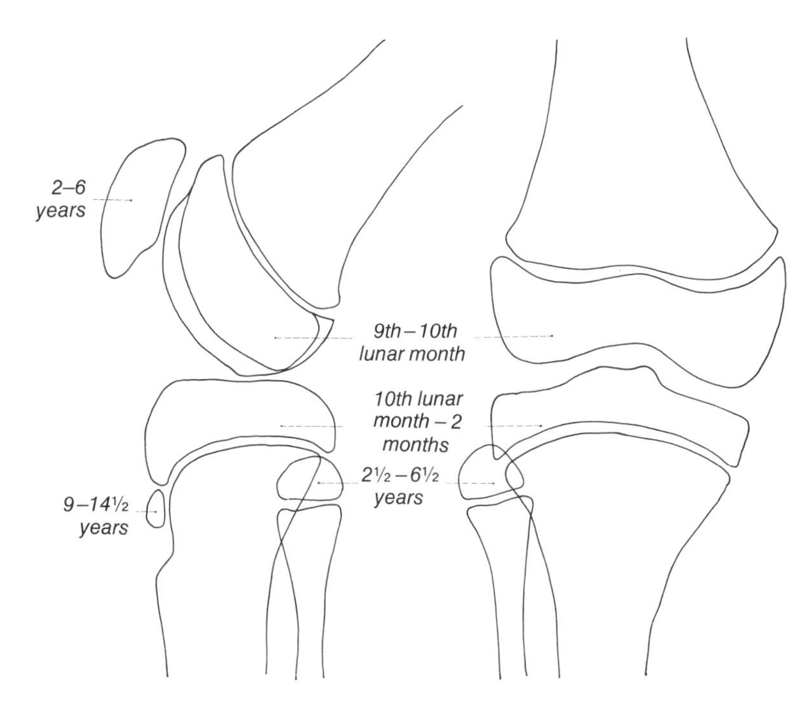

Fig. 1169. Details of the time span in which the osseous nuclei in the region of the knee articulation normally appear.

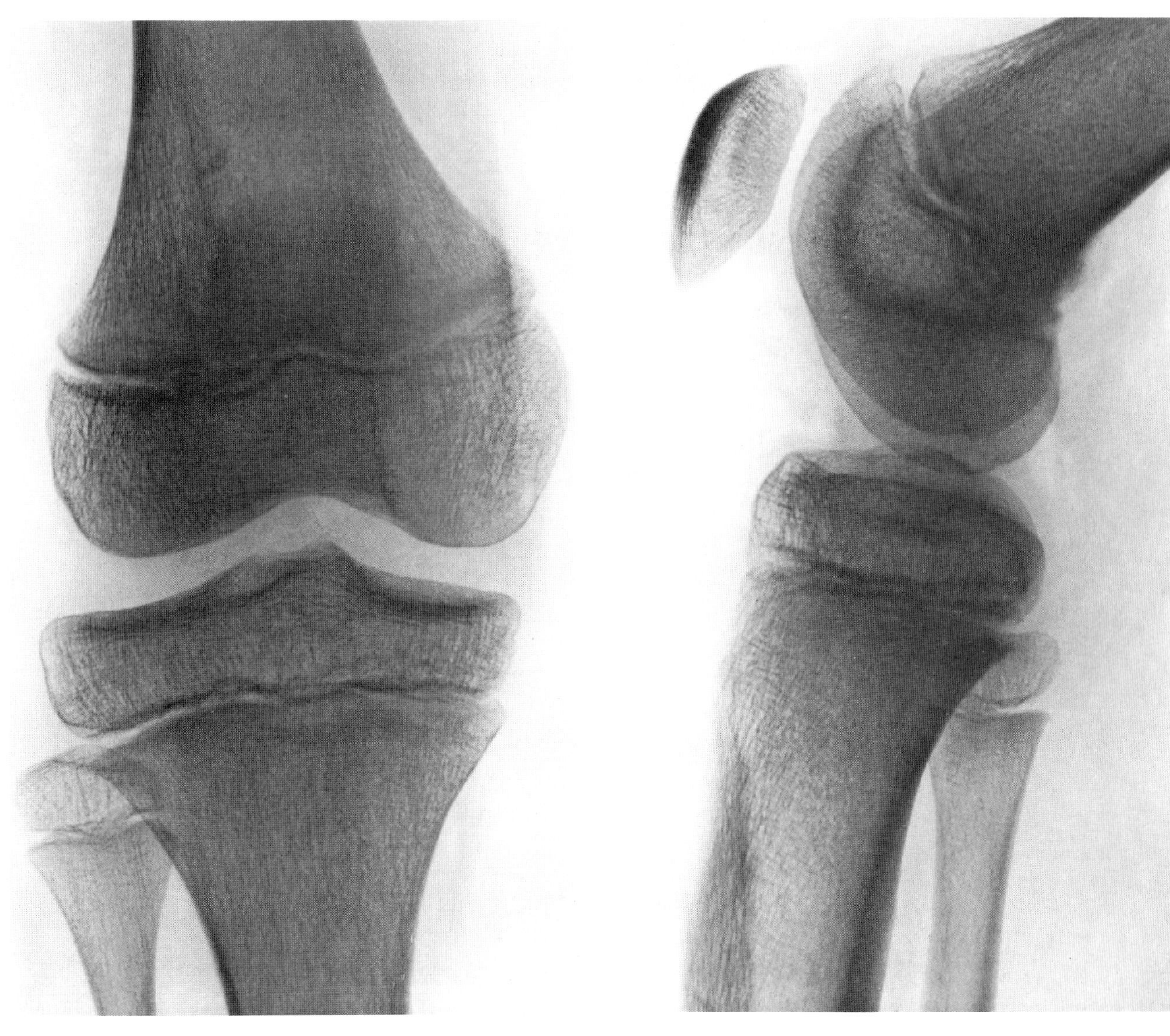

Fig. 1170 a　　**Fig. 1170 b**

Fig. 1170. 12 year old. Right knee articulation, anteroposterior and lateral. Sagitally, the intercondylar eminence shows clearly with a still flat, noticeable intercondylar tubercle. At the place where the tibial tuberosity will later develop, there is a basin-shaped, frequently step-like deepening which later will be filled by the tibial apophysis (not yet visible). The roughness of the epiphyseal and diaphysial extremities becomes smooth. A noticeable loosening of the structure and atrophy of the medial tibial metaphysial edge is seen here. In juveniles between the ages of 7 and 13, it can appear as a type of tibial osteochondrosis deformans (aseptic necrosis) of the medial tibial condyle *(Blount)*. It usually affects one side only and can lead to tibia vara.

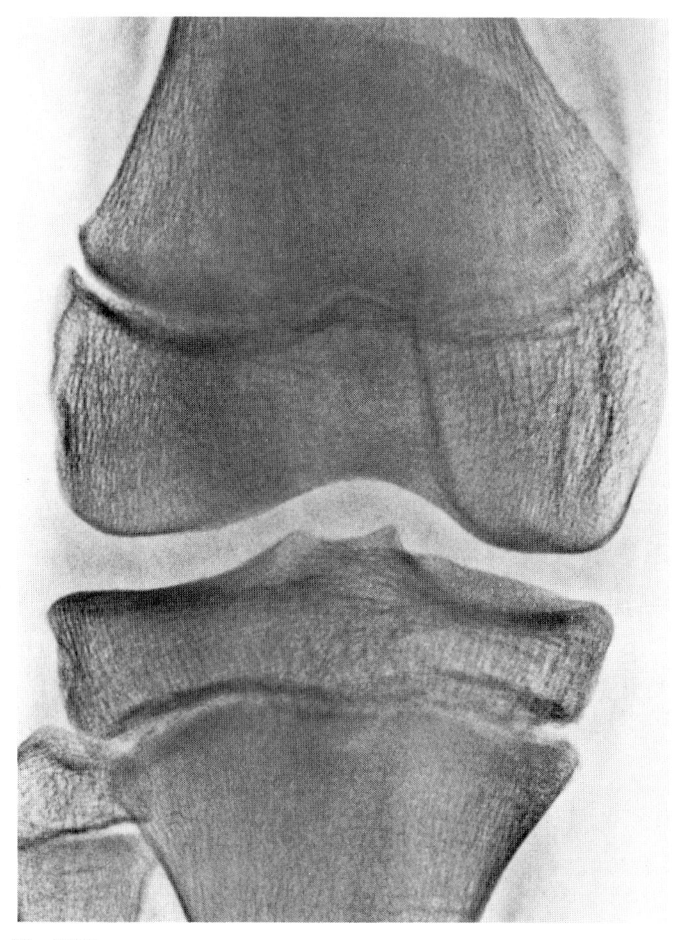

Fig. 1171 a

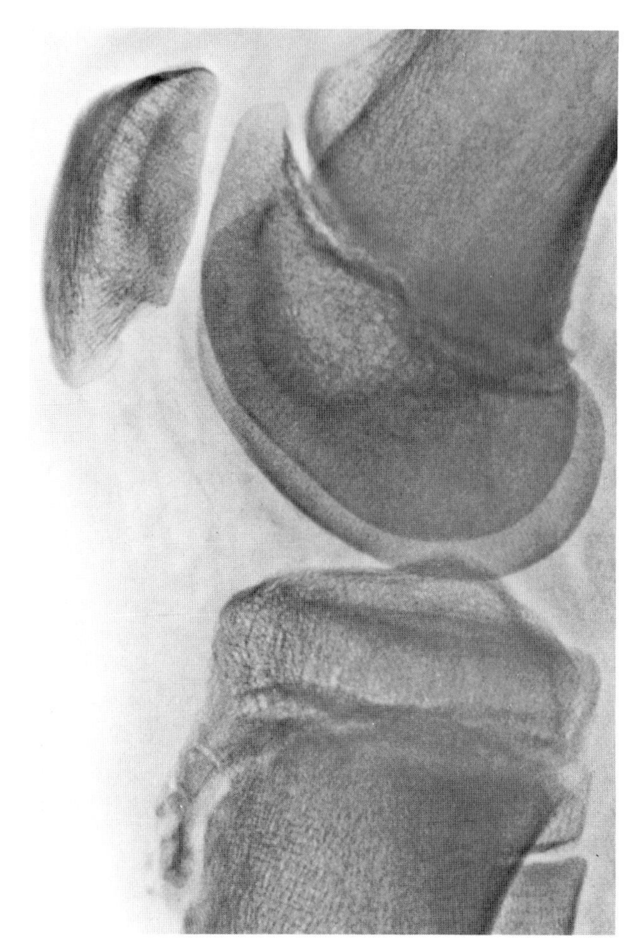

Fig. 1171 b

Fig. 1171. 14 year old. Right knee articulation, anteroposterior and lateral. The beak-shaped anterior process of the proximal tibial apophysis fuses with the still-curved tibial apophysis. The apophyseal nucleus appears at the age of 9 to 14 years and is frequently divided into many parts. It proceeds into a gradual deepening. This finding on the apophyseal nucleus should not be confused with *Osgood-Schlatter*'s, disease, not even in cases of considerable lateral difference. However, the diagnosis of pathological as opposed to normal cases is very difficult. The cruciform ligament humps of the intercondylar eminence are well differentiated.

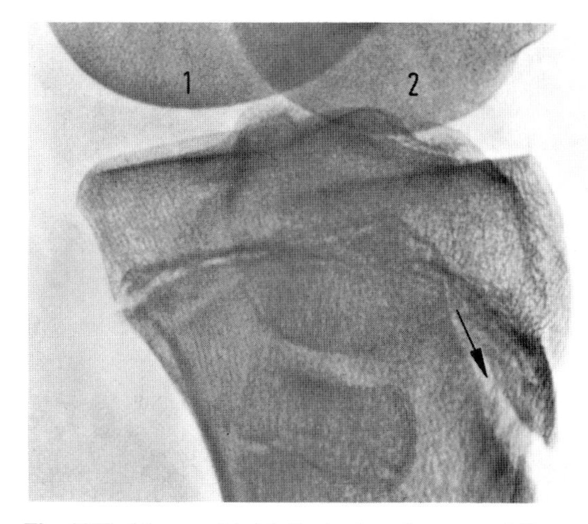

Fig. 1172. 14-year-old girl. Beak-shaped process of the superior tibial apophysis, dorsofibular-tibial.

1 Lateral femoral condyle
2 Medial femoral condyle
↘ Epiphyseal cartilaginous fissure; looks like a fracture. A wider gab of this epiphysis does not necessarily have to be pathological.

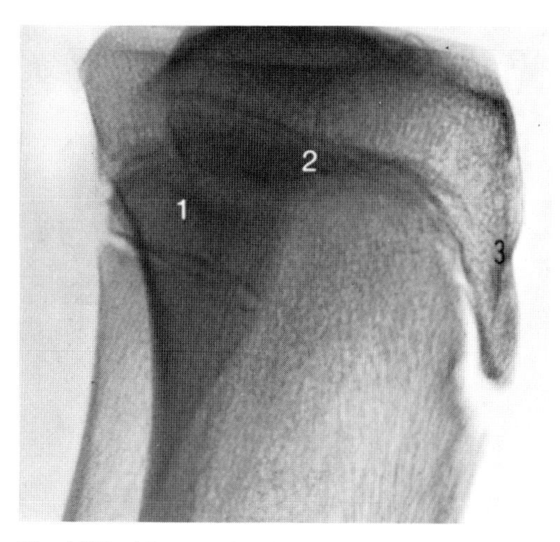

Fig. 1173. 14-year-old girl. Beak-shaped process of the superior tibial epiphysis, fibular-tibial.

1 Fibular epiphysis
2 Superior tibial epiphyseal cartilage
3 Beak-shaped process of the tibial epiphysis

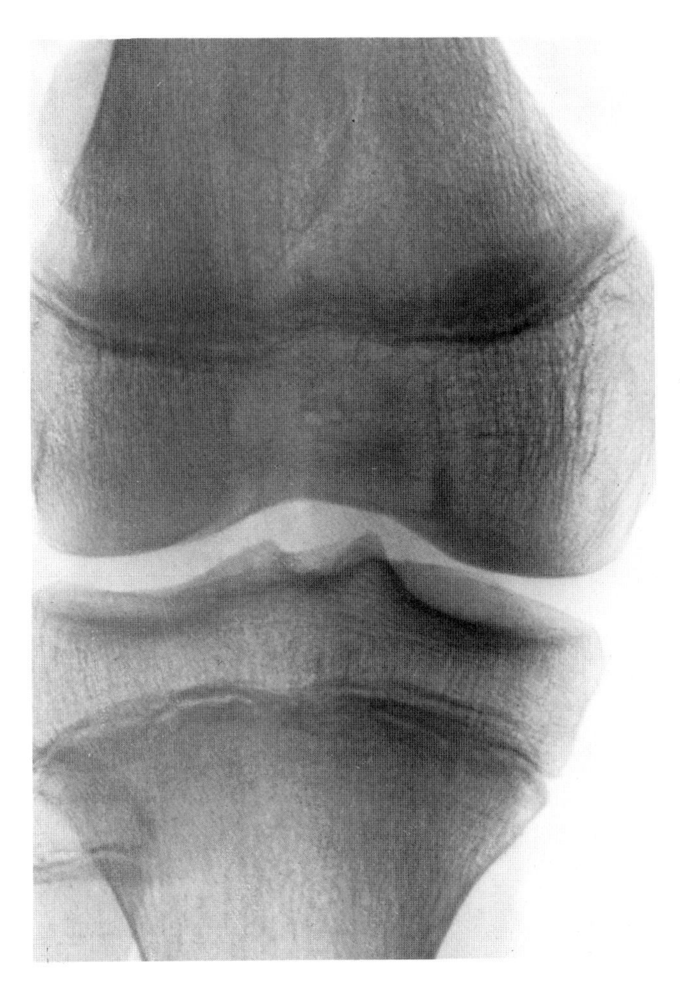

Fig. 1174 a

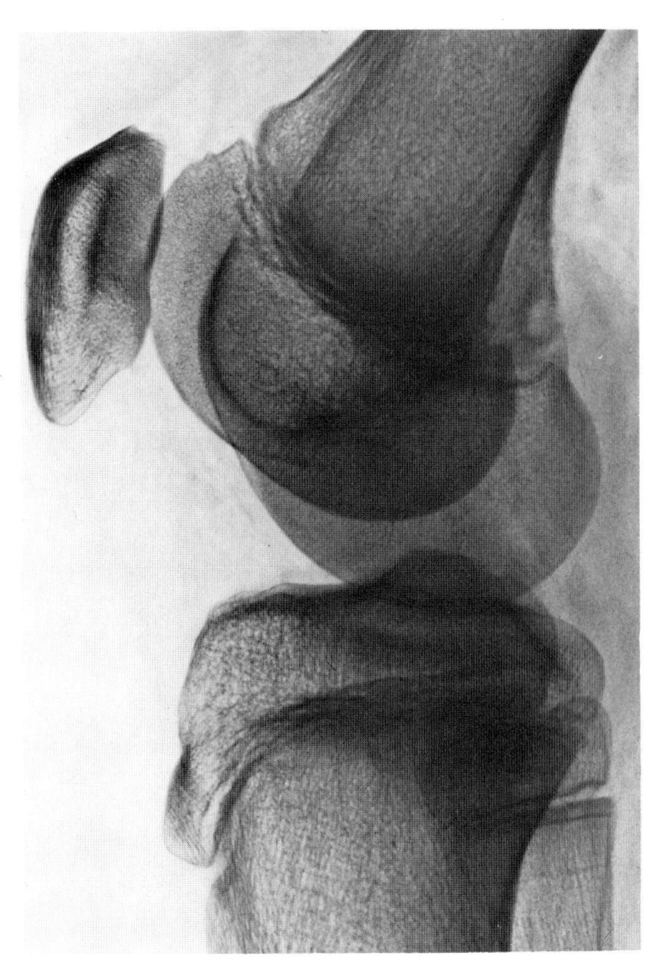

Fig. 1174 b

Fig. 1174. 16 year old. Right knee articulation, anteroposterior and lateral. The epiphyseal fissures are considerably narrower and are about to synostose. In the lateral radiograph, it is possible to recognize the beak-shaped tibial epiphyseal process (see Figs. 1167, 1175).

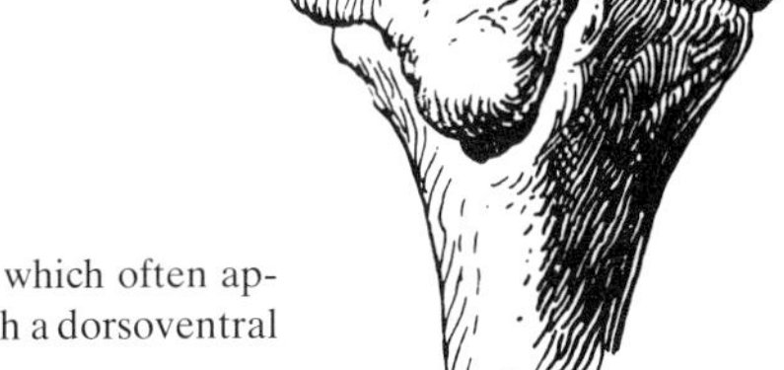

Fig. 1175 shows the **beak-shaped epiphyseal process,** which often appears clearly in a sagittal radiograph also, especially with a dorsoventral course of rays (from *Heitzmann).*

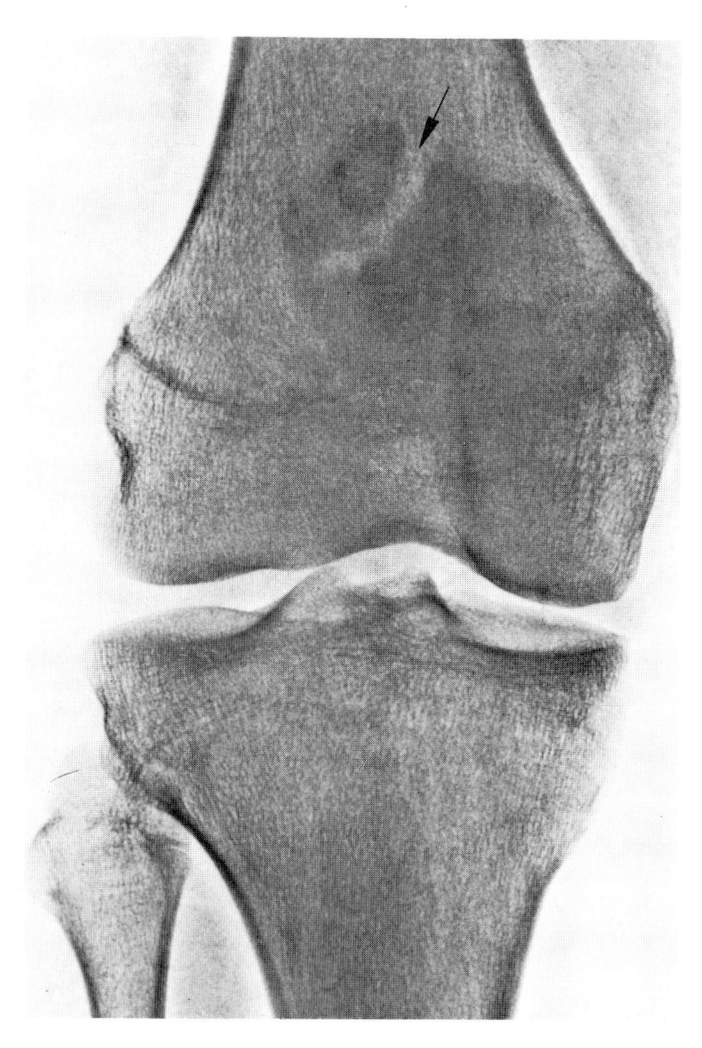

Fig. 1176. 17 year old. Right knee articulation, posteroanterior. A gaping fissure is seen at the point of the arrow. This is a case of a biparted patella (anamnestic trauma is excluded). The epiphyseal sutures are closed. An epiphyseal scar is discernible in the lateral femoral condyle.

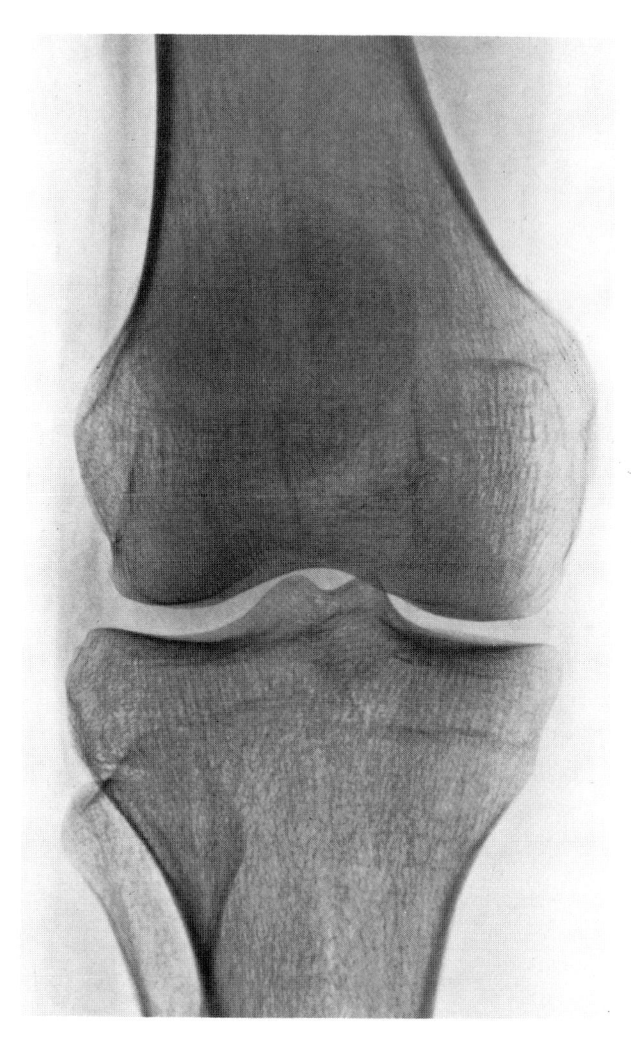

Fig. 1177. 19 year old. Right knee articulation, anteroposterior. The growth in length of the bone ends with the closure of the epiphyseal fissures. A wide "epiphyseal scar" remains in the tibial head; it may disappear and remain only as a diagonal line, but this is infrequent.

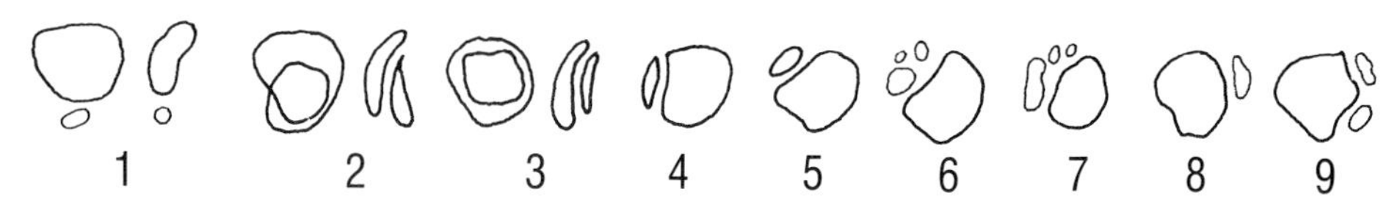

Fig. 1178. Variations of the patella divisions (according to *Hellmer*). The divisions can originate due to ossification anomalies, ossification disorders or diseases (osteochondrosis dissecans, aseptic necrosis). 1 = apical, 2 = frontal, 3 = dorsal, 4–9 marginal partitions.

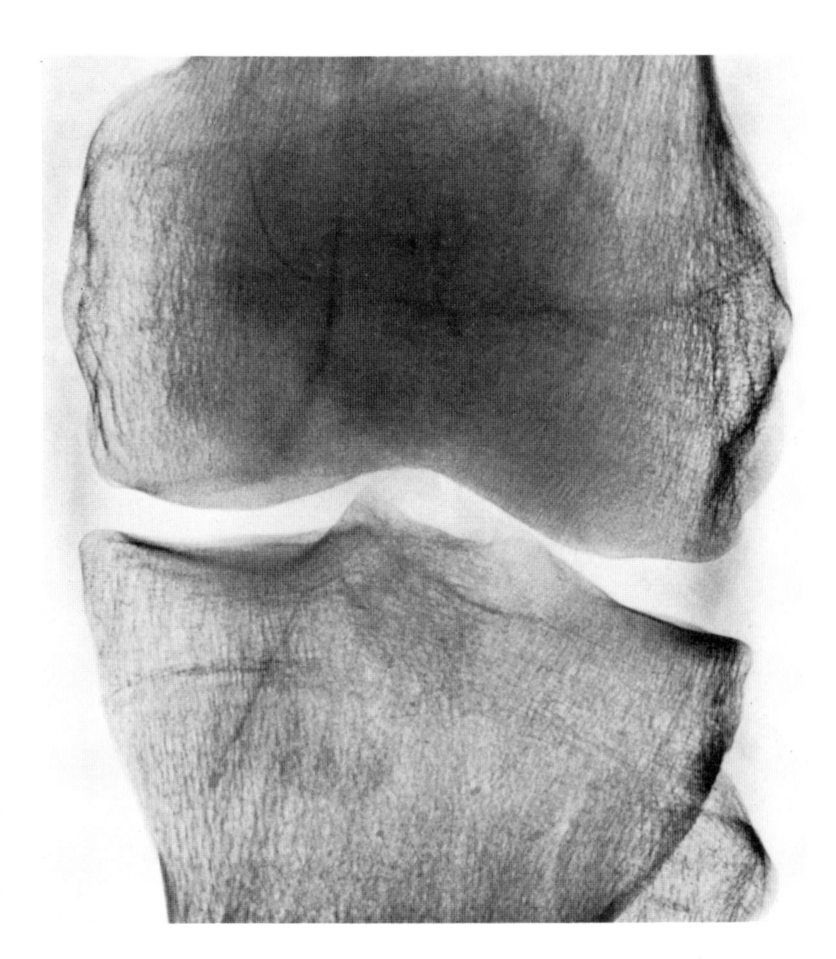

Fig. 1179. 25 year old. Left knee articulation, anteroposterior. Epiphyseal scars are still discernible in the femur and tibia. There is a well-formed intercondylar eminence. All bone edges are smooth. The patella is semidivided with a wide fissure formation, proximal to lateral.

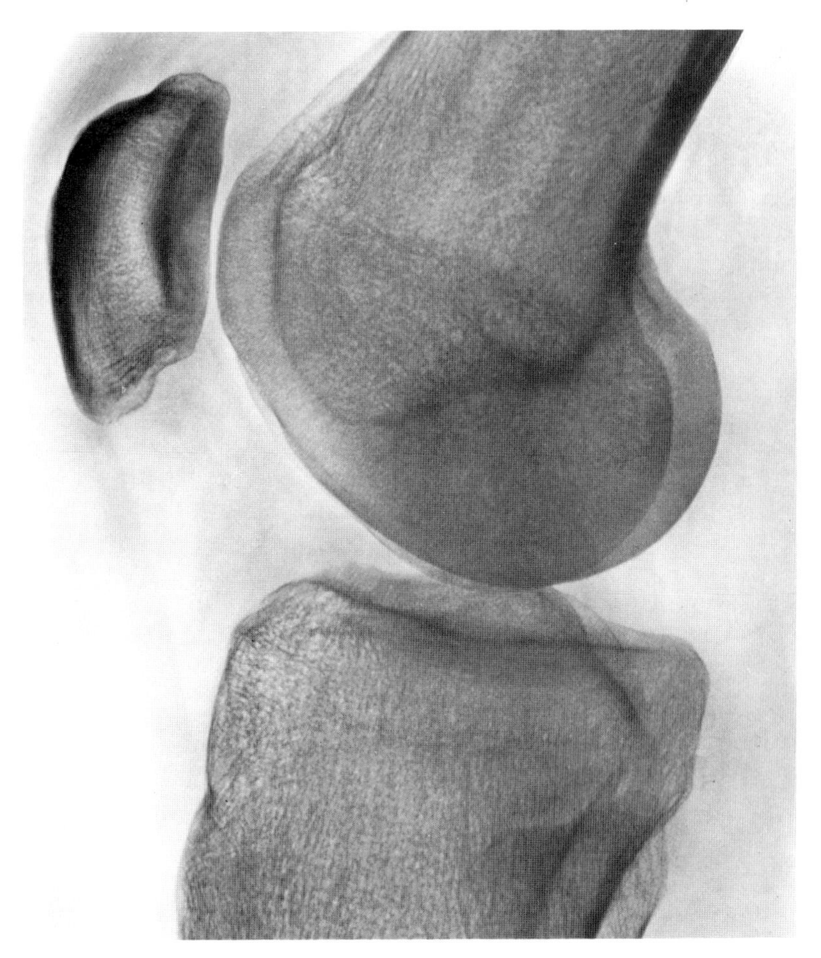

Fig. 1180. 25 year old. Right knee articulation, lateral. The growth in length is completely closed. The characteristic curved line in the distal femoral extremity is caused by the internal condylar contour, which was brought into relief against the intercondylar fossa.

Foot with Ankle Articulation

Two to three osseous nuclei are usually already formed in the tarsal region of the newborn: the nuclei of the calcaneus and the talus, and occasionally the nucleus of the cuboid bone.

The ossification of the foot bones is marked by an especially broad variation and the formation of numerous atypical acessorial ossification centers, as well as the more rapid formation of the osseous nuclei in comparison with the bones of the upper limbs.

Calcaneus. The nucleus of this bone is the first to appear in the tarsal region (around the 5th–7th fetal month). In most cases, there is a formation of two ossification centers *(Hasselwander, Trolle).* The 1st nucleus appears in the 4th to 5th fetal month in a lateral position. This nucleus should become the anlage of the peroneal trochlea. The peroneal trochlea is absent in approximately two thirds of all cases. Around the 7th fetal month it is possible to see the 2nd osseous nucleus, which fuses with the 1st nucleus in the course of the next few months or even after birth. The fused nucleus has an elliptical form in the newborn. It attains an oblong, cylindrical form during the 1st year, and around the 6th year of life it attains its final form.

The posterior calcaneus section is remarkably undular and toothed. Between 6 to 10 years of age, an apophysis (which varies in its form) originates in the joining region of the Achilles tendon. This apophysis originates from single, irregularly arranged ossification centers, and therefore may be formed of numerous jointed segments for many years (see Fig. 1183). This calcaneus apophysis fuses around the 17th to 19th years of life with the calcaneal tuber.

Talus. Its nucleus appears a month after the nucleus of the calcaneus, about the 7th fetal month. Here, too, it is sometimes possible to find two ossification centers. In newborns the nucleus is oblong; a year later it has the form of an hour-glass-like tight lacing. The differentiation of the talus attains its final form up to the ages of 6 or 7.

Cuboid bone. This nucleus is already formed at birth. Its existence, however, is not a reliable birth maturation sign. The cuboid bone can originate from several independent ossification centers, which a half year later, at most, fuse into one round osseous nucleus (frequently normal ossification).

Cuneiform lateral bone (III). This osseous nucleus appears around the middle of the 1st year of life.

Distal tibial epiphysis. In the second half of the 1st year of life, in boys sometimes later, a nucleus appears in the distal tibial epiphysis which develops so quickly that at the age of 4 or 5 it attains the entire width of the diaphysis. At this age it has a wedge-like form with an apex in the direction of the fibula. At the age of 8 or 9, the medial malleolus completes its formation, occasionally with its own nucleus which soon fuses with the tibial epiphysis.

Distal fibular epiphysis. Its nucleus forms slightly later than that of the tibial epiphysis, around the first half of the 2nd year of life.

Medial cuneiform bone (I) and the **intermedial (II)** cuneiform bone, as well as the navicular bone, appear in rapid succession. The chronological order is usually: medial cuneiform, navicular, intermedial cuneiform; however, a modification of this order is frequently noted.

The nuclei of the medial and intermedial cuneiform bones appear between the 2nd and 4th years of life. The medial cuneiform may show a double nucleus anlage. One nucleus is located in the distal superior angle. In the absence of synostosis, bipartition may occur. For ossification of the cuneiform bone, see also *de Cuveland.*

Navicular bone. The nucleus of this bone usually appears as the last foot root bone, around the 4th to 5th years of life; however, there is a large variation range extending from the second half of the 2nd year of life up to the second half of the 6th year of life. Like the medial cuneiform, the navicular bone can also originate from two more nucleus anlagen (see Fig. 875). *Schulte* noted an occurrence of five ossification nuclei.

Diaphyses and epiphyses of the metatarsal and phalanges. Before birth, in the 3rd fetal month, the diaphyses show an ossification nucleus, while the nuclei in the epiphyses are arranged only after birth. The first ossification nucleus appears in the nail process of the big toe in the 9th fetal week. The terminal phalanges of the 2nd, 3rd and 4th toes form their ossification nuclei in the 11th to 12th fetal weeks; the toe basal phalanges are formed in the 14th fetal week.

Thus, at birth, as in the land region, the diaphyses of the tubular bones (metatarsal and phalanges) are formed. The terminal phalanx of the 5th, and occasionally the 4th, toe may be an exception. They may appear much later, and the terminal phalanx of the 5th toe forms only an "appendage" of the middle phalanx.

The first epiphysis to appear is that of the basal phalanx of the big toe (around the 2nd year of life). The epiphyses of the remaining basal phalanges, of the middle phalanges and of the metatarsal bones are formed in the 3rd year of life, whereas the terminal phalanges of the 2nd to 5th toes appear only in the 4th or 5th year of life.

Termination of ossification. The epiphyseal closure at the tibial distal extremity occurs around the 17th to 19th years of life. At almost the same time, occasionally slightly later, the distal fibular epiphysis fuses with the fibular shaft. The osseous fusion of the calcaneal apophysis with the calcaneal tuber also occurs at the same time. The epiphyseal closure, in the region of the metatarsal bones and the phalanges, also occurs in the 17th to 19th years of life. It begins in the terminal phalanx and proceeds proximally; the epiphyses in the metatarsal bones are the last to close in the middle and front foot bone region.

Sesamoid bones of the foot. According to *Kewenter* and *Kassatkin,* the ossification of the sesamoid bone, which lasts one to two years, begins slightly earlier in girls (9th–10th year) than in boys (11th–12th year of life). Ossification from one or several centers is possible during this period, e.g., in the tibial sesamoid bone. It develops and becomes the largest sesamoid bone, and is positioned more distally than the fibular sesamoid bone (see Figs. 843 and 845).

The range of the appearance of the sesamoid bone extends over five years (11th to 16th years of life).

Variations in the development of the foot skeleton (see also Fig. 1122):

Calcaneus bifida. This is only a temporary phenomenon and derives from a developmental disorder with a retarded fusion of both ossification centers in the 1st year of life *(Schlüter, Porstmann* and *Arenz, Smola).* Congenital hereditary connections between the calcaneus and navicular bones are described by *Wray* and *Hernson.*

Calcification of the cartilagenous sutures in the calcaneus. A temporary thickening of the spongiose structure may be discernible in children at the fusion point between the two ossification centers.

An apophysis is sometimes found in the lateral part of the calcaneus, at the peroneal trochlea.

Bipartitum medial cuneiform bone. Since this foot root may originate from two ossification centers, a bipartition is possible in the absence of synostosis of the nucleus *(Böker* and *Müller,* others). See also Fig. 823, No. 183.

Bipartitum Navicular. It is possible for this bone to originate owing to a rather frequent occurrence of several osseous nuclei (Fig. 875) (see Fig. 823, Nb).

One of the variant forms of a child's scaphoid bone, i.e., reduction of the volume of the bone and compression of its structure, is known as *Köhler's* disorder. *Zimmer* showed that after many years it is possible to cure this disorder and to bring the bone back to a normal healthy state. The above disorder mostly affects boys between the ages of 3 and 10. Scaphoid bone tuberculosis should not be confused with this condition, though it may begin with similar changes.

Metatarsal bones. The nuclei of the 2nd to 5th metatarsal heads may appear divided (Fig. 1212). The cup-shaped apophysis at the 5th metatarsal bone may persist (see Fig. 822, No. 172 and Fig. 861). Similarly, the fusion of the distal epiphysis may be absent. The proximal epiphysis of the 1st metatarsal is sometimes fissured in the middle.

Pseudoepiphyses are found in the metatarsal bones, too.

According to *Schinz,* the appearance of an ossification nucleus is connected to the growth in length of the bone. In limited growth, the ossification of the epiphysis begins from the diaphysis; in a more robust growth in length, the ossification begins from an ossification nucleus.

Toes. Variations, especially in the region of the lateral part of the foot, are frequent. Epiphyses are often lacking in the middle phalanges of the 4th and 5th toes, and sometimes of the 2nd and 3rd toes. The ossification then proceeds periostally-enchondrally without epiphysis formation.

A fragmentation of the basal toe epiphysis, especially of the basal phalanx, is attributed to *Thiemann's* disorder *(Thiemann, Krall* and *Krauspe, Liess).* A cavity formation of the foot with an apex occurs in cases of the so-called *Friedreich* foot, a foot deformity in spinal ataxia. In this case the basal articulation of the big toe is overextended. If so-called notchy epiphyses appear, they are discernible in the 2nd to 4th toes in both feet (see Fig. 822) *(Ravelli, Rossmann, Laurent* and *Brombart). Liess* noticed them in hands and feet, and defined them as peripheral dysostoses.

The terminal phalanges may be underdeveloped, especially in the big toe. In 25 to 33% of cases, the terminal and middle phalanges fused into one bone (Fig. 821).

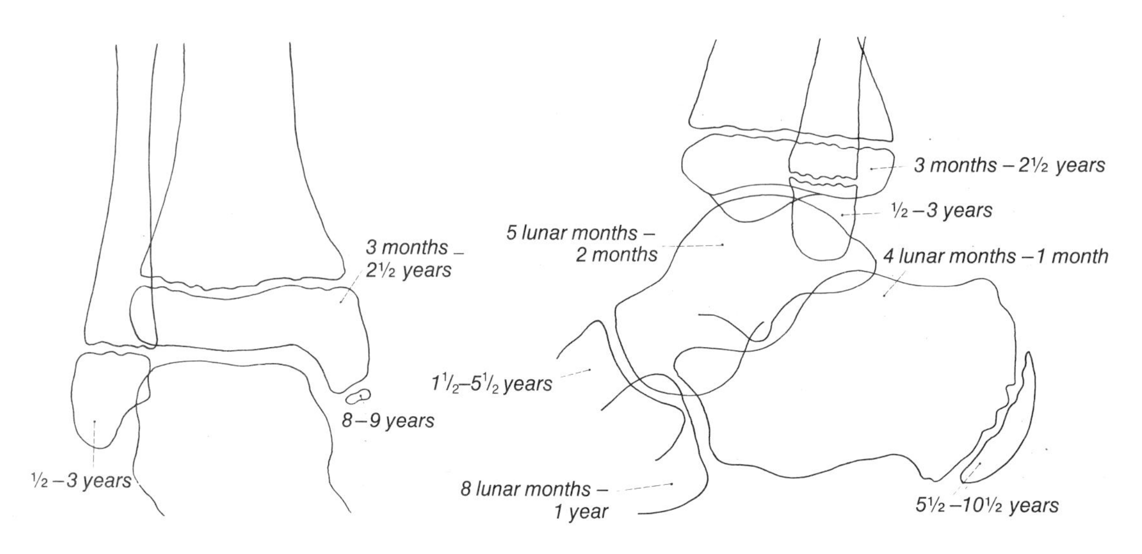

Fig. 1181. Time span in which the osseous nuclei can appear in the ankle articulation.

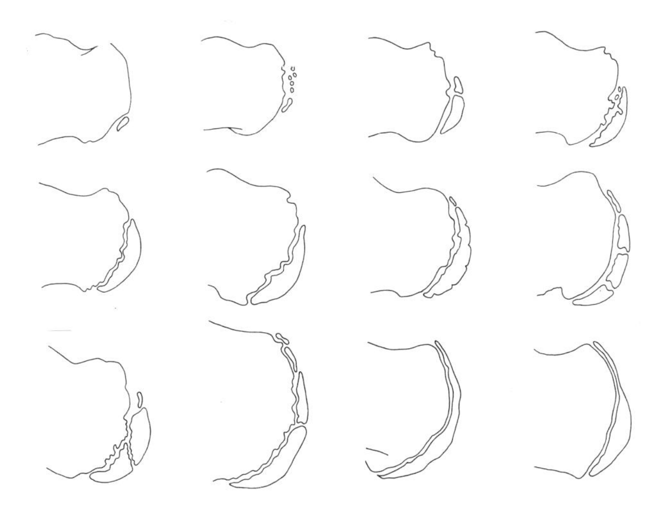

Fig. 1183. Various ossification formations of the apophysis at the calcaneal tuber in 8 to 12-year-old children.

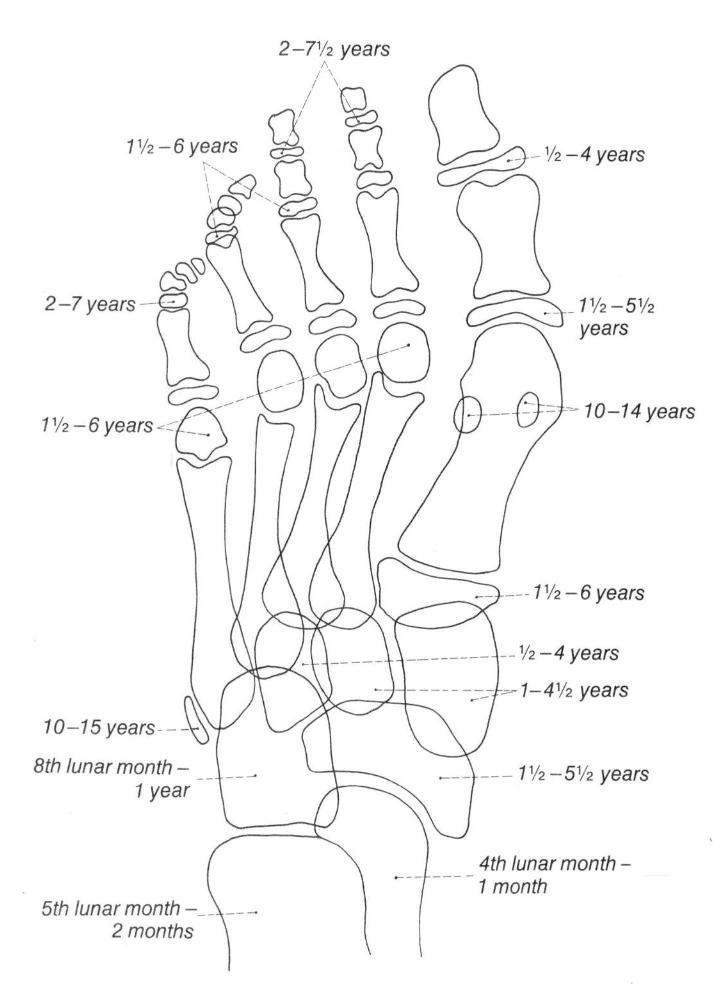

Fig. 1182. Time span in which the osseous nuclei of the bone usually appear.

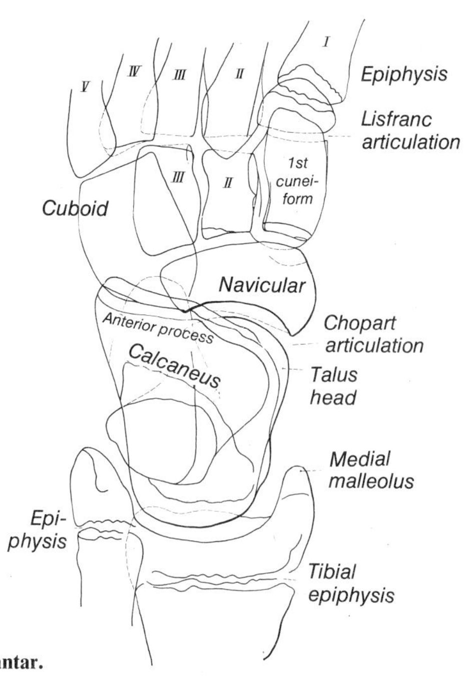

Fig. 1184. 14-year-old boy. Foot, dorsoplantar.

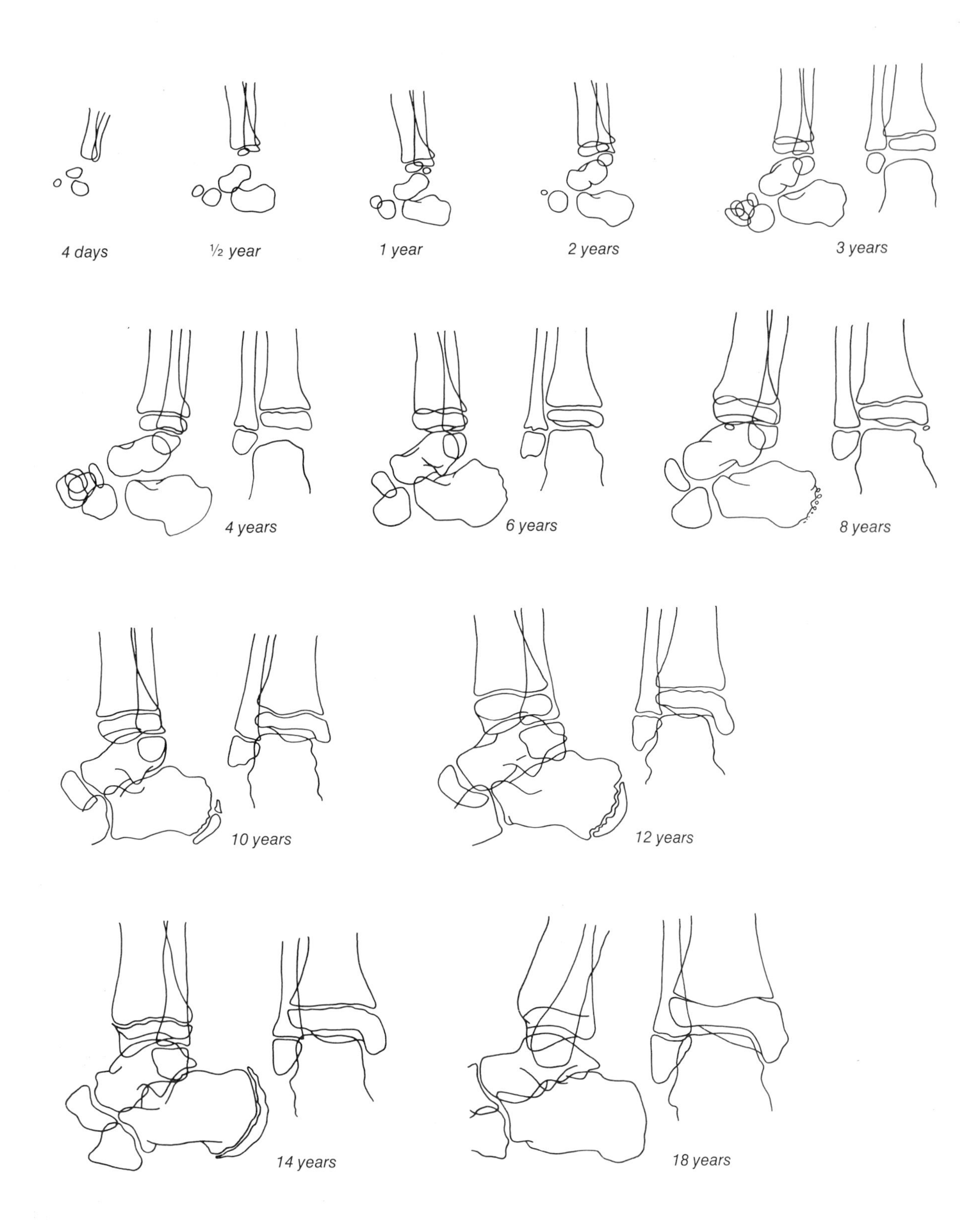

Fig. 1185. Foot articulation in chronological order from newborn to age 18.

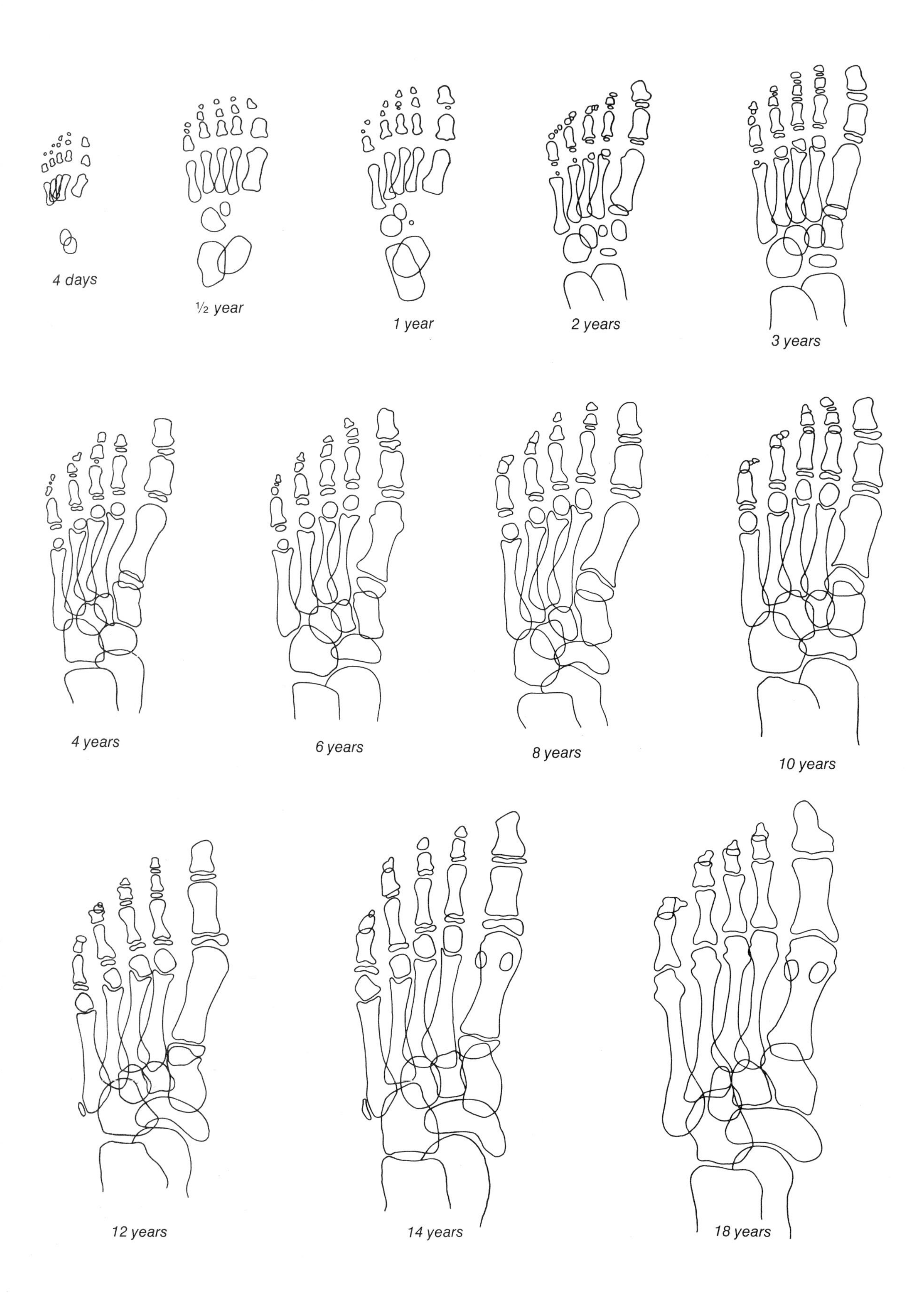

Fig. 1186. The foot, in chronological order from newborn to age 18.

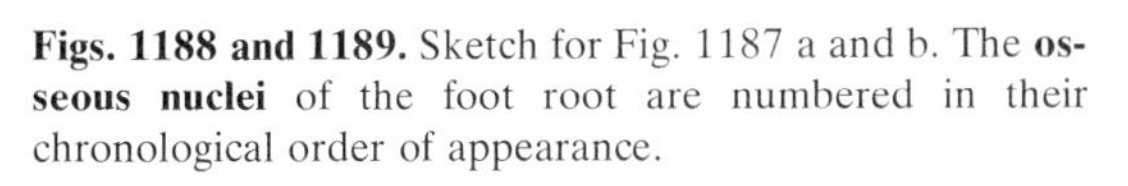

A Series of Radiographs of the Development of the Tibia and Foot from Infancy to Age 17

Figs. 1188 and 1189. Sketch for Fig. 1187 a and b. The **osseous nuclei** of the foot root are numbered in their chronological order of appearance.

1 Calcaneus
2 Talus
3 Cuboid bone
4 Lateral cuneiform bone
5 Tibial epiphysis
6 Fibular diaphysis

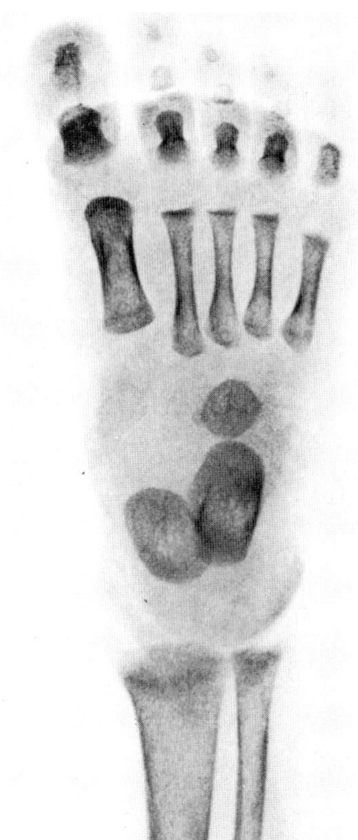

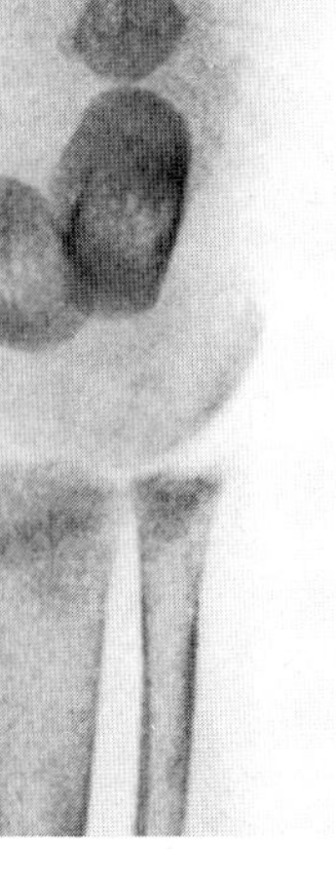

Fig. 1187 a

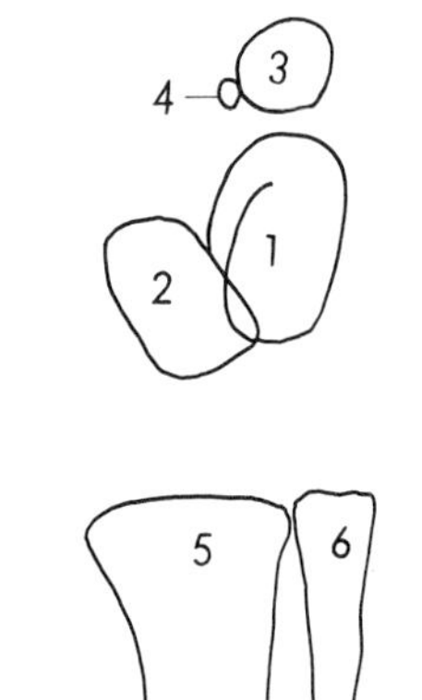

Fig. 1188

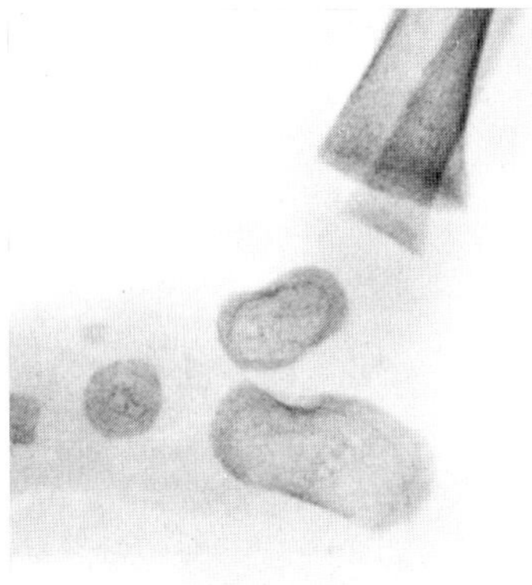

Fig. 1187 b

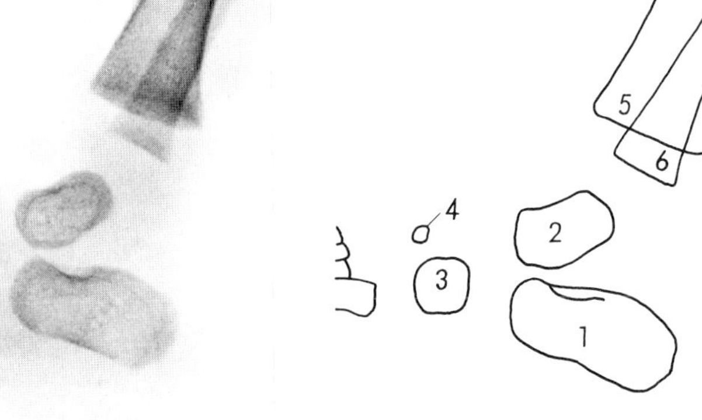

Fig. 1189. Sketch for Fig. 1187b.

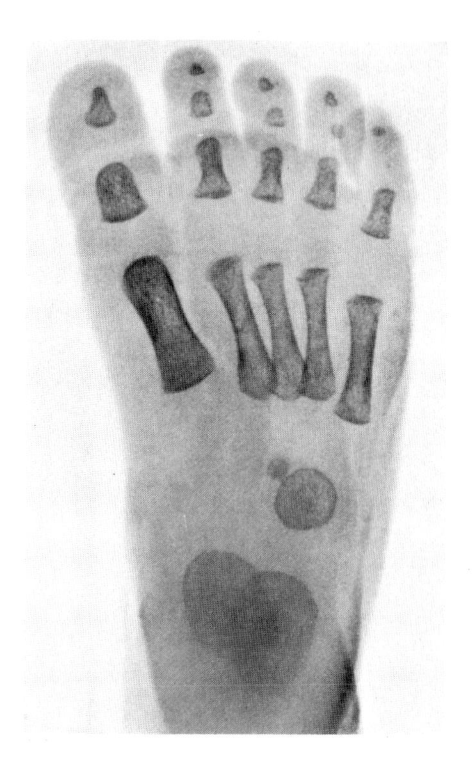

Fig. 1190 a

Fig. 1187. 2 month old. Average norm. Foot and foot root in two levels. The calcaneus (5th–6th lunar months), talus (7th lunar month), as well as the cuboid bone (at birth) are arranged on osseous nuclei of the foot root; they are all well developed. The cuboid bone may originate from several ossification centers. The ossifying nucleus of the lateral cuneiform is already seen in both radiographs from the age of 6 months onwards. The metatarsal and toe bones have no epiphyseal nuclei yet; the diaphyses are osseously arranged.

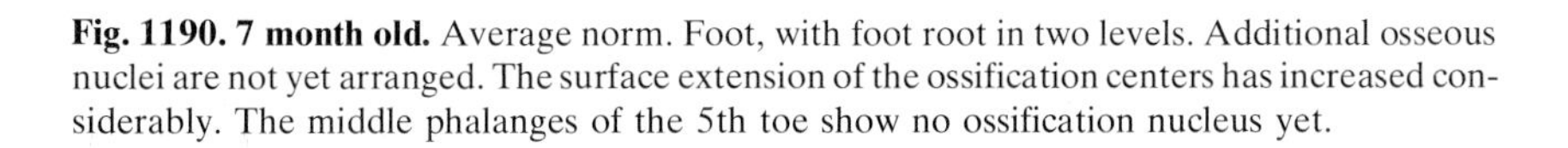

Fig. 1190. 7 month old. Average norm. Foot, with foot root in two levels. Additional osseous nuclei are not yet arranged. The surface extension of the ossification centers has increased considerably. The middle phalanges of the 5th toe show no ossification nucleus yet.

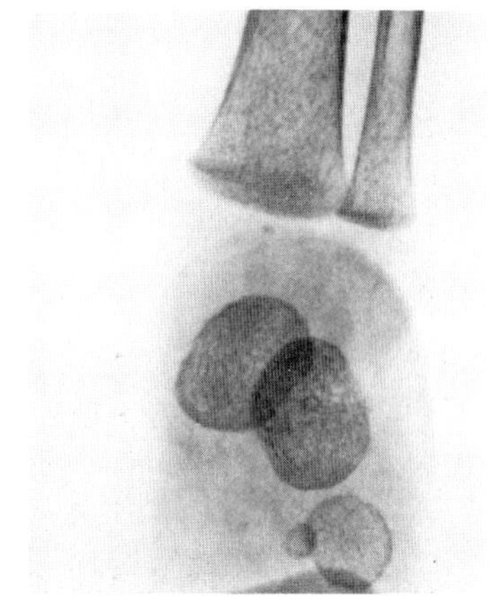

Fig. 1190 b

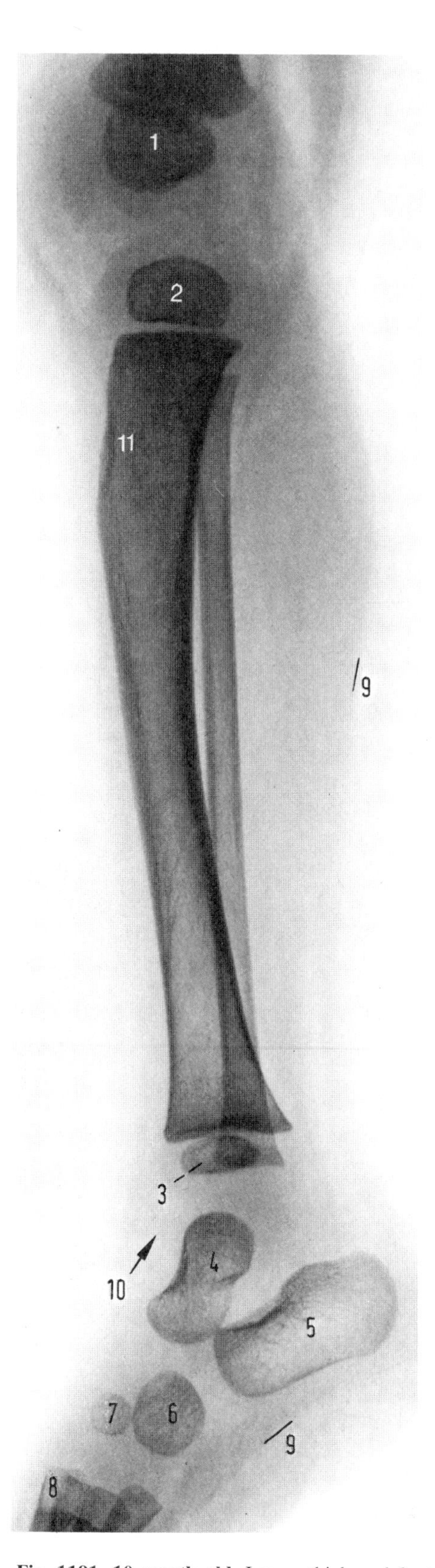

1 Nucleus of the distal epiphysis of the femur
2 Nucleus of the proximal epiphysis of the tibia
} surrounding epiphyseal cartilage clearly visible
3 Nucleus of the distal epiphysis of the tibia
4 Talus
5 Calcaneus
6 Cuboid bone
7 Cuneiform lateral (III)
8 Metatarsal bone (I), epiphysis still absent
9 Border between adipose and muscle layers
10 Flexing tendons
11 Tibial tuberosity

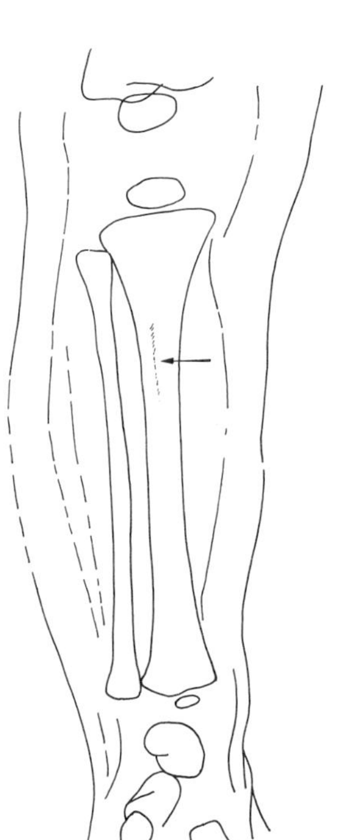

Fig. 1192. Lower thigh, ventrodorsal. At the limit between the superior and middle third, an oblong lightened strip (←): vessel canal.

Fig. 1191. 10 month old. Lower thigh and foot root, fibulotibial.

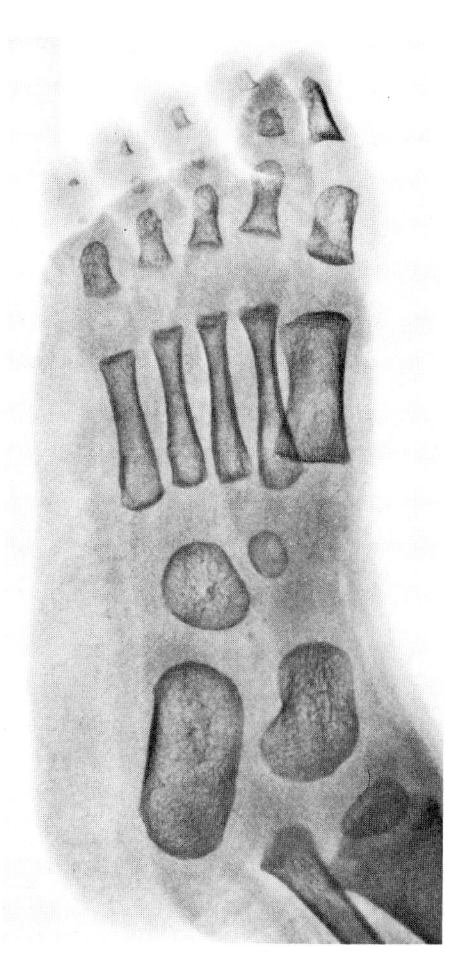

Fig. 1193. 1 year old. Average norm. Foot, with distal extremities of the tibia and fibula. Here, the first ossification center that is arranged is the nucleus of the distal tibial epiphysis. It appears around the second half of the 1st year of life.

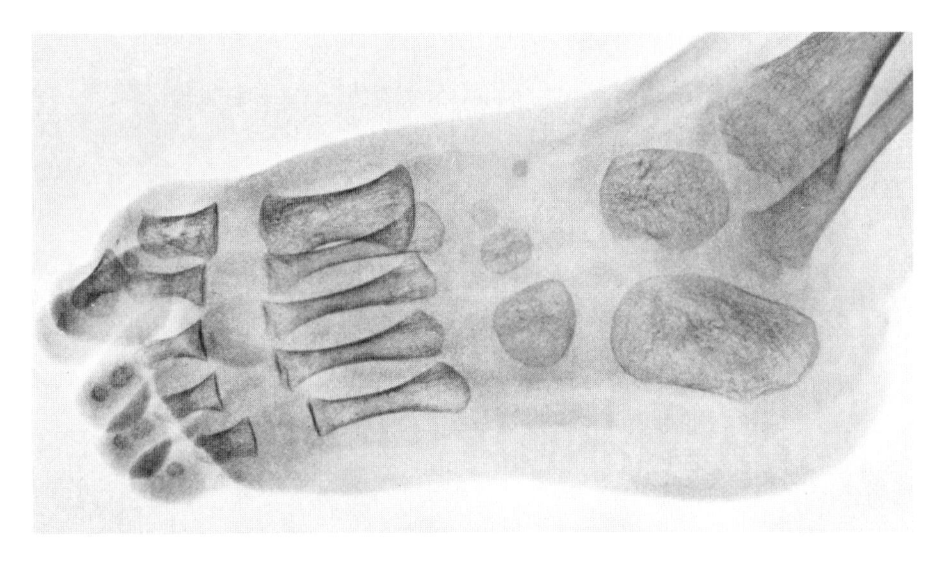

Fig. 1194 a (fibulotibial).

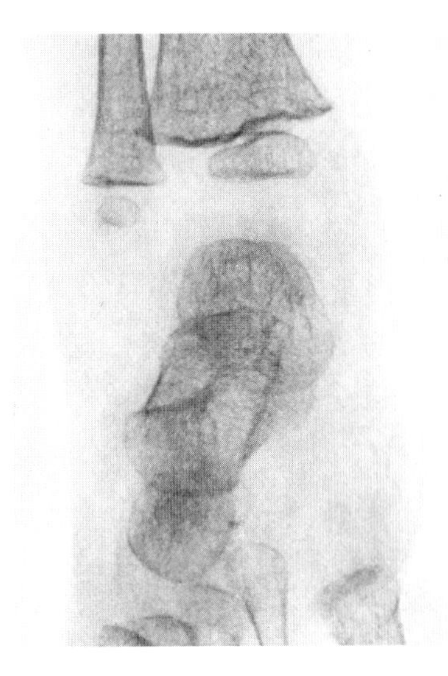

Fig. 1194 b (dorsoplantar).

Fig. 1194. 1 3/4 year old. Average norm. The ossification nuclei in the medial and intermedial cuneiform bones have already appeared in the foot root (2nd to 4th year), as well as the osseous nucleus in the distal fibular epiphysis (in the first half of the 2nd year).

1 Talus
2 Calcaneus
3 Shadow of the cuneiform bones (projected on each other)
4 Cuboid bone
5 Distal epiphysis of the fibula
6 Epiphyseal disk of the tibia, apparently fissured, only in radiograph. New finding: needle fragment

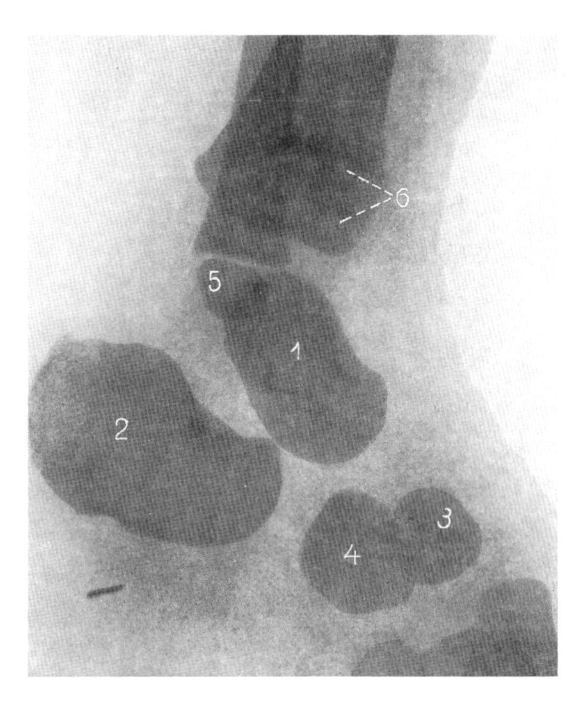

Fig. 1195. 2 3/4 year old. Foot, tibiofibular.

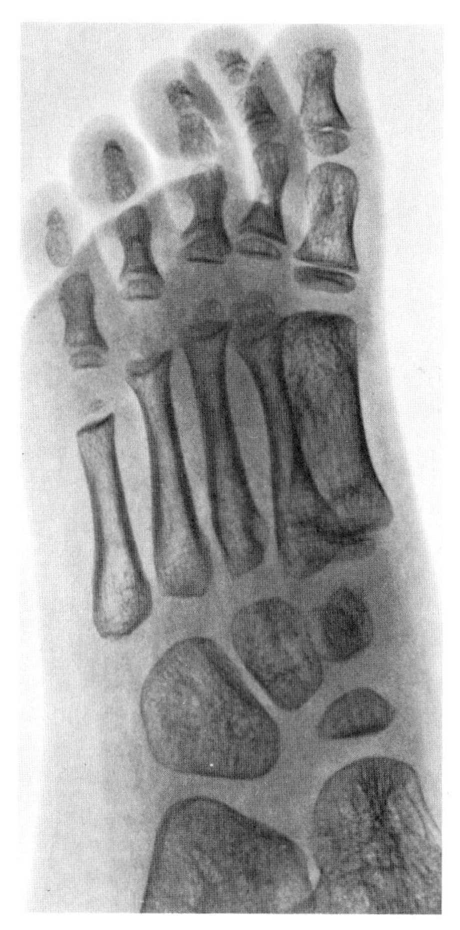

Fig. 1196

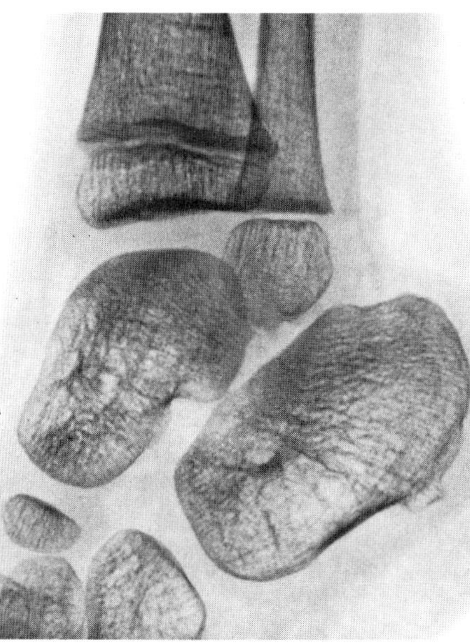

Fig. 1197

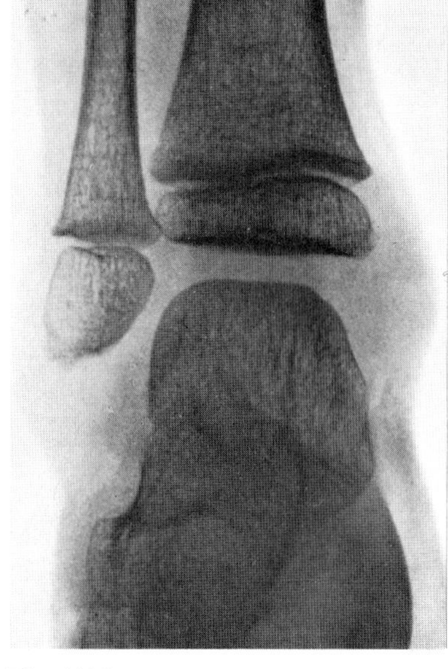

Fig. 1198

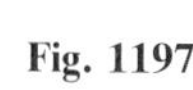

Figs. 1196–1198. 3 year old. Average norm. Foot root on three levels, as well as metatarsus and the forefoot. The last osseous nucleus to appear in the foot root is also the nucleus of the navicular bone (2nd to 5th years, broad time range). The epiphyseal nuclei of the metatarsus (in the 3rd year) as well as the phalanges (end of the 2nd, beginning of the 3rd year) have already appeared. The epiphyseal nuclei of the II-IV terminal phalanges appear slightly later than those of the basal and middle phalanges (3rd to 5th years).

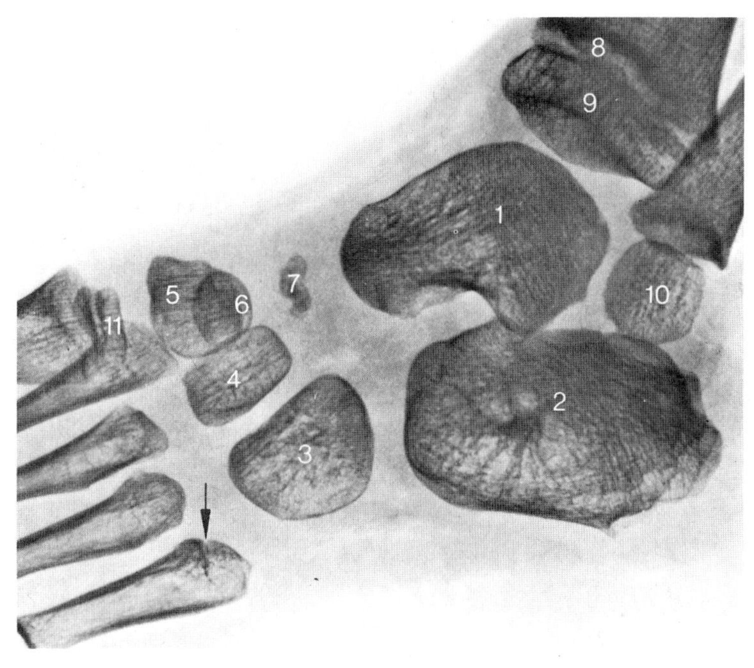

Fig. 1199. 4 year old. Foot diagonal, fibulotibial.

The normal or early appearance of the osseous nucleus of the navicular (normally appears between the ages of 1 1/2 and 5 1/2) is regularly contoured, while the nucleus that first appears at the end of the "normal period" has an irregular contour and can be sequestered. When the navicular bone has a multiplicity of nuclei (Fig. 875), it is possible that there is osteochondrosis dissecans present *(Ueberschär)*.

1 Talus
2 Calcaneus
3 Cuboid
4 Lateral cuneiform
5 Medial cuneiform, and
6 Intermedial cuneiform (projected on each other)
7 Navicular, just formed
8 Distal fibial epiphyseal suture, still strongly undulated
9 Distal tibial epiphysis
10 Distal fibular epiphysis
11 Proximal epiphysis of the I metatarsal
↓ Pseudoepiphysis (fracture simulated)

Fig. 1200. 4 year old. Foot, plantodorsal. Irregular epiphyseal anlage. The first metatarsal shows distally, the 3rd and 4th proximally (←); so-called pseudoepiphyses (this supports the theory that originally all tubular bones of the foot had two epiphyses). The nucleus of the 2nd metatarsal head is divided.

1, 2, 3 Cuneiform bones
4 Cuboid
6 Calcaneus
7, 8 Nuclei of the heads of the 2nd and 3rd metatarsal
9 Middle phalanx of the 5th toe

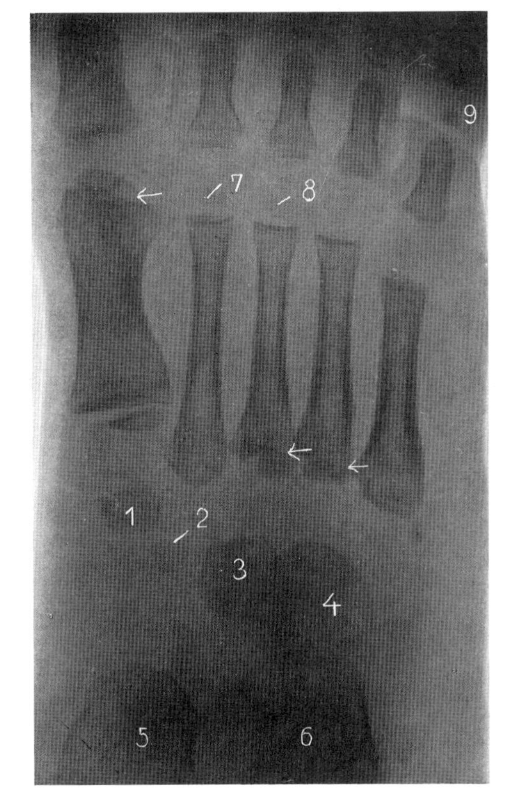

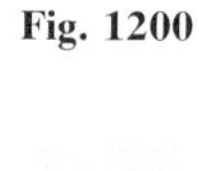

Fig. 1200

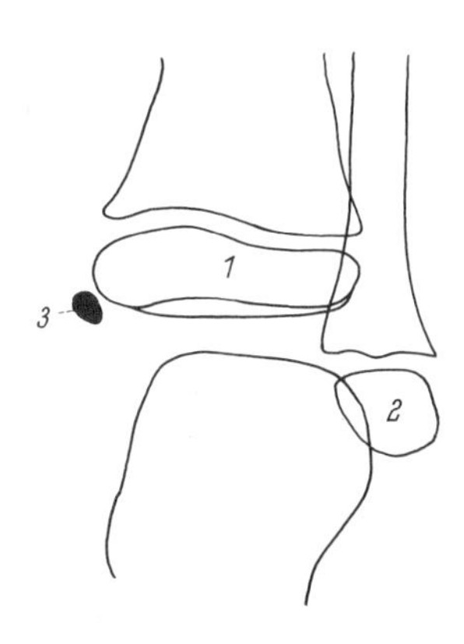

Fig. 1201. 5$^{1}/_{2}$ year old. Besides the epiphyseal nuclei of the tibia and fibula (1, 2), an inconstant nucleus is seen in the medial malleolus (3).

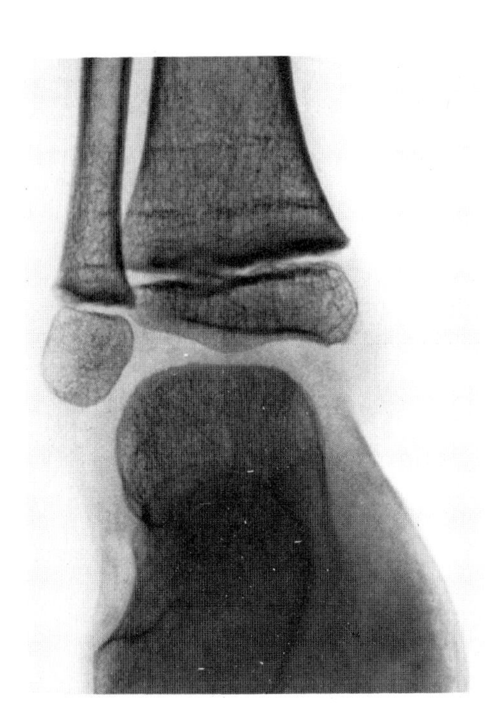

Fig. 1202

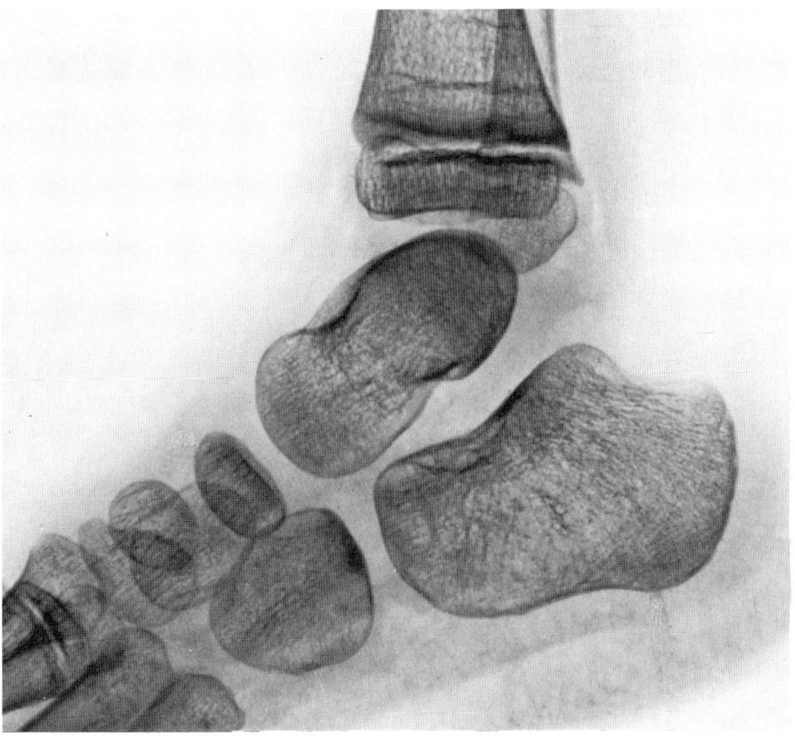

Fig. 1203

Figs. 1202 and 1203. 5 year old. Average norm. The size increase of the ossification centers corresponds to the age. The contours of the foot root bones already show their final form. The tibial epiphysis still has a cuneiform shape. In the distal tibial metaphysis there are so-called diagonal stripes in the bone structure. These are "intermedial stripes." They are a consequence of periodic growth disorders, e.g., rickets or other metabolic or nutritional disorders, and may also occur after infectious diseases. These delays in the growth of the bones can not only be balanced but the ossification process can even be accelerated with treatment of vitamin D in cases of rickets.

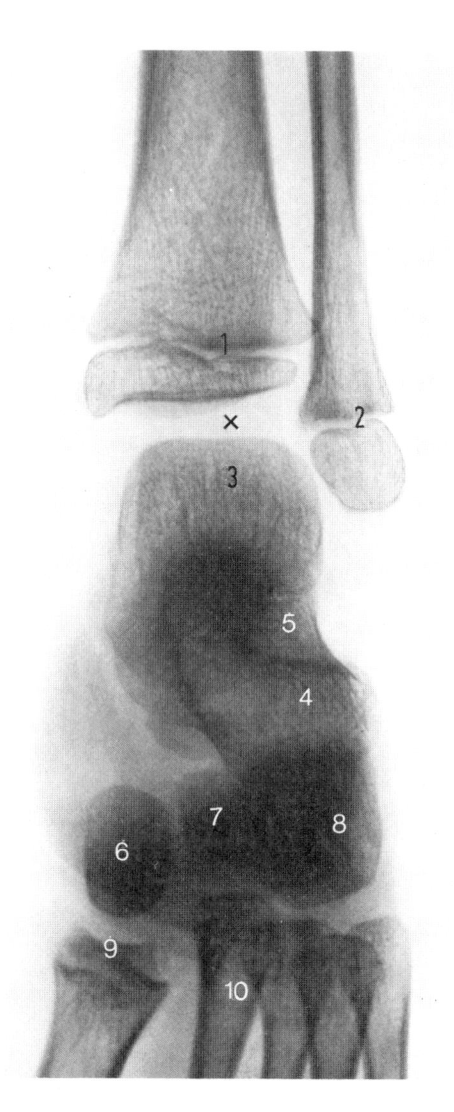

Fig. 1204. 5 1/2 year old. Foot articulation, ventrodorsal. Central radiation: X articulation fissure, middle.

1 Epiphyseal disk of the tibia
2 Epiphyseal disk of the fibula
3 Trochleal talus
4 Calcaneus
5 Tarsal sinus
6 Medial cuneiform bone
7 Intermedial cuneiform bone (the lateral cuneiform bone is covered by the cuboid bone)
8 Cuboid bone
9 Epiphysis of the 1st metatarsal
10 2nd metatarsal

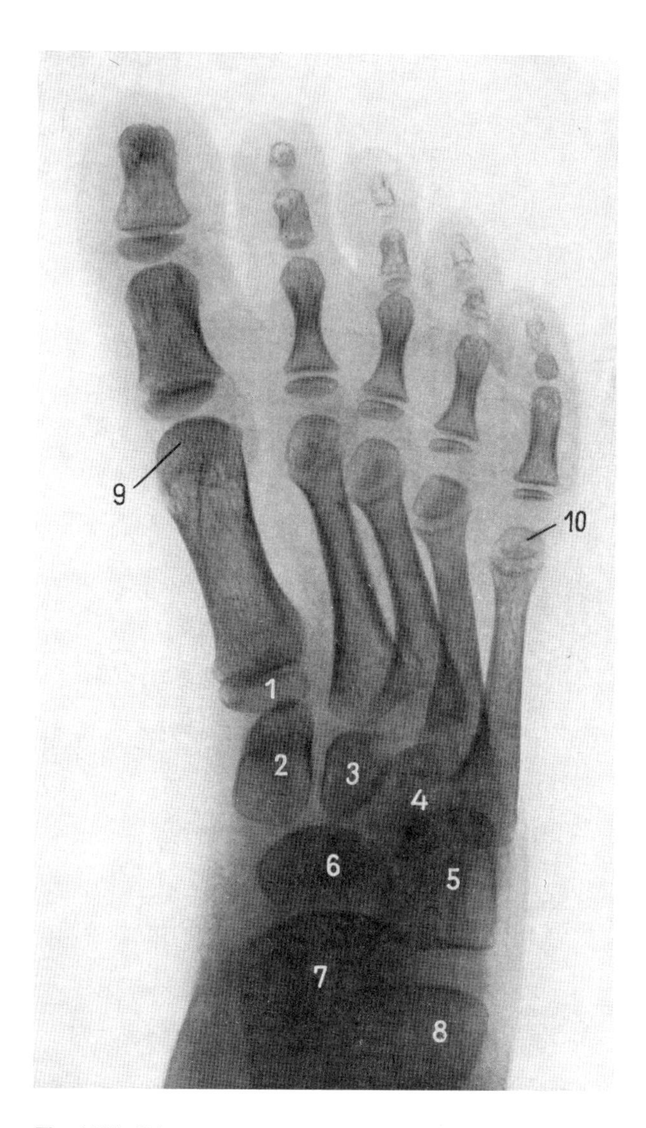

Fig. 1205. 5 1/2 year old. Foot, dorsoplantar.

1 Basal epiphysis of the 1st metatarsal
2 Medial cuneiform bone
3 Intermedial cuneiform bone
4 Lateral cuneiform bone
5 Cuboid bone
6 Navicular bone
7 Talus
8 Calcaneus
9 1st metatarsal head
10 Nucleus of the 5th metatarsal head

In all foot root bones (with the possible exception of the 3rd cuneiform), as well as on all the neighboring metatarsal heads, an osteochondrosis dissecans may appear, even in this stage of growth. The differential diagnosis of necrotic processes, from osteomyelitis or tuberculosis, can be radiographically difficult. Likewise, the differentiation of a primary asepses from a post-traumatic osteochondrosis dissecans may be difficult. Osteochondrosis dissecans of cuneiform bones I and II is diagnostically difficult to assess from the primary juvenile osteochondrosis. Such differences in the 3rd cuneiform bone, which begins to ossify in the 1st year of life, are not discernible because of the rarity of the observations of aseptic necroses.

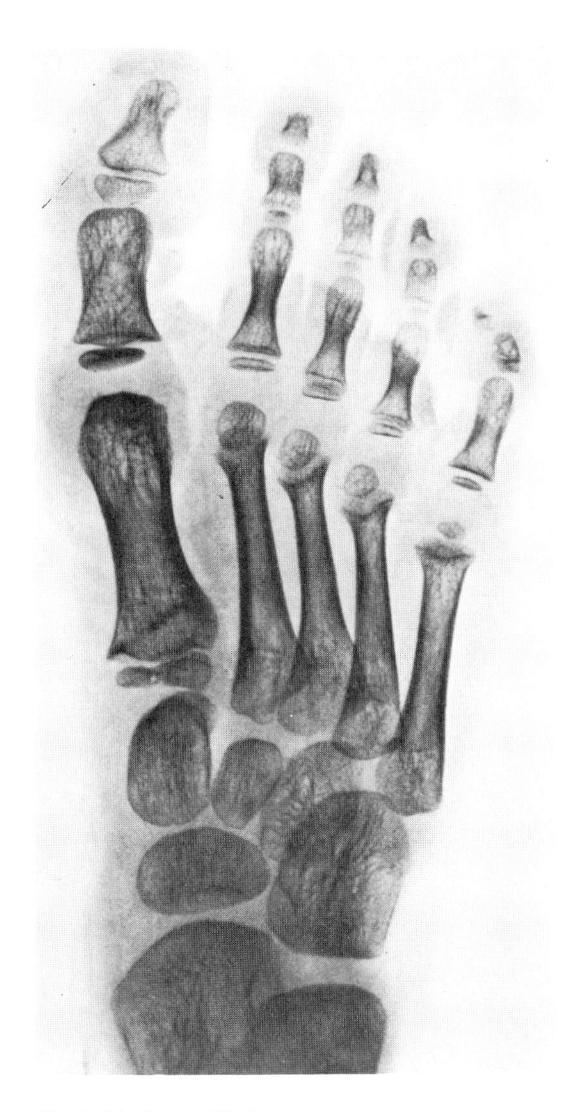

Fig. 1206. 6 year old. Average norm.

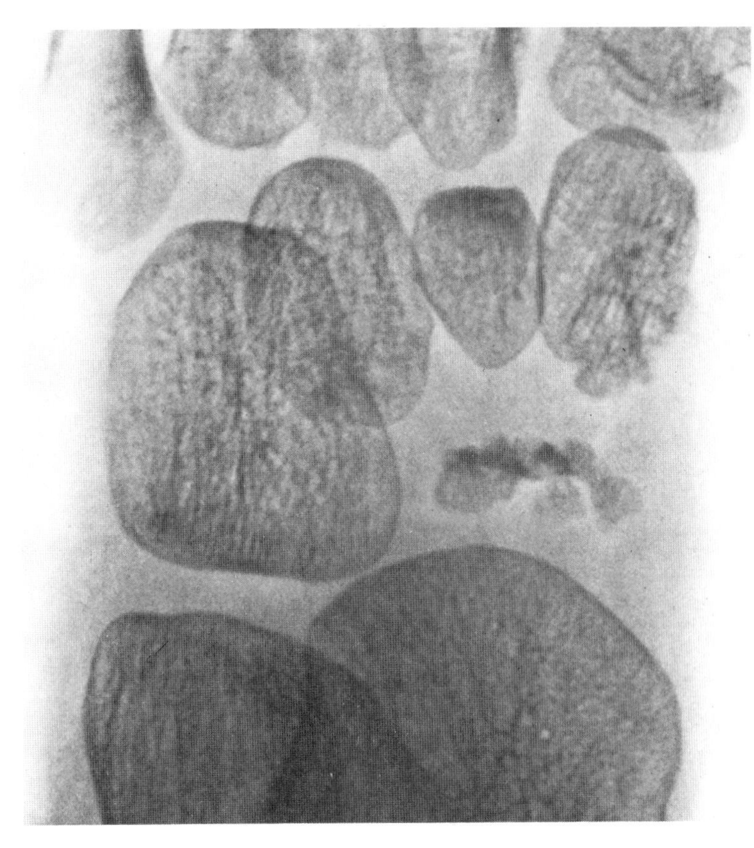

Fig. 1207. 6½ year old. Left foot root, dorsoplantar. This radiograph (from *E. Schulte)* shows a typical ossification of the navicular bone. This finding may be noted in both feet. Two-nuclei anlagen of this bone are frequent; three-nuclei anlagen are seldom found. In this radiograph there are five-nuclei anlagen. The structural development of the scaphoid bone and the special static type of burden on the foot arc cause the navicular to become a very delicate bone as early as the childhood years. (Short distance exposure).

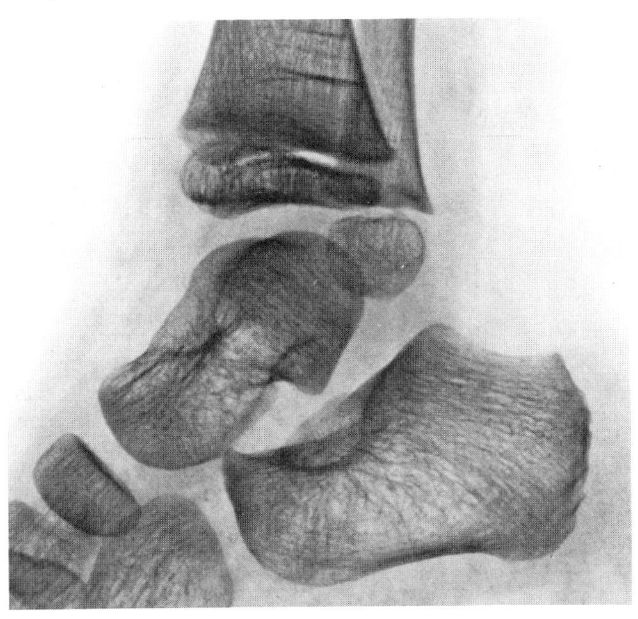

Fig. 1208 a

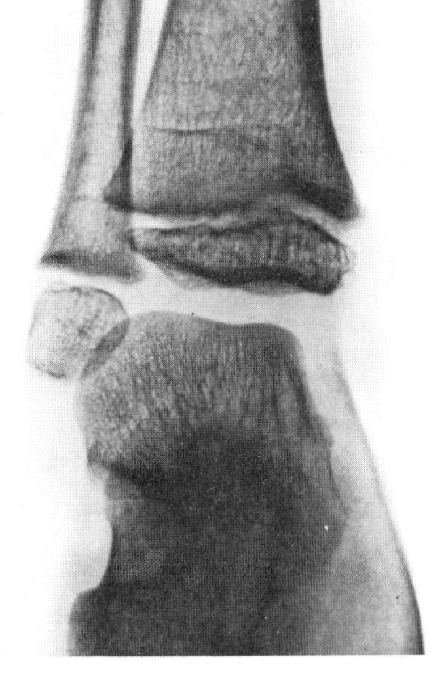

Fig. 1208 b

Fig. 1208. 6 year old. Average norm. Right foot articulation on two levels and foot, dorsoplantar. The rear calcaneal section now shows an undular and notchy contour. An apophysis that is variable in its form originates here at the age of 6 to 10 years in the joining region of the Achilles tendon.

Figs. 1209–1211. 8 year old. Average norm. Right foot articulation on two levels and foot, dorsoplantar; Fig. 1209.
The foot root bones gradually lose their round form, and show their final form. In the lateral picture, the nucleus of the calcaneal apophysis is discernible in its first stage. The medial malleolus begins to develop with an independent nucleus anlage (Fig. 1211). The malleolus, however, soon fuses with the tibial epiphysis.

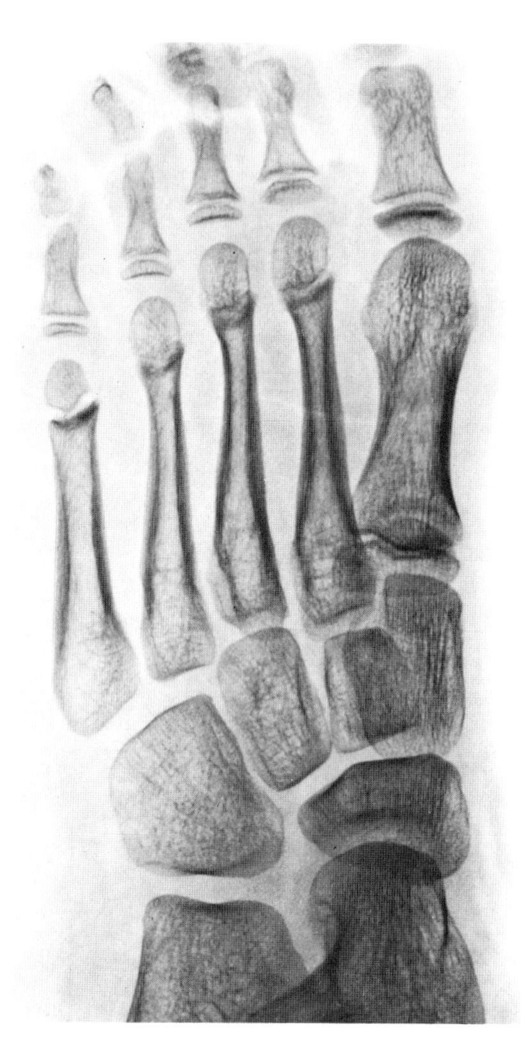

Fig. 1209

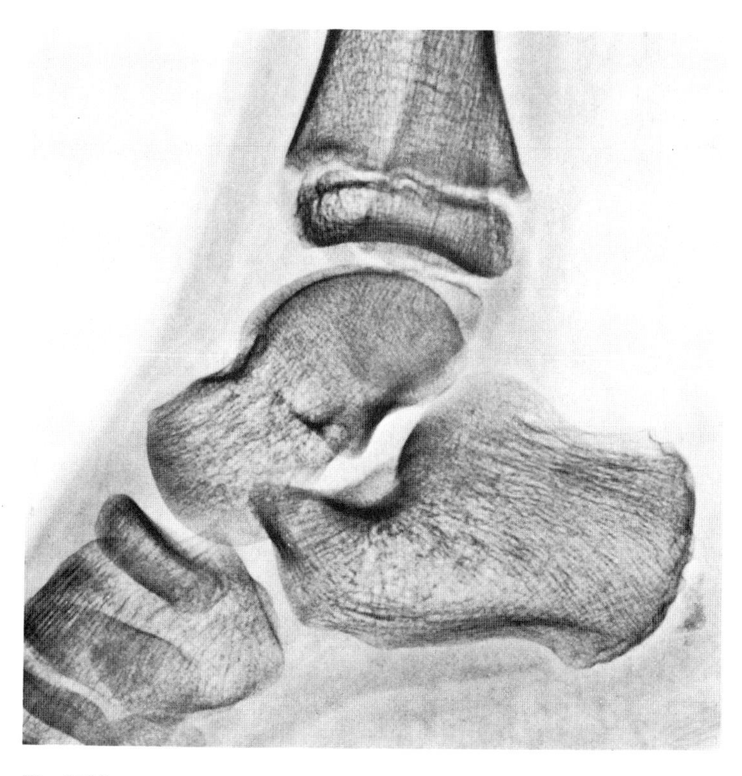

Fig. 1210

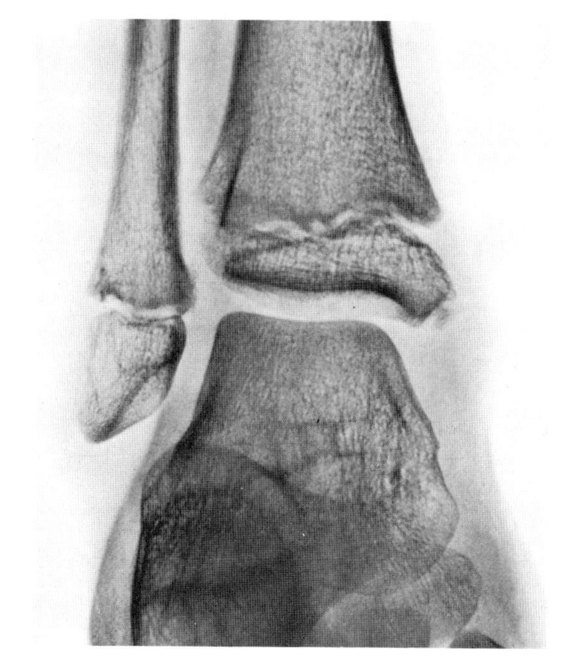

Fig. 1211

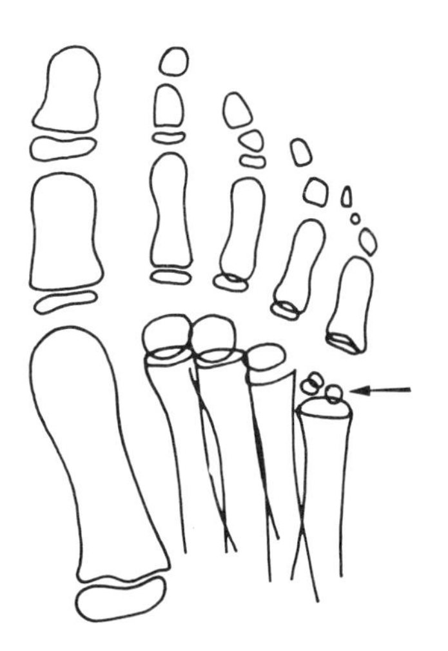

Fig. 1212. Forefoot of a 7-year-old child. The nuclei of the heads of the metatarsal bones can be arranged as a two-part or three-part nucleus.

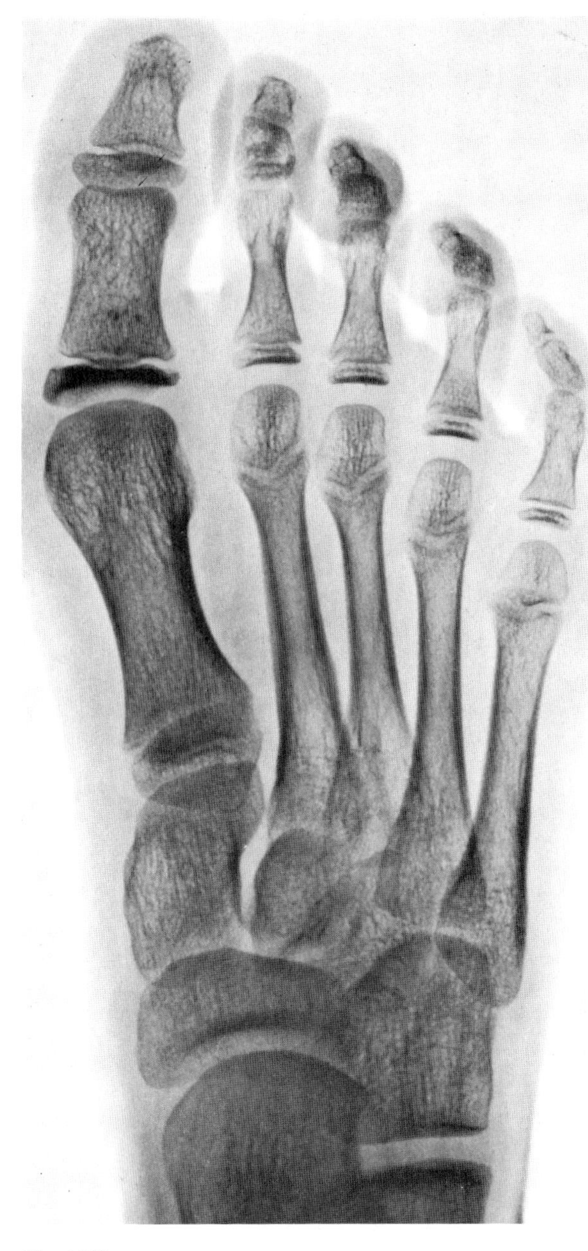

Fig. 1213

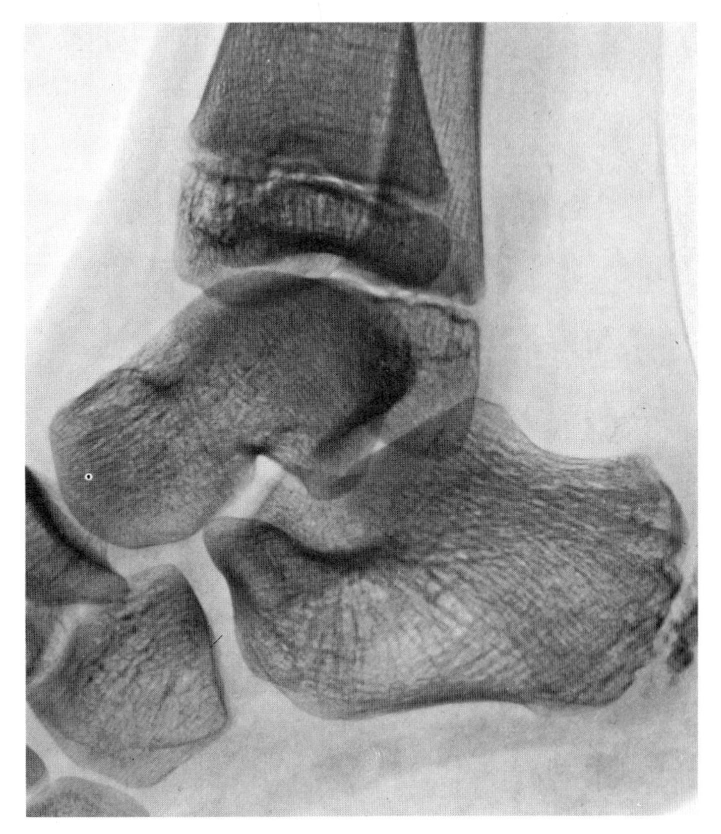

Fig. 1214

Figs. 1213–1215. 10 year old. Right foot, dorsoplantar and foot articulation on two levels. The medial malleolus is already clearly formed, as well as the nucleus of the calcaneal apophysis. In this case there is development of a flat foot with hallux vagus in a noticeable thickening of the basal phalanx epiphysis (probably ossification disorder). Noticeably curved calcaneal apophysis.

The calcaneal apophysis originates only about the 8th year of life, and can consist of many nuclei. It is therefore sensitive to mechanical damage, e.g., stretch deformations ("calcaneal apophysitis"). See *Bergmann.*

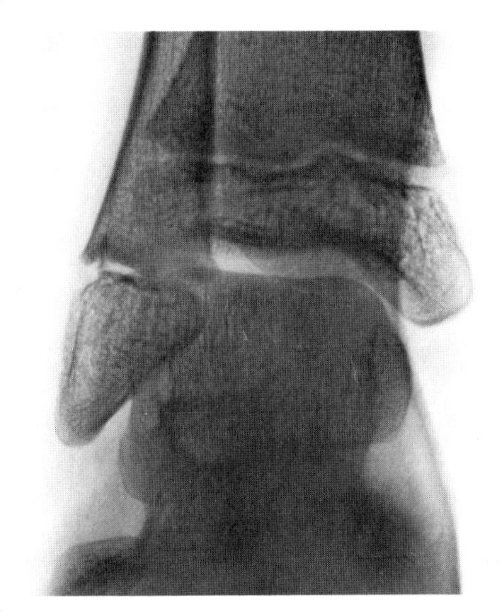

Fig. 1215

Fig. 1216. 9 year old.

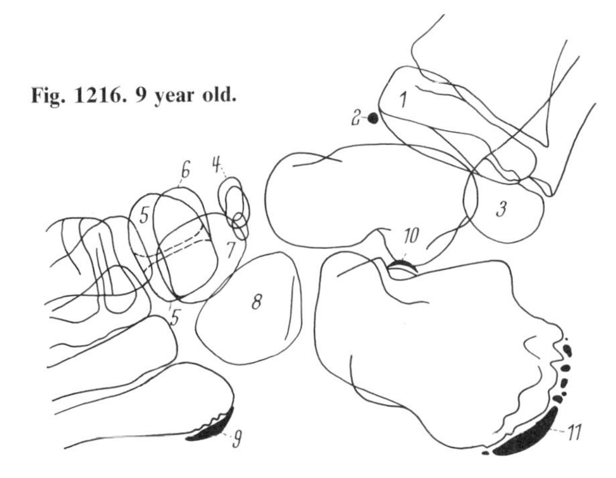

1 Tibial epiphysis
2 Nucleus in the medial malleolus
3 Fibular epiphysis
4 Navicular bone; may have several nuclei
5 Medial bipartitioned cuneiform bone; variants; also as twins (monozygotic) and bilaterally
6, 7 Intermedial and lateral cuneiform bones
8 Cuboid bone
9 Apophyseal nucleus in the 5th metatarsal tuberosity
10 Nucleus of the talus sustentaculum
11 Torn ossification anlage in the calcaneal tuber

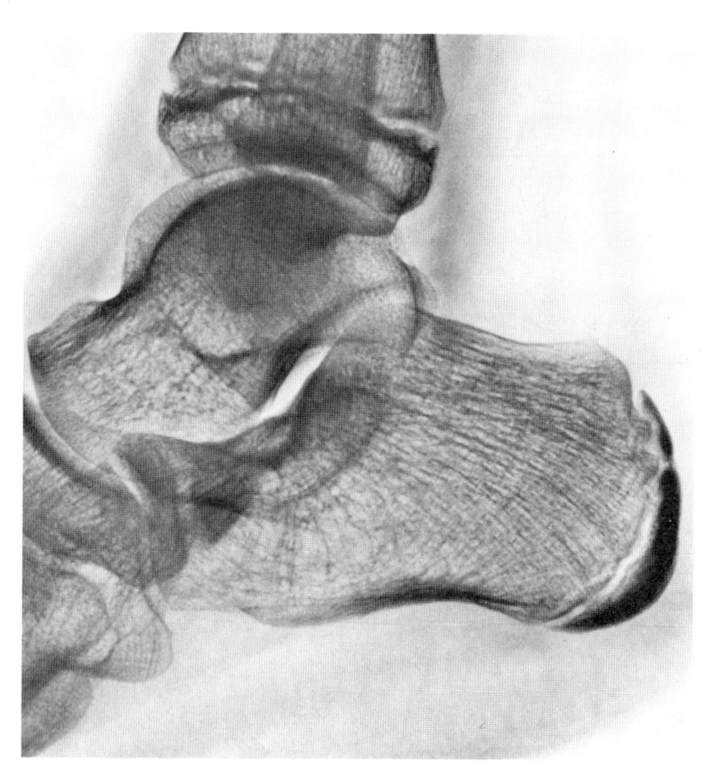

Fig. 1217

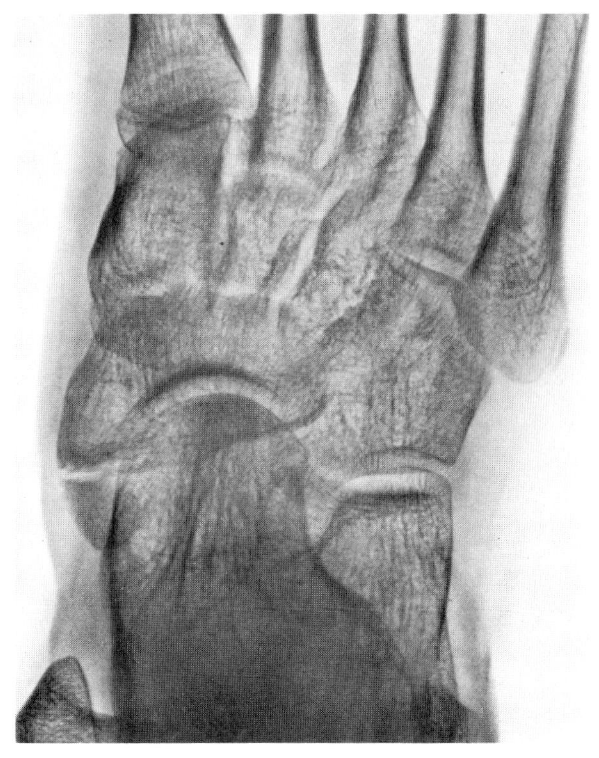

Fig. 1218

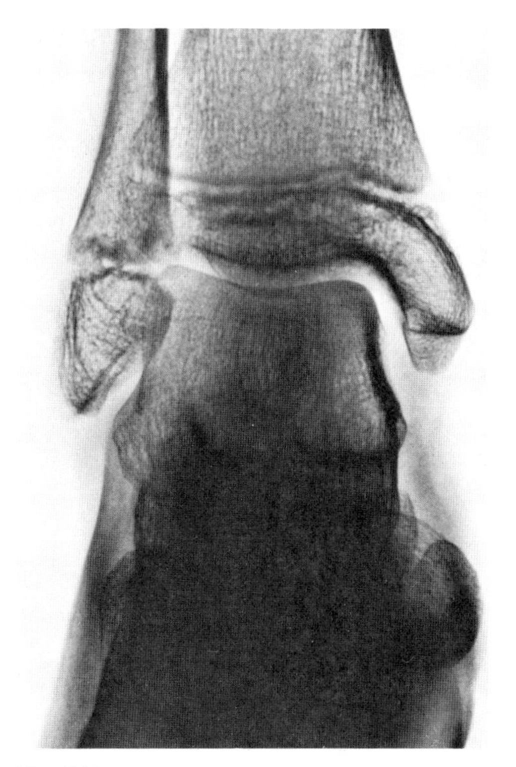

Fig. 1219

Figs. 1217–1219. 12 year old. Right foot articulation on two levels, the right foot root, dorsoplantar. The medial malleolus shows its final form; the calcaneal apophysis is completely ossified. It fuses with the calcaneus around the ages of 17 to 19. In Fig. 1218 a cup-shaped apophyseal nucleus, which may persist, is discernible on the external side of the basis of the 5th metatarsal (Fig. 822, No. 172*). An isolated osseous nucleus is discernible on the inner side of the navicular bone. When this nucleus persists, it is known as the external tibial bone (Fig. 822, No. 170).

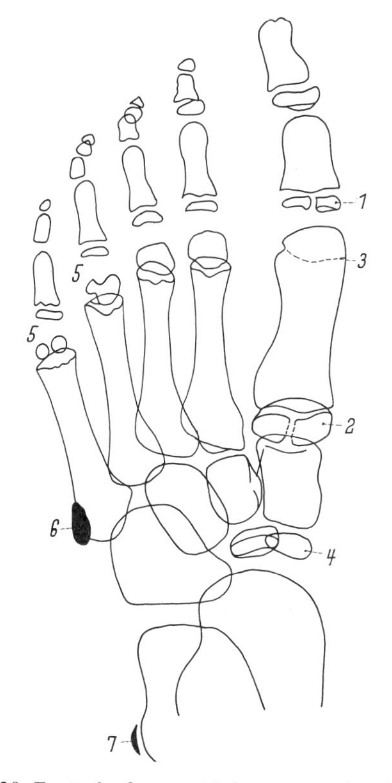

Fig. 1220. Foot of a 9 year old shows several variations.

1 Divided nucleus of the basal epiphyses of the hallux basal bone
2 Similarly in the basis of the 1st metatarsal
3 Pseudoepiphyseal fissure
4 Navicular bone (several nuclei)
5 Divided deformed ossification nuclei in the metatarsal heads. The heads can be divided into three or more parts.
6 Nucleus in the osseous tuberosity of the 5th metatarsal
7 Nucleus in the peroneal trochlea

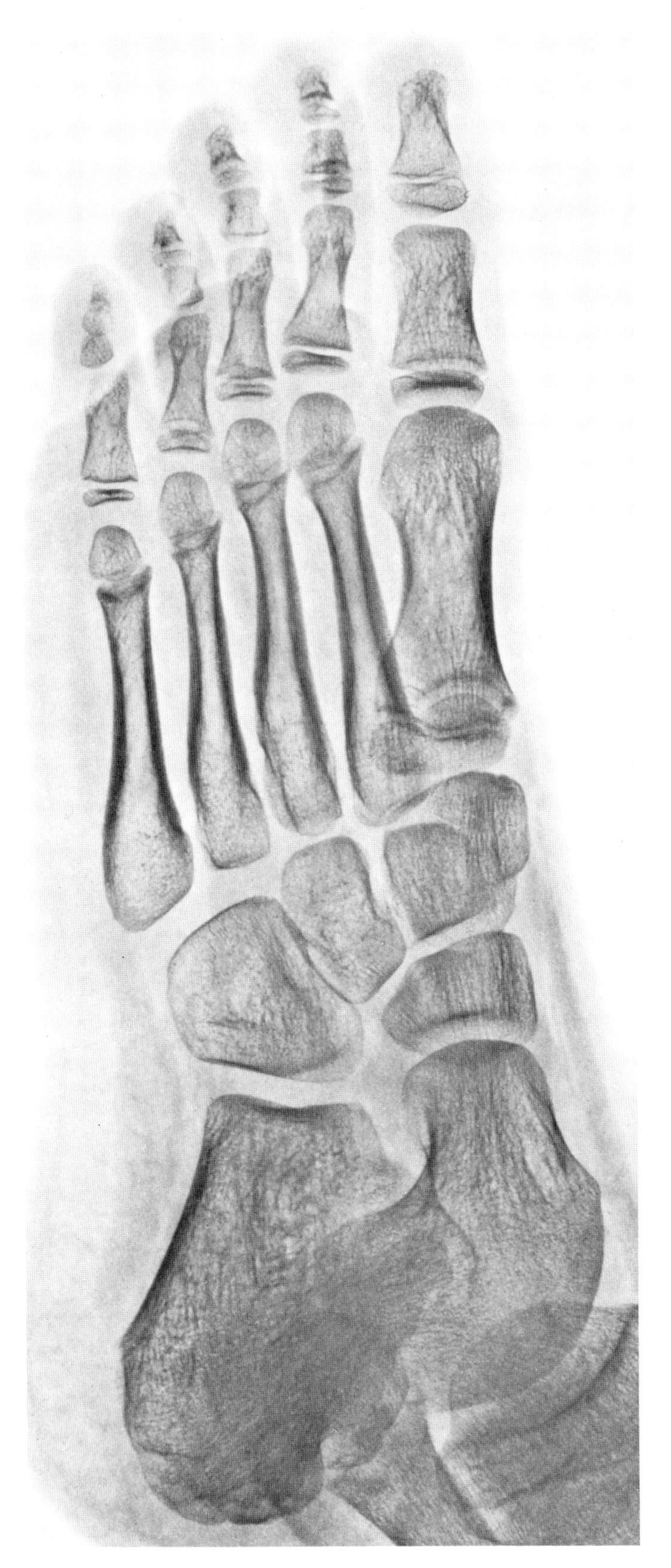

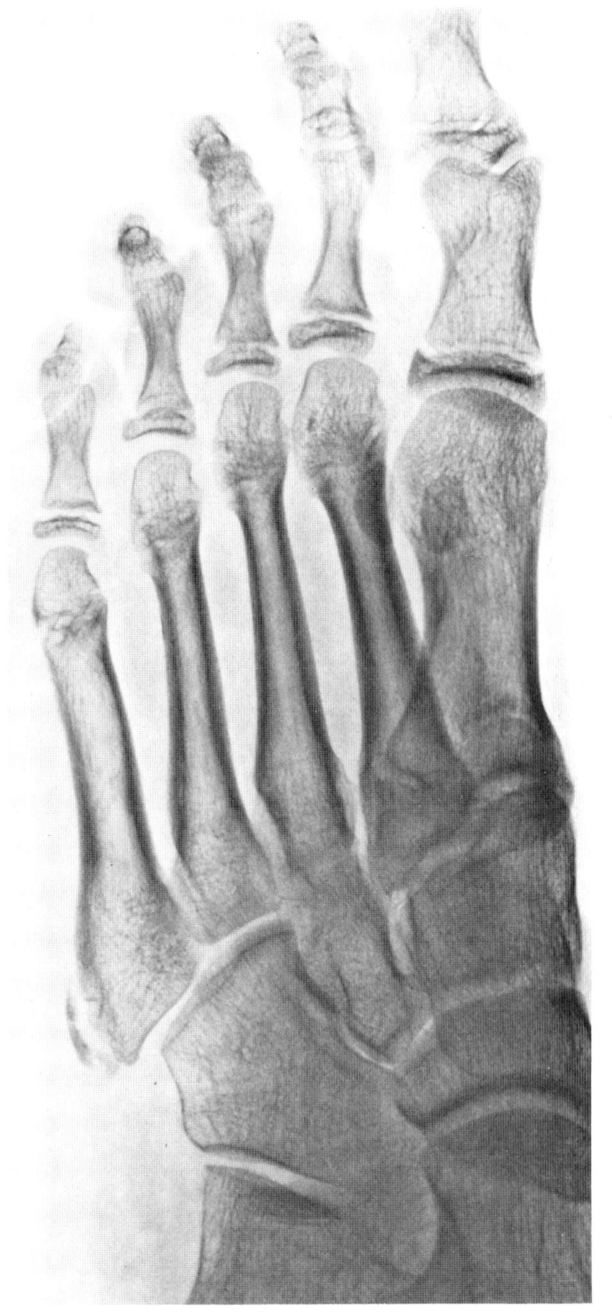

Fig. 1222. 14 year old. Right foot root, plantodorsal. Average norm. The apophyseal nucleus in the basal external part of the 5th metatarsal is well formed but originates from several ossification centers, which then fuse with each other. All epiphyseal fissures begin to narrow at puberty. Sesamoid bones in the 1st metatarsal head are well formed.

Fig. 1221. 13 year old. Left foot, diagonal. Lower norm. In comparison to the preceding radiographs, the foot root bones here show rounded contours. The medial malleolus is formed laterally and diagonally, and is still slightly imprinted. An apophyseal nucleus in the calcaneus is probably absent. In a rotated radiograph, the nucleus already appears to be fused with the calcaneal tuber. No sesamoid bones are discernible yet (9 to 12 years, slightly earlier in girls than in boys).

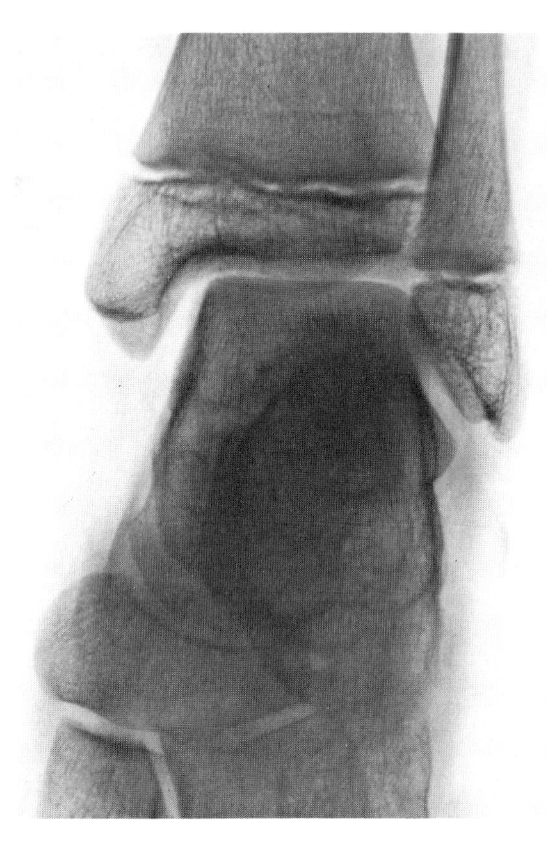

Fig. 1223

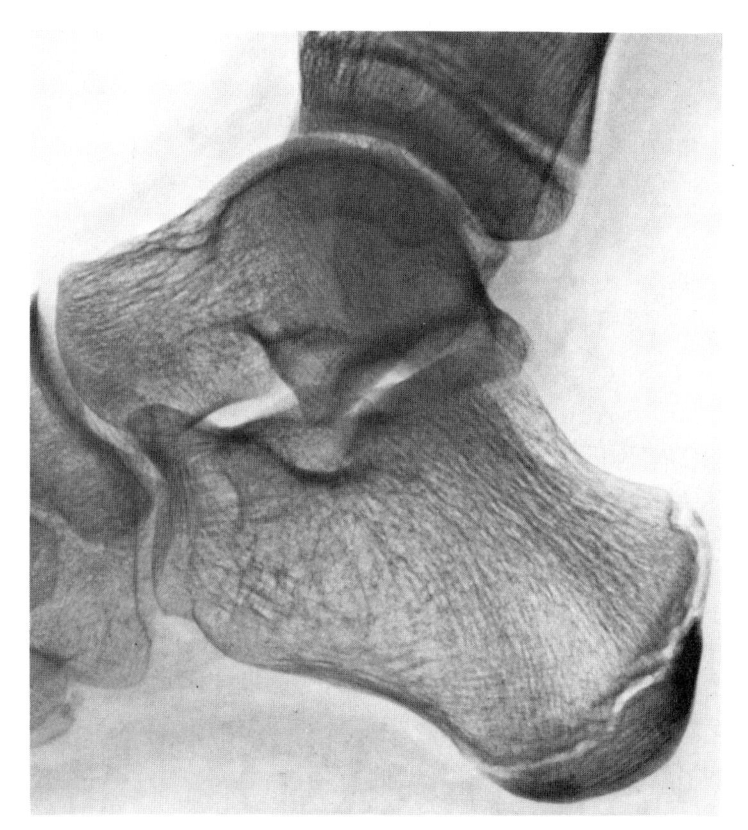

Fig. 1224

Figs. 1223 and 1224. 14 year old. Average norm. Left foot articulation, anteroposterior, and right foot articulation with the calcaneus, lateral.

Figs. 1225–1227. 17 year old. Left foot root with metatarsus, diagonal, and left foot articulation on two levels with the calcaneus, lateral.

The epiphyseal fissures are closed and thus growth has come to a standstill (17th–19th years of life). Thickenings at the distal extremities of the tibia and fibula show the localization of past epiphyseal sutures. A clear marginal fissure is still seen medially and dorsally in the fibular epiphysis. The medial sesamoid bone on the plantar side of the head of the 1st plantar bone is divided into two. The divisions of the sesamoid bones result from anlagen with several nuclei, or in juveniles they are a consequence of osteochondrosis. The clear, oblique division of the medial sesamoid bone and the smooth and regular bone structure indicate the multi-nuclei anlagen of the sesamoid bones.

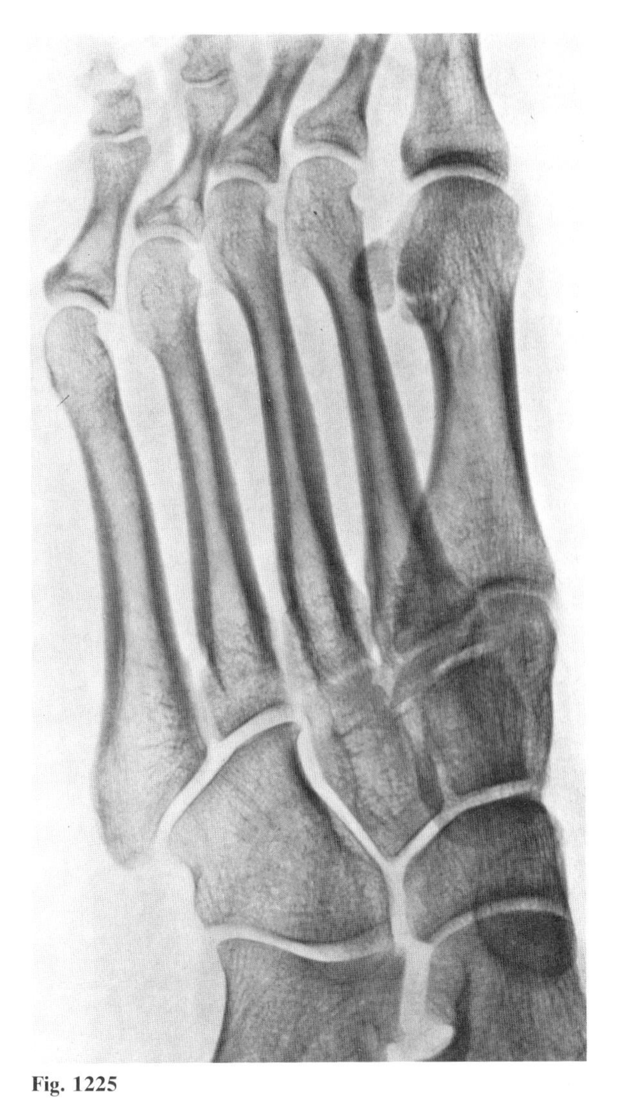

Fig. 1225

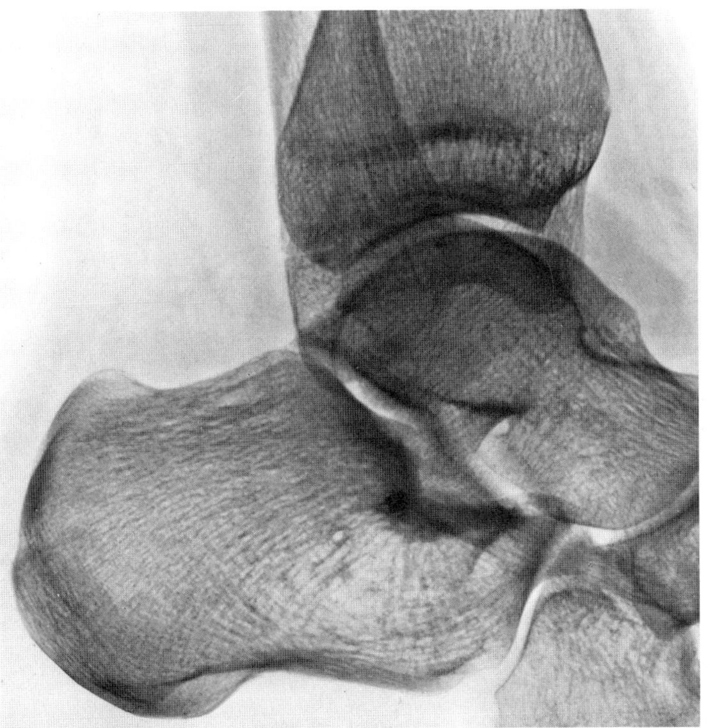

Fig. 1226

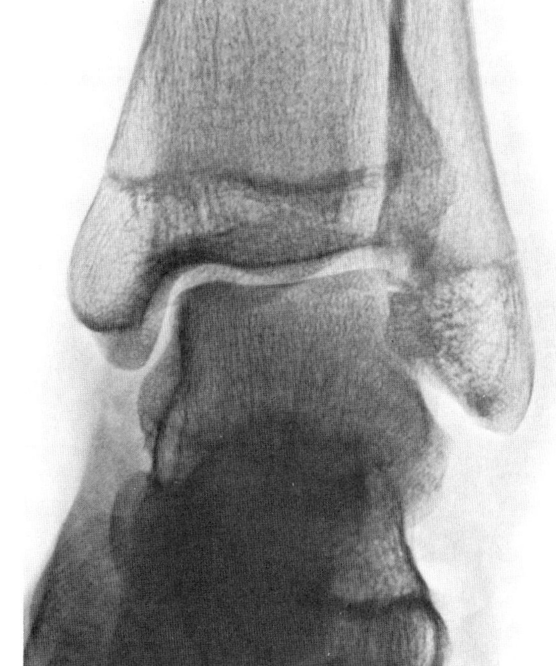

Fig. 1227

VI. Key Aseptic Bone Necroses

Table 17. Survey of the key aseptic bone necroses (from *Swoboda:* Das Skelett des Kindes, 2nd edition, Thieme, Stuttgart, 1956).

Position	*Name of Discoverer*	*Year*	*Disposition According to Age*	*Frequency*
Upper Extremities:				
Humeral head	*Haas*	1921		
Humeral capitulum	*Panner*	1927		
Distal ulnar epiphysis	*Burns*	1921	Mainly	
Scaphoid bone	*Preiser*	1911	adults	rare
Lunate bone	*Kienböck*	1910		
Metacarpal head	*Dietrich*	1932		
Entire carpus	*Caffey*	1945	Children	
Lower Extremities:				
Femoral head and neck	*Calvé-Legg-Perthes*	1909	age 4–10	+ + +
Idiopathic coxa vara			age 6–16	+ +
Patella	*Sinding-Larsen*	1921	age 8–12	+
Tibial apophysis	*Osgood-Schlatter*	1903	age 10–16	+ +
Proximal tibial metaphysis	*Blount*	1937	age 2–14	+
Talus	*Diaz*			
Tibia (external)	*Haglund*	1908		+ +
Calcaneal apophysis	*Haglund*	1902	age 5–15	+ +
Navicular bone	*Köhler (I)*	1903	age 4– 8	+ +
Intermedial cuneiform bone	*Hicks*	1953	age 4– 8	
Metatarsal head II	*Freiberg-Köhler (II)*	1914	age 11–18	
Metatarsal head V	*Iselin*	1912		
Pelvis:				
Ischiopubic synchondrosis	*van Neck*	1924		+ +
Symphyseal synchondrosis	*Pierson*	1929		+
Further Localizations:				
Anterior superior and inferior iliac spine				
Major and minor trochanter				
Ischiadic tuber				
Spinal Column:				
Vertebral body (vertebra plana)	*Calvé*	1925	age 4– 8	+
Vertebral disks and fillets	*Scheuermann*	1921	age 10–18	+ +

References

van Acken, F.: Die Sutura frontalis im Röntgenbild. Fortschr. Röntgenstr. 48 (1933), 209

Agostini, S.: Le fratture dello scafoide carpale. Clin. ortop. 13 (1961), 473

Åkerlund, A.: Entwicklungsreihen in Röntgenbildern von Hand, Fuß und Ellenbogen im Mädchen- und Knabenalter. Fortschr. Röntgenstr. Ergbd. 33 (1918)

Albers-Schönberg, H.: Die Röntgentechnik. 1. u. 2. Bd., Thieme, Leipzig 1940/41

Albert, E.: Über Meniskusganglien. Z. Orthop. 83 (1953), 228

Albert, E.: Veränderungen im Röntgenbild durch Meniskusganglien. Fortschr. Röntgenstr. 82 (1955), 282

Alexander, B.: Die Entwicklung der knöchernen Wirbelsäule. Fortschr. Röntgenstr. Ergbd. 13 (1906)

Alexander, C.: The aetiology of primary protrusio acetabuli. Brit. J. Radiol. 38 (1965), 567

Angerstein, W.: Lexikon der radiologischen Technik in der Medizin. VEB Georg Thieme, Leipzig 1975

Arens, W.: Über die angeborene Synostose zwischen dem Os lunatum und dem Os triquetrum. Fortschr. Röntgenstr. 73 (1950), 772

Arens, W.: Über eine doppelseitige Rückbildung des Kleinfingerstrahles bei zwei Brüdern. Fortschr. Röntgenstr. 74 (1951), 242

Arenz, J.: Seltene Lokalisation von Nebenkernbildungen der Hand. Fortschr. Röntgenstr. 82 (1955), 552

Auer, K.: Beitrag zur Topographie der Kieferhöhlen im Röntgenbild. Z. Laryng. Rhinol. 32 (1953), 206

Aufdermaur, M.: Die Pathogenese der Synchondrose bei der Spondylitis ankylopoetica. Dtsch. med. Wschr. 95 (1970), 110

Aumann, U.: Apophyse am Margo vertebralis scapulae? Fortschr. Röntgenstr. 110 (1969), 409

Baastrup, Ch. I.: Proc. spin. vert. lumb. und einige zwischen diesen liegende Gelenkbildungen mit pathologischen Prozessen in dieser Region. Fortschr. Röntgenstr. 48 (1933), 430

Baensch, W.: Pränatale Röntgendiagnostik des kindlichen Skeletts. Fortschr. Röntgenstr. 90 (1959), 368

Balz, G.: Röntgenologisches Verfahren zur quantitativen Beurteilung des Mineralgehaltes an der Grundphalanx des Daumens. Fortschr. Röntgenstr. 113 (1970), 581

Balz, G. u. R. Birkner: Die Bestimmung des Aluminiumschwächungsgleichwertes von Knochengewebe beim Lebenden. Strahlentherapie 99 (1956), 221

Balz, G., R. Birkner u. J. M. Schmitt-Rohde: Über die calcipenischen Osteopathien und ihre Diagnostik mit Hilfe eines besonderen Röntgenverfahrens. Ärztl. Wschr. 12 (1957), 209 u. 233

Balz, G., R. Birkner u. F. Wachsmann: Experimentelle Untersuchungen über die Absorption von Röntgenstrahlen in verschiedenen Geweben. Strahlentherapie 97 (1955), 382

Bánki, Z.: Apophysenähnliche posttraumatische Verkalkung im Ellengelenk. Fortschr. Röntgenstr. 101 (1964), 96

Bánki, Z.: Über den Processus costalis sterni. Fortschr. Röntgenstr. 102 (1965), 518

Bánki, Z.: Ossifikationsindex der Apophysen des distalen Humerusendes. Fortschr. Röntgenstr. 107 (1967), 791

Bánki, Z.: Die Apophyse mit Fortsatzbildung des Epicondylus medialis humeri. Fortschr. Röntgenstr. 107 (1967), 815

Barclay, M.: A case of duplication of the internal cuneiform bone of the foot. J. Anat. (Lond.) 67 (1932), 175

Barrois, J., J. Piquet et C. Deguine: Confrontation radio-clinique de l'analyse tomographique du rocher. J. belge Radiol. 54 (1971), 293

Bársony, Th. u. K. Winkler: Beiträge zur Röntgenologie der Wirbelsäule. Röntgenpraxis 9 (1937), 601

Bartelheimer, H.: Hyperostosen des Hirnschädels bei Regulationskrankheiten. Fortschr. Röntgenstr. 71 (1949), 118

Bartelheimer, H.: Formen und Entstehungsbedingungen der Entkalkungsosteopathien. Ärztl. Wschr. 6 (1951), 606

Bartelheimer, H.: Mineralhaushalt und Knochen. Klinik. Fortschr. Röntgenstr. 86 (1957), Beih. 39, 59

Bartelheimer, H.: Zur Klinik und Röntgenologie der systemartigen kalzipenischen Osteopathien. Dtsch. med. Wschr. 82 (1957), 1400 u. 1424

Bartelheimer, H. u. J. M. Schmitt-Rohde: Osteoporose als Krankheitsgeschehen. Ergebn. inn. Med. Kinderheilk., N. F. 7 (1956), 454

Bartelink, D. L.: Röntgenschnitte. Fortschr. Röntgenstr. 47 (1933), 399

Barucha, E.: Unsere Erfahrungen über den Wert des *Rauber*schen Röntgenzeichens bei der Meniscusdiagnose. Mschr. Unfallheilk. 63 (1960), 370

Bauer, R.: Beitrag zur Osteochondrosis dissecans patellae. Z. Orthop. 103 (1967), 64

Bažant, B.: Doppelter Ossifikationskern im Fersenbein. Z. Orthop. 98 (1964), 523

Becker, J.: Phalangeale Pseudoepiphysen. Röntgenpraxis 2 (1930), 559

Becker, Th.: Schwerarbeit und degenerativer Wirbelumbau. Dtsch. Gesundh.-Wes. 14 (1959), 1241

Beeler, J. W.: Further evidence on the acquired nature of spondylolysis and spondylolisthesis. Amer. J. Roentgenol. 108 (1970), 796

Bennholdt-Thomsen, C. u. J. Freund: Physiologie und Pathologie der Pubertät. In: Pädiatrie. Springer, Berlin-Göttingen-Heidelberg 1957

Benninghoff-Goerttler: Lehrbuch der Anatomie des Menschen. Bd. I, Urban u. Schwarzenberg, München-Berlin 1968

van de Berg et M. Crèvecoeur: La méniscographie en série du genou. Acta orthop. belg. 19 (1953), 293

Bergerhoff, W.: Wachstum und Bauplan des Schädels im Röntgenbild. Fortschr. Röntgenstr. 79 (1953), 745

Bergerhoff, W.: Über röntgenologische Sellamessungen. Fortschr. Röntgenstr. 85 (1956), 695

Bergerhoff, W. u. W. Höbler: Messungen von Winkeln und Strecken am Röntgenbild des Schädels von Kindern und Jugendlichen. Fortschr. Röntgenstr. 78 (1953), 190

Bergerhoff, W. u. M. Martin: Messungen von Winkeln und Strecken am Röntgenbild des Schädels von Säuglingen und Kleinkindern. Fortschr. Röntgenstr. 80 (1954), 742

Bergmann, E.: Die Calcaneusepiphyse. Arch. klin. Chir. 141 (1926), 463

Bernardeau, M.-M.-J.: L'os acromial. Thèse, Bordeaux 1907

Bernbeck, R.: Einfache klinische Röntgendiagnostik der Femurtorsion bei Luxationshüften. Fortschr. Röntgenstr. 75 (1951), 331

Bernbeck, R.: Kinderorthopädie. Thieme, Stuttgart 1954

Bessler, W.: Die diagnostischen Möglichkeiten der Doppelkontrast-Arthrographie des Kniegelenks. Fortschr. Röntgenstr. 101 (1964), 511

Bessler, W. u. M. E. Müller: Zur Röntgendiagnose der Coxa valga und Coxa vara. Radiol. clin. (Basel) 32 (1963), 538

Billing, L.: Roentgen examination of the proximal femur end in children and adolescents. A standardized technique also suitable for determination of the collum -, anteversion - and epiphysial angles. A study of slipped epiphysis and coxa plana. Acta radiol. (Stockh.) Suppl. 110 (1954)

Bircher, E.: Neue Fälle von Varietäten der Handwurzel und des Fußgelenks. Fortschr. Röntgenstr. 26 (1918/19), 85

Birkner, R.: Der tomographische Horizontalschnitt des Felsenbeins. Klin. Wschr. 26 (1948), 568

Birkner, R.: Der tomographische Horizontalschnitt des Felsenbeins. Fortschr. Röntgenstr. 71 (1949), 349

Birkner, R.: Antwort auf Frage 39 (Fortschr. Röntgenstr. 82, Heft 1, Seite 134). Fortschr. Röntgenstr. 82 (1955), 695

Birkner, R.: Zum Röntgenbild des proximalen Schienbeindrittels. Erwiderung zur gleichnamigen Veröffentlichung von *A. Ravelli.* Fortschr. Röntgenstr. 82 (1955), 542

Birkner, R.: Einseitiges Iliacalhorn. Fortschr. Röntgenstr. 105 (1966), 910

Birkner, R.: Fehldeutungen durch Varia und Pathologica im Röntgenbild des Schädels. Röntgen-Bl. 21 (1968), 555

Birkner, R. u. K. Lagemann: Ausgedehnte Verkalkungen bei Pachymeningitis haemorrhagica interna und Haematoma subdurale. Fortschr. Röntgenstr. 105 (1966), 377

Birkner, R. u. K. Oldenburg: Tabellarische Übersicht über die wichtigsten Daten der Röntgenverordnung vom 1. 3. 1973. Med. Klin. 69 (1974) Nr. 14

Birkner, R. u. K. Consentius: Verknöcherungen in der Wand des Foramen obturatum. Fortschr. Röntgenstr. (im Druck, 1977)

Blank, N. and A. Lieber: The significance of Growing Bone Islands. Radiology 85 (1965), 508

Blankenburg, R.: Die Patella bipartita und ihre Differentialdiagnose. Beitr. Orthop. 13 (1966), 83

Blount, W. P.: Osteochondrosis deformans tibiae. J. Bone Jt Surg. 19 (1937), 1

Böhler, J.: Morphologie der Halswirbelverletzungen nach ätiologischen Gesichtspunkten. H. Unfallheilk. 108 (1971), 10

Böker, H. u. W. Müller: Das Os cuneiforme I bipartitum, eine fortschreitende Umkonstruktion des Quergewölbes im menschlichen Fuß. Anat. Anz. 83 (1936), 193

Boll, I. u. J. M. Schmitt-Rohde: Osteoporose bei der perniciösen Anämie. Ärztl. Wschr. 12 (1957), 419

Boone, M. L., B. E. Swenson and B. Felson: Rib notching: its many causes. Amer. J. Roentgenol. 91 (1964), 1075

Borell, U. and J. Fernström: The diagnostic value of disalignment of the foetal cranial vault bones in intrauterine foetal death. A roentgenologic study. Acta radiol. (Stockh.) 49 (1958), 409

Boulay, du G. and Th. Bostick: Linear tomography in congenital abnormalities of the ear. Brit. J. Radiol. 42 (1969), 161

Boulet, P. et J. Mirouze: Les ostéoses diabétiques. (Ostéoporose et hyperostose) Ann. Méd. 55 (1954), 674

Brat, L.: Klinische Fehldiagnose durch abnorm langen Griffelfortsatz des Felsenbeins. Fortschr. Röntgenstr. 75 (1951), 758

Brauer, W.: Zur posttraumatischen Ossifikation akzessorischer Ossa. Fortschr. Röntgenstr. 90 (1959), 713

Brauer, W. u. C. Coutelle: Verlauf und Histologie einer Melorheostose. Fortschr. Röntgenstr. 105 (1966), 77

Braus, H.: Anatomie des Menschen. 1. Bd. Springer, Berlin-Göttingen-Heidelberg 1954

Breschet, M. G.: Recherches anatomiques, physiologiques et pathologiques sur le système veineux. Villaret, Paris 1829

Brocher, J. E. W.: Mehrfach angeborene Fehlbildungen der Wirbelsäule. Fortschr. Röntgenstr. 58 (1938), 440

Brocher, J. E. W.: Die Okzipito-Zervikal-Gegend. Thieme, Stuttgart 1955

Brocher, J. E. W.: Atlas und Axis. Fortschr. Röntgenstr. 84 (1956), 387

Brocher, J. E. W.: In: Röntgendiagnostik, Ergebnisse 1952 - 1956. Thieme, Stuttgart 1957

Brocher, J. E. W.: Konstitutionell bedingte Veränderungen des Wirbelbogens. Fortschr. Röntgenstr. 92 (1960), 363

Brocher, J. E. W.: Die Wirbelsäulenleiden und ihre Differentialdiagnose. 5. Aufl. Thieme, Stuttgart 1970

Broman, I.: Normale und abnormale Entwicklung des Menschen. Wiesbaden 1911

Broman, I.: Die Entwicklung des Menschen vor der Geburt. München 1927

Bronner, H. u. C. E. Koch: Die Röntgendarstellung der Jochbögen. Röntgenpraxis 2 (1930), 754

Bruch, G., K. A. Bushe u. A. Gregl: Die nichtpathologischen intrakraniellen Verkalkungen. Fortschr. Röntgenstr. 103 (1965), 444

Brünner, S., O. Petersen and P. Stocksted: Tomography of the auditory ossicles. Acta radiol. (Stockh.) 56 (1961), 20

Bruno, G.: Über senile Strukturveränderungen der proximalen Humerusepiphyse. Fortschr. Röntgenstr. 50 (1934), 287

Bucke, B.: Ein Beitrag zum familiären Auftreten der Brachydaktylie. Z. menschl. Vererb.- u. Konstit.- Lehre 37 (1964), 305

Budin, E. and F. Sondheimer: Lateral spread of the atlas without fracture. Radiology 87 (1966), 1095

Buetti-Bäuml, C.: Funktionelle Röntgendiagnostik der Halswirbelsäule. Thieme, Stuttgart 1954

Burrows, F. G. O.: Some aspects of occult spinal dysraphsm: A study of 90 cases. Brit. J. Radiol. 41 (1968), 496

Busch, G.: Verknöcherung des Lig. sacro-spinale. Fortschr. Röntgenstr. 82 (1955), 281

Buse, H.: Beitrag zur Persistenz der Olecranonepiphyse. Fortschr. Röntgenstr. 104 (1966), 867

Butt, W. P. and E. Samuel: Radiologic anatomy of the proximal end of the femur. J. Canad. Ass. Radiol. 17 (1966), 103

Buysch, K. H., J. Drewes u. D. Günther: Synostosen zwischen Multangulum minus und Capitatum. Fortschr. Röntgenstr. 115 (1971), 267

Caffey, J.: On the accessory ossicles of the supraoccipital bone. Some newly recognised roentgen features of the normal infantile skull. Amer. J. Roentgenol. 70 (1953), 401

Caffey, J.: Pediatric X-ray Diagnosis. Year Book Med. Publishers 5. edit., Chicago 1967

Calandriello, B.: Le sinostosi vertebrali intersomatiche. Arch. Putti Chir. Organi Mov. 6 (1955), 109

Camp, J. D.: Significance of intracranial calcification in the roentgenologic of intracranial neoplasms. Radiology 55 (1950), 659

Canigiani, G., J. Wickenhauser u. W. Czech: Beitrag zur Osteochondrosis dissecans im Foramen supratrochleare. Fortschr. Röntgenstr. 117 (1972), 66

Carey, J. P., M. C. u. L. Drexler: Ein atypischer Knochen an der Planta Pedis. Fortschr. Röntgenstr. 86 (1957), 526

Carones, C.: Ein Fall von Mißbildung infolge übertriebener Entwicklung der großen Hörner des Zungenbeines. Rev. méd. del Rosario 17 (1927), 230; ref. Zbl. ges. Radiol. 4 (1928), 481

Carstens, M.: Die Selladiagnostik. Fortschr. Röntgenstr. 71 (1949), 257

Casazza, A.: La sella turcica nei diversi tipi costitutionali cranici. Boll. Soc. ital. Biol. sper. 7 (1932), 1295

Cascelli, G.: Über Rippenanomalien. Röntgenpraxis 12 (1940), 375

Castrucci, A.: Studio stratigrafico dell' osso temporale con apparecchio a traiettoria pluridiregionale. Roentgen-Europ. 2 (1961), 102

Cella, C. e A. Toscano: Osservazione sull'indagine stratigrafica in casi di mastoidite e di petrosite (Riscontro operatio). Ann. Radiol diagn. (Bologna) 24 (1952), 206

Chambers, W. R.: Diastematomyelie. J. Pediat. 45 (1954), 668

Chaussé, C.: Premiers résultats d'une méthode personnelle de radiodiagnostic des tumeurs de l'auditif. Acta otolaryng. 2 (1948), 245

Chobot, R. and E. F. Merill: Bone scarings in normal and allergic children. J. Allergy 8 (1937), 588

Clementschitsch, F.: Die Röntgendarstellung des Gesichtsschädels. 2. Aufl. Urban u. Schwarzenberg, Wien 1950

Climelli, D.: Intorno ad alcuni casi di unione atlo-occipitale. Chir. Organi Mov. 24 (1939), 573

Cocchi, U.: Zur Frage der Epiphysenossifikation des Humeruskopfes. Radiol. clin. (Basel) 19 (1950), 18

Cocchi, U.: Hepatogene Osteoporosen. Radiol. clin. (Basel) 20 (1951), 362

Cockshott, W. P.: Carpal fusions. Amer. J. Roentgenol. 89 (1963), 1260

Cohen, A. S.: The „normal" sacroiliac joint. Amer. J. Roentgenol. 100 (1967), 559

Colin, A.: The aetiology of primary protrusio acetabuli. Brit. J. Radiol. 38 (1965), 567

Collard, M. u. P. Brasseur: Röntgenologischer Nachweis des traumatischen Ursprungs einer Spondylolyse. Fortschr. Röntgenstr. 117 (1972), 647

Colosimo, C.: Xifisterno biforcato ed abnormemente lungo. Radiol. med. (Torino) 26 (1939), 42

Consentius, K.: Die Entwicklung der behandelten Achsenabweichungen an rachitischen unteren Extremitäten. Diss. Berlin 1973

Cook, R. C. M.: Spina bifida and hydrocephalus. Brit. med. J. 4 (1971), 796

Corning, H. K.: Lehrbuch der topographischen Anatomie. 24. Aufl. Springer, Berlin-Göttingen-Heidelberg 1949
Crocellà, A.: Anatomia radiografica delle suture del cranio. Arch. ital. Anat. Embriol. 60 (1955), 201
Csákány, G. u. S. Álmos: Echte Spondylolisthese der Halswirbelsäule. Fortschr. Röntgenstr. 91 (1959), 277
Csákány, G. u. T. Donáth: Vergleichende röntgenanatomische Untersuchung der beiderseitigen Foramina jugularia. Fortschr. Röntgenstr. 88 (1958), 439
Curtius, F.: Spina bifida occulta. Dtsch. med. Wschr. 96 (1971), 709
Cuveland, de E.: Die Apophyse des Metatarsale V und Os vesalianum. Fortschr. Röntgenstr. 82 (1955), 251
Cuveland, de E.: Über eine nicht ausentwickelte, isoliert gebliebene, dorsale Dornfortsatzanlage (Osteochondrom); zugleich ein Beitrag zu den angeborenen Bogenspalten. Fortschr. Röntgenstr. 82 (1955), 416
Cuveland, de E.: Über Beziehungen zwischen vorderer Außenknöchelapophyse und Os subfibulare mit differentialdiagnostischen Erwägungen. Fortschr. Röntgenstr. 83 (1955), 213
Cuveland, de E.: Über das sogenannte Os parasternale. Fortschr. Röntgenstr. 84 (1956), 375
Cuveland, de E.: Über einen abnormen Fortsatz am Darmbein. Fortschr. Röntgenstr. 84 (1956), 379
Cuveland, de E.: Zur Ossifikation des Os naviculare pedis. Fortschr. Röntgenstr. 84 (1956), 710
Cuveland, de E.: Gibt es ein „Os accessorium supracalcaneum"? Fortschr. Röntgenstr. 85 (1956), 58
Cuveland, de E.: Beitrag zu den am medialen Fußrand vorkommenden inkonstanten Skelettelementen. Arch. orthop. Unfall-Chir. 49 (1957), 321
Cuveland, de E.: Inkonstante Skelettelemente (Ossa accessoria) des Fußes. Fortschr. Med. 75 (1957), 351
Cuveland, de E.: Zur Ossifikation des 1. Keilbeines. Z. Orthop. 89 (1957), 266
Cuveland, de E.: Selten beobachtete Ossifikationen am menschlichen Tarsus. Z. Orthop. 89 (1957), 268
Cuveland, de E.: Defekt der lateralen Eminentia-Zacke des Kniegelenks. Ärztl. Prax. 11 (1959), 1891
Cuveland, de E.: Brückenbildungen zwischen den Querfortsätzen von Lendenwirbeln. Ärztl. Forsch. 14 (1960), 449
Cuveland, de E.: Fehlbildung der Großzehengrundphalanx. Fortschr. Röntgenstr. 107 (1967), 570
Cuveland, de E. u. F. Heuck: Osteochondropathie eines akzessorischen Knochenkernes am Malleolus tibiae (des sog. Os subtibiale). Fortschr. Röntgenstr. 79 (1953), 728
Dahm, M.: Zur Problematik einiger Schädeldefekte. Fortschr. Röntgenstr. 76 (1952), 191
Dann, D. S., S. Rubin, I. Birenboim and A. Austin: Value of roentgen study of ethmoid sinuses through the orbital window. Amer. J. Roentgenol. 70 (1953), 226
Davidoff, L. M. and H. Gass: Convolutional markings in the skull roentgenograms of patients with headache. Amer. J. Roentgenol. 61 (1949), 317
Davies, D.: Ankylosing spondylitis and lung fibrosis. Quart. J. Med. 41 (1972), 395
Davies, D. A. and F. G. Parsons: The age order of the appearance and union of the normal epiphyses as seen by X-ray. J. Anat. (Lond.) 62 (1927), 58
Decker, K., H. Fischgold, H. Hacker u. J. Metzger: Entwicklungsstörungen am atlanto-okzipitalen Übergang. Fortschr. Röntgenstr. 84 (1956), 47
Dederich, R.: Kongenitale Synostosen von Handwurzelknochen. Mschr. Unfallheilk. 58 (1955), 112
Delvigne, J.: Une malformation rare de l'apophyse odontoïde de l'axis. J. belge Radiol. 46 (1963), 427
Denisch, E. W.: The cartilage endplates of the human vertebral column (some considerations of postnatal development). Anat. Rec. 169 (1971), 705
Dihlmann, W.: Über ein besonderes Coxarthrosezeichen (Pseudofrakturlinie) im Röntgenbild. (Kritik des sogenannten *Mach*effektes). Fortschr. Röntgenstr. 100 (1964), 383
Dihlmann, W.: Gelenke-Wirbelverbindungen. Thieme, Stuttgart 1972
Dierks, K.: Handwurzelröntgenogramme von Neugeborenen und ihre Bedeutung für die Reife der Frucht. Arch. Gynäk. 150 (1932)
Diethelm, L: Zur Kenntnis der Entwicklungsgeschichte der Wirbelsäule und der Wirbelkörperfehlbildungen. Fortschr. Röntgenstr. 69 (1944), 143
Diethelm, L.: Fehlbildungen des Corpus vertebrae. In Hdb. d. Med. Radiologie. Bd. VI/1, Springer, Berlin - Heidelberg - New York 1974, 190 ff.
Dietzel, F. u. H. F. Schirmer: Doppelseitige Ermüdungsfraktur der ersten Rippe - Entstehung unter typischer Belastung. Fortschr. Röntgenstr. 117 (1972), 228
Dittert, R.: Ungewöhnlicher Sitz einer Peritendinitis calcarea. Fortschr. Röntgenstr. 90 (1959), 523
Djian, A. et P. Scali: Le tomogramme de la base du crâne sur le vivant. J. Radiol. Électrol. 31 (1950), 271
Döhner: Vorgetäuschte Schädelfraktur. Röntgenpraxis 8 (1936), 246
Doesel, H.: Eine ungewöhnlich große Randzacke am Ileosakralgelenk. Fortschr. Röntgenstr. 92 (1960), 466
le Double, A. F.: Traité des variations de la colonne vertébrale de l'homme et de leur signification au point de l'antropologie zoologique. Paris 1912
Drexler, Ch., J. R. Stewart and O. K. Kincaid: Diagnostic implications of rib notching. Amer. J. Roentgenol. 91 (1964), 1064
Dwight, Th.: A Bony supracondyloid Foramen in Man. Amer. J. Anat. 3 (1904), 221
Dyes, O: Os acetabuli persistens bilateralis. Fortschr. Röntgenstr. 39 (1929), 658
Dziallas, P.: Zur Entwicklung und Histogenese der Sternocostalverbindungen und Sternalfugen. Z. Zellforsch. 37 (1952), 127
Ebel, D.: Normales und pathologisches Wachstum des kindlichen Schädels im Röntgenbild. Radiologe 2 (1962), 30
Ebermaier, C.: Über ein seltenes klinisches Symptom bei Blockwirbelbildung der Halswirbelsäule. Röntgenpraxis 10 (1938), 667
Edinger, A., H. Gajewski u. H. Gepp: Röntgen-Ganzaufnahmen der Wirbelsäule. Fortschr. Röntgenstr. 84 (1956), 365
Eggimann, P.: Lunatum bipartitum. Radiol. clin. (Basel) 18 (1949), 203
Eggimann, P.: Zur Bipartition des Lunatum. Radiol. clin. (Basel) 20 (1951), 65
Elingshausen, H. P.: Eine seltene Lokalisation der Osteochondrosis dissecans. Fortschr. Röntgenstr. 82 (1955), 829
Eliot, M., S. P. Souther and E. A. Park: Transverse lines in X-ray plates of the long bones of children. Bull. Johns Hopk. Hosp. 41 (1927), 364
Ellegast, H.: Osteopathien (Sekundäre, systemisierte Osteopathien bei endokrinen und metabolischen Störungen). Hdb. med. Radiol. VII/1, Springer, Berlin-Heidelberg-New York 1963
Elsner, W: Ein Verfahren zur röntgenologischen Darstellung des hinteren Teils des Talokalkanealgelenks und seine klinische und unfallmedizinische Bedeutung. Verh. dtsch. orthop. Ges., Beil.-H. Z. Orthop. 86 (1955), 296
Engel, G.: Über die Häufigkeit einiger Varietäten im Röntgenbild der Halswirbelsäule. Diss. Bonn 1932
Ennevaraa, K.: Painful shoulder joint in rheumatoid arthritis: clinical and radiologic study of 200 cases, with special reference to arthrography of glenohumeral joint. Acta rheum. scand. Suppl. 11 (1967), 11
Epstein, B. S. and L. M. Davidoff: An atlas of skull roentgenograms. Kimpton, London 1953
Epstein, B. S. and J. Sloven: Body-Section radiography. With special reference to the skeleton. Med. Radiogr. Photogr. 32 (1956), 2
Esser, C. Zur Frühdiagnose der Epiphysenlösung des Femurkopfes. Fortschr. Röntgenstr. 84 (1956), 320
Exner, G. u. H. J. Benz: Wirbelgleiten bei Erwachsenen. Dtsch. Ärztebl. 46 (1973), 1391
Faber, A.: Über das Os intermetatarseum. Z. orthop. Chir. 61 (1934), 186
Faber, A.: Erbbiologische Untersuchungen über die Anlage zur „angeborenen" Hüftverrenkung. Z. Orthop. 66 (1937), 140
Faber, A.: Das Hüftgelenk beim Säugling. Z. Orthop. 67 (1938), 251
Fairbank, H. A. T. and E. J. Lloyd: Cysts of external cartilage of knee with erosion of head of tibia. Brit. J. Surg. 22 (1934), 115

Fazekas, P. u. M. Ferjentsik: Lochförmiger Defekt des Schulterblattes mit einer schwalbenschwanzähnlichen Deformität des untersten Abschnitts. Fortschr. Röntgenstr. 121 (1974), 657

Feistmann-Lutterbeck, E.: Verknöcherungen im Ligamentum patellae. Röntgenpraxis 10 (1938), 140

Fick, R.: Handbuch der Anatomie und Mechanik der Gelenke. Fischer, Jena 1911

Fiebelkorn, H.-J.: Über ein wenig bekanntes inkonstantes Skelettelement der Fußwurzel. Fortschr. Röntgenstr. 77 (1952), 624

Fiedler, J.: Osteochondrosis dissecans am oberen Pfannenrand des Hüftgelenkes. Fortschr. Röntgenstr. 74 (1950), 207

Fink, J.: Bedeutung des Schichtbildes in der Otologie. Z. Hals-, Nas.-u. Ohrenheilk. 47 (1941), 499

Finkelnburg, W.: Einführung in die Atomphysik. 5. u. 6. Aufl. Springer, Berlin-Göttingen-Heidelberg 1958

Finze, H.: Exostosen der oberen Felsenbeinpyramide. Fortschr. Röntgenstr. 87 (1957), 415

Fischel, A.: Grundriß der Entwicklung des Menschen. Springer, Berlin 1937

Fischer, E.: Verkalkungsformen der Rippenknorpel. Fortschr. Röntgenstr. 82 (1955), 474

Fischer, E.: Lochförmiger Defekt im Schulterblatt. Fortschr. Röntgenstr. 86 (1957), 530

Fischer, E.: Persistierende Klavikulaapophyse. Fortschr. Röntgenstr. 86 (1957), 532

Fischer, E.: Neues Skelettelement dorsal am Radio-Karpalgelenk. Fortschr. Röntgenstr. 91 (1959), 530

Fischer, E.: Akzessorische freie Knochenelemente in der Umgebung des Foramen magnum. Fortschr. Röntgenstr. 91 (1959), 638

Fischer, E. u. H. Schmidt: Die degenerativen Veränderungen des vorderen atlanto-dentalen Gelenks. Fortschr. Röntgenstr. 111 (1969), 552

Fischer, F.: Über eine traumatisch entstandene Zweiteilung eines sogenannten Os triangulare. Fortschr. Röntgenstr. 83 (1955), 122

Fischer, H.: Beitrag zur Kenntnis der Skelettvarietäten (überzählige Karpalia u. Tarsalia, Sesambeine, Kompaktainseln). Fortschr. Röntgenstr. 19 (1912/13), 43

Fischer, P.: Verknöcherungen von Bändern des Beckenbodens. Fortschr. Röntgenstr. 84 (1956), 765

Fischer-Wasels, J.: Zur Röntgentechnik der Fußwurzeldarstellung. Z. Orthop. 86 (1955), 468

Fischgold, H., M. David et P. Brégeat: La tomographie de la base du crâne en neurochirurgie et neuroophtalmologie. Masson & Cie. Paris 1952

Fischgold, H. u. J. Metzger: Anleitung zur speziellen Röntgenuntersuchung des knöchernen Schädels. In: *K. Decker:* Klinische Neuroradiologie. Thieme, Stuttgart 1960

Fischgold, H., J. Metzger et G. Korach: Tomographie de la région pétro-sphéno-occipitale. Incidence des quatres dernières paires crâniennes. Acta radiol. (Stockh.) 42 (1954), 56

Fleischner, F.: Multiple Epiphysenstörungen an den Händen. Fortschr. Röntgenstr. 31 (1923/24), 206

Fleischner, F.: Rippenanomalien als Quelle diagnostischer Irrtümer und falscher therapeutischer Indikationsstellung. Med. Klin. (1930), 1366

Fochem, K.: Einführung in die geburtshilfliche und gynäkologische Röntgendiagnostik. Thieme, Stuttgart 1967

Fong, E. E.: Iliac horns. Radiology 47 (1946), 517

Fraenkel, E.: Über die Verknöcherung des menschlichen Kehlkopfes. Fortschr. Röntgenstr. 12 (1908), 151

Francillon, M. R.: Zur Anatomie und Klinik des Proc. trochlearis calcanei. Z. orthop. Chir. 57 (1932), 544

Francillon, M. R.: Spondylolysthesis und Unfall. Schweiz. med. Wschr. 80 (1950), 1256

Frasseto, M. F., zit. bei Hiltemann, H.: Fonticulus metopicus und Sutura frontalis persistens mit Hypoplasie der Sinus frontales. Fortschr. Röntgenstr. 81 (1954), 407

Frey, K. W.: Schichtaufnahmen des Felsenbeines mit polyzyklischer Verwischung. Fortschr. Röntgenstr. 85 (1956), 433

Frey, K. W.: Die Tomographie zur Röntgendiagnostik der Gehörknöchelchen. Röntgen-Bl. 17 (1964), 527

Frey, K. W.: Tomographie des Schläfenbeins (Technik, Röntgenanatomie, entzündliche Ohrerkrankungen). Röntgen-Bl. 21 (1968), 347

Friedmann, G. u. J. Seiferth: Entstehung und Bedeutung der Impressiones digitatae des Schädels. Röntgen-Bl. 17 (1964), 80

Frik, W. u. R. Hesse: Die transversale Schichtuntersuchung der Iliosacralgelenke. Fortschr. Röntgenstr. 84 (1956), 671

Fritz, H.: Schädelschichtuntersuchung. Kongr.-Ber. 1. Tagg. Med. Ges. Röntgenol. DDR 1955. Leipzig (1957), 1

Fröhlich, E.: Über die *Haglund*ferse. Röntgenpraxis 12 (1940), 221

Fürmaier, A.: Orthopädische Röntgentechnik. Röntgen- u. Lab.- Prax. 6 (1953), 81 u. 110

Fürmaier, A. u. A. Breit: Über die Röntgenologie des Femoro-Patellargelenkes mit besonderer Berücksichtigung der Diagnose der Chondropathia patellae. Arch. orthop. Unfall-Chir. 45 (1952), 126

Fuhrmann, W., Ch. Steffens u. G. Rompe: Dominant erbliche doppelseitige Dysplasie und Synostose des Ellenbogengelenks. Mit symmetrischer Brachymesophalangie und Brachymetakarpie sowie Synostosen im Finger-, Hand- und Fußwurzelbereich. Humangenetik 3 (1966), 64

Fuhrmann, W., Ch. Steffens, G. Schwarz u. A. Wagner: Dominant erbliche Brachydaktylie mit Gelenksaplasien. Humangenetik 1 (1965), 337

Fullenlove, T. N.: Congenital absence of the odontoid process. Radiology 63 (1954), 72

Gallois, K.: Des causes d'erreur dans la lecture radiographique de la voûte du crâne. Ann. Méd. lég. 110 (1930), 622

Ganz, E.: Fraktur des Processus supracondylicus humeri. Röntgenpraxis 9 (1937), 48

Gardner, E.: Osteogenesis in the human embryo and fetus. In: *Bourne:* The biochemistry and physiology of bone. p. 359, Academic Press, New York 1956

Gassmann, W.: Eine seltene Knochenvarietät am Os occipitale. Fortschr. Röntgenstr. 85 (1956), 633

Gassmann, W.: Ungewöhnlich große Osteophytenbildung an der Synchondrosis sterni. Fortschr. Röntgenstr. 86 (1957), 405

Gebauer, A.: Fehlerquellen im Röntgenschichtbild. Röntgen-Bl. (1961), 145

Gebauer, A., E. Muntean, E. Stutz u. H. Vieten: Das Röntgenschichtbild. Thieme, Stuttgart 1959

Gefferth, K.: Über das Sellaröntgenbild der Frühgeburten. Arch. Kinderheilk. 111 (1937), 87

Geipel, P.: Zur Kenntnis der Spina bifida am Atlas. Fortschr. Röntgenstr. 42 (1930), 583

Geipel, P.: Zur Kenntnis der Spaltbildung des Atlas und Epistropheus. Fortschr. Röntgenstr. 46 (1932), 373

Geipel, P.: Doppelte Spaltbildung des Atlas. Med. Klin. 38 (1936), 1302 u. 1337

Geisler, E. u. M. L. Bannes: Das Röntgenbild des Handskeletts als Hilfsmittel zur Diagnostik zerebraler Schäden von Kindern. Münch. med. Wschr. 102 (1960), 1273

Georgy, H.-U. u. H. Hillger: Beobachtung eines ungewöhnlich großen Os radiale externum. Fortschr. Röntgenstr. 111 (1969), 715

Gersten, A. et S. Lecomte-Ramioul: Étude radiologique des jonctions chondrocostales dans le rachitisme. J. belge Radiol. 37 (1954), 454

Ghislanzoni, R.: Le lacune della volta cranica. Minerva med. (1956), 1148

Ghislanzoni, R. e M. Tasca: Sulla tecnica di esame dei fori di coningazione della colonna cervicale. Radiologia (Roma) 9 (1953), 469

Giles, R. G.: Vertebral anomalies. Radiology 17 (1931), 1262

Giraud, M., P. Bret, A. Anjou, J. Duquesnel et M. Ogier: L'exploration tomographique du rocher et de la mastoïde. J. Radiol. Électrol. 37 (1956), 293

Glauner, R. u. W. Marquardt: Röntgendiagnostik des Hüftgelenkes. Thieme, Stuttgart 1956

Gnilka, G.: Innenknöchelbruch und Abrißbruch am Grundanteil des 5. Mittelfußknochens. Fortschr. Röntgenstr. 78 (1953), 484

Goalwin, H. A.: Die exakte radiographische Darstellung des Canalis opticus. Fortschr. Röntgenstr. 32 (1924), 218

Goalwin, H. A.: One thousand optic canals: Clinical, anatomic and roentgenologic study. J. Amer. med. Ass. 89 (1927), 1745

Gockel, H. P.: Über eine Form von Atlasfehlbildung. Fortschr. Röntgenstr. 88 (1958), 485

Gött, Th.: Die Röntgenuntersuchung in der Kinderheilkunde. In: *Rieder-Rosenthal:* Lehrbuch der Röntgenkunde. Bd. II, Barth, Leipzig 1925

Goldhamer, K.: Welche Skelettvarietäten des Schädels können pathologische und traumatische Veränderungen vortäuschen? Wien. klin. Wschr. (1931), 584

Goldhamer, K. und A. Schüller: Varietäten im Bereich der hinteren Schädelgrube. Fortschr. Röntgenstr. 35 (1926/27), 1163

Gollasch, W.: Das zweigeteilte Kahnbein der Hand, seine Bedeutung für die Erkennung, Behandlung und Begutachtung der Kahnbeinverletzungen. Röntgenpraxis 11 (1939), 564

Gombert, H. J.: Dens-Fraktur mit maximaler dorsaler Luxation des Atlas ohne tödliche Folge. Fortschr. Röntgenstr. 91 (1959), 521

Goodfellow, J.: Aetiology of hallux rigidus. Proc. roy. Soc. Med. 59 (1966), 821

Grant, R. and H. Lanting: An improved technic for roentgenographic examination of the temporo-mandibular joint and condyle. J. oral Surg. 11 (1953), 95

Graser, E.: Handwurzelentwicklung in den ersten Lebensjahren und Rachitis (Röntgenologische Studien). Z. Kinderheilk. 60 (1938), 30

Grashey, R.: Pseudofraktur eines Fingers (Weichteilüberschneidung). Röntgenpraxis 6 (1934), 488

Grashey, R.: Hornförmiger Auswuchs am Os naviculare manus. Röntgenpraxis 7 (1935), 275

Grashey, R.: Ossifikationskerne der Schultergelenksgegend. Röntgenpraxis 7 (1935), 852

Grashey, R.: Pseudoperiostitiden. Röntgenpraxis 8 (1936), 211

Grashey, R.: Vorgetäuschte Schädelfraktur. Röntgenpraxis 8 (1936), 247

Grashey, R.: Dorsale supracondyläre Femurexostose. Röntgenpraxis 9 (1937), 278

Grashey, R.: Articulatio talo-calcanea (Os sustentaculi). Röntgenpraxis 14 (1942), 139

Grashey, R.: Atlas typischer Röntgenbilder vom normalen Menschen. 7. Aufl. Urban & Schwarzenberg, München-Berlin 1950

Grashey, R. u. R. Birkner: Atlas typischer Röntgenbilder vom normalen Menschen. 10. Aufl. Urban u. Schwarzenberg, München-Berlin 1964

Grashey, R. u. R. Birkner: Röntgentafel des Skeletts. 5. Aufl. Urban und Schwarzenberg, München-Berlin-Wien 1966

Graumann, W.: Topogenese der Bindegewebsknochen. Untersuchungen an Schädelknochen menschlicher Embryonen. Z. Anat. Entwickl.-Gesch. 116 (1951), 14

Graumann, W. u. H. Braband: Über Periostveränderungen bei peripheren Durchblutungsstörungen. Fortschr. Röntgenstr. 92 (1960), 337

Greineder, H. W.: Artikulierender Okziputsporn. Fortschr. Röntgenstr. 85 (1956),252

Gremjazkij, M. A.: Über einige Gesetzmäßigkeiten in der Obliterationsreihenfolge der Schädelnähte beim Menschen. Ref. Anat. Ber. 19 (1930)

Greulich, W. W. and S. J. Pyle: Radiographic atlas of skeletal development of the hand and wrist. 2nd ed. Stanford (Calif.), Stanf. Univ. Press 1959

Grob, M: Über die röntgenologischen Nahtverhältnisse der hinteren Schädelgrube beim Kinde mit spezieller Berücksichtigung der Sutura mendosa. Fortschr. Röntgenstr. 57 (1938), 265

Gros, J.: Über die grubige Atrophie des Scheitelbeins. Fortschr. Röntgenstr. 85 (1956), 154

Gros, Ch., J. P. Walter, J. Bloch et P. Bourjat: La paroi labyrinthique normale: aspects tomographiques. J. Radiol. Électrol. 43 (1962), 253

Grossmann, G.: Tomographie I. Röntgenographische Darstellung von Körperschnitten. Tomographie II. Theoretisches über Tomographie. Fortschr. Röntgenstr. 51 (1935), 61 u. 191

Grothe, H.: Betrachtungen zur Patella partita. Wehrmed. Wschr. 10 (1966), 185

Grumbach, A.: Das Handskelett im Lichte der Röntgenstrahlen. Braumüller, Wien-Leipzig 1921

Grundler, E. u. G. Seige: Kinderheilkunde. Thieme, Stuttgart 1960

Günsel, E.: Das Os coracoideum. Fortschr. Röntgenstr. 74 (1951), 112

Günsel, E.: Persistierende Apophyse des Epicondylus medialis humeri. Fortschr. Röntgenstr. 76 (1952), 660

Güntz, E.: Schmerzen und Leistungsstörungen bei Erkrankungen der Wirbelsäule. Enke, Stuttgart 1937

Güntz, E.: Die Kyphose im Jugendalter. In: Die Wirbelsäule in Forschung und Praxis, Bd. 2. Hippokrates, Stuttgart 1957

Guintoli, L. e S. Chiappa: Epoca di comparsa ed evoluzione nel tempo delle calcificazioni paracondiloidee mediali del ginocchio (malattia di *Pellegrini*). Radiologia (Roma) 9 (1953), 857

Haas, E.: Durch Exostose bedingte Bewegungsbehinderung des Kniegelenkes. Zbl. Chir. 67 (1940), 1297

Haas, H.: Posttraumatische Knochenspangenbildung zwischen zwei Lendenwirbelquerfortsätzen. Fortschr. Röntgenstr. 120 (1974), 497

Haas, L.: Verfahren zur sagittalen Aufnahme der Sellagegend. Fortschr. Röntgenstr. 36 (1927), 1198

Haas, L.: Über die klinische Verwertbarkeit der röntgenologischen Nahtdiagnose. Fortschr. Röntgenstr. 41 (1930), 549

Haas, L.: Über die nucho-frontale Aufnahme des Schädels. Fortschr. Röntgenstr. 45 (1932), 532

Haas, L.: Über die Sutura frontalis persistens. Eine röntgenanatomische Studie. Fortschr. Röntgenstr. 48 (1933), 708

Haas, L.: Über die Entwicklung der Nasennebenhöhlen (mit Rücksicht auf die Aplasie der Stirnhöhlen). Fortschr. Röntgenstr. 49 (1934), 203

Haas, L.: Die supraorbitalen Pneumatisationen im Röntgenbilde. Fortschr. Röntgenstr. 50 (1934), 71

Haas, L.: Einzelheiten aus der Röntgendiagnostik der Sella turcica. Fortschr. Röntgenstr. 50 (1934), 465 u. 468

Haas, L.: Einzelheiten über eine Spalte der Tuberculumgegend der Sella turcica. Fortschr. Röntgenstr. 52 (1935), 186 u. 188

Haglund, P.: Beitrag zur Klinik der Achillessehne. Z. orthop. Chir. 49 (1928), 49

Hahn, O.: Scheinbare Spaltbildung der Wirbelkörper in der Adoleszenz. Fortschr. Röntgenstr. 29 (1922), 211

Haid, B.: Beobachtung einer neuen Form des Os intermetatarseum. Z. Orthop. 80 (1950/51), 298

Haines, R. W. and A. McDougall: The anatomy of hallux valgus. J. Bone Jt Surg. 36B (1954), 272

Halgrimsson: Zit. bei *Elsner*

Hamperl, H.: Die anatomischen Grundlagen und die Entstehung der sog. Querschatten in den Metaphysen wachsender Knochen. Z. Kinderheilk. 56 (1934), 324

Hanney, F.: Zur Röntgenkontrastdarstellung der tränenableitenden Wege. Klin. Mbl. Augenheilk. 128 (1956), 336

Hanson, R.: On the development of spinal vertebrae, as seen on skiagrams from the foetal life to the age of fourteen. Acta radiol. (Stockh.) 5 (1926), 112

Harder, J.: Osteochondritis-dissecans-artige Veränderung an einem Processus uncinatus (zugleich Studie über die sog. Uncovertebralgelenke). Fortschr. Röntgenstr. 96 (1962), 423

Harder, D.: Die neuen radiologischen Maßeinheiten *Gray* und *Bequerel*. Med. Welt 26/Heft 44 (1975), 1993

Harris, H. A.: The growth of the long bones in childhood. Arch. intern. Med. 38 (1926), 758

Hartmann, K.: Zur Pathologie der bilateralen Wirbelkörperfehlbildungen und zur normalen Entwicklung der Wirbelkörper. Fortschr. Röntgenstr. 55 (1937), 531

Harzheim, I.: Ein Beitrag zur Bandscheibenverkalkung im Kindesalter. Fortschr. Röntgenstr. 113 (1970), 244

Haslhofer, L.: Luxation und Nekrose des Lunatum in pathologisch-anatomischer Schau. Radiol. Austriaca 7 (1954), 15

Hasselwander, A.: Untersuchungen über die Ossifikation des menschlichen Fußskeletts. Habil.-Schr. Stuttgart 1909

Hasselwander, A.: Atlas der Anatomie des menschlichen Körpers im Röntgenbild. Bergmann, München 1926

Hasselwander, A.: In: Handbuch der Anatomie des Kindes. Bergmann, München 1938

Hayem, F., M. Fortier-Beaulieu, J. Masselot et J.-L. Taillemite: La discopathie calcifiante de l'enfant. Ann. Radiol. 15 (1972), 97

Heckmann, K.: Bivisuelle Röntgenaufnahmen. Röntgen-Bl. 12 (1959), 33

Heidsieck, E.: Os cuneiforme I bipartitum. Röntgenpraxis 8 (1936), 712
Heimerzheim, A.: Über einen seltsamen Knochenbefund am Calcaneus. Dtsch. Z. Chir. 187 (1924), 281
Heitzmann, C.: Atlas der descripitiven Anatomie des Menschen. 9. Aufl., Wien 1902
Hellmer, H.: Röntgenologische Beobachtungen über die Ossifikation der Patella. Acta radiol. (Stockh.), Suppl. 27 (1935)
Helmes, W.: Akzessorische Skelettelemente am Fuß und ihre klinische Bedeutung. Fortschr. Med. 85 (1967), 334
Hennecke, U.: Os radiale externum. Fortschr. Röntgenstr. 78 (1953), 362
Hensel, H.: Das Os tibiale externum, erworben oder angeboren? Diss. Berlin 1939
Henssge, J.: Das sogenannte Naviculare bipartitum pedis - angeborene oder erworbene Knochenteilung. H. Unfallheilk. 93 (1968), 171
Herdner, R.: Traité technique de tomographie osseuse. Masson & Cie. Paris 1953
Heuck, F.: Persistierende Apophyse der Tuberositas tibiae. Fortschr. Röntgenstr. 79 (1953), 781
Heuck, F. u. E. Schmidt: Die quantitative Bestimmung des Mineralgehaltes der Knochen aus dem Röntgenbild. Fortschr. Röntgenstr. 93 (1960), 523
Heuck, F. u. E. Schmidt: Die praktische Anwendung einer Methode zur quantitativen Bestimmung des Kalksalzgehaltes gesunder und kranker Menschen. Fortschr. Röntgenstr. 93 (1960), 761
Hilgenreiner, H.: Zum angeborenen Charakter der sog. angeborenen Hüftverrenkung. Z. Orthop. 65 (1936), 58
Hilgenreiner, H.: Zur Spontannekrose des Schenkelkopfes bei Jugendlichen. Zbl. Chir. (1936), 1266
Hillger, H.: Eine seltene Lokalisation der Osteochondrosis dissecans. Fortschr. Röntgenstr. 81 (1954), 829
Hillger, H. u. H. Schwenkenbecher: Verkalkung im Symphysenknorpel nach Symphysenruptur. Fortschr. Röntgenstr. 85 (1956), 113
Hiltemann, H.: Fonticulus metopicus und Sutura frontalis persistens mit Hypoplasie der Sinus frontales. Fortschr. Röntgenstr. 81 (1954), 407
Hintze, A.: Die Fontanella lumbosacralis und ihr Verhältnis zur Spina bifida occulta. Langenbecks Arch. klin. Chir. 119 (1922), 409
Hinz, P.: Die Verletzung der Halswirbelsäule durch Schleuderung und durch Abknickung. In: Die Wirbelsäule in Forschung und Praxis, Bd. 47, Hippokrates, Stuttgart 1970
Hippe, H.: Seltene proximale tibia-fibulare Synostose. Fortschr. Röntgenstr. 78 (1953), 748
Hippe, H. u. K. Hähle: Tomographie des Warzenfortsatzes. Röntgenpraxis 10 (1938), 393
Hoed den: A separate center of ossification for the tip of the internal malleolus. Brit. J. Radiol. 30 (1925), 67
Hoen, E. u. A. Kaiser: Kritisches zum sog. „Druckschädel". Arch. Kinderheilk. 146 (1953), 109
Hölscher, W.: Die radiologische Bestimmung der Knochendichte zwecks Kontrolle therapeutischer Maßnahmen bei internistischen Erkrankungen des Knochensystems. Diss. Berlin 1958
Hofer, R.: Der Sulcus paraglenoidalis ossis ilei et ossis sacri im Röntgenbild. Fortschr. Röntgenstr. 39 (1929), 1085
Hoff, F.: Klinische Physiologie und Pathologie. 4. Aufl. Thieme, Stuttgart 1954
Hoffmann, D.: Einige seltenere Handwurzelverschmelzungen und andere Mißbildungen des Handskeletts. Röntgenpraxis 12 (1940), 41
Hohl, K.: Das Os odontoideum (partielle Densaplasie). Fortschr. Röntgenstr. 91 (1959), 518
Hohmann, G.: Fuß und Bein. Bergmann, München 1951
Holland, C. u. W. Stolle: Fehlbildungen der Wirbelbogenreihe. Fortschr. Röntgenstr. 112 (1970), 120
Holthusen, H.: In: Medizinische Röntgentechnik II. Physikal.-techn. Teil. Herausgegeben von H. Schoen. 2. Aufl. Thieme, Stuttgart 1958
Horváth, F.: Über die auf dem sternalen Drittel und kaudal befindliche „Usuration" der Klavikula. Fortschr. Röntgenstr. 116 (1972), 836
Hubay, C. A.: Sesamoid bones of the hands and feet. Amer. J. Roentgenol. 61 (1949), 493
Hülshoff, Th.: Eine seltene Rippenanomalie. Fortschr. Röntgenstr. 103 (1965), 231
Hünermann, C.: Die diagnostische Bedeutung der Impressiones digitatae und der Schädelnahtdehiszenzen im Röntgenbild des kindlichen Schädels. Mschr. Kinderheilk. 58 (1933), 415
Iannaccone, G. u. M. Barillà: Die zystenartigen Gebilde am Proximalende der Ulna: Anatomisch-röntgenologisches Bild und dessen Auslegung. Fortschr. Röntgenstr. 84 (1956), 598
Idelberger, K.: Die Erbpathologie der sogenannten angeborenen Hüftverrenkung. Bruns' Beitr. klin. Chir. Sonderbd., Urban u. Schwarzenberg, München-Berlin 1951
Illchmann-Christ, A. u. L. Diethelm: Eine Studie über den sog. genetischen Wirbelsäulenvergleich. Z. menschl. Vererb.-u. Konstit.-Lehre 31 (1953), 431
Imhäuser, G.: Die physiologische intrapelvine Vorragung des Hüftpfannenbodens. Z. Orthop. 81 (1952), 161
Imhäuser, G.: Über Dislokalisation der proximalen Femurepiphyse durch Schädigung der Wachstumszone. (Zugleich ein Beitrag zur Dislokalisation der Hüftkopfepiphyse nach vorn-unten.) Z. Orthop. 96 (1962), 265
Jacobs, Ph.: A note on the diagnosis of early adolescent coxa vara (slipped epiphysis). Brit. J. Radiol. 35 (1962), 619
Jakob, A.: Ein Beitrag zur Differentialdiagnose der enossalen Verkalkung, insbesondere des Knocheninfarktes. Fortschr. Röntgenstr. 74 (1951), 77
Jakob, A.: Knochenveränderungen bei trophischen Störungen am Unterschenkel. Fortschr. Röntgenstr. 82 (1955), 28
Jakob, O.: Über die kindlichen Nebenhöhlen. Diss. Würzburg 1933
Janker, R.: Der Knochenkern der Spina iliaca anterior inferior. Dtsch. Z. Chir. 241 (1933), 477
Janker, R.: Über die Synchondrosis sternalis. Zbl. Chir. (1934), 2775
Janker, R.: Eine anatomische Variante am Querfortsatz des Atlas. Röntgenpraxis 7 (1935), 399
Janker, R.: Der Falxknochen. Fortschr. Röntgenstr. 71 (1949), 114
Janzen, R.: Die versicherungsrechtliche Bedeutung der basilären Impression. Mschr. Unfallheilk. 62 (1959), 361
Jaroschy, W.: Röntgenbefunde bei der sogenannten Kalkaneodynie. Fortschr. Röntgenstr. 43 (1931), 804
Jenkins, F. A.: The evolution and development of the dens of the mammalian axis. Anat. Rec. 164 (1969), 173
Jobstvogt, H.: Die radiologische Bestimmung der Knochendichte zur Feststellung der Kombinationshäufigkeit interner Erkrankungen mit Osteoporose. Diss. Berlin 1958
Johansson, S.: Eine bisher anscheinend unbekannte Erkrankung der Patella. Z. orthop. Chir. 43 (1924), 82
Johnson, V. C.: The value of Roentgen examination of paranasal sinuses. Radiology 32 (1939), 303
Jonasch, E.: Untersuchungen über die Form der Eminentia intercondyloidea tibae im Röntgenbild. Fortschr. Röntgenstr. 89 (1958), 81
Jonasch, E.: Über die röntgenologische Schattenbildung an der Innen- und Außenseite des Kniegelenks. Arch. orthop. Unfall-Chir. 50 (1959), 461
Jonasch, E.: Die Verkalkung der Menisci des Kniegelenks. Arch. orthop. Unfall-Chir. 51 (1960), 659
Jonasch, E.: Die Verknöcherung des Ligamentum popliteum obliquum. Fortschr. Röntgenstr. 99 (1963), 695
Jonasch, E.: Erkennung und Beurteilung der Meniskusverletzung des Kniegelenks durch das gewöhnliche Röntgenbild. Mschr. Unfallheilk. Beih. 90 (1967), 1
Jones u. Hedrick: Zit. bei *Köhler/Zimmer:* Grenzen des Normalen und Anfänge des Pathologischen im Röntgenbild des Skelets. 11. Aufl. Thieme, Stuttgart 1967
Jungblut, R.: Die Knochenkernentwicklung des Processus styloideus ulnae. Fortschr. Röntgenstr. 103 (1965), 499
Junge, H. u. F. Heuck: Die Osteochondropathia ischiopubica. Fortschr. Röntgenstr. 78 (1953), 656
Junghanns, H.: Die Randleisten der Wirbelkörper. Fortschr. Röntgenstr. 42 (1930), 333
Junghanns, H.: Über Wirbelabgleiten, Spondylolisthese, Wirbelverschiebung nach hinten und nach der Seite. Arch. klin. Chir. 159 (1930), 423
Junghanns, H.: Spondylolisthesen ohne Spalt im Zwischengelenkstück („Pseudospondylolisthesen"). Arch. Orthop. 29 (1930), 118

Junghanns, H.: Die Spondylolisthese im Röntgenbild. Fortschr. Röntgenstr. 41 (1930), 239

Junghanns, H.: Spondylolisthese, Pseudospondylolisthese und Wirbelverschiebung nach hinten. Bruns' Beitr. klin. Chir. 151 (1931), 376 u. 394

Junghanns, H.: Die Zwischenwirbelscheiben im Röntgenbild. Fortschr. Röntgenstr. 43 (1931), 275

Junghanns, H.: Die Frühossifikation der Wirbelkörper. Fortschr. Röntgenstr. 68 (1943), 70

Junghanns, H.: Die „funktionelle Röntgenuntersuchung" der Halswirbelsäule. Fortschr. Röntgenstr. 76 (1952), 591

Junghanns, H.: Chondrosis (Osteochondrosis) intervertebralis und Spondylosis deformans in ihren Beziehungen zum Trauma und zur Begutachtung. In: Die Wirbelsäule in Forschung und Praxis, Bd. 11, Hippokrates, Stuttgart 1968

Kamieth, H. u. K. Reinhardt: Der ungleiche Symphysenstand. Ein wichtiges Symptom der Beckenringlockerung. Fortschr. Röntgenstr. 83 (1955), 530

Kamprad, F. u. V. Hasert: Die Tomographie der Kreuzbänder im Doppelkontrast-Arthrogramm des Kniegelenks. Fortschr. Röntgenstr. 112 (1970), 499

Karlas, G. A.: Morphological observations on superior surface of body of sphenoid bone in human adults. Diss. Helsingfors 1948

Kassatkin, S.: Die Sesambeine der Hand und des Fußes beim Menschen. Z. Anat. Entwickl.-Gesch. 102 (1934), 635

Kaufmann, H. J.: Röntgenbefunde am kindlichen Becken bei angeborenen Skelettaffektionen und chromosomalen Aberrationen. Thieme, Stuttgart 1964

Keating, D. R. and J. R. Amberg: A source of potential error in the roentgen diagnosis of cervical ribs. Radiology 62 (1954), 688

Keim, H.: Beitrag zur diagnostischen Verwertung von Abstandsdifferenzen zwischen dem Atlas und dem Dens epistrophei im Röntgenbild. Fortschr. Röntgenstr. 87 (1957), 488

v. Keiser, D.: Cubitus varus und Cubitus valgus. In: Hbd. d. Med. Radiologie Bd IV/2, Springer, Berlin-Heidelberg-New York 1968, 281

Keller, H. L.: Varianten der Arteria carotis interna, der Arteria meningea und der Arteria ophthalmica im Karotisangiogramm. Fortschr. Röntgenstr. 95 (1961), 472

Ken Kuré: Zit. in *F. Hoff:* Klinische Physiologie und Pathologie. 4. Aufl. Thieme, Stuttgart 1954

Kewenter, Y.: Die Sesambeine des I. Metatarsophalangealgelenks des Menschen. Eine röntgenologische, klinische und pathologisch-histologische Studie. Acta orthop. scand., Suppl. II, Kopenhagen (1936), 1

Kewesch, E. L.: Über hereditäre Verschmelzung der Hand- und Fußwurzelknochen. Fortschr. Röntgenstr. 50 (1934), 550

Kienböck, R.: Ellenbogenscheibe (Patella cubiti) und Olecranonfraktur. Fortschr. Röntgenstr. 22 (1914), 89

Kienböck, R.: Anomalie des Ellenbogengelenks. Os sesamoideum cubiti. Presse méd. 45 (1937), 491

Kienböck, R. u. A. Zimmer: Angeborener partieller Kreuz- und Steißbeindefekt. Röntgenpraxis 7 (1935), 111

Kienböck, R. u. G. Desenfans: Über Anomalien am Ellenbogengelenk. Patella cubiti. Bruns' Beitr. klin. Chir. 165 (1937), 524

Kienböck, R. u. W. Müller: Os tibiale externum und Verletzung des Fußes. Z. orthop. Chir. 66 (1937), 257

Kipshoven, H. J.: Die röntgenologische Darstellung der Ossa suprasternalia. Fortschr. Röntgenstr. 74 (1951), 320

Kipshoven, H. J.: Diskontinuitäten im Verlauf der ersten Rippen. Fortschr. Röntgenstr. 74 (1951), 555

Kirchhoff, H. J. u. H. H. Rohwedder: Über Mißbildungen der Wirbelsäule des Säuglings (ein klinischer Beitrag). Arch. Kinderheilk. 148 (1954), 146

Kirschbichler, Th.: Die atlanto-occipitale Dysplasie (Entwicklungsgeschichte, Röntgendiagnose und Klinik an Hand eines seltenen Befundes). Fortschr. Röntgenstr. 111 (1969), 674

Kirschbichler, Th.: Die paarig angelegten Processus odontoidei epistrophei - Eine seltene Fehlbildung im kraniozervikalen Übergangsbereich. Fortschr. Röntgenstr. 117 (1972), 654

Klaus, E.: Röntgendiagnostik der Platybasie und basilären Impression. Fortschr. Röntgenstr. 86 (1957), 460

Kliemann, L.: Die spontane Abbildung des wirklichen Kniegelenkspaltes. Fortschr. Röntgenstr. 76 (1952), 602

Klöppner, K.: Die Sella turcica des Neugeborenen im Röntgenbild (Größe, Kontur, Form und Formvarianten der Sella turcica). Fortschr. Röntgenstr. 60 (1939), 370

Klopfer, F.: Die Protrusio acetabuli. Fortschr. Röntgenstr. 74 (1951), 323

Klümper, A., E. Uehlinger, V. Lohmann, S. Weller u. M. Strey: Femurkopfinfarkte nach Glucocorticoidbehandlung. Dtsch. med. Wschr. 92 (1967), 1108

Knákal, St. u. J. Chvojka: Doppelseitige Kahnbeinaplasie. Fortschr. Röntgenstr. 112 (1970), 837

Knese, K.-H.: Die Ultrastruktur des Knochengewebes. Dtsch. med. Wschr. 84 (1959 b), 1640, 1649

Knese, K.-H.: Struktur und Ultrastruktur des Knochengewebes. In: Handbuch der Medizinischen Radiologie. Bd. IV/1, Springer, Berlin-Heidelberg-New York 1970, 317

Knese, K.-H. u. H. Biermann: Die Knochenbildung an Sehnen- und Bandansätzen im Bereich ursprünglich chondraler Apophysen. Z. Zellforsch. 49 (1958), 142

Knetsch, A.: Beitrag zum Kanalsystem des Schädels (Emissarium frontale im Seitenbild). Fortschr. Röntgenstr. 85 (1956), 761

Knetsch, A.: Wert der axialen Aufnahme bei der Röntgendiagnostik der Nasenbeinfrakturen. Fortschr. Röntgenstr. 85 (1956), 766

Knoll, W.: Über einige im Röntgenbild sichtbare Veränderungen am Fußskelett von Sportsleuten. Dtsch. med. Wschr. 57 (1931), 401

Knutsson, F.: Einiges über Röntgenbilder der Nasenhöhle, deren Nebenhöhlen, des Nasopharynx und des Temporalbeines im ersten Lebensjahr. Nord. med. Hdsk. 13 (1937), 606; ref. Zbl. ges. Radiol. 27 (1938), 677

Knutsson, F.: Wirbelfusionen nach nicht-infektiöser Störung der Wachstumszone. Acta radiol. (Stockh.) 32 (1949), 404; ref. Fortschr. Röntgenstr. 73 (1950), 111

Köhler, A.: Zit in *Lloyd-Roberts, G. C.:* Humerus varus. Report of a case treated by excision of the acromion. J. Bone Jt Surg. 35B (1953), 268

Köhler, A. u. E. A. Zimmer: Grenzen des Normalen und Anfänge des Pathologischen im Röntgenbild des Skelets. 11. Aufl. Thieme, Stuttgart 1967

Kohler, A.: Über Tomographie des Skeletts. Fortschr. Röntgenstr. 56 (1937), 60; Kongreßband

Kohlmann, E. u. G. Neumann: Osteochondrosis dissecans im Foramen supratrochleare beiderseits. Fortschr. Röntgenstr. 94 (1961), 277

Kolář, J. u. R. Vrabec: Der röntgenologische Nachweis von Verkalkungen und Knochenbildung in den gelenknahen Weichteilen nach Verbrennungen. Fortschr. Röntgenstr. 87 (1957), 761

Kopczynska, J.: Détermination radiologique de la maturation osseuse. Amer. Radiol. 7 (1964), 308

Kopylow, M. B.: Ein neues Verfahren zur Darstellung des Canalis nasolacrimalis. Röntgenpraxis 2 (1930), 686

Korkhaus, G.: Zahnärztliche Röntgenologie in diagnostischer und therapeutischer Anwendung. Hauser, München 1955

Kovács, A.: Die sacroiliakale Spaltenaufnahme. Röntgenpraxis 7 (1935), 763

Kovács, A.: Kephalalgia e Subluxatione artic. cervicalis. Fortschr. Röntgenstr. 85 (1956), 142

Krall, J. u. C. Krauspe: Über *Thiemann*sche Erkrankungen. Chirurg 25 (1954), 352

Kraus, R.: Die Arthrosis deformans in den Costotransversalgelenken (eine röntgenologisch-morphologische und histologische Studie). Fortschr. Röntgenstr. 85 (1956), 60

Kremer, W.: Die Darstellung röntgenologisch schwer zugänglicher Skelettabschnitte durch die Tomographie mit mehrseitiger Verwischung. Röntgenpraxis 10 (1938), 26

Kremser, K.: Ein Beitrag zur Kasuistik der Skelettanomalie (Ellenbogenscheibe). Röntgenpraxis 6 (1934), 371

Kremser, K.: Ein weiterer Beitrag zum Kapitel der Ellenbogenscheibe. Röntgenpraxis 10 (1938), 841

Kremser, K.: Atypische Gelenkbildung im Bereich der Wirbelsäule. Fortschr. Röntgenstr. 81 (1954), 832

Kremser, K.: Os accessorium supracalcaneum. Fortschr. Röntgenstr. 82 (1955), 279

Kremser, K.: Os supratalare. Fortschr. Röntgenstr. 85 (1956), 116
Kresse, M. u. Th. Göbbeler: Ungewöhnliche Kalkablagerung im Tentorium cerebelli. Fortschr. Röntgenstr. 109 (1968), 252
Kretschmer, E.: Körperbau und Charakter. 25. Aufl. Springer, Berlin-Heidelberg-New York 1967
Krmpotič, J.: Über ein Erkennungszeichen des 2. Brustwirbels. Z. Anat. Entwickl.-Gesch. 118 (1954), 165
Krokowski, E. u. E. Haasner: Aktuelle Bedeutung der quantitativen Bestimmung des Skelett-Calciumgehaltes. Wehrmed. Mschr. 12 (1968), 229
Kühne, H.: Zur Physiologie der Epiphyse des Knochens. Zbl. Chir. 77 (1952), 2193
Kühne, H.: Über einige röntgenologische Besonderheiten im Kreuzbein- und Symphysenbereich (apophysäre und kommaförmige Ossifikationen). Röntgen-Bl. 19 (1966), 529
Kuhnhenn, W.: Über die Darstellung der Diploevenen im Röntgenbild. Diss. Kiel 1936
Kulka, Z.: Transkranielle Aufnahme des ersten Halswirbels. Röntgenpraxis 9 (1937), 128
Kullnig, G.: Persistierender offener Ductus craniopharyngicus. Fortschr. Röntgenstr. 79 (1953), 127
Laarmann, A.: Die Darstellung des Knieinnern im Röntgenbild. Arch. klin. Chir. 187 (1937), 234
Laarmann, A.: Der Meniscusschatten im Darstellungs-Röntgenbild. Arch. klin. Chir. 192 (1938), 697
Laarmann, A.: Die Darstellung des Kniegelenks im Röntgenbild. Zbl. Chir. 65 (1938), 2830
Laczay, A. u. K. Csapó: Verknöcherungen im Ligamentum patellae und die *Schlatter-Osgood*sche Krankheit. Fortschr. Röntgenstr. 119 (1973), 347
Lagemann, K.: Hintere Längsbandverkalkungen kombiniert mit Wirbelkörperexkavationen. Fortschr. Röntgenstr. 116 (1972), 834
Lahm, W.: Das Röntgenogramm des übertragenen Neugeborenen. Fortschr. Röntgenstr. 37 (1928), 34
Lange, K.: Das Naviculare bipartitum. Röntgenpraxis 11 (1939), 566
Lange, M.: Die Wirbelgelenke. 2. Aufl. Enke, Stuttgart 1936
Langeland, P.: Luxation der 12. Rippe im Costo-Vertebral-Gelenk. Fortschr. Röntgenstr. 84 (1956), 645
Langhof, J.: Zur Differentialdiagnose von Blockbildungen der Wirbelsäule. Zbl. Chir. 79 (1954), 1959
v. Lanz, T. u. W. Wachsmuth: Praktische Anatomie. Springer, Berlin 1935
Lassrich, M. A., R. Prévôt u. K. H. Schäfer: Pädiatrischer Röntgenatlas. Thieme, Stuttgart 1955
Laurent, Y. et M. Brombart: Variation très rare de l'ossification des phalanges des orteils. J. belge Radiol. 36 (1953), 102
Lauven, E.: Kontaktaufnahmen zur Lupenbildausschnitt-Betrachtung in der Röntgendiagnostik. Röntgenpraxis 5 (1933), 602
Lauven, E.: Kontaktaufnahmen in der Röntgen-Knochendiagnostik. Zbl. Chir. 60 (1933), 2418
Lefebvre, J., E. Guy et J. Metzger: Évolution des signes radiographiques des atrophies cérébrales unilatérales. Acta radiol. (Stockh.) 40 (1953), 314
Lefebvre, J., M. R. Klein et C. Faure: La diastématomyélie, à propos d'une observation. Rev. neurol. 94 (1956), 357
Lelong, M., Joseph, R., Canlobre, P. et R. Scholler: Les méthodes d'évaluation du développement osseux. Sem. Hôp. Paris (1955), 1067
v. Lengerke, H.-J.: Kraniometrische Untersuchungen zur normalen Wachstumsrate des intrakraniellen Raums in den ersten 3 Lebensjahren. Fortschr. Röntgenstr. 120 (1974), 300
Lettenbauer, W.: Die Pneumatisation des Felsenbeines. Diss. München 1938
Lichtenstein, L.: Bone Tumors. Mosby, St. Louis 1959
Liechti, A.: Die Röntgendiagnostik der Wirbelsäule und ihre Grundlagen. 2. Aufl. Springer, Wien 1948
Liess, G.: Die Linea innominata des Schädels, ihr anatomisches Substrat und ihre Bedeutung für die Diagnostik der Orbitatumoren. Fortschr. Röntgenstr. 75 (1951), 165
Liess, G.: A-förmige Epiphysen an Händen und Füßen (periphere Dysostosen). Fortschr. Röntgenstr. 81 (1954), 173
Liess, G.: Die Nebenkernbildung bei der normalen und gestörten Epiphysenossifikation und ihre Beziehung zu den aseptischen Nekrosen. Fortschr. Röntgenstr. 80 (1954), 153
Lièvre, J. A. et H. Fischgold: Les lacunes bénignes du crâne. Presse méd. (1953), 919
Lindblom, K.: The contours of the vessels of the calvarium. Acta radiol. (Stockh.) 14 (1933), 658
Lindblom, K.: A roentgenographic study of the vascular channels of the skull, with special references to intracranial tumors and arterio-venous aneurysms. Acta radiol. (Stockh.) Suppl. 30 (1936), 1
Link, R. u. K. Handl: Die Pneumatisation des Schläfenbeines, ein Schutz gegen Lärmschwerhörigkeit. Arch. Ohr.-, Nas.-u. Kehlk.-Heilk. 167 (1955), 610
Lloyd-Roberts, G. C.: Humerus varus. Report of a case treated by excision of the acromion. J. Bone Jt Surg. 35B (1953), 268
Lob, A.: Die Wirbelsäulenverletzungen und ihre Ausheilung. Thieme, Stuttgart 1954
Lob, A.: Die Stellung der Röntgenologie in der Unfallchirurgie. Med. Klin. (1958), 1726 u. 1738
Lob, A.: Handbuch der Unfallbegutachtung. Bd. I, Enke, Stuttgart 1961
Löhr, R. u. W. Hellpap: Der Kniegelenkspalt im Röntgenbild. Fortschr. Röntgenstr. 58 (1938), 45
Loepp, W. u. R. Lorenz: Röntgendiagnostik des Schädels. Thieme, Stuttgart 1971
Loewenhardt, K.: Processus paracondyloideus. Fortschr. Röntgenstr. 122 (1975), 368
Lohmann, Th.: Über eine neue Methode der zahnärztlichen Röntgenaufnahmetechnik. Röntgen-Bl. 15 (1962), 139
Lorenz, K.: Verkalkungen des Plexus chorioideus der Seitenventrikel als Folge kongenitaler Toxoplasmose. Fortschr. Röntgenstr. 73 (1950), 735
Lossen, H.: Chorda dorsalis im Röntgenbild. Anat. Anz. 73 (1931), 168
Lossen, H.: Verknöcherungen im Ligamentum patellae. Röntgenpraxis 5 (1933), 67 u. 215
Lossen, H.: Über vermeintliche und wirkliche Schädeldachverletzungen im Röntgenbild. Röntgenpraxis 9 (1937), 229
Lossen, H. u. R. Hofer: Ossa suprasternalia im Röntgenbild. Röntgenpraxis 3 (1931), 34
Lossen, H. u. R. N. Wegner: Die Knochenkerne der Scapula, röntgenologisch und vergleichend-anatomisch betrachtet. Fortschr. Röntgenstr. 53 (1936), 443
Lucarelli, U. e G. Pompili: Lo studio stratigrafico del condutto uditivo interno. Acta ital. Otol. 72 (1961), 680
Ludloff, K.: Zur Frage der Osteochondritis dissecans am Knie. Arch. klin. Chir. 87 (1908), 552
Lüdeke, H.: Über das gehäufte Vorkommen parostaler Knochenneubildungen bei Querschnittsgelähmten. Fortschr. Röntgenstr. 73 (1950), 564
Lugger, L. J.: Übergroßes Tuberculum ossis scaphoidei. Fortschr. Röntgenstr. 121 (1974), 123
Lutterbeck, G.: Die Bestimmung der Knochendichte durch Schwärzungsmessungen an Röntgenogrammen. Diss. Berlin 1958
Lutz, G.: Die Entwicklung der kleinen Wirbelgelenke. Z. Orthop. 104 (1967), 19
Lyon, E.: Über horizontale Aufhellungen in den Röntgenbildern von Wirbelkörpern. Zbl. Chir. (1932), 1845
Maas, W.: Multiple Pseudoepiphysen bei Dysostosis cleido-cranialis. Fortschr. Röntgenstr. 80 (1954), 788
Maassen, G.: Persistierende Apophyse im Bereich des Margo vertebralis scapulae. Fortschr. Röntgenstr. 108 (1968), 406
Macaulay, D.: Digital markings in the radiographs of the skull in Children. Brit. J. Radiol. 24 (1951), 647
Maes, H. J.: Einseitige vollständige Aplasie des Os scaphoideum. Fortschr. Röntgenstr. 109 (1968), 397
Magnusson, W.: Über die Bedingungen des Hervortretens der wirklichen Gelenkspalte auf dem Röntgenbild. Acta radiol. (Stockh.) 18 (1937), 733
Maier, K.: Über die Möglichkeit einer Verschmelzung des Os trigonum mit dem Kalkaneus. Fortschr. Röntgenstr. 92 (1960), 715
Maier, K.: Beitrag zur Verschmelzung des Os trigonum mit dem Kalkaneus. Fortschr. Röntgenstr. 98 (1963), 644

Mainzer, F.: Herniation of the nucleus pulposus. A rare complication of intervertebral-disk calcification in children. Radiology 107 (1973), 167

Majer, E.: Röntgenologische Betrachtungen der Entwicklung und Ausdehnung der Nasennebenhöhlen. Wien. med. Wschr. (1939), 1162

Mangabeira Albernaz, P. u. M. Dias Da Silva: Röntgendiagnose der Siebbeinregion. (An. da Federacao Brasil de O. R. L., Curtiba, Setembro 1954). Rev. bras. Oto-rino-laring. 23 (1955), 43; ref. Zbl. ges. Radiol. 51 (1956), 202

Mannkopf, H.: Röntgenologische Studien über das Zahn- und Skelettwachstum im Säuglingsalter. I. Mitt. Z. Alternsforsch. 7 (1953), 201

Manns, M.: Über die Verknöcherung der Schädelnähte. Diss. Bonn 1933

Mansfeld, K.: Die Beurteilung der Reifeentwicklung im Schulalter. Öff. Gesundh.-Dienst 25 (1963), 80

Marique, P.: Ostéochondrite dissécante de la rotule. Acta orthop. belg. 18 (1952), 316

Markovits, E: Lehrbuch und Atlas der Röntgendiagnostik. Bd. I, Medica, Stuttgart-Zürich 1956

Marti, Th.: Die Skelettvarietäten des Fußes. Huber, Bern 1947

Marti, Th.: Neuer Beitrag zum Studium der Handwurzelvarietäten. Schweiz. med. Wschr. 83 (1953), 52

Marti, Th.: Os cuneometatarsale I dorsale-fibulare. Fortschr. Röntgenstr. 81 (1954), 830

Marti, Th.: Über den Calcaneus secundarius. Fortschr. Röntgenstr. 82 (1955), 124

Martin, H. O.: Sella turcica und Konstitution. Thieme, Leipzig 1941

Martin, P. L. et J. Duhamel: Quelques applications de la tomographie du crâne. J. Radiol. Électrol. 33 (1952), 190

Martin, R. u. K. Saller: Lehrbuch der Anthropologie. 3. Aufl. Fischer, Stuttgart 1957

Martin-Reith, M.: Über das Emissarium frontale. Fortschr. Röntgenstr. 71 (1949), 127

Marx, H.: Die Verkalkungen des Nucleus pulposus im Kindesalter. Arch. orthop. Unfall-Chir. 46 (1953), 144

Matthiash, H.-H.: Pubertätsverlauf und Störungen der Skelettentwicklung. Z. Orthop. 86 (1955), 410

Maurer, H.-J.: Ungewöhnliche Form eines Tuberculum obturatorium anterius. Fortschr. Röntgenstr. 83 (1955), 889

Maurer, H.-J.: Zur Frage einer Apophyse an der Spitze des Dens axis. Fortschr. Röntgenstr. 87 (1957), 127

Maurer, H.-J.: Zur Frage des Sulcus paraglenoidalis. Fortschr. Röntgenstr. 87 (1957), 253

Maurer, H.-J.: Zur Frage eines Os coronoides ulnae. Fortschr. Röntgenstr. 90 (1959), 264

Maurer, H.-J.: Os coronoides ulnae. Fortschr. Röntgenstr. 96 (1962), 572

Maurer, H.-J.: Symmetrische osteocartilaginäre Exostosen (Osteochondrom) der Patella. Fortschr. Röntgenstr. 98 (1963), 771

Maurer, H.-J.: Die Bedeutung variabler Skelettelemente für die Begutachtung. Arch. orthop. Unfall-Chir. 55 (1963), 578

Mayer, E. G.: Otologische Röntgendiagnostik. Springer, Wien 1930

Mayer, E. G.: Diagnose und Differentialdiagnose in der Schädelröntgenologie. Springer, Wien 1959

Max, J.: Angeborene Fehlbildungen der oberen Extremitäten. Med. Bild (1965), 72

McGann, M. S.: Plesiosectionaltomography of the temporal bone. Amer. J. Roentgenol. 88 (1962), 1183

McMorris, R.O.: Faulty posture. Pediat. Clin. N. Amer. 8 (1961), 213

McRae, D. L.: Bony abnormalities in the region of the foramen magnum; correlation of the anatomic and neurologic findings. Acta radiol. (Stockh.) 40 (1953), 335

McRae, D. L. and A. S. Barnum: Occipitalization of the atlas. Amer. J. Roentgenol. 70 (1953), 23

Meachin, G. and M. S. Cornah: Fine structure of juvenile human nucleus pulposus. J. Anat. 107 (1970), 337

Merkel, F.: Handbuch der topographischen Anatomie. Braunschweig 1885-1907

Merkel, F.: Die Anatomie des Menschen. Wiesbaden 1913 - 1918

Meyer, W.: Die Zahn-, Mund- und Kieferheilkunde. Bd. I. Urban u. Schwarzenberg, München 1957

Meyer-Borstel, H.: Meniscusverkalkungen. Chirurg 3 (1931), 424

Millikan, R. A.: Os subcalcis. Amer. J. Surg. 37 (1937), 116

Milner, R.: Gegen den Begriff und den Mißbrauch des Wortes „Periarthritis humeroscapularis". Zbl. Chir. (1932), 2577

Miyakawa, G.: Congenital absence of the odontoid process. A case report. J. Bone Jt Surg. 34A (1952), 676

Moczkowa, W.: Das normale und pathologische Röntgenbild der Nasennebenhöhlen im Kindesalter. Pol. Przegl. radiol. (1953), 8. Kongreßheft, 49; ref. Fortschr. Röntgenstr. 79 (1953), 799

Mörike, K. D.: Zur Funktion und Herkunft des sogenannten Discus im Sternoclaviculargelenk. Morph. Jb. 108 (1965), 212

Mohing, W. u. P. Polyzoides: Beitrag zur Ätiologie des Fersensporns. Arch. Orthop. Unfall-Chir. 57 (1965), 205

Moll, H.: Das Röntgenbild der Hand im Wachstumsalter. Chir. Praxis 8 (1964), 285

Morrison, A. B.: The os paracuneiforme. J. Bone Jt Surg. 35B (1953), 254

Morrison, A. B.: A study of the hip-joint from the standpoint of the roentgenologist. Amer. J. Roentgenol. 28 (1932), 484

Morscher, E.: Posttraumatische Zapfenepiphyse. Arch. orthop. Unfall-Chir. 61 (1967), 128

Motta, G.: La stratigrafia della regione petro-mastoidea. Radiologia (Roma) 8 (1952), 505

Mükke, G.-Chr. u. W. Poppe: Fenestrae parietales symmetricae unter phylogenetischem Aspekt. Fortschr. Röntgenstr. 111 (1969), 300

Müller, P., Dellenbach, P., Meyer, Ch., Bouryal, P. et S. P. Walter: Étude radiologique de la colonne vertébrale „in utero". Contribition au diagnostic des malformations rachidiennes. J. Radiol. Électrol. 49 (1968), 929

Müller, W.: Malazie der Sesambeinknochen des 1. Metatarsale, ein typisches Krankheitsbild. Bruns' Beitr. klin. Chir. 134 (1925), 308

Müller, W.: Weitere Beobachtungen und Untersuchungen zu der typischen Erkrankung der Sesambeine des 1. Metatarsalknochens. Bruns' Beitr. klin. Chir. 138 (1927), 494

Müller, W.: Über eine typische Gestaltveränderung beim Os naviculare pedis und ihre klinische Bedeutung. Fortschr. Röntgenstr. 37 (1928), 38

Müller, W.: Die angeborenen Fehlbildungen der menschlichen Hand. Thieme, Leipzig 1937

Müller-Miny, H.: Eine seltene Bandverknöcherung. Fortschr. Röntgenstr. 83 (1955), 891

Mündnich, K. u. K. W. Frey: Das Röntgenschichtbild des Ohres. Thieme, Stuttgart 1959

Muntean, E.: Der Wert der Tomographie für die Erkennung pathologischer Veränderungen des Labyrinthes und des Fazialiskanals. Fortschr. Röntgenstr. 64 (1941), 109

Muntean, E.: Der Beitrag der Röntgenschichtuntersuchung zur Frühdiagnose des „Cholesteatoms". Fortschr. Röntgenstr. 65 (1942), 279

Muntean, E.: Zur Frühdiagnose der Lockerung im zervikalen Bewegungssegment. Fortschr. Röntgenstr. 77 (1952), 553

Muntean, E.: In: Das Röntgenschichtbild. Thieme, Stuttgart 1959

Muntean, E. u. J. Fink: Das Röntgenogramm des Felsenbeines. Fortschr. Röntgenstr. 63 (1941), 183

Murczynski, Cz. u. W. Uniecka: Agnesie und Dysraphie des Kreuz- und Steißbeins. Radiol. diagn. (Berl.) 10 (1969), 67

Naumann, E.: Außergewöhnlich großer Calcaneus secundarius mit gelenksähnlicher Verbindung zum Calcaneus und Naviculare. Fortschr. Röntgenstr. 83 (1955), 413

Neiss, A.: Doppelseitige Synostose zwischen dem Os multangulum minus und dem Os capitatum. Fortschr. Röntgenstr. 82 (1955), 825

Neiss, A.: Abrißfraktur eines Processus supracondylicus humeri. Fortschr. Röntgenstr. 83 (1955), 120

Neiss, A.: Die Sellabrücke, eine Erscheinungsform des Foramen caroticoclinoideum. Fortschr. Röntgenstr. 84 (1956), 70

Neiss, A.: Gibt es wirklich eine Apophyse am Margo vertebralis scapulae? Fortschr. Röntgenstr. 84 (1956) 259

Neiss, A.: Skelettvariationen. Röntgendiagnostik, Anthropologie, Personenidentifikationen. Habil.-Schrift, Erlangen-Nürnberg 1964

Neiss, A.: Das Os vesalianum ist eine Konstruktion. Verh. anat. Ges. (Jena) 113, (1964), 228

Neiss, A.: Über den begrifflichen Unsinn: Akzessorische Skelettelemente. Vortr. 47. Tgg. d. Deutschen Röntgenges., Berlin 1966
Neiss, A.: Röntgenidentifikationen. Thieme, Stuttgart 1968
Neumann, G.: Os cuneiforme bipartitum. Diss. Leipzig 1939
Neumann, R.: Das Os praecuneiforme (*Bauhin*) am menschlichen Tarsus. Arch. orthop. Unfall-Chir. 45 (1953), 552
Neumann, W.: Über das „Os acromiale". Fortschr. Röntgenstr. 25 (1917/18), 180
Niemann: Eine seltene Neubildung am Fußskelett. Röntgenpraxis 4 (1932), 249
Nobécourt, P. et J. Haguenau: Caractères radiologiques du crâne et notamment de la selle turcique chez les enfants obèses. Presse méd. (1939), 437
Norley, Th. and W. H. Bickel: Calcification of the Bursae of the Knee. J. Bone Jt Surg. 31A (1949), 417
Oberholzer, J.: Röntgendiagnostik der Gelenke mittels Doppelkontrastmethode. Erg.-Bd. Fortschr. Röntgenstr. 56 (1938), Thieme, Leipzig 1938
Oblak, O.: Über einen seltenen Fall mit mehrfacher okzipito-zervikaler Dysplasie. Fortschr. Röntgenstr. 122 (1975), 565
Ochs, E.: Einseitig persistierende Apophyse am Angulus scapulae superior. Fortschr. Röntgenstr. 78 (1953), 486
Odessky, I. u. L. Melnikowa: Zur Kasuistik der Patella cubiti. Dtsch. Z. Chir. 235 (1932), 807
Oeser, H.: Der mediale Tibiacondylensporn. Röntgenpraxis 10 (1938), 416
Oláh, J. u. Sz. Fehérvári: Heriditäre Onycho-Osteo-Arthrodysplasie. Fortschr. Röntgenstr. 109 (1968), 381
Op den Orth, J.O.: Die Verkalkung bzw. Verknöcherung des Ligamentum longitudinale posterius der Halswirbelsäule. Fortschr. Röntgenstr. 122 (1975), 442
Opitz, H. u. B. de Rudder: Pädiatrie. Springer, Berlin-Göttingen-Heidelberg 1957
Oppenheimer, A.: The apophyseal intervertebral articulations, roentgenologically considered. Radiology 30 (1938), 724
O' Rahilly, R. and M. J. Twohig: Foramina parietalia permagna. Amer. J. Roentgenol. 67 (1952), 551
Ott, W.: Festschrift zur 50-Jahrfeier der Graubündnerischen Zahnärztegesellschaft (GZG), 1961
Overhof, K.: Ungewöhnliche Form von Halsrippen. Fortschr. Röntgenstr. 83 (1955), 279
Pässler, H. W.: Zur normalen und zur pathologischen Anatomie und zur Pathologie des Brustbeins. Beitr. path. Anat. 87 (1931), 659
Pagani, A.: Die Röntgenuntersuchung des Kehlkopfes im Schnittbild. Röntgenpraxis 11 (1939), 137
Pahl, R.: Doppelter Nervenkanal der Klavikula als diagnostische Fehlerquelle. (Zugleich ein Beitrag über das Foramen nervi supraclavicularis). Fortschr. Röntgenstr. 82 (1955), 487
v. Pannewitz, G.: Zur Darstellung der Jochbogenfrakturen. Fortschr. Röntgenstr. 85 (1956), 727
Parma, C.: Die Röntgendiagnostik des Kiefergelenks. Röntgenpraxis 4 (1932), 633
Parnitzke, K. H.: Endokranielle Verkalkungen im Röntgenbild. VEB Thieme, Leipzig 1961
Pauwels, F.: Beitrag zur Klärung der Beanspruchung des Beckens, insbesondere der Beckenfugen. In: Gesammelte Abhandlungen zur funktionellen Anatomie des Bewegungsapparates. Springer, Berlin-Heidelberg-New York 1965
Pawlik, H.-J.: Die Sutura mendosa. Fortschr. Röntgenstr. 84 (1956), 698
Péhu, M et A. Policard: Études d'anatomoradiologie. J. Méd. Lyon (1931), 519
Pendergrass, E. P. and Ph. J. Hodes: The rhomboid fossa of the clavicle. Amer. J. Roentgenol. 38 (1937), 152
Pendergrass, E. P. and O. H. Pepper: Observations on the process of ossification in the formation of persistent enlarged parietal foramina. Amer. J. Roentgenol. 41 (1939), 343
Pernkopf, E.: Topographische Anatomie des Menschen. 2. Aufl. Bd. I. Urban u. Schwarzenberg, Wien 1943
Pessagno, A.: Sui foramina parietalia permagna. Ann. Radiol. diagn. (Bologna) 26 (1953), 250
Petersen, F.: Ossifikationsstörungen an der Tibia und Patella. Fortschr. Röntgenstr. 84 (1956), 259
Petersen, F.: Anomalie der distalen Fibula. Fortschr. Röntgenstr. 85 (1956), 118
Petersen, J.: Persistierende Apophyse am Beckenkamm. Unfallheilk. 55 (1952), 109
Pfeiffer, Kl.: Variationen und Anomalien des Brustbeines sowie Hinweise zu deren Entwicklung. Fortschr. Röntgenstr. 85 (1956), 663
Pfeiffer, Kl.: Über persistierende Gelenkfortsatzapophysen im Lumbalbereich. Fortschr. Röntgenstr. 87 (1957), 628
Pfitzner, W.: Patella cubiti. Schwalbes Morphol. Arb. (1891) 1 (Jena), 575
Pfitzner, W.: Die Variationen im Aufbau des Fußskelettes. Schwalbes Morphol. Arb. (Jena) 6 (1896), 245
Pfitzner, W.: Beiträge zur Kenntnis des menschlichen Extremitätenskeletts. Bd. VIII. Die morphologischen Elemente des menschlichen Handskeletts. Z. Morph. Anthrop. 2 (1900), 365
Pia, H. W.: Megacauda. Eine angeborene Erweiterung des Caudasakkes im Lumbosacralbereich. Langenbecks Arch. klin. Chir. 290 (1959), 429
Pickhan, A.: Röntgenologische und anatomische Beobachtungen über den Verknöcherungsvorgang der Kniescheibe. Fortschr. Röntgenstr. 53 (1936), 458
Pickhan, A.: Auffallende Entwicklung der Querfortsätze des 2. Halswirbels. Fortschr. Röntgenstr. 79 (1953), 777
Pickhan, A.: Rudimentäre Rippe des 3. Halswirbels. Fortschr. Röntgenstr. 82 (1955), 691
Platzer, W.: Zur Anatomie der „Sellabrücke" und ihrer Beziehung zur A. carotis interna. Fortschr. Röntgenstr. 87 (1957), 613
Pöschl, M.: Der tomographische Querschnitt durch das Felsenbein. Fortschr. Röntgenstr. 68 (1943), 174
Pohl, R. W.: Optik und Atomphysik. 9. Aufl. Springer, Berlin-Göttingen-Heidelberg 1954
Politzer, G. u. J. Pick: Über einen röntgenologisch wichtigen Knochenbefund am medialen Kondylus der Tibia. Fortschr. Röntgenstr. 56 (1937), 649
Ponseti, I. V. and B. Friedman: Prognosis in idiopathic scoliosis. J. Bone Jt Surg. 32A (1950), 381
Poppel, M. H. and B. E. Zeitel: Roentgen manifestations of milk drinkers syndrome. Radiology 67 (1956), 195
Porstmann, W. u. J. Arenz: Beitrag zu den akzessorischen Tarsalelementen am Calcaneus. Fortschr. Röntgenstr. 81 (1954), 95
Portmann, J.: Der Forameneffekt am Kreuzbein. Fortschr. Röntgenstr. 96 (1962), 823
Posener, K., E. Walker and G. Weddell: Radiographic studies of the metacarpal and metatarsal bones in children. J. Anat. (Lond.) 74 (1939), 76
Priessnitz, O.: Calcinosis intervertebralis bei einem Zwilling und ihre Beziehungen zur *Scheuermann*schen Krankheit. Arch. orthop. Unfall-Chir. 46 (1954), 565
Probst, J.: Isolierte Interartikulärspaltbildung am Brustwirbel und ihre Darstellung im Röntgenbild. Fortschr. Röntgenstr. 86 (1957), 762
Pschyrembel, W.: Klinisches Wörterbuch. 251. Aufl. de Gruyter, Berlin-New York 1972
Psenner, L.: Die anatomischen Varianten des Hirnschädels. Fortschr. Röntgenstr. 75 (1951), 197
Psenner, L.: Differentialdiagnose der Erkrankungen des Schädelskeletts. Thieme, Stuttgart 1973
Putti, V.: Die angeborenen Deformitäten der Wirbelsäule. Fortschr. Röntgenstr. 14 (1909), 285; Fortschr. Röntgenstr. 15 (1910), 65 u. 243
Putti, V.: Die Anatomie der angeborenen Hüftverrenkung. Enke, Stuttgart 1937
de Quervain, F.: Über Cephalhydrocele traumatica. Bruns' Arch. klin. Chir. 51 (1896), 459
Rabaiotti, A.: Rilievi anatomostratigrafici di una porzione della base cranica con incidenza transbuccale del raggio normale. Ann. Radiol. diagn. (Bologna) 26 (1953), 258
Rahm, H.: Die tibio-fibulare Synostose. Z. orthop. Chir. 43 (1924), 64
Rahm, H.: Zur Frage der Disposition bei der Osteochondritis dissecans capituli humeri. Zbl. Chir. (1934), 2263

v. Ranke, H.: Die Ossifikation der Hand unter Röntgenbeleuchtung. Münch. med. Wschr. 43 (1898), 1365
Raspe, R.: Ein neues Verfahren zur Herstellung von Röntgen-Ganzaufnahmen der Wirbelsäule („3-Phasen-Technik"). Fortschr. Röntgenstr. 85 (1956), 106
Raspe, R.: Was würden Sie diagnostizieren? (sog. *Haglund*sche Exostose) Z. ärztl. Fortbild. 54 (1965)
Rathcke, L.: Über Kalkablagerungen in den Zwischenwirbelscheiben. Fortschr. Röntgenstr. 46 (1932), 66
Rauber, A.: Beitrag zur Frage der Anatomie des Olecranonsporns. Z. Unfallmed. Berufskr. 33 (1939), 83
Rauber, A.: Ein wenig bekanntes Röntgensymptom bei älteren Meniscusaffektionen. Z. Unfallmed. Berufkr. 37 (1944), 168
Rauber-Kopsch: Lehrbuch und Atlas der Anatomie des Menschen. 20. Aufl. Bd. I. Thieme, Stuttgart 1968
Ravelli, A.: Zum Röntgenbild des menschlichen Kniegelenks. Fortschr. Röntgenstr. 71 (1949), 614
Ravelli, A.: Eine seltene Ossifikationsanomalie an den Grundphalangen der Zehen (Zapfenepiphysen). Fortschr. Röntgenstr. 76 (1952), 261
Ravelli, A.: Zur Mondbeinossifikation. Fortschr. Röntgenstr. 76 (1952), 265
Ravelli, A.: Die Richtungslinie der Y-Fuge als Hilfslinie zur Früherkennung der angeborenen Hüftluxation. Z. Orthop. 84 (1953), 28
Ravelli, A.: Zur Messung des Pfannenwinkels bei Neugeborenen. Z. Orthop. 84 (1953), 33
Ravelli, A.: Peritendinitis calcarea an seltenen Stellen. Med. Klin. 48 (1953), 1771
Ravelli, A.: Gefäßkanäle in den Handwurzelknochen. Radiol. clin. (Basel) 22, (1953), 461
Ravelli, A.: Gefäßkanäle in den Fingergliedern. Radiol. clin. (Basel) 22 (1953), 465
Ravelli, A.: Versuch einer entwicklungsgeschichtlichen Deutung bestimmter Einzelheiten am Schlüsselbein und seinen Verbindungen. Z. Anat. Entwickl.-Gesch. 118 (1955), 343
Ravelli, A.: Zur Frage der sogenannten *Friedrich*schen Krankheit. Z. Orthop. 86 (1955), 397
Ravelli, A.: Zum Röntgenbild des proximalen Schienbeindrittels. Fortschr. Röntgenstr. 82 (1955), 48
Ravelli, A.: Zum Bilde der Bandgrube am sternalen Schlüsselbeinende. Fortschr. Röntgenstr. 82 (1955), 804
Ravelli, A.: Fehlbildungen an Bogen und Gelenkfortsätzen der Lendenwirbel. Fortschr. Röntgenstr. 82 (1955), 826
Ravelli, A.: Zur Frage des sog. Os accessorium supracalcaneum. Fortschr. Röntgenstr. 83 (1955), 71
Ravelli, A.: Das Vakuum-Phänomen (*R. Fick*sches Zeichen). Fortschr. Röntgenstr. 83 (1955), 236
Ravelli, A.: Zum anatomischen und röntgenologischen Bild der Tuberositas tibae beim Erwachsenen. Fortschr. Röntgenstr. 83 (1955), 382
Ravelli, A.: Zur Ossikation der Vieleckbeine. Fortschr. Röntgenstr. 83 (1955), 852
Ravelli, A.: Zapfenepiphysen an den Mittelphalangen der Zehen. Fortschr. Röntgenstr. 84 (1956), 498
Ravelli, A.: Nebenkerne an der Basis des Großzehenendglieds. Fortschr. Röntgenstr. 84 (1956), 499
Ravelli, A.: Persistierende Apophyse am Proc. coracoides. Fortschr. Röntgenstr. 84 (1956), 500
Ravelli, A.: Os accessorium supracalcaneum. Fortschr. Röntgenstr. 85 (1956), 121
Ravelli, A.: Das Ossiculum parasternale. Fortschr. Röntgenstr. 85 (1956), 226
Ravelli, A. u. E. Ruckensteiner: Der persistierende Chordakanal in der Schädelbasis (Canalis basilaris medianus). Radiol. Austriaca 9 (1957), 59
Reckling, F.: Eine anlagemäßig bedingte Zweiteilung des Handwurzelkahnbeines. Mschr. Unfallheilk. 46 (1939), 146
Reinhardt, K.: Eine ungewöhnliche Anomalie an den Dornfortsätzen des 5., 6. und 7. Halswirbels. Fortschr. Röntgenstr. 85 (1956), 253
Reinhardt, K.: Das anatomische Substrat lochförmiger Aufhellungen in den unteren Lendenwirbelkörpern und ihre klinische Bedeutung. Fortschr. Röntgenstr. 86 (1957), 222
Reinhardt, K.: Die Anatomie und Pathologie der kleinen Wirbelgelenke im Röntgenbild. Radiol. diagn. (Berl.) 4 (1963), 665
Reinhardt, K.: Der Processus supratrochlearis humeri. Fortschr. Röntgenstr. 105 (1966), 125
Reinhardt, K.: Eine doppelseitige Anomalie am lateralen Klavikuladrittel, bestehend aus einer bogenförmigen Duplikatur des Knochens in Richtung auf das Coracoid und aus akzessorischen Knochenelementen. Fortschr. Röntgenstr. 113 (1970), 527
Reinhardt, K.: Überzählige Wirbelbögen zwischen 4. und 5. Lendenwirbel (sogenanntes Asoma). Fortschr. Röntgenstr. 119 (1973), 252
Reinhardt, K.: Die spina bifida lumbosacralis. In: Hdb. d. Med. Radiologie. Bd. IV/2, Springer, Berlin-Heidelberg-New York 1974, 493
Reinike, A. u. H. Sprenger: Zur Röntgenanatomie des Labyrinths. Z. Laryng. Rhinol. 34 (1955), 361
Reisner, A.: Verknöcherungen im Ligamentum patellae. Angeborene Anomalie? Röntgenpraxis 4 (1932), 84
Reisner, K.: Experimentelle Untersuchungen zur Detailerkennbarkeit im Röntgenschichtbild des Schädels. Fortschr. Röntgenstr. 112 (1970), 332
Reisner, K.: Die Schädeltomographie in transmaxillärer Schrägprojektion. Fortschr. Röntgenstr. 113 (1970), 271
Reisner, K. u. J. Gosepath: Schädeltomographie. Thieme, Stuttgart 1973
Renander, A.: Anomalies roentgenologically observed of the craniovertebral region. Acta radiol. (Stockh.) 10 (1929), 502
Renner, C.: Die *Shenton*sche Linie. Zbl. Chir. 52 (1925), 2875
Retterer: Zit. nach *W. Müller:* Die angeborenen Fehlbildungen der menschlichen Hand. Thieme, Leipzig 1937
Rhese, O. A.: Die chronischen Entzündungen der Siebbeinzellen und der Keilbeinhöhle. Arch. Laryng. Rhinol. (Berlin) 24 (1911), 383
Ribbing, S.: Zur Ätiologie der Osteochondritis dissecans. Acta radiol. (Stockh.) 25 (1944), 732
Rickenbacher, J.: Die Entwicklungsgeschichte der Wirbelsäule. Praxis 58 (1969), 179
Rieder, H. u. J. Rosenthal: Lehrbuch der Röntgenkunde. 2. Aufl. Bd. 2. Barth, Leipzig 1925
Riess, J.: Typische Kniescheibenveränderung beim Morbus *Little,* zweigeteilte Kniescheibe oder Ermüdungsbruch? Fortschr. Röntgenstr. 81 (1954), 221
Rinonapoli, G.: Anomalia rara della rotula. Arch. Med. Chir. (Milano) 2 (1933), 151
Rittweger, W.: Isolierte Apophyse am Margo vertebralis der Scapula. Röntgenpraxis 14 (1942), 227
Riva, G.: Ein Fall von doppelseitigem Os triangulare carpi. Radiol. clin. (Basel) 18 (1949), 78
Roaf, R.: Foramen in the humerus caused by the median nerve. J. Bone Jt Surg. 38B (1957), 748
Rochlin, D. G. u. E. Zeitler: Röntgendiagnostik der Hand und Handwurzel. In: Hdb. d. Med. Radiologie. Bd. IV/2, Springer, Berlin-Heidelberg-New York 1968, 44, 58 f., 100
Rode, J.: Das Röntgen-Nativ-Bild beim Meniskusschaden. Inaug.-Diss. Münster 1971
Roeckerath, W.: Hereditäre Osteo-onycho-dysplasie. Fortschr. Röntgenstr. 75 (1951), 700
Rösli, A.: Über das Vorkommen des zweigeteilten Os radiale dorsale. Radiol. clin. (Basel) 22 (1953), 361
Rösli, A.: Ein Beitrag zur Technik der symmetrischen Jochbogenaufnahme. Radiol. clin. (Basel) 23 (1954), 12
Rokay, Z. E. u. F. Horváth: Exostose seltener Lokalisation. Fortschr. Röntgenstr. 90 (1959), 271
Rosenkranz, A.: Eine seltene Wirbelsäulenmißbildung. Zum Problem des dorsalen Halswirbels. Öst. Z. Kinderheilk. 8 (1953), 291
Ross, E.: Os capitatum bipartitum. Fortschr. Röntgenstr. 81 (1954), 224
Rossmann, B.: Besondere Ossifikationsstörung an den Zehen (Glockenepiphyse). Magy. Radiol. (1955), 235
Rossmann, B.: Einfache röntgenologische Aufnahmetechnik des Säuglingsohres. Fortschr. Röntgenstr. 86 (1957), 741
Rossmann, B.: Über die Röntgendiagnostik des Säuglingsohres. Fortschr. Röntgenstr. 94 (1961), 232 u. 402
Rossmann, B.: Weitere Vereinfachung unserer Aufnahmetechnik bei

der Röntgenuntersuchung des Säuglingsohres. Fortschr. Röntgenstr. 98 (1963), 58
Rowley, R. A.: Coronal cleft vertebra. J. Fac. Radiol. (Lond.) 6 (1955), 267
Rubaschewa, A.: Über den Processus lateralis der Lendenwirbel und spez. über den Processus styloideus im Röntgenbild. Fortschr. Röntgenstr. 47 (1933), 183
Ruckensteiner, E.: Die normale Entwicklung des Knochensystems im Röntgenbild. Thieme, Leipzig 1931
Ruckensteiner, E.: Über multiple Handwurzelknochen. Röntgen-Bl. 4 (1951), 236
Rudder, de B.: Zur Frage nach der Akzelerationsursache. Dtsch. med. Wschr. 85 (1960), 1193
Rühlmann, M., U. Nitschke u. H. Fiehring: Ausgedehnte Nephrokalzinose bei einem 9jährigen Knaben. Fortschr. Röntgenstr. 91 (1959), 815
Rüttimann, A.: Die Doppelkontrastarthrographie des Kniegelenkes. Fortschr. Röntgenstr. 87 (1957), 736
Rump, W.: Elektromedizin und Strahlenkunde. Urban u. Schwarzenberg, München-Berlin 1954
Rumphorst, K.: Über die Knochenkernentwicklung syphilitischer Feten und Neugeborener im Röntgenbild. Fortschr. Röntgenstr. 85 (1956), 76
Rumpold, H.-J.: Beitrag zum Verknöcherungszentrum im proximalen Gelenkanteil der Ulna. Fortschr. Röntgenstr. 99 (1963), 809
Rumpold, H.-J.: Die Persistenz des Verknöcherungszentrums im proximalen Gelenkabschnitt der Ulna (Beitrag zur Abgrenzung gegen dortige Frakturen). Fortschr. Röntgenstr. 100 (1964), 651
Rumpold, H.-J.: Ungewöhnliche Nebenkerne am inneren und äußeren Knöchel (Beitrag zur Fraktur im Nebenkern). Fortschr. Röntgenstr. 102 (1965), 709
Rumpold, H.-J.: Beitrag zu den Distorsionsfrakturen der Fußwurzel (unter besonderer Berücksichtigung des Proc. ant. calcanei). Fortschr. Röntgenstr. 104 (1966), 835
Runge, K.: Über die Knochenkerne der Wirbelkörper. Fortschr. Röntgenstr. 60 (1939), 323
Sabat, B: Intrarektale Radiographie. Fortschr. Röntgenstr. 53 (1936), 143
Sack, G. M.: Os trigonum und *Shepheard*sche Fraktur. Röntgenpraxis 4 (1932), 1028
Sack, G. M.: Über den Kalkaneussporn. Röntgenpraxis 4 (1932), 158
Sander, D.: Die Wichtigkeit der Schichtaufnahmenuntersuchung zur Darstellung von Veränderungen der obersten Halswirbel. Röntgen-Bl. 7 (1954), 70
Santagati, F.: Anatomia radiografica dei solchi e dei canali vascolari del cranio. Radiol. med. (Torino) 26 (1939), 317
Sartorius, W.: Über die Möglichkeit einer objektiven Größenbestimmung der Sella turcica im Kindesalter. Mschr. Kinderheilk. 45 (1929), 259
Saupe, E.: Erweiterung von Knochengefäßkanälen der Tibia bei Unterschenkelvarikosis. Röntgenpraxis 12 (1940), 90
Scarpa, G.: Studio radiologico-statistico dei canali diploici. Arch. ital. Anat. Embriol. 60 (1955), 441
Schaaf, J. u. A. Wagner: Multiplizität von Handwurzelknochen bei drei Geschwistern mit polytoper enchondraler Dysostose. Fortschr. Röntgenstr. 97 (1962), 497
Schaaf, J. u. G. Wilhelm: Über den Canalis craniopharyngeus. Fortschr. Röntgenstr. 86 (1957), 748
Schaefer, H. G.: Zur Klinik der Brüche des Rabenschnabelfortsatzes. Chirurg 22 (1951), 172
Schäfer, H.: Zur röntgenologischen und klinischen Bedeutung der Pseudoepiphysenbildung am kindlichen Handskelett. Kinderärztl. Prax. 20 (1952), 77
Schäfer, K. H., s. Lassrich-Prévôt-Schäfer
Schaer, H.: Die Patella partita. Ergebn. Chir. Orthop. 27 (1934), 1
Schär, W. u. C. Zweifel: Das os acromiale und seine klinische Bedeutung. Bruns' Beitr. klin. Chir. 164 (1936), 101
Scherb, R.: Spondylolisthesis (Spondylolisthesis imminens), Sacrum acutum, Sacrum arcuatum, Regio lumbosacralis fixa als häufige Ursachen von Kreuzschmerzen. Z. orthop. Chir. 50 (1928), 304
Schertel, L., M. Scholz u. H. Kraska: Schläfenbeintomographie (Erfahrungen bei 98 Untersuchungen). Fortschr. Röntgenstr. 121 (1974), 556
Schiffer, K. H.: Cerebrale Frühschädigung und Schädelbasisdysplasie. Fortschr. Röntgenstr. 75 (1951), 54
Schiffer, K. H. u. H. Strubel: Über Störungen der Entwicklungsmechanik des Gehirnschädels beim Mongolismus und andere Konstitutionsanomalien. Nervenarzt 31 (1960), 340
Schillinger, R.: Pneumatisation of the mastoid. A Roentgenstudy. Radiology 33 (1939), 54
Schinz, H. R.: Der Abbruch des Processus styloideus ulnae. Dtsch. Z. Chir. 175 (1922), 81
Schinz, H. R.: Das Foramen supratrochleare humeri. Fortschr. Röntgenstr. 29 (1922), 193
Schinz, H. R.: Altes und Neues zur Beckenossifikation. Fortschr. Röntgenstr. 30 (1922), 66
Schinz, H. R.: Die Schulter, eine anatomische und röntgenologische Studie. Arch. orthop. Unfall-Chir. 22 (1924), 352
Schinz, H. R.: Vererbung und Knochenbau. Schweiz. med. Wschr. 5 (1924), 1176
Schinz, H. R.: Vergleichende Anatomie und Phylogenie des Skeletts in ihrer Bedeutung für den Röntgenologen. Radiol. clin. (Basel) 14 (1945), 19
Schinz, H. R. u. E. Uehlinger: Zur Differentialdiagnose des Knocheninfarktes. Radiol. clin. (Basel) 17 (1948), 57
Schinz, H. R., R. Glauner u. E. Uehlinger: Röntgendiagnostik. Ergebnisse 1952 - 1956, Thieme, Stuttgart 1957
Schinz, H. R., W. E. Baensch, W. Frommhold, R. Glauner, E. Uehlinger u. J. Wellauer: Lehrbuch der Röntgendiagnostik. 5. Aufl. Thieme, Stuttgart 1966
Schlevogt, E.: Die klinische Bedeutung des Os tibiale externum. Diss. Leipzig 1934
Schlitter, H. E.: Skelettanomalien und erworbene Skelettveränderungen bei congenitalen Herz- und Gefäßmißbildungen. Ärztl. Wschr. 12 (1957), 309
Schlüter, A.: Drei Fälle von Calcaneus bipartitus im Kindesalter. Arch. orthop. Unfall-Chir. 45 (1952), 122
Schlüter, K.: Der „Calcaneus bifidus", eine Ossifikationsanomalie des Fersenbeins im Hackenplattfuß. Fortschr. Röntgenstr. 85 (1956), 720
Schmid, F.: Die Handskelettossifikationen als Indikator der Entwicklung. Ergebn. inn. Med. Kinderheilk. 1 (1949), 176
Schmid, F.: Das Handgelenk bei frühinfantilen Affektionen des Zentralnervensystems. Fortschr. Röntgenstr. 86 (1957), 239
Schmid, F. u. L. Halden: Die postfetale Differenzierung der Extremitätenknochenkerne. Fortschr. Röntgenstr. 71 (1949), 975
Schmid, F. u. E. Hoffmann: Die metrische Beurteilung der Handlänge. Fortschr. Röntgenstr. 88 (1958), 450
Schmid, F., N. Homma u. E. Hoffmann: Zusammenhänge zwischen Handwurzelkernentwicklung und Körperlänge. Fortschr. Röntgenstr. 88 (1958), 447
Schmid, F. u. H. Moll: Atlas der normalen und pathologischen Handskelettentwicklung. Springer, Berlin-Göttingen-Heidelberg 1960
Schmid, F. u. G. Weber: Röntgendiagnostik im Kindesalter. Bergmann, München 1955
Schmid, G.: Vertebra plana totalis. Fortschr. Röntgenstr. 76 (1952), 358
Schmidt, H.: Pfannenrandepiphyse und Pfannenrandknochen der Hüfte (Epiphysis acetabuli und Os ad acetabulum). Zbl. allg. Path. Anat. 92 (1954), 271
Schmidt, H.: Okzipitale Dysplasien. Fortschr. Röntgenstr. 90 (1959), 691 (1. Mitteilung)
Schmidt, H.: Die okzipitale Dysplasie. Fortschr. Röntgenstr. 91 (1959), 207 (2. Mitteilung)
Schmidt-Wittkamp, E. u. H. Christians: Die Lückenbildungen der Scheitelbeine. Beobachtungen an 75 Mitgliedern einer Sippe mit gehäuftem Vorkommen von Foramina parietalia permagna. Fortschr. Röntgenstr. 113 (1970), 29
Schmitt, H.: Vorgetäuschter Keilwirbel. Röntgenpraxis 10 (1938), 609
Schmitt, H.: Ein akzessorischer Knochen oberhalb des Kalkaneus (Os accessorium supracalcaneum bilaterale aut unilaterale). Röntgenpraxis 15 (1943), 137

Schmitt, H. G.: Persistierende Apophyse des Olecranons. Fortschr. Röntgenstr. 74 (1951), 241
Schmorl, G. u. H. Junghanns: Die gesunde und die kranke Wirbelsäule in Röntgenbild und Klinik. Thieme, Stuttgart 1968
Schneider, A. J.: Sellabrücken und Konstitution. Thieme, Leipzig 1939
Schneider, F. W.: Bemerkenswerter Fall von Halsrippe. Röntgenpraxis 12 (1940), 162
Schneider, H.: Die Abnützungserkrankungen der Sehnen und ihre Therapie. Thieme, Stuttgart 1959
Schneider, U.: Das akzessorische Iliosakralgelenk (Articulus sacroilicus accessorius) im Röntgenbild. Fortschr. Röntgenstr. 85 (1956), 426
Schneider, V. u. L. Walz: Zur Klinik des Odontoids. Fortschr. Röntgenstr. 115 (1971), 302
Schoen, D.: Über die Ursachen einer auf die unteren Zervikalwirbel projizierten Aufhellungslinie. Fortschr. Röntgenstr. 84 (1956), 763
Schoen, H.: Seltenere akzessorische Knochen am Fußrücken. Röntgenpraxis 7 (1935), 775
Schoen, H.: Das Os vesalianum. Fortschr. Röntgenstr. 75 (1951), 489
Schoen, H.: Medizinische Röntgentechnik. II. Physikalisch-technischer Teil. 2. Aufl. Thieme, Stuttgart 1958
Schoen, H.: Medizinische Röntgentechnik I. 3. Aufl. Thieme, Stuttgart 1960
Schönbauer, H. R.: Zur Röntgentechnik des Schlüsselbeinbruches. Fortschr. Röntgenstr. 86 (1957), 349
Schöneich, R.: Dorsaler Halbwirbel des 1. LWK und Blockwirbelbildung des 12. BWK. Fortschr. Röntgenstr. 82 (1955), 280
Schöneich, R.: Persistierende Epiphyse des rechten Hüftgelenkes. Fortschr. Röntgenstr. 87 (1957), 417
Schönkess, P.: Anomalien der Fußwurzelknochen. Diss. Münster i.W. 1935
Schoeps, J.: Kalkeinlagerungen der Glomi bzw. Plexus chorioidales als Residua und Indikatoren nach spontangeheilter kongenitaler Toxoplasma-Infektion des Zentralnervensystemes. Fortschr. Röntgenstr. 75 (1951), 335
Schreier, K.: Die angeborenen Stoffwechselanomalien. Thieme, Stuttgart 1963
Schrop, F. J.: Zur Genese der primären Meniscusverkalkung. Fortschr. Röntgenstr. 76 (1952), 202
Schüller, A.: Röntgendiagnostik des Kopfes. Hölder, Wien 1912
Schüller, A., E. G. Mayer u. K. B. Amersbach: Schädel-Diagnostik. Fortschr. Röntgenstr. 41 (1930), 793
Schuhknecht, T.: Blockwirbelbildung bei Adoleszenten-Kyphose. Med. Wschr. 6 (1952), 522
Schulte, E.: Atypische Ossifikation des Os naviculare pedis. Fortschr. Röntgenstr. 88 (1958), 371
Schulte, E.: Seltene Skelettanomalie am Schultergürtel. Fortschr. Röntgenstr. 92 (1960), 226
Schulte, E.: Beitrag zum Korakoklavikulargelenk. Fortschr. Röntgenstr. 92 (1960), 463
Schulte, F.: Beitrag zur Kenntnis der primären Meniskusverkalkung. Zbl. Chir. 75 (1950), 214
Schulte, K.-J.: Einige seltenere Knochenbefunde im Bereich des Schultergürtels. Fortschr. Röntgenstr. 86 (1957), 231
Schulte-Brinkmann, W. u. R. M. Konrad: Zur Meßtechnik der Hand- und Fußwurzelknochen bei Kindern. Fortschr. Röntgenstr. 99 (1963), 544
Schulte-Brinkmann, W., R. M. Konrad, P. Schmidt u. F. Ehlers: Der heutige Entwicklungsstand des Hand- und Fußwurzelskeletts bei gesunden und herzkranken Kindern im Schulalter. Arch. Orthop. Unfall-Chir. 62 (1967), 118
Schumann, W.: Doppelseitige Apophysenpersistenz der Tuberositas tibiae bei einem 58jährigen Mann. Fortschr. Röntgenstr. 79 (1953), 247
Schumann, W. u. J. Trautmann: Über röntgenologisch faßbare Veränderungen an den Lendenwirbeldornfortsätzen und ihre Bedeutung für die Pathogenese des Kreuzschmerzes. Fortschr. Röntgenstr. 76 (1952), 579
Schunk, H. and Y. Maruyama: Two vascular grooves of the external table of the skull which simulate fractures. Acta radiol. (Stockh.) 54 (1960). 186
Schwartz, Ch. W.: Anomalies and variations in the normal skull from a roentgenological viewpoint. Amer. J. Roentgenol. 42 (1939), 367
Schwarz, M.: Entwicklung der Nasennebenhöhlen und individuelle Varianten der Pneumatisation beim Menschen. Z. Hals-, Nas.- u. Ohrenheilk. 36 (1934), 296
Sedwick, H. J.: Form, size and position of the maxillary sinus at various ages studied by means of roentgenograms of the skull. Amer. J. Roentgenol. 32 (1934), 154
Seegelken, K. u. G.-A. Schulte: Spaltbildungen des Wirbelbogens (Mitteilung der Beobachtung einer retrosomatischen Spalte). Fortschr. Röntgenstr. 116 (1972), 473
Seibert-Daiker, F. M.: Über eine halbseitige Dornfortsatzhyperplasie des 5. Halswirbels, verbunden mit einer persistierenden Apophyse des 7. Halswirbels. Fortschr. Röntgenstr. 122 (1975), 366
Sever, J. W.: Bifid os calcis. Surg. Gynec. Obstet. 50 (1930), 1012
Seyffarth, G. u. R. Heppe: Die Röntgenaufnahme des Schlüsselbeins in der zweiten Ebene. Beitr. Orthop. 12 (1965), 71
Seyss, R.: Zur Röntgenologie der kindlichen Wirbelsäule. Fortschr. Röntgenstr. 74 (1951), 434
Seyss, R.: Schichtuntersuchungen der Extremitäten mittels Feinstfocus bei entzündlichen Knochenerkrankungen. Arch. orthop. Unfall-Chir. 46 (1954), 251
Seyss, R.: Zu den Verkalkungen der Gelenksbänder. Fortschr. Röntgenstr. 89 (1958), 239
Seyss, R.: Das Vakuumphänomen im Bereich des Hüftgelenks. Fortschr. Röntgenstr. 90 (1959), 140
Seyss, R.: Zu den Verknöcherungen im Bereich des Foramen obturatum. Fortschr. Röntgenstr. 91 (1959), 525
Seyss, R.: Verkalkungen unterhalb der Plantarsehne. Münch. med. Wschr. 102 (1960), 1876
Sèze, de S. u. A. Djian: L'anneau atloïdien de la vertébrale. La déhiscence transversaire de l'axis. Rev. Rhum. 20, Nr. spéc, (1953), 160
Shepheard, F. J.: A hitherto undiscribed fracture of the astragus. J. Anat. Physiol. 17 (1882), 79
Siebert, P.: Processus paracondylicus. Fortschr. Röntgenstr. 111 (1969), 717
Siecke, H.: Beitrag zur Genese des Os peroneum (Beobachtungen an 250 röntgenologisch festgestellten Ossa peronea). Z. Orthop. 98 (1964), 358
Sieckel, L.: Über die persistierenden Knochenkerne am Ellenbogengelenk. Fortschr. Röntgenstr. 85 (1956), 709
Sieckel, L.: Beitrag zur Genese des Os peroneum (Beobachtungen an 250 röntgenologisch festgestellten Ossa peronea). Z. Orthop. 98 (1964), 358
Siegert, F.: Die Osteogenesis chondrodysplastica mit besonderer Berücksichtigung des Pseudoepiphysen-Problems. Fortschr. Röntgenstr. 48 (1933), 666
Siegert, F.: Atlas der normalen Ossifikation der menschlichen Hand. Fortschr. Röntgenstr. Ergbd. 47 (1935)
Silvermann, F. N.: The roentgen manifestations of unrecognized skeletal trauma in infants. Amer. J. Roentgenol. 69 (1953), 413
Silvermann, F. N.: Calcification of the inter-vertebral discs in childhood. Radiology 62 (1954), 801
Simay, A. u. Kl. Murányi: Iliacal-Hörner. Eine familiäre Entwicklungsanomalie. Fortschr. Röntgenstr. 103 (1965), 116
Simon, A.: Erhaltener Kiemenbogen. Röntgenpraxis 3 (1931), 141
Simon, St.: Eine Bandgrube des sternalen Schlüsselbeinendes. Röntgenpraxis 10 (1938), 412
Sirry, A.: The pseudocystic triangle in the normal os calcis. Acta radiol. (Stockh.) 36 (1951), 516
Smola, L.: Der Calcaneus bifidus. Fortschr. Röntgenstr. 85 (1956), 120
Snodgrasse, R. M., S. Dreizen, G. S. Parker and T. D. Spies: Serial sequential development of anomalous metacarpal and phalangeal ossification centers in the human hand. Growth 19 (1955), 307
Sobotta-Becher: Atlas der deskriptiven Anatomie des Menschen. 1. Teil, 15. Aufl. Urban u. Schwarzenberg, München-Berlin 1957
Sonnenkalb, V.: Die Röntgendiagnostik des Nasen- und Ohrenarztes. Fischer, Jena 1914
Sontag, L. W., D. Snell and M. Anderson: Rate of appearance of ossification centers from birth to the age of five years. Amer. J. Dis. Child. 58 (1939), 949
Sorge, F.: Über die Bedeutung der Diploevenen. Arch. klin. Chir. 182 (1935), 289

Spalteholz-Spanner: Handatlas der Anatomie des Menschen. 16. Aufl., Bd. I. Scheltema u. Holkema, Amsterdam 1959

Spiegel, M. B. and G. H. Koiransky: Melorheostosis *Léri.* Review of literature and report of a case. Amer. J. Roentgenol. 64 (1950), 789

Springorum, P. W.: Chronische und eitrige Bursitis. Zbl. Chir. 82 (1957), 2133

Springorum, P. W.: Kontrastdarstellung von Schleimbeuteln. Zbl. Chir. 84 (1959), 721

Stehr, L.: Variationen und Fehlbildungen im Bau des knöchernen Thorax. Fortschr. Röntgenstr. 62 (1940), 67

Stein, H. u. G. Schmidt: Beitrag zu den Spaltbildungen der Wirbelsäule. Arch. Kinderheilk. 163 (1960), 135

Steinhäuser, J. u. G. Merhof: Röntgenstudien an Handgelenken zur sogenannten Minusvariante der Elle (*Hultén*). Z. Orthop. 107 (1969), 11

Stenvers, H. W.: Röntgenologie des Felsenbeines und des bitemporalen Schädelbildes. Mit besonderer Berücksichtigung ihrer klinischen Bedeutung. Bd. 1, Springer, Berlin 1928

Stern, L.: Röntgenologische Betrachtung der Entwicklung und Ausdehnung der Nasennebenhöhlen. Hals-, Nas.- u. Ohrenarzt. 1. Teil (1939), 169

Stettner, E.: Ossifikationsstudien am Handskelett. Z. Kinderheilk. 52 (1931), 1 u. 459

Stieda, A.: Momente aus der Entwicklung des knöchernen Handgelenkes. Verh. dtsch. Röntg.-Ges. 1 (1905), 143

Stieda, L.: Über sekundäre Fußwurzelknochen. Arch. Anat. Physiol. (1869), 108

Stössel, H. G., C. W. Fassbender u. G. Häussler: Die Bedeutung der Übersichtsaufnahme (Leeraufnahme) der Lendenwirbelsäule beim lumbalen Bandscheibenvorfall. Fortschr. Röntgenstr. 91 (1959), 329

Stolze, Th.: Spalten des vorderen und des hinteren Atlasbogens, seltene für den Atlas typische Fehlbildungen. Radiologe 9 (1969), 304

Stuart, H. C. and S. S. Stevenson: Physical growth and development. In: Textbook of pediatrics, 6th edit. Saunders Co., Philadelphia 1954

Stucke, K.: Der Fersenschmerz. Thieme, Stuttgart 1956

Stumme: Über Sesambeine. Fortschr. Röntgenstr. 13 (1908/09), 312

Süsse, H. J.: Gefäßzeichen im Areal der Stirnhöhlen. Fortschr. Röntgenstr. 100 (1964), 215

Süsse, U. u. H. J. Süsse: Über das Emissarium frontale. Fortschr. Röntgenstr. 89 (1958), 202

Swart, B.: De la qualité et des renseignements donnés par les clichés tomographiques dans les divers types de la balayage. Roentgen-Europ. 2 (1961), 2

Swoboda, W.: Das Skelet des Kindes. 1. Aufl. Thieme, Stuttgart 1956 (wiedergegebene Abb. ist in der 2. Aufl. (1969) nicht mehr enthalten!)

Swoboda, W.: Das Skelet des Kindes. 2. Aufl. Thieme, Stuttgart 1969

Swoboda, W. u. H. Wimberger: Röntgenologische Handlängenmessung als Kriterium für das Körperlängenwachstum. Arch. Kinderheilk. 148 (1954), 31

Szántó, D.: Die Verkalkung der Zirbeldrüse bei bösartigen Geschwulsterkrankungen. Röntgen-Bl. 21 (1968), 386

Tänzer, A.: Durch Spalt im vorderen Bogen des Atlas vorgetäuschte Fraktur des Dens epistrophei. Fortschr. Röntgenstr. 86 (1957), 138

Takagi, K.: Über die Deutung und Messung des röntgenologischen Schattens des Türkensattels und der in seiner Nähe sich zeigenden Schatten. Mitt. med. Fak. Tokyo 32 (1925), 251

Tanew, N.: Entwicklung und Anomalien der Stirnhöhlen. Radiol. Austriaca (1948), 113

Tarp, O.: Tomography of temporal bone with polytome. Acta radiol. (Stockh.) 51 (1959), 105

Tatafiore, E.: L' importanza dell' etâ scheletrica nello studio delle alterazioni dell' accrescimento della prima infanzia. Infanzia 3 (1953), 19

Teichert, G.: Beitrag zur Röntgenbild-Analyse des Kniegelenkes. Röntgen-Bl. 8 (1955), 4

Teichert, G.: Schaltknochen der Zwischenwirbelscheiben und Spondylosis deformans. Fortschr. Röntgenstr. 84 (1956), 457

Teichert, G.: Os calcaneocuboideum laterale. Fortschr. Röntgenstr. 84 (1956), 647

Teichert, G.: Verknöcherung im hinteren Kreuzband eine Verletzungsfolge? (Vorkommen mit einem Tuberculum intercondylicum quartum). Fortschr. Röntgenstr. 84 (1956), 766

Teichert, G.: Über Ossifikationsvarianten und Ossifikationsstörungen am Tuber ossis ischii. Arch. orthop. Unfall-Chir. 49 (1957), 169

Teneff, St.: Calcificazione del legamento crociato posteriore del ginocchio. Boll. Soc. piemont. Chir. 7 (1937), 466

Terlep, H.: Os radiale externum. Fortschr. Röntgenstr. 86 (1957), 666

Terrafranca, R. J. and A. Zellis: Congenital Hereditary Cranium Bifidum Occultum Frontalis. Radiology 61 (1953), 60

Thamm, D.: Seltene Bandverknöcherung im Bereich des Foramen obturatum links. Fortschr. Röntgenstr. 116 (1972), 839

Theiler, K.: Embryonale und postnatale Entwicklung des Schädels. In: Handbuch der Medizinischen Radiologie, Bd. VII/1. Springer, Berlin-Göttingen-Heidelberg 1963

Theiler, K.: Onto- und Phylogenese des Skelets, der Gelenke und der Muskulatur. Cytogenese des Bindegewebes, des Knorpels des Knochens und der Muskulatur. In: Handbuch der Kinderheilk. Bd. VI. Springer, Berlin-Heidelberg-New York 1967

Thémido, A.: Un nouveau détail morphologique de l'humérus. Folia anat. (Coimbra) 1 (1926), 3

Thews, K.: Fehldeutung und Fehlbehandlung auf Grund von Varietäten der Handwurzel und Fußwurzel im Röntgenbild. Röntgenpraxis 11 (1939), 184

Thews, K.: Die Entwicklungsstörung des Brustbeins. Röntgenpraxis 11 (1939), 188

Thiemann, H.: Juvenile Epiphysenstörungen. Fortschr. Röntgenstr. 14 (1909/10), 79

Thiemann, H. H.: Zapfenepiphysen in Kombination mit Teilsymptomen des *Marchesani*-Syndroms. Fortschr. Röntgenstr. 93 (1960), 367

Thiemann, R. J., J. Fischer u. G. Mollowitz: Der Beitrag der gezielten Doppelkontrastarthrographie für die Indikationsstellung zur Rearthrotomie des Kniegelenkes. Chirurg 41 (1970), 365

Titze, A.: Über einen akzessorischen Knochenschatten im Bereiche des jugendlichen Kniegelenkes. Fortschr. Röntgenstr. 87 (1957), 668

Tobeck, A.: Über den Verlauf des Facialiskanals im Röntgenbild. Arch. Ohr-, Nas., u. Kehlk.-Heilk. 144 (1938), 276

Tobler, T.: Zur normalen und pathologischen Histologie des Kniegelenkmeniscus. Arch. klin. Chir. 177 (1933), 483

Tompsett, A. C. and S. W. Donaldson: The anterior tubercle of the first cervical vertebra and the hyoid bone: their occurence in newborn infants. Amer. J. Roentgenol. 65 (1951), 582

Töndury, G.: Anatomie und Entwicklungsgeschichte der Wirbelsäule mit besonderer Berücksichtigung der Altersveränderungen der Bandscheiben. Schweiz. med. Wschr. (1955), 825 u. 835

Töndury, G.: Entwicklungsgeschichte und Fehlbildungen der Wirbelsäule. In: Wirbelsäule in Forschung und Praxis. Bd. 7, Hippokrates, Stuttgart 1958, S. 46

Tönnis, W. u. G. Friedmann: Zur Differentialdiagnose der pathologischen intrakraniellen Verkalkungen. Münch. med. Wschr. 101 (1959), 1252 u. 1261

Tönnis, W. u. G. Friedmann: Das Röntgenbild des Schädels bei intrakranieller Drucksteigerung im Wachstumsalter. Springer, Berlin-Heidelberg-Göttingen 1964

Torgersen, J.: A roentgenographic study of the metopic suture. Acta radiol. (Stockh.) 33 (1950), 1

Torgersen, J.: Hereditary factors in the sutural pattern of the skull. Acta radiol. (Stockh.) 36 (1951), 374

Toth, Z.: Lotrechte Röntgenaufnahme des Tränennasenkanals. Klin. Mbl. Augenheilk. 91 (1933), 390

Travers, J. T. and L. C. Wormley: Enlarged parietal foramina. Amer. J. Roentgenol. 40 (1938), 571

Trolle, D.: Accessory bones of the human foot. Munksgaard, Copenhagen 1948

Truchot, P., G. Offret et P. Chauvet: La radiographie normale et pathologique du canal lacrymo-nasal. Arch. Ophtal. (Paris) N. S. 13 (1953), 679

Turpin, R., M. Tisserand et J. Pitou: Gémellité en miroir et double noyau d'ossification du semi-lunaire. Bull. soc. pédiat. (Paris) 36 (1938), 390

Ueberschär, K. H.: Über einen vorgetäuschten „Aufhellungsherd" im Röntgenbild des Femurkopfes. Fortschr. Röntgenstr. 83 (1955), 123

Ueberschär, K. H.: Ossifikationszentren und Nebenkernbildung am Naviculare pedis unter besonderer Berücksichtigung ihrer Folgezustände. Fortschr. Röntgenstr. 87 (1957), 33
Ueda, F. T., T. Ueke, H. O. Kuda, H. Tanaka, M. Suda, Y. Suzuki and Y. Ando: X-ray study of so - called spontaneous healing in congenital dislocalisation of hip-joint. Nagoya med. J. 8 (1962), 5
Unterberg, A.: Sellamessung und Sellaformbestimmung bei Kindern im Alter bis zu 14 Jahren. Mschr. Kinderheilk. 104 (1956), 46
Valentin, B. u. W. Putschar: Dysontogenetische Blockwirbel- und Gibbusbildung (klinische und anatomische Untersuchungen). Z. orthop. Chir. 64 (1936), 338
Vedder, H.: Lochförmige Defekte im Schulterblatt. Fortschr. Röntgenstr. 98 (1963), 62
de Vega-Goicoechea, S.: Estudio radiólogico del laberinto etmoidal. Rev. esp. Oto-neuro-oftal. 10 (1953), 175
Veraguth, O. u. C. Braendli-Wyss: Der Rücken des Menschen. Huber, Bern 1948
Vergau, W., H.-P. Heilmann u. J. Helms: Tomographische Diagnostik des Felsenbeins mit spiraliger Verwischung. Fortschr. Röntgenstr. 116 (1972), 686
zur Verth, M.: Zur Kenntnis der umschriebenen Aufhellungen im Röntgenbild der Hand- und Fußwurzelknochen. Röntgenpraxis 3 (1931), 670
Viehweger, G.: Der Processus paratransversarius, eine Varietät am Atlas. Fortschr. Röntgenstr. 83 (1955), 411
Viehweger, G.: Die Darstellung des medialen Randes der kranialen Gelenkfläche des Atlas auf den Übersichtsaufnahmen der HWS im v.d. Strahlengang. Fortschr. Röntgenstr. 84 (1956), 492
Viehweger, G.: Doppelseitige Hyperplasie des Os pisiforme und des Hamulus ossis hamati. Fortschr. Röntgenstr. 86 (1957), 407
Viehweger, G.: Zur Frage der Entwicklung des Processus styloideus ulnae. Fortschr. Röntgenstr. 86 (1957), 408
Viehweger, G.: Zum Problem der Deutung der knöchernen Gebilde distal des Epicondylus medialis humeri. Fortschr. Röntgenstr. 86 (1957), 643
Viehweger, G.: Oberarm. In: Handbuch der Medizinischen Radiologie, IV/2, Springer, Berlin-Heidelberg-New York 1968, 309, 348 u. 414
Vielberg, H.: Beobachtung seltener Wirbelkörperanomalien an der Lendenwirbelsäule eines Erwachsenen. Diskussionssbeitrag zur gestörten Chordasegmentierung. Fortschr. Röntgenstr. 113 (1970), 60
Villányi, Gy.: Seltener Fall der Verkalkung des Ligamentum coracoclaviculare. Fortschr. Röntgenstr. 112 (1970), 695
Vogel, K.-H.: Doppelseitige Samenblasenverkalkung - ein Beitrag zur Differentialdiagnose von Verkalkungen im kleinen Becken. Fortschr. Röntgenstr. 105 (1966), 127
Voigt, R.: Über die „Fenestrae parietales symmetricae“. Mschr. Kinderheilk. 70 (1937), 224
Volkmann, J.: Das Os subtibiale. Fortschr. Röntgenstr. 48 (1933), 225
Wackenheim, A.: Functional atlanto-occipital block. Neuroradiology 3 (1971), 280
Wackenheim, A.: Fehlbildungen am Schädel-Hals-Übergang. In: Hdb. d. Med. Radiologie, Bd. VI/1. Springer, Berlin-Heidelberg-New York 1974, 391
Waldeyer, A.: Anatomie des Menschen. Erster Teil, de Gruyter, Berlin 1969
Walker, C. S.: Calcification of intervertebral discs in Children. J. Bone Jt Surg. 36B (1954), 601
Wanke, R.: Zur Röntgenkunde der Gefäßkanäle der Diploe. Fortschr. Röntgenstr. 56 (1937), 286
Wanke, R. u. L. Diethelm: Klinische und operative Bedeutung der Schädelnähte. Langenbecks Arch. klin. Chir. 289 (1958), 435
Waschulewski, H.: Submalleoläre inkonstante Skelettelemente und malleoläre Knochenkerne. Fortschr. Röntgenstr. 86 (1957), 492
Watermann, R.: Gefäßdurchtrittsöffnungen und Arthrose am Oberschenkel. Z. Orthop. 98 (1964), 492
Weickmann, F.: Vikariierende Nebenhöhlenhyperplasie bei hypoplastischen Großhirnprozessen. Fortschr. Röntgenstr. 88 (1958), 432
Weidenreich, F.: Knochenstudien über Sehnenverknöcherungen und Faktoren der Knochenbildung. Z. Anat. Entwickl.-Gesch. 69 (1923), 558
Weinert, P.: Ein Beitrag zur Frage der Pseudoepiphysen. Anat. Anz. 99 (1952), 1
Weingraber, H.: Die Funktionsprüfung in der Röntgenfrühdiagnostik der Kiefergelenkserkrankungen. Fortschr. Röntgenstr. 74 (1951), 84
Went, H.: Zur klinischen Bedeutung persistierender Apophysen an den Gelenkfortsätzen der Lendenwirbelsäule. Arch. orthop. Unfall-Chir. 49 (1958), 568
Wentzlik, G.: Zur Einstelltechnik des oberen Sprunggelenkes (Modifikation zur orthograden Darstellung des Spaltes). Fortschr. Röntgenstr. 84 (1956), 362
Wenz, W. u. G. Geipert: Röntgenologie der *Srb*schen Rippen-Sternum-Anomalie. Radiologe 7 (1967), 53
Werkgartner, H.: Über die diagnostische Bedeutung endokranieller Verkalkungen mit besonderer Berücksichtigung der Verkalkung bei Toxoplasmose. Radiol. Austriaca 7 (1954), 141
Werner, K.: Anatomische Schädelschnitte im Röntgenbild als Grundlage des Schädelschichtbildes. Bd. 14, Hüttig, Heidelberg 1961
Werthemann, A.: Die Entwicklungsstörungen der Extremitäten. In: *Henke-Lubarsch-Rössle:* Handbuch der speziellen pathologischen Anatomie und Histologie. Bd. IX, Springer, Berlin-Göttingen-Heidelberg 1952
Wichtl, O.: Tuberculum intercondylicum quartum tibiae. Röntgenpraxis 13 (1941), 397
Wichtl, O.: Über die Bedeutung von Stufenbildungen am fötalen Schädel. Radiol. Austriaca 11 (1961), 115
Wiebrand, H. F. and J. Stehle: Roentgenanatomy of the vestibular canalicle under normal and pathological conditions. XII. Internationaler Kongreß für Radiologie, Madrid 1973
Wieser, W.: Zur Entwicklung der kindlichen Sella unter normalen und pathologischen Verhältnissen. Wien. klin. Wschr. (1933), 1220
Wilhelm, G.: Knöchernes „Intermediärstück“ an der 2. Rippe. Fortschr. Röntgenstr. 86 (1957), 406
Wilk, E. u. Th. Hülshoff: Über eine seltene Rippenanomalie. Fortschr. Röntgenstr. 86 (1957), 531
Wimberger, H.: Klinisch-radiologische Diagnostik von Rachitis, Skorbut und Lues congenita im Kindesalter. Ergebn. inn. Med. Kinderheilk. 28 (1925), 264
Wissler, H.: Fenestrae parietales symmetricae. Arch. Kinderheilk. 115 (1938), 217
Witt, A. N., H. Cotta u. M. Jäger: Die angeborenen Fehlbildungen der Hand und ihre operative Behandlung. Thieme, Stuttgart 1966
Wolf, H. G.: Röntgendiagnostik beim Neugeborenen und Säugling. Maudrich, Wien-Bonn-Bern 1959
Wolf, H. G.: Differenzierung der Extremitätenknochenkerne. Pädiat. Prax. 2 (1963), 89
Wolf, H. G. u. L. Psenner: Pathologisch-anatomische und klinisch-röntgenologische Studien über die sog. Wachstumslinien. Fortschr. Röntgenstr. 80 (1954), 141
Wolfers, H. u. W. Hoeffken: Fehlbildungen der Wirbelbögen. In: Hdb. d. Med. Radiologie Bd. VI/1, Springer, Berlin-Heidelberg-New York 1974, 265
v. Wrangell, U. u. C. W. Fassbender: Zur Verkalkung bzw. Verknöcherung der Falx cerebri. Fortschr. Röntgenstr. 121 (1974), 550
Wray, J. B. and C. N. Hernson: Hereditary transmission of congenital coalition of the calcaneus to the navicular. J. Bone Jt Surg. 45A (1963), 365
Wuensch, K. E.: Ein Fall von „Coalitio vertebrae “ der Halswirbelsäule. Fortschr. Röntgenstr. 121 (1974), 400
Wütschke, J.: Ein Fall von linksseitiger doppelter Patella. Fortschr. Röntgenstr. 78 (1953), 218
Wütschke, J.: Patella partita und Patella duplex. Fortschr. Röntgenstr. 104 (1966), 260
Yoshii, M., T. Sakakura, T. Ishibashi, H. Fukatsu, M. Nakamura and S. Kuwamoto: Studies on the tomography in otorhino-laryngology. Mie med. J. 10 (1960), 133
Zachrisson, C. G.: A comperative study of radiograms and anatomical sections of the temporal bone. Acta radiol. (Stockh.) 19 (1938), 55
Zarfl, M.: Fenestrae parietales symmetricae. Z. Kinderheilk. 57 (1936), 54
Zeller: Zit. bei *Matthiash*
Zetkin-Schaldach: Os centrale carpi. Wörterbuch der Medizin. VEB Volk und Gesundheit, Berlin 1973, S. 561/562

Zetkin-Schaldach: Periarthritis humeroscapularis. Wörterbuch der Medizin. VEB Volk und Gesundheit, Berlin 1973, S. 589

Ziedses des Plantes, B. G.: Eine neue Methode zur Differenzierung in der Röntgenographie (Planigraphie). Acta radiol. (Stockh.) 13 (1932), 182

Ziegler, G.: Ossifikation im Bereich der knorpeligen Gelenkrippe der Schultergelenkpfanne. Fortschr. Röntgenstr. 86 (1957), 270

Zimmer, E. A.: Der normale und der gebrochene Jochbogen in neuen Aufnahmerichtungen. Fortschr. Röntgenstr. 55 (1937), 67

Zimmer, E. A.: Die röntgenologische Untersuchung der Atlasspaltbildung. Acta radiol. (Stockh.) 18 (1937), 842

Zimmer, E. A.: Krankheiten, Verletzungen und Varietäten des Os naviculare pedis. Arch. Orthop. Unfall-Chir. 38 (1938), 396

Zimmer, E. A.: Das Brustbein und seine Gelenke. Fortschr. Röntgenstr. Erg.-Bd. 58 (1939)

Zimmer, E. A.: Zur Darstellung des normalen Kiefergelenkes im Röntgenbild. Radiol. clin. (Basel) 9 (1940), 170

Zimmer, E. A.: Röntgenologische Studien über die Bewegungen des normalen und pathologischen Kiefergelenkes. J. Radiol. Électrol. 34 (1953), 336

Zimmer, E. A. s. a. Köhler/Zimmer: Grenzen des Normalen und Anfänge des Pathologischen im Röntgenbild des Skelets. 11. Aufl. Thieme, Stuttgart 1967

Zimmer, J.: Planigraphie des Schläfenbeines. Acta radiol. (Stockh.) 37 (1952), 419

Zseböck, Z.: Röntgenanatomische Untersuchungen am Beckengürtel des Neugeborenen. Fortschr. Röntgenstr. 87 (1957), 23

Zseböck, Z.: Die Gelenke des Beckengürtels. In: Hdb. d. Med. Radiologie, Bd. IV/2. Springer, Berlin-Heidelberg-New York 1968

Zsernaviczky, J. u. G. Türk: Der ß-Winkel. Ein diagnostisches Zeichen für Frühdiagnose der angeborenen Hüftdysplasie. Fortschr. Röntgenstr. 123 (1975), 131

Zukschwerdt, L., E. Emminger, F. Biedermann u. H. Zettel: Wirbelgelenk und Bandscheibe. Ihre Beziehung zum vertebragenen Schmerz; zugleich eine Stellungnahme zur Chiropraktik und zur Frage der Begutachtung. Hippokrates, Stuttgart 1960

Index

D

E

M

N

O

P

R

S